TEACHING PLAN 1 Breast Self-Exam

- The breast self-exam (BSE) should be done at least once a month. It is best to perform your BSE 1 week after the start of your menstrual period, as your breasts will not be as tender to touch.
- If you do not menstruate, choose a specific time each month to perform the BSE.
- You should examine your breast three different ways: in front of a mirror, in the shower, and when lying flat on your back.

Mirror
Be sure the room is well lit.
- At each step, look for any change in the shape or appearance of your breasts.
  - Arms at your sides
  - Arms over your head
  - Hands on your hips, pressing firmly to flex your chest muscles
  - Bending forward
- Note if there are any skin or nipple changes such as dimpling (orange peel) of the skin.
- Gently squeeze each nipple to see if any fluid comes out of the nipple. If it does, note the color and amount.

Shower
- Soap your hands and use three soapy fingers (index, middle, and ring) to feel the breast tissue in the same systematic pattern (an up-and-down pattern as though you were mowing the yard).
- Raise your right arm above your head and begin to examine your breast.
- Be sure to start at the middle of your chest where your collarbones come together.
- Go up and down the entire breast area and into the armpit. Also examine the area just above your collarbone, because breast tissue is also found in this area on some women.
- Do the same thing on the left breast.

Lying down
- Place a small pillow (or rolled towel) under your right shoulder and place your right hand under your head.
- Use the same steps as in the Shower portion.
- It is best to use the same systematic method each time you perform BSE. That way you won't leave anything out of your exam.
- If you note any unusual lumps, masses, or drainage from your nipples, consult with your health care provider as soon as possible.
- BSE has been proven to be a lifesaver.

TEACHING PLAN 2 Breastfeeding Your Infant

Preparing to breastfeed
- Go to the bathroom.
- Wash your hands with soap and water.
- Wash your breasts with clean, warm water.

Positioning for breastfeeding
- You can be sitting, standing, or lying down to breastfeed your infant.
- The two main types of holds for breastfeeding are cradle and football. With practice, you will find which one works best for you and your infant.
- Your infant's chest should be against your chest with his or her head and neck in a position that appears comfortable for your infant. This allows your infant to latch onto your breast much easier.
- Center your nipple to the nose of your infant with your nipple aimed to the roof of your infant's mouth. You want the lower jaw to latch on first.
- If your infant's mouth is opened wide before latch-on, he or she will be able to latch on much more effectively. To get the infant to open his or her mouth, brush your nipple against the infant's lower lip. A hungry infant will usually open his or her mouth wide with this type of stimulation.

Alternating breasts
- Empty one breast before going to the other breast.
- Alternate the breast you start with on each feeding.
- You can place a safety pin on the bra cup of the breast you last used to remind you with which breast to start the next feeding.

How to tell if your infant is full
- The infant will actively suck and you will hear him or her swallow.
- Your infant should have at least 6 wet diapers a day.
- Your infant will have several stools each day.
- The breast feels full before feeding and feels soft after the infant has fed.

Burping and positioning after feeding
- To break the suction and remove the infant from the breast, gently insert one of your fingers into the corner of your infant's mouth or use your fingers to 'indent' your breast near the infant's mouth.
- Don't pull the baby off your nipple, because this can cause sore nipples.
- Place the infant with his or her head on your shoulder and gently pat the back until your infant burps.

TEACHING PLAN 3 Bathing Your Infant

Preparing
- The room should be warm and free of drafts.
- Your infant can be bathed in a baby bathtub or the bathtub in your home. Whatever you choose to use, be sure it has been cleaned prior to placing your infant and the water has been checked and is not too hot.
- Towel, washcloth, clean clothing, and diaper should be ready to use immediately after the bath.
- Use a mild soap and shampoo, and a comb or brush.
- Remove any jewelry, watches, and roll up long sleeves. This will help prevent any injury to the infant during the bathing process.
- Depending on the type of tub used, place a clean towel on the bottom and on one side of the tub. This helps prevent the infant from slipping while in the tub.

Bathing
- Slowly place your infant into the bath water, being sure to support your infant's head at all times. Be sure you have firm control of one of your infant's arms so the infant won't slip.
- Start bathing your infant at the head. This allows you to move from an area that is cleaner to one that tends not to be as clean. Wet the washcloth and wring it out. Gently wash the eyes starting from the inner to outer corner. Wash the ear, using your index finger inside of the cloth. Gently wash one side of the infant's head and face and then move to the other. To rinse the shampoo, use your free hand to gently cup water and gently pour over the infant's head.
- Continue washing the infant's body. Pay special attention to any skin folds, such as the neck and behind the ears. If soap or shampoo is left on the skin, it can irritate the infant's skin.
- Female infant—spread apart the labia and clean between the skin folds. Be sure to use a front-to-back motion to prevent any stool from being wiped onto the urethra.
- Male infant—gently wash from the tip of the penis to the anus. Again, this prevents any stool from being wiped onto the urethral opening. If your son is not circumcised, do not retract the foreskin. This skin cannot be fully moved down the shaft of the penis until your son is around 3 years of age. If you retract or move the skin down the penis, the skin may not come back to the original position, and this can harm or hurt your son's penis.
- Once you have completed bathing your infant, check his or her skin once more to be sure you have removed all the soap. When done, remove your infant and immediately wrap him or her in a clean towel and gently rub your infant dry. Do not place anything inside the ears of your infant. Diaper and dress your infant and place him or her in the crib or bassinet.
- Empty the tub and clean it thoroughly. Return all supplies to their normal place so they can be easily found when needed.

TEACHING PLAN 4 Skin Care for Infants, Children, and Adolescents

Depending on the age of your child, the type of skin care required may vary.

Infants
- Don't use deodorant soaps or soaps with perfume, because this can cause skin irritation.
- Be careful using products that contain alcohol, because this is very drying to the skin.
- Bathe your infant from the head down to the toes.
- When changing diapers, be sure to wipe from front to back. This will help prevent bladder infections.
- Change diapers whenever they become wet or soiled. This will help prevent diaper rash.
- Whenever going outside of the house, apply sunblock to your infant's skin. Even if it is cloudy, a large amount of sun rays still cut through the clouds, and your infant can still become sunburned.
- Keep your infant's nails trimmed. This will help to prevent scratches.

Child
- Teach your child how to correctly wash his or her hands after going to the bathroom and before eating. This will help decrea spread of infection.
- Clean any wound as quickly as possible, checking to see if there are any fragments such as pebbles, glass, metal, and dirt in wound. Apply antibiotic ointment to the wound using a cotton-tip swab. This will prevent contamination of the ointment tube less painful to the child.
- Apply sunblock any time your child will be playing outdoors for an extended amount of time. If at the beach, lake, or river, the sunblock needs to be reapplied throughout the day, usually every two to three hours.
- Apply lip balm that contains sunblock to prevent chapping and sunburn.

Adolescent
- Teach your son or daughter to wash his or her face at least twice a day. Use a clean cloth each time. Be sure all of the clean agent has been removed as certain ones can cause skin damage.
- Teach your son or daughter not to "pop" a pimple or zit. This can cause infection at the site and scarring.
- The type of skin your adolescent has will determine whether or not a moisturizer lotion is needed. If you are not sure, check health care provider.
- Shaving—both boys and girls need to apply a shaving cream of some type to the area they will be shaving. This helps to soft hair follicle, which in turn helps the razor cut the hair with less trauma to the surrounding skin. This applies to the face, armpi legs.
- Girls—if wearing makeup, it is best to start with one type of product. This way, if she is going to have a skin reaction to it, she know which product to stop using.

PLAN EDUCATIVO 3 Bañando al Bebé

Preparación
- El cuarto debe estar calientito y libre de corrientes de aire.
- Puede bañar al bebé en una bañera o en la tina del baño en su casa. Asegúrese que la bañera esté limpia antes de meterlo al agua, y que el agua no esté muy caliente.
- La toalla, la toallita, ropa limpia y el pañal deben de estar listos para usarlos inmediatamente después del baño.
- Un jabón suave y shampoo, un peine o cepillo para el cabello.
- Quítese la joyería, relojes, y enrolle las mangas largas. Esto ayudará a prevenir daño al bebé durante el baño.
- Dependiendo del tipo de bañera, ponga una toalla limpia en el fondo y otra en el lado de la bañera. Esto previene que el bebé se resbale cuando esté en la bañera.

El Baño
- Despacito, ponga al bebé en el agua, sosténgale la cabeza todo el tiempo que esté en el agua. Cójalo firmemente de un brazo para que el bebé no se resbale.
- Empiece el baño lavando la cabeza. Esto le permite que lave de una area que es más limpia a una que no tiende a estar tan limpia. Moje la toallita y exprímala. Lave los ojos suavemente empezando con el ángulo de enmedio hacia afuera. Lave la oreja cubriendo el dedo índice en una toallita. Lave un lado de la cabeza y de la cara del bebé y luego el otro lado. Para enjuagar la cabeza use la mano libre y póngale agua en la cabeza.
- Continúe lavando el cuerpo. Ponga atención a cualquier doblez de la piel en el cuello y atrás de las orejas. Si deja jabón o shampoo en la piel puede causarle irritación.
- Bebita – Extienda la labia y limpie entre el doblez de la piel. Use un movimiento del frente hacia atrás para prevenir que el excremento entre a la uretra.
- Bebito – Lave suavemente de la punta del pene hasta el ano. Otra vez, esto previene que el excremento entre a la uretra. Si el bebé no está circuncidado, no retracte la piel del prepucio. Esta piel no se debe estirar hacia la base del pene hasta que el niño tenga 3 años de edad. Si estira la piel hacia la base, el pene se puede dañar o lastimar el pene.
- Cuando termine el baño del bebé, chequé la piel una vez más para asegurarse que no tenga jabón. Saque al bebé del agua y envuélvalo inmediatamente en una toalla limpia y séquelo suavemente. No ponga nada en las orejas del bebé. Póngale un pañal, vístalo y acuéstelo en la cuna o cunero.
- Vacíe la bañera y límpiela completamente. Guarde todos los materiales en su lugar para que los pueda usar cuando los necesite.

PLAN EDUCATIVO 4 Cuidado de la Piel de Bebés, Niños, y Adolecentes
Dependiendo de la edad del niño, el tipo de cuidado requerido varía.

Bebés
- No use jabones con desodorantes o perfumes ya que pueden causar irritación en la piel.
- Tenga cuidado al usar productos que contengan alcohol ya que tienden a resecar la piel.
- Bañe al bebé desde la cabeza hasta los pies.
- Cuando cambie el pañal, asegúrese de limpiar del frente hacia atrás. Esto ayuda a prevenir infecciones en la vejiga.
- Cambie el pañal cuando esté mojado o sucio. Esto ayuda a prevenir rozaduras.
- Cuando salga fuera de la casa, aplique bloqueador a la piel del bebé. Aún cuando esté nublado, una gran cantidad de rayos solares pasan por las nubes y pueden causar quemaduras en la piel.
- Mantenga las uñas del bebé cortas. Esto ayuda a prevenir rasguños.

Niño
- Enseñe al niño como lavarse bien las manos después de ir al baño y antes de cada comida. Esto ayuda a disminuir la propagación de infecciones.
- Limpie cualquier herida lo más pronto posible. Cheque si hay fragmentos de piedritas, vidrio, metal, y tierra en la herida. Aplique una pomada antibiótica a la herida usando un palito de algodón. Esto previene la contaminación del envase y es menos doloroso para el niño.
- Aplique bloqueador cuando el niño juegue afuera por períodos largos. Si está en la playa, lago o río, aplicarse durante el día, usualmente cada dos o tres horas.
- Aplique un bálsamo que contenga bloqueador a los labios para prevenir cortaduras o quemaduras causadas por el sol.

Adolecente
- Enseñe a su hijo o hija a lavarse la cara por lo menos dos veces diarias. Use una toalla limpia cada vez. Esto puede causar infección o cicatriz en el area. Asegúrese que todo el agente de limpieza que se usó sea removido ya que le puede causar daño a la piel.
- Enseñe a su hijo o hija a que no se oprima una espinilla o un barro. Esto puede causar infección o cicatriz en la piel.
- El tipo de piel del adolecente determinará si necesita o no una crema humectante. Si no está segura, cheque con su proveedor de cuidados medicos.
- Afeitarse – Los adolecentes (hombres y mujeres) necesitan aplicar crema algún tipo de afeitar. Esto ayuda a suavizar el folículo del pelo que a la vez ayuda al rastrillo a cortar causando menos trauma a la piel. Esto se refiere a la piel de la cara, axilas, y piernas.
- Mujeres adolecentes – Si usa maquillaje, es mejor que empiece con un solo tipo. De esta manera, si tiene una reacción en la piel, ella sabrá cual producto dejar de usar.

PLAN EDUCATIVO 1 Auto Examen de los Senos

- El auto examen de los senos debe hacerse al menos una vez por mes. Es mejor hacerse el auto examen una semana después de que empiece el período menstrual ya que los senos no están tan sensibles al tacto.
- Si ya no menstrua, escoja un día específico en cada mes para hacerse el auto examen.
- Examine los senos de tres maneras diferentes: enfrente del espejo, en la regadera o cuando esté acostada de espaldas.
- Asegúrese de que el cuarto esté bien alumbrado.

Espejo
- En cada paso, vea si hay cambios en la forma o apariencia de los senos:
  - Mantenga los brazos a su lado
  - Extienda los brazos arriba de la cabeza
  - Ponga las manos en la cadera, presione firmemente para flexionar los músculos del pecho
- Note si hay cambios en la piel o en el pezón tal como depresiones pequeñas (apariencia de cascara de naranja).

Regadera
- Apriete suavemente cada pezón para ver si sale líquido. Si sale líquido, note el color y la cantidad.
- Enjabónese las manos y use tres dedos enjabonados (el índice, el del medio, y del anillo) para tocar los tejidos sistemáticamente (de arriba a abajo como si estuviera cortando el césped).
  - Levante el brazo derecho sobre la cabeza y empiece a examinar el seno derecho.
  - Empiece en medio del pecho donde los huesos de la clavícula se juntan.
  - Toque de arriba a abajo toda el area del seno hasta la axila. También examine el area de la clavícula ya que hay mujeres que tienen tejido de los senos en esa area.
  - Repita lo mismo en el seno izquierdo.

Acostada de espaldas
- Ponga una almohadilla (o una toalla enrollada) debajo del hombro derecho y ponga la mano derecha debajo de la cabeza.
  - Use los mismos pasos que usó cuando se examinó en la regadera.
- Es mejor que use el mismo método cada vez que se haga el auto examen. De esta manera no se olvidará ningún paso del examen.
- Si nota cualquier bulto, masas, o líquido que sale del pezón, consulte a su proveedor de cuidados medicos lo más pronto possible.
- El auto examen de los senos ha probado salvar vidas.

PLAN EDUCATIVO 2 Dar Pecho al Bebé

Prepárese para dar pecho
- Vaya al baño.
- Lávese las manos con jabón y agua.
- Lávese los senos con agua limpia y tibia.

Posición para dar pecho
- Puede sentarse, quedarse parada o acostarse para darle pecho al bebé.
- Los dos maneras que puede acostarse para darle pecho al bebé. Con práctica encontrará la mejor manera para usted y el bebé.
- El pecho de bebé debe reposar contra su pecho con la cabeza en una posición que se vea comfortable. Esto le ayuda al bebé a prenderse del pezón más fácilmente.
- Centre el pezón a la nariz del bebé con el pezón apuntando hacia el paladar. Deje que la mandíbula inferior se prenda al pezón primero.
- Si el bebé mantiene la boca bien abierta antes de prenderse, el se prenderá al pezón más fácilmente. Para hacer que el bebé abra la boca, toque el labio inferior del bebé con el pezón. Un bebé que tiene hambre usualmente abre completamente la boca con este tipo de estímulo.

Alternando los senos
- Vacíe un seno antes de pasar al otro.
- Alterne el seno con el que empieza cada vez que da de pecho.
- Puede poner un seguro en la copa del brassier del seno con el que dió de pecho para que le recuerde usar el otro.

Como notar si su bebé está satisfecho
- Puede sentarse, quedarse parada o acostarse para darle pecho al bebé.
- Cuando el bebé chupa el pezón lo escuchará tragar.
- El bebé debe de mojar al menos seis (6) pañales por día.
- El bebé debe tener varios excrementos por día.
- El seno se siente lleno antes de dar pecho y suave después.

Eructar y posicionar después de alimentar
- Para hacer que el bebé deje de chupar el pezón, suavemente, ponga uno de los dedos en un lado de la boca o use el dedo para oprimir el pecho cerca de la boca.
- No jale al bebé del pezón ya que esto puede lastimar el pezón.
- Ponga la cabeza del bebé contra su hombro y déle golpecitos en la espalda hasta que el bebé eructe.

INTRODUCTION TO MATERNITY & PEDIATRIC NURSING

FOURTH EDITION

Gloria Leifer, MA, RN

Associate Professor
Obstetrics, Pediatrics, and
 Trauma Nursing
Riverside Community College
Riverside, California

SAUNDERS
An Imprint of Elsevier Science
Philadelphia   London   New York   St. Louis   Sydney   Tokyo

SAUNDERS
An Imprint of Elsevier Science

11830 Westline Industrial Drive
St. Louis, Missouri 63146

INTRODUCTION TO MATERNITY & PEDIATRIC NURSING ISBN 0-7216-9334-2

NOTICE

Nursing is an ever-changing field. Standard safety precautions must be followed, but as new research and clinical experience broaden our knowledge, changes in treatment and drug therapy may become necessary or appropriate. Readers are advised to check the most current product information provided by the manufacturer of each drug to be administered to verify the recommended dose, the method and duration of administration, and contraindications. It is the responsibility of the licensed prescriber, relying on experience and knowledge of the patient, to determine dosages and the best treatment for each individual patient. Neither the publisher nor the author assumes any liability for any injury and/or damage to persons or property arising from this publication.

The Publisher

FOURTH EDITION

Previous editions copyrighted 1999, 1995, 1990

Vice President, Publishing Director: Sally Schrefer
Acquisitions Editor: Terri Wood
Developmental Editor: Jill Riggin
Publishing Services Manager: Deborah L. Vogel
Project Manager: Jodi M. Willard
Designer: Amy Buxton

CL/PMT

Printed in Hong Kong

Last digit is the print number: 9   8   7   6   5   4   3   2   1

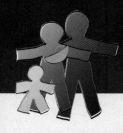

Special Contributor

TRENA L. RICH, RN, MSN, C-ANP
Adult Nurse Practitioner/Nursing
 Supervisor/Occupational Health Program
 Coordinator
Campus Health Center
University of California at Riverside
Riverside, California

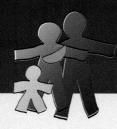

Reviewers

CATHY EDEN AMMERMAN, RN, BSN
Sumner County Practical Nursing Program
Gallatin, Tennessee

COLLEEN BOOTH, RN, MS
Westchester Community College
Valhalla, New York

NELL BRITTON, RN, MSN, CIC, NHA
Trident Technical College
Charleston, South Carolina

JANET K. EKVALL, RN, BSN, MSN
Marshalltown Community College
Marshalltown, Iowa

JUDITH A. GUTSCHENRITTER, RN, BS, MSEd
Mid-Plains Community College
North Platte, Nebraska

KAREN KATHRYN HAAGENSEN, RNC
Howard College
San Angelo, Texas

MILAGROS Y. HALL, RN, BC, CNA
Manhattan School—Adult Practical Nursing
 Program
New York City Board of Education
New York, New York

DOROTHY A. HOGAN-HOWLAND, BSN, RN, MN
Wayne Community College
Goldsboro, North Carolina

STEPHEN P. KILKUS, RN, MSN
Winona State University
Winona, Minnesota

MARY ANN KLOGES, MSN, RN
B.M. Spurr School of Practical Nursing
Glen Dale, West Virginia

MARY MARQUARDT, RN, BA
Central Lakes College
Brainerd, Minnesota

JANET TOMPKINS McMAHON, RN, MSN
Pennsylvania College of Technology
Williamsport, Pennsylvania

MARY R. PRICE, RN, MSN
Vincennes University
Jasper, Indiana

JULIE A. SLACK, RN, MS, ICCE
Mohave Community College
Kingman, Arizona

BEVERLY SMITH, RN, BSN
San Jacinto College, North Campus
Houston, Texas

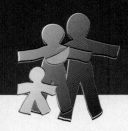

To the Instructor

THE EDUCATION OF THE LICENSED PRACTICAL/VOCATIONAL NURSE

Depth with **simplicity** continues as the theme of this text. This theme is based on current health care reform and the need to adapt to the changes occurring in the twenty-first century in order to maintain quality patient care. The role of the nurse is changing at every level. The curriculum of educational programs preparing the licensed practical/vocational nurse (LPN/LVN) must also change in order to adequately prepare their graduates for entry-level positions. Because of cost containment, more LPNs/LVNs are working in home health and are assuming certain leadership responsibilities in nursing homes with unlicensed staff. Critical thinking skills have become essential and are thus reflected in this text by the inclusion of Critical Thinking Questions in each chapter and detailed rationales in the accompanying Instructor's Manual.

In years past, completion of the LPN/LVN program was considered a terminal certificate. Today, however, many LPN/LVN programs are considered "ladders" into the associate degree nursing (ADN) program. Practical/vocational nurses progressing to the ADN program often do not repeat maternity and pediatric content. This text contains the most accurate, current, and clinically relevant information concerning maternity and pediatrics designed for the LPN/LVN with the depth necessary for those wishing to enter a ladder program of study in nursing.

As in previous editions, maternity and pediatric nursing is presented with an emphasis on how infants and children differ from adults. The fourth edition emphasizes how techniques of care may differ between the traditional adult medical-surgical client and the infant, child, or pregnant adult on the basis of anatomical, physiological, and psychological differences. To limit the size of this book and make it more useful as a reference tool, some content common to medical-surgical nursing is not included, making this a maternity/pediatric content-specific text. Careful consideration of the LPN/LVN Nurse Practice Acts has guided the inclusion of skills and techniques in this text. This organization facilitates the use of this text in a combined maternity/pediatric course, a separate maternity course followed by an independent pediatric course, or a medical-surgical course that integrates the maternity and pediatric patient throughout the curriculum.

ABOUT THE TEXT

This combined maternity and pediatrics text provides comprehensive discussions of family-centered care, wellness, health promotion and illness prevention, women's health issues, and the growth and development of the child *and the parent.* The information forms one continuum of knowledge that flows from conception to adulthood. The concept of studying simple-to-complex and health-to-illness is retained. The systems approach is maintained in presenting physiological illness (other than congenital anomalies that are present at birth and communicable diseases of children).

Today's student is challenged to learn more, often in less time. Therefore a word of explanation is needed about the Complete Bibliography and Reader References list. As in previous editions, the bibliography contains the most up-to-date sources from which information was gathered for this edition. These sources are listed with reader references—sources that will be of value to those who may wish a more in-depth review of a specific topic. In this edition, we have placed all the bibliographies and reader references, sorted by chapter, toward the end of the book. We hope this approach helps the reader focus on the topics of interest in seamless progression. Online Resources related to chapter content are included at the end of each chapter. The chapter websites were chosen because of their correlation with content and the hyperlinks to related topics they provide. With these tools, this textbook is a golden link in the chain of knowledge available to the reader. It is hoped that the essential information necessary for competent nursing practice at the LPN/LVN level provided in this portable, accessible, economical, and well-illustrated text will stimulate the reader to continue self-education with the resources provided, even after the course semester is concluded.

In their 1991 publication *Healthy America: Practitioners for 2005: An Agenda for Action for U.S. Health Professional Schools,* the PEW Health Professions Commission recommended that nursing graduates must "meet the evolving health care needs" of patients and possess the "ability to deal with a racially and culturally diverse society" (p. 18).* These recommendations are reflected in this text as threads of detailed discussions and explanations of diverse cultural health care practices relating to maternity and pediatric care. The LPN/LVN education includes tasks and technology based in acute care hospitals. However, the modern trend of health care reform moves the focus from the institution to the population. The International Childbirth Association states that "Freedom of choice is based upon knowledge of alternatives." The education of all nurses must include alternatives to traditional medicine, and the new chapter on complimentary and alternative therapies as they relate to maternity and pediatric nursing care is designed to increase the awareness of these health care practices, which may impact the care provided by the nurse. An understanding of the trend toward active participation in one's own health care requires knowledge that can help the client use safe self-care practices.

Managed care gave birth to the clinical pathway, and LPN/LVNs must understand their role in that plan of care. The reader is encouraged to approach clinical problems via critical thinking rather than by predetermined habit or memorization of fact. Critical thinking questions are presented with each nursing care plan or at the end of each chapter that does not include a nursing care plan. The four different types of care plan styles presented in this text (standard patient care plan, family care plan, pictorial care plan, and care path or clinical pathway) are designed to assist the reader in adapting to the style used in their area of the country. Nursing Intervention Classifications (NIC), Nursing Outcome Criteria (NOC), and NANDA nursing diagnoses are presented in Chapter 1. NIC and NOC are introduced with a sample nursing care plan in Chapter 1 because the LPN/LVN must understand the concept that will be part of the working environment in some health care settings.

The normal process of growth and development from conception to adulthood is the core of maternity and pediatric knowledge. The presence of a fetus influences the effects of maternal illness and medication. The age of the infant or young child influences the dosage levels of medications, and nothing is "standard" as it is in adult nursing. Illness or injury at a specific phase of growth and development may impact the achievement of normal developmental tasks, and this must be considered in the plan of care. These are the unique aspects of maternity and pediatric nursing. For this reason, the normal process of growth and development is presented

in detail, with a special feature concerning the growth and development of a *parent* that bridges the maternity section with the pediatric section of this text.

In this edition, newborn care is divided into three transitional phases: (1) care in the delivery room, (2) the assessment phase in the first few hours after birth, and (3) couplet care before discharge from the hospital. Nursing responsibilities are outlined in each section.

The women's health section has been expanded at the readers' request. The intent is that the information provided will improve the understanding of women's health problems and therefore help the nurse improve the quality of women's lives by reducing pain, stress, and illness due to delayed treatment or lack of preventive care.

This book, with its theme of **depth** with **simplicity,** is designed both to prepare the LPN/LVN student for mobility in the profession and to enable the LPN/LVN to provide quality maternity and pediatric nursing care to a diverse population in a rapidly changing world.

FEATURES THAT ENHANCE THE STUDENT LEARNING FOCUS

Several user-friendly features incorporated into this edition facilitate learning and enhance review. The *Objectives* of the chapter are identified to help the student focus on the topics to be studied. *Key Terms* are provided to aid the reader in assessing their reading comprehension, and phonetic pronunciations—reviewed by an English as a Second Language (ESL) specialist—are provided for select terms. The terms that were assigned simple phonetic pronunciations were selected because they are either (1) difficult medical, nursing, or scientific terms; or (2) other words that may be difficult for students to pronounce. The goal is to help the student reader with limited proficiency in English to develop a greater command of the pronunciation of scientific and nonscientific English terms. It is hoped that a more general competency in the understanding and use of medical and scientific language may result. All key terms appear in color in the text as they are defined and used, and important concepts are italicized. *Tables* and *boxes* present facts, comparisons, and summaries in outline form to increase reader understanding. *Nursing Tips* within each chapter enhance retention by emphasizing important concepts. *Key Points* at the end of each chapter summarize concepts and serve as a study guide or review for the student. Multiple-choice *Review Questions* at the end of each chapter test comprehension and application of the knowledge learned from the chapter. A new full-color design enhances visual appeal, clarifies concepts, and maintains interest. *Line drawings* are used to identify and emphasize details often hidden in pho-

---

Healthy America: Practitioners for 2005. An agenda for action for U.S. health professional schools. PEW Professional Commission, October 1991.

tographs. There are many new *photographs,* and each photograph provides specific information.

NEW FEATURES

The fourth edition has come of age with 21 new features!

1. The reading level is carefully tuned to the level of the LPN/LVN student. Understandable explanations increase retention of learning.
2. The women's health section has been revised and expanded.
3. Critical thinking scenarios and questions are presented in each chapter.
4. The goals of *Healthy People 2010* are incorporated throughout the text.
5. Cultural practices of childbearing and childrearing are covered in detail.
6. Spanish-English translations of common maternity and pediatric phrases are presented.
7. Spanish-English patient teaching lesson plans are included in a tear-out section.
8. Four different types of care plans are presented: traditional patient care plan, family care plan, pictorial care plan, and clinical pathway. Many chapters offer more than one care plan.
9. NIC, NOC, and NANDA diagnoses are introduced.
10. Maternity- and pediatric-specific skills and techniques are detailed throughout the text and are listed opposite the inside back cover.
11. Key terms, with phonetic pronunciations and page number references, appear in color where defined in the text narrative.
12. New detailed tables outline essential knowledge and help correlate physiology with nursing interventions and rationales.
13. The glossary has been revised and expanded to include more terms essential to maternity and pediatric nursing.
14. Nursing interventions related to end-of-life issues in maternity and pediatrics are discussed.
15. Pain is discussed in detail in maternity and pediatric nursing care.
16. Bioterrorism and the pediatric patient is included in Chapter 31, *The Child with a Communicable Disease,* and in Chapter 5 as it relates to the pregnant patient.
17. A new chapter (Chapter 33) addresses complementary and alternative therapies as they relate to obstetrics, women's health, and pediatrics.
18. A new full-color art program offers hundreds of figures with many new photographs, including a cesarean section collage.
19. Up-to-date bibliography, reader reference, and online resources are provided for each chapter.
20. A soft cover format provides economy and ease of handling.
21. An expanded ancillary package is provided.

TEACHING AND LEARNING PACKAGE

The **Study Guide** to accompany *Introduction to Maternity & Pediatric Nursing,* written by Emily McKinney and Christine Rosner, is a valuable supplement to help students understand and apply the content of the text. *Learning Activities, Thinking Critically, Case Studies, Applying Knowledge, Review Questions,* and *Crossword Puzzles* provide students with various learning tools for reinforcement and exploration of text material. The Study Guide includes text page number references, and answers to selected Study Guide sections appear in the Instructor's Resource.

The **Instructor's Resource (CD-ROM),** available free to adopters of the textbook, includes (1) an **Instructor's Manual** with sample lesson plans, related activities, detailed rationales for the textbook critical thinking questions, answers to selected Study Guide sections, and one open-book quiz for each textbook chapter; (2) an expanded **Computerized Test Bank** with approximately 600 NCLEX-style multiple-choice questions with topic, step of the nursing process, objective, cognitive level, NCLEX category of client need, correct answer, rationale, and text page reference; and (3) **PowerPoint** presentations for each text chapter. Contact your local W.B. Saunders sales representative to obtain a copy of the Instructor's Resource.

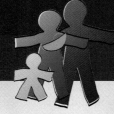

Introduction to Maternity & Pediatric Nursing, 4th edition, shares some features and design elements with other LPN titles on the Mosby and Saunders lists. The purpose of these "LPN Threads" is to make it easier for students and instructors to incorporate multiple books into the relatively brief and demanding LPN curriculum.

The shared features in *Introduction to Maternity & Pediatric Nursing,* 4th edition include the following:

- A **reading level evaluation** was performed on every manuscript chapter during the book's development.
- Cover and internal **design similarities**.
- Numbered lists of **Objectives** that begin each chapter.
- **Key Terms** with phonetic pronunciations and page number references at the beginning of each chapter. The key terms are in color the first time they appear in the chapter. All pronunciations were reviewed by an ESL (English as a Second Language) consultant.
- **Critical Thinking questions** throughout the text. Answers to the critical thinking questions are provided in the Instructor's Manual component of the Instructor's Resource CD-ROM.
- Bulleted lists of **Key Points** at the end of each chapter.

- **Multiple-Choice Review Questions** at the end of each chapter. Answers are provided on the inside back cover of the text, for easy access.
- A **Complete Bibliography and Reader References** list at the end of the text.
- A **Glossary** at the end of the text.
- A **Computerized Test Bank** with the following categories of information: Topic, Step of the Nursing Process, Objective, Cognitive Level, NCLEX Category of Client Need, Correct Answer, Rationale, and Text Page Reference.
- A **PowerPoint slide presentation** in the Instructor's Resource CD-ROM.
- **Open-Book Quizzes** in the Instructor's Manual.
- **Study Guide answer keys** in the Instructor's Manual. The Study Guide itself contains text page number references where students can find the answers.
- **Tips for teaching English as a Second Language (ESL) students** in the Instructor's Manual.
- **Study Hints for English as a Second Language (ESL) students** in the Study Guide.

In addition to content and design threads, these LPN textbooks benefit from the advice and input of the Mosby & Saunders LPN Advisory Board.

LPN Advisory Board

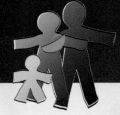

To the Student

Introduction to Maternity & Pediatric Nursing provides a solid foundation in obstetrics and pediatric nursing. New full-color art and photographs, along with many other special features, offer you a valuable learning tool and comprehensive reference.

Objectives list provides a guide to the chapter's essential content and prepares the reader for learning.

All chapters feature a list of **Key Terms** with phonetic pronunciations and page numbers. Key terms appear in color where they are defined in the chapter.

Maternity- and pediatric-specific **skills and techniques** are detailed throughout the text.

Tables and boxes supplement the chapter text by presenting facts, comparisons, and summaries of essential information.

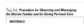
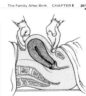

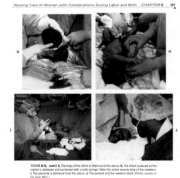

New full-color photographs and illustrations aid in understanding important concepts.

Nursing Tip boxes appear in each chapter and emphasize key concepts.

Nursing Care Plans cover a variety of patient situations with selected nursing diagnoses and provide appropriate outcomes, nursing interventions, and rationales. **Critical Thinking** exercises accompany each care plan.

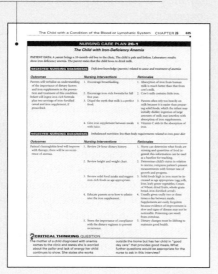

A bulleted list of **Key Points** concludes each chapter.

Online Resources provide additional sources of pertinent information.

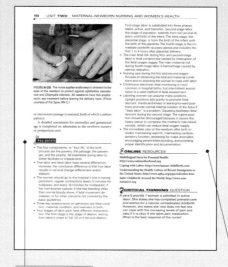

New **full-color photographs with art overlays** illustrate body systems in pediatric chapters.

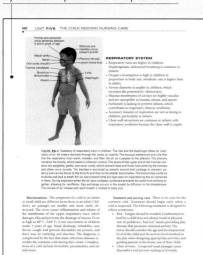

NCLEX-style multiple choice review questions appear at the end of each chapter. Answers are provided on the inside back cover.

STUDY GUIDE
The Study Guide to accompany this textbook includes matching, labeling, and completion activities, critical thinking exercises, case studies, and crossword puzzles.

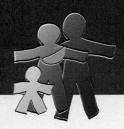

Acknowledgments

Reader confidence in earlier editions of *Introduction to Maternity and Pediatric Nursing* provided the enthusiasm and encouragement for the scope of this revision. I want to thank Ilze Rader, former Senior Nursing Editor at W.B. Saunders Company, and Terri Wood, Senior Nursing Editor, Elsevier Science, for believing in my ability to accomplish this task, for providing insight and inspiration, and for nurturing and allowing the creativity necessary for a text to prepare nurses for practice in the twenty-first century. I am grateful to the educators, clinicians, and students who contributed constructive comments, many of which have influenced the revision of the fourth edition. The project becomes more exciting with each revision because increasing knowledge, new technology, and changing health care delivery systems must be woven into the content as it affects nursing practice.

My first text published by W.B. Saunders Company, *Principles and Techniques in Pediatric Nursing,* was originally published in 1965. Subsequent revisions and the ANA "Book of the Year" award nourished my interest in writing. I continue to publish journal articles, but I am excited to have the opportunity to continue my contributions in the textbook arena.

As a parent, I recognize the value and have experienced the joys of a happy, healthy, loving family. Guiding the growth and development of four tiny children who are now grown and productively contributing to society is a unique experience. I would like to express my gratitude to my children, Heidi, Barnet, Amos, and Eve and David Fleck for their encouragement and patience. They have taught me firsthand what it means to be an anxious parent, thus in a sense providing the basis for content that may enable the student to lessen the anxieties of other parents. This year, my grandchild Zoe contributes to the text as a model and contributes to my understanding of the role of a grandparent in the modern day extended family.

My travels with my husband have made it possible for me to personally investigate the cultural practices and problems of maternity and pediatric clients in developed and undeveloped areas of Africa, the Far East, the Middle East, and Europe, as well as in many parts of the United States, including Alaska. My appreciation is extended to the many members of the medical and nursing professions in these countries for their time and cooperation.

I would also like to thank the medical and nursing staff of Riverside County Regional Medical Center in Moreno Valley, California; the Southern California Kaiser Permanente Medical Center in Fontana, California; Loma Linda University Medical Center in Loma Linda, California; and Arrowhead Regional Medical Center in Colton, California, for their assistance and cooperation in providing access to critical current information and photographs.

I want to thank Trena L. Rich, RN, MSN, C-ANP, for her special contributions and able assistance in the preparation of this manuscript. Pat Spier, RN-C, BSN, staff educator in the Total Care Birth Center at Loma Linda University Medical Center in Loma Linda, California, and labor and delivery nurse at Arrowhead Regional Medical Center in Colton, California, provided special expertise in medical photography that brought concepts into reality in beautiful, full-color pictures. Esperanza Villanueva Joyce, MSN, EdD, CNS, RN, Dean and Professor, Our Lady of the Lake College, Baton Rouge, Louisiana, graciously provided the Spanish translation of the patient teaching plans for the tear-out cards. Emily Slone McKinney, MSN, RN-C, offered a detailed review of the textbook manuscript as she co-wrote the accompanying Study Guide. Her insights and suggestions were greatly appreciated.

Catherine Ott, Senior Editorial Assistant, Elsevier Science, worked wonders with all of the fine details essential to successful publication. Jill Riggin, Associate Developmental Editor, Elsevier Science, was detailed and concise in her approach to the manuscript and was a pleasure to work with. Jodi Willard, Senior Project Manager for Elsevier Science, monitored the precision of the text and ensured that timelines were met. Her expertise and professionalism were invaluable. Thanks also to Amy Buxton, Designer at Elsevier Science, for her exceptional work in creating the new full-color design. I was also blessed with the able assistance of Carolyn Boyd, who provided computer expertise with critical manuscript proofing and competent, constructive suggestions. The blending into one text of traditional, current, and future practices necessary for LPNs/LVNs to function in the twenty-first century was a challenge that required cooperation and compromise. It was a pleasure to work on this team where simple exposition was allowed to develop into a hearty feast of knowledge that will hopefully serve to educate and whet the appetite of the reader for continued education.

Finally, and most important, I would like to thank my nursing students from Fordham School of Nursing, Hunter College of the City University of New York, California State College at Los Angeles, and Riverside Community College for helping me apply and redefine concepts of teaching and learning.

GLORIA LEIFER HARTSTON

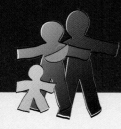

Contents

UNIT **ONE** AN OVERVIEW OF MATERNITY AND PEDIATRIC NURSING

1 The Past, Present, and Future, 1

The Past, 2
  Europe, 2
  The United States, 2
The Present, 4
  Maternity Care, 4
  Child Care, 7
  Health Care Delivery Systems, 10
  Advanced Practice Nurses, 12
  The Nursing Process, 12
  Nursing Care Plans, 13
  Critical Thinking in Nursing, 15
The Future, 16
  Health Care Reform, 16
  Healthy People 2010, 17
  Documentation, 17
  Community-Based Nursing, 18

UNIT **TWO** MATERNAL-NEWBORN NURSING AND WOMEN'S HEALTH

2 Human Reproductive Anatomy and Physiology, 21

Puberty, 21
  The Male, 21
  The Female, 22
Male Reproductive System, 22
  External Genitalia, 22
  Internal Genitalia, 22
Female Reproductive System, 23
  External Genitalia, 23
  Internal Genitalia, 24
  Female Pelvis, 26
  Breasts, 28
Female Reproductive Cycle and Menstruation, 28
Physiology of the Sex Act, 29
  Physiology of the Male Sex Act, 29
  Physiology of the Female Sex Act, 31

3 Prenatal Development, 33

Cell Division and Gametogenesis, 33
Fertilization, 34
  Sex Determination, 34
  Tubal Transport of the Zygote, 34
  Implantation of the Zygote, 34
Development, 34
  Cell Differentiation, 34
  Prenatal Developmental Milestones, 37
Accessory Structures of Pregnancy, 40
  Placenta, 40
  Umbilical Cord, 42
  Fetal Circulation, 42
Prenatal Development and *Healthy People 2010,* 44
Multifetal Pregnancy, 44

4 Prenatal Care and Adaptations to Pregnancy, 47

Goals of Prenatal Care, 47
  Prenatal Visits, 48
  Definition of Terms, 50
  Determining the Estimated Date of Delivery, 51
Diagnosis of Pregnancy, 51
  Presumptive Signs of Pregnancy, 51
  Probable Signs of Pregnancy, 53
  Positive Signs of Pregnancy, 54
Normal Physiological Changes in Pregnancy, 54
  Reproductive System, 54
  Respiratory System, 55
  Cardiovascular System, 55
  Gastrointestinal System, 56
  Urinary System, 57
  Integumentary and Skeletal Systems, 57
Nutrition for Pregnancy and Lactation, 58
  Weight Gain, 60
  Nutritional Requirements, 60
  Recommended Dietary Allowances and Recommended Dietary Intakes, 63
  Special Nutritional Considerations, 64
  Nutrition During Lactation, 65

Exercise During Pregnancy, 65
  Elevated Temperature, 65
  Hypotension, 67
  Cardiac Output, 67
  Hormones, 67
  Other Factors, 67
Common Discomforts in Pregnancy, 68
Psychological Adaptations to
  Pregnancy, 70
  Impact on the Mother, 70
  Impact on the Father, 72
  Impact on the Adolescent, 72
  Impact on the Older Couple, 73
  Impact on the Single Mother, 73
  Impact on the Single Father, 73
  Impact on the Grandparents, 74
Prenatal Education, 74
Physiological and Psychological
  Changes in Pregnancy and Nursing
  Interventions, 74

**5 Nursing Care of Women with
    Complications During
    Pregnancy, 80**
Assessment of Fetal Health, 80
Pregnancy-Related Complications, 81
  Hyperemesis Gravidarum, 81
  Bleeding Disorders of Early
    Pregnancy, 84
  Bleeding Disorders of Late
    Pregnancy, 91
  Hypertension During Pregnancy, 93
  Blood Incompatibility Between the
    Pregnant Woman and the Fetus, 99
Pregnancy Complicated by Medical
  Conditions, 100
  Diabetes Mellitus, 100
  Heart Disease, 106
  Anemia, 107
  Infections, 108
Environmental Hazards During
  Pregnancy, 112
  Bioterrorism and the Pregnant
    Patient, 112
  Substance Abuse, 113
  Trauma During Pregnancy, 115
Effects of a High-Risk Pregnancy on the
  Family, 117
  Disruption of Usual Roles, 117
  Financial Difficulties, 117
  Delayed Attachment to the Infant, 117
  Loss of Expected Birth Experience, 117

**6 Nursing Care During Labor and
    Birth, 119**
Cultural Influence on Birth Practices, 119
Settings for Childbirth, 120
  Hospitals, 120
  Freestanding Birth Centers, 120
  Home, 120
Components of the Birth Process, 124
  The Powers, 124
  The Passage, 126
  The Passenger, 127
  The Pysche, 130
Normal Childbirth, 131
  Signs of Impending Labor, 131
  Mechanisms of Labor, 131
Admission to the Hospital or Birth
  Center, 133
  When to Go to the Hospital or Birth
    Center, 133
  Admission Data Collection, 134
  Admission Procedures, 135
  Nursing Care of the Woman in False
    Labor, 135
Nursing Care Before Birth, 136
  Monitoring the Fetus, 136
  Monitoring the Woman, 141
  Helping the Woman Cope with
    Labor, 142
The Labor Process and the Nurse, 144
  Stages and Phases of Labor, 144
  Vaginal Birth After Cesarean Birth, 144
Nursing Care During Birth, 144
  Nursing Responsibilities During
    Birth, 147
  Immediate Postpartum Period: The Third
    and Fourth Stages of Labor, 148
Nursing Care Immediately After Birth, 148
  Care of the Mother, 148
  Care of the Infant, Phase 1, 151

**7 Nursing Management of Pain
    During Labor and Birth, 156**
Education for Childbearing, 156
  Types of Classes Available, 156
  Variations of Basic Childbirth
    Preparation Classes, 156
  Content of Childbirth Preparation
    Classes, 158
Childbirth and Pain, 158
  How Childbirth Differs from Other
    Pain, 158
  Factors That Influence Labor Pain, 158

Nonpharmacological Pain
  Management, 161
    Advantages of Nonpharmacological
      Methods, 161
    Limitations of Nonpharmacological
      Methods, 161
    Methods of Childbirth Preparation, 161
    Nonpharmacological Techniques, 161
    The Nurse's Role in
      Nonpharmacological Techniques, 164
Pharmacological Pain Management, 164
    Physiology of Pregnancy and Its
      Relationship to Analgesia and
      Anesthesia, 165
    Advantages of Pharmacological
      Methods, 165
    Limitations of Pharmacological
      Methods, 166
    Analgesics and Adjunctive Drugs, 167
    Regional Analgesics and
      Anesthetics, 167
    General Anesthesia, 170
    The Nurse's Role in Pharmacological
      Techniques, 170

8 Nursing Care of Women with
   Complications During Labor and
   Birth, 176
Obstetric Procedures, 176
    Amnioinfusion, 176
    Amniotomy, 176
    Induction or Augmentation of
      Labor, 177
    Version, 180
    Episiotomy and Lacerations, 180
    Forceps and Vacuum Extraction
      Births, 182
    Cesarean Birth, 183
Abnormal Labor, 188
    Problems with the Powers of Labor, 188
    Problems with the Fetus, 192
    Problems with the Pelvis and Soft
      Tissues, 194
    The Psyche, 195
    Abnormal Duration of Labor, 195
Premature Rupture of Membranes, 196
Preterm Labor, 196
    Signs of Impending Preterm Labor, 196
    Tocolytic Therapy, 197
    Stopping Preterm Labor, 197
Prolonged Pregnancy, 198

Emergencies During Childbirth, 198
    Prolapsed Umbilical Cord, 198
    Uterine Rupture, 199
    Uterine Inversion, 200
    Amniotic Fluid Embolism, 201

9 The Family After Birth, 203
Adapting Care to Specific Groups and
  Cultures, 203
    Nursing Considerations for Specific
      Groups of Patients, 203
    Cultural Influences on Postpartum
      Care, 204
Postpartum Changes in the Mother, 204
    Reproductive System, 204
    Cardiovascular System, 209
    Urinary System, 210
    Gastrointestinal System, 210
    Integumentary System, 210
    Musculoskeletal System, 210
    Immune System, 211
    Changes After Cesarean Birth and
      Adaptation of Nursing Care, 211
Emotional Care, 214
    Mothers, 214
    Fathers, 214
    Siblings, 214
    Grandparents, 215
    Grieving Parents, 215
Parenthood, 216
The Family Care Plan, 216
Care of the Newborn, Phase 2, 217
    Admission Care of the Newborn to the
      Postpartum or Nursery Unit, 217
    Hypoglycemia, 221
    Screening Tests, 222
    Skin Care, 222
    Security, 222
    Bonding and Attachment, 222
    Daily Care, 224
Breastfeeding, 224
    Choosing Whether to Breastfeed, 224
    Physiology of Lactation, 225
    Assisting the Mother to Breastfeed, 226
    Preventing Problems, 229
    Special Breastfeeding Situations, 230
    Storing and Freezing Breast Milk, 231
    Maternal Nutrition, 232
    Weaning, 232

Formula Feeding, 232
  Types of Infant Formulas, 232
  Preparation, 233
  Feeding the Infant, 233
Discharge Planning, 234
  Postpartum Self-Care Teaching, 234
  Newborn Discharge Care, 235

10 Nursing Care of Women with Complications Following Birth, 237
Shock, 237
Hemorrhage, 237
  Hypovolemic Shock, 238
  Anemia, 238
  Early Postpartum Hemorrhage, 238
  Late Postpartum Hemorrhage, 242
Thromboembolic Disorders, 243
Puerperal Infection, 244
  Mastitis and Breastfeeding, 246
Subinvolution of the Uterus, 247
Disorders of Mood, 248
  Postpartum Depression, 248
  Postpartum Psychosis, 248
The Homeless Mother and Newborn, 249

11 The Nurse's Role in Women's Health Care, 251
Goals of *Healthy People 2010,* 251
Preventive Health Care for Women, 251
  Breast Care, 252
  Vulvar Self-Examination, 252
  Pelvic Examination, 252
Menstrual Disorders, 254
  Amenorrhea, 254
  Abnormal Uterine Bleeding, 254
  Menstrual Cycle Pain, 254
  Endometriosis, 255
  Premenstrual Dysphoric Disorder, 255
Gynecological Infections, 255
  The Normal Vagina, 256
  Toxic Shock Syndrome, 256
  Sexually Transmitted Diseases, 257
  Pelvic Inflammatory Disease, 261
Family Planning, 261
  Temporary Contraception, 261
  Permanent Contraception, 268
  Emergency Contraception, 269
  Unreliable Contraceptive Methods, 269
Infertility Care, 269
  Social and Psychological Implications, 270

Factors Affecting Infertility, 270
Factors Influencing Infertility, 271
Evaluation of Infertility, 272
Therapy for Infertility, 272
Outcomes of Infertility Therapy, 274
Legal and Ethical Factors in Assisted Reproduction, 274
Nursing Care Related to Infertility Treatment, 274
Hormone Replacement Therapy, 274
  Side Effects and Contraindications, 275
  Complementary Regimens, 275
  Therapy for Osteoporosis, 275
Menopause, 275
  Physical Changes, 276
  Psychological and Cultural Variations, 276
  Treatment Options, 276
  Nursing Care of the Menopausal Woman, 276
Pelvic Floor Dysfunction, 278
  Vaginal Wall Prolapse, 278
  Uterine Prolapse, 279
  Management of Pelvic Floor Dysfunction, 279
  Nursing Care of the Woman with Pelvic Floor Dysfunction, 279
  Urinary Incontinence, 279
Other Female Reproductive Tract Disorders, 279
  Uterine Fibroids, 279
  Ovarian Cysts, 280
Cultural Aspects of Pain Control, 280

12 The Term Newborn, 282
Adjustment to Extrauterine Life, 282
Physical Characteristics and Phase 3 Care of the Newborn, 283
  Nervous System: Reflexes, 283
  Head, 283
  Visual Stimuli and Sensory Overload, 286
  Hearing, 286
  Sleep, 286
  Pain, 287
  Conditioned Responses, 287
  Neonatal Behavioral Assessment Scale, 287
  Respiratory System, 287
  Apgar Score, 288
  Circulatory System, 288
  Providing Warmth, 289

Obtaining Temperature, Pulse, and
Respirations, 289
Musculoskeletal System, 290
Length and Weight, 290
Genitourinary System, 291
Integumentary System, 292
Gastrointestinal System, 295
Preventing Infection, 297
Discharge Planning, 302
Home Care, 302
Furnishings, 302
Clothing, 302

**13 Preterm and Postterm
Newborns, 305**

The Preterm Newborn, 305
Causes, 306
Physical Characteristics, 306
Related Problems, 306
Special Needs, 313
Prognosis, 314
Family Reaction, 317
The Postterm Newborn, 317
Physical Characteristics, 318
Nursing Care, 318
Transporting the High-Risk Newborn, 318

**14 The Newborn with a Congenital
Malformation, 320**

Malformations Present at Birth, 321
Nervous System, 321
Gastrointestinal System, 327
Musculoskeletal System, 329
Metabolic Defects, 334
Phenylketonuria, 334
Maple Syrup Urine Disease, 335
Galactosemia, 335
Chromosomal Abnormalities, 336
Down Syndrome, 336
Perinatal Damage, 338
Hemolytic Disease of the Newborn:
Erythroblastosis Fetalis, 338
Intracranial Hemorrhage, 343
Infant of a Diabetic Mother, 344

**UNIT THREE THE GROWING CHILD
AND FAMILY**

**15 An Overview of Growth,
Development, and Nutrition, 346**

Growth and Development, 346
The Impact of Growth and
Development on Nursing Care, 346
Terminology, 349
Directional Patterns, 349
Some Developmental Differences
Between Children and Adults, 349
Growth Standards, 352
Developmental Screening, 352
Influencing Factors, 352
Personality Development, 356
The Growth and Development of a
Parent, 363
Nutrition, 367
Nutritional Heritage, 367
Family Nutrition, 367
Nutritional Care Plan, 370
Nutrition and Health, 370
Nutrition and Illness, 371
Feeding the Healthy Child, 374
Feeding the Ill Child, 376
Food-Drug Interactions, 378
The Teeth, 378
Play, 382

16 The Infant, 385

General Characteristics, 386
Oral Stage, 386
Motor Development, 386
Emotional Development, 386
Need for Constant Care and
Guidance, 386
Development and Care, 387
Community-Based Care: A
Multidisciplinary Team, 388
Health Maintenance, 395
Illness Prevention, 397
Infant Safety, 402
Car Safety, 402
Fall Prevention, 402
Toy Safety, 403
Summary of Major Developmental
Changes in the First Year, 403

17 The Toddler, 405

General Characteristics, 405
  Physical Development, 405
  Sensorimotor and Cognitive
  Development, 408
  Speech Development, 409
Guidance and Discipline, 410
Daily Care, 411
Toilet Independence, 413
Nutrition Counseling, 414
Day Care, 415
Injury Prevention, 416
  Consumer Education, 416
Toys and Play, 419

18 The Preschool Child, 422

General Characteristics, 422
  Physical Development, 422
  Cognitive Development, 423
  Effects of Cultural Practices, 423
  Language Development, 423
  Development of Play, 425
  Spiritual Development, 425
  Sexual Curiosity, 425
  Bedtime Habits, 427
Physical, Mental, Emotional and Social
  Development, 427
  The Three-Year-Old, 427
  The Four-Year-Old, 428
  The Five-Year-Old, 428
Guidance, 429
  Discipline and Limit Setting, 429
  Jealousy, 430
  Thumb Sucking, 431
  Enuresis, 431
Nursery School, 432
Daily Care, 432
  Clothing, 432
  Accident Prevention, 432
Play in Health and Illness, 433
  Value of Play, 433
  The Nurse's Role, 433
  Types of Play, 434
Nursing Implications of Preschool Growth
  and Development, 435

19 The School-Age Child, 438

General Characteristics, 438
  Physical Growth, 439
  Gender Identity, 440
  Sex Education, 440

Influences from the Wider World, 441
  School-Related Tasks, 441
  Play, 443
  Latchkey Children, 443
Physical, Mental, Emotional, and Social
  Development, 444
  The Six-Year-Old, 444
  The Seven-Year-Old, 445
  The Eight-Year-Old, 445
  The Nine-Year-Old, 446
  Preadolescence, 446
Guidance and Health Supervision, 447
  Health Examinations, 447
  Pet Ownership, 451

20 The Adolescent, 455

General Characteristics, 455
Growth and Development, 456
  Physical Development, 456
  Psychosocial Development, 460
  Cognitive Development, 463
  Peer Relationships, 463
  Career Plans, 464
  Responsibility, 465
  Daydreams, 465
  Sexual Behavior, 465
  Parenting, 467
Health Education and Guidance, 468
  Nutrition, 468
  Personal Care, 470
  Safety, 470
Common Problems of Adolescence, 471
  Substance Abuse, 471
  Depression, 472
The Nursing Approach to
  Adolescents, 472

UNIT **FOUR** ADAPTING CARE TO
THE PEDIATRIC PATIENT

**21 The Child's Experience of
Hospitalization,** 475

Health Care Delivery Settings, 475
  Outpatient Clinic, 475
  Home, 476
  Children's Hospital Unit, 476
The Child's Reaction to
  Hospitalization, 476
  Separation Anxiety, 477
  Pain, 478
  Drug Physiology, 478

Fear, 479
Regression, 479
Cultural Needs, 480
Fostering Intercultural
Communication, 482
The Parents' Reactions to the Child's
Hospitalization, 483
The Nurse's Role in Hospital
Admission, 483
Developing a Pediatric Nursing Care
Plan, 484
Clinical Pathways, 484
Needs of the Hospitalized Child, 486
The Hospitalized Infant, 486
The Hospitalized Toddler, 487
The Hospitalized Preschooler, 489
The Hospitalized School-Age Child, 489
The Hospitalized Adolescent, 490
Confidentiality and Legality, 491
Discharge Planning, 491
Home Care, 492

**22 Health Care Adaptations for the
Child and Family, 494**

Admission to the Pediatric Unit, 494
Informed Consent, 494
Identification, 494
Essential Safety Measures in the
Hospital Setting, 495
Transporting, Positioning, and
Restraining the Infant, 496
Verifying the Child Assessment, 496
Basic Data Collection, 496
The History Survey, 497
The Physical Survey, 497
Collecting Specimens, 505
Urine Specimens, 505
Stool Specimens, 505
Blood Specimens, 506
Lumbar Puncture, 506
Physiological Responses to Medications
in Infants and Children, 507
Absorption of Medications in Infants
and Children, 508
Metabolism of Medications in Infants
and Children, 508
Excretion of Medications in Infants and
Children, 508
Nursing Responsibilities in Administering
Medications to Infants and Children, 508
Calculating Pediatric Drug Dosages, 510
Calculating the Safe Drug Dose, 510
Avoiding Drug Interactions, 511
Administering Oral Medications, 513
Administering Parenteral
Medications, 514
Adaptation of Selected Procedures to
Children, 519
Nutrition, Digestion, and
Elimination, 519
Respiration, 519
Preoperative and Postoperative
Care, 528

UNIT **FIVE** THE CHILD NEEDING NURSING CARE

**23 The Child with a Sensory or
Neurological Condition, 533**

The Ears, 533
Otitis Externa, 535
Acute Otitis Media (AOM), 535
Hearing Impairment, 537
Barotrauma, 538
The Eyes, 538
Visual Acuity Tests, 539
Dyslexia, 540
Amblyopia, 540
Strabismus, 540
Conjunctivitis, 541
Hyphema, 541
Retinoblastoma, 542
The Nervous System, 542
Reye's Syndrome, 542
Sepsis, 545
Meningitis, 546
Encephalitis, 547
Brain Tumors, 548
Seizure Disorders, 549
Other Conditions Causing Decreased
Level of Consciousness, 554
Cerebral Palsy, 554
Cognitive Impairment, 557
Head Injuries, 559
Near-Drowning, 563

**24 The Child with a
Musculoskeletal Condition, 567**

Overview, 567
Observation of the Musculoskeletal
System in the Growing Child, 567
Observation of Gait, 568
Observation of Muscle Tone, 569

Diagnostic Tests and Treatments, 569
Musculoskeletal System Differences
  Between the Child and Adult, 569
Pediatric Trauma, 569
Traumatic Fractures and Traction, 570
Osteomyelitis, 578
Duchenne's or Becker
  (Pseudohypertrophic) Muscular
  Dystrophy, 579
Legg-Calvé-Perthes Disease
  (Coxa Plana), 579
Osteosarcoma, 579
Ewing's Sarcoma, 580
Juvenile Rheumatoid Arthritis, 580
Torticollis (Wry Neck), 581
Scoliosis, 582
Sports Injuries, 583
Family Violence, 584
Child Abuse, 585
  Federal Laws and Agencies, 586
  Nursing Care and Intervention, 586
  Cultural and Medical Issues, 588

**25 The Child with a Respiratory or
     Cardiovascular Disorder, 590**

Respiratory System, 591
  Development of the Respiratory
    Tract, 591
  Normal Respiration, 591
  Ventilation, 591
  Nasopharyngitis, 591
  Acute Pharyngitis, 594
  Sinusitis in Children, 594
  Croup Syndromes, 594
  Respiratory Syncytial Virus, 597
  Pneumonia, 598
  Tonsillitis and Adenoiditis, 599
  Allergic Rhinitis, 600
  Asthma, 602
  Cystic Fibrosis, 608
  Bronchopulmonary Dysplasia, 615
  Sudden Infant Death Syndrome, 615
Cardiovascular System, 616
  Signs Related to Suspected Cardiac
    Pathology, 616
  Congenital Heart Disease, 616
  Acquired Heart Disease, 622
  Rheumatic Fever, 624
  Systemic Hypertension, 627
  Hyperlipidemia, 627
  Kawasaki Disease, 628

**26 The Child with a Condition
     of the Blood, Blood-Forming
     Organs, or Lymphatic
     System, 631**

Anemias, 633
  Iron-Deficiency Anemia, 633
  Sickle Cell Disease, 634
  Thalassemia, 638
Bleeding Disorders, 639
  Hemophilia, 639
  Platelet Disorders, 641
  Idiopathic (Immunological)
    Thrombocytopenic Purpura, 641
Disorders of White Blood Cells, 641
  Leukemia, 641
  Hodgkin's Disease, 645
Nursing Care of the Chronically Ill
  Child, 646
  Chronic Illness, 646
  Developmental Disabilities, 650
  Home Care, 650
  Care of the Chronically Ill Child, 650
Nursing Care of the Dying Child, 650
  Facing Death, 650
  Self-Exploration, 651
  The Child's Reaction to Death, 651
  The Child's Awareness of His or Her
    Condition, 654
  Physical Changes of Impending
    Death, 654
  Stages of Dying, 654

**27 The Child with a
     Gastrointestinal Condition, 656**

Overview, 656
Congenital Disorders, 657
  Esophageal Atresia (Tracheoesophageal
    Fistula, TEF), 657
  Imperforate Anus, 658
  Pyloric Stenosis, 658
  Celiac Disease, 659
  Hirschsprung's Disease (Aganglionic
    Megacolon), 661
  Intussusception, 662
  Meckel's Diverticulum, 663
  Hernias, 663
Disorders of Motility, 664
  Gastroenteritis, 664
  Vomiting, 664
  Gastroesophageal Reflux, 665
  Diarrhea, 665
  Constipation, 666

Fluid and Electrolyte Imbalance, 666
Dehydration, 670
Overhydration, 672
Nutritional Deficiencies, 672
Failure to Thrive, 673
Kwashiorkor, 674
Rickets, 675
Scurvy, 675
Infections, 675
Appendicitis, 675
Thrush (Oral Candidiasis), 676
Worms, 676
Poisoning, 677
General Concepts, 677
Poisonous Plants, 677
Drugs, 677
Lead Poisoning (Plumbism), 680
Foreign Bodies, 681

28 The Child with a Genitourinary Condition, 683

Development of the Urinary Tract, 683
Development of the Reproductive
  Systems, 684
Assessment of Urinary Function, 686
Anomalies of the Urinary Tract, 686
Phimosis, 686
Hypospadias and Epispadias, 687
Exstrophy of the Bladder, 688
Obstructive Uropathy, 688
Acute Urinary Tract Infection, 688
Nephrotic Syndrome (Nephrosis), 690
Acute Glomerulonephritis, 693
Wilms' Tumor, 694
Hydrocele, 694
Cryptorchidism, 697
Impact of Urinary or Genital Surgery on
  Growth and Development, 698

29 The Child with a Skin Condition, 700

Skin Development and Functions, 700
Skin Disorders and Variations, 701
Congenital Lesions, 703
Strawberry Nevus, 703
Port-Wine Nevus, 703
Infections, 703
Miliaria, 703
Intertrigo, 704
Seborrheic Dermatitis, 704
Diaper Dermatitis, 704
Acne Vulgaris, 705

Herpes Simplex Type I, 706
Infantile Eczema, 706
Staphylococcal Infection, 710
Impetigo, 710
Fungal Infections, 711
Pediculosis, 712
Scabies, 713
Injuries, 713
Burns, 713
Frostbite, 720

30 The Child with a Metabolic Condition, 723

Overview, 723
Inborn Errors of Metabolism, 724
Tay-Sachs Disease, 724
Endocrine Disorders, 725
Hypothyroidism, 725
Common Metabolic Dysfunctions, 725
Diabetes Insipidus, 725
Diabetes Mellitus, 727

31 The Child with a Communicable Disease, 741

Communicable Disease, 741
Common Childhood Communicable
  Diseases, 741
Review of Terms, 747
Host Resistance, 747
Types of Immunity, 748
Transmission of Infection, 748
Medical Asepsis and Standard
  Precautions, 748
Protective Isolation, 749
Handwashing, 749
Family Education, 749
Rashes, 749
Worldwide Immunization Programs, 750
Healthy People 2010, 750
The Nurse's Role, 750
Immunization Schedule for
  Children, 751
The Future of Immunotherapy, 753
Bioterrorism and the Pediatric
  Patient, 753
A New Type of Childhood Trauma, 753
Initial Observation, 753
Sexually Transmitted Diseases, 754
Overview, 754
Nursing Care and Responsibilities, 754
HIV/AIDS in Children, 756

32 The Child with an Emotional or Behavioral Condition, 761

The Nurse's Role, 761
Types and Settings of Treatment, 762
Origins of Emotional and Behavioral Conditions, 762
Organic Behavior Disorders, 763
    Childhood Autism, 763
    Obsessive-Compulsive Disorders in Children, 763
Environmental or Biochemical Behavior Disorders, 764
    Depression, 764
    Suicide, 764
    Substance Abuse, 767
    Attention Deficit-Hyperactivity Disorder, 770
    Anorexia Nervosa, 771
    Bulimia, 772
Minimizing the Impact of Behavior Disorders in Children, 773
    Effect of the Illness on Growth and Development, 773
    Effect of the Illness on Siblings, 773

UNIT SIX THE CHANGING HEALTH CARE ENVIRONMENT

33 Complementary and Alternative Therapies in Maternity and Pediatric Nursing, 775

Definition of CAM Therapies, 775
The Nurse's Role in CAM Therapy, 775
Federal Regulations, 776
Overview of Common Alternative Health Care Practices, 778
    Massage, 778
    Osteopathy, 778
    Energy Healing, 778
    Reflexology, 778
    Acupuncture and Acupressure, 778
    Homeopathy, 779
    Ayurveda, 779
    Aromatherapy, 779
    Hypnotherapy, 780
    Hydrotherapy, 780
    Guided Imagery, 780
    Biofeedback, 780
    Chiropractic Care, 781
    Herbal Remedies, 781
    Hyperbaric Oxygen Therapy, 784
    Sauna/Heat Therapy, 784

APPENDIX

A Standard Precautions and Body Substance Isolation Precautions, 787

B Internet Website for Maternal-Child Health Organizations and Foundations, 789

C NANDA-Approved Nursing Diagnoses 2001-2002, 790

D Conversion of Pounds and Ounces to Grams for Newborn Weights, 792

E Temperature Equivalents, 793

F Common Spanish Phrases for Maternity and Pediatric Nurses, 794

G Commonly Used Abbreviations in Maternity and Pediatric Nursing, 799

Complete Bibliography and Reader References, 801

Illustration Credits, 817

Glossary, 821

Index, 835

CHAPTER 1

The Past, Present, and Future

1. Define each key term listed.
2. Contrast present-day concepts of maternity and child care with those of the past.
3. List three environmental stresses on the child-bearing family.
4. List four reasons why statistics are important.
5. Discuss how culture affects childbirth and child care.
6. List the five steps of the nursing process.
7. Recall the contributions of persons in history to the fields of maternity and pediatric care.
8. Name two international organizations concerned with maternity and child care.
9. List three federal programs that assist mothers and infants.
10. Define the role of the community-based nurse as a health care provider to mothers and children.
11. List the organizations concerned with setting standards for the nursing care of maternity and pediatric patients.
12. State the influence of the federal government on maternity and pediatric care.
13. Discuss common terms used in expressing vital statistics.
14. Contrast a nursing care plan with a clinical pathway.
15. Define the Nursing Intervention Classification (NIC) and its relationship to the nursing process.
16. Describe the Nursing Outcome Classification (NOC) and its influence on the nursing process.
17. Compare and contrast nursing and medical diagnosis frameworks with focus on North American Nursing Diagnosis Association (NANDA) taxonomy.
18. Define critical thinking.
19. Discuss the role of critical thinking in the nursing process and in clinical judgment.
20. Discuss the role of critical thinking as it relates to test taking and lifelong learning.
21. Discuss the roles and functions of a school nurse.
22. Describe the role of the community health nurse as a health care provider.

Advanced Practice Nurse (p. 12)
advocate (p. 7)
birthing centers (p. 5)
Clinical Nurse Specialist (CNS) (p. 12)
clinical pathway (p. 6)
cost containment (p. 5)
critical thinking (p. 13)
diagnosis-related grouping (DRG) (p. 10)
documentation (p. 17)
empowerment (p. 2)
family care plan (p. 18)
full inclusion (p. 11)
Health Maintenance Organization (HMO) (p. 11)
Healthy People 2010 (p. 17)
labor, delivery, and recovery (LDR) room (p. 4)
mainstream (p. 11)
midwife (p. 6)
morbidity (mŏr-BĬD-ĭ-tē, p. 2)
mortality (mŏr-TĂL-ĭ-tē, p. 2)
nursing care plan (p. 13)
nursing process (p. 12)
obstetrician (ŏb-stĭ-TRĬSH-ĕn, p. 1)
obstetrics (ŏb-STĔT-rĭks, p. 1)
Pediatric Nurse Practitioner (PNP) (p. 12)
pediatrics (pē-dē-ĂT-rĭks, p. 2)
Preferred Provider Organization (PPO) (p. 11)
puerperium (pū-ĕr-PĒ-rē-ŭm, p. 1)
statistics (stă-TĬS-tĭks, p. 7)

The word obstetrics is derived from the Latin term *obstetrix*, which means "stand by." It is the branch of medicine that pertains to care of women during pregnancy, childbirth, and the postpartum period (puerperium). Maternity nursing is the care given by the nurse to the expectant family before, during, and following birth.

A physician specializing in the care of women during pregnancy, labor, birth, and the postpartum period is an obstetrician. These physicians perform cesarean deliveries and treat women with known or suspected obstetric problems as well as attend normal deliveries. Many family physicians and certified nurse-midwives also deliver babies. The skill and knowledge related to obstetrics have evolved over centuries.

Pediatrics is defined as the branch of medicine that deals with the child's development and care and the diseases of childhood and their treatment. The word is derived from the Greek *pais, paidos* "child" and *iatreia* "cure."

Family-centered care recognizes the strength and integrity of the family as the core of planning and implementing health care. The family as caregivers and decision makers are an integral part of both obstetric and pediatric nursing. The philosophy, goals, culture, and ethnic practices of the family contribute to their ability to accept and maintain *control* over the health care of family members. This control is called empowerment. The nurse's role in maternity and pediatric family-centered care is to enter into a contract or partnership with the family to achieve the goals of health for its members.

THE PAST

EUROPE

The earliest records concerning childbirth are in the Egyptian papyruses (circa 1550 BC). Later advances were made by Soranus, a Greek physician who practiced in second-century Rome and who is known as the father of obstetrics. He instituted the practice of podalic version, a procedure used to rotate a fetus to a breech, or feet-first, position. Podalic version is important in delivering the second infant in a set of twins. In this procedure the physician reaches into the uterus and grasps one or both of the infant's feet to facilitate delivery. Planned cesarean birth is safer and used more often today. Such scientific exploration halted with the decline of the Roman Empire and the ensuing Dark Ages.

During the nineteenth century, Karl Credé (1819-1892) and Ignaz Semmelweis (1818-1865) made contributions that improved the safety and health of mother and child during and after childbirth. In 1884 Credé recommended instilling 2% silver nitrate into the eyes of newborns to prevent blindness caused by gonorrhea. This procedure has basically stayed the same, except that 1% silver nitrate is administered or antibiotic ointments are used. Credé's innovation has saved the eyesight of incalculable numbers of babies.

The classic story of Semmelweis is interesting and tragic. In the 1840s he worked as an assistant professor in the maternity ward of the Vienna general hospital. There he discovered a relationship between the incidence of puerperal fever (or "childbed fever"), which caused many deaths among women in lying-in wards, and the examination of new mothers by student doctors who had just returned from dissecting cadavers. Semmelweis deduced that puerperal fever was septic, contagious, and transmitted by the *unwashed hands* of physicians and medical students. Semmelweis's outstanding work, written in 1861, is titled *The Causes, Understanding, and Prevention of Childbed Fever.* Not until 1890 was his teaching finally accepted.

Louis Pasteur (1822-1895), a French chemist, confirmed that puerperal fever was caused by bacteria and could be spread by improper handwashing and contact with contaminated objects. The simple, but highly effective, procedure of handwashing continues to be one of the most important means of preventing the spread of infection in the hospital and home today. Joseph Lister (1827-1912), a British surgeon influenced by Pasteur, experimented with chemical means of preventing infection. He revolutionized surgical practice by introducing antiseptic surgery.

NURSING **TIP**

Cultural beliefs today, as in the past, affect how a family perceives health and illness. Holistic nursing includes being alert for cultural diversity and incorporating this information into nursing care plans.

THE UNITED STATES

The immigrants who reached the shores of North America brought a wide variety of practices and beliefs about the birth process. Many practices were also contributed by the Native American nations. Most deliveries in the early United States were attended by a midwife or relative. One physician, Samuel Bard, who was educated outside the United States, is credited with writing the first American textbook for midwives in 1807.

Oliver Wendell Holmes (1809-1894), when a young Harvard physician, wrote a paper detailing the contagious nature of puerperal fever but he, like Semmelweis, was widely criticized by his colleagues. Eventually, the "germ theory" became accepted, and more mothers and babies began to survive childbirth in the hospital.

Before the 1900s most babies were born at home. Only very ill patients were cared for in lying-in hospitals. Maternal and child morbidity and mortality rates were high in such institutions because of crowded conditions and unskilled nursing care. Hospitals began to develop training programs for nurses. As the medical profession grew, physicians developed a closer relationship with hospitals. This, along with the advent of obstetric instruments and anesthesia, caused a shift to hospital care during childbirth. By the 1950s hospital practice in obstetrics was well-established. By 1960 more than 90% of births in the United States occurred in hospitals.

However, hospital care did not embrace the family-centered approach. Often the father waited in a separate room during the labor and birth of his child. The mother was often sedated with "twilight sleep" and participated little during labor and delivery. After birth the infant was not reunited with the parents for several hours. Parent-infant bonding was delayed.

Organizations concerned with setting standards for maternity nursing developed. These included the American College of Nurse-Midwives (ACNM), the Association of Women's Health, Obstetric, and Neonatal Nurses (AWHONN), formerly the Nurses Association of the American College of Obstetricians and Gynecologists (NAACOG), and the Division of Maternal Nursing within the American Nurses Association.

Abraham Jacobi (1830-1919) is known as the father of pediatrics because of his many contributions to the field. The establishment of pediatric nursing as a specialty paralleled that of departments of pediatrics in medical schools, the founding of children's hospitals, and the development of separate units for children in foundling homes and general hospitals.

In the Middle Ages the concept of childhood did not exist. Infancy lasted until about age 7 years, at which time the child was assimilated into the adult world. The art of that time depicts the child wearing adult clothes and wigs. Most children did not attend school.

Methods of child care have varied throughout history. The culture of a society has a strong influence on standards of child care. Many primitive tribes were nomads. Strong children survived, whereas the weak were left to die. This practice of infanticide (French and Latin *infans,* "infant," and *caedere,* "to kill") helped to ensure the safety of the group. As tribes became settled, more attention was given to children, but they were still frequently valued only for their productivity. Certain peoples, such as the Egyptians and the Greeks, were advanced in their attitudes. The Greek physician Hippocrates (460-370 BC) wrote of illnesses peculiar to children.

Christianity had a considerable impact on child care. In the early seventeenth century, several children's asylums were founded by Saint Vincent de Paul. Many of these eventually became hospitals, although their original concern was for the abandoned. The first children's hospital was founded in Paris in 1802. In the United States, numerous homeless children were cared for by the Children's Aid Society, founded in New York City in 1853. In 1855 the first pediatric hospital in the United States, The Children's Hospital of Philadelphia, was founded.

By the 1960s a separate pediatric unit in hospitals was common. However, parents were restricted by rigid visiting hours that allowed parent-infant contact for only a few hours each day. When medically indicated,

nursing mothers were allowed to enter the pediatric unit for 1 hour at a time to breastfeed their infants.

NURSING **TIP**
Two nursing journals focusing on maternal and child health are the *Journal of Obstetric, Gynecologic, and Neonatal Nursing (JOGNN)* and the *American Journal of Maternal Child Nursing (MCN).*

Government Influences in Maternity and Pediatric Care

The high mortality rate of mothers and infants motivated action by the federal government to improve care. The Sheppard-Towner Act of 1921 provided funds for state-managed programs for maternity care. Since then, Title V of the Social Security Act has also been providing funds for maternity care. The National Institutes of Health (NIH) support maternity research and education. The Title V amendment of the Public Health Services Act established maternal-infant care centers in public clinics. Title XIX of the Medicaid program increased access to care by indigent women. Head Start programs were established to increase educational exposure of preschool children. The National Center for Family Planning provides contraceptive information, and the Women's, Infant's and Children's (WIC) program provides supplemental food and education for the poor.

The Children's Bureau

Lillian Wald, a nurse who was interested in the welfare of children, is credited with suggesting the establishment of a federal children's bureau.

Once the Children's Bureau was established in 1912, it focused its attention on the problems of infant mortality. This program was then followed by one that dealt with maternal mortality. These programs eventually led to birth registration in all states. In the 1930s the Children's Bureau investigations led to the development of hot lunch programs in many schools.

The Fair Labor Standards Act, passed in 1938, established a general minimum working age of 16 years and a minimum working age of 18 years for jobs considered hazardous. More important, this act paved the way for the establishment of national minimum standards for child labor and provided a means of enforcement.

NURSING **TIP**
Innovative community programs such as foster grandparents, home health or parent aides, and telephone hotlines for children home alone after school are of particular value to dysfunctional or isolated families.

White House Conferences

The First White House Conference on Children and Youth was called by President Theodore Roosevelt in 1909. It continues to meet every 10 years.

In the White House Conference on Child Health and Protection (1930), the Children's Charter was drawn up (Box 1-1). This is considered one of the most important documents in child care history. It lists 17 statements related to the needs of children in the areas of education, health, welfare, and protection. This declaration has been widely distributed throughout the world.

The 1980 White House Conference on Families focused on involving the states at the grass-roots level. A series of statewide hearings were held to identify the most pressing problems of families in the various localities. A tremendous range of viewpoints on many subjects was shared, and specific recommendations were made.

In 1974 and 1975 the government passed the Child Abuse Prevention and Treatment Act. The Education for All Handicapped Children Act provides for support and public education of handicapped children. In 1982 the Community Mental Health Center was funded, and the Missing Children's Act was passed, providing a nationwide clearinghouse for missing children.

International Year of the Child

The year 1979 was designated as the International Year of the Child (IYC). Its purpose was to focus attention on the critical needs of the world's 1.5 billion children and to inspire the nations, the organizations, and the individuals of the world to consider how well they are providing for children (U.S. Commission of the International Year of the Child, 1980). At this time the United Nations reaffirmed the Declaration of the Rights of the Child (Box 1-2).

The Public Health Department

The public health department assumes a great deal of responsibility for the prevention of disease and death during childhood. These preventive efforts are done on national, state, and local levels. The water, milk, and food supplies of communities are inspected. Maintenance of proper sewage and garbage disposal is enforced. Epidemics are investigated, and, when necessary, persons capable of transmitting diseases are isolated. The public health department is also concerned with the inspection of housing.

Laws requiring the licensing of physicians and pharmacists indirectly affect the health of children and of the general public. Protection is also afforded by the Pure Food and Drug Act, which controls medicines, poisons, and the purity of foods. Programs for disaster relief, care and rehabilitation of handicapped children, foster child care, family counseling, family day care, protective services for abused or neglected children, and education of the public are maintained and supported by governmental and private agencies. State licensing bureaus control the regulation of motor vehicles. Car seats for infants and children are currently mandatory. Protection of the public by law enforcement agencies is important because automobile accidents rank among the leading causes of injury and death in children.

THE PRESENT

MATERNITY CARE

Significant changes have occurred in maternity care. In family-centered childbearing the family is recognized as a unique system. Every family member is affected by the birth of a child. Family involvement during pregnancy and birth is seen as constructive and, indeed, necessary for bonding and support. To accommodate family needs, alternative birth centers, birthing rooms, rooming-in units, and mother-infant coupling have been developed. The whole sequence of events may take place in one suite of rooms. These arrangements are alternatives to the previous standard of separate areas for labor and delivery, which made it necessary to transport a mother from one area to another and fragmented her care.

The three separate sections of the maternity unit have merged. The labor-delivery, postpartum, and newborn nursery have become labor, delivery, and recovery (LDR) rooms. The patient is not moved from one area to another, but receives care during labor and delivery and then remains in the same room to recover and care for her new infant. The rooms are often decorated to

box 1-1   *The Children's Charter of 1930**

I. For every child spiritual and moral training to help him or her to stand firm under the pressure of life.

II. For every child understanding and the guarding of personality as a most precious right.

III. For every child a home and that love and security which a home provides; and for those children who must receive foster care, the nearest substitute for their own home.

IV. For every child full preparation for the birth; the mother receiving prenatal, natal, and postnatal care; and the establishment of such protective measures as will make childbearing safer.

V. For every child protection from birth through adolescence, including periodical health examinations and, where needed, care of specialists and hospital treatment; regular dental examinations and care of the teeth; protective and preventive measures against communicable diseases; the ensuring of pure food, pure milk, and pure water.

VI. For every child from birth through adolescence, promotion of health, including health instruction and health programs, wholesome physical and mental recreation, with teachers and leaders adequately trained.

VII. For every child a dwelling place safe, sanitary, and wholesome, with reasonable provisions for privacy; free from conditions which tend to thwart development; and a home environment harmonious and enriching.

VIII. For every child a school which is safe from hazards, sanitary, properly equipped, lighted, and ventilated. For younger children nursery schools and kindergartens to supplement home care.

IX. For every child a community which recognizes and plans for needs; protects against physical dangers, moral hazards, and disease; provides safe and wholesome places for play and recreation; and makes provision for cultural and social needs.

X. For every child an education which, through the discovery and development of individual abilities, prepares the child for life and through training and vocational guidance prepares for a living which will yield the maximum of satisfaction.

XI. For every child such teaching and training as will prepare him or her for successful parenthood, homemaking, and the rights of citizenship and, for parents, supplementary training to fit them to deal wisely with the problems of parenthood.

XII. For every child education for safety and protection against accidents to which modern conditions subject the child—those to which the child is directly exposed and those which, through loss or maiming of the parents, affect the child directly.

XIII. For every child who is blind, deaf, crippled, or otherwise physically handicapped and for the child who is mentally handicapped, such measures as will early discover and diagnose his handicap, provide care and treatment, and so train the child that the child may become an asset to society rather than a liability. Expenses of these services should be borne publicly where they cannot be privately met.

XIV. For every child who is in conflict with society the right to be dealt with intelligently as society's charge, not society's outcast; with the home, the school, the church, the court, and the institution when needed, shaped to return the child whenever possible to the normal stream of life.

XV. For every child the right to grow up in a family with an adequate standard of living and the security of a stable income as the surest safeguard against social handicaps.

XVI. For every child protection against labor that stunts growth, either physical or mental, that limits education, that deprives children of the right of comradeship, of play, and of joy.

XVII. For every rural child as satisfactory schooling and health services as for the city child, and an extension to rural families of social, recreational, and cultural facilities.

*National White House Conference 1930.

look homelike. Freestanding birthing centers outside the traditional hospital setting are popular with low-risk maternity patients. These birthing centers provide comprehensive care, including antepartum, labor-delivery, postpartum, mother's classes, lactation classes, and follow-up family planning. Home birth using midwives is not a current widespread practice because malpractice insurance is expensive and emergency equipment for unexpected complications is not available.

Cost containment influenced maternity care by requiring the discharge of mother and newborn in 24 hours or less. As a result of problems that occurred, current legislation allows a 48-hour hospital stay for vaginal deliveries and 4 days for a cesarean section.

box **1-2** *The United Nations Declaration of the Rights of the Child**

The general assembly proclaims that the child is entitled to a happy childhood and that all should recognize these rights and strive for their observance by legislative and other means:

1. All children without exception shall be entitled to these rights regardless of race, color, sex, language, religion, politics, national or social origin, property, birth, or other status.
2. The child should be protected so that he or she may develop physically, mentally, morally, spiritually, and socially in freedom and dignity.
3. The child is entitled at birth to a name and nationality.
4. The child is entitled to healthy development which includes adequate food, housing, recreation, and medical attention. He or she shall receive the benefits of Social Security.
5. The child who is handicapped physically, mentally, or emotionally shall receive treatment, education, and care according to his or her need.
6. The child is entitled to love and a harmonious atmosphere, preferably in the environment of his or her parents. Particular love, care, and concern need to be extended to children without families and to the poor.
7. The child is entitled to a free education and opportunities for play, recreation, and to develop his or her talents.
8. The child shall be the first one protected in times of adversity.
9. The child shall be protected against all forms of neglect, cruelty, and exploitation. He or she should not be employed in hazardous occupations or before the minimum age.
10. The child shall not be subjected to racial or religious discrimination. The environment should be peaceful and friendly.

*U.N. General Assembly Resolution 1386 (XIV), November 20, 1959.

Clinical pathways, also known as critical pathways or care maps (multidisciplinary action plans), are collaborative guidelines that define multidisciplinary care in terms of outcomes within a timeline. The basis of the pathway is identification of expected progress within a timeline. Expected progress of the patient becomes a standard of care. Therefore clinical pathways are research based rather than tradition based. By setting specific recovery goals of the patient expected each day, deviations are readily identified. These deviations are called *variances.* If the patient's progress is slower than expected, the outcome (goal) is not achieved within the timeline and a *negative variance* occurs, so that discharge from the hospital may be delayed. The use of clinical pathways improves the quality of care and reduces unnecessary hospitalization time. It is an essential component of managed care and promotes coordination of the entire health care team. Sample clinical pathways are presented throughout the chapters.

Current maternity practice focuses on a high-quality family experience. *Childbearing is seen as a normal and healthy event.* Parents are prepared for the changes that take place during pregnancy, labor, and delivery. They are also prepared for the changes in family dynamics. Treating each family according to their individual needs is considered paramount.

During the 1950s the hospital stay for labor and delivery was 1 week. The current stay in uncomplicated cases is 2 days. Routine follow-up of the newborn takes place within 2 weeks. A nurse visits the homes of infants and mothers who appear to be at high risk.

Procedural modifications for the nurse include the institution of standard precautions during delivery (see Appendix A), during umbilical cord care, and in the nursery. More emphasis on data entry and retrieval makes it necessary for nursing personnel to be computer literate.

Sociologically, families have become smaller, the number of single parents is increasing, child and spouse abuse is rampant, and more mothers must work to help support the family. These developments present special challenges to maternal and child health nurses. Careful assessment and documentation to detect abuse are necessary, and nurses must be familiar with community support services for women and children in need. Nurses must also be flexible and promote policies that make health care more available for working parents. Teaching must be integrated into care plans and individually tailored to the family's needs and its cultural and ethnic background.

NURSING TIP

According to standards recommended by the American College of Obstetricians and Gynecologists (ACOG), pregnant women should ideally make about 13 prenatal visits over the course of a normal, full-term pregnancy.

Midwives

Throughout history, women have played an important role as birth attendants or *midwives.* The first school of nurse-midwifery opened in New York City in 1932.

There are many accredited programs across the United States, all located in or affiliated with institutions of higher learning. The certified nurse-midwife (CNM) is a registered nurse who has graduated from an accredited midwife program and is nationally certified by the American College of Nurse-Midwives. The CNM provides comprehensive prenatal and postnatal care and attends uncomplicated deliveries. The CNM assures that each patient has a backup physician who will assume her care should a problem occur.

Role of the Consumer

Consumerism has played an important part in family-centered childbirth. In the early 1960s the natural childbirth movement awakened expectant parents to the need for education and involvement. Prepared childbirth, La Leche League (breastfeeding advocates), and Lamaze classes gradually became accepted. Parents began to question the routine use of anesthesia and the exclusion of fathers from the delivery experience.

Today, a father's attendance at birth is common. Visiting hours are liberal, and extended contact with the newborn is encouraged. The consumer continues to be an important instigator of change. Consumer groups, with the growing support of professionals, have helped to revise restrictive policies once thought necessary for safety. It has been demonstrated that informed parents can make wise decisions about their own care during this period if they are adequately educated and given professional support.

Cross-Cultural Considerations

The cultural background of the expectant family strongly influences its adaptation to the birth experience. Nursing Care Plan 1-1 on pp. 14 and 15 lists nursing interventions for selected diagnoses that pertain to cultural diversity. One way in which the nurse gains important information about an individual's culture is to *ask the pregnant woman* what she considers normal practice. A summary of data collection questions might include the following:

- How does the woman view her pregnancy (as an illness, a vulnerable time, or a healthy time)?
- Does she view the birth process as dangerous? Why?
- Is birth a public or private experience for her?
- In what position does she expect to deliver (i.e., squatting, lithotomy, or some other position)?
- What type of help does she need before and after delivery?
- What role does her immediate or extended family play in relation to the pregnancy and birth?

Such information helps to promote understanding and individualizes patient care. It also increases the satisfaction of patient and nurse with the quality of care provided. Cultural influences on nursing care are discussed in Chapter 6.

CHILD CARE
The Pediatric Nurse as an Advocate

Pediatric nurses are increasingly assuming a role as child advocates. An advocate is a person who intercedes or pleads on behalf of another. Advocacy may be required for the child's physical and emotional health and may include other family members. Hospitalized children frequently cannot determine or express their needs. When nurses feel that the child's best interests are not being met, they must seek assistance. This usually involves taking the problem through the normal chain of command. Nurses must document their efforts to seek instruction and direction from their head nurse, supervisors, or the physician.

Statistics

Statistics refers to the process of gathering and analyzing numerical data. Statistics concerning birth, death (mortality), and illness (morbidity) provide valuable information for determining or projecting the needs of a population or subgroup and for predicting trends. In the United States, vital statistics are compiled for the country as a whole by the National Center for Health Statistics and are published in its annual report, *Vital Statistics of the United States,* and in the pamphlet *Morbidity and Mortality Weekly Report (MMWR).* Statistics are also issued by the various state bureaus of vital statistics. Other independent agencies also supply statistics on various specialties.

A maternity nurse may use statistical data to become aware of reproductive trends, to determine populations at risk, to evaluate the quality of prenatal care, or to compare relevant information from state to state and country to country. Box 1-3 lists some terms used in gathering vital statistics.

Table 1-1 shows 1996 infant death statistics that reveal more than half of all infant deaths resulted from congenital anomalies, preterm status, sudden infant death syndrome (SIDS), and respiratory distress syndrome (RDS). The statistics show that the death rate from all causes declined more than 44% between 1979 and 1996.

Table 1-2 shows the national birth rates for 1998. Statistics show that there may be a relationship between the lack of prenatal care and the infant mortality rates. The occurrence of adolescent and unwed mother birth rates in various areas may indicate a need for public education.

table 1-1 *Infant Deaths and Infant Mortality Rates for the 10 Leading Causes of Infant Death in the United States—1979, 1995, and 1996*

CAUSE OF DEATH	RANK*	1996			1995			1979			PERCENT CHANGE 1979-1996
		NUMBER	PERCENT	RATE	NUMBER	PERCENT	RATE	NUMBER	PERCENT	RATE†	
All causes		28,245	100.0	721.5	29,583	100.0	758.6	45,665	100.0	1306.8	−44.8
Congenital anomalies	1	6463	22.9	165.1	6554	22.2	168.1	8923	19.5	255.4	−35.4
Disorders relating to short gestation and unspecified low birth weight	2	3706	13.1	94.7	3933	13.3	100.9	3495	7.7	100.0	−5.3
Sudden infant death syndrome (SIDS)	3	2906	10.3	74.2	3397	11.5	87.1	5279	11.6	151.1	−50.9
Respiratory distress syndrome	4	1368	4.8	34.9	1454	4.9	37.3	5458	12.0	156.2	−77.7
Newborn affected by maternal complications of pregnancy	5	1212	4.3	31.0	1309	4.4	33.6	1621	3.5	46.4	−33.2
Newborn affected by complications of placenta, cord, and membranes	6	892	3.2	22.8	962	3.3	24.7	970	2.1	27.8	−18.0
Accidents and adverse effects	7	772	2.7	19.7	787	2.7	20.2	1080	2.4	30.9	−36.2
Infections specific to the perinatal period	8	747	2.6	19.1	788	2.7	20.2	981	2.1	28.1	−32.0
Pneumonia and influenza	9	485	1.7	12.4	492	1.7	12.6	1129	2.5	32.3	−61.6
Intrauterine hypoxia and birth asphyxia	10	429	1.5	11.0	475	1.6	12.2	1393	3.1	39.9	−72.4

From American Academy of Pediatrics. (1997). Annual summary of vital statistics, 1996. *Pediatrics, 100*(6), 913.
NOTE: 1996 data are preliminary; 1995 and 1979 data are final. In 1995 infant death from infections specific to the perinatal period was ranked seventh; accidents and adverse effects was eighth. In 1979 respiratory distress syndrome was ranked second; disorders relating to short gestation and unspecified low birth weight, fourth; newborn affected by complications of placenta, cord, and membranes, eleventh; accidents and adverse effects, ninth; infections specific to the perinatal period, tenth; pneumonia and influenza, seventh; and intrauterine hypoxia and birth asphyxia, sixth.
*Rank based on number of deaths.
†Rate per 100,000 live births.

table 1-2 | *Birth Rate Statistics for 1998*

STATE	BIRTHS	BIRTH RATE	TEEN BIRTH RATE	% UNWED MOTHERS	% LOW BIRTH WEIGHT	RATE BY CESAREAN SECTION	% WOMEN RECEIVING PRENATAL CARE FIRST TRIMESTER	INFANT MORTALITY
Alaska	9926	16.2	11.2	31.1	6.0	14.7	81.4	5.9
Arizona	78,243	16.2	15.1	38.4	6.8	17.0	75.1	7.5
Arkansas	36,865	14.5	18.6	35.0	8.9	24.9	77.8	8.9
California	521,661	16.0	11.4	32.8	6.2	21.7	82.4	5.8
Colorado	59,577	15.0	12.1	25.6	8.6	16.4	82.2	6.7
Connecticut	43,820	13.4	8.3	31.2	7.8	20.1	88.0	7.0
Delaware	10,578	14.2	13.1	37.1	8.6	23.2	83.4	9.6
District of Columbia	7686	14.7	15.3	62.9	13.1	20.8	72.0	12.5
Florida	195,637	13.1	13.2	36.6	8.1	22.4	83.6	7.2
Georgia	122,368	16.0	15.0	36.2	8.5	20.8	86.4	8.5
Guam	4318	29.0	14.2	54.2	7.6	14.7	63.0	7.9
Hawaii	17,583	14.7	10.7	31.5	7.5	15.6	85.4	6.9
Idaho	19,391	15.8	12.8	22.0	6.0	15.7	78.7	7.2
Illinois	182,588	15.2	12.4	34.1	8.0	19.4	82.7	8.4
Indiana	85,122	14.4	13.8	33.4	7.9	20.0	79.9	7.6
Iowa	37,282	13.0	10.6	27.2	6.4	19.6	87.3	6.6
Kansas	38,422	14.6	12.6	27.8	7.0	18.6	85.8	7.0
Kentucky	54,329	13.8	15.4	30.1	8.1	22.8	86.4	7.5
Louisiana	66,888	15.3	18.4	44.9	10.1	26.0	82.2	9.1
Maine	13,733	11.0	9.8	30.6	5.8	19.7	88.9	6.3
Maryland	71,972	14.0	10.2	34.4	8.7	21.3	87.8	8.6
Massachusetts	81,411	13.2	7.2	26.1	6.9	20.9	89.5	5.1
Michigan	133,666	13.6	11.6	33.9	7.8	20.6	84.3	8.2
Minnesota	65,202	13.8	8.6	25.6	5.8	18.0	84.5	5.9
Mississippi	42,939	15.6	20.0	45.4	10.1	27.0	80.6	10.1
Missouri	75,358	13.9	13.8	34.1	7.8	20.6	86.1	7.7
Montana	10,795	12.3	12.3	29.9	7.0	18.9	82.3	7.4
Nebraska	23,534	14.2	13.1	26.2	6.5	21.4	83.9	7.3
Nevada	26,699	16.4	13.1	35.0	7.6	21.4	74.6	7.0
New Hampshire	14,429	12.2	7.7	24.1	5.7	18.5	89.7	4.4
New Jersey	114,550	14.1	7.8	28.3	8.0	25.4	81.6	6.4
New Mexico	27,318	15.7	18.2	44.0	7.6	16.4	67.6	7.2
New York	258,207	14.2	8.8	34.9	7.8	22.9	81.2	6.3
North Carolina	111,688	14.8	12.3	32.8	8.8	21.5	84.5	9.3
North Dakota	7932	12.4	9.8	27.0	6.5	19.4	85.6	8.6
Ohio	152,794	13.6	13.0	34.0	7.7	18.9	85.5	8.0
Oklahoma	49,461	14.8	16.3	33.2	7.2	22.8	78.6	8.5
Oregon	45,273	13.8	12.5	29.7	5.4	17.8	80.2	5.4
Pennsylvania	145,899	12.2	10.3	32.8	7.6	19.6	84.8	7.1
Puerto Rico	60,412	15.7	20.5	47.0	10.9	35.1	78.8	10.5
Rhode Island	12,652	12.7	10.5	33.9	7.6	19.5	89.7	7.0
South Carolina	53,877	14.0	16.0	38.8	9.5	23.4	81.4	9.6
South Dakota	10,288	13.9	12.0	32.0	5.8	21.5	82.7	9.1
Tennessee	77,396	14.3	15.9	34.9	9.1	22.6	84.1	8.6
Texas	342,283	17.3	16.1	31.5	7.4	23.5	79.3	6.4
Utah	45,165	25.1	9.8	17.1	6.7	16.0	82.1	5.6
Vermont	6582	11.1	7.9	28.0	6.5	16.5	87.4	7.0
Virginia	91,862	13.9	10.8	29.8	7.9	21.2	85.2	7.7
Washington	79,663	14.0	10.9	27.9	5.7	17.9	83.0	5.7
West Virginia	20,747	11.5	15.7	32.4	8.0	24.1	83.7	8.0
Wisconsin	67,450	12.9	10.5	28.5	6.5	16.0	84.3	7.2
Wyoming	6252	13.0	16.2	29.6	8.9	18.6	81.3	7.2

Data from National Center for Health Statistics (1998); retrieved from http://www.cdc.gov/nchs/fastats.

box 1-3 *Common Vital Statistics Terms*

birth rate The number of live births per 1000 population in 1 year.

fertility rate The number of births per 1000 women ages 15 to 44 years in a given population.

fetal mortality The number of fetal deaths (fetuses weighing 500 g or more) per 1000 live births per year.

infant mortality rate The number of deaths of infants under age 1 year per 1000 live births per year.

maternal mortality rate The number of maternal deaths per 100,000 live births that occurs as a direct result of pregnancy (includes the 42-day postpartum period).

neonatal mortality The number of deaths of infants less than age 28 days per 1000 live births per year.

perinatal mortality Includes both fetal and neonatal deaths per 1000 live births per year.

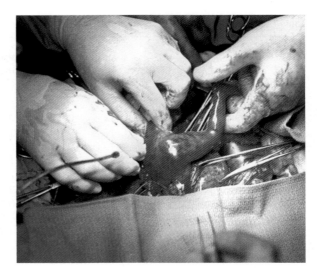

FIGURE **1-1** Fetal surgery can be performed to repair a congenital defect before birth.

Technology

Technological advances have enabled many infants to survive who may have died some years ago (Figure 1-1). High-risk prenatal clinics and the neonatal intensive care unit enable the 1-pound preemie to have an opportunity to survive. Children with heart problems are now treated by a pediatric cardiologist. Much of the complex surgery needed by the newborn with a congenital defect is provided by the pediatric surgeon. Emotional problems are managed by pediatric psychiatrists. Many hospital laboratories are well equipped to test pediatric specimens. Chromosomal studies and biochemical screening have made identification of risks and family counseling more significant than ever. The field of perinatal biology has advanced to the forefront of pediatric medicine (Figure 1-2).

The medical profession and allied health agencies work as a team for the total well-being of the patient. Children with defects previously thought to be incompatible with life are taken to special diagnostic and treatment centers where they receive expert attention and care. After discharge many of these children are being cared for in their homes. The number of chronically disabled children is growing. Some are dependent on sophisticated hospital equipment such as ventilators and home monitors. The nursing care at home may require the suctioning of a tracheostomy, central line care, and other highly technical skills. Parents must be carefully educated and continually supported. Although this type of care is cost-effective and psychologically sound for the child, respite care is extremely important because 24-hour-a-day care is extremely taxing for the family, both physically and psychologically.

The American Nurses Association (ANA) develops standards of care that serve as a guide to meet some current challenges. These standards are used when policies and procedures are established. Also, each state has a nurse practice act that determines the scope of practice for the registered nurse, practical nurse, and certified nurse assistant. Because these descriptions vary from state to state, nurses must keep informed about the laws in the state where they are employed.

HEALTH CARE DELIVERY SYSTEMS

Cost containment is a major motivation in current health care, especially when health costs rise without decreases in morbidity and mortality. Many hospitals are merging to increase their buying power and reduce duplication of services.

Insurance reimbursement has become an important consideration in health care. The federal government has had to revise its Medicare and Medicaid programs. Among other changes it instituted diagnosis-related groupings (DRGs). These refer to a Medicare system that determines payment for a hospital stay based on the patient's diagnosis. This mandate has had a tremendous impact on health care delivery. Patients are being discharged earlier, and more care is being given in skilled nursing facilities and in the home. Some insurance companies are employing nurses in the role of case managers. Nurses remaining in institutions also may be required to assume the role of case managers and to

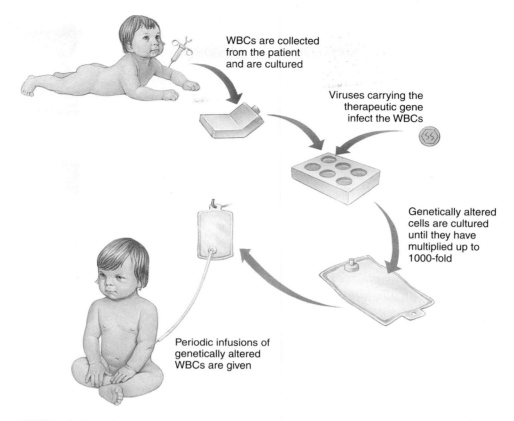

WBCs are collected
from the patient
and are cultured

Viruses carrying the
therapeutic gene
infect the WBCs

Genetically altered
cells are cultured
until they have
multiplied up to
1000-fold

Periodic infusions of
genetically altered
WBCs are given

FIGURE **1-2** Gene therapy. One goal of gene replacement therapy is to alter the existing body cells to eliminate the cause of a genetic disease. The therapeutic or missing gene can be combined with a virus that can enter the infant's system. This is called gene augmentation. In gene replacement therapy, new therapeutic genes are combined with viruses that can enter the human genome.

become more flexible through cross training. Nurses are expected to be concerned with keeping hospital costs down while maintaining quality care. Many suggest that the future of nursing may depend on how well nurses can demonstrate their value and cost-effectiveness.

Health Maintenance Organizations (HMOs) and Preferred Provider Organizations (PPOs) have emerged as alternative medical care delivery systems. Insurers and providers of care have united to hold costs down and yet remain competitive. A two-tiered system has evolved: one tier serves the more financially stable people (private insurance, HMO/PPO), and the other serves the less financially stable people (Medicare and Medicaid). In addition, a large percentage of persons are uninsured or underinsured. This presents problems in access and quality of health care. Box 1-4 defines managed care systems.

Health promotion continues to assume increased importance. Preventing illness or disability is cost-effective; more importantly, it saves the family from stress, disruptions, and financial burden. Healthy children are spending fewer days in the hospital. Many conditions are treated in same-day surgery, ambulatory settings, or emergency rooms. Rather than being distinct, hospital and home care have become interdependent.

Chronically ill children are living into adulthood, creating the need for more support services. Medically fragile and technology-dependent children may change the profile of chronically ill children. The nurse is often the instigator of support services to these patients through education and referral. Ideally these services will assist the child to become as independent as possible, to lead a productive life, and to be integrated into society. In the past the term mainstream was used to describe the process of integrating a physically or mentally challenged child into society. The term full inclusion, an expansion of the mainstream policy, is being used more frequently today. Early infant intervention programs for children with developmental disabilities attempt to reduce or minimize the effects of the disability. These services may be provided in a clinic or in the home. The need for in-home family-centered pediatric

box 1-4 *Health Care Delivery Systems*

managed care Integrates financing with health care for members. For a monthly "capitation" fee, contracts with physicians and hospitals to provide health care with strict utilization review for cost containment.

HMO A health maintenance organization offers health services for a fixed premium.

PPO A preferred provider organization contracts with providers for services on a discounted fee-for-service basis for members.

utilization review Reviews appropriateness of health care services and guidelines for physicians for treatment of illness, controlling management of care to achieve cost containment.

box 1-5 *Advanced Practice Nursing Specialties**

OGNP	Obstetrical/gynecological nurse practitioner
WHNP	Women's health care nurse practitioner
NNP	Neonatal nurse practitioner
FPNP	Family planning nurse practitioner
IBCLC	International board-certified lactation consultant
CDDN	Certified developmental disabilities nurse
CNM	Certified nurse midwife
CPN	Certified pediatric nurse
CPON	Certified pediatric oncology nurse

Data from Hamric, A., Sprouse, J., Hansen, C. (2001). *Advanced practice nursing: An integrative approach* (2nd ed.). Philadelphia: WB Saunders. *CRNA*, Certified registered nurse anesthetist.
*In 1993, the National Council of State Boards of Nursing (NCSBN) stated that "the scope of practice in each of the advanced roles of NP, CRNA, CNM, or CNS is distinguishable from the others. While there is overlapping of activities within these roles, there are activities unique to each role." Core competencies of the APN include masters level nursing education, certification, and a focused area of practice.

care will continue to grow with the number of children with chronic illness who survive.

Quality of life is particularly relevant. Organ transplants have saved some children; however, the complications, limited availability, and expense of these transplants create moral and ethical dilemmas. Older children with life-threatening conditions must be included in planning modified advance directives with their families and the medical team.

These developments, along with the explosion of information, emphasis on individual nurse accountability, new technology, and use of computers in health care, make it especially desirable for nurses to maintain their knowledge and skills at a level necessary to provide safe care. Employers often offer continuing education classes for their employees. Most states require proof of continuing education for the renewal of nursing licenses.

⋆NURSING TIP

Expanded nursing roles include the clinical nurse specialist, the pediatric nurse practitioner, the school nurse practitioner, the family nurse practitioner, and the certified nurse-midwife.

ADVANCED PRACTICE NURSES

In keeping with the current practice of focusing on prevention of illness and maintenance of health rather than the treatment of illness, the specialty of **Pediatric Nurse Practitioner (PNP)** was born. The PNP provides ambulatory and primary care for patients. The school nurse or child life specialist expands the accessibility of preventive health care to the well child.

Clinical Nurse Specialists (CNSs) provide care in the hospital or community to specific specialty patients, such as cardiac, neurological, or oncological care. They con-

duct primary research and facilitate necessary changes in health care management. Often the PNP and the CNS are called **Advanced Practice Nurses,** and they have a degree as a registered nurse (RN) as well as an advanced degree. Advanced practice nurses can specialize in obstetrics or pediatrics. Box 1-5 lists some specialties that have developed in maternal-child care.

THE NURSING PROCESS

The **nursing process** was developed in 1963. This term referred to a series of steps describing the systematic problem-solving approach nurses used to identify, prevent, or treat actual or potential health problems. In 1973 the ANA developed standards relating to this nursing process that have been nationally accepted and include the following:

- *Assessment:* Collection of patient data, both subjective and objective
- *Diagnosis:* Analysis of data in terms of NANDA Nursing Diagnoses (Appendix C)
- *Outcome identification:* Identification of individualized expected patient outcomes
- *Planning:* Preparation of a plan of care designed to achieve stated outcomes
- *Implementation:* Carrying out of interventions identified in the plan of care
- *Evaluation:* Evaluation of outcome progress and redesigning plan if necessary

The nursing process is a framework of action designed to meet the individual needs of patients. It is problem oriented and goal directed and involves the use of critical thinking, problem solving, and decision mak-

table 1-3 *Comparison of Medical and Nursing Diagnoses*

MEDICAL DIAGNOSIS	NURSING DIAGNOSIS
Acquired immuno-deficiency syndrome (AIDS)	Imbalanced nutrition: less than body requirements related to anorexia and evidenced by weight loss
Gestational diabetes (GDM)	Deficient knowledge related to effects of diabetes mellitus on pregnant woman and fetus, manifested by crying, anxiety
Cystic fibrosis (CF)	Ineffective airway clearance related to mucus accumulation manifested by rales, fatigue

ing. The nursing process is expressed in an individualized nursing care plan. Diagnoses approved by NANDA are found in Appendix C. Table 1-3 differentiates between medical and nursing diagnoses.

NURSING CARE PLANS

The nursing care plan is developed as a result of the nursing process. It is a written instrument of communication among staff members that focuses on individualized patient care.

Nursing Care Plan 1-1 is an example of a care plan. Sample care plans for maternity and pediatric nursing are provided throughout the text. Certain terms used in care plans must be understood. Box 1-6 defines these terms.

The Case Study/Care Plan

A nursing care plan is a "picture" of a typical clinical situation that may be encountered by the graduate nurse. Specific data concerning the patient are supplied. These data can be used as clues to solve the mystery or problem concerning the patient (this phase is called *collection*). These clues help the nurse identify the problem of the patient. By organizing all the clues and identifying several problems, the nurse then prioritizes the problems identified. This phase of care planning is called *analysis*. When the priority problem is identified, the nurse can use knowledge, experience, and resources such as doctors' prescriptions, textbooks, journals, or the Internet to decide on a plan of action to solve the problem. This phase is called *planning*. The actual nursing activities necessary to solve the problem are called nursing interventions. The nursing interventions are planned with specific outcomes or goals in mind. An outcome or goal

box 1-6 *Common Terms Used in Nursing Care Plans*

patient An individual, group, family, or community that is the focus of a nursing intervention.

nursing activity An action that implements an intervention to assist the patient toward a desired outcome. (A series of activities may be needed to implement an intervention.)

nursing diagnosis A clinical judgment about a patient's response to an actual or potential health problem. The nursing diagnosis provides the basis for selection of nursing interventions to achieve an outcome for which the nurse is accountable (NANDA, 2001).

nursing intervention Any treatment or nursing activity based on clinical judgment and knowledge that a nurse performs to achieve a specific outcome for the patient. It includes direct or indirect patient care or community or public health activities.

scope of practice Legal authority to perform specific activities related to health care or health promotion. These activities require substantial knowledge or technical skill. Specific activities are listed by the state nurse practice act and nurses must practice within the limitations of the nurse practice act of their state. For example, a LPN/LVN cannot perform surgery; that activity is within the scope of a medical doctor.

standards of care Established minimum criteria for competent nursing care approved by nursing practice organizations such as the state board of nursing, the Joint Committee on the Accreditation of Healthcare Organizations (JCAHO), and the ANA.

is the positive resolving of the patient's problem. The nursing interventions are the basis of the nursing or bedside care provided to the patient. After the nursing care is provided, the nurse reevaluates the original problem to determine if the goal or outcome was met.

The way a nurse solves the problems of a patient is not always found in a textbook or in class lectures. Sometimes the nurse must consider factors individual to the specific patient and affected by specific situations. For example, the cultural background of the patient or the age of the patient influences how effective a specific intervention will be. If the problem is a protein deficiency and the nurse selects the intervention to teach the importance of meat in the diet, the intervention will be ineffective, that is, it will not have a positive outcome, if this patient is a vegetarian because meat will not be eaten. For this reason, critical thinking must enter the picture for optimum nursing care to be provided. Critical thinking involves creativity and ingenuity to solve

NURSING CARE PLAN 1-1

Care of Childbearing Families Related to Potential or Actual Stress Caused by Cultural Diversity

SELECTED NURSING DIAGNOSIS *Impaired verbal communication related to language barriers*

PATIENT DATA: A 22-year-old, para 0 gravida 1, is admitted to the labor room in active early labor. Her partner is with her, and they do not speak English.

Examples of NIC and NOC:
NIC: presence; touch
NOC: communication ability

Outcomes	Nursing Interventions	Rationales
The woman will have an opportunity to share information and states she understands what is explained to her.	1. Arrange for a family or staff member interpreter as needed.	1. Interpreter can provide support for woman and help to lessen her anxieties. Poor communication can result in time delays, errors, and misunderstandings of intent.
	2. Clearly define instructions in woman's language of origin.	2. A shared language is necessary for communication to take place.
	3. Provide written instructions in woman's language whenever possible.	3. Written instructions can be reviewed at a less stressful time by patient. In some cases it is necessary to determine if person can read.
	4. Explain the use and purpose of all instruments and equipment, along with the effects or possible effects on the mother and fetus.	4. Education of family lessens anxiety and provides family with a sense of control.
	5. Provide opportunities for clarification and questions.	5. Learning takes time; repetition of important material promotes learning. Nurse can determine woman's understanding of information and clarify misconceptions.

SELECTED NURSING DIAGNOSIS *Compromised family coping related to isolation, different customs, attitudes, or beliefs*

Examples of NIC and NOC:
NIC: spiritual support
NOC: anxiety control, coping

Outcomes	Nursing Interventions	Rationales
Family members will state that they feel welcome and safe in the environment provided.	1. Encourage orientation visit to the maternity unit before delivery.	1. Families who have clear, accurate information can better participate in labor and delivery. Viewing the delivery setting before using it decreases anxiety about the unknown.
	2. Inform families about routines, visiting hours, significant persons who can assist in labor and delivery, and location of newborn after delivery.	2. Families have different expectations of the health care system. They may hesitate to ask questions because of shyness or fear of "losing face."

NURSING CARE PLAN 1-1—cont'd

Outcomes	Nursing Interventions	Rationales
	3. Determine and respect practices and values of family and incorporate them into nursing care plans as much as possible.	3. Clarification of culturally specific values and practices will avoid misunderstanding and conflict with the nurse's value system. Nursing care plans promote organization of care and communication among staff members.

?CRITICAL THINKING QUESTIONS

The extended family of a patient in the labor room requests permission to stay with the patient and the husband throughout labor. What should be the nurse's response?

A patient admitted to the labor room refuses to let a male physician perform a vaginal examination. What should be the nursing role?

---

box 1-7   **Steps in Preparing a Care Plan**

1. Collect data from chart, medical order sheet, laboratory reports, history and physical examination, progress notes, etc.
2. Review medical diagnosis of patient in text.
3. Assess patient; interview patient.
4. Select appropriate nursing diagnosis from the NANDA list. Note the etiology and evidence related to each choice.
5. Select measurable outcomes (NOC) that are realistic for the patient, stating the timeline for achieving the outcomes.
6. Identify interventions (NIC) that will facilitate outcomes.
7. Identify nursing actions within these interventions.
8. Evaluate outcome; revise care plan as needed.

the problem: combining basic standard principles with data specific to the patient. The basic steps in preparing a care plan (case study) are outlined in Box 1-7.

NIC, NOC, and NANDA

Nursing Interventions Classification (NIC), Nursing Outcome Criteria (NOC), and NANDA (Nursing Diagnoses) are companions that aid in the critical thinking aspect of patient care. They provide a standardization of language concerning patient status and nursing activities that enables nurses to work in the managed care environment, improve quality of care, reduce costs, enable research, and promote the development of a reimbursement system for nursing services rendered.

The codes assigned to NIC and NOC enable computerized data collection for the purposes of research and reimbursement. Nursing Care Plan 1-1 includes NIC and NOC to demonstrate how they are incorporated into the typical care plan. The specific codes assigned to NIC and NOC are not included in this text because the registered nurse is responsible for the coding. However, the licensed practical nurse/licensed vocational nurse (LPN/LVN) is responsible for understanding and working with NIC and NOC.

NIC. NIC specifies actions that nurses perform to help patients toward a goal or outcome. The focus is on the *action* of the nurse.

Physiological interventions such as suctioning and psychosocial interventions such as reducing fears and anxieties are useful in the prevention as well as the treatment of illness. NIC are used together with outcome criteria (NOC) and nursing diagnoses (NANDA). There is a relationship between nursing diagnosis, nursing interventions, and nursing outcomes. Nursing outcomes are different from nursing goals because nursing goals are either met or unmet. Nursing outcomes are described on a continuum. This enables the measurement of *outcomes* as they are influenced by nursing actions.

NOC. NOC was developed to identify outcomes of nursing care that are directly influenced by nursing actions (Johnson, Mass, & Moorhead, 2000). Outcomes are defined as the behaviors and feelings of the patient in *response* to the nursing care given.

CRITICAL THINKING IN NURSING
General Thinking

Nurses have job-specific knowledge and skills they incorporate in their daily nursing practice. General thinking involves random or memorized thoughts. An example of general thinking would be memorizing the steps in a clinical procedure or skill.

Critical Thinking

Critical thinking is purposeful, goal-directed thinking based on scientific evidence rather than assumption or memorization. Critical thinking is an organized approach to discovery that involves the reflection and integration of information that enables the nurse to arrive at a conclusion or make a judgment.

An example of critical thinking would be modifying the steps in a clinical procedure or skill so that the individual patient's needs are met but the basic principles of the skill are not violated (e.g., sterile technique).

With critical thinking, *problem solving* is effective and problem *prevention* occurs. General thinking can occur naturally, but critical thinking is a skill that must be learned.

Because critical thinking is an active process, the regular use of critical thinking can assist in moving general information into long-term memory and can increase creativity. Critical thinking skills help the nurse adapt to new situations that occur every day and aid in clinical decision making about the care given.

Critical thinking can improve the care nurses give to patients, improve test scores (by critically thinking about a scenario in the question), and improve working conditions by enabling the nurse to analyze and find creative ways to improve existing policies and practices.

The Nursing Process and Critical Thinking

The nursing process (assessment, diagnosis, planning, implementation, and evaluation) is a tool for effective critical thinking. When a nurse uses the nursing process in critical thinking, a *clinical judgment* can be made that is specific to the data collected and the clinical situation. In every clinical contact a nurse must identify actual and potential problems and make decisions about a plan of action that will result in a positive patient outcome; know why the actions are appropriate; differentiate between those problems that can be cared for independently and those that require contacting other members of the health care team; and prioritize those actions (Box 1-8).

Differentiating between actions that can be independently carried out and those requiring collaboration with other health care providers is based on the *scope of practice* of the LVN/LPN. The scope of practice of the LVN/LPN is published by the state board of nursing.

Using Critical Thinking to Improve Test Scores

Attending class, reading the text, and studying are the basis of learning, and evaluation of learning is

---

| box 1-8 | *Process of Critical Thinking* |

1. Identify the problem.
2. Differentiate fact from assumption.
3. Check reliability and accuracy of data.
4. Determine relevant from irrelevant.
5. Identify possible conclusions/outcomes.
6. Set priorities and goals.
7. Evaluate response of patient.

---

achieved by testing. Weekly tests evaluate short-term learning. Final examinations evaluate long-term learning or retention of learning. Retained learning is subject to later recall and therefore is most useful in nursing practice after graduation from nursing school. Recalling facts that have been retained enables critical thinking in nursing practice. For a nurse to recognize or analyze *abnormal* findings, the *normal* findings must be recalled and compared. An intervention can then be formulated.

Using critical thinking in studying involves the following:

1. *Understanding* facts before trying to memorize them
2. *Prioritizing* information to be memorized
3. *Relating* facts to other facts (clusters, patterns, groups)
4. *Using all five senses* to study (read, write, draw, listen to tapes, see pictures of symptoms)
5. *Reviewing* before tests
6. *Reading the questions* (identifying key concepts and using critical thinking) seek sample questions during study

THE FUTURE

HEALTH CARE REFORM

The federal government is working to provide a health care reform plan to reduce the cost of health care while making it more accessible to all. Nurses are involved in the health care reform movement as patient advocates to ensure that the patient receives quality care. Health insurance plays an important role in health care delivery. Having health insurance does not ensure access to expensive care, as the insurance company often must "approve" the expenditure before the test or care is provided. Those families who cannot afford health insurance often do not seek preventive health care, such as prenatal care, infant immunizations, and well-baby check-ups. These problems must be dealt with as health care reform evolves. Managed care and utilization review committees who review the appropriateness of health care services have an impact on the management of patients by physicians. Continued study is needed to determine the effect of managed care on the quality and cost containment of health care.

The future role of the nurse will involve providing health care in a variety of settings and working closely with the multidisciplinary health care team. The nurse will function as a caregiver, teacher, collaborator, advocate, manager, and researcher. Competence in care and accountability to the patient, family, community, and profession are core responsibilities of the nurse in the twenty-first century.

The revolution in health care involves the conflict between cost containment and quality care. When health care became big business, cost containment was born and managed care was the result. Managed care openly evaluates care given and, in the right environment, can result in increased quality. Quality assurance committees are investigating the routine management of patients, especially in the area of preventive care and tests. Nurses will take a key role in forming the health care picture of tomorrow.

HEALTHY PEOPLE 2010

Healthy People 2010 is a statement of national health promotion and disease prevention objectives facilitated by the federal government. The objectives are designed to use the vast knowledge and technology of health care that was developed in the twentieth century to improve the health and quality of life of Americans in the twenty-first century. The report identifies objectives in broad categories of effort: health promotion, health protection, preventive services, and the development of surveillance and data systems. The specific goals include increasing the span of healthy life, reducing health disparities among Americans, and achieving access to preventive care for all Americans. Some priority areas include maternal and infant health, immunizations, prevention of sexually transmitted diseases, oral health, nutrition, and physical fitness. It is a "vision for the new century" to achieve a nation of healthy people. An example of the specific contribution of the school nurse to the concept of *Healthy People 2010* is described in Box 1-9.

DOCUMENTATION

Documentation, or charting, has always been a legal responsibility of the nurse. When a medication is given or a treatment is performed, it is accurately documented on the patient's chart. Charting responsibilities also in-

---

| box 1-9 | **Healthy People 2010:** *Specific Contributions of School Nurses*

The expanding role of the school nurse will include the following:

1. Reviewing participation in and effectiveness of physical education programs for normal and disabled students
2. Providing nutritional education and guidance
3. Supervising school nutrition programs
4. Participating in maintaining a drug- and tobacco-free environment for students
5. Providing education in the prevention of sexually transmitted diseases
6. Providing guidance to students and staff concerning prevention of injuries
7. Providing oral health education
8. Providing age-appropriate human immunodeficiency virus (HIV) education
9. Reviewing immunization laws and records
10. Assessing the community needs in relation to the child population and reassessing/revising roles in relation to prevention, screening, monitoring, teaching, and follow-up of health needs or problems

---

clude head-to-toe assessment of the patient and a recording of data pertinent to the diagnosis and response to treatment. There have been many forms of charting required by different hospitals in different areas of the country that guide the nurse toward comprehensive charting. A traditional problem has been with several members of the multidisciplinary health care team accessing the chart at the same time. When the nurse was recording a medication administered, the medication record was "tied-up" until the recording was complete. When a physician was reviewing the chart and progress of the patient, the records were "tied-up" until the conference was completed. With the advent of computers, computerized charting has been fine-tuned and is used by most hospitals in the country. Computerized charting is a paperless method of charting accomplished with a wireless pad and an electronic pen. Security features are usually built in, and prompts encourage accurate and comprehensive charting by "forcing" certain entries before the user can progress through the system. Critical ranges can be programmed into the computer so the nurse is alerted to deviations from the norm as information is recorded. Using computerized charting, all caregivers have access to patient records on all patients at all times from various locations. The adaptation and application of computerized programs to the hospital setting have motivated all nurses to become *basically* computer literate.

COMMUNITY-BASED NURSING

Nursing care within the community and in the home is not a new concept in maternal-child nursing. The work of Lillian Wald, founder of the Henry Street Settlement, brought home health care to poor children. Margaret Sanger's work as a public health nurse accessed care for poor pregnant women and was the seed for the development of modern planned parenthood programs. The community is now the major health care setting for all patients, and the challenge is to provide safe, caring, cost-effective, quality care to mothers, infants, and families. This challenge involves the nurse as a patient advocate to influence government, business, and the community to recognize the need for supporting preventive care of maternal-infant patients to ensure a healthy population for the future. The nurse must work with the interdisciplinary health care team to identify needs within the community and create cost-effective approaches to comprehensive preventive and therapeutic care. The role of the nurse as an educator within the community is facilitated by the use of schools, churches, health fairs, computer web sites, and the media. Some registered nurses are branching out into the community as private practitioners, such as lactation consultants for new mothers. The nursing care plan is expanding to become a family care plan as the nurse is providing care to the patient in the home. Creativity, problem solving, coordination of multidisciplinary caregivers, case management, assessment, and referral are just some of the essential skills required of a nurse providing community-based care to maternal-infant patients.

Preventive care is only one aspect of current and future home care and community-based nursing. Therapeutic care is also provided in the home setting, and the nurse must educate the family concerning the monitoring, care, and need for professional referral when necessary. Specialized care such as fetal monitoring of high-risk pregnant women, apnea monitoring of high-risk newborns, diabetic glucose monitoring, heparin therapy, and total parenteral nutrition can be safely accomplished in the home setting, often with computer or telephone accessibility to a nurse manager.

The home health care team, as advocated by the American Academy of Pediatrics Committee on Children with Disabilities, includes a pediatrician; nurses; occupational, physical, and respiratory therapists; speech therapists; home teachers; social workers; and home health aides. The American Academy of Home Health Care Physicians have expressed a medical commitment to the concept of home care for the future.

key points

- In 1840 Ignaz Semmelweis suggested that hand-washing was an important concept in preventing infection. This simple procedure is still a cornerstone of nursing care.
- The cultural background of the expectant family plays an important role in their adaptation to the birth experience.
- The educational focus for the childbearing family is that childbirth is a normal and healthy event.
- *Statistics* refers to gathering and analyzing numerical data.
- *Birth rate* refers to the number of live births per 1000 population in 1 year.
- In the United States, vital statistics are compiled for the country as a whole by the national Center for Health Statistics.
- The nursing process consists of five steps: assessment, nursing diagnosis, planning, implementation, and evaluation. It is an organized method of nursing practice and a means of communication among staff members.
- The culture of a society has a strong influence on family and child care.
- Lillian Wald, a nurse, is credited with suggesting the establishment of the Children's Bureau.
- The Fair Labor Standards Act, passed in 1938, controls the use of child labor.
- The White House Conferences on Children and Youth investigate and report on matters pertaining to children and their families among all classes of people.
- The Children's Charter of 1930 is considered one of the most important documents in child care history.
- The United Nations Declaration of the Rights of the Child calls for freedom, equality of opportunity, social and emotional benefits, and enhancement of each child's potential.
- The American Nurses Association (ANA) has written standards of maternal-child health practices.
- Diagnosis-related groups (DRGs), a form of cost containment, continue to affect nursing practice.
- Advanced practice nurses are registered nurses with advanced degrees who are certified and specialize, manage care, and conduct research.
- Labor, delivery, and recovery (LDR) rooms provide family-centered birthing and promote early parent-infant bonding.
- Clinical pathways are collaborative guidelines that define multidisciplinary care in terms of outcomes within a timeline.
- The nursing care plan is a written instrument of communication that uses the nursing process to formulate a plan of care for a specific patient. It uses nursing diagnoses and involves critical thinking and problem solving.
- Critical thinking is an active process that involves recall of information that is stored in long-term

memory so that judgments based on facts can be analyzed and prioritized for use in clinical decision making.

- The use of critical thinking skills increases the ability of the nurse to make clinical decisions that meet individual needs of patients. The use of critical thinking skills can also improve test scores. The use of critical thinking also stimulates creativity that can improve quality of care and the work environment.

- *Healthy People 2010* is a statement of national health promotion that is a vision for the new century. The objectives are designed to use twenty-first–century technology and knowledge to improve health care and quality of life.

- Charting is the legal responsibility of the nurse and includes a head-to-toe assessment and data pertinent to the diagnosis and response of the patient to treatment.

- Home health care involves therapy, monitoring, teaching, and referral.

- The nurse must understand the culture and tradition of the family and their influence on health practices.

- Utilization review committees, quality assurance committees, the American Academy of Pediatrics Committee on Children with Disabilities, the American Academy of Home Care Physicians, and the Association of Women's Obstetric and Neonatal Nurses (AWHONN) are some of the organizations that set and maintain standards of maternity and pediatric care.

ONLINE RESOURCES

National Center for Health Statistics:
http://www.cdc.gov/nchs

Division of Intramural Research: Glossary of Genetic Terms:
http://www.nhgri.nih.gov/dir/vip/glossary

National Human Genome Research Institute:
http://www.nhgri.nih.gov/elsi

REVIEW QUESTIONS   *Choose the most appropriate answer.*

1. The number of deaths of infants younger than age 28 days per 1000 live births is termed:
   1. Birth rate
   2. Neonatal birth rate
   3. Neonatal morbidity rate
   4. Neonatal mortality rate

2. The man known as the father of pediatrics is:
   1. Benjamin Spock
   2. Hippocrates
   3. John Semmelweis
   4. Abraham Jacobi

3. An organization that sets standards of care for nursing is the:
   1. American Medical Association
   2. American Nurses Association
   3. Utilization review committee
   4. American Academy of Pediatrics

4. One of the most important documents in child care history formulated by the White House Conference was the:
   1. Fair Labor Practice Act
   2. Children's Charter
   3. Missing Children's Clearinghouse
   4. Education for Handicapped Children Act

5. Which of the following sources would the nurse use to determine if a specific nursing activity is within the scope of practice of a LPN/LVN?
   1. Doctor's prescription record
   2. Hospital procedure book
   3. Head nurse/nurse manager
   4. The nurse practice act

CHAPTER 2

Human Reproductive Anatomy and Physiology

objectives

1. Define each key term listed.
2. Describe changes of puberty in males and females.
3. Identify the anatomy of the male reproductive system.
4. Explain the functions of the external and internal male organs in human reproduction.
5. Describe the influence of hormones in male reproductive processes.
6. Identify the anatomy of the female reproductive system.
7. Explain the functions of the external, internal, and accessory female organs in human reproduction.
8. Explain the menstrual cycle and the female hormones involved in the cycle.
9. Discuss the importance of the pelvic bones to the birth process.

key terms

bi-ischial diameter (p. 28)
climacteric (klī-MĂK-tĕr-ĭk, p. 26)
diagonal conjugate (p. 27)
dyspareunia (dĭs-păh-ROO-nē-ă, p. 24)
embryo (p. 25)
external os (p. 26)
fetus (p. 21)
internal os (p. 26)
menarche (mĕ-NĂR-kē, p. 22)
menopause (MĔN-ō-păwz, p. 29)
obstetric conjugate (p. 27)
ovulation (p. 26)
ovum (p. 26)
puberty (p. 21)
rugae (ROO-jē, p. 25)
semen (p. 23)
smegma (SMĔG-mă, p. 24)
spermatogenesis (spĕr-mă-tō-JĔN-ĕ-sĭs, p. 22)
transverse diameter (p. 27)
zygote (ZĪ-gōt, p. 26)

Understanding childbirth requires an understanding of the structures and functions of the body that make childbearing possible. This knowledge includes anatomy, physiology, sexuality, embryology of the growing fetus, and the psychosocial changes that occur in both the male and the female. This chapter addresses the anatomy and physiology of the male and female reproductive systems.

PUBERTY

Before puberty, male and female children appear very much alike except for their genitalia. Puberty involves changes in the whole body and the psyche as well as in the expectations of society toward the individual.

Puberty is a period of rapid change in the lives of boys and girls during which the reproductive systems mature and become capable of reproduction. Puberty begins when the secondary sex characteristics appear (e.g., pubic hair). Puberty ends when mature sperm are formed or when regular menstrual cycles occur. This transition from childhood to adulthood has been identified and often celebrated by various rites of passage. Some cultures have required demonstrations of bravery, such as hunting wild animals or displays of self-defense. Ritual circumcision is another rite of passage in some cultures and religions. In the United States today, some adolescents participate in religious ceremonies such as bar or bat mitzvah or confirmation, but for others, these ceremonies are unfamiliar. The lack of a "universal rite of passage" to identify adulthood has led to confusion for some contemporary adolescents in many industrialized nations.

THE MALE

Male hormonal changes normally begin between 10 and 16 years of age. Outward changes become apparent when the size of the penis and testes increases and there is a general growth spurt. Testosterone, the primary male hormone, causes the boy to grow taller, become more muscular, and develop secondary sex characteristics such as pubic hair, facial hair, and a deep voice. Testosterone levels are constant, not cyclical like female hormones, although levels may decrease with age to 50% of peak levels by age 80 years. Nocturnal emissions ("wet dreams") may occur without sexual stimulation. These emissions usually do not contain sperm. The voice deepens but is often characterized by squeaks or cracks before reaching its final pitch.

THE FEMALE

The first outward change of puberty in females is development of the breasts (see Figure 2-7). The first menstrual period (menarche) occurs 2 to 2½ years later (age 11 to 15 years). Female reproductive organs mature to prepare for sexual activity and childbearing. The female experiences a growth spurt, but hers ends earlier than the male's. Her hips broaden as her pelvis assumes the wide basin shape needed for birth. Pubic and axillary hair appear. The quantity varies, as it does in males.

MALE REPRODUCTIVE SYSTEM

The male reproductive system consists of external and internal organs (Figure 2-1).

EXTERNAL GENITALIA

The penis and the scrotum, which contains the testes, are the male external genitalia.

Penis

The penis has two functions, as follows:
- To provide a duct to expel urine from the bladder
- To deposit sperm in the female's vagina to fertilize an ovum

The penis comprises the glans and the body. The glans is the rounded, distal end of the penis. It is visible on a circumcised penis but is hidden by the foreskin on an uncircumcised one. At the tip of the glans is an opening called the urethral meatus. The body of the penis contains the urethra (the passageway for sperm and urine) and erectile tissue (the corpus spongiosum and two corpora cavernosa). The usually flaccid penis becomes erect during sexual stimulation when blood is trapped within the spongy erectile tissues. The erection allows the male to penetrate the female's vagina during sexual intercourse.

Scrotum

The scrotum is a sac that contains the testes. The scrotum is suspended from the perineum, keeping the testes away from the body and thereby lowering their temperature. This cooling is necessary for normal sperm production (spermatogenesis).

INTERNAL GENITALIA

The internal genitalia include the testes, vas deferens, prostate, seminal vesicles, ejaculatory ducts, urethra, and accessory glands.

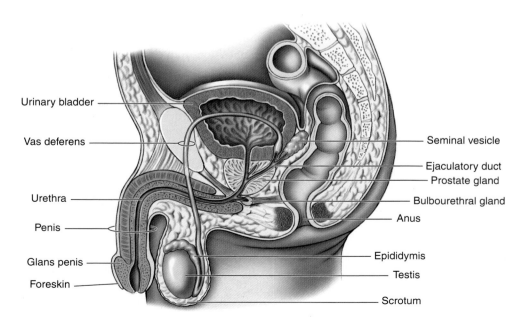

FIGURE **2-1** The male reproductive organs.

Testes

The testes (testicles) are a pair of oval glands housed in the scrotum. They have two functions, as follows:

- Manufacture male germ cells (spermatozoa or sperm)
- Secrete male hormones *(androgens)*

Sperm are made in the convoluted seminiferous tubules that are contained within the testes. Sperm production begins at puberty and continues throughout the life span of the male.

The production of *testosterone,* the most abundant male hormone, begins with the anterior pituitary gland. Under the direction of the hypothalamus, the anterior pituitary gland secretes follicle-stimulating hormone (FSH) and luteinizing hormone (LH). FSH and LH initiate the production of testosterone in the Leydig cells of the testes. Testosterone has the following effects not directly related to sexual reproduction:

- Increases muscle mass and strength
- Promotes growth of long bones
- Increases basal metabolic rate (BMR)
- Enhances production of red blood cells
- Produces enlargement of vocal cords
- Affects the distribution of body hair

These effects result in the greater strength and stature and a higher hematocrit level in males than in females. Testosterone also increases production of sebum, a fatty secretion of the sebaceous glands of the skin, and may contribute to the development of acne during early adolescence. However, as the skin adapts to the higher levels of testosterone, acne generally recedes.

Ducts

Each epididymis, one from each testicle, stores and carries the sperm to the penis. The sperm may remain in the epididymis for 2 to 10 days, during which time they mature and then move on to the vas deferens. Each vas deferens passes upward into the body, goes around the symphysis pubis, circles the bladder, and passes downward to form (with the ducts from the seminal vesicles) the ejaculatory ducts. The ejaculatory ducts then enter the back of the prostate gland and connect to the upper part of the urethra, which is in the penis. The urethra transports both urine from the bladder and *semen* from the prostate to the outside of the body, but not at the same time.

Accessory Glands

The accessory glands are the *seminal vesicles,* the *prostate gland,* and the *bulbourethral glands,* also called *Cowper's glands.* The accessory glands produce secretions (semi-nal plasma). The secretions of these glands accomplish the following:

- Nourish the sperm
- Protect the sperm from the acidic environment of the woman's vagina
- Enhance the motility (movement) of the sperm

The seminal plasma and sperm together are called semen. Semen may be secreted during sexual intercourse *before* ejaculation. Therefore pregnancy may occur even if ejaculation occurs outside the vagina. Increased heat in the environment around the sperm (testes) increases motility but shortens the life of the sperm. A constant increase in temperature around the testes can prevent spermatogenesis and lead to permanent sterility.

FEMALE REPRODUCTIVE SYSTEM

The female reproductive system consists of external genitalia, internal genitalia, and accessory structures such as the mammary glands (breasts). The bony pelvis is discussed in this chapter because of its importance in the childbearing process.

EXTERNAL GENITALIA

The female external genitalia are collectively called the *vulva.* They include the mons pubis, labia majora, labia minora, fourchette, clitoris, vaginal vestibule, and perineum (Figure 2-2).

Mons Pubis

The mons pubis (mons veneris) is a pad of fatty tissue covered by coarse skin and hair. It protects the symphysis pubis and contributes to the rounded contour of the female body.

Labia Majora

The labia majora are two folds of fatty tissue on each side of the vaginal vestibule. Many small glands are located on the moist interior surface.

Labia Minora

The labia minora are two thin, soft folds of erectile tissue that are seen when the labia majora are separated. Secretions from sebaceous glands in the labia are bactericidal to reduce infection and also lubricate and protect the skin of the vulva.

Fourchette

The fourchette is a fold of tissue just below the vagina, where the labia majora and the labia minora meet. Lacerations in this area often occur during childbirth.

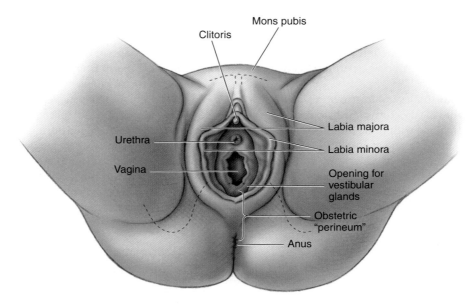

FIGURE **2-2** The external female reproductive organs.

Clitoris

The clitoris is a small, erectile body in the most anterior portion of the labia minora. It is similar in structure to the penis. Functionally, it is the most erotic, sensitive part of the female genitalia, and it produces smegma. Smegma is a cheeselike secretion of the sebaceous glands in the area.

Vaginal Vestibule

The vaginal vestibule is the area seen when the labia minora are separated. The following are the five structures in the vestibule:

- The *urethral meatus* lies approximately 2 cm below the clitoris. It has a foldlike appearance with a slit-type opening, and it serves as the exit for urine.
- *Skene's ducts* (paraurethral ducts) are located on each side of the urethra and provide lubrication for the urethra and the vaginal orifice.
- The *vaginal introitus* is the division between the external and internal female genitalia.
- The *hymen* is a thin elastic membrane that closes the vagina from the vestibule to various degrees.
- The *ducts of the Bartholin glands* (vulvovaginal glands) provide lubrication for the vaginal introitus during sexual arousal and are normally not visible.

Perineum

The perineum is a strong, muscular area between the vaginal opening and the anus. The elastic fibers and connective tissue of the perineum allow stretching to permit the birth of a full-term infant. The perineum is

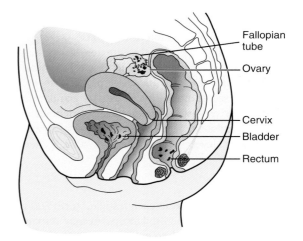

FIGURE **2-3** Side view of the internal female reproductive organs.

the site of the episiotomy (incision) or tears during birth. Pelvic weakness or painful intercourse (dyspareunia) may result if this tissue does not heal properly.

INTERNAL GENITALIA

The internal genitalia are the vagina, uterus, fallopian tubes, and ovaries. Figure 2-3 illustrates the side view of these organs, and Figure 2-4 illustrates the frontal view.

Vagina

The vagina is a tubular structure made of muscle and membranous tissue that connects the external genitalia to the uterus. Because it meets at a right angle with the

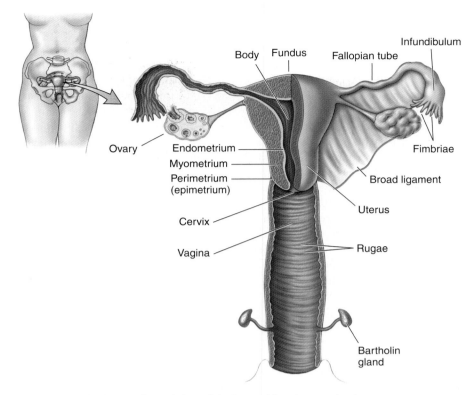

FIGURE **2-4** Frontal view of the internal female reproductive organs.

cervix, the anterior wall is about 2.5 cm (1 inch) shorter than the posterior wall, which varies from 7 to 10 cm (approximately 2.8 to 4 inches). The marked stretching of the vagina during delivery is made possible by the rugae, or transverse ridges of the mucous membrane lining. The vagina is self-cleansing and during the reproductive years maintains a normal acidic pH of 4 to 5. The self-cleansing activity may be altered by antibiotic therapy, frequent douching and excessive use of vaginal sprays, deodorant sanitary pads, or deodorant tampons.

The functions of the vagina are as follows:

- To provide a passageway for sperm to enter the uterus
- To allow drainage of menstrual fluids and other secretions
- To provide a passageway for the infant's birth

Strong pelvic floor muscles stabilize and support the internal and external reproductive organs. The most important of these muscles is the levator ani, which supports the three structures that penetrate it: urethra, vagina, and rectum.

Uterus

The uterus (womb) is a hollow muscular organ in which a fertilized ovum is implanted, an embryo forms, and a fetus develops. It is shaped like an upside-down pear or light bulb. In a mature, nonpregnant female, it weighs approximately 60 g (2 ounces) and is 7.5 cm (3 inches) long, 5 cm (2 inches) wide, and 1 to 2.5 cm (0.4 to 1 inch) thick. The uterus lies between the bladder and the rectum above the vagina.

The uterus is supported by several ligaments. The broad ligament provides stability to the uterus in the pelvic cavity; the round ligament is surrounded by muscles that enlarge during pregnancy and keep the uterus in place; the cardinal ligaments prevent uterine prolapse, and the uterosacral ligaments are surrounded by smooth muscle and contain sensory nerve fibers that may contribute to the sensation of dysmenorrhea (painful menstruation). Stretching of the uterine ligaments as the uterus enlarges during pregnancy can cause minor discomfort to the mother.

NURSING **TIP**

An excellent opportunity to reinforce knowledge about the self-cleansing function of the vagina, menstruation, and reproduction is when teaching women about feminine hygiene or while discussing family planning.

Nerve supply. Because the autonomic nervous system innervates the reproductive system, its functions are not under voluntary (conscious) control. Therefore even a paraplegic woman can have adequate contractions for labor. Sensations for uterine contractions are carried to the central nervous system (CNS) via the eleventh and twelfth thoracic nerve roots. Pain from the cervix and vagina passes through the pudendal nerves. The motor fibers of the uterus arise from the seventh and eighth thoracic vertebrae. This separate motor and sensory nerve supply allows for the use of a local anesthetic without interfering with uterine contractions and is important to pain management during labor.

Anatomy. The uterus is separated into three parts: fundus, corpus, and cervix. The *fundus* (upper part) is broad and flat. The fallopian tubes enter the uterus on each side of the fundus. The *corpus* (body) is the middle portion, and it plays an active role in menstruation and pregnancy.

The fundus and corpus have the following three distinct layers:

- The *perimetrium* is the outermost or serosal layer that envelops the uterus.
- The *myometrium* is the middle muscular layer that functions during pregnancy and birth. It has three involuntary muscle layers: a longitudinal outer layer, a figure-of-eight interlacing middle layer, and circular inner layer that forms sphincters at the fallopian tube attachments and at the internal opening of the cervix.
- The *endometrium* is the inner or mucosal layer that is functional during menstruation and implantation of the fertilized ovum. It is governed by cyclical hormonal changes.

The *cervix* (lower part) is narrow and tubular and opens into the upper vagina. The cervix consists of a cervical canal with an internal opening near the uterine corpus (the internal os) and an opening into the vagina called (the external os). The mucosal lining of the cervix has the following four functions:

- Lubricates the vagina
- Acts as a bacteriostatic agent
- Provides an alkaline environment to shelter deposited sperm from the acidic pH of the vagina
- Produces a mucous plug in the cervical canal during pregnancy

Fallopian Tubes

The fallopian tubes, also called uterine tubes or oviducts, extend laterally from the uterus, one to each ovary (see Figure 2-4). They vary in length from 8 to 13.5 cm (3 to 5.3 inches). Each tube has four sections, as follows:

- The *interstitial* portion runs into the uterine cavity and lies within the wall of the uterus.

- The *isthmus* is a narrow area near the uterus.
- The *ampulla* is the wider area of the tube and is the usual site of fertilization.
- The *infundibulum* is the funnellike enlarged distal end of the tube. Fingerlike projections from the infundibulum called *fimbriae* hover over each ovary and "capture" the ovum (egg) as it is released by the ovary at ovulation.

The four functions of the fallopian tubes are to provide the following:

- A passageway in which sperm meet the ovum
- A site of fertilization
- A safe, nourishing environment for the ovum or zygote (fertilized ovum)
- A means of transporting the ovum or zygote to the corpus of the uterus

Cells within the tubes have *cilia* (hairlike projections) that beat rhythmically to propel the ovum toward the uterus. Other cells secrete a protein-rich fluid to nourish the ovum after it leaves the ovary.

Ovaries

The ovaries are two almond-shaped glands, each about the size of a walnut. They are located in the lower abdominal cavity, one on each side of the uterus, and are held in place by ovarian and uterine ligaments. The ovaries have the following two functions:

- Production of hormones, chiefly estrogen and progesterone
- Maturation of an ovum during each reproductive cycle

At birth, every female infant has all the ova (oocytes) that will be available during her reproductive years (approximately 2 million cells). These degenerate significantly so that by adulthood the remaining oocytes number only in the thousands. Of these, only a small percentage are actually released (about 400 during the reproductive years). Every month one ova matures and is released from the ovary. Any ova that remain after the climacteric (the time surrounding menopause) no longer respond to hormone stimulation to mature.

FEMALE PELVIS

The bony pelvis occupies the lower portion of the trunk of the body. It is formed by the following four bones attached to the lower spine:

- Two innominate bones
- Sacrum
- Coccyx

Each innominate bone is made up of an *ilium, pubis,* and *ischium,* which are separate during childhood but fuse by adulthood. The ilium is the lateral, flaring portion of the hip bone; the pubis is the anterior hip bone.

These two bones join to form the symphysis pubis. The curved space under the symphysis pubis is called the pubic arch. The ischium is *below* the ilium and supports the seated body. An ischial spine, one from each ischium, juts inward to varying degrees. These ischial spines serve as a reference point for descent of the fetus during labor. The posterior pelvis consists of the sacrum and coccyx. Five fused, triangular vertebrae at the base of the spine form the sacrum. The sacrum may jut into the pelvic cavity, causing a narrowing of the birth passageway. Below the sacrum is the coccyx, the lowest part of the spine.

The functions of the bony pelvis are as follows:

- Support and distribute body weight
- Support and protect pelvic organs
- Form the birth passageway

Types of Pelves

There are four basic types of pelves (Figure 2-5). Most women have a combination of pelvic characteristics rather than having one pure type. Each type of pelvis has implications for labor and birth, as follows:

- The *gynecoid* pelvis is the classic female pelvis, with rounded anterior and posterior segments. This type is most favorable for vaginal birth.
- The *android* pelvis has a wedge-shaped inlet with a narrow anterior segment; it is typical of the male anatomy.
- The *anthropoid* pelvis has an anteroposterior diameter that equals or exceeds its transverse diameter. The shape is a long, narrow oval. Women with this type of pelvis can usually deliver vaginally, but their infant is more likely to be born in the occiput posterior (back of the fetal head toward the mother's sacrum) position.
- The *platypelloid* pelvis has a shortened anteroposterior diameter and a flat, transverse oval shape. This type is unfavorable for vaginal birth.

True and False Pelves

The pelvis is divided into the false and true pelves by an imaginary line (the linea terminalis) that proceeds from the sacroiliac joint to the anterior iliopubic prominence. The upper, or false, pelvis supports the enlarging uterus and guides the fetus into the true pelvis. The lower, or true, pelvis consists of the inlet, pelvic cavity, and outlet. The true pelvis is important because it dictates the bony limits of the birth canal.

Pelvic Diameters

The diameters of the pelvis must be adequate for passage of the fetus during birth (Figure 2-6).

Pelvic inlet. The pelvic inlet, just below the linea terminalis, has obstetrically important diameters. The *anteroposterior* diameter is measured between the symphysis pubis and the sacrum and is the shortest inlet diameter. The *transverse* diameter is measured across the linea terminalis and is the largest inlet diameter. The *oblique* diameters are measured from the right or left sacroiliac joint to the prominence of the linea terminalis.

Measurements of the pelvic inlet include the following (Table 2-1):

- **Diagonal conjugate:** The distance between the suprapubic angle and the sacral promontory. This measurement is assessed by the health care provider during a manual pelvic examination.
- **Obstetric conjugate** (the smallest inlet diameter): Estimated by subtracting $1\frac{1}{2}$ to 2 cm from the diagonal conjugate (the approximate thickness of the pubic bone). This measurement determines if the fetus can pass through the birth canal.
- **Transverse diameter:** The largest diameter of the inlet. It determines the inlet's shape.

Pelvic outlet. The *transverse* diameter of the outlet is a measurement of the distance between the inner surfaces of the ischial tuberosities and is known as the

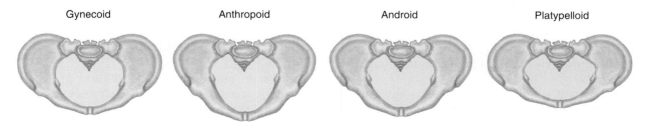

| Gynecoid | Anthropoid | Android | Platypelloid |

FIGURE **2-5** Four types of pelves. The gynecoid pelvis is the typical female pelvis and optimum for passage of the fetal head.

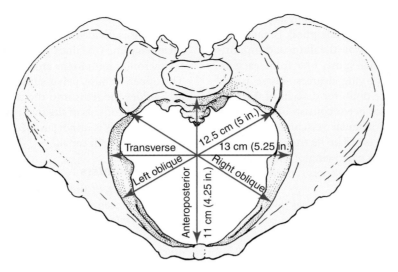

FIGURE **2-6** Four important pelvic inlet diameters are the anteroposterior, the transverse, and the right and left oblique diameters.

table **2-1**	*Average Pelvic Measurements*
MEASUREMENT	**DIAMETER**
INLET	
Diagonal conjugate	11.5 cm
Obstetric conjugate (true)	9.5-10 cm
Transverse	13.5 cm
Oblique	12.75 cm
OUTLET	
Anteroposterior	9.5 cm
Bi-ischial	10-12 cm
Posterior sagittal	7.5 cm

bi-ischial diameter. The anteroposterior measurement of the outlet is the distance between the lower border of the symphysis pubis and the tip of the sacrum. It can be measured by vaginal examination. The *sagittal* diameters are measured from the middle of the transverse diameter to the pubic bone anteriorly and to the sacrococcygeal bone posteriorly. The coccyx can move or break during the passage of the fetal head, but an immobile coccyx can decrease the size of the pelvic outlet and make vaginal birth difficult. A narrow pubic arch can also impact the passage of the fetal head through the birth canal.

Adequate pelvic measurements are essential for a successful vaginal birth. Problems that can cause a pelvis to be small (e.g., a history of a pelvic fracture or rickets) can indicate that delivery may require a cesarean section.

BREASTS

Female breasts (mammary glands) are accessory organs of reproduction. They produce milk after birth to provide nourishment and maternal antibodies to the infant (Figure 2-7). The nipple, in the center of each breast, is surrounded by a pigmented areola. Montgomery's glands (Montgomery's tubercles) are small sebaceous glands in the areola that secrete a substance to lubricate and protect the breasts during lactation.

Each breast is made of 15 to 24 lobes arranged like the spokes of a wheel. The lobes are separated by adipose (fatty) and fibrous tissues. The adipose tissue affects size and firmness and gives the breasts a smooth outline. Breast size is primarily determined by the amount of fatty tissue and is unrelated to a woman's ability to produce milk.

Alveoli (lobules) are the glands that secrete milk. They empty into about 20 separate lactiferous (milk-carrying) ducts. Milk is stored briefly in widened areas of the ducts, called ampullae or lactiferous sinuses.

FEMALE REPRODUCTIVE CYCLE AND MENSTRUATION

The female reproductive cycle consists of regular changes in secretions of the anterior pituitary gland, the ovary, and the endometrial lining of the uterus (Figure 2-8). The anterior pituitary gland, in response to the hypothalamus, secretes FSH and LH. FSH stimulates maturation of a follicle in the ovary that contains a

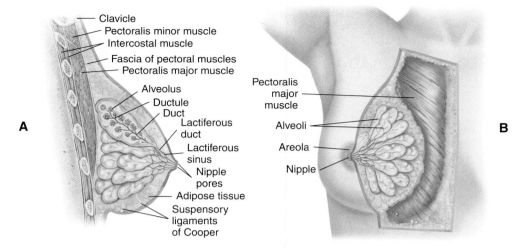

FIGURE **2-7** The female breast. **A,** Side view of a lactating breast. Each lobule of glandular tissue is drained by a lactiferous duct that eventually opens through the nipple. **B,** Anterior view of a lactating breast. Overlying skin and connective tissue has been removed from the medial side to show the internal structure of the breast and underlying skeletal muscle. In nonlactating breasts the glandular tissue is much less prominent, with adipose tissue comprising most of each breast.

single ovum. Several follicles start maturing during each cycle, but only one usually reaches final maturity. The maturing ovum and corpus luteum (the empty follicle after the ovum is released) produce increasing amounts of estrogen and progesterone, which leads to a buildup of the endometrium. A surge in LH stimulates final maturation and the release of an ovum.

Ovulation occurs when a mature ovum is released from the follicle about 14 days before the onset of the next menstrual period. The corpus luteum turns yellow (luteinizing) immediately after ovulation and secretes increasing quantities of progesterone to prepare the uterine lining for a fertilized ovum. Approximately 12 days after ovulation, the corpus luteum degenerates if fertilization has not occurred, and progesterone and estrogen levels decrease. The fall in estrogen and progesterone causes the endometrium to break down, resulting in menstruation. The anterior pituitary gland secretes more FSH and LH, beginning a new cycle.

The beginning of menstruation, called menarche, occurs at about age 11 to 15 years. Early cycles are often irregular and may be anovulatory. Regular cycles are usually established within 6 months to 2 years of the menarche. In an average cycle, the flow (menses) occurs every 28 days, plus or minus 5 to 10 days. The flow itself lasts from 2 to 5 days, with a blood loss of 30 to 40 ml and an additional loss of 30 to 50 ml of serous fluid. Fibrinolysin is contained in the necrotic endometrium

being expelled, and therefore clots are not normally seen in the menstrual discharge.

The *climacteric* is a period of years during which the woman's ability to reproduce gradually declines. Menopause refers to the final menstrual period, although the terms *menopause* and *climacteric* are often casually used interchangeably.

PHYSIOLOGY OF THE SEX ACT

PHYSIOLOGY OF THE MALE SEX ACT

The male psyche can initiate or inhibit the sexual response. The massaging action of intercourse on the glans penis stimulates sensitive nerves that send impulses to the sacral area of the spinal cord and to the brain. Stimulation of nerves supplying the prostate and scrotum enhances sensations. The parasympathetic nerve fibers cause relaxation of penile arteries, which fill the cavernous sinuses of the shaft of the penis that stretch the erectile tissue so that the penis becomes firm and elongated *(erection)*. The same nerve impulses cause the urethral glands to secrete mucus to aid in lubrication for sperm motility. The sympathetic nervous system then stimulates the spinal nerves to contract the vas deferens and cause expulsion of the sperm into the urethra *(emission)*. Contraction of muscle of

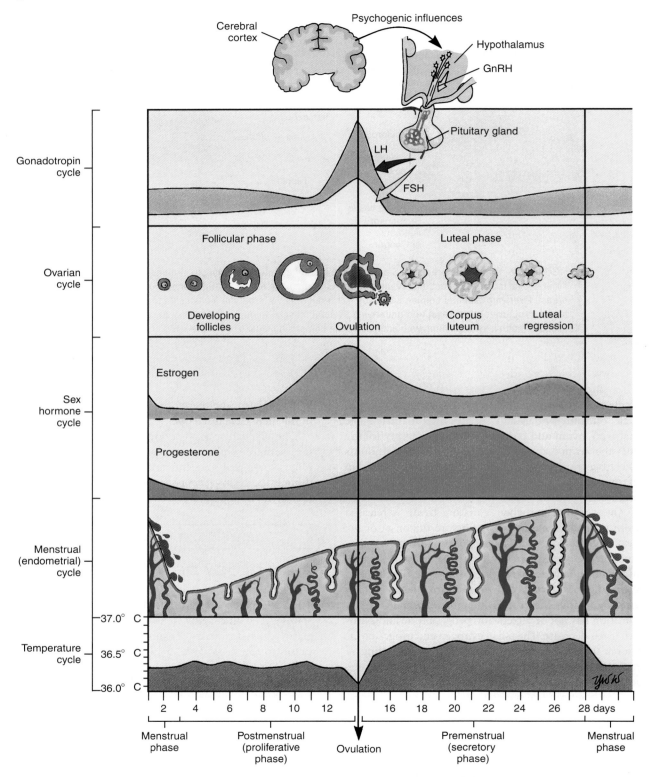

FIGURE **2-8** Female reproductive cycles. This diagram illustrates the interrelationships among the hypothalamic, pituitary, ovarian, and uterine functions throughout a standard 28-day menstrual cycle. The variations in basal body temperature are also illustrated.

the prostate gland and seminal vesicles expels prostatic and seminal fluid into the urethra, contributing to the flow and motility of the sperm. This full sensation in the urethra stimulates nerves in the sacral region of the spinal cord that cause rhythmical contraction of the penile erectile tissues and urethra and skeletal muscles in the shaft of the penis, which expel the semen from the urethra (*ejaculation*). The period of emission and ejaculation is called male *orgasm.*

Within minutes, erection ceases (*resolution*), the cavernous sinuses empty, penile arteries contract, and the penis becomes flaccid. Sperm can reach the woman's fallopian tube within 5 minutes and can remain viable in the female reproductive tract for 4 to 5 days. Of the millions of sperm contained in the ejaculate, a few thousand reach each fallopian tube but only one fertilizes the ovum. The sphincter in the base of the bladder closes during ejaculation so that sperm does not enter the bladder and urine cannot be expelled.

PHYSIOLOGY OF THE FEMALE SEX ACT

The female psyche can initiate or inhibit the sexual responses. Local stimulation by massage to the breasts, vulva, vagina, and perineum creates sexual sensations. The sensitive nerves in the glans of the clitoris send signals to the sacral areas of the spinal cord, and these signals are transmitted to the brain. Parasympathetic nerves from the sacral plexus return signals to the erectile tissue around the vaginal introitus, dilating and filling the arteries and resulting in a tightening of the vagina around the penis. These signals stimulate the Bartholin glands at the vaginal introitus to secrete mucus that aids in vaginal lubrication. The parasympathetic nervous system causes the perineal muscles and other muscles in the body to contract. The posterior pituitary gland secretes oxytocin, which stimulates contraction of the uterus and dilation of the cervical canal. This process (orgasm) is believed to aid in the transport of the sperm to the fallopian tubes. (This process is also the reason why sexual abstention is advised when there is a high risk for miscarriage or preterm labor.)

Following orgasm, the muscles relax (resolution), and this is usually accompanied by a sense of relaxed satisfaction. The egg lives for only 24 hours after ovulation; sperm must be available during that time if fertilization is to occur.

key points

- Testosterone is the principal male hormone. Estrogen and progesterone are the principal female

hormones. Testosterone secretion continues throughout a man's life, but estrogen and progesterone secretions are very low after a woman reaches the climacteric.
- The penis and scrotum are the male external genitalia. The scrotum keeps the testes cooler than the rest of the body, promoting normal sperm production.
- The two main functions of the testes are to manufacture sperm and to secrete male hormones (androgens), primarily testosterone.
- The myometrium (middle muscular uterine layer) is functional in pregnancy and labor. The endometrium (inner uterine layer) is functional in menstruation and implantation of a fertilized ovum.
- The female breasts are composed of fatty and fibrous tissue and of glands that can secrete milk. The size of a woman's breasts is determined by the amount of fatty tissue and does not influence her ability to secrete milk.
- The female reproductive cycle consists of regular changes in hormone secretions from the anterior pituitary gland and the ovary, maturation and release of an ovum, and buildup and breakdown of the uterine lining.
- There are four basic pelvic shapes, but women often have a combination of characteristics. The gynecoid pelvis is the most favorable for vaginal birth.
- The pelvis is divided into a false pelvis above the linea terminalis and the true pelvis below this line. The true pelvis is most important in birth. The true pelvis is further divided into the pelvic inlet, pelvic cavity, and pelvic outlet.

ONLINE RESOURCES

Reproductive System: http://www.cyber-north.com/anatomy/reproduc.htm
Fetal.Com: http://www.fetal.com

CRITICAL THINKING QUESTIONS

A patient is admitted to the labor unit and has not had any prenatal care. Her history reveals that she had a fractured pelvis in an automobile accident several years ago. The patient states she is interested in natural childbirth. What is the nurse's best response?

A male adolescent fears he is becoming incontinent because he notices his pajama pants are wet on occasion when he awakes in the morning. He asks if there is medicine to stop this. What is the best response of the nurse?

REVIEW QUESTIONS   *Choose the most appropriate answer.*

1. Spermatozoa are produced in the:
   1. Vas deferens
   2. Seminiferous tubules
   3. Prostate gland
   4. Leydig cells

2. Production of estrogen from the ovaries occurs under the influence of:
   1. Luteinizing hormone
   2. Growth hormone
   3. Adrenocorticotropic hormone
   4. Follicle-stimulating hormone

3. The typical male pelvic type is the:
   1. Gynecoid
   2. Android
   3. Anthropoid
   4. Platypelloid

4. The muscular layer of the uterus that is the functional unit in pregnancy and labor is the:
   1. Perimetrium
   2. Myometrium
   3. Endometrium
   4. Cervix

5. During a prenatal clinic visit, a woman states that she probably will not plan to breastfeed her infant because she has very small breasts and does not think she can provide adequate milk for a full-term infant. The best response of the nurse would be:
   1. "Ask the physician if he or she will prescribe hormones to build up the breasts."
   2. Provide the woman with exercises that will build up her breast tissue.
   3. "The fluid intake of the mother will determine the milk output."
   4. "The size of the breast has no relationship to the ability to produce adequate milk."

Prenatal Development

objectives

1. Define each key term listed.
2. Describe the process of gametogenesis in human reproduction.
3. Explain human fertilization and implantation.
4. Describe embryonic development.
5. Describe fetal development and maturation of body systems.
6. Describe the development and functions of the placenta, umbilical cord, and amniotic fluid.
7. Compare fetal circulation to circulation after birth.
8. Explain the similarities and differences in the two types of twins.

key terms

age of viability (p. 40)
amniotic sac (p. 36)
autosome (p. 33)
chorion (KŌ-rē-ŏn, p. 34)
decidua (dĕ-SĬD-ū-ă, p. 34)
diploid (DĬP-loid, p. 33)
dizygotic (dī-zī-GŎT-ĭk, p. 44)
fertilization (p. 34)
gametogenesis (găm-ĕ-tō-JĔN-ĕ-sĭs, p. 34)
germ layers (p. 34)
haploid (HĂP-loid, p. 33)
monozygotic (mŏn-ō-zī-GŎT-ĭk, p. 44)
oogenesis (ō-ō-JĔN-ĕ-sĭs, p. 33)
placenta (plă-SĔN-tă, p. 34)
spermatogenesis (spĕr-mă-tō-JĔN-ĕ-sĭs, p. 33)
surfactant (sŭr-FĂK-tănt, p. 39)
teratogen (TĔR-ă-tō-jĕn, p. 33)
Wharton's jelly (p. 42)

The human body contains many millions of cells at birth, but life begins with a single cell created by the fusion of a sperm with an ovum.

Deoxyribonucleic acid (DNA) programs a genetic code into the nucleus of the cell; the nucleus controls the development and function of the cell. Defects in the DNA code can result in inherited disorders. The genes and chromosomes contained within the DNA deter-

mine the uniqueness of the traits and features of the developing person.

Chromosomes begin in pairs, one supplied by the mother and the other by the father. Each body cell contains 46 chromosomes, made up of 22 pairs of autosomes (body chromosomes) and one pair of sex chromosomes that determine the sex of the fetus. Each chromosome contains genes that involve heredity. Cell division then occurs, which is the basis of human growth and regeneration.

Biological development is not isolated. It is influenced by the external environment, such as maternal drug use (teratogens that cause damage to growing cells), maternal undernutrition, or smoking, and it is now known that sounds such as music are heard by the fetus and are recognized by the newborn. All these factors influence prenatal growth and development. Early prenatal care is essential to the optimum outcome of the pregnancy (see Chapter 4).

CELL DIVISION AND GAMETOGENESIS

The division of a cell begins in its nucleus, which contains the gene-bearing chromosomes. The two types of cell division are mitosis and meiosis.

Mitosis is a continuous process by which the body grows and develops and dead body cells are replaced. In this type of cell division, *each daughter cell contains the same number of chromosomes as the parent cell.* The 46 chromosomes in a body cell are called the diploid number of chromosomes. The process of mitosis in the sperm is called spermatogenesis, and in the ovum is called oogenesis.

Meiosis is a different type of cell division in which the reproductive cells undergo two sequential divisions. During meiosis the number of chromosomes in each cell is reduced to half, or 23 chromosomes, each with only one sex chromosome. This is called the haploid number of chromosomes. This process is completed in the sperm before it travels toward the fallopian tube and in the ovum after ovulation if fertilized. At the moment of fertilization (when the sperm and ova unite), the new cell contains 23 chromosomes from the sperm and 23 chromosomes from the ova, thus returning to the diploid number of chromosomes (46); traits are therefore inherited from both the mother and the father. The formation of gametes by this type of cell division is called gametogenesis (Figure 3-1). As soon as fertilization occurs, a chemical change in the membrane around the fertilized ovum prevents penetration by another sperm.

FERTILIZATION

Fertilization occurs when a sperm penetrates an ovum and unites with it, restoring the total number of chromosomes to 46. It normally occurs in the outer third of the fallopian tube, near the ovary (Figure 3-2). The sperm pass through the cervix and uterus and into the fallopian tubes by means of the flagellar (whiplike) activity of their tails and can reach the fallopian tubes within 5 minutes after coitus.

The time during which fertilization can occur is brief because of the short lifespan of mature gametes. The ovum is estimated to survive for up to 24 hours after ovulation. The sperm remains capable of fertilizing the ovum for up to 5 days after being ejaculated in the area of the cervix.

> **NURSING TIP**
> During sexual counseling the nurse should emphasize that the survival time of sperm ejaculated into the area of the cervix may be up to 5 days and that pregnancy can occur with intercourse as long as 5 days before ovulation.

SEX DETERMINATION

The sex of human offspring is determined at fertilization. The ovum always contributes an X chromosome (gamete), whereas the sperm can carry an X *or* a Y chromosome (gamete). When a sperm carrying the X chromosome fertilizes the X-bearing ovum, a female child (XX) results. When a Y-bearing sperm fertilizes the ovum, a male child (XY) is produced (Figure 3-3).

Because sperm can carry either an X or a Y chromosome, the male partner determines the gender of the child. However, the pH of the female reproductive tract and the estrogen levels of the woman's body affect the survival rate of the X- and Y-bearing sperm as well as the speed of their movement through the cervix and fallopian tubes. Thus the female has some influence on which sperm fertilizes the mature ovum.

> **NURSING TIP**
> Both mother and father influence the sex of their offspring, although the father contributes the actual sex chromosome. This fact may reduce blame in some cultures when the child is not of the desired sex.

TUBAL TRANSPORT OF THE ZYGOTE

Fertilization normally occurs in the upper third of the fallopian tube. The *zygote* is the cell formed by the union of the sperm and the ovum, and it is transported through the fallopian tube and into the uterus. During transport through the fallopian tube, the zygote undergoes rapid mitotic division, or *cleavage*. Cleavage begins with two cells, which subdivide into four and then eight cells to form the *blastomere*. The size of the zygote does not increase; rather, the individual cells become smaller as they divide and eventually form a solid ball called the *morula* (see Figure 3-2).

The morula enters the uterus on the third day and floats there for another 2 to 4 days. The cells form a cavity, and two distinct layers evolve. The inner layer is a solid mass of cells called the *blastocyst* (see Figure 3-2), which develops into the embryo and embryonic membranes. The outer layer of cells, called the *trophoblast*, develops into an embryonic membrane, the chorion (see Figure 3-4). Occasionally the zygote does not move through the fallopian tube and instead becomes implanted into the lining of the tube, resulting in a tubal ectopic pregnancy (see Chapter 5).

IMPLANTATION OF THE ZYGOTE

The zygote usually implants in the upper section of the posterior uterine wall. The cells burrow into the prepared lining of the uterus, called the endometrium. The endometrium is now called the decidua; the area under the blastocyst is called the decidua basalis and gives rise to the maternal part of the placenta.

DEVELOPMENT

CELL DIFFERENTIATION

During the week between fertilization and implantation, the cells within a zygote are identical to one another. After implantation the cells begin to differentiate and develop special functions. The chorion, amnion, yolk sac, and primary germ layers appear.

Chorion

The chorion develops from the trophoblast (outer layer of embryonic cells) and envelops the amnion, embryo,

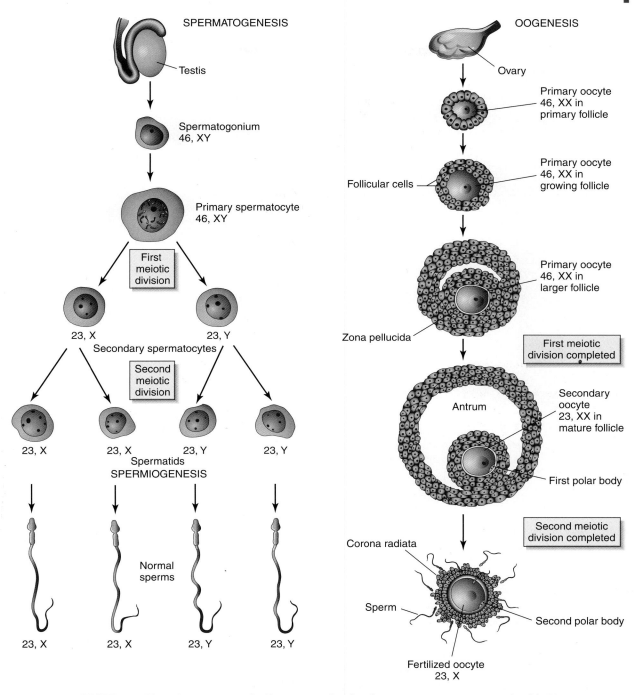

FIGURE **3-1** Normal gametogenesis. Four sperm develop from one spermatocyte, each with 23 chromosomes—with one sex chromosome, either an X or a Y. In oogenesis, one ova develops with 23 chromosomes with one sex chromosome, always an X. An XY combination produces a boy, and an XX combination produces a girl.

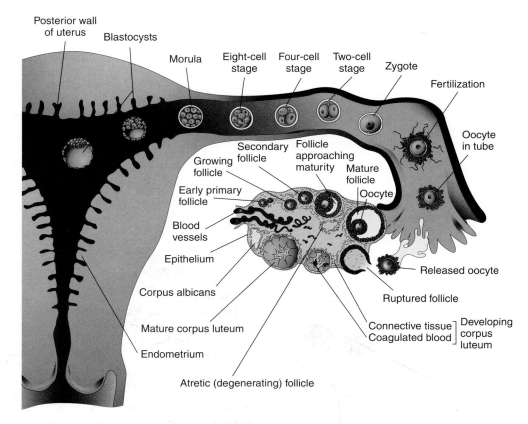

FIGURE **3-2** Ovulation and fertilization. Ovulation occurs; the egg is caught by the fimbria and is guided into the fallopian tube, where fertilization occurs. The zygote continues to multiply (but not grow in size) as it passes through the fallopian tube and implants into the posterior wall of the uterus.

and yolk sac. It is a thick membrane with fingerlike projections called *villi* on its outermost surface. The villi immediately below the embryo extend into the decidua basalis on the uterine wall and form the embryonic/fetal portion of the placenta (see Figure 3-5).

Amnion

The amnion is the second membrane and is a thin structure that envelops and protects the embryo. It forms the boundaries of the amniotic cavity, and its outer aspect meets the inner aspect of the chorion.

The chorion and amnion together form an amniotic sac filled with fluid (bag of waters) that permits the embryo to float freely. Amniotic fluid is clear, has a mild odor, and often contains bits of vernix (fetal skin covering) or lanugo (fetal hair on the skin). The volume of amniotic fluid steadily increases from about 30 ml at 10 weeks of pregnancy to 350 ml at 20 weeks. The volume of fluid is about 1000 ml at 37 weeks. In the latter part of pregnancy the fetus may swallow up to 400 ml of amniotic fluid per day and normally excretes urine into the fluid. The functions of amniotic fluid are as follows:

- Maintain an even temperature
- Prevent the amniotic sac from adhering to the fetal skin
- Allow symmetrical growth
- Allow buoyancy and fetal movement
- Act as a cushion to protect the fetus and umbilical cord from injury

Yolk Sac

On the ninth day after fertilization a cavity called the yolk sac forms in the blastocyst. It functions only during embryonic life and initiates the production of red blood cells. This function continues for about 6 weeks, until the embryonic liver takes over. The umbilical cord then encompasses the yolk sac, and the yolk sac degenerates.

Germ Layers

After implantation the zygote in the blastocyst stage transforms its *embryonic disc* into three primary *germ layers* known as *ectoderm, mesoderm,* and *endoderm.* Each germ layer develops into a different part of the

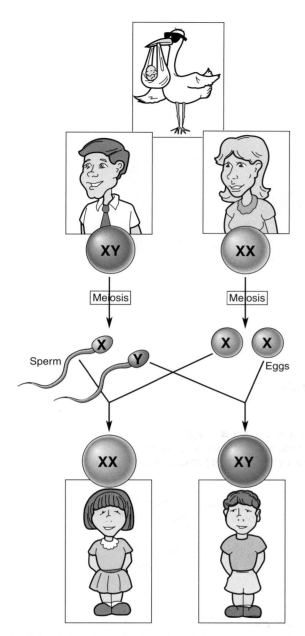

FIGURE **3-3** Sex determination. If an X chromosome from the male unites with an X chromosome from the female, the child will be a female (XX). If a Y chromosome from the male unites with an X chromosome from the female, the child will be a male (XY).

growing embryo. The specific body parts that develop from each layer are listed in Box 3-1.

PRENATAL DEVELOPMENTAL MILESTONES

Table 3-1 follows the developmental milestones during intrauterine development. Developmental milestones exist in fetal growth and development as they do in

box 3-1 *Body Parts That Develop from the Primary Germ Layers*

ECTODERM
Outer layer of skin
Oil glands and hair follicles of skin
Nails and hair
External sense organs
Mucous membrane of mouth and anus

MESODERM
True skin
Skeleton
Bone and cartilage
Connective tissue
Muscles
Blood and blood vessels
Kidneys and gonads

ENDODERM
Lining of trachea, pharynx, and bronchi
Lining of digestive tract
Lining of bladder and urethra

growth and development after birth. Three basic stages characterize prenatal development: the zygote, the embryo, and the fetus. The zygote continues to grow and develop as it passes through the fallopian tube and implants into the wall of the uterus. The second to the eighth week of development is known as the embryonic stage, with the developing infant called an *embryo*. From the ninth week of development until birth the developing infant is called a *fetus*. By the second week after fertilization the ectoderm, endoderm, and amnion begin to develop.

By the third week the mesoderm and neural tube form and the primitive heart begins to pump. It is at this time that some mothers first realize they have "missed" their menstrual period and suspect they are pregnant. It is now known that folic acid supplements can prevent most neural tube defects such as spina bifida. However, in an unplanned pregnancy, it is possible for a neural tube defect to occur before the mother confirms her pregnancy state. For this reason, planned parenthood and early prenatal care with good nutrition and folic acid supplements are desirable so the embryo is protected in the very first days and weeks of development. By 8 weeks' gestation, the ovaries or testes are present, the beginnings of all systems have developed, and there is movement in the extremities. The fetal period begins at the ninth week, and by the tenth week the external genitalia are visible to ultrasound examination. At the

| table **3-1** | **Embryonic and Fetal Development** |

AGE	LENGTH AND WEIGHT	DEVELOPMENT
Week 3 Neural groove / Cut surface of amnion / Neural groove / Neural fold in region of developing spinal cord / Location of primitive streak / Neural fold in region of developing brain / Yolk sac / First pairs of somites / Connecting stalk / Part of chorionic sac — Actual size 2.5 mm	1.5-2.5 mm	*Cardiovascular:* Single tubular heart is formed. *Nervous:* Neural tube forms; primitive spinal cord and brain appear.
Week 4 Forebrain / Heart / Upper limb bud	3.5-4 mm	*Cardiovascular:* Heart pumps blood. *Gastrointestinal (GI):* Esophagus and trachea separate; stomach forms. *Nervous:* Neural tube closes; forebrain forms. *Musculoskeletal:* Upper and lower limb buds appear. *Senses:* Ears and eyes begin to form.
Week 6 External acoustic meatus / Eyelid / Pigmented eye / Nasolacrimal groove / Nasal pit / Umbilical cord / Heart prominence / Auricular hillocks forming auricle of external ear / Digital rays of hand plate / Foot plate — Actual size 11.0 mm	11-13 mm	*Musculoskeletal:* Skull and jaw ossify; hands and elbows differentiate. *Senses:* Auditory canal forms; eye is obvious. *Cardiovascular:* Heart has all four chambers. *GI:* Nasal cavity and upper lip form.

table 3-1 *Embryonic and Fetal Development—cont'd*

AGE	LENGTH AND WEIGHT	DEVELOPMENT
Week 8 Scalp vascular plexus — Auricle of external ear — Eyelid — Eye — Shoulder — Nose — Lower jaw — Mouth — Wrist — Umbilical cord — Arm — Toes separated — Elbow — Sole of foot — Knee Actual size 30.0 mm	30 mm crown-rump 6 g	Embryo has distinct human appearance. Purposeful movements occur. Tail has disappeared. Sex organs form. Beginnings of most external and internal structures are formed. Enters fetal period.
Week 17	150 mm crown-rump 260 g	Genitalia and leg movements are visible on ultrasound and may be felt by the mother. Bones are ossified. Eye movements occur. Fetus sucks and swallows amniotic fluid. Ovaries contain ovum. No subcutaneous fat is present. Thin skin allows blood vessels of scalp to be visible.
Week 25	28 cm (11.2 inches) crown-heel 780 g (1 lb 10 oz)	Wrinkled skin, lean body results from lack of subcutaneous fat. Eyes are open. Fetus is now viable. Mother feels stronger movement (quickening). Fetus has schedule of sleeping and moving. Vernix caseosa is present on skin. Lanugo covers body. Brown fat is formed. Lungs begin to secrete **surfactant.** Fingernails are present. Respiratory movements begin.

Continued

table 3-1 *Embryonic and Fetal Development—cont'd*

AGE	LENGTH AND WEIGHT	DEVELOPMENT
Week 29	38 cm (15 inches) crown-heel 1260 g (2 lb 10 oz)	Fetus assumes stable (cephalic) position in utero. Central nervous system is functioning. Skin is less wrinkled because of the presence of subcutaneous fat. Spleen stops forming blood cells, and bone marrow starts to form blood cells. Increased surfactant is present in lungs.
Week 36	48 cm (19 inches) crown-heel 2500 g (5 lb 12 oz)	Subcutaneous fat is present. Skin is pink and smooth. Grasp reflex is present. Circumferences of head and abdomen are equal. Surge of lung surfactant is produced.

Note: Full-term is considered 38-40 weeks. The crown-heel length is 48-52 cm (18-21 inches), and the weight is 3000-3600 g (6 lb 10 oz-7 lb 15 oz).

fourteenth week the fetus moves in response to external stimuli. By 20 weeks' gestation the lungs have matured functionally enough for the fetus to survive outside the uterus (age of viability), but special care in the neonatal intensive care unit (NICU) would be required. The status of the fetus in utero can be monitored by fetal movements (kick counts). By 28 weeks the eyes open and fetal position in the uterus becomes more stable. The fetus is considered to be full term at 38 to 40 weeks' gestation.

Infant survival at birth depends not only on biological development but also on the response of the parent (see Chapter 15, Table 15-5). The preparation of the parents during pregnancy is vital to the development of a positive, nurturing relationship between the parent and infant. The development of the fetus in Table 3-1 can be correlated with Table 4-7 in Chapter 4, concerning the psychological and physical changes in the mother that occur prenatally.

ACCESSORY STRUCTURES OF PREGNANCY

The placenta, umbilical cord, and fetal circulation support the fetus as it completes prenatal life and prepares for birth.

PLACENTA

The placenta (afterbirth) is a temporary organ for fetal respiration, nutrition, and excretion. It also functions as an endocrine gland.

The placenta forms when the chorionic villi of the embryo extend into the blood-filled spaces of the mother's decidua basalis. The maternal part of the placenta arises from the decidua basalis and has a beefy red appearance. The fetal side of the placenta develops from the chorionic villi and the chorionic blood vessels. The amnion covers the fetal side and umbilical cord and gives them a grayish, shiny appearance at term.

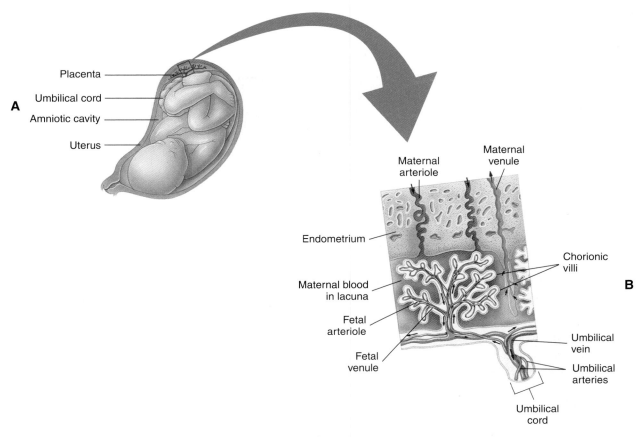

FIGURE **3-4** Maternal-fetal circulation. **A,** Relationship of the fetus and placenta in the uterus. **B,** Close placement of the fetal blood supply to the maternal blood in the placenta. The maternal blood in the lacuna permits the diffusion of nutrients and other substances and has a thin barrier to prevent some harmful substances from passing through. No mixing of fetal or maternal blood occurs.

Placental Transfer

A thin membrane separates the maternal and fetal blood, and the two blood supplies do not normally mix (Figure 3-4). However, separation of the placenta at birth may allow some fetal blood to enter the maternal circulation, which can cause problems with fetuses in subsequent pregnancies if the blood types are not compatible (see Chapter 5). The placenta is divided into 15 to 20 segments called *cotyledons.*

Fetal deoxygenated blood and waste products leave the fetus through the two umbilical arteries and enter the placenta through the branch of a main stem villus, which extends into the intervillus space (lacuna). Oxygenated, nutrient-rich blood from the mother spurts into the intervillus space from the spiral arteries in the decidua (see Figures 3-4 and 3-5). The fetal blood releases carbon dioxide and waste products and takes in oxygen and nutrients before returning to the fetus through the umbilical vein.

The thin placental membrane provides some protection but is not a barrier to most substances ingested by the mother. Many harmful substances such as drugs (therapeutic and abused), nicotine, and viral infectious agents are transferred to the fetus and may cause fetal drug addiction, congenital anomalies, and fetal infection.

Placental Hormones

Four hormones are produced by the placenta: progesterone, estrogen, human chorionic gonadotropin (hCG), and human placental lactogen (hPL).

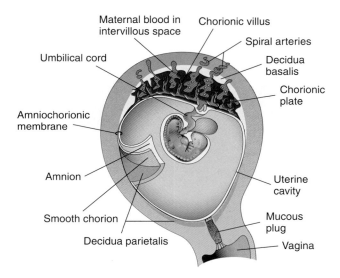

FIGURE **3-5** The pregnant uterus at 4 weeks showing the relationship of the fetal membranes to the decidua of the uterus and the embryo.

Progesterone. Progesterone is first produced by the corpus luteum and later by the placenta. It has the following functions during pregnancy:

- Maintain uterine lining for implantation of the zygote
- Reduce uterine contractions to prevent spontaneous abortion
- Prepare the glands of the breasts for lactation
- Stimulate testes to produce testosterone which aids the male fetus in developing the reproductive tract

Estrogen. Estrogen has the following important functions during pregnancy:

- Stimulate uterine growth
- Increase the blood flow to uterine vessels
- Stimulate development of the breast ducts to prepare for lactation

The effects of estrogen not directly related to pregnancy include the following:

- Increased skin pigmentation (such as the "mask of pregnancy")
- Vascular changes in the skin and the mucous membranes of the nose and mouth
- Increased salivation

Human chorionic gonadotropin. Human chorionic gonadotropin (hCG) is the hormone "signal" sent to the corpus luteum that conception has occurred. The hCG causes the corpus luteum to persist and to continue the production of estrogen and progesterone to sustain pregnancy. hCG is detectable in maternal blood as soon as implantation occurs—usually 7 to 9 days after fertilization—and is the basis for most pregnancy tests.

Human placental lactogen. hPL is also known as human chorionic somatomammotropin (hCS). hPL causes decreased insulin sensitivity and utilization of glucose by the mother, making more glucose available to the fetus to meet growth needs.

UMBILICAL CORD

The umbilical cord develops with the placenta and fetal blood vessels; it is the lifeline between mother and fetus. Two arteries carry blood away from the fetus, and one vein returns blood to the fetus. Wharton's jelly covers and cushions the cord vessels and keeps the three vessels separated. The vessels are coiled within the cord to allow movement and stretching without restricting circulation. The normal length of the cord is about 55 cm (22 inches). The umbilical cord is usually inserted near the center of the placenta.

> **⭐NURSING TIP**
>
> An easy way to remember the number and type of umbilical cord vessels is the woman's name AVA, which stands for "Artery-Vein-Artery."

FETAL CIRCULATION

After the fourth week of gestation, circulation of blood through the placenta to the fetus is well established (see Figure 3-4). Because the fetus does not breathe and the liver does not have to process most waste products, several physiological diversions in the prebirth circulatory

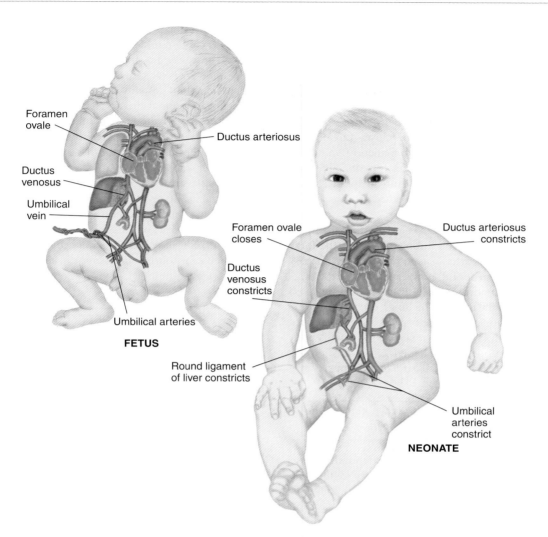

Foramen ovale

Ductus arteriosus

Ductus venosus

Umbilical vein

Umbilical arteries

FETUS

Foramen ovale closes

Ductus venosus constricts

Round ligament of liver constricts

Ductus arteriosus constricts

Umbilical arteries constrict

NEONATE

FIGURE **3-6** Changes in fetal-newborn circulation at birth. The changes in the circulation of the fetus and the neonate are shown. The ductus arteriosus, ductus venosus, and foramen ovale are shunts that close because of the expansion of the lungs and pressure changes within the heart.

route are needed. The three fetal circulatory shunts are as follows:

- *Ductus venosus,* which diverts some blood away from the liver as it returns from the placenta
- *Foramen ovale,* which diverts most blood from the right atrium directly to the left atrium, rather than circulating it to the lungs
- *Ductus arteriosus,* which diverts most blood from the pulmonary artery into the aorta

Circulation Before Birth

Oxygenated blood enters the fetal body through the umbilical vein. About half the blood goes to the liver through the portal sinus, with the remainder entering the inferior vena cava through the *ductus venosus.* Blood in the inferior vena cava enters the right atrium, where most passes directly into the left atrium through the *foramen ovale.* A small amount of blood is pumped to the lungs by the right ventricle. The rest of the blood from the right ventricle joins that from the left ventricle through the *ductus arteriosus.* After circulating through the fetal body, blood containing waste products is returned to the placenta through the umbilical arteries.

Circulation After Birth

Fetal shunts are not needed after birth once the infant breathes and blood is circulated to the lungs. The foramen ovale closes because pressure in the right side of the heart falls as the lungs become fully inflated and there is now little resistance to blood flow. The infant's blood oxygen level rises, causing the ductus arteriosus to constrict. The ductus venosus closes when the flow from the umbilical cord stops (Figure 3-6).

Closure of Fetal Circulatory Shunts

The foramen ovale closes functionally (temporarily) within 2 hours after birth and permanently by age 3 months. The ductus arteriosus closes functionally within 15 hours and closes permanently in about 3 weeks. The ductus venosus closes functionally when the cord is cut and closes permanently in about 1 week. After permanent closure, the ductus arteriosus and ductus venosus become ligaments.

Because they are functionally closed rather than permanently closed, some conditions may cause the foramen ovale or ductus arteriosus to reopen after birth. A condition that impedes full lung expansion (e.g., respiratory distress syndrome) can increase resistance to blood flow from the heart to the lungs, causing the foramen ovale to reopen. Similar conditions often reduce the blood oxygen levels and can cause the ductus arteriosus to remain open. See Chapter 25 for further discussion of newborn congenital cardiac problems.

PRENATAL DEVELOPMENT AND *HEALTHY PEOPLE 2010*

Studies (Barker, 1998) have shown that undernutrition in utero can result in permanent changes in the fetal structure, physiology, and metabolism and can influence the development of conditions such as heart disease and stroke in adult life. Other factors that influence health in later life can be exposure to toxins in utero or factors that occur in the first 3 years of growth and development.

During the first 3 months of fetal life the fetus is most susceptible to external influences such as undernutrition. However, different organs and tissues undergo rapid development at specific times during gestational life and are therefore sensitive to undernourishment or viral and/or toxic influences during these periods.

Infants with intrauterine growth restriction may have a reduced number of cells in their organs and can therefore be predisposed to the development of specific diseases later in life. For example, a reduced number of pancreatic beta cells can impair insulin secretion and result in a health problem as an adult. Obesity, inactivity, and other factors during the life span influence the timing and severity of the adult disease.

It is also possible that in utero changes in vascular or renal structures or hormonal systems resulting from in utero malnourishment can influence the development of hypertension later in life. Studies have also shown that impaired fetal liver growth in late gestation can

permanently impair lipid metabolism and predispose to increased cholesterol levels in adult life. A reduced liver size can be assessed by measuring abdominal circumference at birth. Fetal growth is best assessed when the weight, length of gestation, placental size, and newborn head and abdominal circumference are considered.

The growth of the fetus is limited by the nutrients and oxygen received from the mother. A mother's ability to nourish her fetus is established in her own fetal life and by her adult nutritional experience. Therefore, to prevent illness in the next generation, there must be a focus on the health practices of this generation. A healthy mother can produce a healthy child who is less prone to develop illness. Part of the goal of *Healthy People 2010* is to develop a healthy lifestyle in *all* people so that as parents they can nourish and parent healthy children for the next generation.

MULTIFETAL PREGNANCY

Twins occur once in every 90 pregnancies in North America. When hormones are given to assist with ovulation, twinning and other multifetal births (triplets, quadruplets, and quintuplets) are more likely to occur. The first set of septuplets to survive were born in the United States in 1997.

Dizygotic (DZ) twins (Figure 3-7, *B*), also called fraternal twins, may or may not be of the same sex and develop from *two separate* ova fertilized by *two separate* sperm. Dizygotic twins always have two amnions, two chorions, and two placentas, although their chorions and placentas sometimes fuse. Dizygotic twins tend to repeat in families, and the incidence increases with maternal age. They are about as much alike as any siblings.

Monozygotic (MZ) twins (Figure 3-7, *A*), often called identical twins, are genetically identical, have the same sex, and look alike because they develop from a single fertilized ovum. Physical differences between monozygotic twins are caused by prenatal environmental factors involving variations in the blood supply from the placenta. Most monozygotic twins begin to develop at the end of the first week after fertilization. The result is two identical embryos, each with its own amnion but with a common chorion, placenta, and some common placental vessels. If the embryonic disc does not divide completely, various types of conjoined (formerly called Siamese) twins may form. They are named according to the regions that are joined (e.g., thoracopagus indicates an anterior connection of the thoracic regions). These twins have a single amnion.

Many twin or higher multiples are born prematurely because the uterus becomes overly distended. The pla-

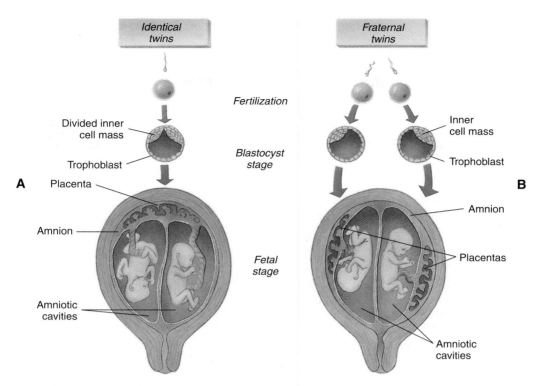

FIGURE **3-7** Multiple births. **A,** Identical (monozygotic) twins develop when the embryonic tissue from a single egg splits to form two individuals. The placenta is shared by the twins. **B,** Fraternal (dizygotic) twins develop when two different ova are fertilized at the same time by two different sperm, producing separate zygotes. Each twin has its own placenta, amnion, and chorion.

centa may not be able to supply sufficient nutrition to both fetuses, resulting in one or both twins being smaller than expected.

key points

- The uniqueness of each individual results from the blending of genes on the 46 chromosomes contained in each body cell and the environment of the embryo and fetus during development.
- Gametogenesis in the male is called spermatogenesis. Each mature sperm has 22 autosomes, plus either an X or a Y sex chromosome, for a total of 23. Gametogenesis in the female is called oogenesis. It begins at ovulation and is not completed until fertilization occurs. The mature ovum has 22 autosomes plus the X sex chromosome, for a total of 23. At conception the total number of chromosomes is restored to 46.
- When the ovum is fertilized by an X-bearing sperm, a female results; when it is fertilized by a Y-bearing sperm, the child will be male.
- After fertilization in the fallopian tube, the zygote enters the uterus, where implantation is complete by 7 days after fertilization. If the zygote fails to

move through the tube, implantation occurs there and a tubal ectopic pregnancy results.
- When implantation occurs in the uterine lining, the cells of the zygote differentiate and develop into the following structures: chorion, amnion, yolk sac, and primary germ layers. The chorion develops into the embryonic/fetal portion of the placenta; the amnion encloses the embryo and the amniotic fluid; the primary germ layers develop into different parts of the growing fetus; and the yolk sac, which functions only during embryonic life, begins to form red blood cells.
- The three germ layers of the embryo are the ectoderm, mesoderm, and endoderm. All structures of the individual develop from these layers.
- All body systems are formed and functioning in a simple way by the end of the eighth week.
- The accessory structures of pregnancy are the placenta, umbilical cord, and fetal circulation.
- These structures continuously support the fetus throughout prenatal life in preparation for birth.
- The placenta is an organ for fetal respiration, nutrition, and excretion. It is also a temporary endocrine gland that produces progesterone, estrogen, human chorionic gonadotropin (hCG), and human placental lactogen (hPL).

- Fetal circulation transports oxygen and nutrients to the fetus and disposes of carbon dioxide and other waste products from the fetus. The temporary fetal circulatory structures are the foramen ovale, ductus arteriosus, and ductus venosus. They divert most blood from the fetal liver and lungs because these organs do not fully function during prenatal life.

ONLINE RESOURCES

Reproductive System: http://www.cyber-north.com/anatomy/reproduc.htm

Genetic Ultrasound: http://www.fetal.com/gen_risk.htm

Intrauterine Growth Restriction: http://www.fetal.com/whyconcern.htm

CRITICAL THINKING QUESTIONS

A patient discusses her family planning decisions. She states that she will come to the clinic for prenatal care and will begin to take prenatal vitamins as soon as she knows she is pregnant. What would be the best response of the nurse?

A patient in the thirty-second week of gestation states she wants to deliver her infant now because she feels so "big and uncomfortable." She states that she knows the infant is fully formed since the first trimester and doesn't mind if it is a little small at birth. What would be the best response of the nurse?

REVIEW QUESTIONS   *Choose the most appropriate answer.*

1. The child's sex is determined by the:
   1. Dominance of either the X or the Y chromosome
   2. Number of X chromosomes in the ovum
   3. Ovum, which contributes either an X or a Y chromosome
   4. Sperm, which contains either an X or a Y chromosome

2. A woman who wants to become pregnant should avoid all medications unless prescribed by a physician who knows she is pregnant because:
   1. The placenta allows most medications to cross into the fetus
   2. Medications often have adverse effects when taken during pregnancy
   3. Fetal growth is likely to be slowed by many medications
   4. The pregnancy is likely to be prolonged by some medications

3. The umbilical cord normally contains:
   1. One artery and one vein
   2. Two arteries and two veins
   3. Two arteries and one vein
   4. Two veins

4. The purpose of the foramen ovale is to:
   1. Increase fetal blood flow to the lungs
   2. Limit blood flow to the liver
   3. Raise the oxygen content of fetal blood
   4. Reduce blood flow to the lungs

5. Twins are often born early because the:
   1. Distended uterus becomes irritable
   2. Amnion and chorion fuse permanently
   3. Woman's body cannot tolerate the weight
   4. Fetuses become too large to deliver vaginally

Prenatal Care and Adaptations to Pregnancy

1. Define each key term listed.
2. Calculate the expected date of delivery and duration of pregnancy.
3. Differentiate among the presumptive, probable, and positive signs of pregnancy.
4. List the goals of prenatal care.
5. Discuss prenatal care for a normal pregnancy.
6. Explain the nurse's role in prenatal care.
7. Describe the physiological changes during pregnancy.
8. Identify nutritional needs for pregnancy and lactation.
9. Describe patient education related to common discomforts of pregnancy.
10. Discuss nursing support of emotional changes that occur in a family during pregnancy.
11. Identify special needs of the pregnant adolescent, the single parent, and the older couple.
12. Discuss the importance and limitations of exercise in pregnancy.
13. Apply the nursing process in developing a prenatal teaching plan.

abortion (p. 50)
antepartum (p. 47)
aortocaval compression (ā-ŏr-tō-KĀ-văl kŏm-PRĔSH-ăn, p. 55)
Braxton Hicks contractions (p. 53)
Chadwick's sign (p. 53)
chloasma (p. 52)
colostrum (kă-LŎS-trŭm, p. 55)
estimated date of delivery (EDD) (p. 48)
gestational age (p. 50)
Goodell's sign (p. 53)
gravida (GRĂV-ĭ-dă, p. 50)
Hegar's sign (p. 53)
lactation (lăk-TĀ-shŭn, p. 55)
last normal menstrual period (LNMP) (p. 48)
lightening (p. 55)

multipara (mŭl-TĬP-ă-ră, p. 50)
Nägele's rule (NĀ-gĕ-lĕz-rōōl, p. 51)
para (PAR-ă, p. 50)
primigravida (prĭ-mĭ-GRĂV-ĭ-dă, p. 50)
primipara (prĭ-MĬP-ă-ră, p. 50)
pseudoanemia (soo-dō-ă-NĒ-mē-ă, p. 56)
quickening (p. 52)
supine hypotension syndrome (p. 55)
trimester (p. 51)

Pregnancy is a temporary, physiological (normal) process that affects the woman physically and emotionally. All systems of her body adapt to support the developing fetus. There are three phases of pregnancy: antepartum or prenatal (before birth), intrapartum (during birth), and postpartum (after birth). The focus of nursing care during pregnancy is to teach the mother how to maintain good health or, in the case of a mother with a condition that places her or her fetus at risk, to improve her health as much as possible. This chapter reviews prenatal care, the physiological and psychological changes of pregnancy, and nursing care to meet the needs of women and families.

GOALS OF PRENATAL CARE

Early and regular prenatal care is the best way to ensure a healthy outcome for both mother and child. Obstetricians, family practice physicians, certified nurse-midwives (CNMs), and nurse practitioners provide prenatal care. Unlike other health care providers, the nurse practitioner does not usually attend the woman at birth. The office or clinic nurse assists the health care provider in evaluating the expectant family's physical, psychological, and social needs and teaches the woman self-care.

The major goals of prenatal care are as follows:
- Ensure a safe birth for mother and child by promoting good health habits and reducing risk factors.
- Teach health habits that may be continued after pregnancy.
- Educate in self-care for pregnancy.

- Provide physical care.
- Prepare parents for the responsibilities of parenthood.

To achieve these goals, health care providers must do more than offer physical care. They must work as a team to create an environment that allows for cultural and individual differences while also being supportive of the entire family.

> ⚡NURSING **TIP**_____
> The major roles of the nurse during prenatal care include data collection from the pregnant woman, identifying and reevaluating risk factors, educating in self-care, providing nutrition counseling, and promoting the family's adaptation to pregnancy.

PRENATAL VISITS

Ideally, health care for childbearing begins before conception. Preconception care identifies risk factors that may be changed before conception to reduce their negative impact on the outcome of pregnancy. For example, the woman may be counseled about how to improve her nutritional state before pregnancy or may receive immunizations to prevent infections that would be harmful to the developing fetus. An adequate folic acid intake before conception can reduce the incidence of congenital anomalies (see p. 37). Some risk factors cannot be eliminated, such as preexisting diabetes, but preconception care helps the woman to begin pregnancy in the best possible state of health.

Prenatal care should begin as soon as a woman suspects that she is pregnant. A complete history and physical examination identify problems that may affect the woman or her fetus. The history should include the following:

- Obstetric history: Number and outcomes of past pregnancies, problems in the mother or infant
- Menstrual history: Usual frequency of menstrual cycles and duration of flow; first day of the last normal menstrual period (LNMP); any "spotting" since the LNMP
- Contraceptive history: Type used; whether an oral contraceptive was taken before the woman realized she might be pregnant; whether an intrauterine device is still in place
- Medical and surgical history: Infections such as hepatitis or pyelonephritis; past surgical procedures; trauma that involved the pelvis or reproductive organs
- Family history of the woman and her partner to identify genetic or other factors that may pose a risk for the pregnancy

- Woman's and partner's health history to identify risk factors (e.g., genetic defects or the use of alcohol, drugs, or tobacco) and possible blood incompatibility between the mother and fetus
- Psychosocial history to identify stability of lifestyle and ability to parent a child; significant cultural practices or health beliefs that affect the pregnancy

The woman has a complete physical examination on her first visit to evaluate her general health, determine her baseline weight and vital signs, evaluate her nutritional status, and identify current physical or social problems. A pelvic examination is performed to evaluate the size, adequacy, and condition of the pelvis and reproductive organs and to assess for signs of pregnancy (see Box 4-3). Her estimated date of delivery (EDD) is calculated based on the LNMP. An ultrasound examination may be done at this visit or at a later visit to confirm the EDD. An assessment for risk factors that may affect the pregnancy is performed during the first visit and updated at subsequent visits.

Several routine laboratory tests are performed on the first or second prenatal visit. Others are done at specific times during pregnancy and may be repeated at certain intervals. Several tests are done for all pregnant women; others are based on the presence of various risk factors. Table 4-1 lists prenatal laboratory tests.

The development of human genome mapping has expanded the prenatal detection of genetic disorders and provides the basis for future therapeutic interventions. The future direction of prenatal testing is to provide early, accurate, noninvasive screening tests.

The recommended schedule for prenatal visits in an uncomplicated pregnancy is as follows:

- Conception to 28 weeks—every 4 weeks
- 29 to 36 weeks—every 2 to 3 weeks
- 37 weeks to birth—weekly

The pregnant woman is seen more often if complications arise. Routine assessments made at each prenatal visit include the following:

- Review of known risk factors and assessment for new ones.
- Vital signs. The woman's blood pressure should be taken in the same arm and in the same posi-

> ⚡NURSING **TIP**_____
> The nurse listens to concerns and answers questions from the expectant family during each prenatal visit. This is a prime time for teaching good health habits, because most women are highly motivated to improve their health.

table 4-1 | *Prenatal Laboratory Tests**

TEST	PURPOSE
FIRST TRIMESTER (ROUTINE)	
Blood type and Rh factor and antibody screen	Determines risk for maternal-fetal blood incompatibility
Complete blood count (CBC)	Detects anemia, infection, or cell abnormalities
Hemoglobin (Hgb) or hematocrit	Detects anemia
VDRL or rapid plasma reagin (RPR)	Syphilis screen mandated by law
Rubella titer	Determines immunity to rubella
Tuberculin skin test	Screening test for exposure to tuberculosis
Hepatitis B screen	Identifies carriers of hepatitis B (recommended by American College of Obstetricians and Gynecologists)
Human immunodeficiency virus (HIV) screen	Detects HIV infection; required by some states (Counseling concerning prevention and risks should be provided to all prenatal patients)
Urinalysis	Detects infection, renal disease or diabetes
Papanicolaou (PAP) test	Screens for cervical cancer (if not done within 6 months before conception)
Cervical culture	Detects group B streptococci or sexually transmitted diseases (STDs) such as gonorrhea, chlamydia
FIRST TRIMESTER (IF INDICATED)	
Hemoglobin electrophoresis	Identifies presence of sickle cell trait or disease (in women of African or Mediterranean descent)
Endovaginal ultrasound	Performed when high risk of fetal loss is suspected
SECOND TRIMESTER (ROUTINE)	
Blood glucose screen:1 hour after ingesting 50 g of glucose liquid	Routine test done at 24-28 weeks' gestation to identify gestational diabetes; results above 135 mg/dl require medical follow-up
Serum alpha-fetoprotein	Optional routine test to identify neural tube or chromosomal defect in fetus
Ultrasonography	An optional noninvasive routine test to identify some anomalies and confirm EDD
SECOND TRIMESTER (IF INDICATED)	
Amniocentesis	Performed at 16-20 weeks' gestation when high risk for problem is suspected
THIRD TRIMESTER (IF INDICATED)	
Real-time ultrasonography	Performed when problem is suspected: • Identifies reduced amniotic fluid, which can result in fetal problem • Identifies excess amniotic fluid, which would indicate fetal anomaly or maternal problem • Confirms gestational age or cephalopelvic disproportion • Determines fetal lung maturity (lecithin and sphingomyelin ratio) with amniocentesis • Confirms presence of anomaly that may require fetal or neonatal surgery
Cervical fibronectin assay	Determines risk of preterm labor when problem is suspected

*Additional prenatal diagnostic tests can be found in Table 5-1.

tion each time for accurate comparison with her baseline value.

- Weight to determine if the pattern of gain is normal. Low prepregnant weight or inadequate gain are risk factors for preterm birth, a low-birth-weight infant, and other problems. A sudden, rapid weight gain is often associated with pregnancy-induced hypertension.
- Urinalysis for protein, glucose, and ketones.
- Blood glucose screening between 24 and 28 weeks' gestation. Additional testing is done if the result of this screening test is 135 mg/dl or higher.
- Fundal height to determine if the fetus is growing as expected and the volume of amniotic fluid is appropriate.
- Leopold's maneuvers to assess the presentation and position of the fetus by abdominal palpation.
- Fetal heart rate. During very early pregnancy, the fetal heart rate is measured with a Doppler transducer; in later pregnancy, it may also be heard with a fetoscope. Beating of the fetal heart can be seen on ultrasound examination as early as 8 weeks after the LNMP.
- Review of nutrition for adequacy of calorie intake and specific nutrients.
- Discomforts or problems that have arisen since the last visit.

The nurse establishes rapport with the expectant family by conveying interest in their needs, listening to their concerns, and directing them to appropriate resources. The health care team must show sensitivity to the family's cultural and health beliefs and incorporate as many as possible into care. For example, Muslim laws of modesty dictate that a woman be covered (hair, body, arms, and legs) when in the presence of an unrelated male, and therefore a female health care provider is often preferred. Latino families expect a brief period of conversation during which pleasantries are exchanged before "getting to the point" of the visit. An Asian woman may nod her head when the nurse teaches her, leading the nurse to believe that she understands and will use the teaching. However, the woman may be showing respect to the nurse rather than agreement with what is taught. Eye contact, which is valued

by many Americans, is seen as confrontational in some cultures.

DEFINITION OF TERMS

The following terms are used to describe the obstetric history of a woman:

- **Gravida:** Any pregnancy, regardless of duration; also, the number of pregnancies, including the one in progress, if applicable.
- Nulligravida: A woman who has never been pregnant.
- **Primigravida:** A woman who is pregnant for the first time.
- Multigravida: A woman who has been pregnant before, regardless of the duration of the pregnancy.
- Para: A woman who has given birth to one or more children who reached the age of viability (20 weeks' gestation), regardless of the number of fetuses delivered and regardless of whether those children are now living.
- Primipara: A woman who has given birth to her first child (past the point of viability), regardless of whether the child was alive at birth or is now living. The term is also used informally to describe a woman before the birth of her first child.
- Multipara: A woman who has given birth to two or more children (past the point of viability), regardless of whether the children were alive at birth or are presently alive. The term is also used informally to describe a woman before the birth of her second child.
- Nullipara: A woman who has not given birth to a child who reached the point of viability.
- **Abortion:** Termination of pregnancy before viability (20 weeks' gestation), either spontaneously or induced.
- **Gestational age:** Prenatal age of the developing fetus calculated from the first day of the woman's LNMP.
- Fertilization age: Prenatal age of the developing fetus calculated from the date of conception; approximately 2 weeks shorter than the gestational age.
- Age of viability: A fetus that has reached the stage (usually 20 weeks) where it is capable of living outside of the uterus.

The gravida number increases by one each time a woman is pregnant, whereas the para number increases *only* when a woman delivers a fetus of at least 20 weeks' gestation. For example, a woman who has had two spontaneous abortions (miscarriages) at 12 weeks' ges-

> **NURSING TIP**
> Early and regular prenatal care is important in reducing the number of low-birth-weight infants born and in reducing mortality and morbidity rates for mothers and newborns.

box 4-1 | *TPALM System to Describe Parity*

T—number of *term* infants born (infants born after at least 37 weeks' gestation)
P—number of *preterm* infants born (infants born before 37 weeks' gestation)
A—number of pregnancies *aborted* (spontaneously or induced)
L—number of children now *living*
M—multiple birth (optional)

EXAMPLE

Name	Gravida	Term	Preterm	Abortions	Living	Multiple
Katie Field	3	1	0	1	1	0
Anna Luz	4	1	1	1	2	0

Katie Field: Gravida 3, para 10110
Anna Luz: Gravida 4, para 11120

box 4-2 | *Nägele's Rule to Determine the Estimated Date of Delivery (EDD)*

- Determine first day of the last normal menstrual period (LNMP).
- Count backward 3 months.
- Add 7 days.
- Correct the year if needed.

EXAMPLE

First day of LNMP: January 27
Count backward 3 months: October 27
Add 7 days: November 3 is EDD

tation, has a 3-year-old son, and is now 32 weeks pregnant would be described as gravida 4, para 1, abortions 2. The TPALM system (Box 4-1) is a standardized way to describe the outcomes of a woman's pregnancies on her prenatal record.

DETERMINING THE ESTIMATED DATE OF DELIVERY

The average duration of a term pregnancy is 40 weeks (280 days) after the first day of the LNMP, plus or minus 2 weeks. Nägele's rule is used to determine the EDD. To calculate the EDD, one identifies the first day of the LNMP, counts backward 3 months, and then adds 7 days (Box 4-2). The year is updated if applicable. The EDD is an *estimated* date; many normal births occur before and after this date. The EDD may also be determined with a gestation wheel, an electronic calculator designed for this purpose, a physical examination, an ultrasound, or a combination of these methods.

Pregnancy is divided into three 13-week parts called trimesters. Predictable changes occur in the woman and the fetus in each trimester. Understanding these developments helps to better provide anticipatory guidance and identify deviations from the expected pattern of development.

DIAGNOSIS OF PREGNANCY

The signs of pregnancy are divided into three general groups: presumptive, probable, and positive, depending on how likely they are to be caused by factors other than pregnancy (Box 4-3).

PRESUMPTIVE SIGNS OF PREGNANCY

The presumptive indications of pregnancy are those from which a definite diagnosis of pregnancy cannot be made. These signs and symptoms are common during pregnancy but often can be caused by other conditions. The presumptive indications are discussed here.

Amenorrhea, the cessation of menses, in a healthy and sexually active woman is often the first sign of pregnancy. However, strenuous exercise, changes in metabolism and endocrine dysfunction, chronic disease, certain medications, anorexia nervosa, early menopause, or serious psychological disturbances may also be the cause.

Nausea and sometimes *vomiting* occur in at least half of all pregnancies. "Morning sickness" describes the symptoms, but they may occur at any time of day. A distaste for certain foods or even their odors may be the main complaint. The nausea begins about 6 weeks after the LNMP and usually improves by the end of the first trimester. Emotional problems or gastrointestinal upsets may also cause nausea and vomiting.

Breast changes include tenderness and tingling as hormones from the placenta stimulate growth of the ductal system in preparation for breastfeeding. Similar breast changes also occur premenstrually in many women. Striae are pink to brown lines that may develop as the breasts enlarge (Figure 4-1).

Pigmentation changes occur primarily in dark-skinned women. They include increased pigmentation of the face (chloasma, or "mask of pregnancy"), breasts (darkening of the areolae), and abdomen (linea nigra, a line extending in the midline of the abdomen from just

box 4-3 | *Signs of Pregnancy*

PRESUMPTIVE
Amenorrhea
Nausea
Breast tenderness
Deepening pigmentation
Urinary frequency
Quickening

PROBABLE
Goodell's sign
Chadwick's sign
Hegar's sign
McDonald's sign
Abdominal enlargement
Braxton Hicks contractions
Ballottement
Striae
Positive pregnancy test

POSITIVE
Audible fetal heartbeat
Fetal movement felt by examiner
Ultrasound visualization of fetus

above the umbilicus to the symphysis pubis). See Figure 4-2 for common skin changes of pregnancy.

Frequency and *urgency of urination* are common in the early months of pregnancy. The enlarging uterus, along with the increased blood supply to the pelvic area, exerts pressure on the bladder. Urinary frequency occurs in the first trimester until the uterus expands and becomes an abdominal organ in the second trimester. The pregnant woman experiences frequency of urination again in the third trimester when the presenting part descends in the pelvis in preparation for birth. Causes of urinary disturbances other than pregnancy are urinary tract infections and pelvic masses.

Fatigue and *drowsiness* are early symptoms of pregnancy. Fatigue is believed to be caused by increased metabolic needs of the woman and fetus. In an otherwise healthy young woman, it is a significant sign of pregnancy. However, illness, stress, or sudden changes in lifestyle may also cause fatigue.

Quickening, fetal movement felt by the mother, is first perceived at 16 to 20 weeks' gestation as a faint fluttering in the lower abdomen. Women who have previously given birth often report quickening at an earlier stage than women who have not. This is an important event to record because it marks the approximate midpoint of the pregnancy and is another reference point to

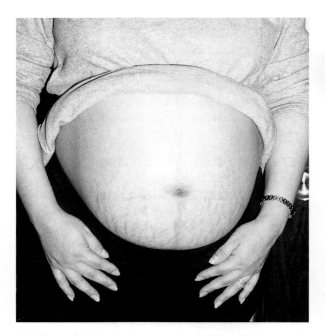

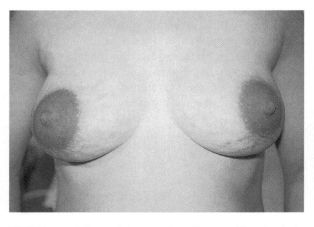

FIGURE **4-1** Striae and pigmentation of breasts. Note the darkened pigmentation of areolae and the pink-white lines at the base of the breasts that are caused by stretching of the elastic tissue as the breasts enlarge. Pigmentation will disappear after pregnancy, and striae will fade into silvery strands.

FIGURE **4-2** Abdominal striae are pinkish white or purple-gray lines that may occur in pregnancy. They may be found on the breasts, abdomen, and thighs. The dark line at the midline is the linea nigra, an area of increased pigmentation most noticeable in dark-skinned women.

verify gestational age. Abdominal gas, normal bowel activity, or false pregnancy (pseudocyesis) are other possible causes.

PROBABLE SIGNS OF PREGNANCY

The probable indications of pregnancy provide stronger evidence of pregnancy. However, these also may be caused by other conditions.

Goodell's sign is the softening of the cervix and the vagina caused by increased vascular congestion. Chadwick's sign is the purplish or bluish discoloration of the cervix, vagina, and vulva caused by increased vascular congestion. Hormonal imbalance or infection may also cause both Goodell's and Chadwick's signs. Hegar's sign is a softening of the lower uterine segment. Because of the softening, it is easy to flex the body of the uterus against the cervix *(McDonald's sign)*.

Abdominal and uterine enlargement occur rather irregularly at the onset of pregnancy. By the end of the twelfth week the uterine fundus may be felt just above the symphysis pubis, and it extends to the umbilicus between the twentieth and twenty-second weeks (Figure 4-3). Uterine or abdominal tumors may also cause enlargement.

Braxton Hicks contractions are irregular, painless uterine contractions that begin in the second trimester. They become progressively more noticeable as term approaches and are more pronounced in multiparas. They may become strong enough to be mistaken for true labor. Uterine fibroids (benign tumors) may also cause these contractions.

Ballottement is a maneuver by which the fetal part is displaced by a light tap of the examining finger on the cervix and then rebounds quickly. Uterine or cervical polyps (small tumors) may cause the sensation of ballottement on the examiner's finger.

Fetal outline may be identified by palpation after the twenty-fourth week. It is possible to mistake a tumor for a fetus.

Abdominal striae (stretch marks) are fine, pinkish white or purplish gray lines that some women develop when the elastic tissue of the skin has been stretched to its capacity (see Figure 4-2). Increased amounts of estrogen cause a rise in adrenal gland activity. This change in addition to the stretching are believed to cause a breakdown and atrophy of the underlying connective tissue in the skin. Striae are seen on the breasts, thighs,

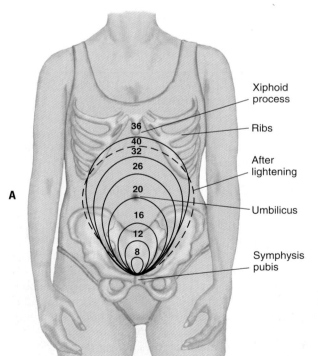

A

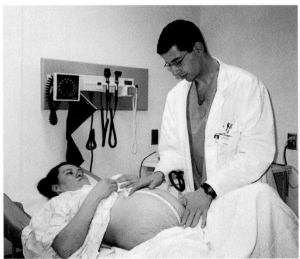

B

Xiphoid process

Ribs

After lightening

Umbilicus

Symphysis pubis

FIGURE **4-3** Height of fundus during gestation. **A,** The numbers represent the weeks of gestation and the circles represent the height of the fundus expected at that stage of gestation. Note the fortieth week is represented by a dotted line to indicate *lightening* has occurred. **B,** A health care provider measures the height of the fundus during a clinic visit. (**B** courtesy of Pat Spier, RN-C.)

abdomen, and buttocks. After pregnancy the striae lose their bright color and become thin, silvery lines. Striae may occur with skin stretching from any cause, such as weight gain.

Pregnancy tests use maternal urine or blood to determine the presence of human chorionic gonadotropin (hCG), a hormone produced by the chorionic villi of the placenta. Home pregnancy tests based on presence of hCG in the urine are capable of greater than 97% accuracy, but the instructions must be followed *precisely* to obtain this accuracy. Professional pregnancy tests are based on urine or blood serum and are more accurate. A highly reliable pregnancy test is the *radioimmunoassay (RIA)*. The RIA accurately identifies pregnancy as early as 1 week after ovulation. Pregnancy tests of all types are probable indicators because several factors may interfere with their accuracy: medications such as antianxiety or anticonvulsant drugs, blood in the urine, malignant tumors, or premature menopause.

POSITIVE SIGNS OF PREGNANCY

Positive signs of pregnancy are caused only by a developing fetus. They include demonstration of fetal heart activity, fetal movements felt by an examiner, and visualization of the fetus with ultrasound.

Fetal heartbeat may be detected as early as 10 weeks of pregnancy by using a Doppler device (Figure 4-4). The examiner can detect the fetal heartbeat using a fetoscope between the eighteenth and twentieth weeks of pregnancy. When the fetal heartbeat is heard with a fetoscope, it is important because it provides another marker of the approximate midpoint of gestation. When assessing the fetal heartbeat with a Doppler device or fetoscope, the woman's pulse must be assessed at the same time to be certain that the fetal heart is what is actually heard. The fetal heart rate at term ranges between a low of 110 to 120 beats/min and a high of 150 to 160 beats/min (AWHONN, 2000). The rate is higher in early gestation and slows as term approaches.

Additional sounds that may be heard while assessing the fetal heartbeat are the uterine and funic souffles. *Uterine souffle* is a soft blowing sound heard over the uterus during auscultation. The sound is synchronous with the mother's pulse and is caused by blood entering the dilated arteries of the uterus. The *funic souffle* is a soft swishing sound heard as the blood passes through the umbilical cord vessels.

Fetal movements can be felt by a trained examiner in the second trimester. Fetal activity must be distinguished by the examiner because, to a prospective mother, normal intestinal movements can appear similar to the faint fetal movements typical of early pregnancy. Fetal movements can be seen with ultrasonography.

Identification of the embryo or fetus by means of ultrasound photography of the gestational sac is possible as early as 4 to 5 weeks' gestation with 100% reliability. This noninvasive method is the earliest positive sign of a pregnancy.

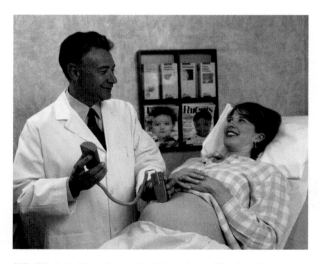

FIGURE **4-4** Listening to fetal heartbeat. The fetal heart rate is checked at each prenatal visit. A Doppler device can be used in early pregnancy. Hearing the infant's heartbeat is reassuring to the expectant mother and helps her accept the reality of her pregnancy.

NORMAL PHYSIOLOGICAL CHANGES IN PREGNANCY

The woman's body undergoes dramatic changes as she houses and nourishes her growing child. Most of these changes reverse shortly after birth.

REPRODUCTIVE SYSTEM
Uterus

The uterus undergoes the most obvious changes in pregnancy. Before pregnancy it is a small, muscular, pear-shaped pelvic organ that weighs about 60 g (2 ounces) and measures 7.5 cm (3 inches) × 5 cm (2 inches) × 2.5 cm (1 inch) and has a capacity of about 10 ml (one third of an ounce). The uterus expands gradually during pregnancy by increasing both the number of myometrial (muscle) cells during the first trimester and the size of individual cells during the second and third trimesters. The uterus becomes a temporary abdominal organ at the end of the first trimester. At term the uterus reaches the woman's xiphoid process and weighs about 1000 g (2.2 pounds). Its capacity is about 5000 ml (5 quarts), enough to house the term fetus, placenta, and amniotic fluid.

Cervix

Soon after conception the cervix changes in color and consistency. Chadwick's and Goodell's signs appear. The glands of the cervical mucosa increase in number and activity. Secretion of thick mucus forms a *mucous plug* that seals the cervical canal. The mucous plug prevents the ascent of vaginal organisms into the uterus. With the beginning of cervical thinning *(effacement)* and opening *(dilation)* near the onset of labor, the plug is loosened and expelled.

Ovaries

The ovaries do not produce ova (eggs) during pregnancy. The *corpus luteum* (empty graafian follicle; see p. 29) remains on the ovary and produces progesterone to maintain the *decidua* (uterine lining) during the first 6 to 7 weeks of the pregnancy until the placenta can perform this function.

Vagina

The vaginal blood supply increases, causing the bluish color of Chadwick's sign. The vaginal mucosa thickens and rugae (ridges) become prominent. The connective tissue softens to prepare for distention as the child is born. Secretions of the vagina increase. In addition, the vaginal pH becomes more acidic to protect the vagina and uterus from pathogenic microorganisms. However, the vaginal secretions also have higher levels of glycogen, a substance that promotes the growth of *Candida albicans,* the organism that causes yeast infections.

Breasts

Hormone-induced breast changes occur early in pregnancy. High levels of estrogen and progesterone prepare the breasts for lactation. The areolae of the breasts usually become deeply pigmented, and sebaceous glands in the nipple (tubercles of Montgomery) become prominent. The tubercles secrete a substance that lubricates the nipples.

In the last few months of pregnancy, thin yellow fluid called colostrum can be expressed from the breasts. This "premilk" is high in protein, fat-soluble vitamins, and minerals but is low in calories, fat, and sugar. Colostrum contains the mother's antibodies to diseases and is secreted for the first 2 to 3 days after birth in the breastfeeding woman.

RESPIRATORY SYSTEM

The pregnant woman breathes more deeply, but her respiratory rate increases only slightly, if at all. These changes increase oxygen and carbon dioxide exchange because she moves more air in and out with each breath. Oxygen consumption increases by 15% during pregnancy. The expanding uterus exerts upward pressure on her diaphragm, causing it to rise about 4 cm (2 inches). To compensate, her rib cage flares, increasing the circumference of the chest about 6 cm (2.5 inches). Dyspnea may occur until the fetus descends into the pelvis (lightening), relieving upward pressure on the diaphragm.

Increased estrogen levels during pregnancy cause edema or swelling of the mucous membranes of the nose, pharynx, mouth, and trachea. The woman may have nasal stuffiness, epistaxis (nosebleeds), and changes in her voice. A similar process occurs in the ears, causing a sense of fullness or earaches.

CARDIOVASCULAR SYSTEM

The growing uterus displaces the heart upward and to the left. The blood volume gradually increases *(hypervolemia)* about 45% over that of the prepregnant state by 32 to 34 weeks' gestation, at which time it levels off or declines slightly. This increase provides added blood for the following:

- Exchange of nutrients, oxygen, and waste products within the placenta
- Needs of expanded maternal tissue
- Reserve for blood loss at birth

Cardiac output increases because more blood is pumped from the heart with each contraction, the pulse rate increases by 10 to 15 beats/min, and the basal metabolic rate (BMR) may increase 20% during pregnancy.

Blood pressure does not increase with the higher blood volume because resistance to blood flow through the vessels decreases. A blood pressure of 140/90 mm Hg or a significant elevation above the woman's baseline requires attention. Supine hypotension syndrome, also called aortocaval compression or vena cava syndrome, may occur if the woman lies on her back (Figure 4-5). The supine position allows the heavy uterus to compress her inferior vena cava, reducing the amount of blood returned to her heart. Circulation to the placenta may also be reduced by increased pressure on the woman's aorta, resulting in fetal hypoxia. Symptoms of supine hypotension syndrome include faintness, lightheadedness, dizziness, and agitation. Displacing the uterus to one side by turning the patient is all that is needed to relieve the pressure. If the woman must remain flat for any reason, a small towel roll placed under one hip will also help to prevent supine hypotensive syndrome.

Orthostatic hypotension may occur whenever a woman rises from a recumbent position, resulting in faintness or lightheadedness. Cardiac output decreases because venous return from the lower body suddenly falls. *Palpitations* (sudden increase in heart rate) may occur from increases in thoracic pressure, particularly if the woman moves suddenly.

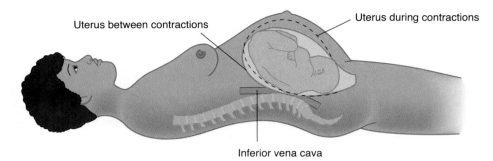

Uterus between contractions

Uterus during contractions

Inferior vena cava

FIGURE **4-5** Supine hypotension syndrome. When a pregnant woman lies on her back (supine), the weight of the uterus with its fetal contents presses on the vena cava and abdominal aorta. Placing a wedge pillow under the woman's right hip helps to relieve compression of these vessels.

| table 4-2 | *Normal Blood Values in Nonpregnant and Pregnant Women* |

VALUE	NONPREGNANT	PREGNANT
Hemoglobin (g/dl)	12-16	11-12
Hematocrit (%)	36-48	33-46
Red blood cells (million/mm^3)	3.8-5.1	4.5-6.5
White blood cells	5000-10,000/mm^3	5000-12,000/mm^3; rises during labor and postpartum up to 25,000/mm^3
Fibrinogen (mg/dl)	200-400	300-600

Although both plasma (fluid) and red blood cells (erythrocytes) increase during pregnancy, they do not increase by the same amount. The fluid part of the blood increases more than the erythrocyte component. This leads to a *dilutional anemia* or pseudoanemia (false anemia). As a result, the normal prepregnant hematocrit level of 36% to 48% may fall to 33% to 46%. Although this is not true anemia, the hematocrit count is reevaluated to determine patient status and needs. The white blood cell (leukocyte) count also increases about 8% (mostly neutrophils) and returns to prepregnant levels by the sixth day postpartum (Table 4-2).

There are increased levels of clotting factors VII, VIII, and X and plasma fibrinogen during the second and third trimesters of pregnancy. This hypercoagulability state helps prevent excessive bleeding after delivery when the placenta separates from the uterine wall. However, these changes increase the possibility of thrombophlebitis during pregnancy and are the reason the pregnant patient requires careful assessment for this risk and specific teaching to prevent the venous stasis that can lead to thrombophlebitis. The current increased interest in physical fitness has resulted in many pregnant women continuing to exercise during pregnancy. Consideration of the effects of exercise on the cardiovascular system that already has an increased blood volume, increased cardiac output, and increased coagulability during pregnancy must be reviewed before an exercise plan is carried out. Venous pressure may increase in the femoral veins as the size and weight of the uterus increase, resulting in varicose veins in the legs of some women.

GASTROINTESTINAL SYSTEM

The growing uterus displaces the stomach and intestines toward the back and sides of the abdomen (Figure 4-6). Increased salivary secretions *(ptyalism)* sometimes affect taste and smell. The mouth tissues may become tender and bleed more easily because of increased blood vessel development caused by high estrogen levels. Contrary to popular belief, teeth are not affected by pregnancy.

The demands of the growing fetus increase the woman's appetite and thirst. The acidity of gastric secretions is decreased; emptying of the stomach and motility (movement) of the intestines are slower. Women often feel bloated and may experience constipation and hemorrhoids. *Pyrosis* (heartburn) is caused by the relaxation of the cardiac sphincter of the stomach, which permits reflux (backward flow) of the acid secretions into the lower esophagus.

Glucose metabolism is altered because of increased insulin resistance during pregnancy. This allows more glucose utilization by the fetus but also places the

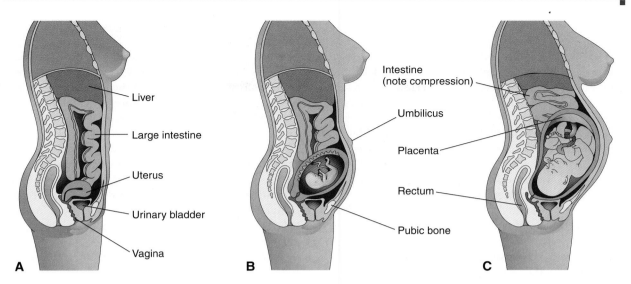

FIGURE **4-6** Compression of abdominal contents as uterus enlarges. The nonpregnant state (**A**) shows the relationship of the uterus to the abdominal contents. As the uterus enlarges at 20 weeks' gestation (**B**) and 30 weeks' gestation (**C**), the abdominal contents are displaced and compressed.

woman at risk for the development of gestational diabetes mellitus. Progesterone and estrogen relax the muscle tone of the gallbladder, resulting in the retention of bile salts, and this can lead to pruritus (itching of the skin) during pregnancy.

URINARY SYSTEM

The urinary system excretes waste products for both the mother and fetus during pregnancy. The glomerular filtration rate of the kidneys rises. The renal tubules increase the reabsorption of substances that the body needs to conserve but may not be able to keep up with the high load of some substances filtered by the glomeruli (e.g., glucose). Therefore glycosuria and proteinuria are more common during pregnancy. Water is retained because it is needed for increased blood volume and for dissolving nutrients that are provided for the fetus.

The relaxing effects of progesterone cause the renal pelvis and ureters to lose tone, resulting in decreased peristalsis to the bladder. The diameter of the ureters and bladder capacity increase because of the relaxing effects of progesterone, causing urine stasis. The combination of urine stasis and nutrient-rich urine makes the pregnant woman more susceptible to urinary tract infection. Consuming at least eight glasses of water each day reduces the risk for urinary tract infection. Although the bladder can hold up to 1500 ml of urine, the pressure of the enlarging uterus causes frequency of urination, especially in the first and third trimesters. Changes in the renal system may take 6 to 12 weeks after delivery to return to the prepregnant state.

Fluid and Electrolyte Balance

The increased glomerular filtration rate in the kidneys increases sodium filtration by 50%, but the increase in the tubular resorption rate results in 99% reabsorption of the sodium. Sodium retention is influenced by many factors, including elevated levels of the hormones of pregnancy. Although much of the sodium is used by the fetus, the remainder is in the maternal circulation and can cause a maternal accumulation of water (edema). This fluid retention may cause a problem if the woman in labor is given intravenous fluids containing oxytocin (Pitocin), which has an *antidiuretic* effect and can result in water intoxication. Agitation and delirium, possible signs of water intoxication, should be recorded and reported, and an accurate intake and output record should be kept during labor and the immediate postpartum phase.

In pregnancy, blood is slightly more alkaline than in the nonpregnant state and this mild alkalemia is enhanced by hyperventilation that often occurs during pregnancy. This status does not impact a normal pregnancy.

INTEGUMENTARY AND SKELETAL SYSTEMS

The high levels of hormones produced during pregnancy cause a variety of temporary changes in the integument (skin) of the pregnant woman. In addition to the pigmentary changes discussed under the presumptive signs of pregnancy, the sweat and sebaceous glands of the skin become more active to dissipate heat from the woman and fetus. Small red elevations of skin with lines radiating from the center, called *spider nevi*, may occur.

The palms of the hands may become deeper red. Most skin changes are reversed shortly after giving birth.

The woman's posture changes as her child grows within the uterus. The anterior part of her body becomes heavier with the expanding uterus, and the lordotic curve in her lumbar spine becomes more pronounced. The woman often experiences low backaches and, in the last few months of pregnancy, rounding of the shoulders may occur along with aching in the cervical spine and upper extremities.

The pelvic joints relax with hormonal changes during late pregnancy and entry of the fetal presenting part into the pelvic brim in the last trimester. A woman often has a "waddling" gait in the last few weeks of pregnancy because of a slight separation of the symphysis pubis.

A change in the center of gravity and joint instability because of the softening of the ligaments predisposes the pregnant woman to problems in balance. Interventions concerning safety should be part of prenatal education.

NUTRITION FOR PREGNANCY AND LACTATION

Good nutrition is essential to establish and maintain a healthy pregnancy and to give birth to a healthy child. Good nutritional habits begun before conception and continued during pregnancy promote adaptation to the maternal and fetal needs. The Food Guide Pyramid should be used as a guide for healthy daily food choices (Figure 4-7). Women who follow this guide before pregnancy will be well nourished at the time of conception. Nursing Care Plan 4-1 lists common nursing diagnoses and interventions for nutrition during pregnancy and lactation.

The woman should be educated to read food labels carefully to promote the intake of calories that are nutrient dense rather than empty. The U.S. Food and Drug Administration (FDA) along with the U.S. Department of Agriculture (USDA) has developed uniform food labels that inform consumers of the contents of packages and canned goods.

During pregnancy and lactation, an adequate dietary intake of docosahexaenoic acid–omega 3 fatty acid (DHA) is essential for the optimum brain development of the fetus and infant. The World Health Organization (WHO) recommends that a full-term infant receive 20 mg of DHA per kilogram per day. Maternal dietary sources of DHA include fish such as mackerel, Atlantic and sockeye salmon, halibut, tuna, flounder, egg yolk, red meat, poultry, canola oil, and soybean oil at two to three servings per week. Frying the above foods negatively alters DHA content (Brooks, Mitchell, & Steffanson, 2000).

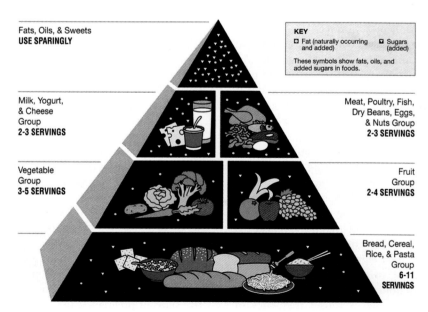

FIGURE **4-7** The Food Guide Pyramid is a daily guide to healthful eating for all people. Pregnant and lactating women can base their diet on the same pyramid.

NURSING CARE PLAN 4-1

Nutrition During Pregnancy and Lactation

PATIENT DATA: Mrs. S is seen in the clinic. She is 35 years old, in the first trimester of her first pregnancy, and appears interested in "starting a health diet" in order to have a healthy pregnancy outcome.

SELECTED NURSING DIAGNOSIS *Deficient knowledge related to importance of nutrition in pregnancy and lactation*

Outcomes	Nursing Interventions	Rationales
Patient will verbalize the need for good nutrition in pregnancy and lactation.	1. Determine age, parity, present weight, prepregnant nutritional status, food preferences and dislikes, food intolerances and general health of pregnant patient. 2. Determine socioeconomic and cultural factors that may influence food choices. Make recommendations to fit specific needs. Consult with a dietitian if the patient's nutritional needs are complex. 3. Review specific nutritional needs and food sources for optimum outcome of pregnancy and successful lactation. 4. Provide written information in the patient's primary language regarding nutrition and food preparation. Modify the information to incorporate cultural practices or food dislikes or intolerances. 5. Encourage questions and provide appropriate answers.	1. Many factors influence nutritional status of patient during pregnancy and lactation; nutrition teaching must be individualized to best meet her pregnancy nutritional needs. 2. Socioeconomic and cultural factors affect the patient's food choices. These factors must be considered to increase the chance that a patient will adhere to dietary recommendations. The assessment may identify the need for referral to programs such as the Women, Infants, and Children (WIC) nutrition program. 3. If patient understands specific nutritional needs of pregnancy and food sources, she is more likely to choose foods that meet these needs. 4. Written information reinforces verbal teaching and helps patient to recall forgotten information. Recommendations must fit within a patient's individualized needs to increase the chance that she will adhere to them. 5. Encouraging the patient's questions allows the nurse to identify and correct areas of inadequate knowledge or misunderstanding.
Patient will implement good nutrition during pregnancy and lactation, as evidenced by a 24-hour diary.	1. Teach the patient the purpose of and how to maintain a 24-hour food diary. Teach the patient to eat normally and to write down everything she eats and drinks, including approximate amounts, for 1 day. 2. Review the 24-hour intake from the diary and make appropriate recommendations for improvement. Refer to a dietitian if nutritional assessment reveals complex needs.	1. A 24-hour food diary helps the nurse to evaluate a patient's usual diet, likes, and dislikes, as well as how to improve her diet. It may identify the need for a dietitian referral. 2. Analysis of usual meals and snacks enables the nurse to identify adequate and inadequate intake of specific nutrients. The 24-hour diary allows the nurse to reinforce areas of adequate intake and concentrate on areas of deficient nutrients.

Continued

NURSING CARE PLAN 4-1—cont'd

Outcomes	Nursing Interventions	Rationales
	3. Teach the patient about the Food Guide Pyramid and how to read food labels.	3. Choices on the Food Guide Pyramid provide essential nutrients on a daily basis. Reading labels helps the patient to select more nutritious items from those available.
Patient will demonstrate a gradual weight gain appropriate for her during pregnancy (25-35 pounds for most women).	1. Maintain a chart to show the patient's actual weight at each visit.	1. Weight chart identifies both the amount and the pattern of weight gain to identify inadequate or excessive gain.
	2. Review progress of weight with patient at each visit and compare it with the recommended amount of gain for that point in pregnancy.	2. Reviewing the patient's weight identifies whether the patient's weight gain is normal and whether additional teaching or exploration of needs is required.

? CRITICAL THINKING QUESTIONS

Mrs. S. states she is anxious to complete this clinic appointment because she wants to "light up a cigarette." What is your major concern about her smoking? What interventions would be appropriate?

Mrs. S. states that her dietary pattern is heavily influenced by her perceived "food cravings," which have occurred increasingly in the past month. What would be your approach to this problem?

★ NURSING TIP

There is a high correlation between maternal diet and fetal health. To ensure that deficiencies do not occur during the critical first weeks of pregnancy, the nurse explains to women of childbearing age the value of eating well-balanced meals so they may start pregnancy in a good nutritional state.

WEIGHT GAIN

In the past a woman's weight gain was restricted during pregnancy. Rickets caused by a deficiency of vitamin D resulted in deformity of women's pelves many years ago. It was thought that minimal weight gain would keep the fetus small and therefore easier to deliver. More recently, low weight gain was thought to reduce the risk for pregnancy-induced hypertension, a theory that has been disproved (Creasy & Resnick, 1999).

Low maternal weight gain is associated with complications such as preterm labor, and recommendations for weight gain during pregnancy have gradually increased. Current recommended weight gains during pregnancy are as follows:

- Women of normal weight: 25 to 35 pounds (11.5 to 16 kg)
- Underweight women: 28 to 40 pounds (12.5 to 18 kg)
- Overweight women: 15 to 25 pounds (7 to 11.5 kg)

Women with multiple fetuses should gain more weight. The adolescent should gain in the upper part of the range currently recommended for adult women.

The pattern of weight gain is also important. The general recommendation is that a woman gain 3.5 pounds (1.6 kg) during the first trimester and just under 1 pound per week (0.44 kg) during the rest of pregnancy. Nausea and vomiting and some transient food dislikes often limit weight gain or cause weight loss during the first trimester, but the weight is usually regained when the gastrointestinal upsets subside.

Women often want to know why they should gain so much weight when their infant weighs only 7 or 8 pounds. The nurse can use the distribution of weight gain during pregnancy shown in Table 4-3 to teach women about all the factors that contribute to weight gain.

NUTRITIONAL REQUIREMENTS

A calorie increase of 300 Calories/day is recommended to provide for the growth of the fetus, placenta, amniotic fluid, and maternal tissues. Three hundred Calories is not a large increase. A banana, a carrot, a piece of whole wheat bread, and a glass of low-fat milk total about 300 Calories. Caloric intake must be nutritious to have beneficial effects on pregnancy. Four nutrients are especially important in pregnancy: protein, calcium, iron, and folic acid. The amounts are specified in Table 4-4.

table **4-3** *Distribution of Weight Gain in Pregnancy*

SOURCE OF WEIGHT GAIN	WEIGHT GAIN IN POUNDS (kg)
Uterus	2.5 (1.1)
Fetus	7.0-7.5 (3.2-3.4)
Placenta	1.0-1.5 (0.5-0.7)
Amniotic fluid	2.0 (0.9)
Breasts	1.5-3.0 (0.7-1.4)
Blood volume	3.5-4.0 (1.6-1.8)
Extravascular fluids	3.5-5.0 (1.6-2.3)
Maternal reserves	4.0-9.5 (1.8-4.3)
TOTAL	25.0-35.0 (11.4-15.9)

Modified from McKinney, E. S., et al. (2000). *Maternal-child nursing.* Philadelphia: W.B. Saunders.

The pregnant woman should use the same Food Guide Pyramid to choose her daily diet. Servings that will supply enough of the additional nutrients needed are presented in Table 4-5. A sample menu for a pregnant woman is shown in Box 4-4.

Protein

Added protein is needed for metabolism and to support the growth and repair of maternal and fetal tissues. An intake of 60 g/day is recommended during pregnancy. The best sources of protein are meat, fish, poultry, and dairy products. Beans, lentils, and other legumes; breads and cereals; and seeds and nuts in combination with another plant or animal protein can provide all the amino acids (components of protein) needed.

Examples of complementary plant protein combinations are corn and beans, lentils and rice, and peanut butter and bread. Plant proteins are also complemented with animal proteins, such as in grilled cheese sandwiches, cereal with milk, and chili made of meat and beans. The complementary foods must be eaten together because all the amino acids necessary for building tissues (essential amino acids) must be present at the same time.

Information about nonmeat sources of protein should be given to women who are vegetarians to ensure that their protein needs are met. The information can also help reduce the family's food budget because many plant protein sources are less expensive than animal sources.

Calcium

Pregnancy and lactation increase calcium requirements by nearly 50%. The recommended daily allowance (RDA) of calcium for pregnant women is 1200 mg. Dairy products are the single most plentiful source of this nutrient. Other sources of calcium include enriched cereals, legumes, nuts, dried fruits, broccoli, green leafy vegetables, and canned salmon and sardines that contain bones. Calcium supplements are necessary for women who do not drink milk (or eat sufficient amounts of equivalent products). Supplements are also necessary for women under 25 years of age because their bone density is not complete. Calcium supplements should be taken separately from iron supplements for best absorption. Nondairy alternatives for women with lactose intolerance are given on p. 65.

Iron

Pregnancy causes a heavy demand for iron because the fetus must store an adequate supply to meet the needs in the first 3 to 6 months after birth. In addition, the pregnant woman increases her production of erythrocytes. The RDA is 15 mg/day for nonpregnant adult women and 30 mg/day for pregnant women. Women who have a known iron deficiency may need more.

It is difficult to obtain this much iron from the diet alone, and most health care providers prescribe iron supplements of 30 mg/day beginning in the second trimester, after morning sickness decreases. Taking the iron on an empty stomach improves absorption, but many women find it difficult to tolerate without food. It should not be taken with coffee or tea or with high-calcium foods such as milk. Vitamin C (ascorbic acid) may enhance iron absorption (Mahan & Escott-Stump, 2000).

Iron comes in two forms, *heme* (found in red and organ meats) and *nonheme* (found in plant products). Heme iron is best absorbed by the body. Nonheme plant foods that are high in iron include molasses, whole grains, iron-fortified cereals and breads, dark green leafy vegetables, and dried fruits.

Folic Acid

Folic acid (folacin or folate) is a water-soluble B vitamin essential for the formation and maturation of both red and white blood cells in bone marrow. This vitamin can also reduce the incidence of neural tube defects such as spina bifida and anencephaly. The RDA for a pregnant woman is 400 μg (0.4 mg) per day. Food sources of folic acid are liver; lean beef; kidney and lima beans; dried beans; fresh, dark green leafy vegetables; potatoes; whole-wheat bread; and peanuts.

Because adequate intake of folic acid *at conception* has a large impact on reducing the incidence of neural tube defects, the Centers for Disease Control and Prevention recommend that all fertile American women consume 400 μg (0.4 mg) of folic acid daily. A higher level of 4 mg/day is recommended for women who have previously had an infant with a neural tube defect and plan to become pregnant again (*Morbidity and Mortality Weekly Report,* 2001).

table 4-4 Recommended Dietary Allowances and Intakes

1997-1998 DIETARY REFERENCE INTAKES (DRI)

AGE (yr)	THIAMIN (mg)	RIBOFLAVIN (mg)	NIACIN (mg NE)	VITAMIN B6 (mg)	FOLATE (µg DFE)	VITAMIN B12 (µg)	PHOSPHORUS (mg)	MAGNESIUM (mg)	VITAMIN D (µg)	PANTOTHENIC ACID (mg)	BIOTIN (µg)	CHOLINE (mg)	CALCIUM (mg)	FLUORIDE (mg)
	RECOMMENDED DIETARY ALLOWANCES (RDA)								ADEQUATE INTAKES (AI)					
MALES														
19-30	1.2	1.3	16	1.3	400	2.4	700	400	5	5.0	30	550	1000	3.8
31-50	1.2	1.3	16	1.3	400	2.4	700	420	5	5.0	30	550	1000	3.8
51-70	1.2	1.3	16	1.7	400	2.4	700	420	10	5.0	30	550	1200	3.8
>70	1.2	1.3	16	1.7	400	2.4	700	420	15	5.0	30	550	1200	3.8
FEMALES														
19-30	1.1	1.1	14	1.3	400	2.4	700	310	5	5.0	30	425	1000	3.1
31-50	1.1	1.1	14	1.3	400	2.4	700	320	5	5.0	30	425	1000	3.1
51-70	1.1	1.1	14	1.5	400	2.4	700	320	10	5.0	30	425	1200	3.1
>70	1.1	1.1	14	1.5	400	2.4	700	320	15	5.0	30	425	1200	3.1
Pregnancy	1.4	1.4	18	1.9	600	2.6	*	+40	*	6.0	30	450	*	*
Lactation	1.5	1.6	17	2.0	500	2.8	*	*	*	7.0	35	550	*	*

1989 RECOMMENDED DIETARY ALLOWANCE (RDA)

AGE (yr)	ENERGY (kcal)	PROTEIN (g)	VITAMIN A (µg RE)	VITAMIN E (mg a-TE)	VITAMIN K (µg)	VITAMIN C (mg)	IRON (mg)	ZINC (mg)	IODINE (µg)	SELENIUM (µg)
MALES										
19-24	2900	58	1000	10	70	60	10	15	150	70
25-50	2900	63	1000	10	80	60	10	15	150	70
51+	2300	63	1000	10	80	60	10	15	150	70
FEMALES										
19-24	2200	46	800	8	60	60	15	12	150	55
25-50	2200	50	800	8	65	60	15	12	150	55
51+	1900	50	800	8	65	60	10	12	150	55
Pregnancy	+300	60	800	10	65	70	30	15	175	65
Lactation										
First 6 months	+500	65	1300	12	65	95	15	19	200	75
Second 6 months	+500	62	1200	11	65	90	15	16	200	75

Modified with permission from *Dietary Recommended Allowances*, 10th Edition, and the first two of the *Dietary Reference Intakes* series, National Academy Press. Copyright 1998 by the National Academy of Sciences. Courtesy of the National Academy Press, Washington, DC.

*Values for these nutrients do not change with pregnancy or lactation. Use the value listed for women of comparable age.

table 4-5 | *Daily Food Pattern for Pregnancy*

FOOD	AMOUNT
Milk, nonfat or low-fat, yogurt, cheese	3-4 cups
Meat (lean), poultry, fish, egg	2 servings (total of 4-6 oz)
Vegetables, cooked or raw: dark green/deep yellow; starchy, including potatoes, dried peas, and beans; all others	3-5 servings, all types, often
Fruits, fresh or canned, dark orange, including apricots, peaches, cantaloupe	2-4 servings, all types, often
Whole grain and enriched breads and cereals	7 or more servings
Fats and sweets	In moderate amounts
Fluids	8-10 glasses (8 oz)

Modified from Mahan, L.K., & Escott-Stump, S. (2000). *Krause's food, nutrition, and diet therapy* (10th ed.). Philadelphia: W.B. Saunders.

Fluids

The woman should drink eight to ten 8-ounce glasses of fluids each day. Water should compose most of this intake. Caffeinated drinks and drinks high in sugar should be limited. Caffeine acts as a diuretic, which counteracts some of the benefit of the fluid intake. The woman should limit her daily caffeine consumption to two cups of coffee or its equivalent.

RECOMMENDED DIETARY ALLOWANCES AND RECOMMENDED DIETARY INTAKES

In the United States the Food and Nutrition Board of the Institute of Medicine, National Academy of Science in cooperation with the USDA and the Department of Health and Human Services, have developed Recommended Dietary Allowances (RDAs) of nutrient intake required to maintain optimal health. The RDAs were most recently revised in 1989, and the nutrients were primarily supplied by foods. In 1994 research by the Food and Nutrition Board found an increasing use of dietary supplements and fortified foods, resulting in the need to describe upper limits of intake levels in order to prevent toxicity. There is no need to provide nutrients in excess of the RDA. The combination of supplements and food fortification must not exceed present upper limits of safety or adverse responses (toxicity) can occur (Table 4-6). When scientific evidence is insufficient to

box 4-4 | *Sample Menu for a Pregnant Woman*

BREAKFAST
Orange juice (½ cup)
Oatmeal (½ cup)
Whole grain or enriched toast (1 slice)
Peanut butter (2 tsp)
Decaffeinated coffee or tea

MIDMORNING SNACK
Apple
High bran cereal (¼ cup)
Nonfat or reduced fat milk (½ cup)

LUNCH
Turkey (2 oz) sandwich on rye or whole-grain bread with lettuce and tomato and 1 tsp mayonnaise
Green salad
Salad dressing (2 tsp)
Fresh peach
Nonfat or low-fat milk (1 cup)

MIDAFTERNOON SNACK
Nonfat or low-fat milk (1 cup)
Graham crackers (4 squares)

DINNER
Baked chicken breast (3 oz)
Baked potato with 2 tbsp sour cream
Peas and carrots (½ cup)
Green salad
Salad dressing (2 tsp)

EVENING SNACK
Nonfat frozen yogurt (1 cup)
Fresh strawberries

This menu assumes that the woman is of normal prepregnancy weight, that her weight gain is appropriate, that her activity is moderate, and that she is carrying only one fetus. Changes would be needed for the underweight or overweight woman, the adolescent, or a woman with a multifetal pregnancy.

Modified from Mahan, L.K., & Escott-Stump, S. (2000). *Krause's food, nutrition, and diet therapy* (10th ed.). Philadelphia: W.B. Saunders.

determine RDA, an adequate intake is probably provided by an adequate diet. Consuming dietary supplements of trace elements can result in toxicity if upper limits of intake are consistently exceeded.

In January 2001 the Committee of the USDA Human Nutrition and Research Center published Recommended Dietary Intakes (RDIs) focusing on specific nutrients. Research is ongoing. Future nutrient recommendations will be expressed as Dietary Reference

table 4-6 | *Preset Upper Limit for Daily Adult Intake of Specific Nutrients*

	RDA	RDI UPPER LIMIT	TOXICITY IF UPPER LIMITS ARE EXCEEDED
Vitamin A	700-1000 µg	3000	Liver damage, birth defects
Iron	15-20 mg	45 mg	Constipation, nausea
Copper	900 µg (3 mg)	10,000 µg (10 mg)	Liver damage
Iodine	150 µg	1100 µg	Hypothyroidism
Manganese	5 mg	11 mg	Neurological damage
Zinc	12-15 mg	40 mg	Copper deficiency by blocking copper absorption
Boron	Trace	20 mg	Reproductive
Nickel	Trace	1 mg	Developmental deficiencies
Vanadium	Trace	1.8 mg	Renal problems
Selenium	65 µg during pregnancy	Not applicable	Deficiency can cause heart pathology in children (usually occurs where soil content is low, such as China)
Molybdenum	45 µg	2 mg	Reproductive and growth problems

Modified from Russell, R. (2001). *Dietary reference intakes.* USDA Human Nutrition Research Center on Aging, Tufts University, Boston Conference, Jan 9, 2001, Washington, DC: National Academy of Science.

Intakes (DRIs). DRI is an umbrella term that includes the RDA and tolerable upper levels of intake. Any RDA for a nutrient not revised to the new DRI will be retained and both RDAs and RDIs will be used until research is completed. Table 4-4 shows current RDA and RDI of nutrients for various age-groups, including pregnancy and lactation.

SPECIAL NUTRITIONAL CONSIDERATIONS
Pregnant Adolescent

Gynecological age is the number of years between the onset of menses and the date of conception. The adolescent who conceives soon after having her first period has greater nutritional needs than one who is more sexually mature. The nurse must consider the adolescent's characteristics of resistance, ambivalence, and inconsistency when planning nutritional interventions. The nurse must also remember that the girl's peer group is of utmost importance to her and help her find nutritious foods that allow her to fit in with her friends.

Inadequate pregnancy weight gain and nutrient deficits are more likely in the pregnant adolescent. The girl's continuing growth plus the growth of the fetus may make it difficult for her to meet her nutritional needs. In addition, a body image in which she sees herself as "fat" at a time when appearance is a high priority, combined with peer pressure to eat "junk" foods, places the pregnant adolescent at special risk.

Even a moderate positive change in diet helps and the nurse should give the girl positive reinforcement for her efforts (Matteson, 2001). Fast foods with poor nutritional content are often the adolescent's foods of choice. However, the nurse can tell the adolescent that many fast food restaurants offer salads, chicken, tacos, baked potatoes, and pizza. These foods provide many important nutrients and allow her to socialize with her peers at mealtime.

Nutritional intervention is necessary early in prenatal care to ensure a healthy mother and child. Many communities offer programs for adolescents that provide social support, education about prenatal care, and nutritional advice. Adolescents often respond well in peer groups. The nurse often refers these young women to programs such as Women, Infants, and Children (WIC) and food stamp programs if needed.

Sodium Intake

The sodium intake of pregnant women was restricted in the past in an attempt to prevent edema and pregnancy-induced hypertension. It is now known that sodium should not be restricted during pregnancy. Sodium intake is essential for maintaining normal sodium levels in plasma, bone, brain, and muscle because both tissue and fluid expand during the prenatal period. However, foods high in sodium should be taken in moderation during pregnancy.

Diuretics to rid the body of excess fluids are not recommended for the healthy pregnant woman because they reduce fluids necessary for the fetus. The added fluid during pregnancy supports the mother's increased blood volume.

Pica

The craving for and ingestion of nonfood substances such as clay, starch, raw flour, and cracked ice is called *pica.* Ingestion of small amounts of these substances may be harmless, but frequent ingestion in large amounts may cause significant health problems. Starch can interfere with iron absorption, and large amounts of clay may cause fecal impaction. Any other nonfood substance ingested in large quantities may be harmful because the necessary nutrients for healthy fetal development will not be available.

Pica is a difficult habit to break, and the nurse often becomes aware of the practice when discussing nutrition, food cravings, and myths with the pregnant woman. The nurse should educate the pregnant woman in a nonjudgmental way about the importance of good nutrition so the pica habit can be eliminated or at least decreased.

Lactose Intolerance

Intolerance to lactose is caused by a deficiency of lactase, the enzyme that digests the sugar in milk. Some women cannot digest milk or milk products, which increases their risk for calcium deficiency. Native Americans, Latinos, and persons of African, Middle Eastern, and Asian descent have a higher incidence of lactose intolerance than Caucasians. Signs and symptoms of lactose intolerance include abdominal distention, flatulence, nausea, vomiting, and loose stools after ingestion of dairy products. In such cases a daily calcium supplement can be taken.

Substitutes for dairy products are listed in the section on calcium. Lactose-intolerant women may tolerate cultured or fermented milk products such as aged cheese, buttermilk, and yogurt. The enzyme lactase (LactAid) is available in tablet form or as a liquid to add to milk. Lactase-treated milk is also available commercially and can be used under a physician's direction.

Gestational Diabetes

Gestational diabetes is first diagnosed during pregnancy rather than being present before pregnancy (see pp. 100 to 106). Calories should be evenly distributed during the day among three meals and three snacks to maintain adequate and stable blood glucose levels. Pregnant diabetic women are susceptible to hypoglycemia (low blood glucose) during the night because the fetus continues to use glucose while the mother sleeps. It is suggested that the final bedtime snack be one of protein and a complex carbohydrate to provide more blood glucose stability. Dietary management may be supervised by a registered dietitian. Glycemic control during the first and second trimesters is most important in preventing complications such as macrosomia (abnormally large newborn).

NUTRITION DURING LACTATION

The caloric intake during lactation should be about 500 Calories more than the nonpregnant woman's RDA. A guide to adequate caloric intake is a stable maternal weight and a gradually increasing infant weight.

The maternal protein intake should be 65 mg/day so the growing infant has adequate protein. Calcium and iron intake is the same as that during pregnancy to allow for the infant's demand on the mother's supply. Vitamin supplements are often continued during lactation.

Fluids sufficient to relieve thirst should be taken. Drinking eight to ten glasses of liquids other than those containing caffeine is adequate intake.

Some foods should be omitted during lactation if they cause gastric upset in the mother or child. The mother will often identify foods that seem to upset her child. Caffeine should be restricted to the equivalent of two cups of coffee each day. Lactating mothers should be instructed that many types of drugs she may take can be secreted in varying amounts in the breast milk. Drugs should be taken only with the health care provider's advice. Alcohol intake should be restricted to an occasional single serving for breastfeeding women.

EXERCISE DURING PREGNANCY

There is evidence that mild to moderate exercise is beneficial during normal pregnancy, but vigorous exercise should be avoided. The nurse should guide the patient concerning exercise during pregnancy based on the understanding that the maternal circulatory system is the lifeline to the fetus and any alteration can affect the growth and survival of the fetus. The maternal cardiac status and fetoplacental reserve should be the basis for determining exercise levels during all trimesters of pregnancy. Current health and fitness lifestyles mandate the inclusion of information concerning exercise during pregnancy in prenatal education programs (Clapp, 2001).

A history of the exercise practices of the patient is important, and gathering such data is the first step in the nursing process. Women who have had prior training may have a higher tolerance for exercise than women who have led a sedentary lifestyle. The goal of exercise during pregnancy should be *maintenance* of fitness, not improvement of fitness or weight loss (Figure 4-8). The following are some basic factors that should be evaluated and discussed.

ELEVATED TEMPERATURE

Exercise can elevate the maternal temperature and result in decreased fetal circulation and cardiac function. Maternal body temperature should not exceed 38° C

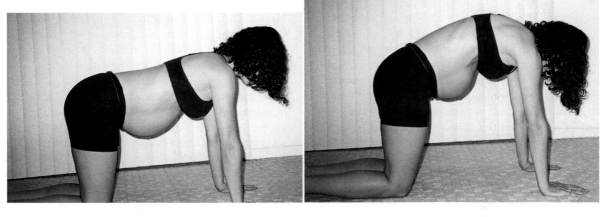

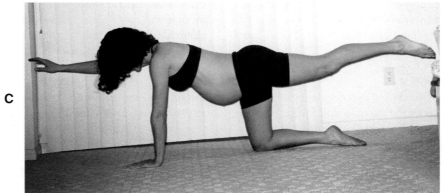

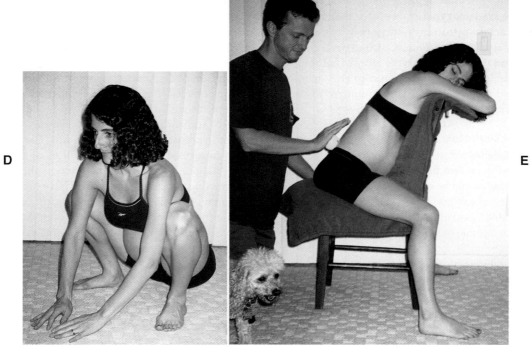

FIGURE **4-8** Exercises during pregnancy. **A** and **B,** The pelvic tilt. **C,** Proper stretch position. **D,** Proper squat position. **E,** Back massage with a tennis ball used as pressure.

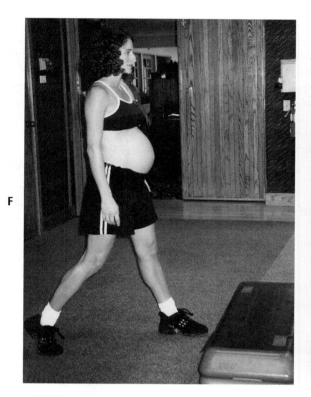

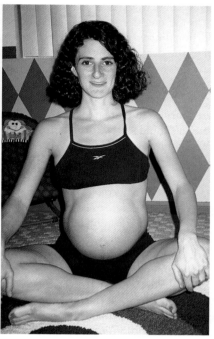

F

G

FIGURE **4-8, cont'd**   **F,** A pregnant woman participating in step aerobics class for moderate exercise. **G,** Tailor sitting position.

(100° F), which rules out the use of hot tubs and saunas during pregnancy. Exercise-related increases in body temperature are somewhat more easily tolerated because of the normal physiology of pregnancy related to increased peripheral blood flow, thermal inertia from weight gain, and peripheral venous pooling. Monitoring the body temperature in addition to the exercise intensity is essential.

HYPOTENSION

When the flat supine position is assumed and the uterus presses on the vena cava, the increasing size and weight of the uterus can cause poor venous return and result in supine hypotensive syndrome. Orthostatic hypotension can also reduce blood flow to the fetus. Certain exercise positions may need to be modified during pregnancy to avoid these problems, which can cause fetal hypoxia.

CARDIAC OUTPUT

Pregnancy increases the workload of the heart. The increase in peripheral pooling during pregnancy results in a decrease in cardiac output reserves for exercise. When exercise is allowed to exceed the ability of the cardiovascular system to respond, blood may be diverted from the uterus, causing fetal hypoxia. Exercise increases catecholamine levels, which the placenta may not be able to filter, resulting in fetal bradycardia and hypoxia. Strenu-

ous and prolonged exercise causes blood flow to be distributed to the skeletal muscles and skin and away from the viscera, uterus, and placenta. If the reduction in uterine blood flow exceeds 50%, serious adverse effects to the fetus may occur. For this reason, moderate exercise is preferred for pregnant women over strenuous or prolonged exercise. Exercise increases maternal hematocrit levels and uterine oxygen uptake, so moderate exercise will not cause decreased oxygen supplies to the fetus.

HORMONES

Exercise can cause changes in oxygen consumption and epinephrine, glucagon, cortisol, prolactin, and endorphin levels. In early pregnancy these hormonal changes can negatively affect implantation of the zygote and vascularization of the uterus. In late pregnancy the increases in catecholamines during exercise can trigger labor. Preterm labor must be avoided. Joint instability caused by hormonal changes can result in injury if the woman engages in deep flexion or extension of joints. Range of motion (ROM) should not be extended beyond prepregnancy abilities.

OTHER FACTORS

In general, moderate exercise several times a week from the eighth week through delivery is advised during pregnancy, with vigorous activity and competitive sports avoided. Vigorous exercise in hot humid weather should be avoided by even the trained woman. Safety measures should be used because of the changes in the body's center of gravity as the uterus enlarges. Liquid and calorie intake should be adjusted to meet the needs of pregnancy as well as the demands of exercise. Mothers who have complications or medical conditions such as diabetes mellitus should consult a health care provider before engaging in any exercise program during pregnancy.

Nursing guidance should include the following:

- The woman should start with a warm-up and end with a cool-down period.
- Women who are beginning an exercise program should not exceed the American College of Obstetricians and Gynecologists (ACOG) recommendations for moderate exercise. Women who have exercised regularly at higher levels before pregnancy may follow more liberal guidelines of weight-bearing exercise for no more than 1 hour three to five times a week.
- Exercise combined with a balanced diet rich in unprocessed, nonroot vegetables, nuts, fruits, and whole-grain breads is beneficial during pregnancy. Eating 2 to 3 hours before exercise and immediately after exercise is recommended.
- The woman should avoid scuba diving below a depth of 30 feet or exercising in altitudes above 8000 feet during pregnancy.
- The woman should avoid getting overheated and should drink plenty of water during exercise.

COMMON DISCOMFORTS IN PREGNANCY

Various discomforts occur during normal pregnancy as a result of physiological changes. The nurse should teach the woman measures to relieve these discomforts. The nurse should also explain signs of problems that can be confused with the normal discomforts of pregnancy. Providing information written in the woman's primary language gives her a reference if she has questions later.

Nausea is a problem chiefly in the first trimester. Persistent nausea with vomiting that significantly interferes with food and fluid intake is not normal and should be reported. Relief measures include the following:

- Eat dry toast or crackers before getting out of bed in the morning.
- Drink fluids between meals instead of with meals.
- Eat small, frequent meals.
- Avoid fried, greasy, or spicy foods and foods with strong odors, such as cabbage and onions.

Vaginal discharge is more noticeable because of the increased blood supply to the pelvic area. A discharge that is yellow, has a foul odor, or is accompanied by itching and inflammation suggests vaginal infection and should be reported. Measures to manage the discharge and reduce the risk for infection include the following:

- Bathe or shower daily.
- Wear loose-fitting cotton panties.
- Do not douche unless specifically ordered by the health care provider.
- Wipe the perineal area from front to back after toileting.

Fatigue may be difficult in the early months of the pregnancy if the mother is working or has other small children. Measures to cope with fatigue include the following:

- Try to get at least 8 to 10 hours of sleep at night.
- Take a nap during the day if possible.
- Use measures such as relaxation techniques, meditation, or a change of scenery.

The extreme exhaustion usually diminishes in the second trimester, and often women then feel exhilarated and full of energy. The tired feeling may return again during the last 4 to 6 weeks of the pregnancy. Again, daytime naps and as much restful nighttime sleep as possible help to provide the energy needed for labor.

Backache occurs because of the spine's adaptation to the back's changing contour as the uterus grows. Relief measures include the following:

- Maintain correct posture with the head up and the shoulders back. Avoid exaggerating the lumbar curve. Wearing low-heeled shoes helps the woman maintain better posture.
- Squat rather than bend over when picking up objects.
- When sitting, support the arms, feet, and back with pillows as needed.
- Exercises include tailor sitting, shoulder circling, and pelvic rocking (see Figure 4-8).

Constipation occurs because of slowed peristalsis, the use of iron supplements, and pressure of the growing uterus on the large intestine. Relief measures include the following:

- Drink at least eight glasses of water each day, not counting coffee, tea, or carbonated drinks.
- Add dietary fiber in foods, such as unpeeled fresh fruits and vegetables, whole-grain cereals, bran muffins, oatmeal, potatoes with skins, and fruit juices.
- Limit cheese consumption if this tends to be constipating.
- Limit sweet foods if they cause flatulence.

- Consult the health care provider if iron supplements cause constipation. Do not stop taking the iron, because a change in the supplement may help.
- Get plenty of exercise. A brisk 1-mile walk is good to stimulate peristalsis.
- Establish a regular time each day for having a bowel movement. Defecate as soon as the urge occurs rather than delaying.
- Take laxatives or enemas *only* under the direction of the health care provider.

Varicose veins are common in the pregnant woman because the large uterus slows venous return, causing the blood to pool especially in her leg veins. This pooling may eventually break down the competence of the valves within the veins, resulting in varicosities. Varicose veins are seen most often on the back of the calves and behind the knees. Excessive weight gain and genetic predisposition affect the occurrence of varicosities and their persistence after the pregnancy. Varicosities may occur on the vulva, especially after the twentieth week of pregnancy. They are usually temporary and subside after the delivery. Measures to relieve the discomfort of varicosities include the following:

- Avoid wearing constricting clothing or crossing the legs at the knees.
- Elevate the legs above hip level when resting.
- Wear support hose or elastic stockings, which increase venous blood flow. For best results, apply them before getting out of bed each morning.
- Avoid standing in one position for prolonged periods. Walk around for a few minutes every 2 hours.

Hemorrhoids are varicosities of the rectum and anus that become more severe with constipation and with descent of the infant's head into the pelvis. They generally decrease or disappear after birth, when pressure is relieved. Relief measures include the following:

- Anesthetic ointments, witch hazel pads, or rectal suppositories
- Sitz baths
- Measures to avoid constipation as previously discussed

Heartburn causes discomfort mainly in late pregnancy, when the uterus presses against the esophagus where it enters the stomach. This pressure may cause a reflux of gastric acids into the esophagus, resulting in a burning feeling in the chest and a bitter taste in the mouth. Suggestions to reduce heartburn include the following:

- Eat small, frequent meals and avoid fatty foods.
- Reduce smoking and caffeine intake.

- Sit upright and sleep with an extra pillow under the head.
- Use deep breathing and take sips of water, both of which may relieve the burning.
- Use antacids if recommended by the health care provider. Those high in sodium (Alka-Seltzer, baking soda) should be avoided.

Nasal stuffiness may occur. Edema of the nasal mucosa is caused by high estrogen levels. Relief can be obtained by saline nasal drops or use of a humidifier.

Dyspnea is often encountered in late pregnancy as the uterus exerts pressure on the diaphragm. Even with mild exercise, many women are unable to breathe deeply. Most women notice improvement in dyspnea with "lightening" (about 2 weeks before birth with the first child). Suggestions for relief include the following:

- Rest with the upper torso propped up.
- Avoid exertion.

Leg cramps may occur in the first 6 weeks of pregnancy but are more often experienced during the third trimester. The superficial calf muscles of the legs involuntarily contract, causing severe pain. Increased uterine weight, increased circulatory load, inadequate rest, and imbalance of the calcium-to-phosphorus ratio are implicated as causes. Intake of phosphorus may exceed the calcium intake, resulting in a calcium-to-phosphorus imbalance. Measures to relieve leg cramps include the following:

- Extend the affected leg, keep the knee straight, and flex the foot. Stand and apply pressure on the affected leg to stretch the muscles in spasm.
- Elevate the legs periodically during the day to improve circulation.
- Consult the health care provider about reducing milk intake or using aluminum hydroxide capsules to restore an ideal calcium-to-phosphorus ratio.

Edema of the lower extremities is common, especially after the twentieth week of pregnancy. It is caused by the increased circulatory load and slower venous return of blood from the legs. Edema in the face and hands may be a sign of pregnancy-induced hypertension and should be reported to the health care provider. Temporary relief measures for lower extremity edema include the following:

- Rest
- Elevation of legs above the heart
- Avoidance of tight restrictive bands around the legs such as garters, knee-highs, or thigh-high stockings

Water aerobics in healthy women can relieve edema because the hydrostatic pressure forces fluid into the circulation, stimulating glomerular filtration and excretion of water. Care should be taken to avoid excessive water temperatures during water aerobics (Kent et al, 1999) (see Exercise During Pregnancy, pp. 65 to 68).

PSYCHOLOGICAL ADAPTATIONS TO PREGNANCY

Pregnancy creates a variety of confusing feelings for all members of the family, whether or not the pregnancy was planned. Both parents may feel ambivalence about the pregnancy and being a parent. First-time parents may be anxious about how the infant will affect their relationship as a couple. Parents who already have a child may wonder how they can stretch their energies, love, and finances to another infant and how the infant will affect their older child or children. The nurse who provides prenatal care helps families to work through this phase in their lives.

Identifying and managing psychosocial problems is essential to the positive outcome of pregnancy. Identifying barriers to accessing care is a primary nursing responsibility. Inadequate health insurance coverage, financial problems, knowledge deficit concerning community resources, lack of transportation, or need for day care for other children or elderly parents are examples of problems that can be referred to a social service worker. Frequent housing relocation may indicate domestic violence, legal problems, or financial difficulties that may need attention to assure compliance with regular prenatal care. Nutritional needs and patterns relating to age, ethnicity, or financial constraints should be discussed. Tobacco or substance abuse should be assessed. Stress in the life of the mother should be reviewed and appropriate referrals to mental health professionals or educational programs should be made to reduce the levels of stress that can affect pregnancy outcome.

IMPACT ON THE MOTHER

In 1984 researcher Reva Rubin noted four maternal tasks that the woman accomplishes during pregnancy as she becomes a mother:

- Seeking safe passage for herself and her fetus. This involves both obtaining health care by a professional and adhering to important cultural practices.
- Securing acceptance of herself as a mother and for her fetus. Will her partner accept the infant?
- Does her partner or family have strong preferences for a child of a particular sex? Will the child be accepted even if he or she does not fit the ideal?

- Learning to give of self and to receive the care and concern of others. The woman will never again be the same carefree girl she was before her infant's arrival. She depends on others in ways she has not experienced before.
- Committing herself to the child as she progresses through pregnancy. Much of the emotional work of pregnancy involves protecting and nurturing the fetus.

Pregnancy is more than a physical event in a woman's life. During the months of pregnancy, she first accepts the fetus as part of her self and gradually moves to acceptance of the child as an independent person. She moves from being a pregnant woman to being a mother. The woman's responses change as pregnancy progresses. These changes will be discussed here within the framework of the three trimesters of pregnancy.

First Trimester

The woman may have difficulty believing that she is pregnant during early pregnancy because she may not feel much different. If a home pregnancy test was positive, the woman often feels "more pregnant" after a professional confirms it, even though her pregnancy is only a few minutes older than it was before that confirmation. An early sonography examination helps the woman to see the reality of the developing fetus within her. Women (and their partners) often show off their sonogram photos to anyone who will look, just as they will show their baby pictures later.

Most women have conflicting feelings about being pregnant (*ambivalence*) during the early weeks. Many, if not most, pregnancies are unplanned. The parents may have wanted to wait longer so they could achieve career or educational goals or to have longer spacing between children. Women who have planned their pregnancies, or even worked hard to overcome infertility, also feel ambivalence. They wonder if they have done the right thing and at the right time. Moreover, the woman often feels that she should not have these conflicting feelings. The nurse can help the woman to express these feelings of ambivalence and reassure her that they are normal.

The woman focuses on herself during this time. She feels many new physical sensations, but none of them seem related to a child. These physical changes and the

> **⟩NURSING TIP**
> Ambivalence about becoming a mother is normal in early pregnancy, and mood swings are common throughout pregnancy. Fathers often experience ambivalence.

higher hormone levels cause her emotions to be more unstable *(labile)*. The nurse can reassure the woman and her partner (who is often confused by her moods) about their cause, that they are normal, and that they will stabilize after pregnancy.

Second Trimester

The fetus becomes real to the woman during the second trimester. Her weight increases and the uterus becomes obvious as it rises up into the abdomen. If she has not already heard the fetal heartbeat or seen it beating on a sonogram, the woman usually will have an opportunity to hear it early in the second trimester. She feels fetal movement, and this is a powerful aid in helping her to distinguish the fetus as a separate person from herself.

The second trimester is a more stable time during pregnancy for most women. They have resolved many of their earlier feelings of ambivalence. They take on the role of an expectant mother wholeheartedly. The mother becomes totally involved with her developing child and her changing body image *(narcissism)*. She often devotes a great deal of time to selecting just the right foods and the best environment to promote her health and that of her infant. She welcomes the solicitous concern of others when they caution her not to pick up a heavy package or work too hard. She may lose interest in work or other activities as she devotes herself to the project of nurturing her fetus. The nurse can take advantage of her heightened interest in healthful living to teach good nutrition and other habits that can benefit the woman and her family long after the child is born.

The woman "tries on" the role of mother by learning what infants are like. She wants to hear stories of what she and her mate were like when they were infants. She often fantasizes about how her child will look and behave or what sex the child will be. She may or may not want to know the sex of the infant if it is apparent on a sonogram, sometimes preferring to be surprised at the birth. The woman who has had a child before undergoes a similar transition as she imagines what this specific child will be like and how he or she will compare to any siblings.

The body changes of pregnancy are now evident. The woman may welcome them as a sign to all that her fetus is well protected and thriving (Figure 4-9). But these same changes may be unwelcome to her because they can be perceived as unattractive and cause her discomfort.

The body changes may alter her sexual relationship with her partner as well. Both partners may fear harming the developing fetus, particularly if there has been a previous miscarriage. Her increasing size, discomforts, and the other changes of pregnancy may make one or

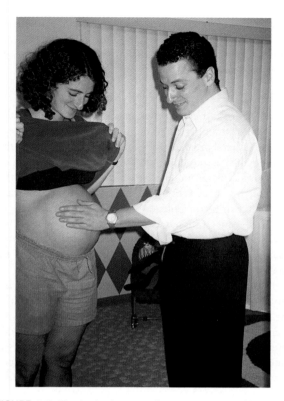

FIGURE **4-9** The body changes of pregnancy are evident, and the woman may welcome them as a sign to all that her pregnancy is real and her fetus is thriving.

both partners have less interest in intercourse. The nurse can assure them that these changes are temporary and help them explore other expressions of love and caring.

Third Trimester

As her body changes even more dramatically, a mother alternates between feeling "absolutely beautiful and productive" and feeling "as big as a house and totally unloved" by her partner. These mood swings reflect her sense of increased vulnerability and dependence on her partner. She becomes introspective about the challenge of labor that is ahead and its outcome. Her moods may again be more labile.

The mother begins to separate herself from the pregnancy and to commit herself to the care of an infant. She and her partner begin making concrete preparations for the infant's arrival. They buy clothes and equipment the infant will need. Many take childbirth preparation classes. The woman's thinking gradually shifts from "I am pregnant" to "I am going to be a mother."

The minor discomforts of pregnancy become tiresome during the last weeks before delivery. It seems that pregnancy will never end. A woman benefits from the gentle understanding of the people near and dear to her. With the support of her family and health care professionals, she can develop inner strength to accomplish the tasks of birth.

IMPACT ON THE FATHER

Responses of fathers vary widely. Some want to be fully involved in the physical and emotional aspects of pregnancy. Others prefer a management role, helping the woman adhere to recommendations of her physician or nurse-midwife. Some fathers want to "be there" for the woman, but prefer not to take an active role during pregnancy or birth. Cultural values influence the role of fathers because pregnancy and birth are viewed exclusively as women's work in some cultures. The nurse should not assume that a father is disinterested if he takes a less active role in pregnancy and birth.

Fathers go through similar processes as expectant mothers. Initially they may also have difficulty perceiving the fetus as real. Ambivalence and self-questioning about their readiness for fatherhood are typical. Fathers who attend prenatal appointments with the woman can see the fetus on ultrasound or hear the fetal heartbeat, making the child seem more like a real person (Figure 4-10).

Pregnancy is considered the beginning of a separate developmental stage called "Growth and Development of a Parent" (see Table 15-5).

Fathers who do not anticipate changes specific to the normal event of pregnancy may be confused or concerned by new feelings or behaviors and the changes that occur in family dynamics. For fathers, the *announcement phase* begins when pregnancy is confirmed. Acceptance of the pregnancy results in strengthening of the family support system and expansion of the social network. Rejection of the pregnancy may result in lack of communication and resentment. The second phase of the father's response is the *adjustment phase*. The father may revise financial plans, become involved in planning the child's room or furniture, and actively listen to the fetal heart and feel fetal movement (see Figure 4-10). Lack of adjustment may result in an increase in outside interests, or developing various symptoms in a struggle to regain attention he may feel has been lost to the fetus. The third phase of the father's response is the *focus phase* where active plans for participation in the labor process, birth, and change in lifestyle result in the partner "feeling like a father" (Box 4-5). The nurse's role is to help the father achieve positive outcomes in each phase (see Table 4-7).

The father is often asked to provide emotional support to his partner while struggling with the issue of fatherhood himself. Too often, he receives the message that his only job is to support the pregnant woman rather than being a parent who is also important and

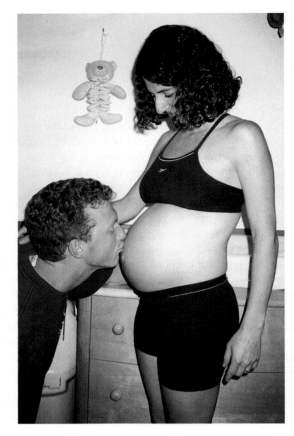

FIGURE **4-10** The father begins to develop a relationship to the fetus as he hears the fetal heart and feels fetal movement.

---

box 4-5	*Developmental Stage of Fatherhood*

- Announcement
- Adjustment
- Focus

---

has needs. The nurse should explore the father's feelings and encourage him during prenatal appointments, childbirth preparation classes, and labor and birth. He is trying to learn the role of father, just as the woman is trying to learn the role of mother.

IMPACT ON THE ADOLESCENT

Pregnant adolescents often have to struggle with feelings they find difficult to express. They are fraught with conflict about how to handle an unplanned pregnancy. Initially, they must face the anxiety of breaking the news to their parents and the father of the child. Denial of the pregnancy until late in gestation is not uncommon. There may be financial problems, shame, guilt, relationship problems with the infant's father, and feelings of low self-esteem. Alcoholism and substance abuse may be a part of the complex picture.

The nurse must assess the girl's developmental and educational level and her support system to best provide care for her. A critical variable is the girl's age. Young adolescents have difficulty considering the needs of others, such as the fetus. The nurse helps the adolescent girl to complete the developmental tasks of adolescence while assuming the new role of motherhood. Ideally, separate prenatal classes tailored to their needs help adolescent girls to learn to care for themselves and assume the role of mother.

NURSING TIP

The nurse must anticipate resistive behavior, ambivalence, and inconsistency in the adolescent. The nurse must consider the girl's developmental level and the priorities typical of her age, such as the importance of her peer group, focus on appearance, and difficulty considering the needs of others.

NURSING TIP

The pregnant adolescent must cope with two of life's most stress-laden transitions simultaneously: adolescence and parenthood.

IMPACT ON THE OLDER COUPLE

Mothers who become pregnant for the first time after age 35 years are called "elderly primips" because they are at a later stage in their childbearing cycle, and they may face special problems during pregnancy and labor. Many factors contribute to the trend of postponing pregnancy until after age 35 years:

- Effective birth control alternatives
- Increasing career options for women
- High cost of living (delays childbearing until financial status is secure)
- Development of fertilization techniques to enable later pregnancy

The "older couple" usually adjusts readily to pregnancy because they are often well-educated, have achieved life experiences that enable them to cope with the realities of parenthood, and are ready for the lifestyle change. Advances in maternal care and delivery practices have decreased the risk of negative pregnancy outcomes, although special problems continue. Women over age 35 years may have a decreased ability to adjust their uterine blood flow to meet the needs of the fetus (Stables, 1999). There may be an increase in multiple pregnancies if fertility drugs were used, which increases fetal risk. The increased risk of a congenital anomaly usually results in the offering of special tests during pregnancy (chorionic

villi sampling, amniocentesis), which increases the cost factor of prenatal care. Although the older couple may adjust to the process of pregnancy and parenthood, they may find themselves "different" from their peers, and this can result in impaired social interaction. Concerns of the older parent relate to age and energy level as the child grows, confronting the issues of their own mortality, and child care requirements. Meeting financial needs of a college-age child at retirement is a special issue that may require discussion and planning. Many older parents are placed in a "high risk" prenatal group that may limit their options for selecting a birth center. However, the pregnancy should be treated as normal unless problems are identified.

IMPACT ON THE SINGLE MOTHER

The single mother may still be an adolescent or she may be a mature woman. She has special emotional needs, especially if the father has left her, if he does not acknowledge the pregnancy, or if she does not care to have a relationship with the father. Some single mothers can turn to their parents, siblings, or close friends for support. Other single women are homosexual and have the support of their female partner. Women who do not have emotional support from significant others will have more difficulty completing the tasks of pregnancy. Their uncertainty in day-to-day living competes with mastering the emotional tasks of pregnancy.

Some single mothers may have conceived by in vitro fertilization because of a strong desire to have a child even in the absence of a stable heterosexual relationship. These women often are nearing the end of their childbearing years and perceive a "now or never" view of motherhood. Single women who plan pregnancies often prepare for the financial and lifestyle changes. Achieving social acceptance is not as difficult today as it was many years ago when single motherhood was taboo and considered a distinct disgrace to the maternal family. The nurse should maintain a nonjudgmental attitude and assist the single mother to successfully achieve the psychological tasks of pregnancy.

IMPACT ON THE SINGLE FATHER

The single father may take an active interest in and financial responsibility for the child. The couple may plan marriage eventually, but it is often delayed. A single father may provide emotional support for the mother during the pregnancy and birth. He often has strong feelings of surprise and accomplishment when he becomes aware of his partner's pregnancy. He may want to participate in plans for the child and take part in infant care after birth. However, his participation is sometimes rejected by the woman.

IMPACT ON THE GRANDPARENTS

Prospective grandparents have different reactions to a woman's pregnancy as well. They may eagerly anticipate the announcement that a grandchild is on the way, or they may feel that they are not ready for the role of grandparent, which they equate with being old. The first grandchild often causes the most excitement in grandparents. Their reaction may be more subdued if they have several grandchildren, which may hurt the excited pregnant couple.

Grandparents have different ideas of how they will be involved with their grandchildren. Distance from the younger family dictates the degree of involvement for some. They may want to be fully involved in the plans for the infant and help with child care, often traveling a great distance to be there for the big event. Other grandparents want less involvement because they welcome the freedom of a childless life again. Many grandparents are in their 40s and 50s, a time when their own career demands and care of their aging parents compete with their ability to be involved with grandchildren.

If grandparents and the expectant couple have similar views of their roles, little conflict is likely. However, disappointment and conflict may occur if the pregnant couple and the grandparents have significantly different expectations of their role and involvement. The nurse can help the young couple understand their parents' reactions and help them to negotiate solutions to conflicts that are satisfactory to both generations.

PRENATAL EDUCATION

Prenatal education is an interactive process that requires input from the patient concerning individual needs and assessment of outcome: a healthy mother and child and an intact family unit.

A plan for prenatal education is based on the desired outcome and includes the development of positive attitudes and perceptions, achievement of knowledge of facts, and the learning of skills to cope with pregnancy, labor, and the transition into parenthood. Examples include the *perception* that pregnancy is a normal process that is enhanced by good nutrition and a healthy lifestyle; the *knowledge* to select the proper diet; and the learning of *skills* to perform exercises, breathing, and relaxation techniques to prepare the woman for labor.

Prenatal education should progress according to the nursing process, as follows:

1. *Assess* the history and cultural needs.
2. *Diagnose* the knowledge deficit.
3. *Plan* the goals and priorities.
4. *Teach* (intervene) the facts and rationales.
5. *Evaluate* the knowledge gained and the goals achieved.

Teaching can occur in formal childbirth education classes or informally during a clinic visit. Every contact a nurse has with a pregnant patient is an opportunity for teaching.

PHYSIOLOGICAL AND PSYCHOLOGICAL CHANGES IN PREGNANCY AND NURSING INTERVENTIONS

Table 4-7 describes the physiological changes that occur during pregnancy, the related signs and symptoms noted in the patient, and some suggested nursing interventions or teaching points appropriate to that phase. The rationales of a nursing care plan can be based on the information within this table.

table **4-7** | *Physiological and Psychological Changes in Pregnancy and Nursing Interventions*

MATERNAL CHANGES	SIGNS AND SYMPTOMS	NURSING INTERVENTIONS
FIRST TRIMESTER		
Fertilization occurs. Increased progesterone results in amenorrhea. Sodium (Na) retention increases. Nitrogen (N) store decreases.	Pregnancy test is positive.	Guide patient regarding nutritional needs and folic acid requirements. Encourage patient to seek early prenatal care. Assess attitude toward this pregnancy and how it affects family.
Blood volume increases. Levels of relaxin hormone increase. Levels of hCG hormone increase.	Fainting is possible. Morning nausea can occur. Relaxation of gastrointestinal (GI) muscles can cause "heartburn". Sensitivity to odors increases.	Teach patient how to rise slowly from prone position. Teach patient how to cope with nausea without medication: • Eat dry crackers before arising • Use acupressure

table 4-7 | *Physiological and Psychological Changes in Pregnancy and Nursing Interventions—cont'd*

MATERNAL CHANGES	SIGNS AND SYMPTOMS	NURSING INTERVENTIONS
Pituitary gland releases melanin-stimulating hormone.	Pigmentation deepens on face (chloasma) and on abdomen (linea nigra).	Discuss body changes and assure patient that pigmentation will fade after puerperium.
Fetus grows. Uterus begins to enlarge.	Abdomen enlarges at end of first trimester when uterus rises out of pelvis. Small weight gain occurs. Enlarged uterus presses on bladder.	Teach methods to minimize fetal problems: • Avoid high temperatures around abdomen (baths and spas). • Discuss the effect of medications and herbs on fetal development. Discuss role of frequency of urination on lifestyle and activities. Facilitate communication with partner concerning relationships during pregnancy. Discuss nutritional and folic acid needs, control of caffeine intake in second and third trimesters, and omega–fatty acid intake.
For fathers, the announcement phase begins when pregnancy is confirmed, followed by an adjustment phase and, finally, the focus phase in third trimester and during labor, when "feeling like a father" develops.	Parents adjust to the reality of pregnancy.	Review father's role as well as mother's responses. Refer to community agencies as needed. Assess for misinformation and knowledge deficit. Help parents identify concerns. Answer questions. Discuss care of siblings, role of grandparents, etc.
SECOND TRIMESTER		
Corpus luteum is absorbed and placenta takes over fetal support (between third and fourth month).	Blood volume increases in placental bed.	Teach patient how to minimize risk of habitual abortion between third and fourth month when placenta begins to take over.
Broad ligament stretches as uterus enlarges.	Occasional pain in groin area occurs.	Teach patient Kegel exercises to strengthen pelvic muscles.
Vascularity of pelvis increases.	Sexual pleasure and desire increases. White discharge may occur.	Discuss modifications of positions for sexual comfort and pleasure. Teach patient to avoid routine douches. Teach patient perineal skin hygiene.
Blood volume and vasomotor lability increases. Cardiac output increases.	Orthostatic hypotension can occur. Physiological anemia may occur.	Teach patient to change positions slowly and to avoid warm, crowded areas. Iron supplements may be prescribed for anemia. Teach patient how to prevent constipation, and teach change in stool color during iron therapy.
Renal threshold decreases.	Perineal itching may occur.	Test for sugar in urine and require glucose tolerance test in second trimester to rule out gestational diabetes. Teach patient hygienic measures when high glucose is present (front to back wiping; wearing cotton panties).

Continued

| table 4-7 | *Physiological and Psychological Changes in Pregnancy and Nursing Interventions—cont'd* |

MATERNAL CHANGES	SIGNS AND SYMPTOMS	NURSING INTERVENTIONS
Uterus rises out of pelvis. Estrogen relaxes sacroiliac joint.	Center of gravity of body changes.	Teach patient proper shoe/heel height to avoid falling. Teach placement of automobile restraints across hips rather than across abdomen. Teach patient to avoid lying supine in bed after the fourth month of pregnancy to prevent supine hypotensive syndrome. Teach posture and pelvic rocking exercises. Instruct that clothes should hang from shoulders.
	Pressure on bladder and rectum increases.	Anticipate urinary frequency during long trips. Teach patient Kegel exercises to strengthen pelvic floor.
Enlarging uterus compresses nerves supplying lower extremities.	Leg muscle spasms occur, especially when reclining.	Nurse checks for Homan's sign. Teach patient how to dorsiflex the foot to help relieve spasms. Massage foot.
Decreased calcium levels and increased phosphorus levels are possible.		Use oral aluminum hydroxide gel to reduce phosphorus levels if elevated (when recommended by health care provider).
Decreasing cardiac reserve and increasing respiratory effort start late in the second trimester.	Physiological stress is possible if exercise levels are not decreased.	Teach patient to monitor pulse (maximum 90 beats/min), and teach patient that inability to converse without taking frequent breaths is a sign of physiological stress. Teach patient to stop exercising if numbness, pain, or dizziness occurs.
Hormonal influence causes *"id"* to come to the surface.	Mood swings occur.	Prepare spouse/significant other and family for mood swings, outspoken behavior, and labile emotions ("speaks before she thinks").
Levels of relaxin hormone increase.	Sphincter of stomach relaxes, and gastrointestinal motility is slowed.	Teach patient how to prevent constipation. Increase fluid intake and avoid gasforming foods.
Increase in estrogen causes increased excretory function of the skin.	Skin itches.	Teach patient to wear loose clothing; shower frequently; and use bland soaps and oils for comfort.
Anterior pituitary secretes melanin-stimulating hormone.	Skin pigmentation deepens.	Prepare patient to anticipate development of spider nevi and skin pigmentation. Reassure patient that most fade after the puerperium.
Estrogen levels increase.	Increased estrogen develops increased vascularity of oral tissues, resulting in gingivitis and stuffy nose.	Teach proper oral hygiene techniques.
	Estrogen levels develop network of increased arterioles.	Edema can occur. Assess blood pressure and report proteinuria.

table 4-7 *Physiological and Psychological Changes in Pregnancy and Nursing Interventions—cont'd*

MATERNAL CHANGES	SIGNS AND SYMPTOMS	NURSING INTERVENTIONS
Pituitary gland secretes prolactin.	Colostrum leaks from nipples and sometimes cakes. Breasts enlarge.	Teach patient to cleanse nipples to keep ducts from being blocked by colostrum. Avoid soaps, ointments, and alcohol that dry skin. Teach patient *not* to stimulate nipples by massage or exercise, because doing so may increase the risk for preterm labor.
Traction on brachial plexus is caused by drooping of shoulders as breast size increases.	Fingers tingle.	Teach patient proper posture. Encourage the use of a supportive maternity bra.
Placental barrier allows certain elements and organisms to pass through to the fetus.	Some medications can pass through the placental barrier and cause fetal defects.	Advise patient not to smoke and not to self-treat with medications. Teach patients that certain jobs should be avoided (e.g., working as a parking attendants, in a dry cleaning plant, and in a chemistry laboratory).
	Traveling to countries that have endemic diseases can have negative effect on fetus; active immunization should be avoided.	Advise patient regarding travel.
Lowered oxygen levels can cause fetal hypoxia.		Most commercial airlines have cabin pressure controlled at or below 5000-foot level and therefore do not pose a risk to the fetus.
Increased levels of platelets	Women are prone to thrombophlebitis if they are inactive for long periods.	Encourage patient to keep hydrated because of low cabin humidity in airplanes and to move around to help prevent thrombophlebitis.
Fetal growth continues.	Mother feels signs of life; fetus moves and kicks.	Teach proper nutrition to foster fetal growth without adding extra "empty" calories. Encourage patient to attend child care/parenting classes.
THIRD TRIMESTER		
Weight gain of 20-25 pounds occurs.	Patient tires easily.	Teach patient the need for rest periods and organization of work.
Colostrum forms.	Colostrum may leak from breasts.	Teach patient care of nipples. Introduce nipple pads. Avoid nipple stimulation to prevent preterm labor.
Increased estrogen levels causes edema of larynx.	Voice changes.	Professional singers may lose voice quality.
Maximum increase in cardiac output (increase in stroke volume) occurs.	Patient tires easily.	Teach patient the need for rest periods.
Edema of hands and wrist is possible.	Risk for carpal-tunnel syndrome increases.	Teach patient signs of pregnancy-induced hypertension (PIH) and assess water retention.

Continued

table 4-7 | *Physiological and Psychological Changes in Pregnancy and Nursing Interventions—cont'd*

MATERNAL CHANGES	SIGNS AND SYMPTOMS	NURSING INTERVENTIONS
Uterus increases in size.	Pressure on stomach occurs. Pressure on diaphragm occurs. Venous congestion increases.	Discuss how to cope with decrease in appetite and shortness of breath. Teach patient how to avoid constipation and leg varicosities. Teach "talk test" for self-evaluation of exercise tolerance to prevent fetal hypoxia (must be able to finish a sentence before taking a breath).
Sensitivity to Braxton Hicks contractions increases.	Fetal head may engage (uterus drops) (lightening).	Teach patient the signs of labor and when to come to hospital. Offer tour of labor and delivery unit.
Hormone levels increase.	"*Id*" is at the surface. Woman becomes self-centered and worries how she will manage labor.	Review labor management learned in prenatal classes. Discuss sibling care and support system.

key points

- Early and regular prenatal care promotes the healthiest possible outcome for mother and infant.
- Determination of the woman's estimated date of delivery is calculated from her last normal menstrual period.
- The length of a pregnancy is 40 weeks after the last normal menstrual period plus or minus 2 weeks. The expected date of delivery is determined by using Nägele's rule.
- Presumptive signs of pregnancy often have other causes. Probable signs more strongly suggest pregnancy, but can still be caused by other conditions. Positive signs have no other cause except pregnancy. The three positive signs of pregnancy include detection of a fetal heartbeat, fetal movements felt by a trained examiner, and visualizing the embryo or fetus on ultrasound.
- The optimal weight gain during pregnancy is 55 to 77 kg (25 to 35 pounds).
- The uterus undergoes the most obvious changes in pregnancy: it increases in weight from approximately 60 g (2 ounces) to 1000 g (2.2 pounds); it increases in capacity from about 10 ml (one third of an ounce) to 5000 ml (5 quarts). Pregnancy affects all body systems.
- The mother's blood volume increases about 45% over her prepregnant volume to perfuse the placenta and extra-maternal tissues. Her blood pressure does not rise because resistance to blood flow in her arteries decreases. The fluid portion of her blood increases more than the cellular portion, resulting in a pseudoanemia.
- The common discomforts of pregnancy occur as a result of hormonal, physiological, and anatomic changes normally occurring during pregnancy. The nurse should teach relief measures and abnormal signs to report to the health care provider.
- Supine hypotension syndrome, also known as aortocaval compression or vena cava syndrome, may occur if the pregnant woman lies flat on her back. Turning to one side or placing a small pillow under one hip can help relieve this hypotension.
- To provide for the growth of the fetus and maternal tissues, the mother needs 300 extra, high-quality calories daily. Important nutrients that must be increased are protein, calcium, iron, and folic acid. Five hundred extra calories a day are needed for lactation.
- Adequate folic acid intake before conception can reduce the incidence of neural tube defects such as anencephaly or spina bifida. The Centers for Disease Control and Prevention recommend that all fertile women consume 400 μg (0.4 mg) of folic acid daily.
- Fathers should be included in prenatal care to the extent they and the woman desire.
- Adaptation to pregnancy occurs in the mother, father, and other family members. Prenatal care involves physical and psychological aspects and should be family centered.
- Childbirth education includes formal classes and informal counseling. Education should include nutrition, prenatal visits, exercise, breathing and relaxation techniques, the birth process, safety issues and beginning parenting skills.

ONLINE RESOURCES

Pregnancy and Childbirth Prenatal Care:
http://www.makewayforbaby.com/prenatalcare.htm

How the Alexander Technique Can Help During Pregnancy, Childbirth and Parenthood:
http://www.alexandertechnique.com/articles/pregnancy

Lamaze International: http://www.lamaze-childbirth.com

The Bradley Method of Natural Childbirth:
http://www.bradleybirth.com/cc.htm

Patient Care Updates: http://www.patientcareonline.com

Journal Articles and Resources:
http://www.nursingcenter.com

REVIEW QUESTIONS   *Choose the most appropriate answer.*

1. A woman is having a prenatal visit at 18 weeks' gestation. Why is it important to ask her about fetal movement?
   1. Absence of fetal movement at this time suggests that the pregnancy is more advanced than her dates indicate
   2. Denial of fetal movement at this stage in pregnancy may indicate that the woman is not accepting her pregnancy
   3. If she has started feeling fetal movement, the fetal heartbeat will be checked with a fetoscope to confirm that the fetus is living
   4. Fetal movement is first felt by the mother about this time and provides a marker for approximate gestational age

2. A pregnant woman complains that she has a large amount of vaginal secretions. The next most appropriate nursing action is to:
   1. Consult her nurse-midwife for a cream or douche
   2. Ask her if the discharge is irritating or causes itching
   3. Advise her to change cotton panties twice daily
   4. Tell her to reduce sexual intercourse for a few weeks

3. During a prenatal examination at 30-weeks gestation, a woman is lying on her back on the examining table. She suddenly complains of dizziness and feeling faint. The most appropriate response of the nurse would be:
   1. Reassure the woman and take measures to reduce her anxiety level
   2. Offer the woman some orange juice or other rapidly absorbed form of glucose
   3. Place a pillow under the woman's head
   4. Turn the woman on to her side

4. A woman is being seen for her first prenatal care appointment. She has a positive home pregnancy test and her chart shows a TPALM recording of gravida 40120. The nurse would understand that:
   1. Minimal prenatal teaching will be required because this is her fourth pregnancy
   2. The woman will need help in planning the care of her other children at home during her labor and delivery
   3. The woman should experience minimal anxiety because she is familiar with the progress of pregnancy
   4. This pregnancy will be considered high risk and measures to reduce anxiety will be needed

5. Prenatal nursing care for the father should emphasize:
   1. Giving him guidance so he can focus on the mother getting through pregnancy
   2. Involving him in the pregnancy as much as he and the mother desire
   3. Encouraging him to attend all prenatal visits with the mother
   4. Making the fact of fatherhood as real as possible to him

CHAPTER 5

Nursing Care of Women with Complications During Pregnancy

1. Define each key term listed.
2. Explain the use of fetal diagnostic tests in women with complicated pregnancies.
3. Describe antepartum complications, their treatment, and their nursing care.
4. Identify methods to reduce a woman's risk for antepartum complications.
5. Discuss the management of concurrent medical conditions during pregnancy.
6. Describe environmental hazards that may adversely affect the outcome of pregnancy.
7. Describe how pregnancy affects care of the trauma victim.
8. Describe psychosocial nursing interventions for the woman who has a high-risk pregnancy and for her family.

key terms

abortion (p. 84)
cerclage (sĕr-KLĂHZH, p. 84)
disseminated intravascular coagulation (DIC) (p. 93)
eclampsia (ĕ-KLĂMP-sē-ă, p. 94)
erythroblastosis fetalis (ĕ-rĭth-rō-blăs-TŌ-sĭs fē-TĂ-lĭs, p. 100)
hydramnios (hī-DRĂM-nē-ŏs, p. 101)
incompetent cervix (ĭn-KŎM-pă-tănt SĔR-vĭkz, p. 84)
isoimmunization (ī-sō-ĭm-ū-nĭ-ZĂ-shŭn, p. 99)
macrosomia (măk-rō-SŌ-mē-ă, p. 101)
preeclampsia (prē-ĕ-KLĂMP-sē-ă, p. 93)
products of conception (POC) (p. 87)
teratogen (TĔR-ă-tō-jĕn, p. 112)
tonic-clonic seizure (p. 95)

Most women have uneventful pregnancies that are free of complications. Others, however, have complications that threaten their well-being and that of their babies. Many problems can be anticipated during prenatal care and thus prevented or made less severe. Others occur without warning.

Women who have no prenatal care or begin care late in pregnancy may have complications that are severe because they were not identified early. Box 5-1 describes the danger signs that should be taught to every pregnant woman and reinforced at each prenatal visit. The woman should be taught to notify her health care provider if any of these danger signs occur. A high-risk pregnancy is defined as one in which the health of the mother or fetus is in jeopardy.

High-risk pregnancies usually have causes characterized by the following:

- Relate to the pregnancy itself
- Occur because the woman has a medical condition or injury that complicates the pregnancy
- Result from environmental hazards that affect her or her fetus
- Arise from maternal behaviors or lifestyles that have a negative effect on the mother or fetus

Early and consistent assessment for risk factors during prenatal visits is essential for a positive outcome for the mother and the fetus.

ASSESSMENT OF FETAL HEALTH

Extraordinary technical advances have enabled the management of high-risk pregnancies so that both the mother and the fetus have positive outcomes. Various tests can be used prenatally to assess the well-being of the fetus. Nursing responsibilities during the assessment of fetal health include preparing the patient properly, explaining the reason for the test, and clarifying and interpreting results in collaboration with other health care providers. The nurse can provide the psychosocial support that will allay or reduce parental anxiety. Figure 5-1 shows amniocentesis, and Table 5-1 reviews common *prenatal* tests to assess the status of the fetus. Fetal assessment techniques used *during labor* are discussed in Chapter 6.

The future of fetal assessment lies in the continued development of new ultrasound technologies and handheld receivers. Ultrasound pictures taken by a portable

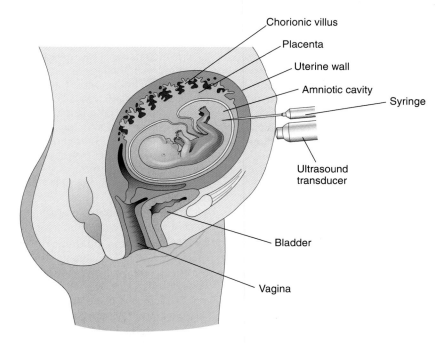

FIGURE **5-1** Amniocentesis. An ultrasound transducer on the abdomen ensures needle placement away from the body of the fetus and the placenta. A needle is inserted into the amniotic cavity, and a sample of amniotic fluid is collected for laboratory examination and fetal assessment.

| box 5-1 | *Danger Signs in Pregnancy* |

- Sudden gush of fluid from vagina
- Vaginal bleeding
- Abdominal pain
- Persistent vomiting
- Epigastric pain
- Edema of face and hands
- Severe, persistent headache
- Blurred vision or dizziness
- Chills with fever over 38.0° C (100.4° F)
- Painful urination or reduced urine output

instrument can be transmitted via the Internet to be interpreted by experts in medical centers. Telemedicine is a growing specialized technology in prenatal care.

PREGNANCY-RELATED COMPLICATIONS

Complications of pregnancy covered in the following sections include hyperemesis gravidarum, bleeding disorders, hypertension, and blood incompatibility between the woman and fetus.

HYPEREMESIS GRAVIDARUM

Mild nausea and/or vomiting are easily managed during pregnancy (see p. 68). In contrast, the woman with hyperemesis gravidarum has excessive nausea and vomiting that can significantly interfere with her food intake and fluid balance. Fetal growth may be restricted, resulting in a low-birth-weight infant. Dehydration impairs perfusion of the placenta, reducing the delivery of blood oxygen and nutrients to the fetus.

Manifestations. Hyperemesis gravidarum differs from "morning sickness" of pregnancy in one or more of the following ways:

- Persistent nausea and vomiting, often with complete inability to retain food and fluids
- Significant weight loss
- Dehydration as evidenced by a dry tongue and mucous membranes, decreased turgor (elasticity) of the skin, scant and concentrated urine, and a high hematocrit
- Electrolyte and acid-base imbalances
- Psychological factors such as unusual stress, emotional immaturity, passivity, or ambivalence about the pregnancy

Treatment. The health care provider will rule out other causes for the excessive nausea and vomiting, such as gastroenteritis, liver, gallbladder, or pancreatic disorders, before making this diagnosis. The medical treat-

table 5-1 **Fetal Diagnostic Tests**

TESTS AND DESCRIPTION	USES DURING PREGNANCY
Ultrasound examination. Uses high-frequency sound waves to visualize structures within the body; the examination may use a transvaginal probe or an abdominal transducer; abdominal ultrasound during early pregnancy requires a full bladder for proper visualization (have the woman drink 1 to 2 quarts of water before the examination). A targeted comprehensive ultrasound detects specific anomalies. Echo/Doppler scan detects fetal heart activity at 6-10 weeks. Three-dimensional (3-D) imaging produces clear detail and features.	Visualize a gestational sac in early pregnancy to confirm the pregnancy. Identify site of implantation (uterine or ectopic). Verify fetal viability or death. Identify a multifetal pregnancy, such as twins or triplets. Diagnose some fetal structural abnormalities. Guide procedures, such as chorionic villus sampling, amniocentesis, percutaneous umbilical blood sampling. Determine gestational age of the embryo or fetus. Locate the placenta. Determine the amount of amniotic fluid. Observe fetal movements.
Amniotic fluid volume (AFV)	This ultrasound scan measures the amniotic fluid pockets in all four quadrants surrounding the mother's umbilicus and produces an amniotic fluid index (AFI). From 5-19 cm is considered normal. Less than 5 cm is known as *oligohydramnios* (decreased amniotic fluid) and is associated with growth restriction and fetal distress during labor because of "kinking" of the cord. A measurement greater than 30 cm is *polyhydramnios* (excess amniotic fluid) and is associated with neural tube defects, gastrointestinal obstruction, and fetal hydrops.
Estimation of gestational age	This ultrasound examination at 8 weeks can measure the gestational sac. Between 7 and 14 weeks the crown-rump length can indicate fetal age. After 12 weeks the biparietal diameter of the fetus and the femur length give an accurate estimation of fetal age. The biparietal diameter of fetus at 36 weeks is 8.7 cm, and at term it is 9.8 cm.
Magnetic resonance imaging (MRI)	Provides a noninvasive radiological view of fetal structures, including placenta. Used when there is a high suspicion of an anomaly.
Kick count (maternal assessment of fetal movement)	Fewer than three fetal kicks within an hour or cessation of fetal movement for 12 hours indicates the need for evaluation. A daily fetal movement record is kept at home once a day and the findings are evaluated during prenatal visits to ensure fetal health. The sleep cycle of the fetus should be considered when selecting a time to evaluate fetal movement.
Doppler ultrasound blood flow assessment. Uses high-frequency sound waves to study the flow of blood through vessels.	Determine adequacy of blood flow through the placenta and umbilical cord vessels in women in whom it is likely to be impaired (such as those with pregnancy-induced hypertension or diabetes mellitus).
Alpha-fetoprotein testing (AFP). Determines the level of this fetal protein in the pregnant woman's serum or in a sample of amniotic fluid; correct interpretation requires an accurate gestational age.	Identify high levels, which are associated with open defects, such as spina bifida (open spine), anencephaly (incomplete development of the skull and brain), or gastroschisis (open abdominal cavity). Identify low levels, which are associated with chromosome abnormalities or gestational trophoblastic disease (hydatidiform mole).

table 5-1 | *Fetal Diagnostic Tests—cont'd*

TESTS AND DESCRIPTION	USES DURING PREGNANCY
Chorionic villus sampling. Obtaining a small part of the developing placenta to analyze fetal cells at 10 to 12 weeks' gestation.	Identify chromosome abnormalities or other defects that can be determined by analysis of cells. Results of chromosome studies are available 24 to 48 hours later. Cannot be used to determine spina bifida or anencephaly (see AFP testing). Higher rate of spontaneous abortion after procedure than after amniocentesis. Reports of limb reduction defects in newborns. $Rh_o(D)$ immune globulin (RhoGAM) is given to the Rh-negative woman.
Amniocentesis. Insertion of a thin needle through the abdominal and uterine walls to obtain a sample of amniotic fluid, which contains cast-off fetal cells and various other fetal products; standard genetic amniocentesis is done at 15 to 17 weeks' gestation; early genetic amniocentesis is done at 11 to 14 weeks' gestation for some disorders (see Figure 5-1).	*Early pregnancy.* Identify chromosome abnormalities, biochemical disorders (such as Tay-Sachs' disease), and level of AFP. A fetus cannot be tested for every possible disorder. Spontaneous abortion following the procedure is the primary risk. *Late pregnancy.* Identify severity of maternal-fetal blood incompatibility and assess fetal lung maturity. $Rh_o(D)$ immune globulin is given to the Rh-negative woman.
Nonstress test (NST). Evaluation with an electronic fetal monitor of the FHR for accelerations of at least 15 beats/min lasting 15 seconds in a 20-minute period. Fetal movements do not need to accompany the accelerations.	Identify fetal compromise in conditions associated with poor placenta function, such as hypertension, diabetes mellitus, or postterm gestation. Adequate accelerations of the FHR are reassuring that the placenta is functioning properly and the fetus is well oxygenated.
Vibroacoustic stimulation test. Procedure similar to the NST; in addition, an artificial larynx device is used to stimulate the fetus with sound; expected response is acceleration of the fetal heart rate, as in the NST.	Clarify (if the NST is questionable) whether the fetus is well oxygenated, thereby reducing the need for more complex testing. Clarify (during labor) questionable FHR patterns.
Contraction stress test (CST). Evaluation of the FHR response to mild uterine contractions by using an electronic fetal monitor; contractions may be induced by self-stimulation of the nipples, which causes the woman's pituitary gland to release oxytocin, or by intravenous oxytocin (Pitocin) infusion. The woman must have at least three contractions at least 40 seconds in duration in a 10-minute period for interpretation of the CST.	Purposes are the same as the NST; the CST may be done if the NST results are nonreassuring (the fetal heart does not accelerate) or if they are questionable. Late decelerations after a contraction can indicate that fetus may not tolerate labor. A negative CST means there are no late decelerations and the fetus can probably tolerate labor.
Biophysical profile (BPP). A group of five fetal assessments: fetal heart rate and reactivity (the NST), fetal breathing movements, fetal body movements, fetal tone (closure of the hand), and the volume of amniotic fluid (AFI). Some centers omit the NST, and others assess only the NST and AFI.	Identify reduced fetal oxygenation in conditions associated with poor placental function, but with greater precision than the NST alone. As fetal hypoxia gradually increases, FHR changes occur first, followed by cessation of fetal breathing movement, gross body movements, and finally loss of fetal tone. Amniotic fluid volume is reduced when placental function is poor (shows pockets of low or absent amniotic fluid).
Percutaneous umbilical blood sampling. Obtaining a fetal blood sample from a placental vessel or from the umbilical cord; may be used to give a blood transfusion to an anemic fetus.	Identify fetal conditions that can be diagnosed only with a blood sample. Blood transfusion for fetal anemia caused by maternal-fetal blood incompatibility, placenta previa, or abruptio placentae.

Continued

table 5-1	*Fetal Diagnostic Tests—cont'd*

TESTS AND DESCRIPTION	USES DURING PREGNANCY
Tests of fetal lung maturity. Tests a sample of amniotic fluid (obtained by amniocentesis or from the pool of fluid in the vagina) to determine substances that indicate fetal lungs are mature enough to adapt to extrauterine life: Lecithin-to-sphingomyelin (L/S) ratio. A 2:1 ratio indicates fetal lung maturity (3:1 ratio desirable for diabetic mother); fluid usually obtained by amniocentesis Presence of phosphatidylglycerol (PG) Presence of phosphatidylinositol (PI) Foam stability index (FSI, or "shake test") Persistence of a ring of bubbles for 15 minutes after shaking together equal amounts of 95% ethanol, isotonic saline, and amniotic fluid	Evaluate whether the fetus is likely to have respiratory complications in adapting to extrauterine life. May be done to determine whether the fetal lungs are mature before performing an elective cesarean birth or inducing labor if the gestational age is questionable. Also used to evaluate whether the fetus should be promptly delivered or allowed to mature further when the membranes rupture and the gestation is less than 37 weeks or if the gestation is questionable.

ment for hyperemesis gravidarum is to correct dehydration and electrolyte or acid-base imbalances with oral or intravenous fluids. Antiemetic drugs may be prescribed after the health care provider informs the woman about any potential risk to the developing infant. Occasionally severe cases require total parenteral nutrition. The woman may need hospital admission to correct dehydration and inadequate nutrition if home measures are not successful. The condition is self-limiting in most women, although it is quite distressing to the woman and her family.

Nursing care. Nursing care focuses on patient teaching because most care occurs in the home. The woman should reduce factors that trigger nausea and vomiting. She should avoid food odors, which may abound in meal preparation areas and tray carts if she is hospitalized. If she becomes nauseated when her food is served, the tray should be removed promptly and offered again later.

Accurate intake and output records are kept to assess fluid balance. Frequent, small amounts of food and fluid keep the stomach from becoming too full, which can trigger vomiting. Easily digested carbohydrates, such as crackers or baked potatoes, are tolerated best. Foods with strong odors should be eliminated. Taking liquids between solid meals helps to reduce gastric distention. Sitting upright after meals reduces gastric reflux (backflow) into the esophagus.

The emesis basin is kept out of sight so that it is not a visual reminder of vomiting. It should be emptied at once if the woman vomits and the amount documented on the intake and output record.

Stress may contribute to hyperemesis gravidarum; stress may also result from this complication. The nurse should provide support by listening to the woman's feel-

ings about pregnancy, child rearing, and living with constant nausea. Although psychological factors may play a role in some cases of hyperemesis gravidarum, the nurse should not assume that every woman with this complication is adjusting poorly to her pregnancy.

BLEEDING DISORDERS OF EARLY PREGNANCY

Several bleeding disorders can complicate early pregnancy, such as abortion (miscarriage) (Figure 5-2), ectopic pregnancy (see Figure 5-3), or hydatidiform mole (see Figure 5-4). Maternal blood loss decreases the oxygen-carrying capacity of the blood, resulting in fetal hypoxia, and places the fetus at risk.

Abortion

Table 5-2 differentiates types of abortions.

Treatment. When a threatened abortion occurs, efforts are made to keep the fetus in utero until the age of viability. In recurrent pregnancy loss, causes are investigated that could include genetic, immunological, anatomic, endocrine, or infectious factors. Cerclage, or suturing an incompetent cervix that opens when the growing fetus presses against it, is successful in most cases. A low human chorionic gonadotropin (hCG) level or low fetal heart rate by 8 weeks' gestation may be an ominous sign.

Termination of pregnancy after 20 weeks' gestation (age of viability) is called *preterm labor* and is discussed in Chapter 13 (see Table 5-3 for procedures used in pregnancy termination). In all cases of pregnancy loss, counseling of the parents is essential. Even when the mother elects to terminate pregnancy, there are emotional responses that should be recognized and addressed.

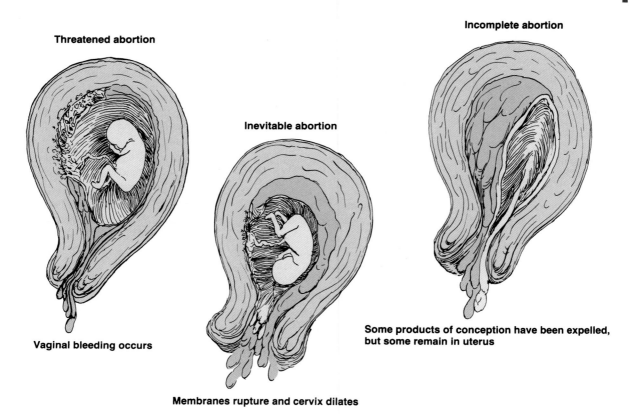

Threatened abortion

Vaginal bleeding occurs

Inevitable abortion

Membranes rupture and cervix dilates

Incomplete abortion

Some products of conception have been expelled, but some remain in uterus

FIGURE **5-2** Three types of spontaneous abortion.

Oxytocin (Pitocin) controls blood loss before and after curettage, much as the drugs do after term birth. $Rh_o(D)$ immune globulin (RhoGAM [300 µg] or the lower-dose MICRhoGAM [50 µg]) is given to Rh-negative women after any abortion to prevent the development of antibodies that might harm the fetus during a subsequent pregnancy.

Nursing care

Physical care. The nurse documents the amount and character of bleeding and saves anything that looks like clots or tissue for evaluation by a pathologist. A pad count and an estimate of how much each is saturated (e.g., 50%, 75%) more accurately documents blood loss. The woman with threatened abortion who remains at home is taught to report increased bleeding or passage of tissue.

The nurse should check the hospitalized woman's bleeding and vital signs to identify hypovolemic shock resulting from blood loss. She should not eat (remain NPO) if she has active bleeding to avoid aspiration if anesthesia is required for dilation and curettage (D&C) treatment. Laboratory tests, such as a hemoglobin and hematocrit, are ordered.

After vacuum aspiration or curettage, the amount of vaginal bleeding is observed. The blood pressure, pulse, and respirations are checked every 15 minutes for 1 hour, then every 30 minutes until discharge from the postanesthesia care unit. The mother's temperature is checked on admission to the recovery area and every 4 hours until discharge to monitor for infection.

Most women are discharged directly from the recovery unit to their home after curettage. Guidelines for self-care at home include the following:

- Report increased bleeding. Do not use tampons, which may cause infection.
- Take temperature every 8 hours for 3 days. Report signs of infection (temperature of 38° C [100.4° F] or higher; foul odor or brownish color of vaginal drainage).
- Take an oral iron supplement if prescribed.
- Resume sexual activity as recommended by the health care provider (usually after the bleeding has stopped).
- Return to the health care provider at the recommended time for a checkup and contraception information.
- Pregnancy can occur before the first menstrual period returns after the abortion procedure.

Emotional care. Society often underestimates the emotional distress spontaneous abortion causes the

| table 5-2 | *Types of Abortions* |

TYPE	DESCRIPTION	TREATMENT
SPONTANEOUS (NONINTENTIONAL) ABORTION	Termination of pregnancy before viability (20 weeks' gestation)	
Threatened abortion	Cramping and backache with light spotting; cervix is closed and no tissue is passed	Ultrasound is used to determine if fetus is living; bed rest is prescribed.
Inevitable abortion	Increased bleeding, cramping; cervix dilates	Patient is placed on bed rest and monitored; awaits natural evacuation of uterus.
Incomplete abortion	Bleeding, cramping, dilation of cervix, passage of tissue	Uterus may be emptied by D&C or vacuum extraction (see Table 5-3).
Complete abortion	Passage of all products of conception; cervix closes; bleeding stops	Patient is monitored and emotional support is given.
Missed abortion	Fetus dies in utero but is not expelled; uterine growth stops, sepsis can occur	If fetus is not expelled, uterus is evacuated by D&C (see Table 5-3).
Recurrent abortion	Two or more consecutive spontaneous abortions (habitual abortion) usually caused by incompetent cervix or inadequate progesterone levels necessary to maintain pregnancy	Incompetent cervix is treated with *cerclage,* a reinforcement of cervix with a surgical suture; the patient is then monitored for early signs of labor at term to prevent uterine rupture.
INDUCED ABORTION	Intentional termination of pregnancy before age of viability	
Therapeutic abortion	Intentional termination of pregnancy to preserve the health of the mother	Induced abortion is currently legal in the United States when performed by a qualified health care provider.
Elective abortion	Intentional termination of pregnancy for reasons other than the health of the mother (such as fetal anomaly)	Septic abortion (hemorrhage and infection) is a risk to the mother; counseling is advised even if the mother elects to abort.

D&C, Dilation and curettage.

woman and her family. Even if the pregnancy was not planned or not suspected, they often grieve for what might have been. Their grief may last longer and be deeper than they or other people expect. The nurse listens to the woman and acknowledges the grief she and her partner feel. Table 5-4 contains information about communicating with the family experiencing pregnancy loss. Spiritual support of the family's choice and community support groups may help the family work through the grief of any pregnancy loss. Nursing Care

Plan 5-1 suggests interventions for families experiencing early pregnancy loss.

Ectopic Pregnancy

Ectopic pregnancy occurs when the fertilized ovum (zygote) is implanted outside the uterine cavity (Figure 5-3). Of all ectopic pregnancies, 95% occur in the fallopian tube (tubal pregnancy). An obstruction or other abnormality of the tube prevents the zygote from being transported into the uterus. Scarring or deformity of the

table 5-3 | *Procedures Used in Pregnancy Termination*

PROCEDURE AND DESCRIPTION	COMMENTS
Vacuum aspiration (vacuum curettage). Cervical dilation with metal rods or laminaria (a substance that absorbs water and swells, thus enlarging the cervical opening) followed by controlled suction through a plastic cannula to remove all products of conception (POC)	Used for first-trimester abortions; also used to remove remaining POC after spontaneous abortion; may be followed by curettage (see dilation and curettage); paracervical block (local anesthesia of the cervix) or general anesthesia needed; conscious sedation with midazolam (Versed) may be used
Dilation and curettage (D&C). Dilation of the cervix as in vacuum curettage followed by gentle scraping of the uterine walls to remove POC	Used for first-trimester abortions and to remove all POC after a spontaneous abortion; greater risk of cervical or uterine trauma and excessive blood loss than with vacuum curettage; paracervical block or general anesthesia needed
Mifepristone (RU486)	An oral medication that may be taken up to 5 weeks' gestation; often used with a prostaglandin agent that causes bleeding and termination of pregnancy within 5 days
Methotrexate	An oral or intramuscular medication given with misoprostol, a prostaglandin analog, applied intravaginally causes termination of pregnancy within 1 or 2 days
Prostaglandins	In gel form or intrauterine injection can be used in the second trimester to terminate pregnancy; unpleasant side effects can occur
Hypertonic uterine infusion	Causes uterine contractions to occur within 12-24 hours; in early second trimester, drugs such as misoprostol (Cytotec) and oxytocin expedite the process; complications include sepsis and bleeding

table 5-4 | *Communicating with a Family Experiencing Pregnancy Loss*

INEFFECTIVE TECHNIQUES	EFFECTIVE TECHNIQUES
Do not give the woman/family any information.	Keep the family together.
Separate family members.	Wait quietly with family: "being there."
Discourage expressions of sadness; for example, expecting the father to be strong for the mother's sake.	Say "I'm sorry" or "I'm here if you need to talk."
Avoid interacting with the family and talking about their loss.	Touch (may not be appreciated by some people or in some cultures).
Act uncomfortable with the family's expressions of grief.	Refer to spontaneous abortion as "miscarriage" rather than the harsher sounding "abortion."
Minimize the importance of the pregnancy by comments such as "You're young—you can always have more children," "At least you didn't lose a real baby," "It was for the best; the baby was abnormal," or "You have another healthy child at home."	Provide mementos as appropriate (lock of hair, photograph, footprint); save keepsakes for later retrieval if the family does not want them immediately.
Say, "I know how you feel"; self-disclosure of your similar experience must be used carefully and only if it is likely to be therapeutic to the patient.	Alert other hospital personnel to the family's loss to prevent hurtful comments or questions.
Encourage the family not to cry.	Allow the family to see the fetus if they wish; prepare them for the appearance of the fetus.
	Reduce the number of staff with whom the family must interact.
	Summon a chaplain, minister, or rabbi.
	Make referrals to support groups in the area.

NURSING CARE PLAN 5-1

The Family Experiencing Early Pregnancy Loss

PATIENT DATA: A woman is admitted at 18 weeks' gestation and within a few hours delivers a fetus that does not survive. The woman asks what she has done wrong to cause this loss.

SELECTED NURSING DIAGNOSIS *Grieving related to loss of anticipated infant*

Outcomes	Nursing Interventions	Rationales

The woman and family will express grief to significant others.
 	
The woman and family will complete each stage of the grieving process within individual time frames.
	1. Promote expression of grief by providing privacy, eliminating time restrictions, allowing support persons of choice to visit, and recognizing individualized grief expressions and cultural norms.
	
	2. Use the four stages of grief as a basis for nursing interventions:
	  a. Stage 1: shock and disbelief at loss; characterized by numbness, apathy, impaired decision making
	  b. Stage 2: seeking answers for why loss happened; characterized by crying, tears, guilt, loss of appetite, insomnia, blame placing
	  c. Stage 3: disorganization; characterized by feelings of purposelessness and malaise; gradual resumption of normal activities
	  d. Stage 4: reorganization; characterized by sad memories, but daily functioning returns
	
	3. Use open communication techniques such as:
	  a. Quiet presence
	  b. Expression of sympathy ("I'm sorry this happened")
	  c. Open-ended statements ("This must be really sad for you")
	  d. Reflection of patient's expressed feelings ("You feel guilty because you didn't stay in bed constantly?")
	
	4. Reinforce explanations given by the health care provider or others (e.g., what the problem was, why it occurred); use simple language.
		1. Grief is an individual process and people react to it in different ways; these measures encourage woman and family to express grief and begin resolving it.
		
		2. Knowledge of normal stages of grieving helps the nurse identify whether it is progressing normally or if there is dysfunctional grieving in any family member. Stages help the nurse better interpret patients' behavior; for example, blame placing is a normal part of grieving and is not necessarily directed at the nurse or caregivers; allows the nurse to reassure the patient that feelings are normal without diminishing the intensity of their feelings.
		
		3. Presence, empathy, and open communication encourage the family to express feelings about the loss, which is the first step in resolving them. Refer as needed to community agency or multidisciplinary health care team.
		
		4. Grieving people often do not hear or understand explanations the first time they are given because their concentration is impaired.

❓CRITICAL THINKING QUESTION

If you were the patient who had an early pregnancy loss, how should your nurse best support you during your hospital stay?

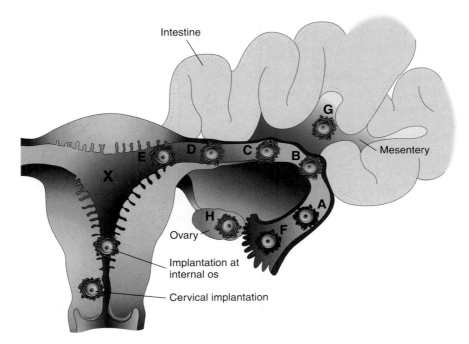

Intestine

G

Mesentery

E D C B

X

A

H

Ovary

F

Implantation at
internal os

Cervical implantation

FIGURE **5-3** The uterus and fallopian tubes illustrating various abnormal implantation sites. *A* to *F* are tubal pregnancies (the most common); *G* is an abdominal pregnancy; *X* indicates the wall of the uterus where normal implantation should occur.

fallopian tubes or inhibition of normal tubal motion to propel the zygote into the uterus may result from the following:

- Hormonal abnormalities
- Inflammation
- Infection
- Adhesions
- Congenital defects
- Endometriosis (uterine lining outside the uterus)

Use of an intrauterine device for contraception may contribute to ectopic pregnancy, because these devices promote inflammation within the uterus. A woman who has had a previous tubal pregnancy or a failed tubal ligation is also more likely to have an ectopic pregnancy.

A zygote that is implanted in a fallopian tube cannot survive for long because the blood supply and size of the tube are inadequate. The zygote or embryo may die and be reabsorbed by the woman's body, or the tube may rupture with bleeding into the abdominal cavity, creating a surgical emergency.

Manifestations. The woman often complains of lower abdominal pain, sometimes accompanied by light vaginal bleeding. If the tube ruptures, she may have sudden severe lower abdominal pain, vaginal bleeding, and signs of hypovolemic shock (Box 5-2). The amount of

vaginal bleeding may be minimal because most blood is lost into the abdomen rather than externally through the vagina. Shoulder pain is a symptom that often accompanies bleeding into the abdomen (referred pain).

Treatment. A sensitive pregnancy test for hCG is done to determine if the woman is pregnant. Transvaginal ultrasound examination determines whether the embryo is growing within the uterine cavity. Culdocentesis (puncture of the upper posterior vaginal wall with removal of peritoneal fluid) may occasionally be done to identify blood in the woman's pelvis, which suggests tubal rupture. A laparoscopic examination may be done to view the damaged tube with an endoscope (lighted instrument for viewing internal organs).

The physician attempts to preserve the tube if the woman wants other children, but this is not always possible. The priority medical treatment is to control blood loss. Blood transfusion may be required for massive hemorrhage. One of the following three courses of treatment is chosen, depending on the gestation and the amount of damage to the fallopian tube:

- No action if the pregnancy is being reabsorbed by the woman's body
- Medical therapy with methotrexate (if the tube is not ruptured), which inhibits cell division in the embryo and allows it to be reabsorbed

- Surgery to remove the pregnancy from the tube if damage is minimal; severe damage requires removal of the entire tube and occasionally the uterus

Nursing care. Nursing care includes observing for hypovolemic shock as in spontaneous abortion. Vaginal bleeding is assessed, although most lost blood may remain in the abdomen. The nurse should report increasing pain, particularly shoulder pain, to the physician.

If the woman has surgery, preoperative and postoperative care is similar to that for other abdominal surgery, as follows:

- Vital signs to identify hypovolemic shock; temperature to identify infection.
- Assessment of lung and bowel sounds.
- Intravenous fluid. Blood replacement may be ordered if the loss was substantial.
- Antibiotics as ordered.
- Pain medication, often with patient-controlled analgesia (PCA) after surgery.
- NPO preoperatively. Oral intake usually resumes after surgery, beginning with ice chips, then clear liquids, and it is advanced as bowel sounds resume.
- Indwelling catheter as ordered. Urine output is a significant indicator of fluid balance and will fall or stop if the woman hemorrhages. The minimal urine output is 30 ml/hr.
- Bed rest before surgery; progressive ambulation postoperatively. The nurse should have adequate assistance when the woman first ambulates because she is more likely to faint if she lost a significant amount of blood.

In addition to physical preoperative and postoperative care the nurse provides emotional support because the woman and her family may experience grieving similar to that accompanying spontaneous abortion. Loss of a fallopian tube threatens future fertility and is another source of grief.

> ### NURSING **TIP**
> Supporting and encouraging the grieving process in families who suffer a pregnancy loss, such as a spontaneous abortion or ectopic pregnancy, allows them to resolve their grief.

Hydatidiform Mole

Hydatidiform mole (gestational trophoblastic disease, also known as a molar pregnancy) occurs when the chorionic villi (fringelike structures that form the placenta) abnormally increase and develop vesicles (small sacs) that resemble tiny grapes (Figure 5-4). The mole may be complete, with no fetus present, or partial, in which only part of the placenta has the characteristic vesicles. Hydatidiform mole may cause hemorrhage, clotting abnormalities, hypertension, and later development of cancer (choriocarcinoma). Chromosome abnormalities are found in many cases of hydatidiform mole. It is more likely to occur in women at the age ex-

| box 5-2 | **Signs and Symptoms of Hypovolemic Shock**

- Fetal heart rate changes (increased, decreased, less fluctuation)
- Rising, weak pulse (tachycardia)
- Rising respiratory rate (tachypnea)
- Shallow, irregular respirations; air hunger
- Falling blood pressure (hypotension)
- Decreased (usually less than 30 ml/hr) or absent urine output
- Pale skin or mucous membranes
- Cold, clammy skin
- Faintness
- Thirst

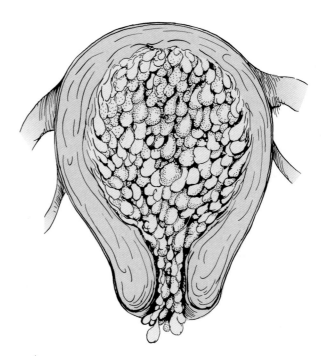

FIGURE **5-4** A hydatidiform mole (gestational trophoblastic disease).

tremes of reproductive life, and a woman who has had one molar pregnancy has a 1% chance of another molar pregnancy in the future.

Manifestations. Signs associated with hydatidiform mole appear early in pregnancy and can include the following:

- Bleeding, which may range from spotting to profuse hemorrhage; cramping may be present
- Rapid uterine growth and a uterine size that is larger than expected for the gestation
- Failure to detect fetal heart activity
- Signs of hyperemesis gravidarum (see p. 81)
- Unusually early development of pregnancy-induced hypertension (see p. 94)
- Higher than expected levels of hCG
- A distinctive "snowstorm" pattern on ultrasound but no evidence of a developing fetus in the uterus

> ⭐ NURSING **TIP**
> The nurse should teach the woman to promptly report any danger signs that occur during pregnancy.

Treatment. The uterus is evacuated by vacuum aspiration and D&C. The level of hCG is tested until it is undetectable, and the levels are followed for at least 1 year. Persistent or rising levels suggest that vesicles remain or that malignant change has occurred. The woman should delay conceiving until follow-up care is complete because a new pregnancy would confuse tests for hCG. $Rh_o(D)$ immune globulin is prescribed for the Rh-negative woman.

Nursing care. The nurse observes for bleeding and shock; care is similar to that given in spontaneous abortion and ectopic pregnancy. If the woman also experiences hyperemesis or preeclampsia, the nurse incorporates care related to those conditions as well. The woman has also lost a pregnancy, so the nurse should provide care related to grieving, similar to that for a spontaneous abortion. The need to delay another pregnancy may be a concern if the woman is nearing the end of her reproductive life and wants a child, therefore the need for follow-up examinations is reinforced. The woman is encouraged and taught how to use contraception (see Chapter 11).

BLEEDING DISORDERS OF LATE PREGNANCY

Bleeding in late pregnancy is often caused by placenta previa or abruptio placentae (Table 5-5).

Placenta Previa

Placenta previa occurs when the placenta develops in the lower part of the uterus rather than in the upper part. There are three degrees of placenta previa, depending on the location of the placenta in relation to the cervix (Figure 5-5, *A*):

- Marginal: placenta reaches within 2 to 3 cm of the cervical opening
- Partial: placenta partly covers the cervical opening
- Total: placenta completely covers the cervical opening

A low-lying placenta is implanted near the cervix but does not cover any of the opening. This variation is not a true placenta previa and may or may not be accompanied by bleeding. The low-lying placenta may be discovered during a routine ultrasound examination in early pregnancy. It also may be diagnosed during late pregnancy because the woman has signs similar to those of a true placenta previa.

Manifestations. Painless vaginal bleeding, usually bright red, is the main characteristic of placenta previa. The woman's risk of hemorrhage increases as term approaches and the cervix begins to *efface* (thin) and *dilate* (open). These normal prelabor changes disrupt the pla-

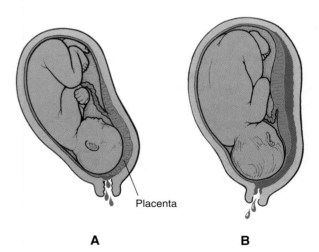

A   **B**

FIGURE **5-5 A,** Placenta previa. The placenta *(purple in this illustration)* is implanted low in the uterus. Detachment of the placenta from the uterine wall occurs as the cervix dilates, resulting in bleeding. **B,** Abruptio placentae. The placenta *(purple)* is implanted normally in the uterus but separates from the uterine wall. If the fetal head is engaged, bleeding *(red in this illustration)* may accumulate in the uterus instead of being expelled externally.

| table 5-5 | *Comparison of Placenta Previa and Abruptio Placentae* |

PLACENTA PREVIA	ABRUPTIO PLACENTAE
Abnormal implantation of the placenta in the lower uterus *Marginal:* Approaches, but does not reach, the cervical opening (≤3 cm) *Partial:* Partially covers the cervical opening *Total:* Completely covers the cervical opening	Premature separation of the normally implanted placenta *Partial:* Detachment of part of the placenta *Total:* Complete detachment of the placenta *Marginal:* Detachment at the edge of the placenta *Central:* Detachment of the center surface of the placenta; edges stay attached
BLEEDING	
Obvious vaginal bleeding, usually bright; may be profuse	Visible dark vaginal bleeding and/or concealed bleeding within the uterus; enlargement of uterus suggests that blood is accumulating within the cavity
PAIN	
None, other than from normal uterine contractions if in labor	Gradual or abrupt onset of pain and uterine tenderness; possibly low back pain
UTERINE CONSISTENCY	
Uterus soft; no abnormal contractions or irritability	Uterus firm and boardlike; may be irritable, with frequent, brief contractions
FETUS	
Fetus may be in an abnormal presentation, such as breech or transverse lie (see Chapter 8)	Fetal presentation usually normal
BLOOD CLOTTING	
Normal	Often accompanied by impaired blood clotting More likely to occur if the woman recently ingested cocaine
POSTPARTUM COMPLICATIONS	
Infection: Placental site is near the nonsterile vagina	*Infection:* Bleeding into uterine muscle fibers predisposes to bacterial invasion
Hemorrhage: Lower uterine segment does not contract as effectively to compress bleeding vessels	*Hemorrhage:* Bleeding into uterine muscle fibers damages them, inhibiting uterine contraction after birth
Signs of fetal compromise if maternal shock or extensive placental detachment occur	Signs of fetal compromise, depending on amount and location of the placental surface that is disrupted
Fetal/neonatal anemia may occur because of blood loss	Fetal/neonatal anemia may occur because of blood loss

cental attachment. The fetus is often in an abnormal presentation (e.g., breech or transverse lie) because the placenta occupies the lower uterus, which often prevents the fetus from assuming the normal head-down presentation.

The fetus or neonate may have anemia or hypovolemic shock because some of the blood lost may be fetal blood. Fetal hypoxia may occur if a large disruption of the placental surface reduces the transfer of oxygen and nutrients.

The woman with placenta previa is more likely than others to have an infection or hemorrhage after birth for the following reasons:

- Infection is more likely to occur because vaginal organisms can easily reach the placental site,

which is a good growth medium for microorganisms.

- Postpartum hemorrhage may occur because the lower segment of the uterus, where the placenta was attached, has fewer muscle fibers than the upper uterus. The resulting weak contraction of the lower uterus does not compress the open blood vessels at the placental site as effectively as would the upper segment of the uterus.

Treatment. Medical care depends on the length of gestation and amount of bleeding. The goal is to maintain the pregnancy until the fetal lungs are mature enough that respiratory distress is less likely (about 34 weeks). Delivery will be done if bleeding is sufficient to jeopardize the mother or fetus, regardless of gestational age.

The woman should lie on her side or have a pillow under one hip to avoid supine hypotension. If bleeding is extensive or the gestation is near term, cesarean delivery is done for partial or total placenta previa. The woman with a low-lying placenta or marginal placenta previa may be able to deliver vaginally unless the blood loss is excessive.

Nursing care. The priorities of nursing care include observation of vaginal blood loss and of signs and symptoms of shock. Vital signs are taken every 15 minutes if the woman is actively bleeding, and oxygen is often given to increase the amount delivered to the fetus. Vaginal examination is *not* done because it may precipitate bleeding if the placental attachment is disrupted. The fetal heart rate is monitored continuously. The nurse implements care for a cesarean delivery, as needed (see Chapter 8). The parents of the infant are often fearful for their child, particularly if a preterm delivery is required. Supportive care should be given.

> ⚡NURSING **TIP**_____
> If a vaginal examination is done when placenta previa is suspected, the physician will perform it with preparations for both vaginal and cesarean delivery (a double setup) in place.

Abruptio Placentae

Abruptio placentae is the premature separation of a placenta that is normally implanted. Predisposing factors include the following:

- Hypertension
- Cocaine or alcohol use
- Cigarette smoking and poor nutrition
- Blows to the abdomen, such as might occur in battering or accidental trauma
- Prior history of abruptio placentae
- Folate deficiency

Abruptio placentae may be partial or total (Figure 5-5, *B*); it may be marginal (separating at the edges) or central (separating in the middle). Bleeding may be visible or concealed behind the partially attached placenta.

> ⚡NURSING **TIP**_____
> Pain is an important symptom that distinguishes abruptio placentae from placenta previa.

Manifestations. Bleeding accompanied by abdominal or low back pain is the typical characteristic of abruptio placentae. Unlike the bleeding in placenta previa, most or all of the bleeding may be concealed behind the placenta. Obvious dark-red vaginal bleeding occurs when blood leaks past the edge of the placenta. The woman's uterus is tender and unusually firm (boardlike) because blood leaks into its muscle fibers. Frequent, cramplike uterine contractions often occur (uterine irritability).

The fetus may or may not have problems, depending on how much placental surface is disrupted. As in placenta previa, some of the blood lost may be fetal, and the fetus or neonate may have anemia or hypovolemic shock.

Disseminated intravascular coagulation (DIC) is a complex disorder that may complicate abruptio placentae. The large blood clot that forms behind the placenta consumes clotting factors, which leaves the rest of the mother's body deficient in these factors. Clot formation and anticoagulation (destruction of clots) occur simultaneously throughout the body in the woman with DIC. She may bleed from her mouth, nose, incisions, or venipuncture sites because the clotting factors are depleted.

Postpartum hemorrhage may also occur because the injured uterine muscle does not contract effectively to control blood loss. Infection is more likely to occur because the damaged tissue is susceptible to microbial invasion.

Treatment. The treatment of choice, immediate cesarean delivery, is done because of the risk for maternal shock, clotting disorders, and fetal death. Blood and clotting factor replacement may be needed because of DIC. The mother's clotting action quickly returns to normal after birth because the source of the abnormality is removed.

Nursing care. Preparation for cesarean section and close monitoring of vital signs and fetal heart are essential. Observation for shock and for bleeding from the nose, gums, or other unexpected sites should be promptly reported. Rapid increase in the size of the uterus suggests that blood is accumulating within it. The uterus is usually very tender and hard. Nursing care after delivery is similar to that with placenta previa.

The fetus sometimes dies before delivery (see Nursing Care Plan 5-1 for nursing care related to fetal death [stillbirth] and support of the grieving family). Many therapeutic communication techniques outlined in Table 5-4 are appropriate.

HYPERTENSION DURING PREGNANCY

Hypertension may exist before pregnancy (chronic hypertension), but it often develops as a pregnancy complication (*pregnancy-induced hypertension [PIH]*). Table 5-6 compares the different types of hypertension during pregnancy. The term preeclampsia may be used when PIH includes proteinuria. Preeclampsia pro-

table 5-6 *Hypertensive Disorders of Pregnancy*

DISORDER	CHARACTERISTICS
Pregnancy-induced hypertension (PIH)	Development of hypertension (blood pressure over 140/90 mm Hg) in a previously normotensive woman after 20 weeks' gestation
Preeclampsia	As above, with renal involvement leading to proteinuria
Eclampsia	As above, with central nervous system involvement causing seizures
HELLP (*h*emolysis, *e*levated *l*iver enzymes, *l*ow *p*latelets)	Liver and coagulation abnormalities dominate the clinical picture
Chronic hypertension	Presence of hypertension before 20 weeks' gestation and perhaps after delivery
Transient gestational hypertension	Hypertension with other signs of preeclampsia not present; blood pressure returns to normal 12 weeks postpartum

Modified from National High Blood Pressure Education Program. (2001). Working group on high blood pressure in pregnancy. *Contemporary Obstetrics and Gynecology, 46*(2), 16.

gresses to eclampsia when convulsions occur. One sometimes hears the word *toxemia,* an old word for PIH.

The cause of PIH is unknown, but birth is its cure. It usually develops after the twentieth week of gestation. Vasospasm (spasm of the arteries) is the main characteristic of PIH. Although the cause is unknown, any of several risk factors increases a woman's chance of developing PIH (Box 5-3).

There has been a gradual increase in the number of women delaying pregnancy until over age 30 years, and the chances of chronic hypertension complicating pregnancy has increased. Chronic hypertension is considered moderate if the systolic reading is below 160 mm Hg and diastolic reading is below 110 mm Hg. However, blood pressure normally decreases during the first two trimesters. Therefore when a baseline blood pressure is not known before a woman becomes pregnant, the chronic hypertension may not be revealed early and she may be diagnosed as having PIH.

Hypertension is closely related to the development of complications, such as abruptio placentae, fetal growth restriction, preeclampsia, prematurity, and stillbirth, so special care of the pregnant woman with hypertension is essential. The approach to chronic hypertension during pregnancy is complex because many drugs used to treat hypertension, such as atenolol, cause a drop in mean arterial blood pressure and can result in restricted fetal growth and other problems. For this reason, antihypertensive medication is not given for mild to moderate levels of high blood pressure. Instead, frequent prenatal visits, urinalysis to detect proteinuria, and fetal assessments are protocol, and medication is started if the blood pressure exceeds the

box 5-3 *Risk Factors for Pregnancy-Induced Hypertension*

- First pregnancy
- Obesity
- Family history of pregnancy-induced hypertension (PIH)
- Age over 40 years or under 19 years
- Multifetal pregnancy (e.g., twins)
- Chronic hypertension
- Chronic renal disease
- Diabetes mellitus

Modified from Creasy, R. & Resnick, R. (1999). *Maternal-fetal medicine* (4th ed.). Philadelphia: WB Saunders.

moderate range. Drugs of choice include methyldopa (Aldomet), alpha- and beta-adrenergic blockers (labetalol), and calcium channel blockers (nifedipine) in some cases of hypertensive crisis.

Manifestations of pregnancy-induced hypertension. Vasospasm impedes blood flow to the mother's organs and placenta, resulting in one or more of these signs: (1) hypertension, (2) edema, and (3) proteinuria (protein in the urine). Severe PIH can also affect the central nervous system, eyes, urinary tract, liver, gastrointestinal system, and blood clotting function. See Table 5-7 for a summary of laboratory tests that aid in diagnosis.

Hypertension. Despite an increase in blood volume and cardiac output, most pregnant women do not experience a rise in blood pressure because they have a resistance to factors that cause vasoconstriction. In addition, the resistance to blood flow in their vessels (peripheral vascular resistance) decreases because of the effects of

table **5-7**	*Laboratory Tests for Patients with Pregnancy-Induced Hypertension*
TEST	**RATIONALE**
Hemoglobin and hematocrit	Detects hemoconcentration to indicate severity of pregnancy-induced hypertension (PIH)
Platelets	Thrombocytopenia suggests PIH
Urine for protein	Proteinuria confirms PIH when hypotension is present
Serum creatinine	Elevated creatinine and oliguria suggest PIH
Serum uric acid	Elevated uric acid suggests PIH
Serum transaminase	Elevated transaminase confirms liver involvement in PIH

Modified from National High Blood Pressure Education Program. (2001). Working group on high blood pressure in pregnancy. *Contemporary Obstetrics and Gynecology, 46*(2), 22.

hormonal changes. A blood pressure of 140/90 mm Hg or above is considered hypertensive in pregnancy.

Edema. Edema can occur because fluid leaves the blood vessels and enters the tissues. Although total body fluid is increased, the amount within the blood vessels is reduced (hypovolemia), further decreasing blood flow to the maternal organs and placenta. It is likely to be the first sign the woman notices but is not essential to the diagnosis.

Sudden excessive weight gain is the first sign of fluid retention. Visible edema follows the weight gain. Edema of the feet and legs is common during pregnancy, but edema above the waist suggests PIH. The woman may notice facial swelling or stop wearing rings because they are hard to remove. Edema is severe if a depression remains after the tissue is compressed briefly with the finger ("pitting").

Edema resolves quickly after birth as excess tissue fluid returns to the circulation and is excreted in the urine. Urine output may reach 6 L daily and often exceeds fluid intake.

Proteinuria. Proteinuria develops as reduced blood flow damages the kidneys. This damage allows protein to leak into the urine. A clean-catch (midstream) or catheterized urine specimen is used to check for proteinuria because vaginal secretions might give a false-positive result.

Other manifestations of preeclampsia. Other signs and symptoms occur with severe preeclampsia. All are related to decreased blood flow and edema of the organs involved.

Central nervous system. A severe, unrelenting headache may occur because of brain edema and small cerebral hemorrhages. The severe headache often precedes a convulsion. Deep tendon reflexes become hyperactive because of central nervous system irritability.

Eyes. Visual disturbances such as blurred or double vision or "spots before the eyes" occur because of arterial spasm and edema surrounding the retina. Visual disturbances often precede a convulsion.

Urinary tract. Decreased blood flow to the kidneys reduces urine production and worsens hypertension.

Respiratory system. Pulmonary edema (accumulation of fluid in the lungs) may occur with severe PIH.

Gastrointestinal system and liver. Epigastric pain or nausea occurs because of liver edema, ischemia, and necrosis and often precedes a convulsion. Liver enzyme levels are elevated because of reduced circulation, edema, and small hemorrhages.

Blood clotting. HELLP syndrome is a variant of PIH that involves *h*emolysis (breakage of erythrocytes), *e*levated *l*iver enzymes, and *l*ow *p*latelets. Hemolysis occurs as erythrocytes break up when passing through small blood vessels damaged by the hypertension. Obstruction of hepatic blood flow causes the liver enzyme levels to become elevated. Low platelet levels occur when the platelets gather at the site of blood vessel damage, reducing the number available in the general circulation. Low platelet levels cause abnormal blood clotting.

Eclampsia. Progression to eclampsia occurs when the woman has one or more generalized tonic-clonic seizures. Facial muscles twitch; this sign is followed by generalized contraction of all muscles (tonic phase), then alternate contraction and relaxation of the muscles (clonic phase). *An eclamptic seizure may result in cerebral hemorrhage, abruptio placentae, fetal compromise, or death of the mother or fetus.*

Effects on fetus. PIH reduces maternal blood and nutrition flow through the placenta and decreases the oxygen available to the fetus. Fetal hypoxia may result in meconium (first stool) passage into the amniotic fluid or in fetal distress. The fetus may have intrauterine growth restriction and at birth may be long and thin with peeling skin if the reduced placental blood flow has been prolonged. Fetal death sometimes occurs.

Treatment. Medical care focuses on prevention and early detection of PIH. Drugs are sometimes needed to prevent convulsions and to reduce a dangerously high blood pressure.

Prevention. Correction of some risk factors reduces the risk for PIH. For example, improving the diet, particularly of the pregnant adolescent, may prevent PIH and promote normal fetal growth. Other risk factors, such as family history, cannot be changed. Early and regular prenatal care allows PIH to be diagnosed promptly so that it is more effectively managed.

Management. Treatment of PIH depends on the severity of the hypertension and on the maturity of the fetus. Treatment focuses on (1) maintaining blood flow to the woman's vital organs and the placenta, and (2) preventing convulsions. Birth is the cure for PIH. If the fetus is mature, pregnancy is ended by labor induction or cesarean birth. If PIH is severe, the fetus is often in greater danger from being in the uterus than from being born prematurely.

Some women with mild PIH can be managed at home if they can comply with treatment and if home nursing visits are possible (Box 5-4). If the woman has severe PIH or cannot comply with treatment, or if home nursing visits are not available, she is usually admitted to the hospital. Conservative treatment, whether at home or in the hospital, includes the following:

- Activity restriction to allow blood that would be circulated to skeletal muscles to be conserved for circulation to the mother's vital organs and the placenta. The woman should remain on bed rest on her side to improve blood flow to the placenta.
- Maternal assessment of fetal activity ("kick counts"). She should report a decrease in movement or if none occur during a 4-hour period.
- Blood pressure monitoring two to four times per day in the same arm and in the same position. A family member must be taught the technique if the woman can safely remain at home.
- Daily weight on the same scale, in the same type of clothing, and at the same time of day to observe for sudden weight gain.
- Checking urine for protein with a dipstick using a first-voided, clean-catch specimen.

Diuretics and sodium restriction are not prescribed for PIH. They are not effective for the treatment of PIH and may aggravate it because they further deplete the woman's blood volume. Aspirin therapy or dietary sup-

---

box 5-4 | *Protocol for Chronic Hypertension in Pregnancy*

- Exercise may need to be curtailed.
- Avoid weight loss programs.
- Discontinue smoking and alcohol.
- Primary management is without drugs since blood pressure normally falls in the first two trimesters of pregnancy.

---

plements such as calcium have not been shown to be helpful in managing PIH. The intake of high-salt foods is discouraged. The woman's diet should have adequate calories and protein (see Chapter 4 for prenatal dietary guidelines). Fetal assessment tests that may be done are reviewed in Table 5-1.

Drug therapy. Several drugs may also be used to treat PIH, as described in the following sections.

Magnesium sulfate is an anticonvulsant given to prevent seizures. It also may slightly reduce the blood pressure, but its main purpose is as an anticonvulsant. It is usually given by intravenous infusion (controlled with an infusion pump). Administration continues for at least 12 to 24 hours after birth because the woman remains at risk for seizures.

Magnesium is excreted by the kidneys. Poor urine output (less than 30 ml/hr) may allow serum levels of magnesium to reach toxic levels. Excess magnesium first causes loss of the deep tendon reflexes, which is followed by depression of respirations; if levels continue to rise, collapse and death can occur. *Calcium gluconate* reverses the effects of magnesium and should be available for immediate use when a woman receives magnesium sulfate.

The therapeutic serum level of magnesium is 4 to 8 mg/dl, which would be an abnormal level in a person not receiving this therapy. The woman with this serum level is slightly drowsy but retains all her reflexes and has normal respiratory function; the level is high enough to prevent convulsions.

Magnesium inhibits uterine contractions. Most women receiving the drug must also receive oxytocin to strengthen labor contractions (see Chapter 8). They are at increased risk for postpartum hemorrhage because the uterus does not contract firmly on bleeding vessels after birth. This contraction-inhibiting effect of magnesium makes it useful to stop preterm labor. The nurse should alert the newborn nursery staff when magnesium sulfate has been administered during labor, because if the newborn is treated with aminoglycosides (such as kanamycin [Kantrex] or neomycin), an interaction can occur and result in paralysis of the newborn.

Antihypertensive drugs are used to reduce blood pressure when it reaches a level that might cause intracranial bleeding, usually higher than 160/100 mm Hg. Severe hypertension can harm the fetus by causing abruptio placentae or placental infarcts (death of placental tissue). The goal of antihypertensive therapy is a gradual reduction of blood pressure to normal levels. The nurse should observe for untoward signs such as sudden hypotension. Hydralazine and labetalol are the drugs most often used. Nifedipine is not currently approved by the Food and Drug Administration (FDA) for hypertensive control. Sodium nitroprusside may be used in hypertensive crisis, but prolonged use can cause fetal complications.

Nursing care. Nursing care focuses on (1) assisting women to obtain prenatal care, (2) helping them cope with therapy, (3) caring for acutely ill women, and (4) administering medications. Nursing Care Plan 5-2 gives common interventions for women with PIH.

Promoting prenatal care. Nurses can promote awareness of how prenatal care allows risk identification and early intervention if complications arise. Nurses can help the woman to feel like an individual—especially in busy clinics, which often seem impersonal—thus encouraging her to return regularly.

Coping with therapy. Daily weights identify sudden weight gain that precedes visible edema. The weight should be checked early in the morning, after urination, and in similar clothes each day.

The nurse helps the woman to understand the importance of bed rest and to find ways to manage it. Activity diverts blood from the placenta, reducing the infant's oxygen supply, so the nurse must impress upon the woman how important rest is to her child's well-being. See preterm labor (Chapter 8) for more information about care related to bed rest.

Caring for the acutely ill woman. The acutely ill woman requires intensive nursing care directed by an experienced registered nurse. A quiet, low-light environment reduces the risk of seizures. The woman should remain on bed rest on her side, often the left side, to promote maximum fetal oxygenation. Side rails should be padded and raised to prevent injury if a convulsion occurs. Stimulation such as loud noises or bumping of the bed should be avoided. Visitors are limited, usually to one or two support persons. Suction equipment is available for immediate use.

If a seizure occurs, the nursing focus is to prevent injury and restore oxygenation to the mother and fetus. If the woman is not already on her side, the nurse should try to turn her before the seizure begins. The nurse does not forcibly hold the woman's body but prevents her from injury due to striking hard surfaces.

Breathing can stop during a seizure. An oral airway, inserted *after* the seizure, facilitates breathing and suc-

tioning of secretions. Aspiration of secretions can occur during a seizure, so the health care provider may order chest radiographs and arterial blood gas measurements. Oxygen by face mask improves fetal oxygenation. The woman is reoriented to the environment when she regains consciousness. Labor may progress rapidly after a seizure, often while the woman is still drowsy and the fetus is monitored continuously (see Chapter 6 for signs of impending birth).

Administering medications. Magnesium sulfate is administered by an experienced registered nurse. A licensed practical nurse/licensed vocational nurse (LPN/LVN) may assist. Hospital protocols provide specific guidelines for care when magnesium sulfate is given. Common protocols include the following:

- Blood pressure, pulse, respirations hourly; temperature every 4 hours
- Deep tendon reflexes every 1 to 4 hours
- Intake and output (often hourly); an indwelling Foley catheter may be ordered
- Checking urine protein with a reagent strip (dipstick) at each voiding
- Laboratory blood levels of magnesium every 4 hours

Deterioration of the maternal or fetal condition is promptly reported. Signs and symptoms of deterioration include the following:

- Increasing hypertension, particularly if blood pressure is 160/100 mm Hg or higher
- Signs of central nervous system irritability, such as facial twitching or hyperactive deep tendon reflexes
- Decreased urine output, especially if less than 25 ml/hr
- Abnormal fetal heart rates
- Symptoms such as severe headache, visual disturbances, or epigastric pain, which often immediately precede a convulsion

The registered nurse reports the following signs of possible magnesium toxicity or factors that may cause magnesium toxicity to the physician and prepares calcium gluconate to reverse this toxicity:

- Absent deep tendon reflexes
- Respiration rate under 12 breaths/min
- Urine output less than 30 ml/hr (allows accumulation of excess magnesium in the blood)
- Serum magnesium levels above 8 mg/dl

Postpartum care. PIH is of concern to the prenatal patient and the fetus and continues to be a threat in the postpartum period. Women with chronic hypertension are at risk for pulmonary edema, renal failure, and convulsions. Close monitoring for 48 hours after delivery is essential. Patients requiring antihypertensive drugs

> ⚡NURSING **TIP**
> Positioning the patient on her side during bed rest helps to improve blood flow to the placenta and more effectively provides oxygen and nutrients to the fetus.

NURSING CARE PLAN 5-2

The Woman with Pregnancy-Induced Hypertension

PATIENT DATA: A woman is admitted with signs of mild pregnancy-induced hypertension (PIH), and plans are made for discharge to the home with careful follow-up. The woman asks what she can do to avoid further complications and problems.

SELECTED NURSING DIAGNOSIS *Deficient knowledge related to home care of mild PIH*

Outcomes	Nursing Interventions	Rationales
The woman will restate correct home care measures related to PIH. The woman will keep prescribed prenatal appointments.	1. Ask the woman what she knows about hypertension during pregnancy; include family members if present.	1. Allows the nurse to build on woman's existing knowledge, reinforcing it and correcting any misunderstandings of the woman or family.
	2. Teach the woman the importance of keeping prenatal appointments, which will be more frequent because she has mild PIH.	2. PIH can quickly become more severe between prenatal care visits. If the woman understands why she should keep appointments, she is more likely to do so.
	3. Reinforce to the woman the prescribed measures to care for herself at home:	3. If woman understands these measures to limit the severity of PIH, she may be more motivated to maintain them:
	a. Remain on bed rest, spending most of the time on her side (may walk to the bathroom and eat meals at table in most cases).	a. Bed rest reduces the flow of blood to the skeletal muscles, thus making more available to placenta; this enhances fetal oxygenation.
	b. Eat a well-balanced, high-protein diet; limit high-sodium foods such as potato chips, salted nuts, pickles, and many snack foods; include high-fiber foods and at least eight glasses of noncaffeine drinks each day; consider food preferences and economic restraints when helping the woman choose appropriate foods.	b. Women with PIH lose protein in their urine, which must be replaced to maintain nutrition and fluid balance; severe sodium restriction may increase severity of PIH, but a high sodium intake may worsen hypertension and decrease the woman's blood volume; fiber and fluids help to reduce constipation, which is more likely when activity is restricted.
	c. Discuss quiet activities the woman enjoys that can be done while she is on bed rest.	c. Bed rest can lead to boredom, and the woman may not maintain the prescribed activity if she is unaware of which activities she can do.
	4. Teach the woman to report signs that indicate worsening PIH promptly: headache; visual disturbances (blurring, flashes of light, "spots" before the eyes); gastrointestinal symptoms (nausea, pain); worsening edema, especially of the face and fingers; noticeable drop in urine output.	4. PIH can worsen despite careful home management and patient compliance; if the woman has these symptoms, she needs to be evaluated and possibly hospitalized to prevent progression to eclampsia.

NURSING CARE PLAN 5-2—cont'd

SELECTED NURSING DIAGNOSIS   *Effective therapeutic regimen management related to PIH*

Outcomes	Nursing Interventions	Rationales
Blood pressure will remain within normal limits. Fetal heart rate will remain in a reassuring pattern. There will be an absence of peripheral facial and abdominal edema. Weight gain will be within normal limits. Seizures will not occur.	1. Monitor and record baseline vital signs. 2. Monitor changes in fetal heart rate (FHR). 3. Monitor urine protein (proteinuria). 4. With severe preeclampsia, keep the room quiet with minimal stimulation in environment. 5. Monitor weight gain and fluid intake and output and edema above the waist.	1. Compare baseline data to changes that occur which may indicate fetus is in jeopardy. 2. FHR reflects fetal status. 3. Protein of 3+ or more may be a sign of impending eclampsia. 4. Environmental stimulants can precipitate seizure. 5. Weight gain exceeding 0.5 kg per week is indicative of PIH. Urine output of less than 30 ml/hr may indicate renal shutdown. Edema may indicate increasing complications.

?CRITICAL THINKING QUESTION

A woman in the prenatal clinic states that high blood pressure runs in her family, and she has been taking medication for a slightly elevated blood pressure for many years. She states she has had most success with the medication she is currently taking (atenolol) and would like to continue this regimen during her pregnancy. What is the best response of the nurse?

postpartum who are breastfeeding are usually given methyldopa or labetalol. Other antihypertensive drugs may have adverse effects on the breastfeeding infant. Diuretics decrease milk production and are generally not administered.

BLOOD INCOMPATIBILITY BETWEEN THE PREGNANT WOMAN AND THE FETUS

The placenta allows maternal and fetal blood to be close enough to exchange oxygen and waste products without actually mixing (see Chapter 3). However, small leaks that allow fetal blood to enter the mother's circulation may occur during pregnancy or when the placenta detaches at birth.

No problem occurs if maternal and fetal blood types are compatible. However, if the maternal and fetal blood factors differ, the mother's body will produce antibodies to destroy the foreign fetal red blood cells (RBCs, or erythrocytes). These antibodies will pass through the placenta to the fetus and destroy the Rh-positive blood cells in the fetus.

Rh and ABO Incompatibility

People either have the Rh blood factor on their erythrocytes or they do not. If they have the factor, they are Rh positive; if not, they are Rh negative. An Rh-positive person can receive Rh-negative blood (if all other factors are compatible) because in Rh-negative blood this factor is *absent*. However, the reverse is not true for the Rh-negative person. Rh incompatibility between the woman and fetus can occur *only* if the woman is Rh negative and the fetus is Rh-positive.

The Rh-negative blood type is an autosomal recessive trait, which means that a person must receive a gene for this characteristic from both parents. The Rh-positive blood type is a dominant trait. The Rh-positive person may have inherited two Rh-positive genes or may have one Rh-positive and one Rh-negative gene. This explains why two Rh-positive parents can conceive a child who is Rh-negative.

A person with Rh-negative blood is not born with antibodies against the Rh factor. However, exposure to Rh-positive blood causes the person to make antibodies to destroy Rh-positive erythrocytes. The antibodies remain ready to destroy any future Rh-positive erythrocytes that enter the circulation (sensitization).

If fetal Rh-positive blood leaks into the mother's circulation, her body may respond by making antibodies to destroy the Rh-positive erythrocytes. This process is called isoimmunization. Because this leakage usually occurs at birth, the first Rh-positive child is rarely seriously affected. However, the woman's blood levels of antibodies increase rapidly each time she is exposed to more Rh-positive blood (in subsequent pregnancies with Rh-positive fetuses). Antibodies against Rh-positive blood cross the placenta and destroy the fetal Rh-positive erythrocytes before the infant is born. A similar response occurs with ABO incompatibility when the mother is type O and the infant's blood type is type A or type B.

Manifestations. The woman has no obvious effects if her body produces anti-Rh antibodies. Increased levels of these antibodies in her blood are revealed by rising antibody titers in laboratory tests.

When these maternal anti-Rh antibodies cross the placenta and destroy fetal erythrocytes, erythroblastosis fetalis results (Figure 5-6). The effect on the newborn is discussed in Chapter 14.

Treatment and nursing care. The primary management is to prevent the manufacture of anti-Rh antibodies by giving $Rh_o(D)$ immune globulin (RhoGAM) to the Rh-negative woman at 28 weeks' gestation and within 72 hours after birth of an Rh-positive infant or abortion (see Chapter 14). It is also given after amniocentesis and to women who experience bleeding during pregnancy, because fetal blood may leak into the mother's circulation at these times. If the fetal blood type is unknown (as in abortion), $Rh_o(D)$ immune globulin is given to the Rh-negative mother. $Rh_o(D)$ immune globulin has greatly decreased the incidence of infants with Rh incompatibility problems. However, some women are still sensitized, usually because they did not receive $Rh_o(D)$ immune globulin after childbirth or abortion. $Rh_o(D)$ immune globulin will not be effective if sensitization has already occurred.

The woman who is sensitized to destroy Rh-positive blood cells is carefully monitored during pregnancy to determine if too many fetal erythrocytes are being destroyed. Several fetal assessment tests may be used, including the Coombs' test, amniocentesis, or percutaneous umbilical blood sampling (see Table 5-1).

An intrauterine transfusion may be done for the severely anemic fetus. The Rh factor should be documented on the chart and the health care provider notified if the woman is Rh negative.

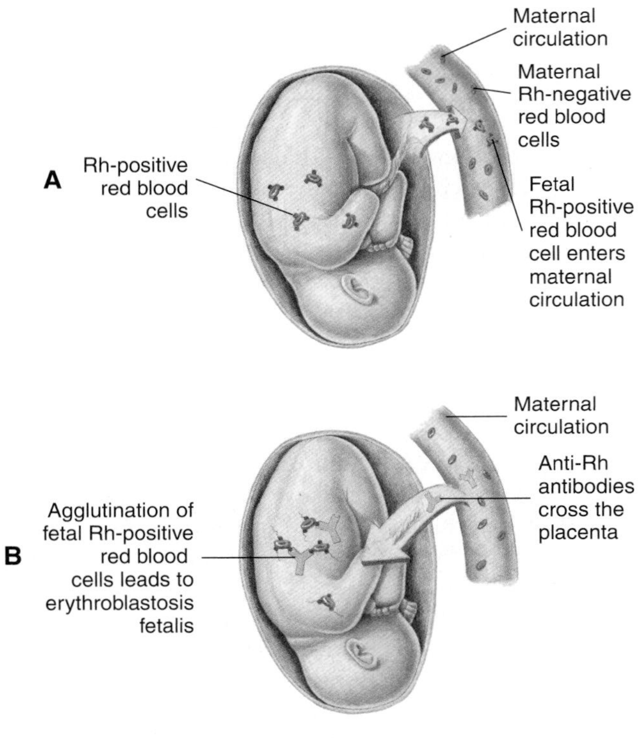

> **NURSING TIP**
>
> Most cases of Rh incompatibility between an Rh-negative mother and an Rh-positive fetus can be prevented with the administration of $Rh_o(D)$ immune globulin (RhoGAM) every time it is indicated.

FIGURE **5-6** Erythroblastosis fetalis. **A,** A few fetal Rh-positive red blood cells enter the circulation of the Rh-negative mother during pregnancy or at birth, causing mother to produce antibodies against Rh-positive blood cells. **B,** The Rh-positive antibodies from the maternal circulation cross the placenta, enter the fetal circulation, and destroy fetal Rh-positive blood cells.

PREGNANCY COMPLICATED BY MEDICAL CONDITIONS

Health problems that are present before pregnancy can influence the outcome of pregnancy and require special management. Chronic health problems discussed in this section include the following: diabetes mellitus, heart disease, anemia, and infections.

DIABETES MELLITUS

Diabetes mellitus (DM) can be classified according to whether it preceded pregnancy or had its onset during pregnancy. Types of DM include the following:

- Preexisting diabetes mellitus, which includes insulin-dependent (type I) and non–insulin-dependent (type II) diabetes with onset before pregnancy
- Gestational diabetes mellitus (GDM), which occurs only during pregnancy and is first identified during pregnancy

A medical-surgical nursing text should be consulted for a more detailed discussion of diabetes in the non-pregnant person.

Pathophysiology of Diabetes Mellitus

Diabetes mellitus is a disorder in which there is inadequate insulin to move glucose from the blood into body cells. It occurs because the pancreas produces no insulin or insufficient insulin or because cells resist the effects of insulin.

In the woman with diabetes, cells are essentially starving because they cannot obtain glucose. To compensate, the body metabolizes protein and fat for energy, which causes ketones and acids to accumulate (keto-acidosis). The person loses weight despite eating large amounts of food (polyphagia). Fatigue and lethargy accompany cell starvation. To dilute excess glucose in the blood, thirst increases (polydipsia) and fluid moves from the tissues into the blood. This results in tissue dehydration and the excretion of large amounts (polyuria) of glucose-bearing urine (glycosuria).

Effect of Pregnancy on Glucose Metabolism

Pregnancy affects a woman's metabolism (whether or not she has diabetes mellitus) to make ample glucose available to the growing fetus. Hormones (estrogen and progesterone), an enzyme (insulinase) produced by the placenta, and increased prolactin levels have two effects:

- Increased resistance of cells to insulin
- Increased speed of insulin breakdown

Most women respond to these changes by secreting extra insulin to maintain normal carbohydrate metabolism while still providing plenty of glucose for the fetus. If the woman cannot increase her insulin production, she will have periods of *hyperglycemia* (increased blood glucose levels) as glucose accumulates in the blood. Because the fetus continuously draws glucose from the mother, maternal *hypoglycemia* (low blood sugar) can occur between meals and during the night. There is also a normally increased tissue resistance to maternal insulin action in the second and third trimesters, and the fetus is then at risk for organ damage resulting from hyperglycemia.

Women who are diabetic before pregnancy must alter the management of their condition. The time of major risk for congenital anomalies to occur from maternal hyperglycemia is during the embryonic period of development in the first trimester. Therefore women who are diabetic *before* pregnancy have a greater risk for a newborn with a congenital anomaly than a woman who develops gestational diabetes, which is usually manifested after the first trimester. With careful management, most diabetic women can have successful pregnancies and healthy babies. Nevertheless, there are many potential complications of diabetes (Box 5-5).

Gestational Diabetes Mellitus

GDM is common and resolves quickly after birth; however, some women develop overt diabetes later in life. The following factors in a woman's history are linked to gestational diabetes:

- Maternal obesity (over 90 kg or 198 pounds)
- Large infant (over 4000 g or about 9 pounds [Figure 5-7], macrosomia)
- Maternal age older than 25 years
- Previous unexplained stillbirth or infant having congenital abnormalities
- History of GDM in a previous pregnancy
- Family history of DM
- Fasting glucose over 135 mg/dl or postmeal glucose over 200 mg/dl

Nursing Care Plan 5-3 lists specific interventions for the pregnant woman with GDM.

---

box 5-5 | *Effects of Diabetes in Pregnancy*

MATERNAL EFFECTS

Spontaneous abortion
Pregnancy-induced hypertension
Preterm labor and premature rupture of the membranes
Hydramnios (excessive amniotic fluid; also called polyhydramnios)
Infections
- Vaginitis
- Urinary tract infections
Complications of large fetal size
- Birth canal injuries
- Forceps-assisted or cesarean birth
Ketoacidosis

FETAL AND NEONATAL EFFECTS

Congenital abnormalities
Macrosomia (large size)
Intrauterine growth restriction
Birth injury
Delayed lung maturation
Neonatal hypoglycemia
Neonatal hypocalcemia
Neonatal hyperbilirubinemia and jaundice
Neonatal polycythemia (excess erythrocytes)
Perinatal death

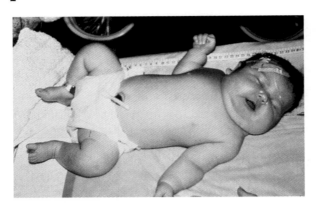

FIGURE **5-7** Macrosomic infant. A newborn with macrosomia caused by maternal diabetes mellitus during pregnancy. This infant weighed 5 kg (11 pounds) at birth. Newborns with macrosomia often have respiratory and other problems.

Treatment

The nonpregnant woman is treated with a balance of insulin or an oral hypoglycemic drug (agent that reduces blood glucose level), diet, and exercise. Some people with mild diabetes do not need drugs and control their condition by diet and exercise alone. Medical therapy during pregnancy includes identification of gestational diabetes, diet, monitoring of blood glucose levels, insulin, exercise, and selected fetal assessments.

Identification of gestational diabetes mellitus. If the woman does not have preexisting diabetes, a prenatal screening test to identify GDM is routinely done between 24 and 28 weeks' gestation. The woman drinks 50 g of an oral glucose solution (fasting is not necessary), and a blood sample is analyzed for glucose 1 hour later. If the blood glucose level is 140 mg/dl or higher, a more complex 3-hour glucose tolerance test is done.

Diet. The woman is counseled to avoid single large meals with high amounts of simple carbohydrates. A balanced food intake is divided among three meals and at least two snacks throughout the day to maintain stable blood glucose levels. The timing and content of meals and snacks may require adjustment to avoid early-morning hypoglycemia. Foods that release glucose slowly are preferred to avoid rapid changes in blood glucose.

Monitoring of blood glucose levels. To ensure a successful pregnancy the woman must keep her blood glucose levels as close to normal as possible. For self-monitored glucose, these levels are as follows:

- Fasting: not under 70 mg/dl
- Premeal: 70 to 95 mg/dl
- 1 hour postmeal: under 130 mg/dl after 1 hour; under 120 mg/dl after 2 hours

The pregnant diabetic woman monitors her blood glucose levels several times a day as directed by the health care provider. Blood glucose self-monitoring is discussed in Chapter 30. Glycosylated hemoglobin (HgA$_1$C) is an indication of long-term (4- to 6-week) glucose control and can indicate successful glucose management of the pregnant diabetic, but it cannot be used as a guide to adjust daily insulin needs during pregnancy.

Ketone monitoring. Urine ketones may be checked to identify the need for more carbohydrates. If the woman's carbohydrate intake is insufficient, she may metabolize fat and protein to produce glucose, resulting in ketonuria. However, ketonuria that is accompanied by hyperglycemia requires prompt evaluation for diabetic ketoacidosis. Ketoacidosis can be rapidly fatal to the fetus. It is more likely to occur if the woman has preexisting diabetes or if she has an infection.

Insulin. Most oral hypoglycemic agents are not used during pregnancy because they can cross the placenta, possibly resulting in fetal birth defects or neonatal hypoglycemia. Glyburide is the only oral hypoglycemic agent that can be considered for use after the first trimester when the benefits outweigh the risks for the mother and fetus. Insulin is the preferred drug prescribed to lower blood glucose levels during pregnancy because it does not cross the placenta. GDM may be controlled by diet and exercise alone, or the woman may require insulin injections. The dose and frequency of insulin injections are tailored to a woman's individual needs. Insulin is often given on a sliding scale, in which the woman varies her dose of insulin based on each blood glucose level.

The insulin regimen of a diabetic woman is different during pregnancy than in the nonpregnant state. Typically, insulin dosage may need to be reduced to avoid hypoglycemia in the first trimester, when nausea decreases appetite and physical activity may be reduced. In the second trimester, increasing placental hormones increases insulin resistance (see p. 56), and the dosage of insulin may need to be increased. Insulin requirements may drop again at 38 weeks' gestation. GDM resolves promptly after birth, when the insulin-antagonistic (diabetogenic) effects of pregnancy cease.

NPH or Lente insulin is not given at dinnertime because hypoglycemia during the night can occur. Humalog or lispro insulin is a fast-acting insulin that is highly effective if given before meals. The use of an insulin pump has proved to be of great value for glucose control in pregnant and nonpregnant patients with DM. (See Chapter 30 for the discussion of insulin administration and insulin pumps.)

Exercise. A pregnant woman with preexisting diabetes may have vascular damage, and exercise may then

NURSING CARE PLAN 5-3

The Pregnant Woman with Gestational Diabetes Mellitus

PATIENT DATA: A woman, para 0 gravida 1, is diagnosed with gestational diabetes mellitus. She states that she has no diabetes in her family history and has never been on any type of restricted diet. She is discharged home to receive home care and close follow-up.

SELECTED NURSING DIAGNOSIS   *Risk for ineffective therapeutic regimen management related to lack of knowledge about new diagnosis*

Outcomes	Nursing Interventions	Rationales
The woman will identify appropriate and inappropriate food choices. The woman will demonstrate correct self-care techniques for assessing blood glucose and administering insulin. The woman will verbalize symptoms of hypoglycemia and hyperglycemia, including correct self-care.	1. Determine knowledge of diabetes and its management, including family members if appropriate.	1. Allows nurse to identify correct and incorrect information and relate new knowledge to what the woman already knows, thus promoting individualized teaching.
	2. Assist the registered nurse to teach prescribed diet; provide written information; have the woman identify appropriate foods and the best time to eat them; general guidelines are as follows: a. Avoid simple sugars, such as cakes, candies, and ice creams because they are quickly converted to glucose, causing wide fluctuations in blood glucose levels. b. Eat complex, high-fiber carbohydrates such as grains, breads, and pasta; these foods are converted to glucose slowly, thus maintaining stable blood glucose levels. c. Eat three meals a day plus at least two snacks to balance insulin and provide sustained release of glucose to prevent hypoglycemia during late afternoon and evening.	2. A woman who understands diet requirements is more likely to follow them carefully; written information helps to refresh her memory if she forgets verbal teaching. Verbalizing food choices allows the nurse to determine if the woman has correctly learned the information.
	3. Consult with a dietitian to help maintain cultural food patterns.	3. A dietitian specializes in foods and nutrition and can help the woman to select foods that are acceptable within her dietary limits and that meet her preferences and cultural needs.
	4. Assist the registered nurse to teach the woman how to perform blood glucose monitoring; have her perform a return demonstration and/or verbalize the regimen. Common teaching includes testing frequency, accurate technique, and responses to low or high levels.	4. Insulin requirements fluctuate during pregnancy, generally increasing as pregnancy progresses. Frequent blood glucose monitoring allows adjustment of insulin, thus maintaining stable blood glucose levels; stable blood glucose levels are associated with better outcomes for mother and infant. Return demonstration of skills or verbalizing information helps the nurse determine if the woman has learned information.

Continued

Outcomes	Nursing Interventions	Rationales
	5. Assist the registered nurse to teach insulin self-administration (see Chapter 30 for additional information); have woman give a return demonstration and/or verbalization of each step; teaching includes when to take insulin and how to administer it.	5. Correct insulin administration maintains the most stable blood glucose levels; see point 4 for rationale for return demonstration and verbalization.
	6. Teach signs and symptoms of hypoglycemia and hyperglycemia (see Table 5-8); teach appropriate responses to these signs and symptoms.	6. Persistence of low or high blood glucose levels requires adjustment of insulin dose and/or food intake; in addition, hyperglycemia may be an early sign of infection in the diabetic woman. A woman who understands the signs, symptoms, and corrective actions is likely to see the care needed to maintain optimal blood glucose levels.
	7. Explain that gestational diabetes usually resolves quickly after birth but may recur in future pregnancies or in midlife.	7. Advance information about possible future diabetes improves ongoing health monitoring.

SELECTED NURSING DIAGNOSIS   *Deficient knowledge related to complications of diabetes during pregnancy*

Outcomes	Nursing Interventions	Rationales
The woman will verbalize correct responses to potential complications of gestational diabetes.	1. Teach danger signs in pregnancy (see Box 5-1) and reinforce them at each prenatal visit.	1. Increases likelihood that woman will seek prompt treatment for all pregnancy complications, including those relating to diabetes.
	2. Teach the signs and symptoms of urinary tract infection and vaginal infection, especially candidiasis or yeast infection (see Chapter 11).	2. Candidiasis is common in women with diabetes mellitus; urinary tract infections are common and can also lead to maternal sepsis or preterm labor.
	3. Explain the importance of keeping prenatal appointments.	3. Prenatal visits at prescribed intervals can prevent or allow early intervention for complications.
	4. Teach about fetal diagnostic tests done; for example, biophysical profile evaluates how well placenta is delivering oxygen and nutrients to fetus.	4. Fetal diagnostic tests allow for early identification and prompt intervention for problems; knowledge decreases woman's anxiety related to the unknown. If the woman does not understand the reason for doing diagnostic tests, she may incorrectly assume that she or her infant is in danger.

❓ CRITICAL THINKING QUESTION

A 25-year-old primigravida has been diagnosed with gestational diabetes mellitus at 25 weeks' gestation and has been managing her condition at home with diet, exercise, and insulin. During a clinic visit early in her *third* trimester, she states her mother had large infants and "everything was just fine" and does not feel any extra tests or monitoring or changes in her insulin regimen is necessary. What would be the best response of the nurse to ensure patient compliance with the prescribed regimen?

table 5-8 *Comparison of Hypoglycemia and Hyperglycemia in the Diabetic Woman*

HYPOGLYCEMIA	HYPERGLYCEMIA
Caused by excess insulin, excess exercise, and/or inadequate food intake	Caused by inadequate insulin, reduced activity, and/or excessive food intake; more likely if the woman has an infection, because this increases her need for insulin
Blood glucose below normal (usually under 60 mg/dl)	Blood glucose above normal (greater than 120 mg/dl)
Urine glucose absent	Glucosuria (glucose in the urine); possibly ketonuria (ketones in the urine)
Behavioral and physiological manifestations: hunger, trembling; weakness; faintness; lethargy; headache; irritability; sweating; pale, cool, moist skin; blurred vision; loss of consciousness	Behavioral and physiological manifestations: fatigue; headache; flushed, hot skin; dry mouth; thirst; dehydration; frequent urination; weight loss; nausea and vomiting; rapid, deep respirations (Kussmaul's respirations); acetone odor to the breath; depressed reflexes
Measures to correct: Drink a glass of milk or juice; eat a piece of fruit or two crackers; recurrent hypoglycemia requires adjustment of insulin or food intake	Measures to correct: Evaluate food intake; emphasize that patient be honest if she "cheats" to avoid inappropriate adjustment of insulin dose; identify and treat infections; insulin dose often adjusted throughout pregnancy to maintain normal glucose levels

result in ischemia (decreased circulation) to the placenta and hypoxia (decreased oxygen) to the fetus. The level of exercise should be prescribed by the health care provider and blood glucose levels monitored closely. In GDM, however, exercise can help control blood glucose levels, and diet and exercise can minimize the need for insulin. The woman with GDM should be counseled that exercise after meals is preferred because glucose levels are high. Hypoglycemia can occur if the exercise occurs when the effects of the last insulin dose are at peak. Hyperglycemia can occur if exercise occurs when the effects of the last dose of insulin have decreased. Therefore blood glucose levels should be monitored before, during, and after exercise (Table 5-8).

Fetal assessments. Assessments (see Table 5-1) may be done to identify fetal growth and the placenta's ability to provide oxygen and nutrients. Ultrasound examinations are used to identify intrauterine growth restriction, macrosomia, excess amniotic fluid (polyhydramnios) in the poorly controlled diabetic woman, or decreased amniotic fluid (oligohydramnios) in placental failure.

Diabetes can affect the blood vessels that supply the placenta, impairing the transport of oxygen and nutrients to the fetus and the removal of fetal wastes. The nonstress test, contraction stress test, and biophysical profile provide information about how the placenta is functioning. Tests of fetal lung maturity are common if early delivery is considered.

Care during labor. Labor is work (exercise) that affects the amount of insulin and glucose needed. Some women receive an intravenous infusion of a dextrose solution plus regular insulin as needed. Regular insulin is the *only* type given intravenously. Blood glucose levels are assessed hourly and the insulin dose is adjusted accordingly. Because *macrosomia* (large fetal size) is a common complication of GDM, close monitoring of the fetus during labor is essential, and cesarean delivery may be indicated. (See Chapter 8 for care of a woman requiring cesarean section.)

Care of the neonate. Infant complications after birth may include hypoglycemia, respiratory distress, and injury caused by macrosomia. Some infants have growth restriction because the placenta functions poorly. Neonatal nurses and a neonatologist (a physician specializing in care of newborns) are often present at the birth. (See Chapter 14 for a discussion of these neonatal problems.)

Nursing Care

Nursing care of the pregnant woman with diabetes mellitus involves helping her to learn to care for herself and providing emotional care to meet the demands imposed by this complication. Care during labor primarily involves careful monitoring for signs of fetal distress.

Self-care. Most women with preexisting diabetes already know how to check their blood glucose level and administer insulin. They should be taught why diabetic management changes during pregnancy. The woman

box 5-6 | *Signs of Congestive Heart Failure During Pregnancy*

- Persistent cough, often with expectoration of mucus that may be blood-tinged
- Moist lung sounds because of fluid within lungs
- Fatigue or fainting on exertion
- Difficulty breathing on exertion
- Orthopnea (having to sit upright to breathe more easily)
- Severe pitting edema of the lower extremities or generalized edema
- Palpitations
- Changes in fetal heart rate indicating hypoxia or growth restriction if placental blood flow is reduced

with newly diagnosed GDM must be taught these self-care skills.

The woman is taught how to select appropriate foods for the prescribed diet. She is more likely to maintain the diet if her caregivers are sensitive to her food preferences and cultural needs. A dietitian can determine foods to meet her needs and find solutions to problems in adhering to the diet.

The woman who takes insulin may experience episodes of hypoglycemia (low blood sugar) or hyperglycemia (high blood sugar) (see Table 5-8). The woman is taught to recognize and respond to each condition, and family members are included in the teaching. Maintaining glycemic control during pregnancy is essential to prevent later complications such as macrosomia.

Emotional support. Pregnant women with diabetes often find that living with the glucose monitoring, diet control, and frequent insulin administration is bothersome. The expectant mother may be anxious about the outcome for herself and her child. Therapeutic communication helps her to express her frustrations and fears. For example, to elicit her feelings about her condition the nurse might say, "Many women find that all the changes they have to make are demanding. How has it been for you?" It may help to emphasize that the close management is usually temporary, especially if she has GDM.

A woman who is actively involved in her care is more likely to maintain the prescribed therapy. Referral to a diabetes management center is often helpful. As she learns to manage her care, liberal praise motivates the woman to maintain her therapy.

Breastfeeding. Studies have shown that newborns who have been exclusively breastfed have a lower incidence of developing diabetes later in life. Breastfeeding should be encouraged if the newborn does not have

perinatal complications related to maternal diabetes, such as macrosomia, respiratory problems, or anomalies. Blood glucose levels of newborns are monitored closely in the first 24 hours of life. Breastfeeding uses glucose reserves in the mother, and glucose monitoring of the mother after breastfeeding is important. Fluids or food intake during breastfeeding may be desirable.

HEART DISEASE

Heart disease affects a small percentage of pregnant women. During a normal pregnancy, an increase in heart rate, blood volume, and cardiac output places a physiological strain on the heart that may not be tolerated in a woman with preexisting heart disease. Cardiac failure can occur prenatally, during labor or in the postpartum period.

Manifestations. Increased levels of clotting factors predispose a woman to thrombosis (formation of clots in the veins). If her heart cannot meet these increased demands of pregnancy, congestive heart failure (CHF) results and the fetus suffers from reduced placental blood flow. See Box 5-6 for signs and symptoms of CHF.

During labor, each contraction temporarily shifts 300 to 500 ml of blood from the uterus and placenta into the woman's circulation, possibly overloading her weakened heart. Excess interstitial fluid rapidly returns to the circulation after birth, predisposing the woman to circulatory overload during the postpartum period. She remains at an increased risk for CHF after birth until her circulating blood volume returns to normal levels in the postpartum period.

> ≯NURSING **TIP**
> The nurse should observe the woman with heart disease for signs of congestive heart failure, which can occur before, during, or after birth.

Treatment. The pregnant woman with heart disease is usually under the care of both a cardiologist and an obstetrician. She needs more frequent antepartum visits to determine how her heart is coping with the increased demands of pregnancy. Excessive weight gain must be avoided because it adds to the demands on her heart. Preventing anemia with adequate diet and supplemental iron prevents a compensatory rise in the heart rate, which would add to the strain on the woman's heart. The priority of care is limiting physical activity to decrease the demands made on the heart. The limitation of activity can range from frequent rest periods to strict bed rest depending on the degree of heart impairment. A woman on prolonged bed rest for any reason has a greater risk for forming venous thrombi (blood clots).

Drug therapy may include heparin to prevent clot formation. Anticoagulants such as warfarin (Coumadin) may cause birth defects and are not given during pregnancy.

Beta-adrenergic blocking drugs used to treat hypertension and arrhythmia can cause fetal bradycardia (slow heartbeat), respiratory depression, and hypoglycemia. Thiazide diuretics can cause harmful effects on the fetus, especially if given in the third trimester. Angiotensin-converting enzyme (ACE) inhibitors are contraindicated during pregnancy.

A vaginal birth is preferred over cesarean delivery because it carries less risk for infection or respiratory complications that would further tax the impaired heart. Forceps or a vacuum extractor may be used to decrease the need for maternal pushing (see Chapter 8).

Nursing care. A woman with heart disease may already be familiar with its management. She should be taught needed changes, such as the change from warfarin anticoagulants to subcutaneous heparin, and should be instructed in how to inject the drug. Laboratory tests include partial thromboplastin time (PTT), activated partial thromboplastin time (aPTT), and platelet counts. She should promptly report signs of excess anticoagulation, such as bruising without reason, petechiae (tiny red spots on the skin), nosebleeds, or bleeding from the gums when brushing her teeth.

The woman is taught signs that may indicate CHF so that she can promptly report them. The nurse helps her to identify how she can obtain rest to minimize the demands on her heart. She should avoid exercise in temperature extremes. She should be taught to stop an activity if she experiences dyspnea, chest pain, or tachycardia.

The woman may need help to plan her diet so that she has enough calories to meet her needs during pregnancy but without gaining too much weight. She should be taught about foods that are high in iron and folic acid to prevent anemia. She should avoid foods high in sodium, such as smoked meats and potato chips. Foods high in vitamin K should be avoided in patients receiving heparin therapy.

Stress can also increase demands on the heart. The nurse should discuss stressors in the woman's life and help her to identify ways to reduce them. During hospitalization the health care provider should be notified if the pulse exceeds 100 beats/min or respirations are greater than 25 breaths/min at rest. Signs of dyspnea (difficulty in breathing), coughing, and abnormal breath sounds should be recorded and reported. Postpartum bradycardia (slowed heart rate) should be reported to the health care provider because the heart may fail as a result of the increased blood volume that occurs after delivery.

ANEMIA

Anemia is the reduced ability of the blood to carry oxygen to the cells. Hemoglobin levels lower than 10.5 to 11 g/dl indicate anemia during pregnancy. Four anemias are significant during pregnancy: two nutritional anemias (iron-deficiency anemia and folic acid-deficiency anemia), and two anemias resulting from genetic disorders (sickle cell disease and thalassemia).

Nutritional Anemias

Most women with anemia have vague symptoms, if any. The anemic woman may fatigue easily and have little energy. Her skin and mucous membranes are pale. Shortness of breath, a pounding heart, and a rapid pulse may occur with severe anemia. The woman who develops anemia gradually has fewer symptoms than the woman who becomes anemic abruptly, such as through blood loss.

Iron-deficiency anemia. The pregnant woman needs additional iron for her own increased blood volume, for transfer to the fetus, and for a cushion against the blood loss expected at birth. The RBCs are small (microcytic) and pale (hypochromic) in iron-deficiency anemia. The tannic acid in tea and bran may decrease absorption of iron from foods eaten at the same meal.

Prevention. Iron supplements are commonly used to meet the needs of pregnancy and maintain iron stores. Vitamin C may enhance the absorption of iron. Iron should not be taken with milk or antacids because calcium impairs absorption.

Treatment. The woman with iron-deficiency anemia needs extra iron to correct the anemia and replenish her stores. She is treated with oral doses of *elemental iron* and continues this dose for about 3 months after the anemia has been corrected.

Folic acid-deficiency anemia. Folic acid (also called folate or folacin) deficiency is characterized by large, immature RBCs (megaloblastic anemia). Iron-deficiency anemia is often present at the same time. Anticonvulsants, oral contraceptives, sulfa drugs, and alcohol can decrease the absorption of folate from meals.

Prevention. Folic acid is essential for normal growth and development of the fetus. Folic acid deficiency has been associated with neural tube defects in the newborn. A supplement of 400 µg (0.4 mg) each day ensures adequate folic acid and is now recommended for all women of childbearing age.

Treatment. Treatment of folate deficiency is with folic acid supplementation, 1 mg/day (over twice the amount of the preventive supplement). The dose of preventive folic acid supplementation may be higher for women who have had a previous child with a neural tube defect.

Genetic Anemias

Sickle cell disease. Unlike nutritional anemias, people with sickle cell disease have abnormal hemoglobin that causes their erythrocytes to become distorted in a sickle (crescent) shape during episodes of hypoxia or acidosis. It is an autosomal recessive disorder, meaning that the person receives an abnormal gene from each parent. The abnormally shaped blood cells do not flow smoothly, and they clog small blood vessels. The sickle cells are destroyed faster, resulting in chronic anemia. Approximately one out of 12 African-Americans have the trait (HgbAS). (See Chapter 26 for further discussion of sickle cell disease.)

Pregnancy may cause a sickle cell crisis with massive erythrocyte destruction and occlusion of blood vessels. The main risk to the fetus is occlusion of vessels that supply the placenta, leading to preterm birth, growth retardation, and fetal death.

The woman should have frequent evaluation and treatment for anemia during prenatal care. Fetal evaluations concentrate on fetal growth and placental function. Oxygen and fluids are given continuously during labor to prevent sickle cell crisis. Genetic counseling should be offered.

Thalassemia. Thalassemia is a genetic trait that causes an abnormality in one of two chains of hemoglobin, the alpha (α) or beta (β) chain. The β chain variety is most often encountered in the United States. The person can inherit an abnormal gene from each parent, causing β-thalassemia major, or Cooley's anemia. If only one abnormal gene is inherited, the person will have β-thalassemia minor.

The woman with β-thalassemia minor usually has few problems other than mild anemia, and the fetus does not appear to be affected. However, administration of iron supplements may cause iron overload in a woman with β-thalassemia because the body absorbs and stores iron in higher than usual amounts.

Nursing Care for Anemias During Pregnancy

The woman is taught which foods are high in iron and folic acid to prevent or treat anemia (Box 5-7). She is taught how to take the supplements so that they are optimally effective. For example, the nurse explains that although milk is good to drink during pregnancy, it should not be taken at the same time as the iron supplement or the iron will not be absorbed as easily. Vitamin C foods may enhance absorption.

The woman is taught that when she takes iron, her stools will be dark green to black and that mild gastrointestinal discomfort may occur. She should contact her physician or nurse-midwife if these side effects trouble

---

> **box 5-7**   *Foods Recommended in Pregnancy*
>
> **FOODS HIGH IN IRON**
>
> Meats, chicken, fish, liver, legumes, green leafy vegetables, whole or enriched grain products, nuts, blackstrap molasses, tofu, eggs, dried fruits
>
> **FOODS HIGH IN FOLIC ACID**
>
> Green leafy vegetables, asparagus, green beans, fruits, whole grains, liver, legumes, yeast
>
> **FOODS HIGH IN VITAMIN C (MAY ENHANCE ABSORPTION OF IRON)**
>
> Citrus fruits and juices, strawberries, cantaloupe, cabbage, green and red peppers, tomatoes, potatoes, green leafy vegetables

---

her; another iron preparation may be better tolerated. She should not take antacids with iron.

The woman with sickle cell disease requires close medical and nursing care. She should be taught to avoid dehydration and activities that cause hypoxia. The woman with β-thalassemia is taught to avoid situations in which infections are more likely (e.g., avoid crowds during flu season) and to report any symptoms of infection promptly. See Chapter 26 for a discussion of sickle cell anemia and thalassemia.

> **NURSING TIP**
>
> To prevent or correct nutritional anemias, such as iron and folic acid deficiencies, the nurse should teach all women appropriate food sources of those nutrients.

INFECTIONS

The acronym TORCH has been used to describe infections that can be devastating for the fetus or newborn. The letters stand for the first letters of these four infections or infectious agents: *t*oxoplasmosis, *r*ubella, *c*ytomegalovirus, and *h*erpes simplex virus; the *o* is sometimes used to designate "other" infections. However, there are many more infections that may be devastating for the mother, fetus, or newborn. Some of these are damaging any time they are acquired, whereas others are relatively harmless except when acquired during pregnancy.

Viral Infections

Viral infections often have no effective therapy and may cause serious problems in the mother and/or fetus or newborn. Immunizations can prevent some of these infections. Some are sexually transmitted diseases, although they have other routes of transmission.

Cytomegalovirus. Cytomegalovirus (CMV) infection is widespread and commonly occurs during the childbearing years. The infection is often asymptomatic in the mother. However, an infected infant may have serious problems, as follows:

- Mental retardation
- Seizures
- Blindness
- Deafness
- Dental abnormalities
- Petechiae (often called a "blueberry muffin" rash)

Treatment and nursing care. There is no effective treatment for CMV infection. Therapeutic pregnancy termination may be offered if CMV infection is discovered during early pregnancy.

Rubella. Rubella is a mild viral disease with a low fever and rash. However, its effects on the developing fetus can be destructive. Rubella occurring in very early pregnancy can disrupt the formation of major body systems, whereas rubella acquired later is more likely to damage organs that are already formed. Some effects of rubella on the embryo/fetus include the following:

- Microcephaly (small head size)
- Mental retardation
- Congenital cataracts
- Deafness
- Cardiac defects
- Intrauterine growth restriction (IUGR)

Treatment and nursing care. Immunization against rubella infection has been available for some time, but some women of childbearing age are still susceptible. When a woman of childbearing age is immunized, she should not get pregnant for at least 3 months after the immunization. The vaccine is offered during the postpartum period to nonimmune women. It is *not* given during pregnancy because it is a live attenuated (weakened) form of the virus.

NURSING TIP

Rubella is a cause of birth defects that is almost completely preventable by immunization before childbearing age. The nurse should check each postpartum woman's chart for rubella immunity and notify her physician or nurse-midwife if she is not immune.

Herpesvirus. There are two types of herpes viruses, types 1 and 2. Type 1 is more likely to cause fever blisters or cold sores. Type 2 is more likely to cause genital herpes.

After the primary infection the virus becomes dormant in the nerves and may be reactivated later as a recurrent (secondary) infection. Initial infection during the first half of pregnancy may cause spontaneous abortion, IUGR, and preterm labor. Most pregnancies are affected by recurrent infections rather than primary infections. The infant is infected by one of the following ways:

- The virus ascends into the uterus after the membranes rupture.
- The infant has direct contact with infectious lesions during vaginal delivery.

Neonatal herpes infection can be either localized or disseminated (widespread). Disseminated neonatal infection has a high mortality rate and survivors may have neurological complications.

Treatment and nursing care. Neonatal herpes infection can be prevented by avoiding contact with the lesions. If the woman has active genital herpes lesions when the membranes rupture or labor begins, a cesarean delivery may be required to avoid fetal contact during birth or ascending infection. Cesarean birth is not necessary if there are no active genital lesions. The mother and infant do not need to be isolated as long as direct contact with lesions is avoided (see Appendix A). Breastfeeding is safe if there are no lesions on the breasts.

Hepatitis B. The virus that causes hepatitis B infection can be transmitted by blood, saliva, vaginal secretions, semen, and breast milk; it can also cross the placenta. The woman may be asymptomatic or acutely ill with chronic low-grade fever, anorexia, nausea, and vomiting. Some become chronic carriers of the virus. The fetus may be infected transplacentally or by contact with blood or vaginal secretions at birth. The infant may become a chronic carrier and a continuing source of infection. Box 5-8 lists those who are at greater risk of having hepatitis B infection.

Treatment and nursing care. All women should be screened for hepatitis B during prenatal care, and the screening should be repeated during the third trimester for women in high-risk groups. Infants born to women who are positive for hepatitis B should receive a single dose of hepatitis B immune globulin (for temporary immunity right after birth) followed by hepatitis B vaccine (for long-term immunity). The Centers for Disease Control and Prevention (CDC) recommend routine immunization with hepatitis B vaccine for all newborns (those born to carrier mothers and to noncarrier mothers) at birth, 1 to 2 months, and 6 to 18 months. Immunization during pregnancy is contraindicated. If possible, injections should be delayed until after the infant's first bath, so that blood and other potentially infectious secretions are removed to avoid introducing them

box 5-8 | *Persons at Higher Risk for Hepatitis B Infection*

- Intravenous drug users
- Persons with multiple sexual partners
- Persons with repeated infection with sexually transmitted diseases
- Health care workers with occupational exposure to blood products and needle sticks
- Hemodialysis patients
- Recipients of multiple blood transfusions or other blood products
- Household contact with hepatitis carrier or hemodialysis patient
- Persons arriving from countries where there is a higher incidence of the disease

box 5-9 | *High-Risk Factors for Human Immunodeficiency Virus (HIV)*

- Intravenous drug abuse and needle sharing
- Multiple sexual partners
- Prostitution
- Blood transfusion before 1985
- History of sexually transmitted diseases
- Immigration from area where infection is endemic, such as Haiti or Central Africa
- Sexual partner in a high-risk group
- Sexual partner with HIV infection

under the skin. Because they have occupational exposure to blood and other infectious secretions, health care staff should be immunized against hepatitis B.

Human immunodeficiency virus. Human immunodeficiency virus (HIV) is the causative organism of acquired immunodeficiency syndrome (AIDS). The virus eventually cripples the immune system, making the person susceptible to infections that eventually can result in death. There is no known immunization or curative treatment. (See Chapter 11 or a medical-surgical text for further discussion of AIDS, infections associated with the syndrome, and treatment.)

Although first identified in homosexual males, the incidence of HIV infection and AIDS continues to rise in women. HIV infection is acquired one of the following three ways:

- Sexual contact (anal or vaginal) with an infected person
- Parenteral or mucous membrane exposure to infected body fluids
- Perinatal exposure (infants)

The infant may be infected in one of the following ways:

- Transplacentally
- Through contact with infected maternal secretions at birth
- Through breast milk

The infected woman has a 20% to 40% chance of transmitting the virus to her fetus perinatally. Infants born to HIV-positive women will be HIV-positive at birth because maternal antibodies to the virus pass through the placenta to the infant. From 3 to 6 months are needed to identify the infants who are truly infected.

Nursing care. Counseling should be provided to all women concerning behaviors that place them at risk for developing AIDS (Box 5-9). HIV testing is recom-

mended for all prenatal patients. HIV-positive women should be educated that the transmission of HIV infection to the newborn can be greatly reduced by appropriate drug therapy. Pregnant women with AIDS are more susceptible to infection, and the fetus may develop an impaired immune system that increases the risk of opportunistic infections after birth. Breastfeeding may be contraindicated for mothers who are actively HIV-positive.

The fetus and the woman are monitored closely during the antepartum period. All infants born to HIV-positive women are presumed to be HIV-positive, and standard care precautions (see Appendix A) are initiated for both mother and infant. The infant may receive drug therapy during the first 6 weeks of life. The nurse should anticipate and help the mother cope with the anxiety that is almost certain to occur about whether the neonate is infected. Social services can help the family with the care of the child at home. Women should be taught about the risks of sharing needles, the importance of using condoms, and the need to avoid oral sex.

>NURSING **TIP**_____

The nurse should wear protective equipment, such as gloves, with *every* potential exposure to a patient's body secretions. This practice protects the nurse from direct exposure to many pathogenic organisms.

Nonviral Infections

Toxoplasmosis. Toxoplasmosis is caused by *Toxoplasma gondii*, a parasite that may be acquired by contact with cat feces or raw meat and transmitted through the placenta. The woman usually has mild symptoms. Congenital toxoplasmosis includes the following possible signs in the newborn:

- Low birth weight
- Enlarged liver and spleen

- Jaundice
- Anemia
- Inflammation of eye structures
- Neurological damage

Treatment and nursing care. Specific treatment for toxoplasmosis is controversial. Therapeutic abortion may be offered to the woman who contracts the infection during the first half of pregnancy. Nurses can teach women the following measures to reduce the likelihood of acquiring the infection:

- Cook all meat thoroughly.
- Wash hands and all kitchen surfaces after handling raw meat.
- Avoid touching the mucous membranes of the eyes or mouth while handling raw meat.
- Avoid uncooked eggs and unpasteurized milk.
- Wash fresh fruits and vegetables well.
- Avoid materials contaminated with cat feces, such as litter boxes, sand boxes, and garden soil.

Group B streptococcus infection. Group B streptococcus (GBS) is a leading cause of perinatal infections that have a high neonatal mortality rate. The organism is found in the woman's rectum, vagina, cervix, throat, or skin. Although she is colonized with the organism, the woman is usually asymptomatic, but the infant may be infected through contact with vaginal secretions at birth. The risk is greater if the woman has a long labor or premature rupture of membranes. GBS is a significant cause of maternal postpartum infection (endometritis, or infection of the uterine interior), especially after cesarean birth. Symptoms include an elevated temperature within 12 hours after delivery, rapid heart rate (tachycardia), and abdominal distention. Diagnosis of GBS is confirmed by culture.

GBS infection can be deadly for the infant. A newborn may have either early-onset (before 7 days) or late-onset (after 7 days) GBS infection.

Treatment. A culture of the woman's rectum and vagina for the presence of GBS should be taken at 35 to 37 weeks' gestation. All positive cultures require immediate penicillin treatment. High risk factors such as previous history of GBS infection, prolonged rupture of the membranes, or fever above 37.7° C (100° F) during labor require penicillin treatment to prevent GBS infection. Any GBS-positive urine culture is considered a cause for antibiotic treatment during pregnancy, and the newborn is treated with antibiotics at birth. See Chapter 9 for more information about neonatal GBS infection.

Tuberculosis. The incidence of tuberculosis is rising in the United States, and drug-resistant strains of the bacterium are emerging. Pregnant women are screened as other patients (refer to a medical-surgical nursing text). If the screening test is positive, they should have a chest radiograph (x-ray) with the abdomen shielded with a lead apron. Sputum specimens that are positive for the bacterium confirm the diagnosis.

The adult with tuberculosis experiences fatigue, weakness, loss of appetite and weight, fever, and night sweats. The newborn may acquire the disease by contact with an untreated mother after birth.

Treatment and nursing care. Isoniazid and rifampin are usually prescribed for 9 months. Pregnant women who are taking isoniazid should also take pyridoxine to reduce the risk of peripheral neuritis. Ethambutol may be given if drug-resistant tuberculosis is suspected. The infant may have preventive therapy with isoniazid for 3 months. The health care staff, including nurses, must teach the family how the organism is transmitted and the importance of continuing the antitubercular drugs consistently for the full course of therapy. Incompletely treated tuberculosis is a significant cause of drug-resistant organisms. Modern antitubercular drugs usually render the sputum negative within 2 weeks so that home care is the protocol, with health department follow-up.

Sexually Transmitted Diseases

Sexually transmitted diseases (STDs) are those for which a common mode of transmission is sexual intercourse, although several can also be transmitted in other ways. Herpesvirus and HIV infections have been discussed. Other infections that are typically transmitted sexually are syphilis, gonorrhea, chlamydia, trichomoniasis, and condylomata acuminata (genital warts).

Changes in the vaginal secretions that occur during pregnancy can increase the risk of developing a vaginal infection. The high estrogen levels present during pregnancy thicken the vaginal mucosa and increase secretions that have a high glycogen content. This makes the woman susceptible to yeast infections and other problems. Later in pregnancy the pH of the vagina decreases, resulting in a protective effect.

All sexual contacts of persons infected with a disease that can be sexually transmitted should be informed and treated; otherwise the cycle of infection and reinfection will continue. Consistent use of a latex condom, including the female condom, helps to reduce the sexual spread of STDs. STDs and vaginal infections are discussed in detail in Chapter 11.

Urinary Tract Infections

Urinary tract infections (UTIs) are common in females because of the short urethra, contamination of the urethra from the rectum, and contamination from the vagina during sexual activity.

The urinary tract is normally self-cleaning because acidic urine inhibits the growth of microorganisms and flushes them out of the body with each voiding. Pregnancy alters this self-cleaning action because pressure on urinary structures keeps the bladder from emptying completely and because the ureters dilate and lose motility under the relaxing effects of the hormone progesterone. Urine that is retained in the bladder becomes more alkaline, providing a favorable environment for the growth of microorganisms.

Some women have excessive microorganisms in their urine but no symptoms (asymptomatic bacteriuria). The asymptomatic infection may eventually cause cystitis (bladder infection) or pyelonephritis (kidney infection). The woman with cystitis has the following signs and symptoms:

- Burning with urination
- Increased frequency and urgency of urination
- A normal or slightly elevated temperature

If not treated, cystitis can ascend in the urinary tract and cause pyelonephritis. Pyelonephritis is a particularly serious infection in pregnancy and is accompanied by the following signs and symptoms:

- High fever
- Chills
- Flank pain or tenderness
- Nausea and vomiting

Maternal hypertension, chronic renal disease, and preterm birth may occur with pyelonephritis during pregnancy. The high maternal fever is dangerous for the fetus because it increases the fetal metabolic rate, which in turn increases fetal oxygen needs to levels that the mother cannot readily supply.

Treatment. UTIs are treated with antibiotics, often ampicillin. Asymptomatic bacteriuria is treated with oral antibiotics for 10 days, cystitis for 1 to 2 weeks. Pyelonephritis is treated with multiple antibiotics, initially administered intravenously. Cystitis in pregnant women is treated with a full 7 days of antibiotic therapy.

> ✴NURSING **TIP**
> The nurse should teach all females measures to reduce their risk for urinary tract infections.

Nursing care. All females should be taught how to reduce the introduction of rectal microorganisms into the bladder. For example, a front-to-back direction should be used when wiping after urination or a bowel movement, when doing perineal cleansing, or when applying and removing perineal pads. The nurse can begin teaching during the woman's prenatal visits and rein-force it during the postpartum stay. The mother should be taught how to clean and diaper an infant girl to avoid fecal contamination of her urethra.

Adequate fluid intake promotes frequent voiding. At least eight glasses of liquid per day, excluding caffeine-containing beverages, helps to flush urine through the urinary tract regularly. Cranberry juice may make the urine more acidic and therefore less conducive to the growth of infectious organisms.

Sexual intercourse mildly irritates the bladder and urethra, which can promote a UTI. Urinating before intercourse reduces irritation; urinating afterward flushes urine from the bladder. Using water-soluble lubricant during intercourse can also reduce periurethral irritation related to intercourse.

Pregnant women should be taught the signs and symptoms of cystitis and pyelonephritis so that they will know to seek treatment at once.

ENVIRONMENTAL HAZARDS DURING PREGNANCY

A teratogen is a substance that causes an adverse effect on the developing embryo or fetus. Some birth defects are caused by a combination of genetic and environmental factors. The specific anomaly that develops depends on the time of exposure to the environmental teratogen in relation to the stage of development of the embryo. In the first weeks of life the vital organs are developing and exposure to an environmental teratogen may cause miscarriage. Exposure to a teratogen in later pregnancy might result in growth restriction. The four main teratogens of concern during pregnancy are drugs, chemicals, infectious agents, and radiation.

BIOTERRORISM AND THE PREGNANT PATIENT

The concepts learned in a microbiology class come to life when nurses discuss the current threat of bioterrorism. In general, there are three categories of biological agents:

- Category A: Can be easily transmitted from person to person (such as smallpox, anthrax, or tularemia)
- Category B: Can be spread via food and water (such as Q fever, brucellosis, and *Staphylococcus* enterotoxin B [SEB])
- Category C: Can be spread via manufactured weapons designed to spread disease (such as Hantavirus and tick-borne encephalitis)

Even diseases not normally transmitted by airborne means can be altered to make them transmissible by air.

Therefore routine knowledge of an illness related to bioterrorist attacks does not always indicate all possible methods of transmission.

The obstetrical nurse must be observant for unusual symptoms present in large numbers of young, healthy pregnant patients who come to the clinic or emergency department. This unusual increase should trigger suspicion of a bioterrorism-related illness and be reported to the charge nurse or unit manager. These suspicions should then be promptly reported to the local health department or to the CDC to ensure that appropriate safety protocols are activated. A laboratory test, Rapid Antigen Detection for influenza, can be performed on these patients. A positive result on this test rules out symptoms that mimic influenza but may be an early sign of a bioterrorist infection.

The approach to the care of a pregnant patient who is a victim of a bioterrorist attack may follow protocols similar to those presented in this section of general trauma during pregnancy. Other general protocols relate to the use of standard precautions (see Appendix A), the maintenance of a safe food and water supply to ensure adequate nutrition and hydration, and the maintenance of a safe air supply to prevent further transmission of disease (Box 5-10). The use of available vaccines for the pregnant patient can adversely affect the fetus and must be carefully evaluated, and informed consent must be obtained. The choice of antibiotics must also be weighed according to the risks to the fetus and the mother whenever possible.

Nurses should participate in community emergency preparedness programs that set up response protocols for patients of all ages and provide shelters, supportive services, intensive care units, emergency supplies, and communication services. Continuing education units (CEUs) are now available to help the nurse stay current in this area of nursing. *Morbidity and Mortality Weekly Report* (MMWR) is a publication available to health care professionals via the Internet to monitor for any unusual biological or chemical outbreaks across the nation and worldwide (http://www.cdc.gov/mmwr).

---

box 5-10 | ***Precautions Required for Common Bioterrorist Agents***

- Botulism, anthrax, tularemia: Standard precautions
- Smallpox, tuberculosis: Airborne precautions
- Plague: Droplet precautions
- Hemorrhagic fever: Airborne, droplet, and contact precautions

SUBSTANCE ABUSE

The use of illicit or recreational drugs during pregnancy has an adverse effect on both the mother and the fetus. Often multiple drugs are used, and lifestyle factors such as malnutrition, poor prenatal care, and STDs also may exist. Prescribed drugs are assigned a "pregnancy risk category" by the FDA that are published in most drug reference books. Classifications range from A (no risk) to D (positive evidence of risk) and X (contraindicated in pregnancy).

It is well established that several legal and illicit substances are harmful to the developing fetus (Figure 5-8). Many environmental substances are most harmful to the fetus early in pregnancy, perhaps before the woman realizes she is pregnant. Table 5-9 reviews some substances that are harmful to the fetus.

> NURSING **TIP**
>
> When questioning about substance use during pregnancy, the nurse should focus on how the information will help nurses and physicians provide the safest and most appropriate care to the pregnant woman and her infant.

Treatment and Nursing Care

Care focuses on identifying the substance-abusing woman early in pregnancy, educating her about their

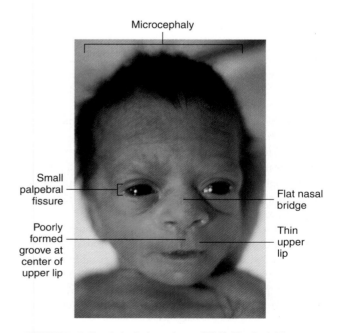

FIGURE **5-8** Fetal alcohol syndrome (FAS). The facial features of an infant with FAS include short palpebral (eye) fissures; a flat nasal bridge; a thin, flat upper lip; a poorly formed groove at the center of the upper lip; and a small head (microcephaly).

table 5-9 | **Substances Harmful to the Fetus**

SUBSTANCE	EFFECTS
Alcohol	Alcohol is the most commonly abused substance by women of childbearing age. Fetal alcohol syndrome (FAS) is well documented (see Figure 5-8) and includes growth restriction, mental retardation, and facial abnormalities. No "safe" level of alcohol ingestion during pregnancy is known.
Cocaine	Cocaine is a powerful central nervous system (CNS) stimulant that causes vasoconstriction that may precipitate preterm labor. It can cause hypertension, seizures, and stroke in the mother, fetal anomalies, and addiction in the newborn.
Marijuana	Harmful effects of marijuana use during pregnancy are not clearly identified but cannot be ruled out. Marijuana users may ingest other substances, and this lifestyle may be harmful to the fetus.
Tobacco	Smoking can cause fetal growth restriction. Nicotine causes vasoconstriction that reduces blood flow to the placenta. Nicotine patches also expose the fetus to this substance. Poor pregnancy outcome has been linked to smoking.
Heroin	The heroin-addicted woman is likely to be exposed to HIV because the drug is taken intravenously and may include the use of dirty needles and a lifestyle of high-risk behaviors. Withdrawal syndrome (agitation, cramps, diarrhea, rhinorrhea [runny nose]) occurs if drug is stopped suddenly. Neonatal abstinence syndrome occurs within 24 hours of birth (high-pitched cry, tremors, seizures, and disrupted sleep-wake cycles). Serious maternal and fetal effects occur.
Anticoagulants	Warfarin (Coumadin) can cross the placenta and cause spontaneous abortion, growth restriction, CNS problems, and facial defects (fetal warfarin syndrome). Heparin does not cross the placenta and is the drug of choice when an anticoagulant is required; however, it can cause premature labor.
Antibiotics	A few antibiotics have an adverse effect on the fetus, although no anomalies have been reported. Tetracycline exposure after the fourth month of gestation can cause yellowing of the deciduous teeth and hyperplasia of the enamel. To avoid tooth discoloration, tetracycline is not advised for children under age 7 years. Drugs such as streptomycin and kanamycin are associated with damage to the eighth cranial nerve and hearing loss in the newborn.

effects, and encouraging her to reduce or eliminate their use. Appropriate referrals should be made.

A partnership should be created with the woman, and a plan for compromises and treatment should be developed. Dietary support, monitoring of their weight gain, and fetal assessment promote better pregnancy outcomes.

In the case of therapeutic drugs, the woman's need for the drug is weighed against the potential for fetal harm it may cause and the fetal or maternal harm that may occur if the woman is not treated. In general, the health care provider will choose the least teratogenic drug that is effective and prescribe it in the lowest effective dose.

Educating females about the effect of drugs on a developing fetus is best done before pregnancy. Because drug use is prevalent in schools, preadolescence is not too soon to begin this education. Women should be taught to eliminate the use of any unnecessary substance before becoming pregnant. A woman is encouraged to tell her health care provider if she thinks she is pregnant (or is trying to conceive) before having a non-emergency radiograph, being prescribed a drug, or taking herbal or food supplements.

A trusting, therapeutic nurse-patient relationship makes it more likely that a woman will be truthful about the use of substances, both legal and illicit. The nurse who collects data must use a nonjudgmental approach and treat the problem as a health problem rather than a moral problem. The nurse should support the woman who is trying to reduce her drug use. The nurse should praise her efforts to improve her overall health and to have a successful pregnancy.

A multidisciplinary approach is needed to plan for the care of a mother and newborn that includes referral to community agencies after discharge or child protec-

table 5-9	*Substances Harmful to the Fetus—cont'd*
SUBSTANCE	**EFFECTS**
Anticonvulsants	Dilantin (diphenylhydantoin) can cause craniofacial abnormalities and mental retardation in the fetus and may be carcinogenic. The woman must be counseled concerning the risk of medication and the benefits of seizure control during pregnancy. Trimethadione (Tridione) and paramethadione (Paradione) are used to treat petit mal epilepsy and are contraindicated in pregnancy because of the high risk for major anomalies. Pregnant women who must take valproic acid (Depakene) or carbamazepine (Tegretol) should have fetal assessments for skeletal anomalies and neural tube defects. The use of phenobarbital has not been associated with the development of anomalies, but neonatal withdrawal may occur.
Isotretinoin (Accutane) and vitamin A derivatives	Isotretinoin and etretinate are used for skin disorders and are clearly associated with fetal anomalies and are contraindicated in pregnancy. Birth control is advised for a minimum of 3 months after isotretinoin therapy.
Diethylstilbestrol (DES)	DES can cause uterine malformation, vaginal carcinoma, and testicular abnormalities in the newborn.
ACE inhibitors (captopril, enalapril)	ACE inhibitors can cause fetal kidney anomalies, growth restriction, and oligohydramnios (decreased amniotic fluid).
Folic acid antagonists (methotrexate, amethopterin)	Folic acid antagonists cause spontaneous abortion and serious fetal anomalies.
Lithium	Lithium is associated with the development of congenital heart disease. It can also be toxic to the thyroid and kidneys of the fetus.
Radiation	Radiation exposure before 6 weeks' gestation can cause serious fetal damage that includes leukemia, eye and CNS anomalies, and fetal loss. Doses for diagnostic tests are small, and the risk to the fetus is small; however, abdominal protection with lead aprons is advised. Therapeutic radiation is contraindicated during pregnancy.

tive services if needed. The American Academy of Pediatrics has listed drugs that are contraindicated during breastfeeding (Lewis, 2000). This should be used as a guide in counseling mothers concerning breastfeeding.

TRAUMA DURING PREGNANCY

There is a high incidence of trauma during the childbearing years. The incidence of trauma during pregnancy may continue to rise because women are increasingly employed during their pregnancy and there is a trend toward a more violent society. Automobile accidents, homicide, and suicide are the three leading causes of traumatic death. Although pregnant women usually are more careful to protect themselves from harm, increased stress from pregnancy may lead to injury both in and out of the home. Falls are not uncommon because of the woman's altered sense of balance. The pregnant woman also needs to be especially careful when stepping in and out of the bathtub or when using a ladder or stepstool.

The automobile is another hazard. The woman needs to wear a seat belt every time she is in a car, both as a driver and as a passenger. The lap portion of the belt is placed low, just below her protruding abdomen. The pregnant woman and her fetus are more likely to suffer severe injury or death because of not being restrained during a crash than they are to be injured by the restraint itself. Air bags are a *supplemental* restraint and are intended for use in addition to seat belts. No one should ride with anyone who has been drinking alcohol or whose judgment is impaired for other reasons.

Physical trauma is usually blunt trauma (falls or blows to the body) but may be penetrating trauma (knife or gunshot wounds). Physical abuse against women (battering) is a significant cause of trauma, and the violence often escalates during pregnancy.

Battering occurs in all ethnic groups and all social strata. It often begins or becomes worse during pregnancy. The abuser is usually her male partner, but he may be another male, such as the father of a pregnant adolescent. Men who abuse women are also likely to abuse children in the relationship.

Women abused during pregnancy are more likely to have miscarriages, stillbirths, and low-birth-weight babies. They often enter prenatal care late, if at all. The risk of homicide escalates during pregnancy.

Abuse during pregnancy, as at other times, may take many forms. It is not always physical abuse; many women are abused emotionally. Emotional abuse makes leaving the relationship especially difficult because it lowers the woman's self-esteem and isolates her from sources of help. The time of greatest danger to the abused woman occurs when she leaves her abuser.

Manifestations of Battering

In addition to having late or erratic prenatal care, the battered woman may have bruises or lacerations in various stages of healing. A radiograph may reveal old fractures. The woman tends to minimize injury or "forget" its severity. She may assume responsibility for the trauma, as evidenced by remarks such as, "If I had only kept the children quiet, he wouldn't have gotten so mad." Her abuser is often unusually attentive after the battering episode.

Treatment and Nursing Care of the Pregnant Woman Experiencing Trauma

Nurses must be aware that any woman may be in an abusive relationship. Therapeutic, nonjudgmental communication helps establish a trusting relationship. Nonabused women, including nurses, often cannot understand why a woman would stay in a harmful relationship. The abuser has usually isolated the woman by controlling whom she sees, where she goes, and how she spends money. Emotional abuse often supplements physical abuse, making the woman feel that she is "stupid" or "no good" and that she is "lucky that he loves her because no one else would ever love her." She usually feels that she has no choice but to stay in the abusive relationship. She may assume part of the blame, believing that her abuser will stop hurting her if she tries harder.

The woman being assessed for abuse is taken to a private area. The nurse determines whether there are factors that increase the risk for severe injuries or homicide, such as drug use by the abuser, a gun in the house, use of a weapon, or violent behavior by the abuser outside the home. The nurse also determines whether the children are being hurt. *It is vital that the abuser not find out that the woman has reported the abuse or that she intends to leave.*

> ⭐ NURSING **TIP**
>
> If a woman confides that she is being abused during pregnancy, this information must be kept absolutely confidential. Her life may be in danger if her abuser learns that she has told anyone. She should be referred to local shelters, but the decision to leave her abuser is hers alone.

Nurses can refer women to shelters and other services if they wish to leave the abuser. However, the decision about whether to end the relationship rests with the woman. Abuse of children must be reported to appropriate authorities.

Nursing care for the acutely injured pregnant woman supplements medical management: the focus is on stabilizing the mother's condition when life-threatening injuries occur. Placing a small pillow under one hip tilts the heavy uterus off the inferior vena cava to improve blood flow throughout the woman's body and to the placenta. An assessment of vital signs and urine output reflects blood circulation to the kidneys. Urine output should average at least 30 ml/hr. Bloody urine may indicate damage to the kidneys or bladder.

The nurse assesses for uterine contractions or tenderness, which may indicate onset of labor or abruptio placentae. Continuous electronic fetal monitoring (see Chapter 6) is usually instituted if the fetus is viable and near maturity.

In cases of severe trauma and blood loss, the nurse must relate the increased blood volume of pregnancy to the probable need for increased fluid and blood intake for stabilizing the pregnant trauma patient. Peripheral vasoconstriction that normally occurs as a response to shock will cause a decreased flow of oxygen to the fetus. Placing a pillow under one hip to prevent pressure of the uterus on the vena cava is essential. Because of the increased coagulation status of the pregnant woman, the aftermath of trauma can result in a high risk for blood-clotting problems such as thrombophlebitis. Values of fibrinogen of 200 to 400 mg/100 ml may be normal for a nonpregnant patient but are indicative of the development of disseminated intravascular coagulation (DIC) in the pregnant woman, who normally has a fibrinogen level of 400 to 650 mg/100 ml. A fractured pelvis may result in cephalopelvic disproportion (CPD) and require cesarean delivery. Dopamine, a drug routinely used to achieve hemodynamic stability in trauma patients, causes uteroplacental vasoconstriction and may lead to fetal death.

The use of tocolytics to delay labor may be contraindicated in some types of trauma such as burns. Magnesium sulfate is a vasodilator and also may be contraindicated in some types of trauma and shock. Electrical shock injuries can be more serious to the fetus even though the mother does not seem to be seriously injured because amniotic fluid offers low resistance to the passage of the electrical current to the fetus. In general, it is important for the nurse to understand and correlate the physiology of pregnancy in order to help the mother and fetus who are victims of trauma.

EFFECTS OF A HIGH-RISK PREGNANCY ON THE FAMILY

Normal pregnancy can be a crisis because it is a time of significant change and growth. The woman with a complicated pregnancy has stressors beyond those of the normal pregnancy. Her family is also affected by the pregnancy and impending birth.

DISRUPTION OF USUAL ROLES

The woman who has a difficult pregnancy must often remain on bed rest at home or in the hospital, sometimes for several weeks. Others must assume her usual roles in the family, in addition to their own obligations. Finding caregivers for young children in the family may be difficult if extended family live far away. Placing the children in day care may not be an option if financial problems exist.

Nurses can help families adjust to these disruptions by identifying sources of support to help maintain reasonably normal household function.

FINANCIAL DIFFICULTIES

Many women work outside the home, and their salary may stop if they cannot work for an extended period. At the same time, their medical costs are rising. Social service referrals may help the family cope with their expenses.

DELAYED ATTACHMENT TO THE INFANT

Pregnancy normally involves gradual acceptance of and emotional attachment to the fetus, especially after the woman feels fetal movement. Fathers feel a similar attachment, although at a slower pace. The woman who has a high-risk pregnancy often halts planning for the child and may withdraw emotionally to protect herself from pain and loss if the outcome is poor.

LOSS OF EXPECTED BIRTH EXPERIENCE

Couples rarely anticipate problems when they begin a pregnancy. Most have specific expectations about how their pregnancy, particularly the birth, will proceed.

A high-risk pregnancy may result in the loss of their expected experience. They may be unable to attend childbirth preparation classes or to have a vaginal birth. Nurses can help incorporate as many of the couple's plans as possible, particularly at the time of birth.

key points

- Hyperemesis gravidarum is persistent nausea and vomiting of pregnancy and often interferes with nutrition and fluid balance.
- The most common reason for early spontaneous abortion is abnormality of the developing fetus or placenta.
- If a woman has a tubal rupture from an ectopic pregnancy, the nurse should observe for shock.
- Because of hemorrhage into the abdomen, vaginal blood loss may be minimal, whereas intraabdominal blood loss can be massive in a tubal rupture.
- The woman who has gestational trophoblastic disease (hydatidiform mole) should have follow-up medical care for 1 year to detect the possible development of choriocarcinoma. She should not get pregnant during this time.
- Placenta previa is the abnormal implantation of the placenta in the lower part of the uterus.
- Abruptio placentae is the premature separation of the placenta that is normally implanted.
- The three main manifestations of preeclampsia are hypertension, edema, and proteinuria.
- Eclampsia occurs when the woman has a seizure.
- A positive nonstress test (NST) indicates heart accelerations and is reassuring of fetal health.
- A negative contraction stress test (CST) indicates there are no late decelerations after a uterine contraction and denotes fetal health.
- An abortion is the termination of pregnancy before the fetus is viable.
- Positioning the mother on her left side during bed rest helps improve blood flow to the placenta and avoid pressure on the vena cava.
- A blood pressure of 140/90 mm Hg or above is considered hypertension in the pregnant patient.
- A routine, noninvasive ultrasound examination can confirm pregnancy, detect some anomalies, and reveal the sex of the fetus.
- Rh_o(D) immune globulin (RhoGAM) can be given to an Rh-negative mother to prevent blood incompatibilities between the mother and an Rh-positive fetus (erythroblastosis fetalis).
- Gestational diabetes mellitus first occurs during pregnancy and resolves after pregnancy. The newborn may be excessively large (macrosomia), and the mother may develop diabetes mellitus later in life. Control of blood glucose level is essential to protect the fetus.

- TORCH diseases of pregnancy include *t*oxoplasmosis, *r*ubella, *c*ytomegalovirus, and *h*erpes, with the *o* for *o*thers.
- The nurse must consider the physiological changes during pregnancy to understand and care for the pregnant trauma victim. Both the mother and fetus must be monitored closely.
- Urinary tract infections are more common during pregnancy because compression and dilation of the ureters result in urine stasis. Preterm labor is more likely to occur if a woman has pyelonephritis.
- The fetus of the woman who takes drugs (legal or illicit) or drinks alcohol is exposed to higher levels of the substance for a longer time because the substances become concentrated in the amniotic fluid and the fetus ingests the fluid.
- Drugs and alcohol consumed by the mother can cross the placenta and adversely effect the developing fetus.

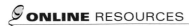

ONLINE RESOURCES

Pregnancy and Exercise: http://www.familydoctor.org/handouts/305.html

Violence Against Women: http://www.ojp.usdoj.gov/vawo

REVIEW QUESTIONS   *Choose the most appropriate answer.*

1. A woman has an incomplete abortion followed by vacuum aspiration. She is now in the recovery room and is crying softly with her husband. Select the most appropriate nursing action.
   1. Leave the couple alone, except for necessary recovery room care
   2. Tell the couple that most abortions are for the best because the infant would be abnormal
   3. Tell the couple that spontaneous abortion is very common and does not mean they cannot have other children
   4. Express your regret at their loss and remain nearby if they want to talk about it

2. A woman is admitted with a diagnosis of "possible ectopic pregnancy." Select the nursing assessment that should be promptly reported.
   1. Absence of vaginal bleeding
   2. Complaint of shoulder pain
   3. Stable pulse and respiratory rate; rise in blood pressure more than 10 mm Hg systolic
   4. Temperature of 99.6° F (37.6° C)

3. It is important to emphasize that a woman who has gestational trophoblastic disease (hydatidiform mole) should continue to have follow-up medical care after initial treatment because:
   1. Choriocarcinoma sometimes occurs after the initial treatment
   2. She has lower levels of immune factors and is vulnerable to infection
   3. Anemia complicates most cases of hydatidiform mole
   4. Permanent elevation of her blood pressure is more likely

4. Select the primary difference between the symptoms of placenta previa and abruptio placentae.
   1. Fetal presentation
   2. Presence of pain
   3. Abnormal blood clotting
   4. Presence of bleeding

5. During the prenatal clinic visit, your intervention with an abused woman is successful if you have assessed the status of the woman and:
   1. Persuaded her to leave her abusive partner
   2. Informed her of her safety options
   3. Convinced her to notify the police
   4. Placed her in a shelter for abused women

Nursing Care During Labor and Birth

1. Define each key term listed.
2. Describe the four components ("four *P*s") of the birth process: powers, passage, passenger, and psyche.
3. Describe how the four *P*s of labor interrelate to result in the birth of a infant.
4. Explain the normal processes of childbirth: premonitory signs, mechanisms of birth, and stages and phases of labor.
5. Explain how false labor differs from true labor.
6. Compare the advantages and disadvantages for each type of childbearing setting: hospital, freestanding birth center, and home.
7. Determine appropriate nursing care for the intrapartum patient, including the woman in false labor and the woman having a vaginal birth after a cesarean birth (VBAC).
8. Explain common nursing responsibilities during the birth.
9. Discuss specific cultural beliefs the nurse may encounter when providing care to a woman in labor.
10. Describe the care of the newborn immediately after birth.

acrocyanosis (ăk-rō-sī-ă-NŌ-sĭs, p. 152)
amnioinfusion (ăm-nē-ō-ĭn-FŪ-zhăn, p. 140)
amniotomy (ăm-nē-ŌT-ŏ-mē, p. 141)
bloody show (p. 131)
cold stress (p. 151)
crowning (p. 144)
doula (DŪ-lă, p. 143)
efface (ĕ-FĀS, p. 124)
episiotomy (ĕ-pēz-ē-ŎT-ō-mē, p. 135)
fontanel (FŎN-tă-nĕl, p. 127)
lie (p. 127)
molding (p. 127)
neutral thermal environment (p. 151)
Nitrazine test (p. 141)
nuchal cord (NŪ-kăl kŏrd, p. 140)
ophthalmia neonatorum (ŏf-THĂL-mē-ă nē-ō-nă-TŌR-ăm, p. 153)

station (p. 131)
suture (p. 127)
uteroplacental insufficiency (ū-tăr-ō-plă-SĔN-tăl ĭn-să-FĬSH-ăn-sē, p. 140)
vaginal birth after cesarean (VBAC) (p. 144)

Childbirth is a normal physiological process that involves the health of the mother and a fetus, who will become part of our next generation. The nursing care is unique because every nursing intervention involves the welfare of two patients and the use of skills from medical-surgical and pediatric nursing, psychosocial and communication skills, and specific skills involved in obstetrical care. In addition, labor and delivery are often a family affair, with fathers, grandparents, and others closely involved. The details of this experience are often remembered for a long time by each family participant.

The privacy and rights of the mother must be protected, the policies and procedures of the institution must be considered, and the nurse must be familiar with the scope of practice set out by the state board of nursing. Recent changes in the management of labor and delivery include practices related to induction and augmentation of labor, fetal monitoring techniques, maternal positions, types of analgesia offered, and assistive devices such as vacuum extraction.

This chapter provides information concerning the birth process and the nursing responsibilities during labor and delivery. A chart correlating the physiology of the four stages of labor with the related nursing interventions can be used as a guide in planning the care of the woman during labor and delivery.

CULTURAL INFLUENCE ON BIRTH PRACTICES

The needs of the woman may be influenced by her cultural background, which may be very different from that of the nurse but must be understood and respected. In a multicultural environment, nothing is routine. Patient and cultural preferences require flexibility on the

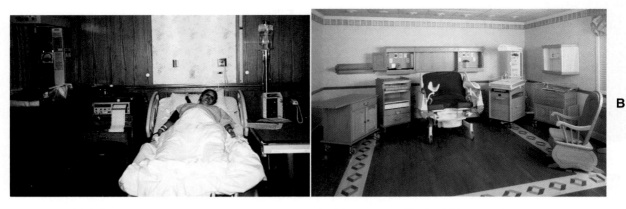

FIGURE **6-1 A,** Typical labor, delivery, and recovery (LDR) room. Homelike furnishings can be quickly adapted to provide essential equipment **(B)** when woman enters active phase of labor.

part of the nurse. Most cultures prefer the presence of a support person at all times during labor and delivery, and that can include the father or family as well as professional staff. The United States is a multicultural society. Table 6-1 lists common traditional birth practices of selected cultures. The practices of these cultural groups may vary depending on the amount of time they have been in the United States and the degree of "westernization" they have achieved.

SETTINGS FOR CHILDBIRTH

Depending on facilities available in their area and the risks for complications, a woman can choose among three settings in which to deliver her child. Most women give birth in the hospital, whereas others choose freestanding birth facilities or their own home with a nurse-midwife.

HOSPITALS

The woman who chooses a hospital birth may have a "traditional" setting, in which she labors, delivers, and recovers in separate rooms. After the recovery period, she is transferred to the postpartum unit.

A more common setting for hospital maternity care is the birthing room, often called a labor-delivery-recovery (LDR) room. The woman labors, delivers, and recovers in this room. She is then transferred to the postpartum unit for continuing care.

The appearance of the birthing room is more homelike than institutional. The fully functional birthing bed has wood trim that hides its utilitarian purpose (Figure 6-1). The beds have receptacles for various fittings, such as a "squat bar," which facilitates squatting during second-stage labor. The foot of the bed can be detached or rolled away to reveal foot supports or stirrups.

Another hospital birth setting is a single-room maternity care arrangement, often called a labor-delivery-recovery-postpartum (LDRP) room. It is similar to the LDR room, but the mother and infant remain in the same room until discharge.

Advantages of hospital-based birth settings include the following:

- Preregistration, which allows important information to be available on admission
- Easy access to sophisticated services and specialized personnel if complications develop
- Ability to provide family-centered care for the woman who has a complicated pregnancy

FREESTANDING BIRTH CENTERS

Some communities have birth centers that are separate from, although usually near, hospitals. These settings are similar to outpatient surgical centers. Many birth centers are operated by full-service hospitals and are close enough for easy transfer if the mother, fetus, or newborn develops complications. Certified nurse-midwives often attend the births.

Advantages of freestanding birth centers include the following:

- A homelike setting for the low-risk woman
- Lower costs because the freestanding center does not require expensive departments such as emergency or critical care

Disadvantages include the following:

- A slight but significant delay in emergency care if the mother or child develops life-threatening complications

HOME

Some women give birth at home. Many factors enter their decision, and most families have carefully weighed the pros and cons of their choice.

table 6-1 | *Birth Practices of Selected Cultural Groups*

ROLE OF WOMAN IN LABOR AND DELIVERY	ROLE OF FATHER/PARTNER IN LABOR AND DELIVERY
AMERICAN INDIAN	
Is stoic	Husband avoids eating meat during perinatal phase.
May have indigenous plants in room	Husband may provide support during labor.
May wear special necklaces	
May commonly use meditation chants	
Prefers water at room temperature to drink	
Prefers chicken soup and rice postpartum	
ARABIC	
Is passive but expressive	Husband is not expected to participate but remains in control.
Views keeping body covered as important	Female family member is preferred as coach.
May wear protective amulets	Husband must be present if male health care provider examines woman.
May have low pain tolerance	Husband may whisper praises in newborn's ear.
Values male newborn more than female	
Expects 20 days of bed rest after birth	
AFRICAN-AMERICAN	
Participates actively	Female attendants are usually preferred.
Is vocal in labor	
Wants only sponge bath postpartum	
Avoids hair washing until lochia ceases	
CAMBODIAN (KHMER)	
Is stoic in labor	Individual family preference decides if father is present during delivery.
If walking during labor, must not pause in doorway (thought to delay birth)	
Does not want head touched without permission	
Colostrum discarded	
Will not nurse after delivery or eat vegetables in first week	
CENTRAL AMERICA (GUATEMALA, NICARAGUA, SALVADOR)	
Is vocal and active during labor	Husband is expected to present for support, but female family members participate more.
May prefer to wear red (a protective color)	
If more affluent, prefers bottle feeding	
Prefers chicken soup, banana, meat, and herbal tea and showers postpartum	
Avoids "cold foods"	
CHINESE	
May be vocal during labor	Husband usually do not play an active role in labor and delivery, but oldest male makes decisions.
Must not pause in doorway if walking during labor (thought to delay birth)	Woman's mother may participate.
All doors and windows to be unlocked (thought to ease passage of infant)	
Do not use first name of woman	
May not shower for 30 days postpartum	
Covers ears to prevent air from entering body	
Prefers breastfeeding	
Needs to be encouraged to ask questions	
CUBAN	
Is vocal but passive during labor and delivery	Mother of woman preferred as coach.
Uses formal name at introduction	Husband are not usually involved in labor but must be informed first of problems and progress.
Must stay at home 41 days postpartum and sheltered from stress	

Data from Nichols, F.H.; & Zwelling, E. (1997). *Maternal-newborn nursing: theory and practice.* Philadelphia: WB Saunders; Minark, P.A., Lipson, J.G., & Dibble, S.L. (1996). *Culture and nursing care.* San Francisco: University of California, San Francisco, School of Nursing; Lowdermilk, D.L., Perry, S.E., & Bobak, I.M. (2000). *Maternity and women's health care* (7th ed.). St Louis: Mosby; Lipson, J.G., & Steiger, N.J. (1996). *Self-care nursing in a multicultural context.* Thousand Oaks, Calif: Sage Publications; Wong, D.L., Perry, S.E., & Hockenberry-Eaton, M. (2002). *Maternal and child nursing care* (2nd ed.). St Louis: Mosby; Murasaki, S. (1996). *Diary of Lady Murasaki.* New York: Penguin Books.

NOTE: Use professional translators whenever possible. Family members may not convey taboo topics accurately. *Continued*

table 6-1 | *Birth Practices of Selected Cultural Groups—cont'd*

ROLE OF WOMAN IN LABOR AND DELIVERY	ROLE OF FATHER/PARTNER IN LABOR AND DELIVERY
ERITREAN/ETHIOPIAN	
Is stoic but takes active role	Traditionally, husbands are not allowed to be present
Modesty very important, must remain covered	during labor and delivery.
Prefers breastfeeding for 2 years	
Remains in seclusion 40 days postpartum	
All food and drinks during puerperium must be warm	
FILIPINO	
Prefers slippery foods (such as eggs) so infant will "slip through birth canal"	Husband is not usually with woman during labor.
Prefers midwife support	
Assumes active role in labor	
Prefers sponge baths postpartum	
FALKLAND ISLANDS	
Places keys (unlock) and combs (untangle) under pillow of labor bed	Husband is expected to be supportive.
HINDU, SIKH, MUSLIM, NEPALESE, FIJI, PAKISTAN	
Assumes passive role and follows directions of trained professionals	Female coach is preferred, although father waits near labor room for consultation.
May keep head covered during labor	Husband must be present if male physician examines woman.
Prenatal care started on one hundred twentieth day of gestation	Ceremony of "A qiqah" involves father shaving head of newborn and whispering praises into ear of newborn.
Should not reveal sex of newborn until after placenta is delivered (to avoid upsetting the mother if the sex is not of her preference)	Coach may chant scriptures during birth.
Takes sponge baths postpartum	
Remains in seclusion 40 days postpartum	
HMONG (LAOS, BURMA, THAILAND)	
Is usually quiet and passive	Husband is usually present and makes all decisions.
Avoids multiple caregivers	
Avoids internal examinations	
Views full genital exposure as unacceptable	
Prefers squat position	
Do not remove amulets on wrists or ankles	
Do not use first name initially	
Prefers chicken, white rice, and warm fluids postpartum	
Bottle feeding popular	
ISRAELI (ORTHODOX JEWISH)	
Prefers nurse-midwife	Husband may not participate in prenatal classes.
Maintains modesty	Husband may not touch wife during labor, view perineum, or view infant as it is born.
Must not be intimate with husband until 7 days after lochia stops	Husband may participate from afar with verbal encouragement during labor.
Males are circumcised on the eighth day	Woman's mother participates in birth process.
Females named on first Saturday after birth	
JAPANESE	
Prefers north part of room	Chants and rice throwing ward off evil spirits.
May cut hair and take special vows	Modern-day husbands present and participate during labor and delivery.
Is assertive during labor but may not ask for pain relief	

Data from Nichols, F.H.; & Zwelling, E. (1997). *Maternal-newborn nursing: theory and practice.* Philadelphia: WB Saunders; Minark, P.A., Lipson, J.G., & Dibble, S.L. (1996). *Culture and nursing care.* San Francisco: University of California, San Francisco, School of Nursing; Lowdermilk, D.L., Perry, S.E., & Bobak, I.M. (2000). *Maternity and women's health care* (7th ed.). St Louis: Mosby; Lipson, J.G., & Steiger, N.J. (1996). *Self-care nursing in a multicultural context.* Thousand Oaks, Calif: Sage Publications; Wong, D.L., Perry, S.E., & Hockenberry-Eaton, M. (2002). *Maternal and child nursing care* (2nd ed.). St Louis: Mosby; Murasaki, S. (1996). *Diary of Lady Murasaki.* New York: Penguin Books.
NOTE: Use professional translators whenever possible. Family members may not convey taboo topics accurately.

table 6-1 | *Birth Practices of Selected Cultural Groups—cont'd*

ROLE OF WOMAN IN LABOR AND DELIVERY	ROLE OF FATHER/PARTNER IN LABOR AND DELIVERY
JAPANESE—*cont'd*	
Modesty is important Will bathe and shower postpartum Infant may be bathed twice each day for a week with loud noise and music to ward off evil spirits	In modern Japan, husbands are compliant with health education.
KOREAN	
Is compliant with health care provider Avoids ice water Is an active participant in labor Do not address by first name initially Prefers sponge bath postpartum May breastfeed but needs instruction on pumping and storage of milk May not wish to ambulate early	Husband participates in labor and delivery. Husband prefers not to be told in advance of fetal prognosis. Family makes medical decisions.
MEXICAN AMERICAN	
Believes supine position is best for fetus Decides her selected coach Prefers privacy Accepts pain but is active in labor Will not shower postpartum and ambulates only to bathroom Avoids beans postpartum Uses alternative therapies for mother and infant (see Chapter 33)	Husband is in control of decisions but is not present during labor. Female relatives provide support. Husband prefers not to be told in advance of serious fetal prognosis.
PUERTO RICAN	
Is active in labor Prefers hospital care Keeps body covered Does not eat beans, starch, or eggs if breastfeeding Will not wash hair for 40 days postpartum Prefers sponge bath and lotions	Husband assumes supportive role during labor and delivery. If not present during delivery, husband expects to be kept informed.
SOUTH AMERICAN (BRAZILIAN)	
May not participate in coping techniques during delivery Needs to be offered pain relief options Stays at home for 40 days postpartum except for medical appointments	Presence of husband in delivery room is discouraged.
VIETNAMESE	
Woman expected to "suffer in silence" Offer options for pain relief Prefers upright position for labor and delivery Prefers warm fluids to drink Sponge bathes only for 2 weeks postpartum Newborn is not praised to protect from jealousy	Female family member is preferred. Husband is expected to remain nearby. Sexual intercourse is prohibited during pregnancy and puerperium.
WEST INDIAN (TRINIDAD, JAMAICA, BARBADOS)	
Prefers midwife Maintains passive role and follows instructions Prefers bed rest for 1 week postpartum Do not address by first name initially	Female relative or friend as coach is preferred. Husband is not present in area.

Advantages of a home birth include the following:

- Control over persons who will or will not be present for the labor and birth, including children
- No risk of acquiring pathogens from other patients
- A low-technology birth, which is important to some families

Disadvantages may include the following and vary with the location within the country:

- Limited choice of birth attendants. Most physicians and nurse-midwives will not attend home births. In many communities, only lay midwives (whose training and abilities vary widely) attend home births. Lay midwives may not be licensed in every state.
- Significant delay in reaching emergency care if the mother or child develops life-threatening complications.
- There may not be a preestablished relationship with a physician if an emergency arises that requires the woman or newborn to be transferred to a hospital.

COMPONENTS OF THE BIRTH PROCESS

Four interrelated components, often called the "four *P*s," make up the process of labor and birth: the powers, the passage, the passenger, and the psyche. These factors are discussed in detail in the following sections.

Other factors that influence the progress of labor include *preparation,* such as attendance at prenatal classes; *position,* horizontal or vertical; *professional help,* such as knowledgeable nurses in attendance who explain and coach; the *place* or setting, because a lack of privacy and changes in shift personnel can interrupt rapport; *procedures,* such as internal examinations; and *people,* such as the presence of supportive family members (Vande-Vusse, 1999).

THE POWERS

The powers of labor are forces that cause the cervix to open and that propel the fetus downward through the birth canal. The two powers are (1) the uterine contractions and (2) the mother's pushing efforts.

Uterine Contractions

Uterine contractions are the primary powers of labor during the first stage (from onset until full dilation of the cervix). Uterine contractions are involuntary smooth muscle contractions; the woman cannot consciously cause them to stop or start. However, their intensity and effectiveness are influenced by a number of factors, such as walking, drugs, maternal anxiety, and vaginal examinations.

Effect of contractions on the cervix. Contractions cause the cervix to efface (thin) and *dilate* (open) to allow the fetus to descend in the birth canal (Figure 6-2). Before labor begins, the cervix is a tubular structure about 2 cm long. Contractions simultaneously push the fetus downward as they pull the cervix upward (an action similar to pushing a ball out the cuff of a sock). This causes the cervix to become thinner and shorter. Effacement is determined by a vaginal examination and is described as a percentage of the original cervical length. When the cervix is 100% effaced, it feels like a thin, slick membrane over the fetus.

Dilation of the cervix is determined during a vaginal examination. Dilation is described in centimeters, with full dilation being 10 cm (Figure 6-3). Both dilation and effacement are estimated by touch rather than being precisely measured.

Phases of contractions. Each contraction has the following three phases (Figure 6-4):

- Increment, the period of increasing strength
- Peak, or acme, the period of greatest strength
- Decrement, the period of decreasing strength

Contractions are also described by their average frequency, duration, intensity, and interval.

Frequency. Frequency is the elapsed time from the beginning of one contraction until the beginning of the next contraction. Frequency is described in minutes and fractions of minutes, such as "contractions every 4½ minutes." *Contractions occurring more often than every 2 minutes may reduce fetal oxygen supply and should be reported.*

Duration. Duration is the elapsed time from the beginning of a contraction until the end of the same contraction. Duration is described as the average number of seconds for which contractions last, such as "duration of 45 to 50 seconds." *Persistent contraction durations longer than 90 seconds may reduce fetal oxygen supply and should be reported.*

Intensity. Intensity is the approximate strength of the contraction. In most cases, intensity is described in words such as "mild," "moderate," or "strong," which are defined as follows:

- *Mild contractions.* Fundus is easily indented with the fingertips; the fundus of the uterus feels similar to the tip of the nose.
- *Moderate contractions.* Fundus can be indented with the fingertips but with more difficulty; the fundus of the uterus feels similar to the chin.
- *Firm contractions.* Fundus cannot be readily indented with the fingertips; the fundus of the uterus feels similar to the forehead.

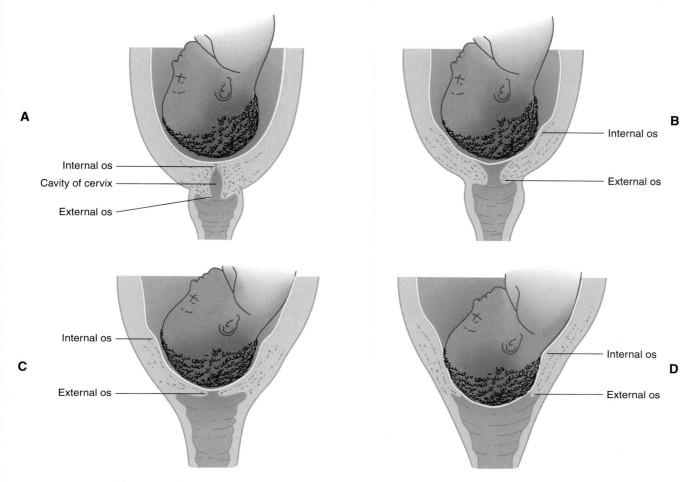

FIGURE 6-2 Cervical effacement and dilation. **A,** No effacement, no dilation. **B,** Early effacement and dilation. **C,** Complete effacement, some dilation. **D,** Complete dilation and effacement.

Interval. The interval is the amount of time the uterus relaxes between contractions. Blood flow from the mother into the placenta gradually decreases during contractions and resumes during each interval. The placenta refills with freshly oxygenated blood for the fetus and removes fetal waste products. *Persistent contraction intervals shorter than 60 seconds may reduce fetal oxygen supply.*

⚡ NURSING **TIP**_____
Report to the registered nurse any contractions that occur more frequently than every 2 minutes, last longer than 90 seconds, or have intervals shorter than 60 seconds.

Maternal Pushing

When the woman's cervix is fully dilated, she adds voluntary pushing to involuntary uterine contractions. The combined powers of uterine contractions and voluntary maternal pushing propel the fetus downward through the pelvis.

Most women feel a strong urge to push or bear down when the cervix is fully dilated and the fetus begins to descend. However, factors such as maternal exhaustion or sometimes epidural analgesia (see p. 168) may reduce or eliminate the natural urge to push. Some women feel a premature urge to push before the cervix is fully dilated because the fetus pushes against the rectum. This should be discouraged because it may contribute to maternal exhaustion and fetal hypoxia.

⚡ NURSING **TIP**_____
Provide emotional support to the laboring woman so she is less anxious and fearful. Excessive anxiety or fear can cause greater pain, inhibit the progress of labor, and reduce blood flow to the placenta/fetus.

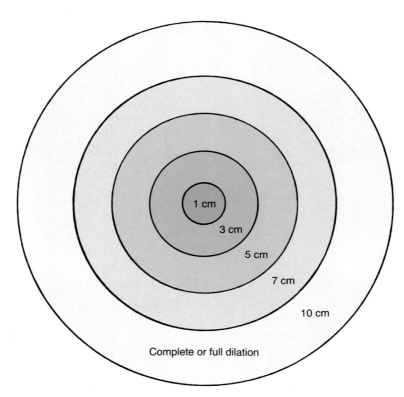

FIGURE **6-3** Cervical dilation in centimeters. Full dilation is 10 cm (1 cm is approximately one finger's width).

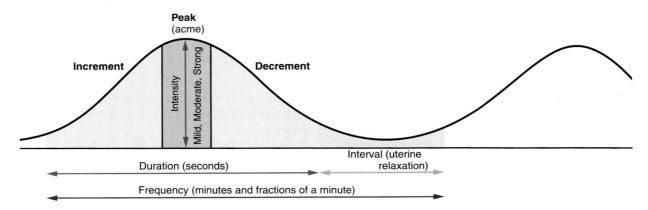

FIGURE **6-4** Contraction cycle. Each contraction can be likened to a bell shape, with an increment, peak (acme), and decrement. The *frequency* of contractions is the average time from the beginning of one to the beginning of the next. The *duration* is the average time from the beginning to the end of one contraction. The *interval* is the period of uterine relaxation between contractions.

THE PASSAGE

The passage consists of the mother's bony pelvis and the soft tissues (cervix, muscles, ligaments, fascia) of her pelvis and perineum (see Chapter 2 for a review of the structure of the bony pelvis).

Bony Pelvis

The pelvis is divided into two major parts: (1) the false pelvis (upper, flaring part), and (2) the true pelvis (lower part). The true pelvis is directly involved in childbirth. The true pelvis is further divided into the inlet at

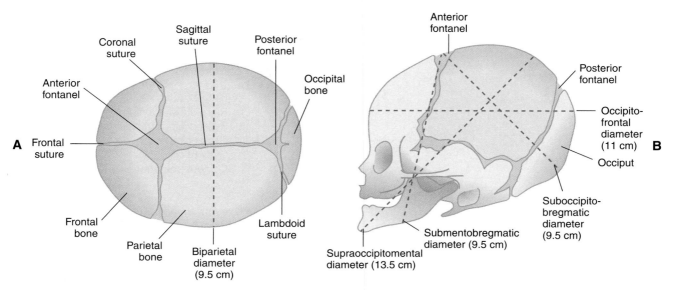

FIGURE **6-5** The fetal skull, showing sutures, fontanels, and important measurements. **A,** Superior view. Note that the anterior fontanel has a diamond shape; the posterior fontanel is triangular. The biparietal diameter is an important fetal skull measurement. **B,** Lateral view. The measurements of the fetal skull are important to determine if cephalopelvic disproportion will be a problem. The mechanisms of labor allow the fetal head to rotate so that the smallest diameter of the head passes through the pelvis as it descends.

the top, the midpelvis in the middle, and the outlet near the perineum. It is shaped somewhat like a curved cylinder or a wide, curved funnel. The measurements of the maternal bony pelvis must be adequate to allow the fetal head to pass through or cephalopelvic disproportion (CPD) will occur and a cesarean birth may be indicated.

Soft Tissues

In general, women who have had previous vaginal births deliver more quickly than women having their first births because their soft tissues yield more readily to the forces of contractions and pushing efforts. This advantage is not present if the woman's prior births were cesarean. Soft tissue may not yield as readily in older mothers or after cervical procedures that have caused scarring.

THE PASSENGER

The passenger is the fetus, along with the placenta (afterbirth), amniotic membranes, and amniotic fluid. Because the fetus usually enters the pelvis head first (cephalic presentation), the nurse should understand the basic structure of the fetal head.

Fetal Head

The fetal head is composed of several bones separated by strong connective tissue, called sutures (Figure 6-5). A wider area called a fontanel is formed where the su-

tures meet. The following two fontanels are important in obstetrics:

- The *anterior fontanel,* a diamond-shaped area formed by the intersection of four sutures (frontal, sagittal, and two coronal)
- The *posterior fontanel,* a tiny triangular depression formed by the intersection of three sutures (one sagittal and two lambdoid)

The sutures and fontanels of the fetal head allow it to change shape as it passes through the pelvis (molding). They are important landmarks in determining how the fetus is oriented within the mother's pelvis during birth.

The main transverse diameter of the fetal head is the *biparietal diameter,* which is measured between the points of the two parietal bones on each side of the head. The anteroposterior diameter of the fetal head can vary depending on how much the head is flexed or extended.

Lie

Lie describes how the fetus is oriented to the mother's spine (Figure 6-6). The most common orientation is the longitudinal lie (over 99% of births), in which the fetus is parallel to the mother's spine. The fetus in a transverse lie is at right angles to the mother's spine. The transverse lie may also be called a shoulder presentation. In an oblique lie the fetus is between a longitudinal lie and a transverse lie.

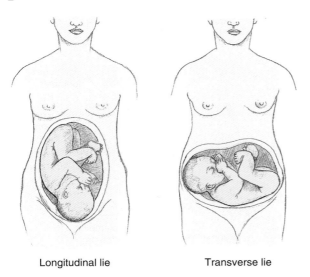

Longitudinal lie   Transverse lie

FIGURE **6-6** Lie. In the longitudinal lie the fetus is parallel to the mother's spine. In the transverse lie, the fetus is at right angles to the mother's spine. The shoulder presents at the cervix.

box 6-1 *Classifications of Fetal Presentations and Positions**

CEPHALIC PRESENTATIONS	
Vertex	
LOA	Left occiput anterior
ROA	Right occiput anterior
ROT	Right occiput transverse
LOT	Left occiput transverse
OA	Occiput anterior
OP	Occiput posterior
Face	
LMA	Left mentum anterior
RMA	Right mentum anterior
LMP	Left mentum posterior
RMP	Right mentum posterior
BREECH PRESENTATIONS	
LSA	Left sacrum anterior
RSA	Right sacrum anterior
LSP	Left sacrum posterior
RSP	Right sacrum posterior

*Abbreviations that designate brow, military, and shoulder presentations are not included here because they occur infrequently.

Attitude

The fetal attitude is normally one of flexion, with the head flexed forward and the arms and legs flexed. The flexed fetus is compact and ovoid and most efficiently occupies the space in the mother's uterus and pelvis. Extension of the head, arms, and/or legs sometimes occurs, and labor may be prolonged.

Presentation

Presentation refers to the fetal part that enters the pelvis first. The cephalic presentation is the most common. Any of the following four variations of cephalic presentations can occur, depending on the extent to which the fetal head is flexed (Figure 6-7):

- The *vertex presentation,* with the fetal head fully flexed, is the most favorable cephalic variation because the smallest possible diameter of the head enters the pelvis. It occurs in about 96% of births.
- The *military presentation* is one in which the fetal head is neither flexed nor extended.
- The *brow presentation* is one in which the fetal head is partly extended. The longest diameter of the fetal head is presenting. This presentation is unstable and tends to convert to either a vertex or a face presentation.
- The *face presentation* is one in which the head is fully extended and the face presents.

The next most common presentation is the breech, which can have the following three variations (Figure 6-7, E to G):

- The *frank breech,* with the fetal legs flexed at the hips and extending toward the shoulders, is the most common type of breech presentation. The buttocks present at the cervix.
- The *full or complete breech* is a reversal of the cephalic presentation, with flexion of the head and extremities. Both feet and the buttocks present at the cervix.
- The *footling breech* is one in which one or both feet present first at the cervix.

Many women with a fetus in the breech presentation have cesarean births because the head, which is the largest single fetal part, is the last to be born and may not pass through the pelvis easily because flexion of the fetal head cannot occur. After the fetal body is born, the head must be delivered quickly so the fetus can breathe; at this point, part of the umbilical cord is outside the mother's body and the remaining part is subject to compression by the fetal head against the bony pelvis.

When the fetus is in a transverse lie, the fetal shoulder enters the pelvis first. A fetus in this orientation must be born by cesarean delivery because it cannot safely pass through the pelvis.

Position

Position refers to how a reference point on the fetal presenting part is oriented within the mother's pelvis. The

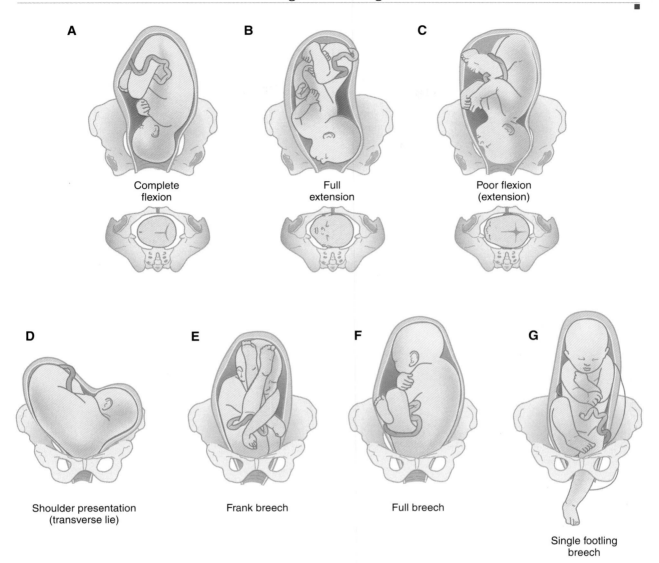

A Complete flexion

B Full extension

C Poor flexion (extension)

D Shoulder presentation (transverse lie)

E Frank breech

F Full breech

G Single footling breech

FIGURE **6-7** Fetal presentations. **A,** Cephalic vertex. **B,** Cephalic face. **C,** Cephalic brow. **D,** Shoulder. **E,** Frank breech. **F,** Full or complete breech. **G,** Footling breech (can be single or double). The vertex presentation in which the fetal chin is flexed on the chest is the most common and favorable for a vaginal birth because it allows the smallest diameter of the head to go through the bony pelvis of the mother. Note how the anterior and posterior fontanels can be used to determine fetal presentation and position in the pelvis.

term *occiput* is used to describe how the head is oriented if the fetus is in a cephalic vertex presentation. The term *sacrum* is used to describe how a fetus in a breech presentation is oriented within the pelvis. The shoulder and back are reference points if the fetus is in a shoulder presentation.

The maternal pelvis is divided into four imaginary quadrants: right and left anterior and right and left posterior. If the fetal occiput is in the left front quadrant of the mother's pelvis, it is described as *left occiput anterior*. If the sacrum of a fetus in a breech presentation is in the

mother's right posterior pelvis, it is described as *right sacrum posterior*.

Abbreviations describe the fetal presentation and position within the pelvis (Box 6-1). Three letters are used for most abbreviations:

- *First letter:* Right or left side of the woman's pelvis. This letter is omitted if the fetal reference point is directly anterior or posterior, such as occiput anterior (OA).
- *Second letter:* Fetal reference point (occiput for vertex presentations; mentum [chin] for face

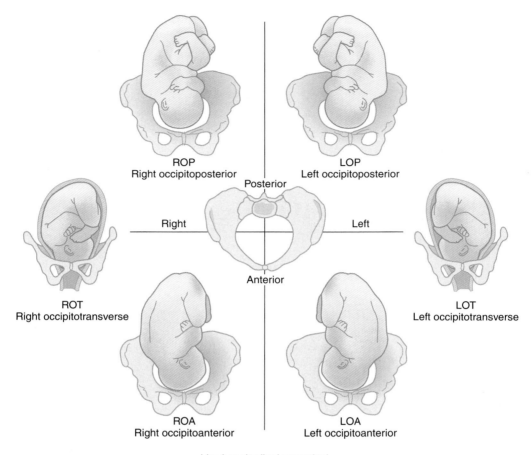

Lie: Longitudinal or vertical
Presentation: Vertex
Reference point: Occiput
Attitude: Complete flexion

FIGURE **6-8** Fetal position. The right occiput anterior *(ROA)* or left occiput anterior *(LOA)* are most favorable for normal labor. When the occiput faces the posterior section of the women's pelvis, a longer, "back labor" birth process is anticipated.

presentations; and sacrum for breech presentations).

- *Third letter:* Front or back of the mother's pelvis (anterior or posterior). Transverse (T) denotes a fetal position that is neither anterior nor posterior.

Figure 6-8 shows various fetal presentations and positions.

THE PSYCHE

Childbirth is more than a physical process; it involves the woman's entire being. Women do not recount the births of their children in the same manner that they do surgical procedures. They describe births in emotional terms, such as those they use to describe marriages, an-

niversaries, religious events, or even deaths. Families often have great expectations about the birth *experience.* The nurse can promote a positive childbearing experience by incorporating as many of the family's birth expectations as possible.

A woman's mental state can influence the course of her labor. For example, the woman who is relaxed and optimistic during labor is better able to tolerate discomfort and work with the physiological processes. By contrast, marked anxiety can increase her perception of pain and reduce her tolerance of it. Anxiety and fear also cause the secretion of stress compounds from the adrenal glands. These compounds, called catecholamines, inhibit uterine contractions and divert blood flow from the placenta.

A woman's cultural and individual values influence how she views and copes with childbirth (see Table 6-1).

NORMAL CHILDBIRTH

The specific event that triggers the onset of labor remains unknown. Many factors probably play a part in initiating labor, which is an interaction of the mother and fetus. These factors include stretching of the uterine muscles, hormonal changes, placental aging, and increased sensitivity to oxytocin. Labor normally begins when the fetus is mature enough to adjust easily to life outside the uterus yet still small enough to fit through the mother's pelvis. This point is usually reached between 38 and 42 weeks after the mother's last menstrual period.

SIGNS OF IMPENDING LABOR

Signs and symptoms that labor is about to start may occur from a few hours to a few weeks before the actual onset of labor.

Braxton Hicks Contractions

Braxton Hicks contractions are irregular contractions that begin during early pregnancy and intensify as full term approaches. They often become regular and somewhat uncomfortable, leading many women to believe that labor has started (see the discussion of true and false labor later in this chapter). Although Braxton Hicks contractions are often called "false" labor, they play a part in preparing the cervix to dilate and in adjusting the fetal position within the uterus.

Increased Vaginal Discharge

Fetal pressure causes an increase in clear and nonirritating vaginal secretions. Irritation or itching with the increased secretions is not normal and should be reported to the physician or certified nurse-midwife (CNM) because these symptoms are characteristic of infection.

Bloody Show

As the time for birth approaches, the cervix undergoes changes in preparation for labor. It softens ("ripens"), effaces, and dilates slightly. When this occurs, the mucous plug that has sealed the uterus during pregnancy is dislodged from the cervix, tearing small capillaries in the process. Bloody show is thick mucus mixed with pink or dark brown blood. It may begin a few days before labor, or a woman may not have bloody show until labor is underway. Bloody show may also occur if the woman has had a recent vaginal examination or intercourse.

Rupture of the Membranes

The amniotic sac (bag of waters) sometimes ruptures before labor begins. Infection is more likely if many hours elapse between rupture of membranes and birth because the amniotic sac seals the uterine cavity against organisms from the vagina. In addition, the fetal umbilical cord may slip down and become compressed between the mother's pelvis and the fetal presenting part. For these two reasons, women should go to the birth facility when their membranes rupture, even if they have no other signs of labor.

Energy Spurt

Many women have a sudden burst of energy shortly before the onset of labor ("nesting"). The nurse should teach women to conserve their strength, even if they feel unusually energetic.

Weight Loss

Occasionally a woman may notice that she loses 1 to 3 pounds shortly before labor begins because hormone changes cause her to excrete extra body water.

MECHANISMS OF LABOR

As the fetus descends into the pelvis, it undergoes several positional changes so that it adapts optimally to the changing pelvic shape and size. Many of these *mechanisms*, also called *cardinal movements*, occur simultaneously (Figure 6-9).

Descent

Descent is required for all other mechanisms of labor to occur and for the infant to be born. Station describes the level of the presenting part (usually the head) in the pelvis. Station is estimated in centimeters from the level of the ischial spines in the mother's pelvis (a zero station). Minus stations are above the ischial spines; plus stations are below the ischial spines (Figure 6-10). As the fetus descends, the minus numbers get smaller (e.g., -2, -1) and the plus numbers get higher (e.g., $+1$, $+2$).

Engagement

Engagement occurs when the biparietal diameter of the fetal head reaches the level of the ischial spines of the mother's pelvis (presenting part is at a zero station or lower). Engagement often occurs before the onset of labor in a woman who has not previously given birth (a nullipara); if the woman has had prior vaginal births (a multipara), engagement may not occur until well after labor begins.

Flexion

The fetal head should be flexed to pass most easily through the pelvis. As labor progresses, uterine contrac-

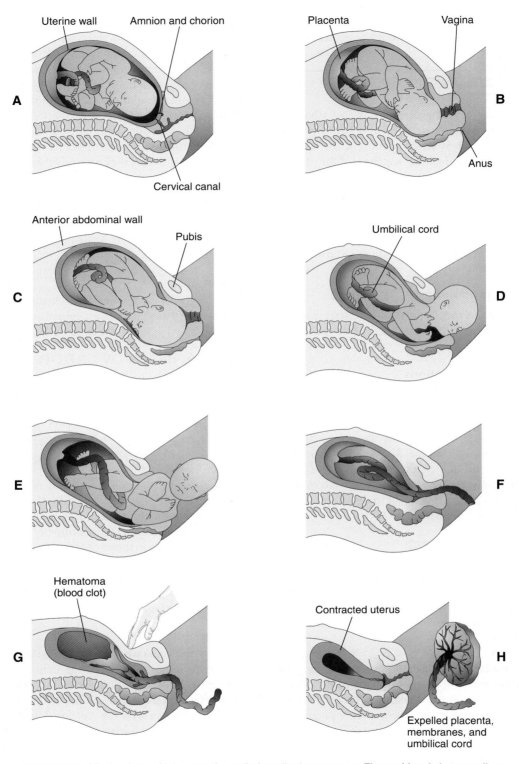

FIGURE **6-9** Mechanisms of labor are also called cardinal movements. The positional changes allow the fetus to fit through the pelvis with the least resistance. **A,** Engagement, descent, and flexion. **B,** Internal rotation. **C,** Beginning extension. **D,** Birth of the head by complete extension. **E,** External rotation, birth of shoulders and body. **F,** Separation of placenta begins. **G,** Complete separation of placenta from uterine wall. **H,** Placenta is expelled and uterus contracts.

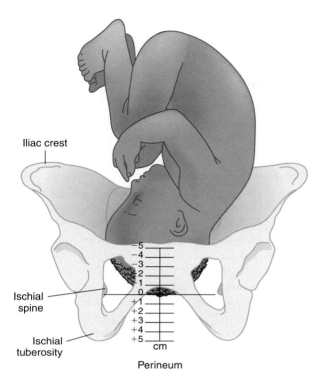

Iliac crest

Ischial spine

Ischial tuberosity

Perineum

−5
−4
−3
−2
−1
0
+1
+2
+3
+4
+5
cm

FIGURE **6-10** Station. The station describes the level of the presenting part in relation to the ischial spines of the mother's pelvis. The "minus" stations are above the ischial spines and the "plus" stations are below the ischial spines.

tions increase the amount of fetal head flexion until the fetal chin is on the chest.

Internal Rotation
When the fetus enters the pelvis, the head is usually oriented so the occiput is toward the mother's right or left side. As the fetus is pushed downward by contractions, the curved, cylindrical shape of the pelvis causes the fetal head to turn until the occiput is directly under the symphysis pubis (occiput anterior [OA]).

Extension
As the fetal head passes under the mother's symphysis pubis, it must change from flexion to extension so it can properly negotiate the curve. To do this, the fetal neck stops under the symphysis, which acts as a pivot. The head swings anteriorly as it extends with each maternal push until it is born.

External Rotation
When the head is born in extension, the shoulders are crosswise in the pelvis and the head is somewhat twisted in relation to the shoulders. The head spontaneously turns to one side as it realigns with the shoulders (resti-

tution). The shoulders then rotate within the pelvis until their transverse diameter is aligned with the mother's anteroposterior pelvis. The head turns farther to the side as the shoulders rotate within the pelvis.

Expulsion
The anterior shoulder and then the posterior shoulder are born, quickly followed by the rest of the body.

ADMISSION TO THE HOSPITAL OR BIRTH CENTER

Intrapartum nursing care begins before admission by educating the woman about the appropriate time to come to the facility. Nursing care includes admission assessments and the initiation of needed procedures. Many women have false labor and are discharged after a short observation period; nursing care of these patients is included.

WHEN TO GO TO THE HOSPITAL OR BIRTH CENTER
During late pregnancy the woman should be instructed about when to go to the hospital or birth center. This is *not* an exact time, but the general guidelines areas follows:
- *Contractions.* The woman should go to the hospital or birth center when the contractions have a pattern of increasing frequency, duration, and intensity. The woman having her first child is usually advised to enter the facility when contractions have been regular (every 5 minutes) for 1 hour. Women having second or later children should go sooner, when regular contractions are 10 minutes apart for a period of 1 hour.
- *Ruptured membranes.* The woman should go to the facility if her membranes rupture or if she thinks they may have ruptured.
- *Bleeding other than bloody show.* Bloody show is a mixture of blood and thick mucus. Active bleeding is free flowing, bright red, and not mixed with thick mucus.
- *Decreased fetal movement.* The woman should be evaluated if the fetus is moving less than usual. Many fetuses become quiet shortly before labor, but decreased fetal activity can also be a sign of fetal compromise or fetal demise (death).
- *Any other concern.* Because these guidelines cannot cover every situation, the woman should contact her health care provider or go to the birth facility for evaluation if she has any other concerns.

ADMISSION DATA COLLECTION

The nurse should observe the appropriate infection control measures when providing care in any clinical area. Water-repellent gowns, eye shields, and gloves are worn in the delivery area, and the newborn infant is handled with gloves until after the first bath. General guidelines for wearing protective clothing in the intrapartal area can be found in Appendix A.

When a woman is admitted, the nurse establishes a therapeutic relationship by welcoming her and her family members. The nurse continues developing the therapeutic relationship during labor by determining the woman's expectations about birth and assists in achieving these expectations. Some women have a written birth plan that they have discussed with their health care provider and the facility personnel. Her partner and other family members she wants to be part of her care are included. From the first encounter the nurse conveys confidence in the woman's ability to cope with labor and give birth to her child.

Three major assessments are performed promptly on admission: (1) fetal condition, (2) maternal condition, and (3) nearness to birth.

Fetal Condition

The fetal heart rate (FHR) is assessed with a fetoscope (stethoscope for listening to fetal heart sounds), a handheld Doppler transducer, or the external fetal monitor (see p. 136).

When the amniotic membranes are ruptured, the color, amount, and odor of the fluid are assessed and the FHR is recorded (see Box 6-4).

Maternal Condition

The temperature, pulse, respirations, and blood pressure are assessed for signs of infection or hypertension (see p. 141).

Impending Birth

The nurse continually observes the woman for behaviors that suggest she is about to give birth. Examples of these behaviors include the following:

- Sitting on one buttock
- Making grunting sounds
- Bearing down with contractions
- Stating "The baby's coming"
- Bulging of the perineum or the fetal presenting part visible at the vaginal opening

If it appears that birth is imminent, the nurse does not leave the woman but summons help or uses the call bell. Gloves should be applied in case the infant is born quickly. Emergency delivery kits (called "precip trays" for "precipitous birth") containing essential equipment are in all delivery areas. The student should locate this tray early in the clinical experience because one cannot predict when it will be needed. (See Box 6-2 for emergency birth procedures.)

NURSING TIP

It is unlikely that a nursing student must deliver an infant during an unexpected birth, but the process should be reviewed in case it does occur.

Additional Data Collection

If the maternal and fetal conditions are normal and if birth is not imminent, other data can be gathered in a more leisurely way. Most birth facilities have a preprinted form to guide admission assessments. Women who have had prenatal care should have a prenatal record on file for retrieval of that information. Examples of assessment data needed are as follows:

- Basic information such as the woman's reason for coming to the facility, the name of her health care provider, medical and obstetric history, allergies,

---

| box 6-2 | *Assisting with an Emergency Birth* |

- The priorities of nursing care are to prevent injury to the mother and child.
- Get the emergency delivery tray ("precip tray").
- Do not leave the woman if she exhibits any signs of imminent birth, such as grunting, bearing down, perineal bulging, or a statement that the baby is coming. Summon the experienced nurse with the call bell and try to remain calm.
- Put on gloves. Either clean or sterile is acceptable because no invasive procedures will be done. Gloves are used primarily to protect the nurse from secretions while supporting the infant.
- Support the infant's head and body as it emerges. Wipe secretions from the face.
- Use a bulb syringe to remove secretions from the mouth and nose, then clamp and cut the cord.
- Dry the infant quickly and wrap in blankets or place in skin-to-skin contact with the mother to maintain the infant's temperature.
- Observe the infant's color and respirations. The cry should be vigorous and the color pink (bluish hands and feet are acceptable).
- Observe for placental detachment and bleeding. After the placenta detaches, observe for a firm fundus. If the fundus is not firm, massage it. The infant can suckle at the mother's breast to promote the release of oxytocin, which causes uterine contraction.

food intake, any recent illness, and medications (including illicit substances).

- Woman's plans for birth.
- Status of labor. A vaginal examination is done by the registered nurse, CNM, or physician to determine cervical effacement and dilation, fetal presentation, position, and station. Contractions are assessed for frequency, duration, and intensity by palpation and/or with an electronic fetal monitor.
- General condition. A brief physical examination is done to evaluate the woman's general condition. Any edema, especially of the fingers and face, and abdominal scars should be further explored. Fundal height is measured (or estimated by an experienced nurse) to determine if it is appropriate for her gestation. Reflexes are checked to identify hyperactivity that may occur with pregnancy-induced hypertension (PIH).

ADMISSION PROCEDURES

Several procedures may be done when a woman is admitted to a birth facility. Some common procedures are described in the following sections.

Permits

The mother signs permissions/consents for care of herself and her infant during labor, delivery, and the post-birth period. Permission for an emergency cesarean delivery may be included. All signatures must be witnessed by the health care provider and the nurse who confirms that proper information was given to the patient.

Laboratory Tests

Blood for hematocrit and a midstream urine specimen for glucose and protein are common. The hematocrit is often omitted if a woman has had regular prenatal care and a recent evaluation. The woman who did not have prenatal care will have additional tests that may include a complete blood count, urinalysis, drug screen, tests for sexually transmitted diseases, and others as indicated.

Intravenous Infusion

An intravenous (IV) line is started to allow the administration of fluids and drugs. The woman may have a constant fluid infusion, or venous access may be maintained with a saline lock to permit greater patient mobility in early labor.

Shave Prep

A perineal shave prep is occasionally done to remove pubic hair that would interfere with the repair of a laceration or episiotomy. Its use has declined because it

does not prevent infection as was once thought. If done, it is restricted to a small area of the perineum (a "mini-prep"). The woman who has a cesarean birth will usually have an abdominal shave prep.

Enema

An enema is occasionally administered if the woman has been constipated or if the nurse notes a significant amount of stool in the rectum when doing a vaginal examination. Small-volume enemas, such as Fleets, are typical. Extra lubrication of the enema tip avoids irritating hemorrhoids (varicose veins in the rectum), which are common in pregnant and postpartum women.

NURSING CARE OF THE WOMAN IN FALSE LABOR

True labor is characterized by changes in the cervix (effacement and dilation), which is the key distinction between true and false labor. See Table 6-2 for other characteristics of true and false labor.

A better term for false labor might be *prodromal labor,* because these contractions help prepare the woman's body and the fetus for true labor. Many women are observed for a short while (1 to 2 hours) if their initial assessment suggests that they are not in true labor and their membranes are intact. The mother and fetus are assessed during observation as if labor were occurring. Most facilities run an external electronic fetal monitor strip for at least 20 minutes to document fetal well-being (see Figure 6-12). The woman can usually walk about when not being monitored. If she is in true labor, walking often helps to intensify the contractions and to cause cervical effacement and dilation to occur.

After the observation period the woman's labor status is reevaluated by the health care provider, who performs another vaginal examination. If there is no change in the cervical effacement or dilation, the woman is usually sent home to await true labor. Sometimes, if it is her first child and she lives nearby, the woman in very early labor is sent home because the latent phase of most first labors is quite long.

Each woman in false labor (or early latent-phase labor) is evaluated individually. Factors to be considered include the number and duration of previous labors, distance from the facility, and availability of transportation.

> NURSING **TIP**
> Encourage the woman in false labor to return when she thinks she should. It is better to have another "trial run" than to wait at home until she is in advanced labor.

table 6-2 *Comparison of True Labor and False Labor*

FALSE LABOR (PRODROMAL LABOR OR PRELABOR)	TRUE LABOR
Contractions are irregular or do not increase in frequency, duration, and intensity.	Contractions gradually develop a regular pattern and become more frequent, longer, and more intense.
Walking tends to relieve or decrease contractions.	Contractions become stronger and more effective with walking.
Discomfort is felt in the abdomen and groin.	Discomfort is felt in the lower back and lower abdomen; often feels like menstrual cramps at first.
Bloody show is usually not present.	Bloody show is often present, especially in women having their first child.
There is no change in effacement or dilation of the cervix.	Progressive effacement and dilation of the cervix occur.

If her membranes are ruptured, she is usually admitted even if labor has not begun because of the risk for infection or a prolapsed umbilical cord (see p. 198).

The woman in false labor is often frustrated and needs generous reassurance that her symptoms will eventually change to true labor. No one stays pregnant forever, although it sometimes feels that way to a woman who has had several false alarms and is tired of being pregnant. Guidelines for coming to the facility should be reinforced before she leaves.

NURSING CARE BEFORE BIRTH

After admission to the labor unit, nursing care consists of the following elements:

- Monitoring the fetus
- Monitoring the laboring woman
- Helping the woman cope with labor

MONITORING THE FETUS

Intrapartum care of the fetus includes assessment of FHR patterns and the amniotic fluid. In addition, several observations of the mother's status, such as vital signs and contraction pattern, are closely related to fetal well-being because they influence fetal oxygen supply.

Fetal Heart Rate

The FHR can be assessed by intermittent auscultation, a fetoscope or Doppler transducer, or continuous electronic fetal monitoring. (See Box 6-4 for the procedure for assessing FHR.) Electronic fetal monitoring is more widely used in the United States, but intermittent auscultation is a valid method of intrapartum fetal assessment when performed according to established intervals and with a 1:1 nurse-patient ratio.

The guidelines for a normal FHR at term are as follows:

- Lower limit of 110 to 120 beats/min
- Upper limit of 150 to 160 beats/min

Intermittent Auscultation

Intermittent auscultation allows the mother greater freedom of movement, which is helpful during early labor and is the method used during home births and in most birth centers. However, unlike continuous monitoring, intermittent auscultation does not provide a written recording.

Intermittent auscultation of the FHR should be performed as noted in Box 6-3. Figure 6-11 shows the approximate location of the fetal heart sounds when the fetus is in various presentations and positions. *Any FHR outside the normal limits or slowing of the FHR that persists after the contraction ends is promptly reported to the health care provider.*

Continuous Electronic Fetal Monitoring

Continuous electronic fetal monitoring (EFM) allows the nurse to collect more data about the fetus than intermittent auscultation. FHR and uterine contraction patterns are continuously recorded. Most hospitals use continuous EFM because the permanent written recording becomes part of the mother's chart.

Some monitors have telemetry, allowing the woman to walk while a transmitter sends the data back to the monitor at her bedside for recording (like a cordless telephone). Intermittent monitoring is a variation that promotes walking during labor. An initial recording of at least 20 minutes is obtained, and then the fetus is remonitored for 15 minutes at regular intervals of 30 to 60 minutes (Box 6-4).

EFM can be performed with external or internal devices. Internal devices require that the membranes be

box 6-3 | *When to Auscultate and Document the Fetal Heart Rate*

Use these guidelines for charting the FHR when the woman has intermittent auscultation or continuous electronic fetal monitoring.

LOW-RISK WOMEN

Every hour in the latent phase
Every 30 minutes in the active phase
Every 15 minutes in the second stage

HIGH-RISK WOMEN

Every 30 minutes in the latent phase
Every 15 minutes in the active phase
Every 5 minutes in the second stage

ROUTINE AUSCULTATIONS

When the membranes rupture (spontaneously or artificially)
Before and after ambulation
Before and after medication or anesthesia administration or a change in medication
At the time of peak action of analgesic drugs
After a vaginal examination
After the expulsion of enema
After catheterization
If uterine contractions are abnormal or excessive

Modified from Nurses' Association of the American College of Obstetricians and Gynecologists (NAACOG). (1990). *Fetal heart rate auscultation.* Washington, DC: Author. With permission of the Association of Women's Health, Obstetric and Neonatal Nurses; American College of Obstetricians and Gynecologists (ACOG). (1995). *Technical Bulletin Number 207: Fetal heart rate patterns: Monitoring, interpretation, and management.* Washington, DC: Author.

box 6-4 | *Procedure for Determining Fetal Heart Rate*

1. *Location.* Identify where the clearest fetal heart sounds will most likely be found, over the fetal back and usually in the lower abdomen (see Figure 6-11 and Chapter 8).
2. *Fetoscope.* Place the head attachment (if there is one) over your head and the earpieces in your ear. Place the bell in the approximate area of the fetal back and press firmly while listening for the muffled fetal heart sounds. When they are heard, count the rate for 1 minute. Count the rate in 6-second increments for at least 1 minute. Multiply the low and high numbers by 10 to compute the average range of the rate (for example, 130 to 140 beats/min). Assess rate before and after at least one full contraction cycle. Check the mother's pulse at the same time if uncertain whether the fetal heart sounds are being heard; the rates and rhythms will be different.
3. *Doppler transducer.* Put water-soluble gel on the head of the hand-held transducer. Put the earpieces in your ear, or connect the transducer to a speaker. Turn the switch on and place the transducer head over the approximate area of the fetal back. Count as instructed in step 2. If earpieces are used, let the parents hear the fetal heartbeat.
4. *External fetal monitor.* Read manufacturer's instructions for specific procedures. Connect cable to correct socket on monitor unit. Put water-soluble gel on the transducer and apply as instructed in step 3. Either belts, a wide band of stockinette, or an adhesive ring is used to secure the transducers for external fetal monitoring. The rate is calculated by the monitor and displayed on an electronic panel. The displayed number will change as the machine recalculates the rate.
5. *Chart the rate.* Promptly report rates below 110 beats/min or above 160 beats/min for a full-term fetus. Report slowing of the rate that lingers after the end of a contraction. Report a lack of variability in the rate (see Figures 6-12, 6-13, and 6-14).

ruptured and the cervix be dilated 1 to 2 cm to insert the devices. Internal devices are disposable to reduce transmission of infection. A small spiral electrode applied to the fetal presenting part allows internal FHR monitoring. Two types of devices are used for internal contraction monitoring. One uses a fluid-filled catheter connected to a pressure-sensitive device on the monitor. The other uses a solid catheter with an electronic pressure sensor in its tip.

External fetal heart monitoring is done with a Doppler transducer, which uses sound waves to detect motion of the fetal heart and calculate the rate, just as the hand-held model does. Contractions are sensed externally with a tocotransducer (a "toco"), which has a pressure-sensitive button. The toco is positioned over the mother's upper uterus (fundus), about where the nurse would palpate contractions by hand (Figure 6-12).

Evaluating fetal heart rate patterns. The FHR is recorded on the upper grid of the paper; the uterine contraction pattern is recorded on the lower grid. Both grids must be evaluated together for accurate interpretation of FHR patterns.

The FHR is evaluated for baseline, variability, and periodic changes. The *baseline rate* is the rate between contractions and between periodic changes. *Variability* describes fluctuations, or constant changes, in the baseline

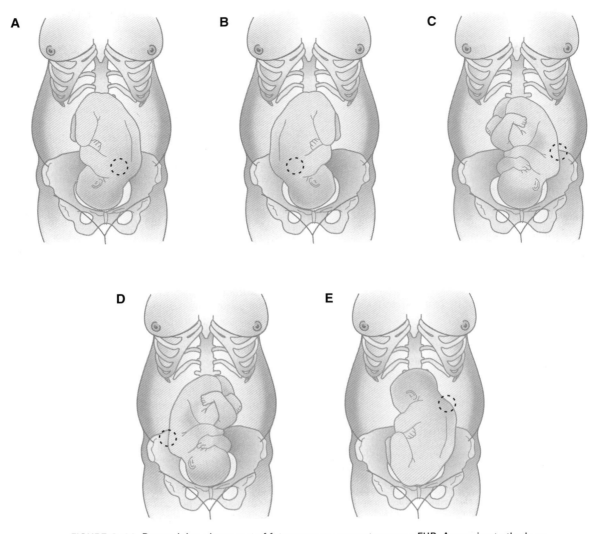

FIGURE **6-11** Determining placement of fetoscope or sensor to assess FHR. Approximate the location of the strongest fetal heart sound when the fetus is in various positions and presentations. The fetal heart sounds are heard best in the lower abdomen in a cephalic (vertex) presentation and higher on the abdomen when the fetus is in a breech presentation (**E**). **A,** LOA; **B,** ROA; **C,** LOP; **D,** ROP; **E,** LSA.

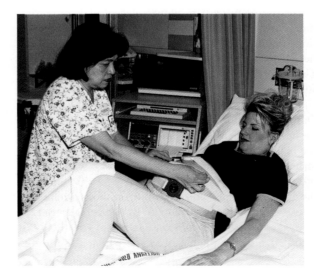

FIGURE **6-12** External electronic fetal monitoring. The nurse applies the sensors on the mother's abdomen. One sensor is placed over the fundus of the uterus to record uterine contractions; one sensor is placed over the location of the strongest fetal heart sound to record the FHR. This woman has twins and requires two fetal heart sensors.

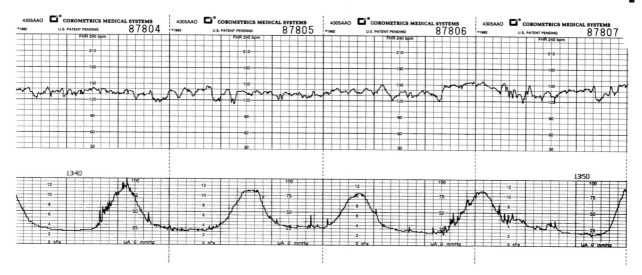

FIGURE **6-13** Recording of the FHR in the upper grid and the uterine contractions in the lower grid. Note the sawtooth appearance of the FHR tracing because of the constant changes in the rate (variability).

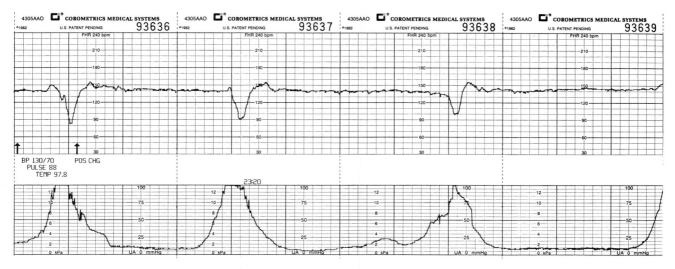

FIGURE **6-14** Variable decelerations, showing their typically abrupt onset and offset. They are caused by umbilical cord compression. The first response to this pattern is to reposition the mother to relieve pressure on the cord.

rate (Figure 6-13). Variability causes the recording of the FHR to have a fine sawtooth appearance with larger, undulating wavelike movements. Variability is desirable, but it may be depressed by narcotics given to the woman and may normally be absent if the fetus is preterm.

Periodic changes are temporary changes in the baseline rate. Periodic changes include *accelerations* (rate increases) or one of three types of *decelerations* (rate decreases).

Accelerations. Accelerations are rate increases of at least 15 beats/min over the baseline rate that last approximately 15 seconds. This pattern suggests a fetus that is well oxygenated and is known as a "reassuring pattern."

Early decelerations. Early decelerations are rate decreases during contractions; they always return to the baseline rate by the end of the contractions. This results from compression of the fetal head and is a reassuring sign of fetal well-being.

Variable decelerations. Variable decelerations begin and end abruptly; they are V, W-, or U-shaped (Figure 6-14). They do not always exhibit a consistent pattern in

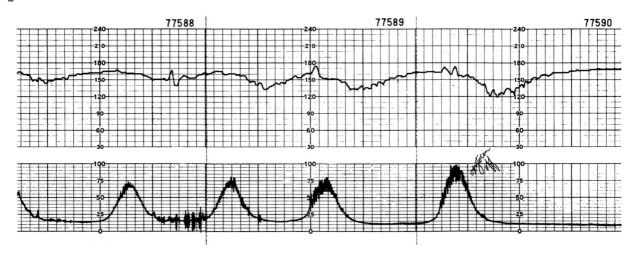

FIGURE **6-15** Late decelerations, showing their pattern of slowing, which persists after the contraction ends. The usual cause is reduced blood flow from the placenta (uteroplacental insufficiency [UPI]). Measures to correct this include repositioning the woman, giving oxygen, increasing nonmedicated intravenous fluid and stopping administration of oxytocin if it is being given, and giving drugs to reduce uterine contractions.

| box 6-5 | *Reassuring and Nonreassuring Fetal Heart Rate and Uterine Activity Patterns* |

REASSURING PATTERNS

Stable rate with a lower limit of 110 to 120 beats/min and an upper limit of 160 beats/min (term fetus)

Variability present

Accelerations of rate

Contraction frequency greater than every 2 minutes; duration less than 90 seconds; relaxation interval of at least 60 seconds

NONREASSURING PATTERNS

Tachycardia: rate over 160 beats/min for 10 minutes or longer

Bradycardia: rate under 110 beats/min for 10 minutes or longer

Decreased or absent variability: little fluctuation in rate

Late decelerations: begin after the contraction starts and persist after the contraction is over

Variable decelerations: rate abruptly falls when deceleration occurs, returns abruptly to the baseline; may or may not occur in a consistent relationship with contractions

Absence of variability

NURSING TIP_____

Report any questionable FHR or contraction pattern to the experienced labor nurse for complete evaluation.

relation to contractions. Variable decelerations suggest that the umbilical cord is being compressed, often because it is around the fetal neck (a nuchal cord) or because there is inadequate amniotic fluid to cushion it well.

Late decelerations. Late decelerations of the FHR look similar to early decelerations, except that they do not return to the baseline FHR until after the contraction ends (Figure 6-15). Late decelerations suggest that the placenta is not delivering enough oxygen to the fetus (uteroplacental insufficiency). This is known as a "nonreassuring pattern."

Nursing response to monitor patterns. The nursing response depends on the pattern identified (Box 6-5). Accelerations and early decelerations are reassuring and thus require no intervention other than continued observation.

Repositioning the woman is usually the first response to a pattern of variable decelerations. Changing the mother's position can relieve pressure on the umbilical cord and improve blood flow through it. The woman is turned to her side. Other positions, such as the knee-chest or a slight Trendelenburg (head-down) position, may be tried if the side-lying positions do not restore the pattern to a reassuring one. If membranes have ruptured, an amnioinfusion technique, in which IV fluid is infused into the amniotic cavity through the intrauterine pressure catheter, may be done to add a fluid cushion around the cord.

Late decelerations are initially treated by measures to increase maternal oxygenation and blood flow to the placenta. The specific measures depend on the most likely cause of the pattern and may include the following:

- Repositioning to prevent supine hypotension (see Figure 4-5)
- Giving oxygen by facemask to increase the amount in the mother's blood
- Increasing the nonadditive IV fluid to expand the blood volume and make more available for the placenta; this is often needed if regional analgesia or anesthesia causes hypotension
- Stopping oxytocin (Pitocin) infusion because the drug intensifies contractions and reduces placental blood flow
- Giving tocolytic drugs to decrease uterine contractions

The health care provider is notified of any nonreassuring pattern after initial steps are taken to correct it.

Inspection of Amniotic Fluid

The membranes may rupture spontaneously, or the health care provider may rupture them artificially in a procedure called an amniotomy. The color, odor, and amount of fluid are recorded. The normal color of amniotic fluid is clear, possibly with flecks of white vernix (fetal skin protectant). The amount of amniotic fluid is usually estimated as scant (only a trickle), moderate (about 500 ml), or large (about 1000 ml or more). Green-stained fluid may indicate the fetus has passed meconium (the first stool) before birth, a situation associated with fetal compromise that can cause respiratory problems at birth. Cloudy or yellow amniotic fluid with an offensive odor may indicate an infection and should be reported immediately.

The FHR should be assessed for at least 1 full minute after the membranes rupture and must be recorded and reported. Marked slowing of the rate or variable decelerations suggest that the fetal umbilical cord may have come down with the fluid gush and is being compressed.

A Nitrazine test or fern test may be performed if it is not clear whether the mother's membranes have ruptured. Nitrazine paper is a pH paper; alkaline amniotic fluid turns it dark blue-green or dark blue. In the fern test a sample of amniotic fluid is spread on a microscope slide and allowed to dry. It is then viewed under the microscope; the crystals in the fluid look like tiny fern leaves.

MONITORING THE WOMAN

Intrapartum care of the woman includes assessing her vital signs, contractions, progress of labor, intake and output, and responses to labor.

Vital Signs

The temperature is checked every 4 hours, or every 2 hours if it is elevated or if the membranes have rup-

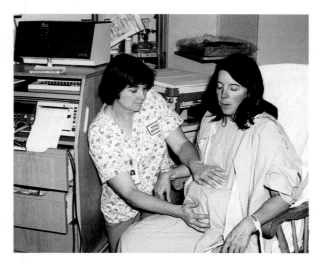

FIGURE **6-16** The nurse helps the mother maintain control and use breathing techniques during active labor. The use of an electronic monitor for fetal heart and contractions is *not* a substitute for personal hands-on care during labor. Note that the nurse places the entire hand on the fundus to determine the intensity of the contraction.

tured (frequency varies among facilities). A temperature of 38° C (100.4° F) or higher should be reported. If the temperature is elevated, the amniotic fluid is assessed for signs of infection. IV antibiotics are usually given to a woman who has a fever because of the risk that the infant will acquire group B streptococcus (GBS) infection. The pulse, blood pressure, and respirations are assessed every hour. Maternal hypotension (particularly if the systolic pressure is below 90 mm Hg) or hypertension (above 140/90 mm Hg) can reduce blood flow to the placenta.

Contractions

Contractions can be assessed by palpation and/or by continuous EFM. Some women have sensitive abdominal skin, especially around the umbilicus. When palpation is used to evaluate contractions, the entire hand is placed lightly on her uterine fundus (Figure 6-16). The nurse should keep the fingers still when palpating contractions. Moving the fingers over the uterus can stimulate contractions and give an inaccurate idea of their true frequency (Box 6-6).

Progress of Labor

The health care provider does a vaginal examination periodically to determine how labor is progressing. The cervix is evaluated for effacement and dilation. The descent of the fetus is determined in relation to the ischial spines (station) (see Figure 6-10). There is no set interval for doing vaginal examinations. The observant

---

box 6-6 *Procedure for Determining Contractions by Palpation*

1. Place the fingertips of one hand lightly on the upper uterus. Keep the fingers relatively still, but move them occasionally so that mild contractions can be felt.
2. Palpate at least three to five contractions for an accurate estimate of their average characteristics.
3. Note the time when each contraction begins and ends. Calculate the *frequency* by counting the elapsed time from the beginning of one contraction to the beginning of the next. Calculate the *duration* by determining the number of seconds from the beginning to the end of each contraction.
4. Estimate the *intensity* by trying to indent the uterus at the contraction's peak. If it is easily indented (like the tip of the nose), the contraction is mild; if it is harder to indent (like the chin), it is moderate; if nearly impossible to indent (like the forehead), it is firm.
5. Chart the average frequency (in minutes and fractions), duration (in seconds), and intensity.
6. Report contractions more frequent than every 2 minutes or lasting longer than 90 seconds or intervals of relaxation shorter than 60 seconds.

---

nurse watches for physical and behavioral changes associated with progression of labor to reduce the number of vaginal examinations needed. Vaginal examinations are limited to prevent infection, especially if the membranes are ruptured. They are also uncomfortable.

Intake and Output

Women in labor do not usually need strict measurement of intake and output, but the time and approximate amount of each urination are recorded. The woman may not sense a full bladder; she should be checked every 1 or 2 hours for a bulge above the symphysis pubis. A full bladder is a source of vague discomfort and can impede fetal descent. It often causes discomfort that persists after an epidural block has been initiated.

Policies about oral intake vary among birth facilities. Ice chips are usually allowed to moisten the mouth, unless it is likely that the woman will have a cesarean birth. Many facilities allow Popsicles or hard sugarless lollipops.

Response to Labor

The nurse assesses the woman's response to labor, including her use of breathing and relaxation techniques,

and supports adaptive responses. Nonverbal behaviors that suggest difficulty coping with labor include a tense body posture and thrashing in bed. The health care provider is notified if the woman requests added pain relief, such as epidural analgesia.

Signs that suggest rapid labor progress are promptly addressed. Bloody show may increase markedly, and the perineum may bulge as the fetal head stretches it. The student nurse should summon a registered nurse with the call signal if bloody show or perineal bulging increases or if the woman exhibits behaviors typical of imminent birth (listed earlier in this chapter). *Do not leave the woman if birth is imminent!*

HELPING THE WOMAN COPE WITH LABOR

The nurse must understand the physiology of the normal process of labor to recognize abnormalities. The nurse collects, records, and interprets data during labor, such as FHR responses to uterine contractions (see discussion of electronic fetal monitoring, pp. 136-141), maternal physical responses (e.g., vital signs and duration of contractions), and psychological responses (e.g., anxiety and tension). The nurse also maintains open communication with the health care provider and provides general hygiene and comfort measures for the mother according to the needs presented.

In addition to consistent assessment of the fetal and maternal conditions, the nurse helps the woman to cope with labor by comforting, positioning, teaching, and encouraging her (Figure 6-17). Another aspect of intrapartum nursing is care of the woman's partner (see Table 6-3).

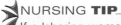

NURSING **TIP**
If a laboring woman says her baby is coming, *believe* her.

Teaching

Teaching the laboring woman and her partner is an ongoing task of the intrapartum nurse. Even women who attended prepared childbirth classes often find that the measures they learned are inadequate or need to be adapted. Positions or breathing techniques different from those learned in class can be tried. A woman should usually try a change in technique or position for two or three contractions before abandoning it.

Many women are discouraged when their cervix is about 5 cm dilated because it has taken many hours to reach that point. They think they are only halfway through labor (full dilation is 10 cm). However, a 5 cm

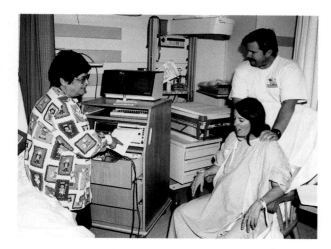

FIGURE **6-17** The nurse explains the external electronic fetal monitor to the woman. The uterine activity sensor is placed on her upper abdomen, over the uterine fundus. The Doppler transducer is placed over her lower abdomen, or wherever the FHR is clearest. The woman and partner are kept informed of progress.

dilation signifies that about two thirds of the labor is over because the rate of progress increases. Laboring women often need support and reassurance to overcome their discouragement at this point.

The nurse must often help the woman avoid pushing before her cervix is fully dilated. She can be taught to blow out in short puffs when the urge to push is strong before the cervix is fully dilated. Pushing before full dilation can cause maternal exhaustion and fetal hypoxia, thus slowing progress rather than speeding it.

When the cervix is fully dilated, the nurse teaches or supports effective pushing techniques. If the woman is pushing effectively and the fetus is tolerating labor well, the nurse should not interfere with her efforts. The woman takes a deep breath and exhales at the beginning of a contraction. She then takes another deep breath and pushes with her abdominal muscles while exhaling. Prolonged breath holding while pushing can impair fetal blood circulation (the Valsalva maneuver). She should push for about 4 to 6 seconds at a time. If she is in a semi-sitting position in bed, she should pull back on her knees, behind her thighs, or use the hand-holds on the bed.

> **NURSING TIP**
> Regular changes of position make the laboring woman more comfortable and promote the normal processes of labor.

> **NURSING TIP**
> Teaching the father/partner. The father/partner should be taught the following:
> - How labor pains affect the woman's behavior/attitude
> - How to adapt responses to the woman's behavior
> - What to expect in his own emotional responses as the woman becomes introverted or negative
> - Effects of epidural analgesia

Providing Encouragement

Encouragement is a powerful tool for intrapartum nursing care because it helps the woman to summon inner strength and gives her courage to continue. After each vaginal examination, she is told of the progress in cervical change or fetal descent. Liberal praise is given if she successfully uses techniques to cope with labor. Her partner needs encouragement as well; labor coaching is a demanding job. Some women may use a doula, a person whose only job is to support and encourage the woman in the task of giving birth.

The nurse's caring presence cannot be overlooked as a source of support and encouragement for the laboring woman and her partner. Many women feel dependent during labor and are more secure if the nurse is in their room or nearby. Just being present helps, even if no specific care is given, because they see the nurse as the expert.

Supporting the Partner

Partners, or coaches, vary considerably in the degree of involvement with which they are comfortable. The labor partner is most often the infant's father but may be the woman's mother or friend. Some partners are truly coaches and take a leading role in helping the woman cope with labor (Figure 6-18). Others are willing to assist if they are shown how, but they will not take the initiative. Still other couples are content with the partner's encouragement and support but do not expect him or her to have an active role. The partner should be permitted to provide the type of support comfortable for the couple. The nurse does not take the partner's place but remains available as needed.

The partner should be encouraged to take a break and periodically eat a snack or meal. Many partners are reluctant to leave the woman's bedside, but they may faint during the birth if they have not eaten. A chair or stool near the bed allows the partner to sit down as much as possible.

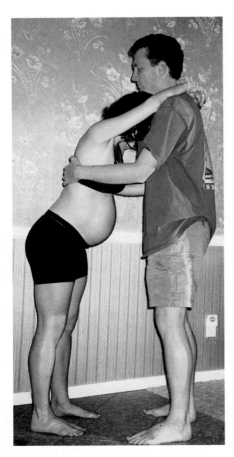

FIGURE **6-18** Standing and walking during early labor and leaning on the partner during contractions uses gravity to aid in fetal descent, reduces back pain, and stimulates contractions.

THE LABOR PROCESS AND THE NURSE

STAGES AND PHASES OF LABOR

Women giving birth display common physical and behavioral characteristics in each of the four stages of labor. Those who receive an epidural analgesic during labor may not exhibit the behaviors and sensations associated with each stage and phase. The nurse must also realize that women are individuals and that each responds to labor in her own way. Table 6-3 summarizes the stages and phases of labor, the related behavior changes, and the nursing care responsibilities.

> **NURSING TIP**
> The bedside nurse in the labor and delivery unit bridges the gap between sophisticated technology and the individual patient's needs, providing a positive outcome both physically and psychologically.

> **NURSING TIP**
> If a woman suddenly loses control and becomes irritable, suspect that she has progressed to the transition phase of labor.

VAGINAL BIRTH AFTER CESAREAN BIRTH

It was once thought that a woman who had a cesarean delivery for one infant must have a surgical birth for every subsequent infant. Today, physicians carefully select women who are appropriate candidates for vaginal birth after cesarean (VBAC). See p. 183 for more information about cesarean birth and subsequent vaginal births.

Nursing care for women who plan to have a VBAC is similar to that for women who have had no cesarean births. The main concern is that the uterine scar will rupture (see p. 199), which can disrupt the placental blood flow and cause hemorrhage. Observation for signs of uterine rupture should be part of the nursing care for all laboring women, regardless of whether they have had a previous cesarean birth.

Women having a VBAC often need more support than other laboring women. They are often anxious about their ability to cope with labor's demands and to deliver vaginally, especially if they have never done so. If their cesarean birth occurred during rather than before labor, they may become anxious when they reach the same point in the current labor. The nurse must provide empathy and support to help the woman cross this psychological barrier. However, the nurse cannot promise the woman that a repeat cesarean birth will not be needed, because one may be required for many reasons.

> **NURSING TIP**
> The woman who is having a vaginal birth after cesarean delivery needs special emotional support. She is often anxious, and a cesarean procedure may seem like the easiest way to give birth.

NURSING CARE DURING BIRTH

There is no exact time when the woman should be prepared for delivery. In general, the woman having her first child is prepared when about 3 to 4 cm of the fetal head is visible (crowning) at the vaginal opening. The multipara is usually prepared when her cervix is fully dilated but before crowning has occurred. If the woman must be transferred to a delivery room rather than give birth in a LDR, she should be moved early enough to avoid a last-minute rush.

table 6-3 *The Labor Process and the Nurse*

CHARACTERISTICS	PATIENT BEHAVIOR	NURSING INTERVENTIONS
FIRST STAGE—STAGE OF DILATION AND EFFACEMENT		
Latent Phase (4-6 hours)		
1-4 cm dilation of cervix.	Cooperative	Establish positive relationships.
Amniotic membranes may be intact.	Alert	Encourage alternating ambulation and rest.
There may be "bloody show."	Talkative	Review breathing and relaxation techniques with coach.
Contractions: q 20 minutes decreasing to q 5 minutes	Welcomes diversions	Assess fetal heart rate.
Duration: 15-40 seconds	Urinary frequency	Time contractions.
Intensity: mild to moderate	Thirsty	Document color of vaginal discharge.
		Assess for distended bladder.
		Provide opportunity to void.
		May provide lollipops for mother to hold and suck on between contractions for carbohydrate and fluid intake.
		Assess vital signs q 2 hours.
		Woman may take showers.
		Teach what to expect as labor progresses.
Active Phase (2-6 hours)		
4-7 cm dilation of cervix.	Apprehensive	Help coach apply coping strategies learned in prenatal classes (breathing, relaxation).
Amniotic membranes may rupture.	Anxious	Continue maternal and fetal assessments.
Effacement of cervix occurs.	Introverted	Reassure woman.
Contractions: 2-5 minutes apart	Less social	Praise progress.
Duration: 40-60 seconds	Focused on breathing	Provide back massage.
Intensity: Moderate to firm	Perspires	Facilitate position changes (avoid lying flat on back).
	Facial flushing	If taking nothing orally (NPO), moisten mouth.
	Requests pain relief	Maintain communication with health care provider.
	Fears losing control	Monitor IV fluid intake.
	May need epidural analgesia at this time	Watch for bladder distention.
		Encourage voiding.
		Report color, odor, amount of vaginal discharge; report if meconium is seen.
		Maintain warmth.
		Woman may shower if allowed.
		Provide general comfort measures.
Transition Phase (30 minutes-2 hours)		
Cervix dilation 7-10 cm; cervix fully effaced.	Irritable	Provide firm coaching of breathing and relaxation techniques, focusing.
Amniotic membranes rupture.	Rejects support person	Support coach.
Contractions: q 2-3 minutes	Introverted	Praise and reassure woman.
Duration: 60-90 seconds	Wants to give up	Assess monitor strips of fetal heart rate and contractions.
Intensity: firm	Restless	Assess color of vaginal discharge.
	Tremor of legs	Keep woman informed as to progress with each contraction.
	Fears losing control	Accept negative comments from woman.
	Requests medication	Maintain positive approach.

Continued

table 6-3 | *The Labor Process and the Nurse—cont'd*

CHARACTERISTICS	PATIENT BEHAVIOR	NURSING INTERVENTIONS
SECOND STAGE—STAGE OF EXPULSION (30 minutes-2 hours)		
Cervix dilation 10 cm *Contractions:* q 1½-3 minutes *Duration:* 60-80 seconds *Intensity:* firm Episiotomy may be performed by health care provider. Second stage ends with birth of infant.	Bulging perineum Mother may pass stool Uncontrollable urge to push States "baby is coming" Exhaustion after each contraction Unable to follow directions easily Excitement concerning imminent birth	Assist woman to assume position that helps her push. Assist with open glottis pushing technique and coping strategies. Support coach. Maintain communication with health care provider. Monitor contractions and fetal heart rate q 5 minutes. Assess perineum and vaginal discharge. Report bulging or crowning. Observe for bladder distention. Prepare sterile supplies for delivery. Prepare infant resuscitation equipment. Provide feedback to woman and partner.
THIRD STAGE—EXPULSION OF PLACENTA		
Duration: 5-30 minutes *Contractions:* intermittent *Intensity:* mild to moderate Umbilical cord is cut. Signs of placental separation include the following: • Lengthening of cord • Uterine fundus rises and becomes firm • Fresh blood expelled from vagina Placenta is expelled by Schultze mechanism (shiny fetal side first) or by Duncan's mechanism (dull, rough maternal side first) (see Figure 6-21). Uterus contracts to size of grapefruit. Episiotomy is sutured by health care provider.	Elation Relief Tremors Increased physical energy Curiosity about infant Desire to nurse infant Pain is minimal as placenta is expelled	Observe and document blood loss. Document delivery of placenta. Examine placenta to determine if all of it was expelled (retained placenta causes hemorrhage because it prevents uterus from contracting). Monitor mother's vital signs q 15 minutes. Assess vaginal discharge. Massage uterus until it is firm in midline at or below level of umbilicus. Administer oxytocin to mother as ordered. Obtain cord blood if needed. Note parent/infant interaction. Dry newborn and place in radiant warmer. Attach heart and temperature monitor. Assess and provide immediate newborn care (see p. 151). Perform Apgar evaluation. Apply proper identification to mother, infant, and partner.
FOURTH STAGE—RECOVERY		
Uterus remains midline, firmly contracted at or below umbilicus level. Lochia rubra saturates perineal pad (no more than one pad per hour). Cramping may occur. Woman may have shaking chills that may be a thermoregulation response.	A get-acquainted period between woman, partner, and infant Mother breastfeeds infant	Provide proper identification of mother, partner, and newborn. Obtain cord blood if needed. Assess woman's vital signs q 15 minutes. Assess maternal voiding. Monitor heart rate and temperature of newborn. Provide warmth to newborn. Assess newborn for anomalies. Assess fundus and massage to maintain firm contraction (a fundus that is displaced to the side indicates a full bladder is pressing against it). Assess lochia (no more than one saturated pad per hour). Change mother's gown and underpads. Encourage breastfeeding. Encourage bonding between parent and infant.

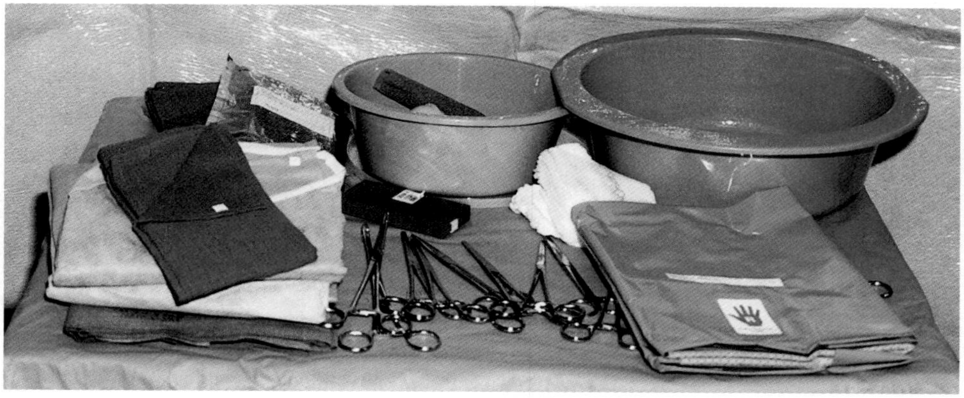

FIGURE **6-19** The table contains the sterile instruments that the health care provider will use for delivery. The table is kept covered with a sterile sheet in the LDR room until it is ready for use.

If the woman does not have full sensation or movement of the legs because of an epidural anesthetic, padded stirrups may be used and the woman observed closely for excess pressure behind the knee, which can cause thrombophlebitis (blood clot).

A woman can give birth in many different positions. The "traditional" position, semi-sitting and using foot supports, improves access to her perineum but may not be the most comfortable for her or the best one to expel the infant. She may give birth in a side-lying position, squatting, standing, or other positions.

NURSING **TIP**
Support the woman's partner so that he or she can be the most effective coach possible during labor.

NURSING RESPONSIBILITIES DURING BIRTH

Health care providers do not usually need a scrub nurse during the birth. The registered nurse who cares for the woman during labor usually continues to do so in a "circulating" capacity during delivery. Typical delivery responsibilities include the following:

- Preparing the delivery instruments and infant equipment (Figure 6-19)
- Doing the perineal scrub prep (Figure 6-20)
- Administering drugs to the mother or infant
- Providing initial care to the infant, such as suctioning the airway with a bulb syringe, drying the skin, and placing the infant in a radiant warmer to maintain body heat
- Assessing the infant's Apgar score (see Table 6-4)
- Assessing the infant for obvious abnormalities (A note is made if the infant has a stool or urinates.)

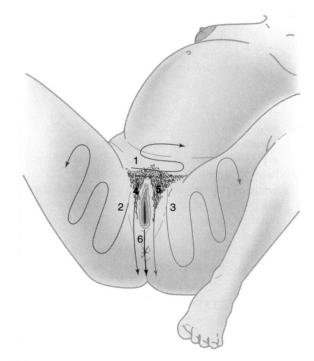

FIGURE **6-20** Perineal scrub preparation is done just before birth. Numbers and arrows indicate the order and the direction of each stroke. A clean sponge is used for each step.

- Examining the placenta to be sure it is intact and recording if it was expelled via the Schultze or Duncan mechanisms (Figure 6-21)
- Identifying the mother and infant with like-numbered identification bands (The father or other support person usually receives a band as well; infant footprints and the mother's fingerprints are often obtained.)

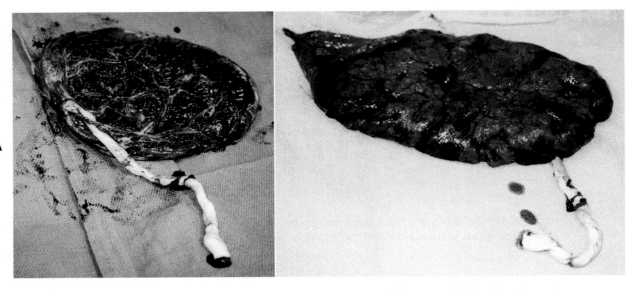

FIGURE **6-21** The placenta after delivery. **A,** Duncan's delivery. The maternal side of the placenta, which is dull and rough, is delivered first. **B,** Schultze delivery. The fetal side of the placenta, which is shiny and smooth, is delivered first. (Photos courtesy of Pat Spier, RN-C.)

- Promoting parent-infant bonding and initial breastfeeding by encouraging parents to hold and explore the infant while maintaining the infant's body temperature (Observe for eye contact, fingertip or palm touch of the infant, and talking to the infant, all of which are associated with initial bonding; these observations continue throughout the postpartum period.)

Figure 6-22 shows an infant being born in the vertex presentation in a spontaneous vaginal birth.

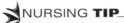
NURSING **TIP**

An easy way to remember placental delivery is **D**uncan: **D**ull; **S**chultze: **S**hiny.

IMMEDIATE POSTPARTUM PERIOD: THE THIRD AND FOURTH STAGES OF LABOR

The third stage of labor is the expulsion of the placenta. The nurse examines the placenta and monitors the woman's vital signs (see Table 6-3).

The fourth stage of labor is the first 1 to 4 hours after birth of the placenta or until the mother is physiologically stable. Nursing care during the fourth stage of labor includes the following general care:
- Identifying and preventing hemorrhage
- Evaluating and intervening for pain

- Observing bladder function and urine output
- Evaluating recovery from anesthesia
- Providing initial care to the newborn infant
- Promoting bonding and attachment between the infant and family

NURSING CARE IMMEDIATELY AFTER BIRTH

CARE OF THE MOTHER

Facility protocols will vary, but a common schedule for assessing the mother during the fourth stage is every 15 minutes for 1 hour, every 30 minutes during the second hour, and hourly until transfer to the postpartum unit. After transfer to the postpartum unit, applicable routine assessments are made every 4 to 8 hours. Assessments that should be made each time during the fourth stage include the following:
- Vital signs (temperature may be taken hourly if normal)
- Skin color
- Location and firmness of the uterine fundus (see Chapter 9)
- Amount and color of lochia (see Chapter 9)
- Presence and location of pain
- IV infusion and medications
- Fullness of the bladder or urine output from a catheter

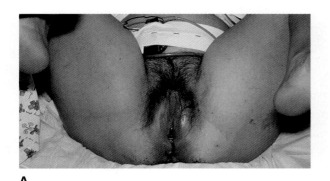
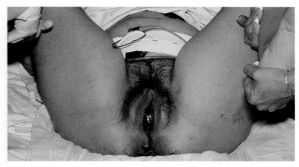

A

B

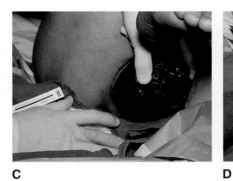
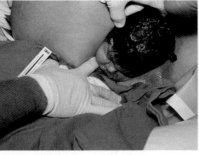
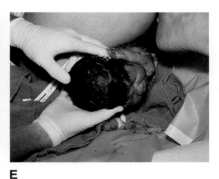

C

D

E

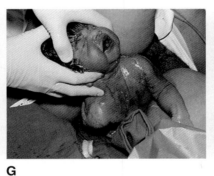
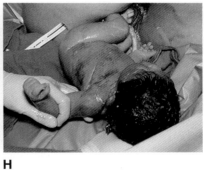

F

G

H

FIGURE **6-22** Vaginal birth of a fetus in vertex presentation. **A** and **B,** Bulging of the perineum. **C,** Crowning. **D,** Head born by extension. **E,** External rotation. **F,** Delivery of the shoulders; infant is suctioned. **G,** Delivery of posterior shoulder and chest. **H,** Expulsion of newborn.

Continued

- Condition of the perineum for vaginal birth
- Condition of dressing for cesarean birth or tubal ligation
- Level of sensation and ability to move lower extremities if an epidural or spinal block was used

Observing for Hemorrhage

The uterine fundus is assessed for firmness, height in relation to the umbilicus, and position (midline or deviated to one side). Refer to Chapter 9 for assessment of the fundus. Vaginal bleeding should be dark red (lochia rubra). No more than one pad should be saturated in an

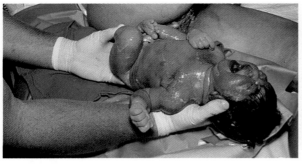

I

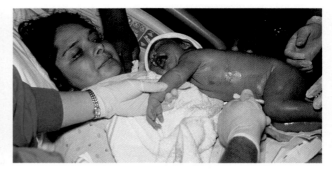

J

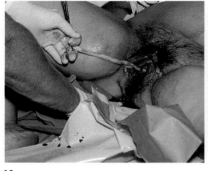

K

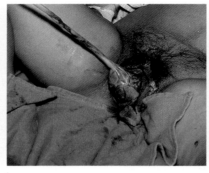

L

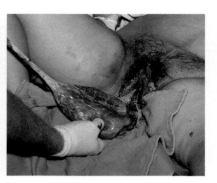

M

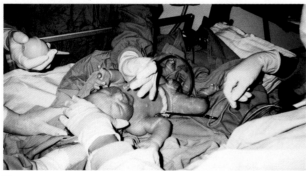

N

FIGURE **6-22,** cont'd **I,** Newborn cries; color is cyanotic. **J,** Newborn placed on mother's abdomen and cord is cut. **K** to **M,** Delivery of placenta. **N,** Newborn is given whiffs of oxygen and suctioned with bulb syringe while in radiant warmer. Note that the caregivers are wearing gloves while caring for the unwashed newborn.

hour, and the woman should not pass large clots. A continuous trickle of bright red blood suggests a bleeding laceration. The blood pressure, pulse, and respirations are taken to identify a rising pulse or falling blood pressure, which suggest shock. An oral temperature is taken and reported if it is 38° C (100.4° F) or higher or if the woman has a higher risk for infection.

The bladder is assessed for distention, which may occur soon after birth. The woman often does not feel the urge to urinate because of the effects of the anesthetic, perineal trauma, and loss of fetal pressure against the bladder. If her bladder is full, the uterus will be higher than expected and often displaced to one side. A full bladder inhibits uterine contraction and can lead to hemorrhage. Catheterization will be needed if the woman cannot urinate.

Promoting Comfort

Many women have a shaking chill after birth yet deny that they are cold. A warm blanket over the woman makes her feel more comfortable until the chill subsides. The warm blanket also maintains the infant's warmth while parents get acquainted.

An ice pack may be placed on the mother's perineum to reduce bruising and edema. A glove can be filled with ice and wrapped in a wash cloth. Perineal pads that incorporate a chemical cold pack are often used. These pads do not absorb as much lochia as those without the cold pack, and this must be considered in evaluating the quantity of bleeding. Cold applications are continued for at least 12 hours. A warm pack pad may be used after the first 12 to 24 hours to encourage blood flow to the area.

CARE OF THE INFANT

The infant usually stays with the parents during recovery if there are no complications. The priority care involves promoting respiratory function and maintaining the temperature. (See Chapter 9 for care of the newborn after the fourth stage of labor and Chapter 12 for an in-depth discussion of the normal newborn.)

Care of the Newborn Immediately After Delivery

Care of the newborn after delivery is divided into the following three "transition phases" that are involved in adapting to extrauterine life:

- First phase: the immediate care after birth; from birth to 1 hour (usually in delivery room) (discussed in the next section)
- Second phase: from 1 to 3 hours after birth; usually in the transition nursery or postpartum unit (see Chapter 9)
- Third phase: from 2 to 12 hours after birth; usually in the postpartum unit if rooming-in with the mother (see Chapter 12)

Phase 1

Initial care of the newborn includes the following:

- Maintaining thermoregulation
- Maintaining cardiorespiratory function
- Observing for urination and/or passage of meconium
- Identifying the mother, father, and newborn
- Performing a brief assessment for major anomalies
- Encouraging bonding/breastfeeding

The infant will be covered in blood and amniotic fluid at birth. All caregivers should wear gloves when handling the newborn until after the first bath.

Maintaining thermoregulation in the newborn. A critical factor in the transition of the newborn is maintaining a neutral thermal environment in which heat loss is minimal and oxygen consumption needs are the lowest. *Hypothermia* (low body temperature) can cause hypo-

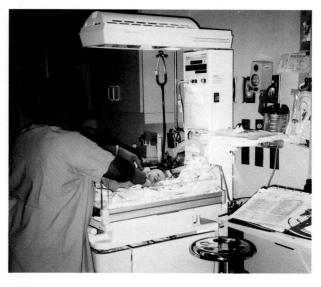

FIGURE **6-23** The nurse applies the sensor and assesses the newborn in the radiant warmer. Note: This nurse is wearing purple nitrite (latex-free) gloves when handling the newborn. (Some newborns can be allergic to latex.)

glycemia (low blood sugar) because glucose is used by the infant's body to generate heat. Hypoglycemia is associated with the development of neurological problems in the newborn. Hypothermia can also cause cold stress, in which the increased metabolic rate required to generate body heat causes increased respiratory rate and oxygen consumption. If the infant cannot supply the increased demand for oxygen, hypoxia will result and cause further problems.

Essential nursing interventions to maintain a neutral thermal environment include the following:

- *Drying the infant* with a towel to avoid heat loss caused by evaporation of amniotic fluid on the skin. The body and head should be gently dried with a warm towel.
- *Placing infant in radiant warmer.* A skin probe can be placed on the right upper abdomen (over the spleen or liver) to act as a thermostat to the radiant warmer so that the proper setting of heat will be supplied (Figure 6-23).
- *Placing a hat on the infant's head* after the head is dried. The head is the largest body surface area in the newborn, and significant heat loss can occur if the moist head is left open to room air.
- *Wrapping the infant* in warm blankets when taken out of the warmer. Skin to skin (kangaroo) contact between mother and newborn during bonding or breastfeeding can also prevent heat loss (see Figure 13-8).

An incubator may be necessary if the infant is unable to stabilize body temperature. The first bath is delayed until the infant's temperature is stabilized at 36.5° to 37° C.

Maintaining cardiorespiratory function. Physiological changes in the cardiopulmonary circulation in the newborn are discussed in Chapter 12.

Respiratory support immediately after delivery includes the following:

- Gentle wiping of the face, nose, and mouth to remove mucus and excess amniotic fluid.
- Gentle bulb suctioning of nose and mouth to clear airways. At birth the infant may be placed on the mother's abdomen. Suctioning may be initiated by the health care provider before cutting the cord. Further need for suctioning is determined when the infant is placed in the radiant warmer.
- A cord clamp is applied when the infant is stabilized in the radiant warmer (Figure 6-24).

Spontaneous breathing usually begins within a few seconds after birth. The infant's color at birth may be cyanotic (blue) but quickly turns pink (often except for the hands and feet). As the infant cries, the skin color will be pink. Acrocyanosis is the bluish color of hands and feet of the newborn that is normal and is caused by sluggish peripheral circulation. Oxygen by facemask may be given until the infant is crying vigorously. Some signs of respiratory distress that should be immediately reported include the following:

- Persistent cyanosis (other than the hands and feet)
- Grunting respirations: a noise heard without a stethoscope as the infant exhales
- Flaring of the nostrils
- Retractions: under the sternum or between the ribs
- Sustained respiratory rate higher than 60 breaths/min
- Sustained heart rate above 160 beats/min or below 110 beats/min

Narcan (naloxone) is kept on hand to reverse narcotic-induced respiratory depression.

Performing Apgar scoring. Dr. Virginia Apgar devised a system for evaluating the infant's condition and need for resuscitation at birth (Table 6-4). Five factors are evaluated at 1 minute and 5 minutes after birth and are ranked in order of importance, as follows:

- Heart rate
- Respiratory effort
- Muscle tone
- Reflex response to suction or gentle stimulation on the soles of the feet
- Skin color

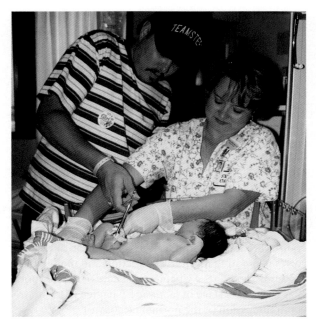

FIGURE **6-24** The nurse assists the father in cutting the umbilical cord to a proper length so the umbilical clamp can be applied. Note the identification band on the father's wrist.

The Apgar score is not a predictor of future intelligence or abilities/disabilities. It was meant to identify only the condition and need for neonatal resuscitation measures. Equipment, medications, and personnel must be readily available for resuscitation at any birth, however, because the need cannot always be anticipated.

Identifying the infant. Wristbands with preprinted numbers are placed on the mother, the infant, and often the father or other support person in the birthing room as the primary means of identifying the infant. The nurse should check to be sure that all numbers in the set are identical. Other identifying information is completed, such as mother's name, birth attendant's name, date and time of birth, sex of the infant, and usually the mother's hospital identification number. The bands are applied relatively snugly on the infant and have only a finger's width of slack because infants lose weight after birth.

The nurse must check the preprinted wristband numbers to see that they match every time the infant returns to the mother after a separation or the mother goes to the nursery to retrieve her infant. The nurse should either look at the numbers to see that they are identical or have the mother read her own band number while looking at the infant's band.

Footprints of the infant and one or both index fingerprints of the mother are often taken. Many birth facilities take a photograph of the infant in the birthing room or very soon after admission and record birth-

table 6-4 | *Apgar Scoring System*

SIGN	0	1	2
Heart rate	Absent	Below 100 beats/min	100 beats/min or higher
Respiratory effort	No spontaneous respirations	Slow; weak cry	Spontaneous, with a strong, lusty cry
Muscle tone	Limp	Minimal flexion of extremities; sluggish movement	Active spontaneous motion; flexed body posture
Reflex irritability	No response to suction or gentle slap on soles	Minimal response (grimace) to stimulation	Prompt response to suction with a gentle slap to sole of foot with cry or active movement
Color	Blue or pale	Body pink, extremities blue	Completely pink (light skin) or absence of cyanosis (dark skin)

NOTE: The nurse evaluates each sign in the Apgar and totals the score to determine what interventions the infant needs. A score of 8 to 10 requires no action other than continued observation and support of the infant's adaptation. A score from 4 to 7 means the infant needs gentle stimulation such as rubbing the back; the possibility of narcotic-induced respiratory depression should also be considered. Scores of 3 or lower mean that the infant needs active resuscitation.

marks or unique features. This is primarily for identification of the infant in the event of an abduction and for keepsake purposes.

Observing urinary function/passage of meconium. Newborns may not urinate for as long as 24 hours after delivery. If the infant voids in the LDR, it must be documented on the chart. Meconium, the first stool of the newborn, may be passed anytime within 12 to 24 hours. If meconium is passed in the LDR, it should be documented in the chart. The infant cannot be discharged to the home until documentation that the gastrointestinal and genitourinary tracts are functioning. Passing meconium and voiding help determine the status of these systems.

Promoting maternal-infant bonding. Every attempt should be made to facilitate maternal-infant contact. As soon as the infant is dried and warmed and cardiorespiratory function is stable, the infant should be warmly wrapped and placed in the mother's arms or in skin-to-skin contact with the mother. The infant is alert in the first hour of life, and therefore this is the best time to initiate breastfeeding and bonding. Breastfeeding is discussed in Chapter 9.

After the first hour of life the infant begins a sleep pattern with decreased motor activity. This is the best time for medication administration before leaving the delivery room. Referral to a nurse who is a lactation specialist may be initiated if the mother needs assistance with breastfeeding.

Administering medications

Eye care. All newborn infants are given specific eye care to prevent ophthalmia neonatorum, which is caused by *Neisseria gonorrhoeae*. The American Academy of Pediatrics also recommends protection against *Chlamydia trachomatis*. Therefore erythromycin eye ointment (administered from individual dose tubes) is placed in each eye (Figure 6-25). Eye care is given 1 hour *after* birth (so that the infant and mother can bond in that first hour), but it must be given and charted *before* leaving the delivery room.

Vitamin K (AquaMEPHYTON). Newborns need vitamin K to assist in blood clotting. Vitamin K is naturally produced from intestinal flora, which is absent in the newborn. One single dose of vitamin K is injected into the vastus lateralis muscle (thigh) before the infant leaves the delivery room, usually at age 1 hour.

Observing for major anomalies. The nurse notes signs of injury or anomalies while performing other assessments and care. The infant's movements and facial expressions during crying are observed for symmetry and equality of movement. The head and face should be assessed for trauma, especially if forceps were used. A small puncture wound is usually apparent on the scalp if an internal spiral electrode was used for fetal monitoring. If the infant was born vaginally in a breech presentation, the buttocks may be bruised.

Many anomalies, such as spina bifida (open spine) or a cleft lip (see Chapter 14), are immediately obvious. The fingers and toes should be counted to identify abnormal numbers or webbing. The feet are observed for straightness; if deviated, it should be determined if the feet can be returned to the straight position. Length equality of arms and legs should be checked. Urination

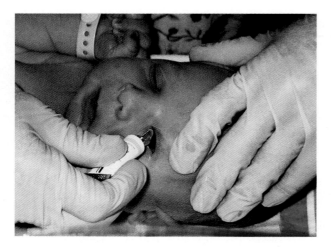

FIGURE **6-25** The nurse applies erythromycin ointment to the eyes of the newborn to protect against ophthalmia neonatorum and *Chlamydia* infection. All newborns have this prophylactic eye treatment before leaving the delivery room. (Photo courtesy of Pat Spier, RN-C.)

or meconium passage is assessed, both of which confirm patency.

A detailed assessment for anomalies and gestational age is completed on admission to the newborn nursery or postpartum unit.

key points

- The four components, or "four *P*s," of the birth process are the powers, the passage, the passenger, and the psyche. All interrelate during labor to either facilitate or impede birth.
- True labor and false labor have several differences. However, the conclusive difference is that true labor results in cervical change (effacement and/or dilation).
- The woman should go to the hospital if she is having persistent, regular contractions (every 5 minutes for nulliparas, and every 10 minutes for multiparas); if her membranes rupture; if she has bleeding other than normal bloody show; if fetal movement decreases; or for other concerns not covered by the basic guidelines.
- Three key assessments on admission are fetal condition, maternal condition, and nearness to birth.
- Four stages of labor each have different characteristics. The first stage is the stage of dilation, lasting from labor's onset to full (10 cm) cervical dilation.

First-stage labor is subdivided into three phases: latent, active, and transition. Second-stage labor, the stage of expulsion, extends from full cervical dilation until birth of the infant. The third stage, the placental stage, is from the birth of the infant until the birth of the placenta. The fourth stage is the immediate postbirth recovery period and includes the first 1 to 4 hours after placental delivery.

- The main fetal risk during first- and second-stage labor is fetal compromise caused by interruption of the fetal oxygen supply. The main maternal risk during fourth-stage labor is hemorrhage caused by uterine relaxation.
- Nursing care during the first and second stages focuses on observing the fetal and maternal conditions and on assisting the woman to cope with labor.
- Continuous electronic fetal monitoring is most common in hospital births, but intermittent auscultation is a valid method of fetal assessment.
- Laboring women can assume many positions. Upright positions add gravity to promote fetal descent. Hands-and-knees or leaning-forward positions promote normal internal rotation of the fetus if "back labor" is a problem. Squatting facilitates fetal descent during the second stage. The supine position should be discouraged because it causes the heavy uterus to compress the mother's main blood vessels, which can reduce fetal oxygen supply.
- The immediate care of the newborn after birth includes maintaining warmth, maintaining cardiorespiratory function, assessing for major anomalies, encouraging parent-infant bonding, and providing proper identification and documentation.

ONLINE RESOURCES

Multilingual Facts for Prenatal Health:
http://www.safemotherhood.org

Coping with Labor: http://www.lamaze-childbirth.com

Understanding the Health Culture of Recent Immigrants to the United States: http://www.apha.org/ppp/red/other.htm

Safer Childbirth Around the World: http://www.asia-initiative.org

CRITICAL THINKING QUESTION

A para 0 gravida 1 woman is admitted in active labor. She states she has completed prenatal care and wishes for a natural, unmedicated childbirth. However, she states she now does not feel she can cope with the increasing levels of pain and asks if it is okay if she takes pain medication. What is the best response of the nurse?

REVIEW QUESTIONS   *Choose the most appropriate answer.*

1. To determine the frequency of uterine contractions, the nurse should note the time from the:
   1. Beginning to end of the same contraction
   2. End of one contraction to the beginning of the next contraction
   3. Beginning of one contraction to the beginning of the next contraction
   4. Contraction's peak until the contraction begins to relax

2. Excessive anxiety and fear during labor may result in:
   1. An ineffective labor pattern
   2. An abnormal fetal presentation or position
   3. A release of oxytocin from the pituitary gland
   4. A rapid labor and uncontrolled birth

3. A woman who is pregnant with her first child phones an intrapartum facility and says her "water broke." The nurse should tell her to:
   1. Wait until she has contractions every 5 minutes for 1 hour
   2. Take her temperature every 4 hours and come to the facility if it is over 38° C (100.4° F)
   3. Come to the facility promptly, but safely
   4. Call an ambulance to bring her to the facility

4. A laboring woman suddenly begins making grunting sounds and bearing down during a strong contraction. The student nurse should initially:
   1. Go and get an experienced nurse to assess the woman
   2. Look at her perineum for increased bloody show or perineal bulging
   3. Ask her if she needs pain medication
   4. Tell her that these are common sensations in late labor

5. To assess contractions by palpation, the nurse should palpate the:
   1. Fetal head
   2. Mother's cervix
   3. Uterine fundus
   4. Lower abdomen

Nursing Management of Pain During Labor and Birth

1. Define each key term listed.
2. Describe factors that influence a woman's comfort during labor.
3. List the common types of classes offered to childbearing families.
4. Describe the methods of childbirth preparation.
5. Discuss the advantages and limitations of nonpharmacological methods of pain management during labor.
6. Discuss the advantages and limitations of pharmacological methods of pain management.
7. Explain nonpharmacological methods of pain management for labor, including the nursing role for each.
8. Explain each type of pharmacological pain management, including the nursing role for each.

blood patch (p. 170)
Bradley method (p. 161)
cleansing breath (p. 163)
effleurage (ĕf-loo-RĂHZH, p. 162)
endorphin (ĕn-DŌR-fĭn, p. 160)
focal point (p. 162)
opioid (Ō-pē-oid, p. 167)
pain threshold (p. 158)
pain tolerance (p. 158)
vaginal birth after cesarean (VBAC) (p. 156)

Pregnant women are usually interested in how labor will feel and want to know how they can manage the experience, especially the pain. Women can manage labor pain by using nonpharmacological (nondrug) or pharmacological (drug) methods. Most use a combination of the two. Because preparation for childbirth is an important part of nonpharmacological pain management, it is also discussed in this chapter. General labor comfort measures, such as adjustment of the environment and maternal positioning, were discussed in Chapter 6.

EDUCATION FOR CHILDBEARING

Various classes are offered to women during pregnancy by most hospitals and freestanding birth centers to help women adjust to pregnancy, cope with labor, and prepare for life with an infant (Figure 7-1). Women who plan a home birth usually prepare intensely because they want to avoid medications and other interventions associated with hospital births.

TYPES OF CLASSES AVAILABLE

Classes during pregnancy focus on topics that contribute to good outcomes for the mother and infant (Box 7-1). Special classes prepare other family members for the birth and new infant. Other classes are sometimes available, such as the following:

- Gestational diabetes mellitus classes
- Early pregnancy classes
- Exercise classes for pregnant women
- Infant care classes
- Breastfeeding classes
- Sibling classes
- Grandparent classes

VARIATIONS OF BASIC CHILDBIRTH PREPARATION CLASSES

Refresher Classes

Refresher classes consist of one to three sessions to review the material learned during a previous pregnancy. Ways to help siblings adjust to the new baby and a review of infant feeding are often included.

Cesarean Birth Classes

Classes for women who expect a cesarean birth help the woman and her support person to understand the reasons for this method of delivery and anticipate what is likely to occur during and after surgery.

Vaginal Birth After Cesarean Classes

Women in vaginal birth after cesarean (VBAC) classes may need to express unresolved feelings about their

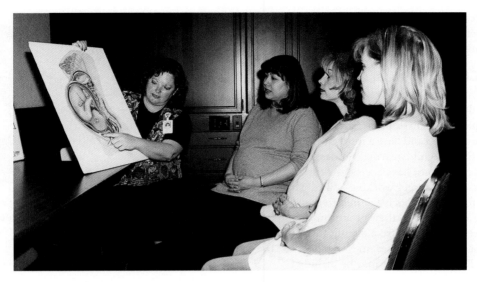

FIGURE **7-1** The nurse teaching this prenatal class discusses the movement of the fetus through the pelvis.

---

box 7-1 | *Types of Prenatal Classes*

CHILDBIRTH PREPARATION CLASSES
Changes of pregnancy
Fetal development
Prenatal care
Hazardous substances to avoid
Good nutrition for pregnancy
Relieving common pregnancy discomforts
Working during pregnancy and parenthood
Coping with labor and delivery
Care of the infant, such as feeding methods, choosing a pediatrician, and selecting clothing and equipment
Early growth and development

EXERCISE CLASSES
Maintaining the woman's fitness during pregnancy (see Chapter 4)
Postpartum classes for toning and fitness
Positions and environments to avoid

GESTATIONAL DIABETES MELLITUS
Monitoring blood sugar levels
Diet modifications
Need for frequent prenatal visits
Preventing infection and complications

SIBLING CLASSES
Helping children to prepare realistically for their new brother or sister

Helping children to understand that feelings of jealousy and anger are normal
Giving parents tips about helping older children adjust to the new baby after birth

GRANDPARENT CLASSES
Trends in childbirth and parenting styles
Importance of grandparents to a child's development
Reducing conflict between the generations

BREASTFEEDING CLASSES
Processes of breastfeeding
Feeding techniques
Solving common problems
Some classes continue after birth with lactation specialists

INFANT CARE CLASSES
Growth, development, and care of the newborn
Needed clothing and equipment
Adolescent classes for birth and parenthood preparation

VBAC CLASSES
What to expect during labor when previous childbirth was cesarean section

VBAC, Vaginal birth after cesarean.

previous cesarean birth. Depending on the reason for the cesarean delivery, they may be more anxious about the forthcoming labor.

Adolescent Childbirth Preparation Classes

A pregnant adolescent's needs are different from those of an adult. Adolescents are therefore usually uncomfortable in regular childbirth preparation classes. They are often single mothers and have a more immature perception of birth and child rearing. Some are not old enough to drive or do not have access to a car and cannot attend classes that target working adults. The content of classes for adolescents is tailored to their special needs. Because acceptance by their peer group is important to adolescents, the girls are a significant source of support for each other. Classes may be held in the school setting. Expectant fathers may be included.

CONTENT OF CHILDBIRTH PREPARATION CLASSES

Regardless of the specific method taught, most classes are similar in basic content. Box 7-2 highlights several techniques that may be taught in childbirth classes. Many of the techniques can also be used to help the unprepared woman during labor.

The woman who learns about the changes produced by pregnancy and childbirth is less likely to respond with fear and tension during labor. Information about cesarean birth is usually included.

The Benefits of Exercise

Conditioning exercises, such as the pelvic rock, tailor sitting, and shoulder circling, prepare the woman's muscles for the demands of birth (see Chapter 4). These exercises also relieve the back discomfort common during late pregnancy.

Pain Control Methods for Labor

The woman and her partner learn a variety of techniques that may be used during labor as needed (Figure 7-2). Examples of these include the following:

- Skin stimulation, such as effleurage (see Figure 7-3)
- Diversion/distraction
- Breathing techniques

These techniques are most effective if learned before labor begins. Box 7-2 reviews selected nonpharmacological pain relief techniques.

CHILDBIRTH AND PAIN

Pain is an unpleasant and distressing symptom that is personal and subjective. No one can feel another's pain,

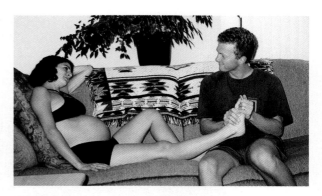

FIGURE **7-2** The partner massages the foot of the pregnant woman. Massage can provide an effective technique of pain relief during labor (see also Chapter 33).

but empathic nursing care helps to alleviate pain and helps the woman cope with it.

HOW CHILDBIRTH PAIN DIFFERS FROM OTHER PAIN

Childbirth pain differs from other types of pain in the following ways:

- It is part of a normal birth process.
- The woman has several months to prepare for pain management.
- It is self-limiting and rapidly declines after birth.

Pain is usually a symptom of injury or illness, yet pain during labor is almost a universal part of the normal process of birth. Although excessive pain is detrimental to the labor process, pain can also be beneficial. It may cause a woman to feel vulnerable and seek shelter and help from others. Pain often motivates her to assume different body positions, which can facilitate the normal descent of the fetus. Birth pain lasts for hours, as opposed to days or weeks. Labor ends with the birth of an infant, followed by a rapid and nearly total cessation of pain.

FACTORS THAT INFLUENCE LABOR PAIN

Several factors cause pain during labor and influence the amount of pain a woman experiences. Other factors influence a woman's response to and ability to tolerate labor pain.

Pain Threshold and Pain Tolerance

Two terms are often used interchangeably to describe pain, although they have different meanings. Pain threshold, also called pain perception, is the least amount of sensation that a person perceives as painful. Pain threshold is fairly constant, and it varies little under different conditions. Pain tolerance is the amount of pain one is willing to endure. Unlike the pain threshold, one's pain tolerance can change under different

box 7-2 *Selected Nonpharmacological Pain Relief Measures*

PROGRESSIVE RELAXATION

- The woman contracts and then consciously releases different muscle groups.
- Technique helps the woman to distinguish tense muscles from relaxed ones.
- The woman can assess and then release muscle tension throughout her body.
- Technique is most effective if practiced before labor.

NEUROMUSCULAR DISSOCIATION (DIFFERENTIAL RELAXATION)

- The woman contracts one group of muscles strongly and consciously relaxes all others.
- The coach checks for unrecognized tension in muscle groups other than the one contracted.
- This prepares the woman to relax the rest of her body while the uterus is contracting.
- Technique is most effective if practiced before labor.

TOUCH RELAXATION

- The woman contracts a muscle group and then relaxes it when her partner strokes or massages it.
- The woman learns to respond to touch with relaxation.
- Technique is most effective if practiced before labor.

RELAXATION AGAINST PAIN

- The woman's partner exerts pressure against a tendon or large muscle of the arm or leg, gradually increasing the pressure and gradually decreasing pressure to simulate the gradual increase, peak, and decrease in contraction strength.
- The woman consciously relaxes despite this deliberate discomfort.
- This gives the woman practice in relaxation against pain.
- Technique is most effective if practiced before labor.

EFFLEURAGE

- The abdomen or other areas are massaged during contractions.
- Massage interferes with transmission of pain impulses, but prolonged continuous use reduces effectiveness (habituation). The pattern or area massaged should be changed when it becomes less effective.
- Massaging in a specific pattern (such as circles or a figure eight) also provides distraction.

OTHER MASSAGE

- Massage of the feet, hands, or shoulders often helps relaxation.
- Habituation may occur in any type of massage. Change the area massaged if it occurs.

SACRAL PRESSURE

- Technique helps to reduce the pain of back labor.
- Obtain the woman's input about the best position. Moving the pressure point a fraction of an inch or changing the amount of pressure may significantly improve effectiveness.
- Pressure may also be applied by tennis balls in a sock, a warmed plastic container of intravenous solution, or other means (see Figure 7-4).

THERMAL STIMULATION

- Technique stimulates temperature receptors that interfere with pain transmission.
- Either heat or cold applications may be beneficial. Examples are cool cloths to the face and ice in a glove to the lower back.

POSITIONING

- Any position except the supine position is acceptable if there is no need for a specific position.
- Upright positions favor fetal descent.
- Hands-and-knees positions help to reduce the pain of back labor.
- Change positions about every 30 to 60 minutes to relieve pressure and muscle fatigue.

DIVERSION/DISTRACTION

- Technique increases mental concentration on something besides the pain. It may take many forms:
  Focal point: concentrating on a specific object or other point
  Imagery: creating an imaginary mental picture of a pleasant environment or visualizing the cervix opening and the infant descending
  Music: serves as a distraction or provides "white noise" to obscure environmental sounds

HYDROTHERAPY

- Water delivered by shower, tub, or whirlpool relieves tired muscles and relaxes the woman.
- Nipple stimulation by shower can increase contraction because it stimulates the pituitary to release oxytocin.

conditions. A primary nursing responsibility is to modify as many factors as possible so that the woman can tolerate the pain of labor.

Sources of Pain During Labor

The following physical factors contribute to pain during labor:

- Dilation and stretching of the cervix
- Reduced uterine blood supply during contractions (ischemia)
- Pressure of the fetus on pelvic structures
- Stretching of the vagina and perineum

Physical Factors That Modify Pain

Several physical factors influence the amount of pain a woman feels or is willing to tolerate during labor.

Central nervous system factors

Gate control theory. The gate control theory explains how pain impulses reach the brain for interpretation. It supports several nonpharmacological methods of pain control. According to this theory, pain is transmitted through small-diameter nerve fibers. However, the stimulation of large-diameter nerve fibers temporarily interferes with the conduction of impulses through small-diameter fibers. Techniques to stimulate large-diameter fibers and "close the gate" to painful impulses include massage, palm and fingertip pressure, and heat and cold applications.

> **NURSING TIP**
> Stroking or massage, palm or foot rubbing, pressure, or gripping a cool bed rail stimulate nerve fibers that interfere with the transmission of pain impulses to the brain.

Endorphins. Endorphins are natural body substances similar to morphine. Endorphin levels increase during pregnancy and reach a peak during labor. Endorphins may explain why women in labor often need smaller doses of an analgesic or anesthetic than might be expected in a similarly painful experience.

> **NURSING TIP**
> Laboring women often tolerate more pain than usual because they have high levels of endorphins and because they are concerned about the infant's well-being.

Maternal condition

Cervical readiness. The mother's cervix normally undergoes prelabor changes that facilitate effacement and dilation in labor (see p. 178). If her cervix does not make these changes (ripening), more contractions are needed to cause effacement and dilation.

Pelvis. The size and shape of the pelvis significantly influence how readily the fetus can descend through it. Pelvic abnormalities can result in a longer labor and greater maternal fatigue. In addition, the fetus may remain in an abnormal presentation or position, which interferes with the mechanisms of labor.

Labor intensity. The woman who has a short, intense labor often experiences more pain than the woman whose birth process is more gradual. Contractions are intense and frequent, and their onset may be sudden. The cervix, vagina, and perineum stretch more abruptly than during a gentler labor. Contractions come so fast that the woman cannot recover from one before another begins. In addition, a rapid labor limits the woman's choices for pharmacological pain control.

Fatigue. Fatigue reduces pain tolerance and a woman's ability to use coping skills. Many women are tired when labor begins because sleep during late pregnancy is difficult. The active fetus, frequent urination, and shortness of breath when lying down all interrupt sleep.

Fetal presentation and position. The fetal presenting part acts as a wedge to efface and dilate the cervix as each contraction pushes it downward. The fetal head is a smooth, rounded wedge that most effectively causes effacement and dilation of the round cervix. The fetus in an abnormal presentation or position applies uneven pressure to the cervix, resulting in less effective effacement and dilation, thus prolonging the labor and delivery process.

The fetus usually turns during early labor so that the occiput is in the front left or right quadrant of the mother's pelvis (occiput anterior positions; see Figures 6-7 and 6-8). If the fetal occiput is in a posterior pelvic quadrant, each contraction pushes it against the mother's sacrum, resulting in persistent and poorly relieved back pain (back labor). Labor is often longer with this fetal position.

Interventions of Caregivers

Although they are intended to promote maternal and fetal safety, several common interventions may add to pain during labor. Examples include the following:

- Intravenous lines
- Continuous fetal monitoring, especially if it hampers mobility
- Amniotomy (artificial rupture of the membranes)
- Vaginal examinations or other interruptions

Psychosocial Factors That Modify Pain

Several psychosocial variables alter the pain a woman experiences during labor. Many of these variables interrelate with one another and with physical factors.

Culture. Culture influences how a woman feels about pregnancy and birth and how she reacts to pain during childbirth. See Table 6-1 for selected traditional cultural practices during labor and delivery.

NONPHARMACOLOGICAL PAIN MANAGEMENT

Nonpharmacological pain control methods are important, even if the woman receives medication or an anesthetic. Most pharmacological methods cannot be instituted until labor is well established because they tend to slow the progress of labor. Nonpharmacological methods help the woman to cope with labor before it has advanced far enough to give her medication. In addition, most medications for labor do not *eliminate* pain, and the woman will need nonpharmacological methods to manage the discomfort that remains. Nonpharmacological methods are usually the only realistic option if the woman comes to the hospital in advanced labor.

ADVANTAGES OF NONPHARMACOLOGICAL METHODS

There are several advantages to nonpharmacological methods if pain control is adequate. Poorly relieved pain increases fear and anxiety, thus diverting blood flow from the uterus and impairing the normal labor process. It also reduces the pleasure of this extraordinary experience. Nonpharmacological methods do not harm the mother or fetus. They do not slow labor if they provide adequate pain control. They carry no risk for allergy or adverse drug effects.

LIMITATIONS OF NONPHARMACOLOGICAL METHODS

For best results, nonpharmacological methods should be rehearsed before labor begins. They can be taught to the unprepared woman, preferably during early labor, when she is anxious enough to be interested yet comfortable enough to learn.

The nurse may help the woman use several key techniques of nonpharmacological pain control during labor. If the woman and her partner attended childbirth preparation classes, the nurse builds on their knowledge during labor.

METHODS OF CHILDBIRTH PREPARATION

Most childbirth preparation classes are based on one of several methods. The basic method is often modified to meet the specific needs of the women who attend.

Dick-Read Method

Grantly Dick-Read was an English physician who introduced the concept of a fear-tension-pain cycle during labor. He believed that fear of childbirth contributed to tension, which resulted in pain. His methods include education and relaxation techniques to interrupt the cycle.

Bradley Method

The Bradley method was originally called "husband-coached childbirth" and was the first to include the father as an integral part of labor. It emphasizes slow abdominal breathing and relaxation techniques.

Lamaze Method

The Lamaze method, also called the psychoprophylactic method, is the basis of most childbirth preparation classes in the United States. It uses mental techniques that condition the woman to respond to contractions with relaxation rather than tension. Other mental and breathing techniques occupy her mind and limit the brain's ability to interpret labor sensations as painful. The Lamaze breathing technique should be no slower than half of the woman's baseline respiratory rate and no faster than twice the baseline rate.

NONPHARMACOLOGICAL TECHNIQUES
Relaxation Techniques

The ability to release tension is a vital part of the expectant mother's "tool kit." Relaxation techniques require concentration, thus occupying the mind while reducing muscle tension.

Promoting relaxation is basic to all other methods, both nonpharmacological and pharmacological. The nurse should adjust the woman's environment and help her with general comfort measures as discussed in Chapter 6. Water in a tub or shower helps to refresh her and promotes relaxation.

To reduce anxiety and fear, the woman is oriented to the labor area, any procedures that are done, and what is happening in her body during the normal process of birth. A partnership style of nurse-patient-labor partner is usual in maternity settings.

Looking for signs of muscle tension and teaching her partner to do so help the woman who is not aware of becoming tense. She can change position or guide her partner to massage the area where muscle tension is

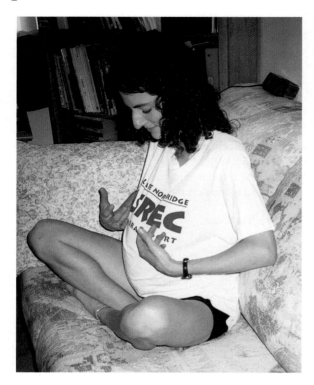

FIGURE **7-3** Effleurage. This woman is practicing effleurage, stroking the abdomen with the fingertips in a circular motion. This technique stimulates large-diameter nerve fibers, thus interfering with pain transmission. Fingertip pressure should be firm enough to avoid a tickling sensation.

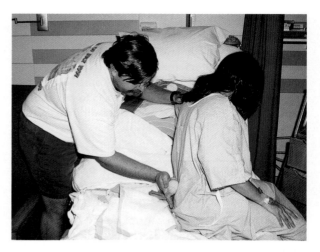

FIGURE **7-4** The partner applies firm pressure on the lower back of the woman in labor. Using a tennis ball enhances the effect (see also Chapter 33).

Sacral pressure. Firm pressure against the lower back helps relieve some of the pain of back labor. The woman should tell her partner where to apply the pressure and how much pressure is helpful (Figure 7-4).

Thermal stimulation. Heat can be applied with a warm blanket or glove filled with warm water. Warmth can also be applied in the form of a shower if there is no contraindication against doing so. Most women appreciate a cool cloth on the face. Two or three moistened washcloths are kept at hand and changed as they become warm.

Positioning

Frequent changing of position relieves muscle fatigue and strain. In addition, position changes can promote the normal mechanisms of labor.

Diversion/Distraction

Several methods may be used to stimulate the woman's brain, thus limiting her ability to perceive sensations as painful. All methods direct her mind away from the pain.

Focal point. The woman fixes her eyes on a picture, an object, or simply a particular spot in the room. Some women prefer to close their eyes during contractions and focus on an internal focal point.

Imagery. The woman learns to create a tranquil mental environment by imagining that she is in a place of relaxation and peace. Preferred mental scenes often involve warmth and sunlight, although some women imagine themselves in a cool environment. During la-

noted. The laboring woman is guided to release the tension specifically, one muscle group at a time, by saying, for example, "Let your arm relax; let the tension out of your neck . . . your shoulders . . . ." Specific instructions are repeated until she relaxes each body part.

Skin Stimulation

Several variations of massage are often used during labor. Most can be taught to the woman and partner who did not attend childbirth preparation classes.

Effleurage. Effleurage stimulates the large-diameter nerve fibers that inhibit painful stimuli traveling through the small-diameter fibers. The woman strokes her abdomen in a circular movement during contractions (Figure 7-3). If fetal monitor belts are on her abdomen, she can massage between them or on her thigh, or she can trace circles or a figure eight on the bed. She can use one hand when on her side. The woman should change methods at intervals because constant use of a single technique reduces its effectiveness (habituation).

bor the woman can imagine her cervix opening and allowing the infant to come out, as a flower opens from bud to full bloom. The nurse can help to create a tranquil mental image, even in the unprepared woman.

Music. Favorite music or relaxation recordings divert the woman's attention from pain. The sounds of rainfall, wind, or the ocean contribute to relaxation and block disturbing sounds.

Television. Women often enjoy the diversion of television, especially during early labor. The woman may not watch the program, but it provides background noise that reduces intrusive sounds. Some labor rooms have videotape players, and the woman can bring her own tapes to watch during labor.

Breathing

Like other techniques, breathing techniques are most effective if practiced before labor. The woman should not use them until she needs them, generally when she can no longer walk or talk through a contraction. She may become tired if she uses them too early or if she moves to a more advanced technique sooner than she must. If the woman has not had childbirth preparation classes, each technique is taught as she needs it.

Each breathing pattern begins and ends with a cleansing breath, which is a deep inspiration and expiration, similar to a deep sigh. The cleansing breaths help the woman to relax and focus on relaxing.

First-stage breathing

Slow-paced breathing. The woman begins with a technique of slow-paced breathing. She starts the pattern with a cleansing breath, then breathes slowly, as during sleep (Figure 7-5, *A*). A cleansing breath ends the contraction. An exact rate is not important, but about six to nine breaths a minute is average. The rate should be at least half her usual rate to ensure adequate fetal oxygenation and prevent hyperventilation.

Modified paced breathing. This pattern begins and ends with a cleansing breath. During the contraction the woman breathes more rapidly and shallowly (Figures 7-5, *B* and *C*). The rate should be no more than twice her usual rate. She may combine slow-paced with modified paced breathing. In this variation she begins with a cleansing breath and breathes slowly until the peak of the contraction, when she begins rapid, shallow breathing. As the contraction abates, she resumes slow, deep breathing and ends with a cleansing breath.

Hyperventilation is sometimes a problem when the woman is breathing rapidly. She may complain of dizziness, tingling, and numbness around her mouth and may have spasms of her fingers and feet. Box 7-3 lists measures to combat hyperventilation.

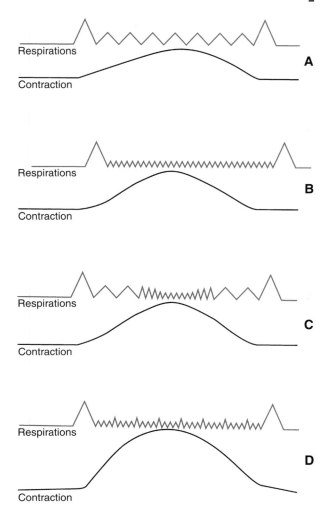

FIGURE **7-5 A,** Slow-paced breathing. The pattern starts with a cleansing breath as the contraction begins. The woman breathes slowly, at about half her usual rate, and ends with a second cleansing breath at the end of the contraction. **B,** As labor intensifies, the woman may need to use modified paced breathing. The pattern begins and ends with a cleansing breath. The woman breathes rapidly, no faster than twice her usual respiratory rate, during the peak of the contraction. She ends with another cleansing breath. **C,** In this variation of modified paced breathing the woman begins with slow-paced breathing at the first of the contraction, switching to faster breathing during its peak. A cleansing breath also begins and ends this pattern. **D,** Patterned paced breathing begins and ends with a cleansing breath. During the contraction the woman emphasizes the exhalation of some breaths. She may use a specific pattern or may randomly emphasize the blow.

box 7-3 | *How to Recognize and Correct Hyperventilation*

SIGNS AND SYMPTOMS
Dizziness
Tingling of hands and feet
Cramps and muscle spasms of hands
Numbness around nose and mouth
Blurring of vision

CORRECTIVE MEASURES
Breathe slowly, especially in exhalation
Breathe into cupped hands
Place a moist washcloth over the mouth and nose
    while breathing
Hold breath for a few seconds before exhaling

Patterned paced breathing. Patterned paced breathing is more difficult to teach the unprepared laboring woman because it requires her to focus on the pattern of her breathing. It begins with a cleansing breath, which is followed by rapid breaths punctuated with an intermittent slight blow (Figure 7-5, *D*), often called pant-BLOW, or "hee hoo" breathing. The woman may maintain a constant number of breaths before the blow or may vary the number in a specific pattern, as follows:

- Constant pattern: pant-pant-pant-BLOW, pant-pant-pant-BLOW, etc.
- Stairstep pattern: pant-BLOW, pant-pant-BLOW, pant-pant-pant-BLOW, pant-pant-BLOW, pant-BLOW

In another variation her partner calls out random numbers to indicate the number of pants to take before a blow.

If she feels an urge to push before her cervix is fully dilated, the woman is taught to blow in short breaths to avoid bearing down. Pushing before full cervical dilation may cause cervical edema or lacerations, especially with her first child, because the cervix is not as stretchable as it is after one or more births.

Second-stage breathing. When it is time for the woman to push, she takes a cleansing breath, then takes another deep breath and pushes down while exhaling to a count of 10. She blows out, takes a deep breath, and pushes again while exhaling (open glottis pushing).

NURSING **TIP**
If a woman is successfully using a safe, nonpharmacological pain control technique, do not interfere.

THE NURSE'S ROLE IN NONPHARMACOLOGICAL TECHNIQUES

When a woman is admitted, the nurse determines whether she had childbirth preparation classes and works with what the woman and her partner learned. The nurse helps them to identify signs of tension so the woman can be guided to release it.

If the woman did not have childbirth preparation classes, the nurse teaches her the simple breathing and relaxation techniques. If the woman is extremely anxious and out of control, she will not be able to comprehend verbal instructions. It may be necessary to make close eye contact with her and to breathe with her through each contraction until she can regain control.

The nurse minimizes environmental irritants as much as possible. The lights should be lowered and the woman kept reasonably dry by regularly changing the underpads on the bed. The temperature should be adjusted; the nurse provides a warm blanket if that offers the most comfort. (See Chapter 6 for other general comfort measures during labor.)

The nurse should be cautious not to overestimate or underestimate the amount of pain a woman is experiencing. The quiet, stoic woman may need analgesia yet be reluctant to ask. A tense body posture or facial grimacing may indicate that she needs additional pain relief measures.

PHARMACOLOGICAL PAIN MANAGEMENT

Pharmacological pain management methods include analgesics, adjunctive drugs to improve the effectiveness of analgesics or to counteract their side effects, and anesthetics. Analgesics are systemic drugs (affecting the entire body) that reduce pain without loss of consciousness. Anesthetics cause a loss of sensation, especially to pain. Regional anesthetics block sensation from a localized area without causing a loss of consciousness. General anesthetics are systemic drugs that cause a loss of consciousness and sensation to pain. Tables 7-1 and 7-2 summarize intrapartum analgesics, adjunctive drugs, and anesthetic methods.

Anesthetics are administered by various clinicians depending on the type of drug. Local anesthetics are given by the physician or nurse-midwife at the time of birth. Other anesthetics may be given by a specialist in anesthetic administration.

There are two types of anesthesia clinicians: an anesthesiologist is a physician who specializes in giving anesthesia, and a certified nurse anesthetist (CRNA) is a reg-

| table 7-1 | *Intrapartum Analgesics and Related Drugs* |

DRUG	USE/EFFECTS
NARCOTICS	
Meperidine (Demerol)	Given to mothers in labor either intravenously with a 5- to 10-minute peak of action or intramuscularly with a 50-minute peak of action
	Maternal responses may include hypotension, sedation, nausea and vomiting, and pruritus; fetal responses can include decrease in fetal heart variability
	Can cause respiratory depression and sedation in newborn if delivery occurs within 2 hours after the last dose is administered
Fentanyl (Sublimaze)	Rapid onset and short duration of action
	NOTE: fentanyl, sufentanil, and alfentanil are *not* the same drug
	Can cause respiratory depression
	Often used with epidural analgesia
COMBINATION OPIOID AGONIST/ANTAGONIST	
Butorphanol (Stadol)	Mixed narcotic and narcotic antagonist effect
	Both drugs reduce pain and are thought to cause less respiratory depression than meperidine
Nalbuphine (Nubain)	Should not be used in women who are drug addicts
OPIOID ANTAGONIST	
Naloxone (Narcan)	An opioid antagonist that acts within minutes to help resuscitate a newborn who has respiratory depression because of narcotic sedation of the mother during labor; also relieves the maternal itching side effect of narcotics
	Duration of action is 1 to 2 hours, so the vital signs of the newborn should continue to be observed
	May cause withdrawal symptoms if administered to a woman who regularly uses illicit drugs (e.g., tremors, perspiration, anxiety, irritability, and seizures)
ATARACTICS (ANALGESIC POTENTIATORS)	
Promethazine (Phenergan)	Reduce anxiety and potentiate the effects of narcotic drugs, resulting in a lower dose of narcotic needed for pain relief
Hydroxyzine (Vistaril)	Also have antinausea and antiemetic effects
	May decrease beat-to-beat variability in fetal heart rate

NOTE: Consult drug guide for safe doses of drugs.

istered nurse who has advanced training in anesthetic administration. State licensing laws and individual facility policies affect which anesthetic methods each clinician may use.

PHYSIOLOGY OF PREGNANCY AND ITS RELATIONSHIP TO ANALGESIA AND ANESTHESIA

Specific factors in the physiology of pregnancy affect the pregnant woman's response to analgesia and anesthesia:

- The pregnant woman is at a higher risk for hypoxia caused by the pressure of the enlarging uterus on the diaphragm.
- The sluggish gastrointestinal tract of the pregnant woman can result in increased risk for vomiting and aspiration.
- Aortocaval compression (pressure on the abdominal aorta by the heavy uterus when the woman is in supine position) increases the risk of hypotension and the development of shock.
- The effect on the fetus must be considered.

ADVANTAGES OF PHARMACOLOGICAL METHODS

Methods that use drugs for reducing pain during birth can help the woman to be a more active participant in birth. They help her relax and work with contractions.

table 7-2 | *Types of Anesthesia for Childbirth*

ANESTHETIC METHOD	NURSING IMPLICATIONS
Local infiltration. Injection of the perineum with a local anesthetic drug just before vaginal birth; administered by nurse-midwife or physician to site of episiotomy on perineum	Injection may burn until the area becomes numb; adverse effects are rare; check for allergies to *-caine* drugs or for allergies to dental anesthetics.
Pudendal block. Injection of the pudendal nerves with local anesthetic just before vaginal birth; local infiltration of the perineum is also usually done; may be used for some forceps births; administered by nurse-midwife or physician	Similar to local infiltration; warn the woman that the long needle is needed to reach the nerve and is shielded by the needle guide or "trumpet"; observe for hematoma (collection of blood within tissues), which may become evident during the recovery period and is evidenced by excessive perineal or pelvic pain; pelvic infection sometimes occurs but is uncommon.
Epidural block. Injection of local anesthetic drug into the epidural space, which blocks transmission of pain impulses to brain; epidural narcotics are often added to reduce the amount of anesthetic needed and reduce the adverse effects; used for pain relief during labor and vaginal birth, also for cesarean birth; administered by physician (obstetrician or anesthesiologist) or by nurse anesthetist when cervix is at least 4 cm dilated	Observe for hypotension and urinary retention; assist the woman to maintain position as needed by anesthesia clinician; initially record blood pressure every 5 minutes after the block is begun and after each reinjection until stable; record fetal heart rates, usually with continuous electronic fetal monitoring; a full bladder may require catheterization if the woman cannot feel the urge to void; ambulate carefully because sensation will be reduced.
Subarachnoid (spinal) block. Injection of local anesthetic drug under the dura and arachnoid membranes to block transmission of pain impulses to brain; used primarily for cesarean birth; usually administered by anesthesiologist	Observe for hypotension and urinary retention as in epidural block (interventions are the same); suspect postspinal headache (usually during postpartum period) if woman complains of a headache that is worse when she is in an upright position; give oral fluids and analgesics as ordered.

General anesthesia. Uses a combination of IV and inhalational drugs to produce a loss of consciousness; rarely used for vaginal births; used for cesarean births under some conditions:
    Woman's refusal of regional block
    Contraindication for regional block
    Emergency cesarean when there is not time to establish a regional block
	Regurgitation, with aspiration of gastric contents is the primary risk; IV drugs to reduce gastric acidity or speed up stomach emptying may also be given by the anesthesia clinician; assistant gives cricoid pressure until the woman is intubated to prevent any regurgitated stomach contents from reaching her trachea; anesthesia is light and woman may move on the operating table; postanesthesia recovery care includes observation of level of consciousness, vital signs, oxygen saturation, plus postcesarean birth care; infant is likely to be born with respiratory depression and require aggressive resuscitation.

Drugs do not usually relieve *all* pain and pressure sensations.

The pain of labor may cause a "stress response" in the mother that results in an increase in autonomic activity, a release of catecholamines, and a decrease in platelet perfusion. This stress response results in fetal acidosis. The pain can also cause maternal hyperventilation and lead to respiratory alkalosis, then a compensating metabolic acidosis. Metabolic acidosis in the woman results in further fetal acidosis. Therefore appropriate pain re-

lief during labor can play an important role in the positive outcome of pregnancy for mother and infant.

LIMITATIONS OF PHARMACOLOGICAL METHODS

Pharmacological methods are effective, but they do have limits. One important limitation is that two persons are medicated—the mother and her fetus. Any drug given to the mother can affect the fetus, and the effects may be prolonged in the infant after birth. The drug may directly affect the fetus, or it may indirectly affect the fetus because of effects in the mother (such as hypotension).

Several pharmacological methods may slow labor's progress if used early in labor. Some complications during pregnancy limit the pharmacological methods that are safe. For example, a method that requires the infusion of large amounts of intravenous (IV) fluids might overload the woman's circulation if she has heart disease. If she takes other medications (legal or illicit), they may interact adversely with the drugs used to relieve labor pain.

ANALGESICS AND ADJUNCTIVE DRUGS
Narcotic (Opioid) Analgesics

Systemic opioids are the most common means of labor analgesia in the United States. They are used in small doses to avoid fetal respiratory depression. Opioids do *not* provide complete pain relief during labor, but they do help the woman cope with a tolerable level of intermittent labor pains. Drugs used are reviewed in Table 7-1.

In general, narcotic analgesics are avoided if birth is expected within an hour. An attempt is made to time administration so the drug does not reach its peak at the time of birth. However, small doses are sometimes given in late labor if the fetus has no problems. The nurse must be prepared to support the respiratory efforts of all infants at birth, regardless of whether the mother received narcotics during labor.

Narcotic Antagonist

Naloxone (Narcan) is used to reverse respiratory depression, usually in the infant, caused by opioid drugs such as meperidine. It is not effective against respiratory depression from other causes, such as intrauterine hypoxia. It can be given by the IV route, or it may be given through the endotracheal tube during resuscitation. IV naloxone can be given to the neonate immediately after birth via the umbilical cord vein. The use of naloxone in a woman who is drug dependent can cause withdrawal syndrome in the mother or neonate.

Adjunctive Drugs

Adjunctive drugs enhance the pain-relieving action of analgesics and reduce nausea. Hydroxyzine is given only by the intramuscular route using a Z-track technique.

REGIONAL ANALGESICS AND ANESTHETICS

The membranes around the spinal cord are called the meninges. The meninges have three layers:
- Dura mater
- Arachnoid mater
- Pia mater

The *epidural space* is located between the dura mater and the inside bony covering of the brain or spinal cord. The *subdural space* is located between the dura mater and the arachnoid mater, and the *subarachnoid* space is located between the arachnoid mater and the pia mater. Regional anesthesia in obstetrics usually involves the placement of an anesthetic in the epidural or subarachnoid space.

An analgesic blocks pain, whereas an anesthetic blocks both pain and motor responses. For example, an epidural block may provide analgesia and allow the woman to ambulate with assistance, but spinal anesthesia prevents ambulation. The role of the nurse in caring for a woman with regional analgesia/anesthesia is to monitor her responses and the status of the fetus. Starting or managing intermittent dosages of a regional anesthetic is not within the nursing scope of practice (Association of Woman's Health, Obstetric, and Neonatal Nurses, 2001).

Regional anesthetics block sensation to varying degrees, depending on the type of regional block used, the quantity of medication, and the drugs injected. The woman still feels pressure and may feel some pain. The major advantage of regional anesthetics is that they provide satisfactory pain relief yet allow the woman to be awake and participate in the birthing process (see Table 7-2).

Local and pudendal blocks are given in the vaginal-perineal area. Epidural and subarachnoid blocks and intrathecal narcotics are given by injecting anesthetic drugs so they bathe the nerves as they emerge from the spinal cord. The spinal cord and nerves are not directly injected.

Local anesthetic agents for childbirth are related to those for dental work. On admission, the nurse should ask each woman if she is allergic to or has had problems with dental anesthesia. If so, her physician or nurse-midwife should be alerted to enable her to have the safest pain relief measures.

Local Infiltration

Injection of the perineal area for an episiotomy is done just before birth, when the fetal head is visible. It may also be done after placental expulsion to repair a perineal laceration. There is a short delay between injection of the anesthetic agent and the loss of pain sensation. The physician or nurse-midwife allows the anesthetic to become effective before beginning the episiotomy. There are virtually no risks if the woman is not allergic to the drug.

Pudendal Block

The pudendal block is used for vaginal births, although its use has become less common as the popularity of the

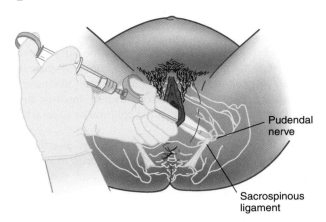

FIGURE **7-6** Pudendal block anesthesia. The two pudendal nerves on each side of the pelvis are injected to numb the vagina and perineum. The illustration shows the technique of inserting the needle beyond the needle guard and passing through the sacrospinous ligament to reach the pudendal nerve.

epidural block has increased. It provides adequate anesthesia for an episiotomy and for most low forceps births. It does not block pain from contractions and, like local infiltration, is given just before birth. There is a delay of a few minutes between injection of the drug and the onset of numbness (paresthesia).

The physician or nurse-midwife injects the pudendal nerves on each side of the mother's pelvis (Figure 7-6). The nerves may be reached through the vagina or by injection directly through her perineum. A long needle (13 to 15 cm [5 to 6 inches]) is needed to reach the pudendal nerves, which are near the mother's ischial spines. If the injection is done through the vagina, a needle guide ("trumpet") is used to protect the mother's tissues. The needle is injected only about 1.3 cm (0.5 inch) into the woman's tissues. The perineum is also infiltrated because the pudendal block alone does not completely anesthetize the perineum.

Adverse effects of pudendal block. The pudendal block has few adverse effects if the woman is not allergic to the drug. A vaginal hematoma (collection of blood within the tissues) sometimes occurs. An abscess may develop, but this is not common.

Epidural Block

The epidural space is a small space just outside the dura (outermost membrane covering the brain and spinal cord). The woman is in a sitting or side-lying position for the epidural block. Her back is relatively straight rather than sharply curved forward to avoid compressing the tiny epidural space, which is about 1 mm (the thickness of a dime).

The physician or nurse anesthetist penetrates the epidural space with a large needle (16- to 18-gauge). A fine catheter is threaded into the epidural space through the bore of the needle (Figure 7-7). A test dose (2 to 3 ml) of local anesthetic agent is injected through the catheter. The woman is not expected to have effects from the test dose if the catheter is in the right place. Numbness or loss of movement after the small test dose indicates that her dura mater was probably punctured and the drug was injected into the subarachnoid space (as in a subarachnoid block) rather than in the epidural space. Numbness around the mouth, ringing in the ears (tinnitus), visual disturbances, or jitteriness are symptoms that suggest injection into a vein. The test dose is small enough to avoid long-term adverse effects.

If the test dose is normal (no effects), a larger amount of anesthetic agent is injected to begin the block. A few minutes are needed before the onset of the block. If an epidural block is being used for surgery, such as cesarean delivery or tubal ligation, the anesthesiologist or CRNA will test for the level of numbness before surgery begins.

Local anesthetic drugs are usually combined with a small dose of an opioid analgesic such as fentanyl (Sublimaze). The combination of drugs allows quicker and longer-lasting pain relief with less anesthetic agent and minimal loss of movement. An epidural block for labor is more accurately termed *analgesia* (reducing pain) than *anesthesia* (obliterating all sensation).

The woman can sometimes ambulate when a combination-drug epidural is used because the local anesthetic dose is much lower. She can assume any position with this type of block, although any pregnant woman should avoid the supine position.

To maintain pain relief during labor, the anesthetic drug is constantly infused into the catheter via an infusion pump. Alternatively, repeat intermittent injections of the drug may be given.

Dural puncture. The dura lies just below the tiny epidural space. This membrane is sometimes punctured accidentally ("wet tap") with the epidural needle or the catheter that is inserted through it. If a dural puncture occurs, a relatively large amount of spinal fluid can leak from the hole and may result in a headache.

Limitations of epidural block. Although it is a popular method of intrapartum pain relief, an epidural block is not used if the woman has any of the following:

- Abnormal blood clotting
- An infection in the area of injection or a systemic infection
- Hypovolemia (inadequate blood volume)

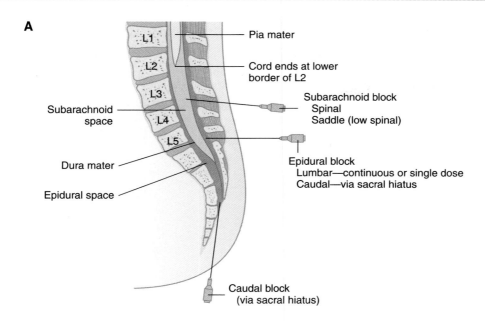

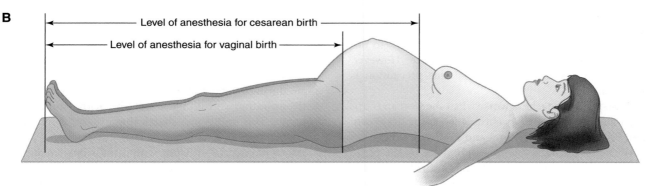

FIGURE **7-7** Epidural and spinal anesthesia. **A,** The insertion sites for the needle in epidural, subarachnoid, or spinal blocks. **B,** Levels of anesthesia for vaginal birth compared with minimum level required for cesarean birth.

Adverse effects of epidural block. The most common side effects are maternal hypotension, which can compromise fetal oxygenation, and urinary retention. To counteract hypotension, a large quantity (500 to 1000 ml or more) of IV solution such as Ringer's lactate is infused rapidly before the block is begun.

The large quantity of IV fluids combined with reduced sensation may result in urinary retention. The nurse should palpate the suprapubic area for a full bladder every 2 hours or more often if a large quantity of IV solution was given. The woman will need catheterization if she is unable to void.

The woman may feel less of an urge to push in the second stage of labor when she has an epidural block, depending on the drugs used for her block. Therefore this stage may be longer if a woman has an epidural block. Maternal and fetal conditions are monitored closely.

>NURSING **TIP**
> Assess the woman for bladder distention regularly if she has received an epidural or subarachnoid block. A full bladder can delay birth and can cause hemorrhage after birth.

Subarachnoid (Spinal) Block

The woman's position for a subarachnoid block is similar to that for the epidural block except that her back is curled around her uterus in a C shape. The dura is punctured with a thin (25- to 27-gauge) spinal needle. A few drops of spinal fluid confirms entry into the subarachnoid space (see Figure 7-7). The local anesthetic drug is then injected. A much smaller quantity of drug is needed to achieve anesthesia in the subarachnoid block than in the epidural block. Anesthesia occurs quickly and is more profound than the epidural block; the woman loses movement and sensation below the block.

The subarachnoid block is a "one-shot" block because it does not involve placing a catheter for reinjection of the drug. It is not often used for vaginal births today but remains common for cesarean births. Its limitations are essentially the same as for an epidural block.

Adverse effects of subarachnoid block. Hypotension and urinary retention are the main adverse effects of subarachnoid block, as in the epidural block. They are managed as in the epidural block. Hypotension is often more severe with a subarachnoid block.

A postspinal headache sometimes occurs, most likely because of spinal fluid loss. The woman may be advised to remain flat for several hours after the block to decrease the chance of postspinal headache. However, there is no absolute evidence that this precaution is effective.

Postspinal headache is worse when the woman is upright and often disappears entirely when she lies down. Bed rest, analgesics, and oral and IV fluids help to relieve the headache. A blood patch, done by the nurse anesthetist or anesthesiologist, may provide dramatic relief from postspinal headache. The woman's blood (10 to 15 ml) is withdrawn from her vein and injected into the epidural space in the area of the subarachnoid puncture (Figure 7-8). The blood clots and forms a gelatinous seal that stops spinal fluid leakage. The clot later breaks down and is reabsorbed by the body.

GENERAL ANESTHESIA

General anesthesia is rarely used for vaginal births or for most cesarean births. Regional blocks are preferred for cesarean births, if possible. General anesthesia may be necessary in the following circumstances:

- Emergency cesarean birth, when there is not time to establish either an epidural or a subarachnoid block
- Cesarean birth in the woman who refuses or has a contraindication to epidural or subarachnoid block

Combinations of general anesthetic drugs (balanced anesthesia) allow for a quick onset of anesthesia, minimal fetal effects, and prompt maternal wakening once the drug is stopped.

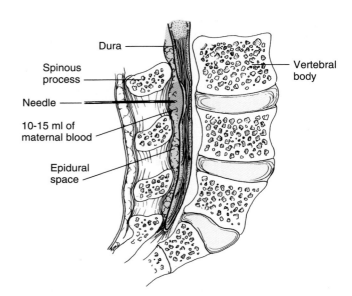

FIGURE **7-8** Epidural blood patch. An epidural blood patch may provide dramatic relief from postspinal headache.

Adverse Effects in the Mother

The major adverse effect of general anesthesia is the same during birth as at any other time: regurgitation with aspiration (breathing in) of the acidic stomach contents. This results in a chemical injury to the lungs, *aspiration pneumonitis.* It can be fatal.

Many women begin labor with a full stomach, and their gastric action slows during labor. In addition, the full uterus exerts upward pressure against the stomach. Therefore every pregnant woman is presumed to have a full stomach for purposes of anesthesia.

Adverse Effects in the Neonate

Respiratory depression is the main neonatal risk because drugs given to the mother may cross the placenta. To reduce this risk, the time from induction of anesthesia to clamping of the umbilical cord is kept as short as possible. The woman is prepped and draped for surgery, and all personnel are scrubbed, gowned, and gloved before anesthesia begins. In addition, the anesthesia is kept as light as possible until the cord is clamped. Aggressive resuscitation of the newborn may be necessary.

THE NURSE'S ROLE IN PHARMACOLOGICAL TECHNIQUES

The nurse's responsibility in pharmacological pain management begins at admission (see Nursing Care Plan 7-1). The woman should be closely questioned about allergy to foods, drugs, including dental anesthetics, or latex to identify pain relief measures that may not

NURSING CARE PLAN 7-1

The Woman Needing Pain Management During Labor

PATIENT DATA: A woman, para 1 gravida 2, is in active labor and is 4 cm dilated. She is thrashing in bed and is not cooperating with the coaching of her partner.

SELECTED NURSING DIAGNOSIS   *Acute pain related to uterine contractions and descent of fetus in pelvis*

Outcomes	Nursing Interventions	Rationales

The woman will state that her discomfort is manageable during labor using techniques learned in childbirth preparation classes and/or taught by the nurse. The woman will have a relaxed facial and body appearance between contractions.	1. Determine presence and character of pain continuously during labor:
	  a. Statement of pain (assess nature of pain, such as location, intensity, whether intermittent or constant)
	  b. Crying, moaning during and/or between contractions
	  c. Tense, guarded body posture or thrashing with contractions
	  d. "Mask of pain" facial expression
		1. These are common verbal and nonverbal signs of pain; assessment enables the nurse to identify if pain is normal for woman's labor status and to choose the best interventions for pain relief (nonpharmacological and/or pharmacological measures); evaluating verbal and nonverbal communication helps the nurse to evaluate the need for pain relief in women who may not directly communicate their need for pain relief or who do not speak prevailing language.

	2. Provide general comfort measures, such as the following:
	  a. Adjust the room temperature and light level for comfort.
	  b. Reduce irritants, such as wet underpads.
	  c. Provide ice chips, Popsicles, or juices to relieve dry mouth.
	  d. Avoid bumping the bed.
		2. These general measures reduce outside irritants that make it harder for the woman to use childbirth preparation techniques and are themselves a source of discomfort. A comfortable environment is conducive to relaxation.

	3. Encourage the woman to assume positions she finds most comfortable, other than supine.	3. Position changes promote comfort and help the fetus adapt to the size and shape of woman's pelvis; supine position can result in supine hypotensive syndrome, which reduces placental blood flow and fetal oxygenation.
	4. Observe for a full bladder every 1 to 2 hours, or more often if the woman receives large amounts of oral or IV fluids.	4. A full bladder is a source of discomfort and can prolong labor by inhibiting fetal descent; it may cause pain that lingers after epidural analgesia is begun.

	5. Promote the use of childbirth preparation techniques, including labor partner as appropriate:
	  a. Do not stand in front of her focal point.
	  b. Offer a back rub or firm sacral pressure; ask her about the best location and amount of pressure; use powder to prevent skin irritation.
		5. These are examples of how to assist the woman and her partner in using methods they learned most effectively. The use of nonpharmacological pain relief avoids problems associated with pharmacological interventions and supplements any drug therapy used. They also give the woman and her partner a sense of control and mastery that enhances the perception of birth as a positive experience.

Continued

NURSING CARE PLAN 7-1—cont'd

Outcomes	Nursing Interventions	Rationales
	c. Encourage the woman to switch to more complex patterns only when simpler ones are no longer effective. d. Breathe along with the woman if she has trouble maintaining patterns; make eye contact. 6. If the woman has signs of hyperventilation (dizziness, numbness or tingling sensations, spasms of the hands and feet), have her breathe into her cupped hands, a small bag, or a washcloth placed over her mouth and nose. 7. Tell the woman and her partner when labor progresses; for example, if she is pushing and her infant's head becomes visible, let her see or feel it.	 6. Hyperventilation often occurs when woman uses rapid breathing patterns because she exhales too much carbon dioxide. These measures help her to conserve carbon dioxide and rebreathe it to correct excess loss. 7. Labor does not last forever; knowing that her efforts are having the desired results gives her courage to continue and helps her to tolerate pain.

SELECTED NURSING DIAGNOSIS *Deficient knowledge related to unfamiliar procedures and expected effects of epidural block*

Outcomes	Nursing Interventions	Rationales

After explanations, the woman will state that she understands what will happen during and after epidural block is begun.	1. Explain what to expect as the epidural block is begun (reinforcing explanations of the anesthesiologist or nurse anesthetist):
	  a. An IV line will be started and she will receive fluids to offset the tendency of her blood pressure to fall.
	  b. The fetus will be monitored by electronic fetal monitoring.
	  c. The nurse anesthetist or anesthesiologist will position her; she should remain still and in this position for insertion of catheter.
	  d. A small plastic catheter will be taped to her back to allow constant infusion of medication (or reinjection).
	  e. Her blood pressure will be checked every 5 minutes when the block is first begun.
	
	2. If she needs to remain flat briefly to allow the drug to disperse, put a small pillow under her right hip.
		1. This list reflects a common sequence of events for starting an epidural block. The anesthesia clinician explains the procedure and expected effects; the nurse reinforces explanations as needed because the woman in pain may not be able to concentrate. Knowledge reduces anxiety and fear of the unknown. If the woman understands that these procedures are a normal part of an epidural block, she is less likely to interpret them as abnormal.
		
		2. Placing a pillow under her hip avoids supine hypotensive syndrome.

NURSING CARE PLAN 7-1—cont'd

Outcomes	Nursing Interventions	Rationales
	3. Explain that she will feel less pain but will feel pressure; movement and sensation in her legs and feet will vary.	3. Explanations help the woman to understand that the epidural block is not expected to abolish the pain of labor. Leg movement and sensation are affected to varying degrees. If she understands this variation in effects, she is less likely to interpret them as abnormal or as evidence that the block is not working.

SELECTED NURSING DIAGNOSIS *Risk for injury related to loss of sensation*

Outcomes	Nursing Interventions	Rationales
The woman will not have an injury, such as a muscle strain or fall, while her epidural block is in effect. The fetus will not be born in an uncontrolled delivery.	1. Check for movement, sensation, and leg strength before ambulating; ambulate cautiously with an assistant. Assist the woman to change positions regularly.	1. A fall is more likely if the woman does not have sensation and control over her movements. A change of position prevents muscle strain.
	2. Observe for signs that birth may be near: increase in bloody show, perineal bulging, or crowning.	2. Loss of sensation varies among women having an epidural block. Labor may progress more rapidly than expected. These are signs associated with imminent birth that should be evaluated by the experienced nurse, nurse-midwife, or physician.

?CRITICAL THINKING QUESTION

A woman, para 1 gravida 2, is in active labor. The last examination revealed that her cervix was 7 cm dilated and 75% effaced. She states that her contraction pains are almost unbearable, even with the medication she has received.

Because getting up and walking helped her earlier and she needs to go to the bathroom now, she asks the nurse to help her out of bed to walk to the nearby bathroom. What would be the best response of the nurse?

---

be advisable. She should be questioned about her preferences for pain relief. Factors that may impact the choice of pain relief should be noted, such as back surgery, infection in the area where an epidural block would be injected, or blood pressure abnormalities.

The nurse keeps the side rails up if the woman takes pain relief drugs. Narcotics may cause drowsiness or dizziness. Regional anesthetics reduce sensation and movement to varying degrees, and therefore the woman may have less control over her body. Side rails on the bed may be necessary for safety.

The nurse reinforces the explanations given by the anesthesia clinician regarding procedures and the expected effects of the selected pain management method. Women often receive these explanations when they are very uncomfortable and do not remember everything they were told. The woman is helped to assume and hold the position for the epidural or subarachnoid block. The nurse tells the anesthesia clinician if the woman has a contraction because it might prevent her from holding still. The anesthetic drug is usually injected between contractions.

The woman is observed for hypotension if an epidural or subarachnoid block is given. Hospital protocols vary, but blood pressure is usually measured every 5 minutes after the block begins (and with each reinjection) until her blood pressure is stable. An automatic blood pressure monitor is often used. Some facilities add a pulse oximeter to monitor oxygen saturation. At the same time the nurse observes the fetal monitor for signs associated with fetal compromise (see pp. 136 to 141), because maternal hypotension can reduce placental blood flow.

The epidural block is given during labor and may reduce the mother's sensation of rectal pressure. The nurse coaches her about the right time to start and stop pushing with each contraction if needed. The nurse also observes for signs of imminent birth, such as increased bloody show and perineal bulging, because the woman may not be able to feel the sensations clearly.

Nursing responsibilities related to general anesthesia include assessment and documentation of oral intake and administration of medications to reduce gastric acidity. The woman should be told that all preparations for surgery will be performed *before* she is put to sleep. The nurse should reassure her that she will be asleep before any incision is made. Having a familiar nurse in the operating room full of new people is reassuring to the woman before surgery.

The woman who has received a general anesthetic is usually awake enough to move from the operating table to her bed after surgery. Her respiratory status is observed every 15 minutes for 1 to 2 hours. A pulse oximeter provides constant information about her blood oxygen level. She is given oxygen by facemask or other means until she is fully awake. Her uterine fundus and vaginal bleeding are observed as for any other postpartum woman. Her urine output from the indwelling catheter should be observed for quantity and color at least hourly for 4 hours. The nurse should ambulate the woman cautiously and with assistance to prevent potential falling.

If the woman receives narcotic drugs, the nurse observes her respiratory rate for depression. Because respiratory depression is more likely to occur in the neonate than in the mother, the neonate is closely observed after birth. Narcotic effects in the infant may persist longer than in an adult. The nurse has naloxone on hand in case it is needed to reverse respiratory depression in the mother or neonate.

The nurse observes the woman for late-appearing respiratory depression and excessive sedation if she received epidural narcotics after cesarean birth. This may be up to 24 hours after administration, depending on the drug given. The woman's vital signs are monitored hourly, and a pulse oximeter may be applied. Facilities often use a scale to assess for sedation so that all caregivers use the same criteria for assessment and documentation. Additional analgesics are given cautiously and strictly as ordered. If mild analgesics do not relieve the pain, the health care provider is contacted for additional orders.

key points

- Pain during childbirth is different from other types of pain because it is part of a normal process that results in the birth of an infant. The woman has time to prepare for it, and the pain is self-limiting.
- A woman's pain threshold is fairly constant. Her pain tolerance varies, and nursing actions can increase her ability to tolerate pain. Irritants can reduce her pain tolerance.
- The pain of labor is caused by cervical dilation and effacement, uterine ischemia, and stretching of the vagina and perineum.
- Poorly relieved pain can be detrimental to the labor process.
- Childbirth preparation classes give the woman and her partner pain management tools they can use during labor. Some tools, such as breathing techniques and effleurage, can also be taught to the unprepared woman.
- The nurse should do everything possible to promote relaxation during labor because it enhances the effectiveness of all other pain management methods, both nonpharmacological and pharmacological.
- Any drug taken by the expectant mother may cross the placenta and affect the fetus. Effects may persist in the infant much longer than in an adult.
- The use of narcotic antagonist drugs for women who have a drug dependency can cause withdrawal syndrome in the mother or neonate.
- Observe the mother and/or infant for respiratory depression if the mother received opioids, including epidural narcotics, during the intrapartum period.
- Regional anesthetics are the most common for birth because they allow the mother to remain awake, including for cesarean birth.
- Closely question the woman about drug allergies when she is admitted. Because drugs used for regional anesthesia are related to those used in dentistry, ask her about reactions to dental anesthetics.
- Observe the mother's blood pressure and the fetal heart rate after epidural or spinal block to identify hypotension or fetal compromise. Urinary retention is also more likely.

ONLINE RESOURCES

Association of Women's Health, Obstetric and Neonatal Nurses: http://www.awhonn.org

All About Pregnancy: http://www.gowingo.com/health

NURSING **TIP**

The following are important admission assessments related to pharmacological pain management: last oral intake (time and type), adverse reactions to drugs (especially dental anesthetics), other medications taken, and any food allergies or latex allergy.

REVIEW QUESTIONS   *Choose the most appropriate answer.*

1. The narcotic drug of choice for pain relief during labor when the cervix is less than 4 cm dilated is:
   1. Morphine
   2. Meperidine
   3. Lidocaine
   4. Narcan

2. Which technique is likely to be most effective for "back labor"?
   1. Stimulating the abdomen by effleurage
   2. Applying firm pressure in the sacral area
   3. Blowing out in short breaths during each contraction
   4. Rocking from side to side at the peak of each contraction

3. What drug should be immediately available for emergency use when a woman receives narcotics during labor?
   1. Fentanyl (Sublimaze)
   2. Diphenhydramine (Benadryl)
   3. Lidocaine (Xylocaine)
   4. Naloxone (Narcan)

4. Choose the most important nursing assessment immediately after a woman receives an epidural block.
   1. Bladder distention
   2. Intravenous site
   3. Respiratory rate
   4. Blood pressure

5. Spinal headache after epidural anesthesia may be relieved by:
   1. Positioning woman on her side supported by pillows
   2. Epidural injection of a blood patch at the puncture site
   3. Avoiding ambulation for 12 hours
   4. Paced breathing techniques

Nursing Care of Women with Complications During Labor and Birth

objectives

1. Define each key term listed.
2. Describe each obstetric procedure discussed in this chapter.
3. Explain the nurse's role in each obstetric procedure.
4. Describe factors that contribute to an abnormal labor.
5. Explain each intrapartum complication discussed in this chapter.
6. Explain the nurse's role in caring for women having each intrapartum complication.

key terms

artificial rupture of membranes (AROM) (p. 176)
cephalopelvic disproportion (sĕf-ăh-lō-PĔL-vĭk dĭs-prō-PŎR-shŭn, p. 183)
chignon (SHĔN-yŏn, p. 183)
chorioamnionitis (kō-rē-ō-ăm-nē-ō-NĪ-tĭs, p. 196)
dysfunctional labor (p. 188)
dystocia (dĭs-TŌ-sē-ă, p. 188)
fibronectin test (fī-brō-NĔK-tĭn tĕst, p. 196)
hydramnios (hī-DRĂM-nē-ŏs, p. 177)
laminaria (lăm-ĭ-NĀ-rē-ăh, p. 178)
macrosomia (măk-rō-SŌM-ē-ă, p. 192)
oligohydramnios (ŏl-ĭ-gō-hī-DRĂM-nē-ŏs, p. 176)
shoulder dystocia (SHŌL-dĕr dĭs-TŌ-sē-ă, p. 193)
spontaneous rupture of membranes (SROM) (p. 177)
tocolytic (tō-kō-LĬT-ĭk, p. 178)
version (p. 180)

Childbirth is a normal, natural event in the life of most women and their families. When the many factors that affect the birth process function in harmony, complications are unlikely. However, some women experience complications during childbirth that threaten their well-being or that of the infant.

OBSTETRIC PROCEDURES

Nurses assist with several obstetric procedures during birth; they also care for women after the procedures. Some procedures, such as amniotomy or *amnioinfusion*, are performed to prevent complications during birth. Other procedures are needed when the woman has a complication that requires an intervention in order to promote a positive outcome for the mother and fetus.

AMNIOINFUSION

An amnioinfusion is the injection of warmed sterile saline or lactated Ringer's solution into the uterus via an intrauterine pressure catheter during labor after the membranes have ruptured. Indications for this procedure include the following:

- Oligohydramnios (decrease in amniotic fluid)
- Umbilical cord compression resulting from lack of amniotic fluid
- Reducing recurrent variable decelerations in fetal heart rate
- To dilute meconium-stained amniotic fluid

Amnioinfusion replaces the "cushion" for the umbilical cord and relieves the variable decelerations of the fetal heart rate that may occur during contractions when decreased amniotic fluid is present. It can be administered as a one-time bolus for 1 hour or as a continuous infusion. Continuous monitoring of uterine activity and fetal heart rate is essential. The nurse should change the underpads on the bed as needed to maintain patient comfort and should document the color, amount, and any odor of the fluid expelled via the vagina.

AMNIOTOMY

Amniotomy is the *artificial rupture of membranes* (amniotic sac) (AROM) by using a sterile sharp instrument. It is performed by a physician or nurse-midwife. The nurse assists the health care provider with the procedure and cares for the woman and fetus afterward.

Amniotomy is done to stimulate contractions. It may provide enough stimulation to start labor before it begins naturally, but more often it is done to enhance contractions that have already begun. It may be done to permit internal fetal monitoring (see pp. 136 to 141). The amniotomy stimulates prostaglandin secretion, which stimulates labor, but the loss of amniotic fluid may result in umbilical cord compression.

Technique

To determine if amniotomy is safe and indicated, the health care provider does a vaginal examination to assess the cervical effacement and dilation and the station of the fetus. A disposable plastic hook (Amnihook) is passed through the cervix, and the amniotic sac is snagged to create a hole and release the amniotic fluid.

Complications

Three complications associated with amniotomy may also occur if a woman's membranes rupture spontaneously (*spontaneous rupture of membranes* [SROM]). These complications are prolapse of the umbilical cord, infection, and abruptio placentae.

Prolapse of the umbilical cord. Prolapse may occur if the cord slips downward with the gush of amniotic fluid (p. 198).

Infection. Infection may occur because the membranes no longer block vaginal organisms from entering the uterus. An amniotomy commits the woman to delivery. The physician or nurse-midwife delays amniotomy until he or she is reasonably certain that birth will occur before the risk of infection markedly increases.

Abruptio placentae. Abruptio placentae (separation of the placenta before birth) is more likely to occur if the uterus is overdistended with amniotic fluid (*hydramnios*) when the membranes rupture. The uterus becomes smaller with the discharge of amniotic fluid, but the placenta stays the same size and no longer fits its implantation site (see p. 93 for more information about abruptio placentae).

Nursing Care

The nursing care after amniotomy is the same as that after spontaneous membrane rupture: observing for complications and promoting the woman's comfort.

> **NURSING TIP**
> Observe for wet underpads and linens after the membranes rupture. Change them as often as needed to keep the woman relatively dry and to reduce the risk for infection or skin breakdown.

Observing for complications. The fetal heart rate is recorded for at least 1 minute after amniotomy. Rates outside the normal range of 110 to 160 beats/min for a term fetus suggest a prolapsed umbilical cord. A large quantity of fluid increases the risk for prolapsed cord, especially if the fetus is high in the pelvis.

The color, odor, amount, and character of amniotic fluid are recorded. The fluid should be clear, possibly with flecks of vernix (newborn skin coating) and should not have a bad odor. Cloudy, yellow, or malodorous fluid suggests infection.

The woman's temperature is taken every 2 to 4 hours after her membranes rupture according to facility policy. A maternal temperature of 38° C (100.4° F) or higher suggests infection. An increase in the fetal heart rate, especially if above 160 beats/min, may precede the woman's temperature increase.

Green fluid means that the fetus passed the first stool (meconium) into the fluid before birth. Meconium-stained amniotic fluid may occur and is associated with fetal compromise during labor and infant respiratory distress after birth.

Promoting comfort. When amniotomy is anticipated, several disposable underpads are placed under the woman's hips to absorb the fluid that continues to leak from the woman's vagina during labor. Disposable underpads are changed often enough to keep her reasonably dry and to reduce the moist, warm environment that favors the growth of microorganisms.

INDUCTION OR AUGMENTATION OF LABOR

Induction of labor is the initiation of labor before it begins naturally. *Augmentation* is the stimulation of contractions after they have begun naturally.

Labor involves the complex interaction between fetus and mother. Before labor is induced, it is important that fetal maturity be confirmed by ultrasound or amniotic fluid analysis (L/S ratio) (see Chapter 5), and the status of the cervix is determined. *Bishop's score* is used to assess the status of the cervix in determining its response to induction (Table 8-1). A score of 6 or more indicates a favorable prognosis for induction. Continuous uterine activity and fetal heart monitoring during labor induction is essential.

Indications for Labor Induction

Labor is induced if continuing the pregnancy is hazardous for the woman or fetus. The following are examples of indications for labor induction:

- Pregnancy-induced hypertension (see p. 94)
- Ruptured membranes without spontaneous onset of labor

| table 8-1 | *Bishop's Scoring System* |

SCORE	0	1	2	3
Dilation of cervix (cm)	0	1-2	3-4	5-6
Consistency of cervix	Firm	Medium	Soft	—
Length of cervical canal (cm)	>2	1-2	0.5-1	<0.5
Cervical effacement (%)	0-30	40-50	60-70	80
Position of cervix	Posterior	Midline	Anterior	—
Station of presenting part related to ischial spines	−3	−2	−1	+1, +2

From Stables, D., & Novak, B. (1999). *Physiology in childbearing: With anatomy and related biosciences.* St Louis: Mosby.

- Infection within the uterus
- Medical problems in the woman that worsen during pregnancy, such as diabetes, kidney disease, or pulmonary disease
- Fetal problems, such as slowed growth, prolonged pregnancy, or incompatibility between fetal and maternal blood types (see p. 99)
- Placental insufficiency
- Fetal death

Convenience for the health care provider or family is not an indication for inducing labor. However, the woman who has a history of rapid labors and lives a long distance from the birth facility may have her labor induced because she has a higher risk of giving birth en route if she awaits spontaneous labor.

Contraindications

Labor is *not* induced in the following conditions:
- Placenta previa (see p. 91)
- Umbilical cord prolapse (see p. 198)
- Abnormal fetal presentation
- High station of the fetus, which suggests a preterm fetus or a small maternal pelvis
- Active herpes infection in the birth canal, which the infant can acquire during birth
- Abnormal size or structure of the mother's pelvis
- Previous classic (vertical) cesarean incision (see p. 183)

The physician may attempt to induce labor in a preterm pregnancy if continuing the pregnancy is more harmful to the woman and/or fetus than the hazards of prematurity would be to the infant.

Technique

Amniotomy may be the only method used to initiate labor, but it is more likely to be used in addition to oxytocin (Pitocin) to stimulate contractions. Induction and augmentation of labor may rely on both pharmacological and nonpharmacological methods.

Pharmacological methods to stimulate contractions

Cervical ripening. Induction of labor is easier if the woman's cervix is soft, partially effaced, and beginning to dilate. These prelabor cervical changes occur naturally in most women. Methods to hasten the changes, or "ripen" the cervix, ease labor induction because oxytocic drugs have no effect on the cervix.

Prostaglandin in the form of a gel or commercially prepared vaginal insert softens the cervix when applied before labor induction. The procedure should be explained to the woman and her family. A fetal heart rate baseline is recorded. An intravenous (IV) line with saline or heparin sodium (Hep-Lock) may be placed in case uterine hyperstimulation occurs and IV tocolytics (drugs that stop labor) are needed. After insertion of the prostaglandin gel, the woman remains on bed rest for 1 to 2 hours and is monitored for uterine contractions. Vital signs and fetal heart rates are also recorded. Oxytocin induction can be started when the insert is removed—usually after 6 to 12 hours. Signs of uterine hyperstimulation include uterine contractions that last longer than 90 seconds and/or more than five contractions in 10 minutes. The vaginal insert can be removed by pulling on the netted string that protrudes from the vaginal orifice. The contractions and fetal heart rate are monitored, and oxytocin may be started as needed. Some women who receive cervical ripening products begin labor without additional oxytocin stimulation. The use of misoprostol (Cytotec) is under study.

An alternative to prostaglandin for cervical ripening is insertion of one or more laminaria into the cervix (Quilligan & Zuspan, 2000). A laminaria is a narrow cone of a substance that absorbs water. The laminaria swells inside the cervix, thus beginning cervical dilation. Oxytocin induction follows, usually on the next day.

Oxytocin induction and augmentation of labor. Initiation or stimulation of contractions with oxytocin (Pitocin) is the most common method of labor induction and augmentation. Oxytocin is administered by registered nurses with additional training in the induction of labor and electronic fetal monitoring. Augmentation of labor with oxytocin follows a similar procedure.

Oxytocin for induction or augmentation of labor is diluted in an IV solution. The oxytocin solution is a secondary (piggyback) infusion that is inserted into the primary (nonmedicated) IV solution line so it can be stopped quickly while an open IV line is maintained.

The infusion of oxytocin solution is regulated with an infusion pump. Administration begins at a very low rate and is adjusted upward or downward according to how the fetus responds to labor and to the woman's contractions. The dose is individualized for every woman. When contractions are well established, it is often possible to reduce the rate of oxytocin. Augmentation of labor usually requires less total oxytocin than induction of labor because the uterus is more sensitive to the drug when labor has already begun.

Continuous electronic monitoring is the usual method to assess and record fetal and maternal responses to oxytocin. Many health care providers prefer internal methods of monitoring when oxytocin is used because these techniques are more accurate, especially for contraction intensity.

Nonpharmacological methods to stimulate contractions

Walking. Many women benefit from a change in activity if their labor slows. Walking stimulates contractions, eases the pressure of the fetus on the mother's back, and adds gravity to the downward force of contractions. If she does not feel like walking, other upright positions often improve the effectiveness of each contraction. She can sit (in a chair, on the side of the bed, or in the bed), squat, kneel while facing the raised head of the bed for support, or maintain other upright positions.

Nipple stimulation of labor. Stimulating the nipples causes the woman's posterior pituitary gland to secrete natural oxytocin. This improves the quality of contractions that have slowed or weakened, just as synthetic IV oxytocin does. The woman can stimulate her nipples by doing the following:

- Pulling or rolling them, one at a time
- Gently brushing them with a dry washcloth
- Using water in a whirlpool tub or a shower
- Applying suction with a breast pump

If contractions become too strong with these techniques, the woman simply stops stimulation.

Complications of Oxytocin Induction and Augmentation of Labor

The most common complications related to overstimulation of contractions are fetal compromise and uterine rupture. Fetal compromise can occur because blood flow to the placenta is reduced if contractions are excessive. Most placental exchange of oxygen, nutrients, and waste products occurs between contractions. This exchange is likely to be impaired if the contractions are too long, too frequent, or too intense. See p. 199 for discussion of uterine rupture.

Water intoxication sometimes occurs because oxytocin inhibits the excretion of urine and promotes fluid retention. Water intoxication is not likely with the small amounts of oxytocin and fluids given intravenously during labor, but it is more likely to occur if large doses of oxytocin and fluids are given intravenously *after* birth.

Oxytocin is discontinued, or its rate reduced, if signs of fetal compromise or excessive uterine contractions occur. Fetal heart rates outside the normal range of 110 to 160 beats/min, late decelerations, and loss of variability (see p. 139) are the most common signs of fetal compromise. Excessive uterine contractions are most often evidenced by contractions closer than every 2 minutes, durations longer than 90 seconds, or resting intervals shorter than 60 seconds. The resting tone of the uterus (muscle tension when it is not contracting) is often higher than normal. Internal uterine activity monitoring allows determination of peak uterine pressures and uterine resting tone.

In addition to stopping the oxytocin infusion, the registered nurse chooses one or more of the following measures to correct adverse maternal or fetal reactions:

- Increasing the nonmedicated intravenous solution
- Changing the woman's position, avoiding the supine position
- Giving oxygen by facemask at 8 to 10 L/min

The health care provider is notified after corrective measures are taken. A tocolytic (drug that reduces uterine contractions) may be ordered if contractions do not quickly decrease after oxytocin is stopped.

Nursing Care

Nursing care in labor induction and augmentation is directed by the registered nurse and by hospital policies. Baseline maternal vital signs are assessed and a fetal monitor tracing is performed to identify contraindications to induction or augmentation before the procedure begins.

During induction or augmentation the principal nursing observations are the fetal heart rate and character of uterine contractions. If abnormalities are noted in either, the nurse stops the oxytocin and begins measures to reduce contractions and increase placental blood flow.

The woman's blood pressure, pulse, and respirations are measured every 30 to 60 minutes. Her temperature is taken every 2 to 4 hours. Recording her intake and output identifies potential water intoxication.

> ✦ NURSING **TIP**
> Women who have oxytocin stimulation of labor may find that their contractions are difficult to manage. Help them to stay focused on breathing and relaxation techniques with each contraction.

VERSION

Version is a method of changing the fetal presentation, usually from breech to cephalic. There are two methods: external and internal. External version is the more common one. A successful version reduces the likelihood that the woman will need cesarean delivery.

Risks and Contraindications

Few maternal and fetal risks are associated with version, especially external version. Version is not indicated if there is any maternal or fetal reason why vaginal birth should not occur, because that is its goal. The following are examples of maternal or fetal conditions that are contraindications for version:

- Disproportion between the mother's pelvis and fetal size
- Abnormal uterine or pelvic size or shape
- Abnormal placental placement
- Previous cesarean birth with a vertical uterine incision
- Active herpesvirus infection
- Inadequate amniotic fluid
- Poor placental function
- Multifetal gestation

Version may not be attempted in a woman who has a higher risk for uterine rupture, such as several prior cesarean births or high parity. It is not usually attempted if the fetal presenting part is engaged in the pelvis.

The main risk to the fetus is that it will become entangled in the umbilical cord, thus compressing the cord. This is more likely to happen if there is not adequate room to turn the fetus, such as in multifetal gestation (e.g., twins) or when the amount of amniotic fluid is small. Version is not done if there are signs that the placenta is not functioning normally.

Technique

External version is done after 37 weeks' gestation but before the onset of labor. The procedure begins with a nonstress test or biophysical profile (see Table 5-1) to determine if the fetus is in good condition and if there is adequate amniotic fluid to perform the version. The woman receives a tocolytic drug to relax her uterus during the version.

Using ultrasound to guide the procedure, the physician pushes the fetal buttocks upward out of the pelvis while pushing the fetal head downward toward the pelvis in either a clockwise or counterclockwise turn. The fetus is monitored frequently during the procedure. The tocolytic drug is discontinued after the external version is completed (or the effort abandoned). Rh-negative women receive a dose of $Rh_o(D)$ immune globulin (RhoGAM).

Internal version is an emergency procedure. The physician usually performs internal version during a vaginal birth of twins to change the fetal presentation of the second twin.

Nursing Care

Nursing care of the woman having external version includes assisting with the procedure and observing the mother and fetus afterward for 1 to 2 hours. Baseline maternal vital signs and a fetal monitor strip (part of the nonstress test or biophysical profile) are taken before the version. The mother's vital signs and the fetal heart rates are observed to ensure return to normal levels after the version is complete.

Vaginal leaking of amniotic fluid suggests that manipulating the fetus caused a tear in the membranes, and this is reported. Uterine contractions usually decrease or stop shortly after the version. The physician is notified if they do not. The nurse reviews signs of labor with the woman because version is performed near term, when spontaneous labor is expected.

EPISIOTOMY AND LACERATIONS

Episiotomy is the surgical enlargement of the vagina during birth. Either the physician or a nurse-midwife performs and repairs an episiotomy. A laceration is an uncontrolled tear of the tissues that results in a jagged wound. Lacerations of the perineum and episiotomy incisions are treated similarly.

Perineal lacerations and often episiotomies are described by the amount of tissue involved:

- *First degree:* involves the superficial vaginal mucosa or perineal skin
- *Second degree:* involves the vaginal mucosa, perineal skin, and deeper tissues of the perineum
- *Third degree:* same as second degree, plus involves the anal sphincter

- *Fourth degree:* extends through the anal sphincter into the rectal mucosa

Women with third- and fourth-degree lacerations may have more discomfort postpartum if they are constipated after birth.

Indications

Fetal indications for an episiotomy are similar to those for forceps or vacuum extraction (see p. 182). Additional maternal indications include the following:

- Better control over where and how much the vaginal opening is enlarged
- An opening with a clean edge rather than the ragged opening of a tear

Routine episiotomy has been challenged by several recent studies that do not support many of its supposed benefits. Nevertheless, it is so common that the nurse can expect to give postpartum care to many women with episiotomies. Perineal massage and stretching exercises before labor are becoming popular techniques to decrease the need for episiotomy during birth.

> ✷NURSING **TIP**
> Pay special attention to a woman's diet and fluids if she had a third- or fourth-degree laceration. A high-fiber diet and adequate fluids help to prevent constipation that might result in a breakdown of the perineal area where the laceration was sutured.

Risks

As in other incisions, infection is the primary risk in an episiotomy or laceration. An additional risk is extension of the episiotomy with a laceration into or through the rectal sphincter (third or fourth degree), which can cause prolonged perineal discomfort and stress incontinence.

Technique

The episiotomy is performed with blunt-tipped scissors just before birth. One of the following two directions is chosen (Figure 8-1):

- *Median (midline),* extending directly from the lower vaginal border toward the anus
- *Mediolateral,* extending from the lower vaginal border toward the mother's right or left

A median episiotomy is easier to repair and heals neatly. The mediolateral incision provides more room, but greater scarring during healing may cause painful sexual intercourse. A laceration that extends a median episiotomy is more likely to go into the rectal sphincter than one that extends the mediolateral episiotomy.

Nursing Care

Nursing care for an episiotomy or laceration begins during the fourth stage of labor. Cold packs should be applied to the perineum for at least the first 12 hours to reduce pain, bruising, and edema. After 12 to 24 hours

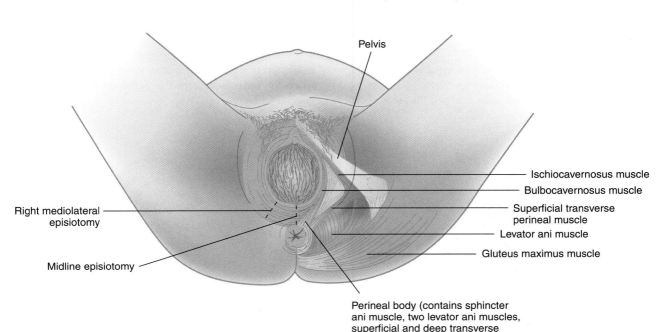

Pelvis

Right mediolateral episiotomy

Midline episiotomy

Ischiocavernosus muscle

Bulbocavernosus muscle

Superficial transverse perineal muscle

Levator ani muscle

Gluteus maximus muscle

Perineal body (contains sphincter ani muscle, two levator ani muscles, superficial and deep transverse perineal muscles, and the bulbocavernosus muscle)

FIGURE **8-1** Episiotomies. The two common types of episiotomies are midline and mediolateral.

of cold applications, warmth in the form of heat packs or sitz baths increases blood circulation, enhancing comfort and healing. Mild oral analgesics are usually sufficient for pain management. (See Chapter 9 for postpartum nursing care of the woman with an episiotomy or laceration.)

FORCEPS AND VACUUM EXTRACTION BIRTHS

Obstetric forceps and vacuum extractors are used by an obstetrician to provide traction and rotation to the fetal head when the mother's pushing efforts are insufficient to accomplish a safe delivery.

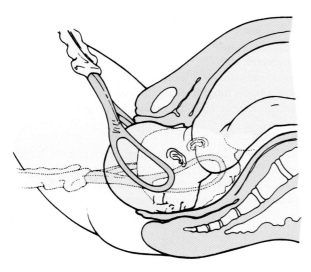

FIGURE **8-2** Forceps to assist the birth of the fetal head. After applying the forceps to each side of the fetal head and locking the two blades, the physician pulls, following the pelvic curve.

Forceps are instruments with curved blades that fit around the fetal head without unduly compressing it (Figure 8-2). Several different styles are available to assist the birth of the fetal head in a cephalic presentation or the after-coming head in a breech delivery. Forceps may also help the physician extract the fetal head through the incision during cesarean birth.

A vacuum extractor uses suction applied to the fetal head so the physician can assist the mother's expulsive efforts (Figure 8-3). The vacuum extractor is used only with an occiput presentation. One advantage of the vacuum extractor is that it does not take up room in the mother's pelvis, as forceps do.

Indications

Forceps or vacuum extraction may be used to end the second stage of labor if it is in the best interest of the mother and/or fetus. The mother may be exhausted, or she may be unable to push effectively. Women with cardiac or pulmonary disorders often have forceps or vacuum extraction births because prolonged pushing can worsen these conditions. Fetal indications include conditions in which there is evidence of an increased risk to the fetus near the end of labor. The cervix must be fully dilated, the membranes ruptured, the bladder empty, and the fetal head engaged and at +2 station for optimum outcome.

Contraindications

Forceps or vacuum extraction cannot substitute for cesarean birth if the maternal or fetal condition requires a quicker delivery. These techniques are not done if they would be more traumatic than cesarean birth, such as when the fetus is high in the pelvis or too large for a vaginal delivery.

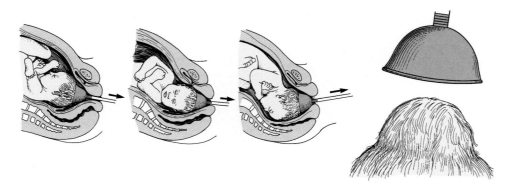

FIGURE **8-3** Use of the vacuum extractor to rotate the fetal head and assist with delivery. The arrows indicate the direction of traction on the vacuum cup. The vacuum cup is positioned on the midline, near the posterior fontanel.

Risks

Trauma to maternal and/or fetal tissues is the main risk when forceps or vacuum extraction is used. The mother may have a laceration or hematoma (collection of blood in the tissues) in her vagina. The infant may have bruising, facial or scalp lacerations or abrasions, cephalhematoma (see Chapter 12), or intracranial hemorrhage. The vacuum extractor causes a harmless area of circular edema on the infant's scalp (chignon) where it was applied.

Technique

The health care provider catheterizes the woman to prevent trauma to her bladder and to make more room in her pelvis. After the forceps are applied, the physician pulls in line with the pelvic curve. An episiotomy is usually done. After the fetal head is brought under the mother's symphysis, the rest of the birth occurs in the usual way.

Birth assisted with the vacuum extractor follows a similar sequence. The health care provider applies the cup over the posterior fontanel of the fetal occiput, and suction is created with a machine to hold it there. Traction is applied by pulling on the handle of the extractor cup.

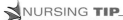

NURSING **TIP**
Many parents are concerned about the marks made by forceps. Reassure them that these marks are temporary and usually resolve without treatment.

Nursing Care

If the use of forceps or vacuum extraction is anticipated, the nurse places the sterile equipment on the delivery instrument table.

After birth, care is similar to that for episiotomy and perineal lacerations. Ice is applied to the perineum to reduce bruising and edema. The physician is notified if the woman has signs of vaginal hematoma, which include severe and poorly relieved pelvic or rectal pain.

The infant's head is examined for lacerations, abrasions, or bruising. Mild facial reddening and molding (alteration in shape) of the head are common and require no treatment. Cold treatments are not used on neonates because they would cause hypothermia.

Pressure from forceps may injure the infant's facial nerve. This is evidenced by facial asymmetry (different appearance of right and left sides), which is most obvious when the infant cries. Facial nerve injury usually resolves without treatment. The scalp chignon from the vacuum extractor requires no intervention and resolves quickly.

CESAREAN BIRTH

Cesarean birth is the surgical delivery of the fetus through incisions in the mother's abdomen and uterus. Cesarean birth rates in the United States are 23.5% (National Center for Health Statistics, 2001), and the goal of *Healthy People 2010* is to reduce cesarean sections to 15%. This is the basis for some of the changes in the management of the second stage of labor, such as the following:

- Position (upright or horizontal)
- Epidural analgesia and subarachnoid analgesia that allows ambulation and delivery in squatting position
- Oxytocin (Pitocin) augmentation of labor
- Spontaneous open glottis pushing when fetus is +1 station
- Use of vacuum-assisted delivery rapidly replacing forceps delivery
- Trial of labor before repeat cesarean (vaginal birth after cesarean [VBAC])
- Electronic fetal and uterine monitoring

In 1997 the World Health Organization (WHO) recommended minimal intervention with maximum patience, support, and tender loving care (TLC).

Indications

Several conditions may require cesarean delivery:
- Abnormal labor
- Inability of the fetus to pass through the mother's pelvis (cephalopelvic disproportion)
- Maternal conditions such as pregnancy-induced hypertension or diabetes
- Active maternal herpesvirus, which may cause serious or fatal infant infection
- Previous surgery on the uterus, including the classic type of cesarean incision
- Fetal compromise, including prolapsed umbilical cord and abnormal presentations
- Placenta previa or abruptio placentae

Contraindications

There are few contraindications to cesarean birth, but it is not usually done if the fetus is dead or too premature to survive or if the mother has abnormal blood clotting.

Risks

Cesarean birth carries risks to both mother and fetus. Maternal risks are similar to those of other types of surgery and include the following:
- Risks related to anesthesia (see Chapter 7)
- Respiratory complications
- Hemorrhage

- Blood clots
- Injury to the urinary tract
- Delayed intestinal peristalsis (paralytic ileus)
- Infection

Risks to the newborn may include the following:

- Inadvertent preterm birth
- Respiratory problems because of delayed absorption of lung fluid
- Injury, such as laceration or bruising

To avoid the unintentional birth of a preterm fetus, the physician often performs amniocentesis before a planned cesarean birth to determine if the fetal lungs are mature (see Chapter 5).

Technique

Cesarean birth may occur under planned, unplanned, or emergency conditions. The preparation is similar for each and include routine preoperative care such as obtaining informed consent. If the woman wears eyeglasses, they should accompany her to the operating room because she is usually awake to bond with the infant after birth.

Preparations for cesarean birth. As with other surgery, several laboratory studies are done to identify anemia or blood-clotting abnormalities. Complete blood count, coagulation studies, and blood typing and screening are common. One or more units of blood may be typed and crossmatched if the woman is likely to need a transfusion. The baseline vital signs of the mother and fetal heart rate are recorded.

The woman receives an IV drug to reduce gastric acidity and speed stomach emptying. Antibiotic doses may be ordered for the woman who has an increased risk for infection (such as prolonged ruptured membranes), displays signs of infection, or is positive for group B streptococcus (GBS).

If a vertical skin incision is expected, the woman's abdomen may be shaved from just above her umbilicus to her mons pubis, where her thighs come together. If a Pfannenstiel (transverse, or "bikini") skin incision is planned, the upper border of the shave is about 3 inches above her pubic hairline.

An indwelling Foley catheter is inserted to keep the bladder empty and prevent trauma to it. The catheter bag is placed near the head of the operating table so the anesthesiologist can monitor urine output, an important indicator of the woman's circulating blood volume. The circulating nurse scrubs the abdomen by using a circular motion that goes outward from the incisional area. The husband or partner of the woman may don a hat, mask, and gown and provide support to the mother at the head of the table (see Figure 8-5).

Types of incisions. There are two incisions in cesarean birth: a skin incision and a uterine incision. The directions of these incisions are not always the same.

Skin incisions. The skin incision is done in either a vertical or a transverse direction. A vertical incision allows more room if a large fetus is being delivered, and it is usually needed for an obese woman. In an emergency, the vertical incision can be done more quickly. The transverse, or Pfannenstiel, incision is nearly invisible when healed but cannot always be used in obese women or in women with a large fetus.

Uterine incisions. The more important of the two incisions is the one that cuts into the uterus. There are three types of uterine incisions (Figure 8-4): low transverse, low vertical, and classic.

Low transverse incision. A low transverse incision is preferred because it is not likely to rupture during another birth, causes less blood loss, and is easier to repair. It may not be an option if the fetus is large or if there is a placenta previa in the area where the incision would be made. This type of incision makes VBAC possible for subsequent births.

Low vertical incision. A low vertical incision produces minimal blood loss and allows delivery of a larger fetus. However, it is more likely to rupture during another birth, although less so than the classic incision.

Classic incision. The classic incision is rarely used because it involves more blood loss and is the most likely of the three types to rupture during another pregnancy. However, it may be the only choice if the fetus is in a transverse lie or if there is scarring or a placenta previa in the lower anterior uterus.

Sequence of Events in Cesarean Birth

After the woman has been given a spinal anesthetic, scrubbed, and draped, the physician makes the skin incision. After making the uterine incision, the physician ruptures the membranes (unless they are already ruptured) with a sharp instrument. The amniotic fluid is suctioned from the operative area, and its amount, color, and odor are noted.

The physician reaches into the uterus to lift out the fetal head or buttocks. Forceps or vacuum extraction may be used to assist birth of the head. The infant's mouth and nose are quickly suctioned to remove secretions, and the cord is clamped. The physician hands the infant to the nurse, who receives the infant into sterile blankets and places the child into a radiant warmer. A pediatrician is usually available for resuscitation.

After the birth of the infant, the physician scoops out the placenta and examines it for intactness. The uterine cavity is sponged to remove blood clots and other debris. The uterine and skin incisions are then sutured in layers (Figure 8-5).

Nursing Care

The registered nurse assumes most of the preoperative and postoperative care of the woman. This includes obtaining the required laboratory studies, administering medications, performing preoperative teaching, and preparing for surgery.

Women who have cesarean birth usually need greater emotional support than those having vaginal births. They are usually happy and excited about the newborn but may also feel grief, guilt, or anger because the expected course of birth did not occur. These feelings may linger and resurface during another pregnancy.

Emotional care of the partner and family is essential; they are included in explanations of the surgery as much as the woman wishes. The partner may be frightened when an emergency cesarean is needed but may not express these feelings because the woman needs so much support. The partner may be almost as exhausted as the woman if a cesarean birth is performed after hours of labor. The thoughtful nurse includes the partner and promotes his or her emotional and physical well-being.

The nurse informs the partner of when he or she may enter the operating room because ½ hour or more may be needed to administer a regional anesthetic and for surgical preparations if there is no emergency. The partner dons surgical attire during this time.

The mother, neonate, and partner are kept together as much as possible after birth, just as in a vaginal birth. The woman and her partner are encouraged to talk about the cesarean birth so they can integrate the experience. The nurse answers questions about events surrounding the birth. The focus is on the *birth* rather than on the surgical aspects of cesarean delivery.

Nursing assessments after cesarean birth are similar to those after vaginal birth, including assessment of the uterine fundus. Assessments are done every 15 minutes for the first 1 or 2 hours according to hospital policy. Recovery room assessments after cesarean birth include the following:

- Vital signs to identify hemorrhage or shock; a pulse oximeter is used to better identify depressed respiratory function
- IV site and rate of solution flow
- Fundus for firmness, height, and midline position
- Dressing for drainage
- Lochia for quantity, color, and presence of clots
- Urine output from the indwelling catheter

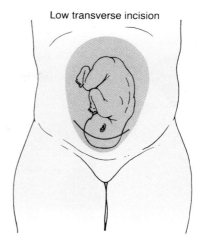

Low transverse incision

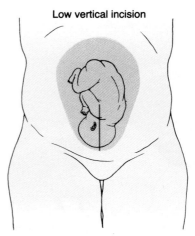

Low vertical incision

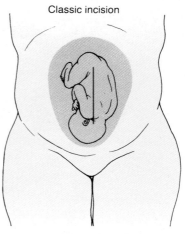

Classic incision

FIGURE **8-4** Three types of uterine incisions for cesarean birth. The low transverse uterine incision is preferred because it is not likely to rupture during a subsequent birth, allowing vaginal birth after a cesarean birth. The low vertical and classic incisions may occasionally be used. The skin incision and uterine incision do not always match.

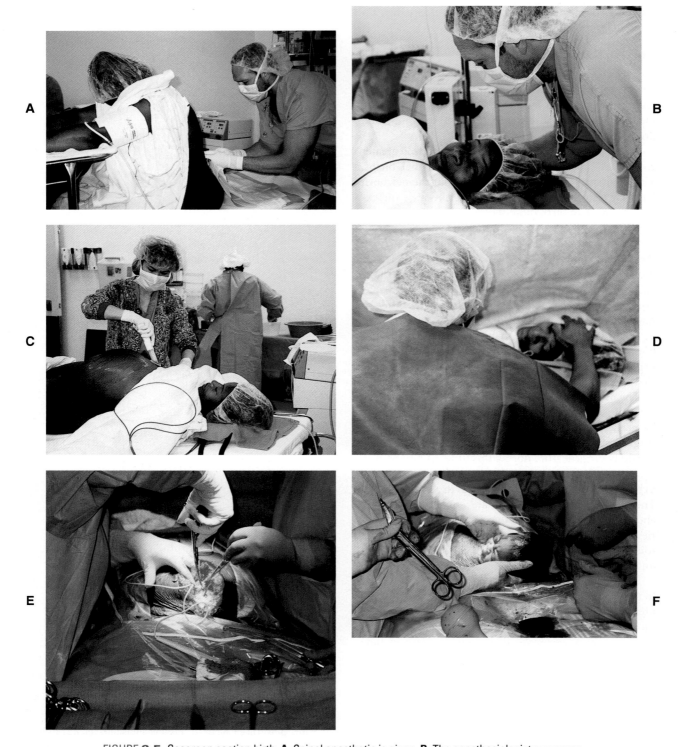

FIGURE **8-5** Cesarean section birth. **A,** Spinal anesthetic is given. **B,** The anesthesiologist reassures the woman. **C,** The nurse preps the abdomen. **D,** The partner encourages the woman. **E,** A vertical incision is made. **F,** The head of the infant is lifted out of the uterus.

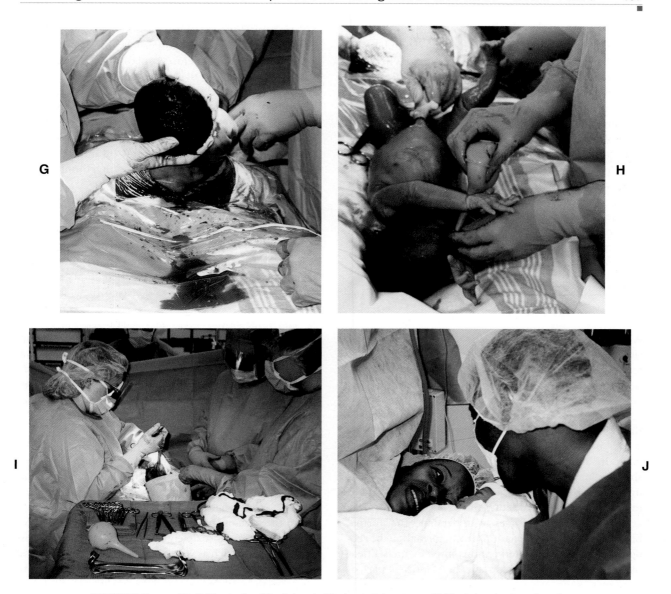

FIGURE **8-5, cont'd G,** The body of the infant is lifted out of the uterus. **H,** The infant is placed on the mother's abdomen and suctioned with a bulb syringe. Note the active muscle tone of the newborn. **I,** The placenta is delivered from the uterus. **J,** The parents and the newborn bond. (Photos courtesy of Pat Spier, RN-C.)

The fundus is checked as gently as possible. The woman flexes her knees slightly and takes slow, deep breaths to minimize the discomfort of fundal assessments. While supporting the lower uterus with one hand, the fingers of the other hand are gently "walked" from the side of the uterus toward the midline. Massage is not needed if the fundus is already firm.

NURSING **TIP**

Although assessing the uterus after cesarean birth causes discomfort, it is important to do so regularly. The woman can have a relaxed uterus that causes excessive blood loss, regardless of how she delivered her child.

The woman is told to take deep breaths at each assessment and to cough to move secretions from her airways. A small pillow or folded blanket supports her incision when she coughs or moves, which reduces pain. Changing her position every 1 or 2 hours helps expand her lungs and also makes her more comfortable.

Pain relief after cesarean birth may be by patient-controlled analgesia (PCA) pump or by intermittent injections of narcotic analgesics. Epidural narcotics provide long-lasting pain relief but are associated with delayed respiratory depression and itching (see p. 168), which vary with the drug injected. The woman is changed to oral analgesics after about the first 24 hours. Nursing Care Plan 8-1 details interventions for selected nursing diagnoses that pertain to the woman with an unplanned cesarean birth.

ABNORMAL LABOR

A normal labor is labor that evidences a regular progression in cervical effacement, dilation, and descent of the fetus. Abnormal labor, called dysfunctional labor, does not progress. Dystocia is a term used to describe a difficult labor.

The "four Ps" of labor (see p. 124) interact constantly throughout the birth. Abnormalities in the powers, passenger, passage, or psyche may result in a dysfunctional labor. In addition, the length of labor may be unusually short or long. Labor abnormalities may require forceps or cesarean delivery, and they are more likely to result in injury to the mother or fetus.

It is essential for nurses to understand the normal birth process so that deviations from normal can be recognized and prompt interventions implemented. Effective support for the woman and her family is part of competent and compassionate care. Risk factors for dysfunctional labor include the following:
- Advanced maternal age
- Obesity
- Overdistention of uterus (hydramnios or multifetal)
- Abnormal presentation
- Cephalopelvic disproportion (CPD)
- Overstimulation of the uterus
- Maternal fatigue, dehydration, fear
- Lack of analgesic assistance

PROBLEMS WITH THE POWERS OF LABOR

A woman may have contractions that are hypertonic or hypotonic. She may not have adequate pushing efforts to bring about fetal descent.

Hypertonic Labor Dysfunction

Hypertonic labor dysfunction usually occurs during the latent phase of labor (before 4 cm of cervical dilation).

Hypertonic labor dysfunction is characterized by contractions that are frequent, cramplike, and poorly coordinated. They are painful but nonproductive. The uterus is tense, even between contractions, which reduces blood flow to the placenta. It is less common than hypotonic dysfunction. Box 8-1 summarizes the differences between hypertonic and hypotonic labor dysfunction.

Medical treatment. Medical treatment may include mild sedation to allow the woman to rest. *Tocolytic drugs* (see p. 197) such as terbutaline (Brethine) may be ordered.

Nursing care. Women with hypertonic dysfunction are uncomfortable and frustrated. Anxiety about the lack of progress and fatigue impair their ability to tolerate pain. They may lose confidence in their ability to give birth.

The nurse should accept the woman's frustration and that of her partner. Both may be exhausted from the near-constant discomfort. It is important not to equate the amount of pain a woman reports with how much she "should" feel at that point in labor. The nurse provides general comfort measures that promote rest and relaxation.

Hypotonic Labor Dysfunction

A woman has hypotonic labor if her contractions are too weak to be effective during active labor. The woman begins labor normally, but contractions diminish during the active phase (after 4 cm of cervical dilation), when the pace of labor is expected to accelerate. Hypotonic labor is more likely to occur if the uterus is overdistended, such as with twins, a large fetus, or excess amniotic fluid (hydramnios). Uterine overdistention stretches the muscle fibers and thus reduces their ability to contract effectively.

Medical treatment. The physician usually does an amniotomy if the membranes are intact. Augmentation of labor with oxytocin or by nipple stimulation increases the strength of contractions. IV or oral fluids may improve the quality of contractions if the woman is dehydrated.

Nursing care. The woman is reasonably comfortable but frustrated because her labor is not progressing. In addition to providing care related to amniotomy and labor augmentation, the nurse gives emotional support to the woman and her partner. She is allowed to express her frustrations. The nurse tells her when she makes progress to encourage continuing her efforts.

Position changes may help to relieve discomfort and enhance progress. Contractions are usually stronger and

NURSING CARE PLAN 8-1

The Woman with an Unplanned Cesarean Birth

PATIENT DATA: A woman, para 0 gravida 1, has been using breathing, relaxation, and imagery techniques during the first stage of labor, and her husband has been helpful and supportive. However, the labor is not progressing, and there are signs of fetal distress. The physician orders that the patient be prepared for an emergency cesarean section.

SELECTED NURSING DIAGNOSIS   *Anxiety related to development of complications*

Outcomes	Nursing Interventions	Rationales
The woman and her partner will express decreased anxiety after explanations about the planned surgery.	1. Determine stress level and learning needs.	1. Provides a database to build on to provide information that will decrease anxiety.
	2. Reinforce all explanations given by physician, expressing them in simpler terms if needed.	2. Anxiety tends to narrow attention; although physician may have explained the need for surgery, the woman and her partner may not have comprehended everything they were told.
	3. Encourage the woman to continue using the breathing and relaxation techniques she learned in prepared childbirth classes as long as contractions continue.	3. Learned pain management techniques increase the woman's sense of control. Control over a situation reduces feelings of helplessness and decreases anxiety.
	4. Tell the woman what the operating room looks like and who will be present. Explain basic equipment, such as catheter, narrow table, monitors for her heart and blood pressure, anesthetic machine, and large overhead lights. Explain that personnel will wear protective equipment such as masks, eye protection, gowns, gloves, hats, and shoe covers.	4. Commonplace equipment and attire in an operating room can be intimidating for someone who has not seen them before. Unfamiliarity increases anxiety; preparation reduces anxiety and fear of the unknown.
	5. Describe the usual postoperative care: assessment of the vital signs, fundus, vaginal bleeding, dressing, and catheter. Tell her she will be asked to take deep breaths and change position regularly.	5. If woman understands common postoperative care, she is more likely to cooperate with it, even if assessments are uncomfortable.
	6. Encourage her partner to be with her during surgery, and do not separate family afterward, if possible.	6. Companionship of familiar persons helps to reduce anxiety; keeping new family together promotes attachment to the newborn.
	7. Stay with the woman. Encourage verbalization and support her coping mechanisms.	7. The presence of a professional person reduces anxiety.

Continued

NURSING CARE PLAN 8-1—cont'd

SELECTED NURSING DIAGNOSIS *Impaired comfort related to decreased coping ability*

Outcomes	Nursing Interventions	Rationales
The woman will verbalize reduced discomfort or will be able to use effective techniques to decrease perception of pain.	1. Determine the nature, duration, and location of pain.	1. Never assume that the pain is related to a contraction. Locating the site of pain helps identify complications that may be occurring (e.g., embolism). Assessing pain and contractions can help identify a prolonged contraction that can cause fetal hypoxia.
	2. Encourage the woman to continue using coping mechanisms learned during prenatal classes. Use therapeutic touch to increase comfort.	2. A feeling of loss of control can increase the perception of pain. Reduction of tension can promote comfort.
	3. Maintain a calm manner and environment.	3. A calm manner calms the parents and reduces anxieties and tensions that elevate pain perception.

?CRITICAL THINKING QUESTION

What are the advantages and disadvantages of a transverse abdominal incision compared to the classic midline incision?

---

box 8-1 | **Differences Between Hypertonic Labor and Hypotonic Labor Dysfunction**

HYPERTONIC LABOR

Contractions are poorly coordinated, frequent, and painful.
Uterine resting tone between contractions is tense.
It is less common than hypotonic labor dysfunction.
It is more likely to occur during latent labor, before 4 cm of cervical dilation.
Medical management includes mild sedation and tocolytic drugs.
Nursing interventions include acceptance of the woman's discomfort and frustration and the provision of comfort measures.

HYPOTONIC LABOR

Contractions are weak and ineffective.
It is more common than hypertonic labor dysfunction.
It occurs during the active phase, after 4 cm of cervical dilation.
It is more likely if the uterus is overly distended or if the woman has had many other births.
Medical management includes amniotomy, oxytocin augmentation, and adequate hydration.
Nonpharmacological stimulation methods include walking, other upright positions, and nipple stimulation.
Other nursing interventions include position changes and encouragement.

---

more effective when the woman assumes an upright position or lies on her side, although they may be less frequent. Walking or nipple stimulation may intensify contractions. Nursing Care Plan 8-2 details interventions for selected nursing diagnoses that pertain to the woman with hypotonic labor dysfunction.

Ineffective Maternal Pushing

The woman may not push effectively during the second stage of labor because she does not understand which techniques to use or fears tearing her perineal tissues. Epidural or subarachnoid blocks (see pp. 168 and 169) may depress or eliminate the natural urge to push. An exhausted woman may be unable to gather her resources to push appropriately.

Nursing care. Nursing care focuses on coaching the woman about the most effective techniques for pushing. If she cannot feel her contractions because of a regional block, the nurse tells her when to push as each contraction reaches its peak.

NURSING CARE PLAN 8-2

The Woman with Hypotonic Labor Dysfunction

PATIENT DATA: A woman, para 0 gravida 1, is admitted at 7 PM because of premature rupture of the membranes. Contractions remain irregular at 7 AM the next morning. The woman appears anxious and fearful concerning her lack of progress.

SELECTED NURSING DIAGNOSIS   *Risk for infection related to loss of barrier (ruptured membranes)*

Outcomes	Nursing Interventions	Rationales
The woman's temperature will remain under 38° C (100.4° F), and the amniotic fluid will remain clear with a mild odor.	1. Take the woman's temperature every 2 to 4 hours or more often if elevated. At the same time, assess the amniotic fluid drainage for color, clarity, and odor.	1. Elevated temperature is a sign of infection; cloudy, yellow, or foul-odored fluid suggests infection; and meconium (green) staining suggests fetal compromise but is also seen with prolonged pregnancy.
	2. Observe fetal heart rates (see p. 136).	2. Fetal tachycardia (rate >160 beats/min) may be the first sign of infection. Poor fetal oxygenation may also occur, especially with abnormal labor.
	3. Assist the woman to maintain good perineal hygiene (wiping front to back). Keep underpads clean and dry.	3. Good hygiene reduces the possibility of introducing bacteria into the birth canal.
	4. Monitor IV line, electrode sites, and incision sites for signs of redness, edema, pain, and drainage.	4. These are the primary sites where infection can occur.
	5. After birth, continue to assess the woman's temperature at least every 4 hours. Assess the lochia (postbirth vaginal drainage) for a foul odor or brown color.	5. The woman may not show these signs of infection until after birth.
	6. Observe the neonate for a temperature below 36.2° C (97° F) or over 38° C (100.4° F). Observe for poor feeding, lethargy, irritability, or "not looking right."	6. The neonate may become infected in utero and display these signs of infection after birth. Neonatal sepsis may occur with prolonged rupture of membranes and is a potentially fatal infection.

SELECTED NURSING DIAGNOSIS   *Ineffective coping related to frustration with slow labor and delayed birth*

Outcomes	Nursing Interventions	Rationales
The woman will use breathing and relaxation techniques that she and her partner learned in prepared childbirth class. The woman will verbalize an understanding of what is happening and how she can still participate in the birth process.	1. If there is no contraindication, encourage the woman to walk or to sit upright in bed or chair. Walking may not be wise if the membranes are ruptured and the fetus is high.	1. Upright positions enhance fetal descent. Walking strengthens labor contractions; walking when membranes are ruptured and fetal station is high could lead to umbilical cord prolapse.

Continued

NURSING CARE PLAN 8-2—cont'd

Outcomes	Nursing Interventions	Rationales
	2. Help the woman to use natural methods to stimulate contractions, such as nipple stimulation. Encourage a shower or whirlpool if available and not contraindicated.	2. Nipple stimulation causes the woman's posterior pituitary gland to secrete natural oxytocin, which strengthens contractions. Water may help the woman relax, which improves labor. All nonpharmacological methods to stimulate labor enhance her sense of control.
	3. Assist the registered nurse with oxytocin augmentation if it is ordered. Observe contractions for excessive frequency (more frequent than every 2 minutes), duration (over 90 seconds), or inadequate rest interval (under 60 seconds). Observe fetal heart rate for rates outside the normal 110 to 160 beats/min.	3. The primary risks of oxytocin augmentation or induction of labor relate to overstimulating the uterus. Excessive contractions can reduce fetal oxygen supply. These are signs of potential uterine overstimulation.
	4. Explain to the woman how each method is expected to help her labor advance. Tell her any time she makes progress, either in improved contractions or increasing cervical dilation.	4. If the woman understands the reason for any interventions, she will more likely cooperate with them and feel more in control. Knowing that her efforts are having the desired effect encourages her to continue with her learned coping methods.
	5. Help the woman relax and use the breathing techniques she learned in prepared childbirth class. Praise and support her when she uses them.	5. Relaxation promotes normal labor. Praise encourages the woman to continue efforts at managing contractions.
	6. Reposition frequently. Acknowledge the reality of discomfort.	6. Feeling supported enhances coping.

CRITICAL THINKING QUESTION

A woman, para 0 gravida 1, has been admitted with ruptured membranes. Contractions are irregular and ineffective, and progress in dilation and effacement of the cervix is very slow. An oxytocin IV infusion is started after 15 hours. What could happen if the health care provider decided not to augment labor?

The exhausted woman may benefit from pushing only when she feels a strong urge. The fearful woman may benefit from explanations that sensations of tearing or splitting often accompany fetal descent but that her body is designed to accommodate the fetus. Promoting relaxation, relieving fatigue, changing position, and increasing hydration can help the woman's energy level needed for effective pushing.

PROBLEMS WITH THE FETUS

Several fetal conditions can contribute to abnormal labor, including fetal size, presentation, or position. Mul-

tifetal pregnancies are associated with difficult labor. Some birth defects alter the fetal body in such a way as to impede birth.

Fetal Size

A large fetus (macrosomia) is generally considered to be one that weighs more than 4000 g (8.8 pounds) at birth. The large fetus may not fit through the woman's pelvis. A very large fetus also distends the uterus and can contribute to hypotonic labor dysfunction.

Sometimes a single part of the fetus is too large. For example, the fetus may have hydrocephalus (an abnormal amount of fluid in the brain). In that case the fetal body size and weight may be normal, but the head is too large to fit through the pelvis. These infants are often in an abnormal presentation as well. Hydrocephalus is discussed in Chapter 14.

Shoulder dystocia may occur, usually when the fetus is large. The fetal head is born, but the shoulders become impacted above the mother's symphysis pubis. A shoulder dystocia is an emergency because the fetus needs to breathe. The head is out, but the chest cannot expand. The cord is compressed between the fetus and the mother's pelvis. The health care provider may request that the nurse apply firm downward pressure just above the symphysis (suprapubic pressure) to push the shoulders toward the pelvic canal. Squatting or sharp flexion of the thighs against the abdomen may also loosen the shoulders.

Nursing care. If the woman successfully delivers a large infant, both mother and child should be observed for injuries after birth. The woman may have a large episiotomy or laceration. The large infant is more likely to have a fracture of one or both clavicles (collarbones). The infant's clavicles are felt for crepitus (crackling sensation) or deformity of the bones, and the arms are observed for equal movement (unilateral Moro reflex). The woman is more at risk for uterine atony and postpartum hemorrhage because her uterus does not contract well after birth to control bleeding at the placental site.

Abnormal Fetal Presentation or Position

Labor is most efficient if the fetus is in a flexed, cephalic presentation and in one of the occiput anterior positions (see p. 128). Abnormalities of fetal presentation and position prevent the smallest diameter of the fetal head to pass through the smallest diameter of the pelvis for the effective progress of labor.

Abnormal presentations. The fetus in an abnormal presentation, such as the breech or face presentation, does not pass easily through the woman's pelvis (see Chapter 6) and interferes with the most efficient mechanisms of labor (p. 131).

In the United States most fetuses in the breech presentation are born by cesarean delivery. During vaginal birth in this presentation, the trunk and extremities are born before the head. After the fetal body delivers, the umbilical cord can be compressed between the fetal head and the mother's pelvis. The head, which is the single largest part of the fetus, must be quickly delivered so the infant can breathe. Figure 8-6 illustrates the sequence of delivery for a vaginal breech birth.

Intrapartum nurses must be prepared to assist with a breech birth, because a woman sometimes arrives at the birth facility in advanced labor with her fetus in a breech presentation.

External version is being used to avoid some cesarean deliveries for a breech presentation. However, external version is not always successful, and the fetus sometimes returns to the abnormal presentation.

Abnormal positions. A common cause of abnormal labor is a fetus that remains in a persistent occiput posterior position (left [LOP] or right [ROP]). The fetal occiput occupies either the left or right posterior quadrant of the mother's pelvis. In most women the fetal head rotates in a clockwise or counterclockwise direction until the occiput is in one of the anterior quadrants of the pelvis (left [LOA] or right [ROA]).

Labor is likely to be longer when rotation does not occur. Intense and poorly relieved back and leg pain characterizes labor when the fetus is in the occiput posterior position. Women with a small or average-size pelvis may have difficulty delivering infants who remain in an occiput posterior position. The physician may use forceps to rotate the fetal head into an occiput anterior position.

Nursing care. During labor the nurse should encourage the woman to assume positions that favor fetal rotation and descent. These positions also reduce some of the back pain. Good positions for back labor include the following:

- Sitting, kneeling, or standing while leaning forward
- Rocking the pelvis back and forth while on hands and knees (Figure 8-7) to encourage rotation
- Side-lying (on the left side for an ROP position, on the right side for an LOP position)
- Squatting (for second-stage labor)
- Lunging by placing one foot in a chair with the foot and knee pointed to that side; lunging sideways repeatedly during a contraction for 5 seconds at a time

After birth, the mother and infant are observed for signs of birth trauma. The mother is more likely to have a hematoma of her vaginal wall if the fetus remained in the occiput posterior position for a long time. The infant may have excessive molding (alteration in shape) of the head, caput succedaneum (scalp edema, see Chapter 12), and possibly injury from forceps or the vacuum extractor.

Multifetal Pregnancy

If the woman has more than one fetus, dysfunctional labor is likely for the following reasons:

- Uterine overdistention contributes to poor contraction quality.

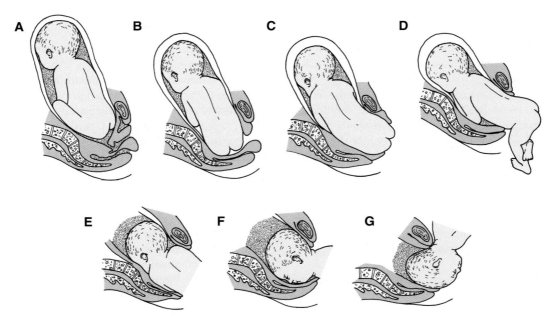

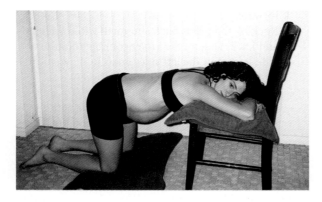

FIGURE **8-6** The mechanism of labor in a breech birth. **A,** Breech before onset of labor. **B,** Engagement and internal rotation of buttocks. **C,** Lateral flexion. **D,** External rotation and restitution of buttocks. **E,** Internal rotation of shoulders and head. **F,** Face rotates to sacrum. Note that there is no flexion of the head so that the smallest diameter of the fetal head is not passing through the pelvis. The umbilical cord is compressed between the fetal head and the bony pelvis. **G,** The head is born as the fetal body is elevated.

FIGURE **8-7** The hands-and-knees position can help the fetus rotate from an occiput posterior to an occiput anterior position. Gravity causes the fetus to float downward toward the pool of amniotic fluid. This position can be practiced before labor.

- Abnormal presentation or position of one or more fetuses interferes with labor mechanisms.
- Often one fetus is delivered as cephalic and the second as breech unless a version is done.

Because of the difficulties inherent in multifetal deliveries, cesarean birth is common. Birth is almost always cesarean if three or more fetuses are involved.

Nursing care. When the woman has a multifetal pregnancy, each fetus is monitored separately during labor. An upright or side-lying position with the head slightly elevated aids breathing and is usually most comfortable. Labor care is similar to that for single pregnancies, with observations for hypotonic labor.

The nursery and intrapartum staffs prepare equipment and medications for every infant expected. An anesthesiologist and a pediatrician are often present at birth because of the potential for maternal and/or neonatal problems. One nurse is available for each infant. Another nurse focuses on the mother's needs.

PROBLEMS WITH THE PELVIS AND SOFT TISSUES

The woman's pelvic size or shape and the characteristics of her soft tissues can either facilitate or impede birth.

Bony Pelvis

Some women have a small or abnormally shaped pelvis, thus impeding the normal mechanisms of labor. The gynecoid pelvis is the most favorable for vaginal birth.

Absolute pelvic measurements are rarely helpful to determine whether a woman's pelvis is adequate for birth. A woman with a "small" pelvis may still deliver vaginally if other factors are favorable. She often delivers vaginally if her fetus is not too large, the head is well flexed, contractions are good, and her soft tissues yield easily to the forces of labor.

In contrast, some women have vaginally delivered several infants well over 9 pounds but cannot deliver one weighing 10 pounds. Obviously, the pelvis of each was "adequate," or even "large," according to standard measurements. However, the pelvis was not large enough for her largest infant. The ultimate test of a woman's pelvic size is whether her child fits through it at birth. A trial of labor may be indicated, and a cesarean delivery is done if necessary.

Soft Tissue Obstructions

The most common soft tissue obstruction during labor is a full bladder. The woman is encouraged to urinate every 1 or 2 hours. Catheterization may be needed if she cannot urinate, especially if a regional anesthetic and/or large quantities of IV fluids were given, which fills her bladder quickly yet reduces her sensation to void.

Less common soft tissue obstructions include pelvic tumors such as benign (noncancerous) fibroids. Some women have a cervix that is scarred from previous infections or surgery. The scar tissue may not readily yield to labor's forces to efface and dilate.

THE PSYCHE

Labor is stressful. However, women who have had prenatal care and have adequate social and professional support usually adapt to this stress and can labor and deliver normally. The most common factors that can increase stress and cause dystocia include lack of analgesic control of excessive pain, absence of a support person or coach to assist with nonpharmacological pain relief measures, immobility and restriction to bed, and a lack of ability to carry out cultural traditions.

The increased anxiety releases hormones such as epinephrine, cortisol, and adrenocorticotropic hormone that reduce contractility of the smooth muscle of the uterus. The body responds to stress with a "fight-or-flight" reaction that impedes normal labor. For example, the fight-or-flight reaction does the following:

- Uses glucose the uterus needs for energy
- Diverts blood from the uterus
- Increases tension of the pelvic muscles, which impedes fetal descent
- Increases perception of pain, creating greater anxiety and stress and thus worsening the cycle

Nursing care. Promoting relaxation and helping the woman conserve her resources for the work of childbirth are the principal nursing goals. The nurse uses every opportunity to spare her energy and promote her comfort. See Chapter 7 for more information about promoting comfort.

ABNORMAL DURATION OF LABOR

An unusually long or short labor can cause problems in the mother or in her fetus.

Prolonged Labor

Any of the previously discussed factors may be associated with a long or difficult labor (dystocia). The average rate of cervical dilation during the active phase of labor is about 1.2 cm/hr for the woman having her first child and about 1.5 cm/hr if she has had a child before. Descent is expected to occur at a rate of at least 1.0 cm/hr in a first-time mother and 2.0 cm/hr in a woman who has had a child before. A *Friedman curve* is often used to graph the progress of cervical dilation and fetal descent. The graph can help identify normal progress and the type of abnormal labor progress.

Prolonged labor can result in several problems, such as the following:

- Maternal or newborn infection, especially if the membranes have been ruptured for a long time (usually about 24 hours)
- Maternal exhaustion
- Postpartum hemorrhage (see Chapter 10)
- Greater anxiety and fear in an ensuing pregnancy

In addition, mothers who have difficult and long labors are more likely to be anxious and fearful about their next labor.

Nursing care. Nursing care focuses on helping the woman conserve her strength and encouraging her as she copes with the long labor. The nurse should observe for signs of infection during and after birth in both the mother and the newborn.

See Chapter 10 for further information about postpartum infection and Chapter 9 for discussion of neonatal infection.

Precipitate Birth

A precipitate birth is completed in less than 3 hours and there may be no health care provider present. Labor often begins abruptly and intensifies quickly, rather than having a more subtle onset and gradual progression. Contractions may be frequent and intense, often from the onset. If the woman's tissues do not yield easily to the powerful contractions, she may have uterine rupture, cervical lacerations, or hematoma.

Fetal oxygenation can be compromised by intense contractions because the placenta is resupplied with oxygenated blood between contractions. In precipitate labor this interval may be very short. Birth injury from rapid passage through the birth canal may become evident in the infant after birth. These injuries can include intracranial hemorrhage or nerve damage. Women who experience precipitous birth may have panic responses about the possibility of not getting to the hospital in time or having their health care provider present. Although they are relieved after birth, they require continued support and reassurance concerning the deviation from their expected experience.

After birth the nurse observes the mother and infant for signs of injury. Excessive pain or bruising of the woman's vulva is reported. Cold applications limit pain, bruising, and edema. Abnormal findings on the newborn's assessment (see Chapter 12) are reported to the physician.

PREMATURE RUPTURE OF MEMBRANES

Premature rupture of membranes (PROM) is spontaneous rupture of the membranes at term (38 or more weeks' gestation) at least 1 hour before labor contractions begin. A related term, *preterm premature rupture of membranes* (PPROM), is rupture of the membranes before term (before 38 weeks' gestation) with or without uterine contractions. Vaginal or cervical infection may cause prematurely ruptured membranes; it has been associated with nutritional deficiency involving copper and ascorbic acid (Hacker & Moore, 1998).

Diagnosis is confirmed by testing the fluid with Nitrazine paper, which turns blue in the presence of amniotic fluid. A sample of vaginal fluid placed on a slide and sent to the laboratory will show a ferning pattern under the microscope, confirming that it is amniotic fluid. Treatment is based on weighing the risks of early delivery of the fetus against the risks of infection in the mother (chorioamnionitis, or inflammation of the fetal membranes) and sepsis in the newborn. An ultrasound determines gestational age, and oligohydramnios is confirmed if the amniotic fluid index (AFI) is less than 5 cm. Oligohydramnios in a gestation less than 24 weeks can lead to fetal pulmonary and skeletal defects. If PROM occurs at 36 weeks' gestation or later, labor is induced within 24 hours. Because the cushion of amniotic fluid is lost, the risk for umbilical cord compression is great.

Nursing care. The nurse should observe, document, and report maternal temperature above 38° C (100.4° F), fetal tachycardia, and tenderness over the uterine area. Antibiotic and steroid therapy may be anticipated, cul-

tures may be ordered, and labor may be induced or a cesarean section may be indicated.

Nursing care for the woman who is not having labor induced right away primarily involves monitoring and teaching the woman. Teaching combines information about infection and preterm labor and includes the following:

- Report a temperature that is above 38° C (100.4° F).
- Avoid sexual intercourse or insertion of anything in the vagina, which can increase the risk for infection.
- Avoid orgasm, which can stimulate contractions.
- Avoid breast stimulation, which can stimulate contractions because of natural oxytocin release.
- Maintain any activity restrictions prescribed.
- Note any uterine contractions, reduced fetal activity, or other signs of infection (discussed under Amniotomy).
- Record fetal kick counts daily and report less than 10 kicks in a 12-hour period.

PRETERM LABOR

Preterm labor occurs after 20 and before 38 weeks' gestation. The main risks are the problems of immaturity in the newborn. One goal of *Healthy People 2010* is that 90% of all women will receive prenatal care starting in the first trimester. Preterm delivery is a major cause of perinatal morbidity and mortality and has a major medical and economic impact on the rising costs of health care. Early prenatal care can prevent premature labor or identify women at risk (Box 8-2).

Early prenatal care allows women to be educated concerning signs of preterm labor so that interventions can occur early. Home uterine activity monitoring can be initiated for women at risk for preterm labor.

SIGNS OF IMPENDING PRETERM LABOR

A transvaginal ultrasound showing a shortened cervix at 20 weeks' gestation may be predictive for impending preterm labor. The ultrasound may be advised for high-risk women. A cervical or vaginal fetal fibronectin test has been approved by the Food and Drug Administration (FDA) (Hacker & Moore, 1998) for clinical use in the United States. Fibronectin is a protein produced by the fetal membranes that can leak into vaginal secretions if uterine activity, infection, or cervical effacement occurs. The presence of fibronectin in vaginal secretions between 22 and 24 weeks' gestation is predictive of preterm labor. Maternal corticotropin-releasing hormone (CRH) increases significantly in the weeks before preterm labor.

box 8-2 | *Some Risk Factors for Preterm Labor*

- Exposure to diethylstilbestrol (DES)
- Underweight
- Chronic illness such as diabetes or hypertension
- Dehydration
- Preeclampsia
- Previous preterm labor or birth
- Previous pregnancy losses
- Uterine or cervical abnormalities or surgery
    Uterine distention
    Abdominal surgery during pregnancy
- Infection
- Anemia
- Preterm premature rupture of the membranes
- Inadequate prenatal care
- Poor nutrition
- Age under 18 or over 40 years
- Low education level
- Poverty
- Smoking
- Substance abuse
- Chronic stress
- Multifetal presentation

Stress reduction and improved nutrition are indicated if CRH levels are high. Diagnosis of preterm labor is based on cervical effacement and dilation of more than 2 cm.

Maternal symptoms of preterm labor include the following:

- Contractions that may be either uncomfortable or painless
- Feeling that the fetus is "balling up" frequently
- Menstrual-like cramps
- Constant low backache
- Pelvic pressure or a feeling that the fetus is pushing down
- A change in the vaginal discharge
- Abdominal cramps with or without diarrhea
- Pain or discomfort in the vulva or thighs
- "Just feeling bad" or "coming down with something"

Laboratory tests include glucose level, electrolyte level, urinalysis and culture, and an ultrasound of the fetus to determine maturity, position, and other problems that may exist. Treatment of preterm labor is more aggressive at 28 weeks' gestation than at 34 weeks' gestation.

TOCOLYTIC THERAPY

The goal of tocolytic therapy is to stop uterine contractions and keep the fetus in utero until the lungs are mature enough to adapt to extrauterine life. *Magnesium*

sulfate is the drug of choice for initiating therapy to stop labor. A continuous IV infusion is given and therapeutic levels are monitored. Oral magnesium therapy may continue after contractions stop. The woman should be informed that a warm flush may be perceived during the initiation of therapy. Overdose can affect the cardiorespiratory system, and vital signs are recorded every hour. If the fetus is born during magnesium therapy, drowsiness may be present and resuscitation may be required. The nursery staff should be notified if magnesium sulfate therapy was used before delivery, because interaction with aminoglycoside drugs prescribed for neonatal infection can result in weakness or paralysis in the newborn (Briggs, 2001).

β-adrenergic drugs such as terbutaline (Brethine) are given subcutaneously to stop uterine contractions. Cardiac side effects such as increased pulse and blood pressure can occur. Propranolol should be available to counter the effects of the drug. Ritodrine (Yutopar) may be given intravenously to stop preterm labor. Hypotension, cardiac arrhythmia, and pulmonary edema may occur. Women with diabetes who are receiving these drugs must be closely monitored.

Prostaglandin synthesis inhibitors such as indomethacin is another type of drug used to stop labor contractions and can be given orally or rectally. The drug causes a reduction in amniotic fluid, which is helpful when polyhydramnios is a problem. However, it can stimulate the ductus arteriosus to close prematurely, causing fetal death. Close fetal monitoring is essential.

Calcium channel blockers such as nifedipine (Procardia) can be given orally to stop labor contractions. Because the drug causes vasodilation, maternal flushing and hypotension could be a side effect.

Antibiotic therapy is often initiated in women with preterm labor because studies have shown (Hacker & Moore, 1998) that there often is a subclinical chorioamnionitis. Preventing this from spreading to the newborn improves the outcome of therapy.

Contraindications to tocolytic therapy. Tocolytics should not be used in women with preeclampsia, placenta previa, abruptio placenta, chorioamnionitis, and fetal demise. In these cases it would not improve the obstetric outcome to delay birth of the fetus.

STOPPING PRETERM LABOR

The initial measures to stop preterm labor include identifying and treating infection, activity restriction, and hydration.

Speeding fetal lung maturation. If it appears that preterm birth is inevitable, the physician may give the woman steroid drugs (glucocorticoids) to increase fetal lung maturity if the gestation is between 24 and 34 weeks.

Betamethasone may be given for this purpose in two intramuscular injections 24 hours apart.

Thyroid hormones in the form of thyroid-releasing hormone (tRH) have been found to enhance pulmonary maturation in fetuses younger than 28 weeks (Hacker & Moore, 1998).

Activity restrictions. Bed rest was often prescribed for women at risk for preterm birth. However, the benefits of bed rest are not clear, and many adverse maternal effects can occur. Therefore total bed rest is prescribed less frequently than in the past. Activity restrictions are often more moderate, such as resting in a semi-Fowler's position or partial bed rest.

Nursing care. Nurses should be aware of the symptoms of preterm labor because they may occur in any pregnant woman, with or without risk factors. Symptoms are taught and regularly reinforced for women who have increased risk factors.

Nursing care includes positioning the woman on her side for better placental blood flow, assessing vital signs frequently, and notifying the health care provider if tachycardia occurs. Signs of pulmonary edema (chest pains, cough, crackles, or rhonchi) and intake and output should be closely monitored. If the woman is monitored at home, appropriate activities and restrictions are identified and arrangements for household responsibilities such as child care should be made with family or with the help of social services. If delivery occurs, monitoring the fetal heart rate is essential and preparation for admission to the neonatal intensive care unit is initiated. Full emotional support of the parents is offered because they may be grieving the loss of the normal birth process.

PROLONGED PREGNANCY

Prolonged pregnancy lasts longer than 42 weeks. Other terms that are often used interchangeably for prolonged pregnancy include *postmature, postdate,* or *postterm.* The term *postmature* most accurately describes the infant whose characteristics are consistent with a prolonged gestation (see Chapter 13).

Risks. The greatest risks of prolonged pregnancy are to the fetus. As the placenta ages, it delivers oxygen and nutrients to the fetus less efficiently. The fetus may lose weight, and the skin may begin to peel; these are the typical characteristics of postmaturity. Meconium may be expelled into the amniotic fluid, which can cause severe respiratory problems at birth. Low blood sugar is a likely complication after birth.

The fetus with placental insufficiency does not tolerate labor well. Because the fetus has less reserve than needed, the normal interruption in blood flow

during contractions may cause excessive stress on the infant.

If the placenta continues functioning well, the fetus continues growing. This can lead to a large fetus and the problems accompanying macrosomia.

There is little physical risk to the mother other than laboring with a large fetus if placental function remains normal. Psychologically, however, she often feels that pregnancy will never end. She becomes more anxious about when labor will begin and when her health care provider will "do something."

Medical treatment. The physician or nurse-midwife will evaluate whether the pregnancy is truly prolonged or if the gestation has been miscalculated. If she had early and regular prenatal care, ultrasound examinations have usually clarified her true gestation. If the woman's pregnancy has definitely reached 42 weeks, labor is usually induced by oxytocin. Prostaglandin application to ripen the cervix before oxytocin administration makes induction more likely to be successful.

Nursing care. Nursing care involves careful observation of the fetus during labor to identify signs associated with poor placental blood flow, such as late decelerations (see p. 140). After birth, the newborn is observed for respiratory difficulties and hypoglycemia.

EMERGENCIES DURING CHILDBIRTH

Several intrapartum conditions can endanger the life or well-being of the woman or her fetus. They require prompt nursing and medical action to reduce the likelihood of damage. Nursing and medical management often overlap in emergencies.

PROLAPSED UMBILICAL CORD

The umbilical cord prolapses if it slips downward in the pelvis after the membranes rupture. In this position, it can be compressed between the fetal head and the woman's pelvis, interrupting blood supply to and from the placenta. It may slip down immediately after the membranes rupture, or the prolapse may occur later.

A prolapsed cord can be classified in the following ways (Figure 8-8):

- *Complete.* The cord is visible at the vaginal opening.
- *Palpated.* The cord cannot be seen but can be felt as a pulsating structure when a vaginal examination is done.
- *Occult.* The prolapse is hidden and cannot be seen or felt; it is suspected on the basis of abnormal fetal heart rates.

Risk factors. Prolapse of the umbilical cord is more likely if the fetus does not completely fill the space in the

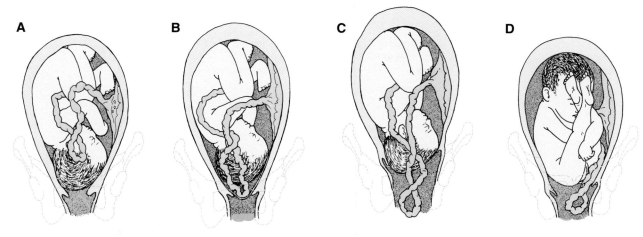

FIGURE **8-8** Prolapsed umbilical cord. Note the pressure of the presenting part on the umbilical cord, which will interfere with oxygenation of the fetus. **A,** Occult (hidden) prolapse of cord. The cord will be compressed between the fetal head and the mother's bony pelvis. **B,** Complete prolapsed cord. Note that the membranes are intact. **C,** Cord presenting in front of the fetal head and may be seen in the vagina. **D,** Frank breech presentation with prolapsed cord.

pelvis or if fluid pressure is great when the membranes rupture. These conditions are more likely to occur when the following happen:

- Fetus high in the pelvis when the membranes rupture (presenting part is not engaged)
- Very small fetus, as in prematurity
- Abnormal presentations, such as footling breech or transverse lie
- Hydramnios (excess amniotic fluid)

Medical treatment. The main risk of a prolapsed cord is to the fetus. When a prolapsed cord occurs, the first action is to displace the fetus upward to stop compression against the pelvis. Maternal positions such as the knee-chest or Trendelenburg (head down) can accomplish this displacement (Figure 8-9). Placing the mother in a side-lying position with her hips elevated on pillows also reduces cord pressure. The experienced physician may push the fetus upward from the vagina. Oxygen and a tocolytic drug such as terbutaline may be given. The primary focus is to deliver the fetus by the quickest means possible, usually cesarean delivery.

Nursing care. In addition to prompt corrective actions and assisting with emergency procedures, the nurse should remain calm to avoid increasing the woman's anxiety. Prolapsed cord is a sudden development; anxiety and fear are inevitable reactions in the woman and her partner. Calm, quick actions on the part of nurses help the woman and her family to feel that she is in competent hands.

After birth the nurse helps the woman to understand the experience. She may need several explanations of what happened and why.

UTERINE RUPTURE

A tear in the uterine wall occurs if the muscle cannot withstand the pressure inside the organ. The three variations of uterine rupture are as follows:

- *Complete rupture.* There is a hole through the uterine wall, from the uterine cavity to the abdominal cavity.
- *Incomplete rupture.* The uterus tears into a nearby structure, such as a ligament, but not all the way into the abdominal cavity.
- *Dehiscence.* An old uterine scar, usually from a previous cesarean birth, separates.

Risk factors. Uterine rupture is more likely if the woman has had previous surgery on her uterus, such as a previous cesarean delivery. The low-transverse uterine incision (see Figure 8-4) is least likely to rupture. Because the classic uterine incision is prone to rupture, a vaginal birth after this type of incision is not recommended.

Uterine rupture may occur in the unscarred uterus in the following cases:

- The woman has had many other births (grand multiparity).
- The woman has intense labor contractions, as with oxytocin stimulation.
- The woman has had blunt abdominal trauma, such as from a vehicle accident or battering.

Characteristics. The woman may have no symptoms, or she may have sudden onset of severe signs and symptoms, as follows:

- Shock caused by bleeding into the abdomen (vaginal bleeding may be minimal)
- Abdominal pain

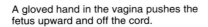

A gloved hand in the vagina pushes the fetus upward and off the cord.

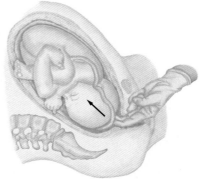

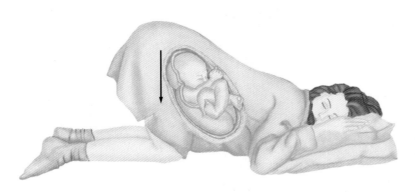

Knee-chest position uses gravity to shift the fetus out of the pelvis. The woman's thighs should be at right angles to the bed and her chest flat on the bed.

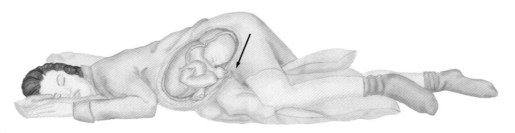

The woman's hips are elevated with two pillows; this is often combined with the Trendelenburg (head down) position.

FIGURE **8-9** Positioning of the mother when the umbilical cord prolapses. These positions can be used to relieve pressure on the prolapsed umbilical cord until delivery can take place.

- Pain in the chest, between the scapula (shoulder blades), or with inspiration
- Cessation of contractions
- Abnormal or absent fetal heart tones
- Palpation of the fetus outside the uterus because the fetus has pushed through the torn area

Medical treatment. If the fetus is living when the rupture is detected and/or if blood loss is excessive, the physician performs surgery to deliver the fetus and to stop the bleeding. Hysterectomy (removal of the uterus) is likely for an extensive tear. Smaller tears may be surgically repaired.

Nursing care. The nurse should be aware of women who are at high risk for uterine rupture. Women who are having a trial of labor after a previous cesarean section (VBAC) and women who are receiving oxytocin are at highest risk for uterine rupture and must be monitored closely during labor. When uterine rupture occurs the woman is prepared for immediate cesarean sec-

tion. Measures to allay anxiety in the woman and her partner are necessary as emergency measures are being initiated.

Uterine rupture is sometimes not discovered until after birth. In these cases the woman does not have dramatic symptoms of blood loss. However, she may have continuous bleeding that is brighter red than the normal postbirth bleeding. A rising pulse and falling blood pressure are signs of hypovolemic shock, which may occur if blood loss is excessive.

UTERINE INVERSION

Uterine inversion occurs if the uterus turns inside out after the infant is born. The incidence is approximately 1:2500 births (American College of Obstetricians and Gynecologists, 1995a). Inversion may be partial or complete. The physician may note a small depression in the top of the uterus or may discover that the uterus is not in the abdomen and protrudes from the vagina with its inner surface showing. Rapid onset of shock is common.

Uterine inversion is more likely to occur if the uterus is not firmly contracted, especially if the health care provider pulls on the umbilical cord to deliver the placenta. Inversion can also occur during vigorous fundal massage when the uterus is not firm and is pushed downward toward the pelvis.

Medical treatment. The physician will try to replace the inverted uterus while the woman is under general anesthesia. The anesthetic agent is chosen to cause uterine relaxation; tocolytic drugs also may be used. After the uterus is replaced, oxytocin is given to contract the uterus and control bleeding. If replacement of the uterus is not successful, the woman may require a hysterectomy.

Nursing care. Nursing care during the emergency supplements medical management. Two IV lines are usually established to administer fluids and medications and to combat shock.

During the recovery period the woman's uterus is assessed at least every 15 minutes for firmness, height, and deviation from the midline; the lower uterus is supported at each assessment (see Figures 9-2 and 9-4). Her vital signs and the amount of vaginal bleeding are assessed. An indwelling catheter may be used to keep her bladder empty so that the uterus can contract well. The catheter is assessed for patency and the output recorded; output may fall below 25 or 30 ml/hr with shock. The patient should take nothing orally until her condition is stable and the health care provider orders oral intake.

After birth the nurse provides explanations and emotional support to the woman and her partner.

AMNIOTIC FLUID EMBOLISM

Amniotic fluid embolism occurs when amniotic fluid, with its particles such as vernix, fetal hair, and sometimes meconium, enters the woman's circulation and obstructs small blood vessels in her lungs. It is more likely to occur during a very strong labor because the fluid is "pushed" into small blood vessels that rupture as the cervix dilates.

Amniotic fluid embolism is characterized by abrupt onset of hypotension, respiratory distress, and coagulation abnormalities triggered by the thromboplastin contained in the amniotic fluid.

Treatment includes providing respiratory support with intubation and mechanical ventilation as necessary, treating shock with electrolytes and volume expanders, and replacing the coagulation factors such as platelets and fibrinogen. Packed red blood cells are sometimes given intravenously.

The woman's intake and output are monitored closely. A pulse oximeter monitors oxygen saturation. The woman may be transferred to the intensive care unit for closer monitoring and nursing care.

key points

- The nurse observes the character of the amniotic fluid and fetal heart rate when the membranes are ruptured. Fluid should be clear and mild odored; the fetal heart rate should remain near its baseline level and between 110 and 160 beats/min at term.
- The nurse observes the fetal condition and character of contractions if any methods to stimulate labor are used. These methods may include walking, nipple stimulation, amniotomy, or oxytocin infusion.
- After version, the nurse observes for leaking amniotic fluid and for a pattern of contractions that may indicate labor has begun. Before discharge, signs of labor are reviewed with the woman so she will know when to return to the birth center.
- Nursing care after episiotomy or perineal lacerations includes comfort measures such as cold applications and analgesics.
- Nursing care after cesarean birth is similar to that after vaginal birth with the addition of assessing the wound, indwelling catheter patency, and intravenous flow. The woman and her partner may need extra emotional support after cesarean birth.
- Nursing measures such as encouraging position changes, aiding relaxation, and reminding the woman to empty her bladder can promote a more normal labor.
- Nursing care after births involving instruments (forceps or vacuum extraction) and after abnormal labor and birth includes observations for maternal and newborn injuries or infections. Infection is the most common hazard after membranes rupture prematurely, especially if there is a long interval before delivery.
- Nurses should be aware of the subtle symptoms a woman may have at the beginning of preterm labor and encourage her to seek care at the hospital promptly.
- After any type of emergency, the woman and her family need emotional support, explanations of what happened, and patience with their repeated questions.

ONLINE RESOURCES

Healthy People 2010: http://www.health.gov/healthypeople/document/tableofcontents.htm

National Center for Health Statistics: http://www.cdc.gov/nchs/fastats

Preterm Labor: http://www.merck.com/pubs/mmanual/section18/chapter253/253b.htm

REVIEW QUESTIONS *Choose the most appropriate answer.*

1. The nurse notes that a woman's contractions during oxytocin induction of labor are every 2 minutes; the contractions last 95 seconds, and the uterus remains tense between contractions. What action is expected based on these assessments?
   1. No action expected; the contractions are normal
   2. Rate of oxytocin will be increased slightly
   3. Pain medication or an epidural block will be offered
   4. Infusion of oxytocin will be stopped

2. Select the appropriate nursing intervention during the early recovery period to increase the woman's comfort if she had a forceps-assisted birth and a median episiotomy.
   1. Application of a cold pack to her perineal area
   2. Encouragement of perineal stretching exercises
   3. Application of warm, moist heat to the perineum
   4. Administration of stool softeners

3. A woman has an emergency cesarean delivery after the umbilical cord was found to be prolapsed. She repeatedly asks similar questions about what happened at birth. The nurse's interpretation of her behavior is that she:
   1. Cannot accept that she did not have the type of delivery she planned
   2. Is trying to understand her experience and move on with postpartum adaptation
   3. Thinks the staff is not telling her the truth about what happened at birth
   4. Is confused about events because the effects of the general anesthetic are persisting

4. What nursing intervention during labor can increase space in the woman's pelvis?
   1. Promote adequate fluid intake
   2. Position her on the left side
   3. Assist her to take a shower
   4. Encourage regular urination

5. A woman is being observed in the hospital because her membranes ruptured at 30 weeks' gestation. While giving morning care, the nursing student notices that the draining fluid has a strong odor. The priority nursing action is to:
   1. Caution the woman to remain in bed until her physician visits
   2. Ask the woman if she is having any more contractions than usual
   3. Take the woman's temperature; report it and the fluid odor to the registered nurse
   4. Help to prepare the woman for an immediate cesarean delivery

The Family After Birth

objectives

1. Define each key term listed.
2. Describe how to individualize postpartum and newborn nursing care for different patients.
3. Describe specific cultural beliefs that the nurse may encounter when providing postpartum and newborn care.
4. Describe postpartum changes in maternal systems and the nursing care associated with those changes.
5. Modify nursing assessments and interventions for the woman who has a cesarean birth.
6. Explain the emotional needs of postpartum women and their families.
7. Describe nursing care of the normal newborn.
8. Describe nursing interventions to promote optimal infant nutrition.
9. Identify signs and symptoms that may indicate a complication in the postpartum mother or infant.
10. Plan appropriate discharge teaching for the postpartum woman and her infant.

key terms

afterpains (p. 205)
attachment (p. 222)
bonding (p. 222)
colostrum (kă-LŌS-trŭm, p. 226)
diastasis recti (dī-ĂS-tăh-sĭs RĔK-tī, p. 210)
fundus (p. 205)
galactagogue (găh-LĂK-tō-gŏg, p. 226)
involution (ĭn-vō-LOO-shŭn, p. 204)
let-down reflex (p. 225)
lochia (LŌ-kē-ăh, p. 205)
postpartum blues (p. 214)
puerperium (pū-ĕr-PĒ-rē-ŭm, p. 203)
suckling (p. 228)

The postpartum period, or *puerperium* is the 6 weeks following childbirth. This period is often referred to as the fourth trimester of pregnancy. This chapter addresses the physiological and psychological changes in the mother and her family and the initial care of the newborn.

ADAPTING CARE TO SPECIFIC GROUPS AND CULTURES

The nurse must adapt care to a person's circumstances, such as those of the single or adolescent parent, the poor, families who have a multiple birth, and families from other cultures.

NURSING CONSIDERATIONS FOR SPECIFIC GROUPS OF PATIENTS

Adolescents, particularly younger ones, need help to learn parenting skills. Their peer group is very important to them, so the nurse must make every effort during both pregnancy and the postpartum period to help them to fit in with their peers. They are often passive in caring for themselves and their infants. They may also be single and poor. Poor, young adolescent mothers often have several children in a short time, which compounds their social problems.

A single woman may have problems making postpartum adaptations if she does not have a strong support system. She often must return to work very soon because she is the sole provider for her family.

Poor families may have difficulty meeting their basic needs before a new infant arrives, and a new family member adds to their strain. Women may have inadequate or sporadic prenatal care, which increases their risk for complications that extend into the puerperium and to their child. They may need social service referrals to direct them to public assistance programs or other resources.

Families who add twins (or more) face different challenges. The infants are more likely to need intensive care because of preterm birth, which delays the parents' attachment and assumption of newborn care. It is also more difficult for the parents to see the individuality of each infant rather than attaching to them as a set. The infants may require care at a distant hospital if their problems are severe. Financial strains mount with each added problem.

CULTURAL INFLUENCES ON POSTPARTUM CARE

The United States has a diverse population. Special cultural practices are often most evident at significant life events such as birth and even death. The nurse must adapt care to fit the health beliefs, values, and practices of that specific culture to make the birth a meaningful emotional and social event as well as a safe physical event. See Chapter 6 for specific cultural practices during labor, delivery, and postpartum.

Using Translators

The nurse may need an interpreter to understand and provide optimal care to the woman and her family. If possible, the interpreter should not be a family member if sensitive information is discussed. That person may interpret selectively. The interpreter should not be of a group that is in social or religious conflict with the patient and her family, as is the case in many Middle Eastern cultures. It is also important to remember that an affirmative nod from the woman may be a sign of courtesy to the nurse rather than a sign of understanding or agreement. Cultural preferences influence the presence of partners, parents, siblings, and children in the labor and delivery room (Figure 9-1).

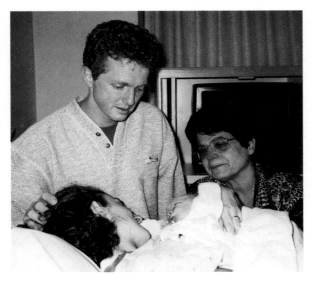

FIGURE **9-1** Mother, husband, and grandmother share relief as they get to see the newborn soon after birth in the delivery room.

Dietary Practices

Some cultures adhere to the "hot" and "cold" theory of diet after childbirth. Temperature has nothing to do with which foods are hot and which are cold; it is the intrinsic property of the food itself that classifies it. For example, "hot" foods include eggs, chicken, and rice. Women may also prefer their drinking water hot rather than cool or cold.

Other hot/cold dietary practices include a balance between *yin* foods (e.g., bean sprouts, broccoli, and carrots) and *yang* foods (e.g., broiled meat, chicken, soup, and eggs).

POSTPARTUM CHANGES IN THE MOTHER

Box 9-1 summarizes nursing assessments for the postpartum woman. See Chapter 10 for additional information about postpartum complications.

REPRODUCTIVE SYSTEM

Following the third stage of labor, there is a fall in the blood levels of placental hormones, human placental lactogen, human chorionic gonadotropin, estrogen, and progesterone that help return the body to the prepregnant state. The most dramatic changes after birth occur in the woman's reproductive system. These changes are discussed in the following sections, with nursing care discussed for each area as applicable.

Uterus

Involution refers to changes that the reproductive organs, particularly the uterus, undergo after birth to return them to their prepregnancy size and condition. The uterus undergoes a rapid reduction in size and weight after birth. The uterus should return to the prepregnant size by 5 to 6 weeks after delivery.

Uterine lining. The uterine lining (called the *endometrium* when not pregnant and the *decidua* during pregnancy) is shed when the placenta detaches. A basal layer of the lining remains to generate new endometrium to prepare for future pregnancies. The placental site is fully healed in 6 to 7 weeks.

Descent of the uterine fundus. The uterine fundus (the upper portion of the body of the uterus) descends at a predictable rate as the muscle cells contract to control bleeding at the placental insertion site and as the size of each muscle cell decreases. Immediately after the placenta is expelled, the uterine fundus can be felt as a firm mass, about the size of a grapefruit. After 24 hours the fundus begins to descend about 1 cm (one finger's width) each day. By 10 days postpartum, it should no longer be palpable. A full bladder interferes with uterine contraction because it pushes the fundus up and causes it to deviate to one side, usually the right side (Figure 9-2).

> **NURSING TIP**
> If the mother's uterus is soft, massage it (supporting the lower segment), then expel clots so it will remain contracted. If her bladder is also full, massage the uterus until firm, then address emptying the bladder. Control bleeding first, then keep it controlled by emptying the bladder.

Afterpains. Intermittent uterine contractions may cause afterpains similar to menstrual cramps. The discomfort is self-limiting and decreases rapidly within 48 hours postpartum. Afterpains occur more often in multiparas or in women whose uterus was overly distended. Breastfeeding mothers may have more afterpains because infant suckling causes their posterior pituitary to release oxytocin, a hormone that contracts the uterus. Mild analgesics may be prescribed. Aspirin is not used postpartum because it interferes with blood clotting.

> **NURSING TIP**
> The nurse should assess the fundus for descent each shift and teach the mother the expected changes.

Lochia. Vaginal discharge after delivery is called lochia. It is composed of endometrial tissue, blood, and lymph. Lochia gradually changes characteristics during the early postpartum period:

- *Lochia rubra* is red because it is composed mostly of blood; it lasts for about 3 days after birth.

| box 9-1 | *Summary of Nursing Assessment Postpartum* |

Routine assessments are usually done every 4 to 6 hours unless risk factors exist.

Vital signs	Report temperature above 38° C (100.4° F) or abnormal heart or respiratory rates.
Fundus	Evaluate firmness, height, and location.
Lochia	Observe for character, color, amount, odor, and presence of clots.
Perineum	Observe for hematoma, edema, and episiotomy using REEDA scale; note hemorrhoids and degree of discomfort.
Bladder	Observe for fullness, output, burning, and pain.
Breasts	Check for engorgement, nipple tenderness, and breastfeeding.
Bowels	Determine passage of flatus, bowel sounds, and defecation.
Pain	Determine location, character, severity, use of relief measures, and need for analgesics.
Extremities	Observe for signs of thrombophlebitis, ability to ambulate, and Homan's sign.
Emotional state	Evaluate family interaction, support, and signs of depression.
Attachment	Observe for interest in newborn, eye contact, touch contact, ability to respond to infant cries.
Cultural variations	Observe for cultural practices that the staff can incorporate into a plan of care.

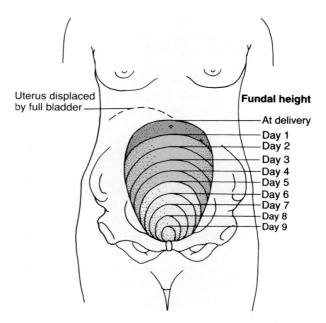

FIGURE **9-2** Changes in the height of the uterine fundus each day as involution progresses.

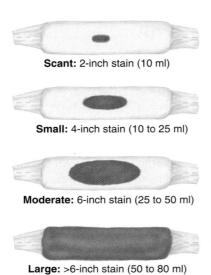

Scant: 2-inch stain (10 ml)

Small: 4-inch stain (10 to 25 ml)

Moderate: 6-inch stain (25 to 50 ml)

Large: >6-inch stain (50 to 80 ml)

FIGURE **9-3** Estimating volume of lochia on the perineal pad; different brands of peripads absorb in different patterns: some soak down, some spread out. The nurse should be familiar with the pattern of the peripad used at the facility in order to standardize documentation.

- *Lochia serosa* is pinkish because of its blood and mucus content. It lasts from about the third through the tenth day after birth.
- *Lochia alba* is mostly mucus and is clear and colorless or white. It lasts from the tenth through the twenty-first day after birth.

Lochia has a characteristic fleshy or menstrual odor; it should not have a foul odor. The nurse assesses lochia for quantity, type, and characteristics. A guideline to estimate and chart the amount of flow on the menstrual pad in 1 hour is as follows (Figure 9-3):

- Scant: less than a 2-inch (5-cm) stain
- Light: less than a 4-inch (10-cm) stain
- Moderate: less than a 6-inch (15-cm) stain
- Large or heavy: larger than a 6-inch stain or one pad saturated within 2 hours
- Excessive: saturation of a perineal pad within 15 minutes

Many facilities use perineal pads that contain cold or warm packs. These pads absorb less lochia, and that fact must be considered when estimating the amount. If a mother has excessive lochia, a clean pad should be applied and checked within 15 minutes. The number of peripads applied during a given time period are counted or weighed to help determine the amount of vaginal discharge. One gram of weight equals about 1 ml of blood. The nurse should assess the underpads on the bed to determine if bleeding has overflowed onto the

bed linen. The woman's fundus should be checked for firmness, because an uncontracted uterus allows blood to flow freely from vessels at the placenta insertion site.

Lochia is briefly heavier when the mother ambulates because lochia pooled in the vagina is discharged when she assumes an upright position. A few small clots may be seen at this time, but large clots should not be present. Lochia may briefly increase when the mother breastfeeds because suckling causes uterine contraction. Lochia increases with exercise. Women who had a cesarean birth have less lochia during the first 24 hours because the uterine cavity was sponged at delivery. The absence of lochia is not normal and may be associated with blood clots retained within the uterus or with infection.

Nursing care. The fundus is assessed for firmness, location, and position (see Figure 9-2) in relation to the midline at routine intervals (Box 9-2). Women who have a higher risk for postpartum hemorrhage (see Chapter 10) should be assessed more often. While doing early assessments, the nurse explains the reason they are done and teaches the woman how to assess her fundus. If her uterus stops descending, she should report that to her birth attendant.

A poorly contracted (soft or boggy) uterus should be massaged until firm to prevent hemorrhage (Figure 9-4). Lochia may increase briefly as the uterus contracts and expels it. It is essential *not* to push down on an uncontracted uterus to avoid inverting it (see p. 200). If a full bladder contributes to poor uterine contraction, the mother should be assisted to void in the bathroom or on a bedpan if she cannot ambulate. Catheterization may be necessary if she cannot void.

Medications that may be given to stimulate uterine contraction include the following:

- Oxytocin (Pitocin), often routinely given in an intravenous infusion after birth
- Methylergonovine (Methergine), given intramuscularly or orally

An infant suckling at the breast has a similar effect because natural oxytocin release stimulates contractions.

Mild analgesics relieve afterpains adequately for most women. The breastfeeding mother will get maximum pain relief if she takes an analgesic immediately after breastfeeding to minimize sedation and side effects passing to the newborn. Afterpains persisting longer than the expected time should be reported.

The woman should be taught the expected sequence for lochia changes and the amount she should expect. The woman should report any of the following abnormal characteristics:

- Foul-smelling lochia, with or without fever
- Lochia rubra that persists beyond the third day

box 9-2 *Procedure for Observing and Massaging the Uterine Fundus and for Giving Perineal Care*

MATERIALS

Clean gloves
Peribottle filled with warm water
Perineal pad

METHOD

1. Identify the need for fundal massage. The uterus will be soft and usually higher than the umbilicus. A firm fundus does not need massage.
2. Place the woman in a supine position with the knees slightly flexed. Lower the perineal pad to observe lochia as the fundus is palpated.
3. Place the outer edge of nondominant hand just above the symphysis pubis, and press downward slightly to anchor the lower uterus.
4. Locate and massage the uterine fundus with the flat portion of the fingers of the dominant hand in a firm circular motion.
5. When the uterus is firm, gently push downward on the fundus, toward the vaginal outlet, to expel blood and clots that have accumulated inside the uterus. *Keep the other hand on the lower uterus to avoid inverting it.*
6. If a full bladder contributes to uterine relaxation, have the mother void. Catheterize her (with a health care provider's order) if she cannot void.
7. Document the consistency and location of the fundus before and after massage.
8. Give any medications, such as oxytocin, to maintain uterine contraction. Have the mother nurse her infant if she is breastfeeding to stimulate the secretion of natural oxytocin.
9. Report a fundus that does not stay firm.

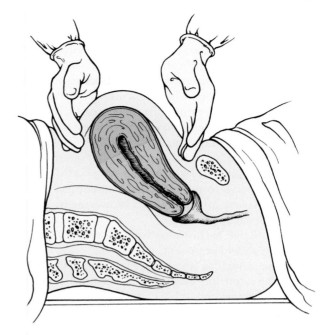

FIGURE **9-4** When assessing or massaging the fundus, the nurse keeps one hand firmly on the lower uterus, just above the symphysis pubis. The uterus is massaged in a firm, circular motion. After the uterus becomes firm, the nurse pushes toward the vagina to expel accumulated blood. A firm fundus does not need massage.

- Unusually heavy lochia
- Lochia that returns to a bright red color after it has progressed to serosa or alba

Cervix

The cervix regains its muscle tone but never closes as tightly as during the prepregnant state. Some edema persists for a few weeks after delivery. A constant trickle of brighter red lochia is associated with bleeding from lacerations of the cervix or vagina, particularly if the fundus remains firm.

Vagina

The vagina undergoes a great deal of stretching during childbirth. The *rugae,* or vaginal folds, disappear, and the walls of the vagina become smooth and spacious. The rugae reappear 3 weeks postpartum. Within 6 weeks the vagina has regained most of its prepregnancy form, but it never returns to the size it was before pregnancy.

Couples often are hesitant to ask questions concerning resumption of sexual activity after childbirth, and many resume activity before the 6-week checkup. It is important for the nurse to teach the woman that it is considered safe to resume sexual intercourse when bleeding has stopped and the perineum (episiotomy) has healed. However, the vagina does not lubricate well in the first 6 weeks after childbirth (or longer in the breastfeeding mother). A water-soluble gel such as K-Y or a contraceptive gel can be used for lubrication to make intercourse more comfortable. Instructing the woman to correctly perform the Kegel exercise strengthens muscles involved in urination, bowel function, and vaginal sensations during intercourse.

Perineum

The perineum is often edematous, tender, and bruised. An *episiotomy* (incision to enlarge the vaginal opening) may have been done or a perineal laceration may have occurred. Women with hemorrhoids often find that these temporarily worsen during the pressure of birth.

The perineum should be assessed for normal healing and signs of complications. The following REEDA acronym helps the nurse remember the five signs to assess:

- *Redness.* Redness without excessive tenderness is probably the normal inflammation associated with healing, but pain with the redness is more likely to be infection.
- *Edema.* Mild edema is common, but severe edema interferes with healing.
- *Ecchymosis* (bruising). A few small superficial bruises are common. Larger bruises interfere with normal healing.
- *Discharge.* No discharge from the perineal suture line should be present.
- *Approximation* (intactness of the suture line). The suture line should not be separated. If intact, it is almost impossible to distinguish the laceration or episiotomy from surrounding skin folds.

The REEDA acronym is also useful when assessing a cesarean incision for healing.

Nursing care. Comfort and hygienic measures are the focus of nursing care and patient teaching. An ice pack or chemical cold pack is applied for the first 12 to 24 hours to reduce edema and bruising and numb the perineal area. A disposable rubber glove filled with ice chips and taped at the wrist can also be used. The cold pack should be covered with a paper cover or a washcloth. When the ice melts, the cold pack is left off for 10 minutes before applying another for maximum effect. In some cultures, women believe that heat has healing properties and may resist the use of an ice pack.

After 24 hours, heat in the form of a chemical warm pack, a bidet, or a sitz bath increases circulation and promotes healing. The sitz bath may circulate either cool or warm water over the perineum to cleanse the area and increase comfort. Sitting in 4 to 5 inches of water in a bathtub has a similar effect.

The woman is taught to do perineal care after each voiding or bowel movement to cleanse the area without trauma. A plastic bottle (peribottle) is filled with warm water, and the water is squirted over the perineum in a front-to-back direction. The perineum is blotted dry. Perineal pads should be applied and removed in the same front-to-back direction to prevent fecal contamination of the perineum and vagina.

Topical and systemic medications may be used to relieve perineal pain. Topical perineal medications reduce inflammation or numb the perineum. Commonly prescribed medications include the following:

- Hydrocortisone and pramoxine (Epifoam)
- Benzocaine (Americaine or Dermoplast)

In addition to these topical medications, witch hazel pads (Tucks) and sitz baths reduce the discomfort of hemorrhoids.

To reduce pain when sitting, the mother can be taught to squeeze her buttocks together as she lowers herself to a sitting position and then to relax her buttocks. An air ring, or "donut," takes pressure off the perineal area when sitting. The mother should inflate the ring about halfway. (If it is inflated fully, she tends to topple off when she sits on it.) A small eggcrate pad is an alternative to the air ring.

Return of Ovulation and Menstruation

The production of placental estrogen and progesterone stops when the placenta is delivered, causing a rise in the production of follicle-stimulating hormone and the return of ovulation and menstruation. Menstrual cycles resume in about 6 to 8 weeks if the woman is not breastfeeding. The early menstrual periods may or may not be preceded by ovulation. Return of ovulation is delayed longer in the breastfeeding mother. However, *ovulation may occur at any time after birth, with or without menstrual bleeding, and pregnancy is possible.* Therefore pregnancy can occur unless birth control is practiced. Regular oral contraceptives are not used during early breastfeeding, but a mini-pill can be used effectively.

Breasts

Both nursing and nonnursing mothers experience breast changes after birth. Assessments for both types of mothers are similar, but nursing care differs.

Changes in the breasts. For the first 2 or 3 days the breasts are full but soft. By the third day the breasts become firm and lumpy as blood flow increases and milk production begins. Breast engorgement may occur in both nursing and nonnursing mothers. The engorged breast is hard, erect, and very uncomfortable. The nipple may be so hard that the infant cannot easily grasp it. The breasts of the nonnursing mother return to their normal size in 1 to 2 weeks.

Nursing care. At each assessment the nurse checks the woman's breasts for consistency, size, shape, and symmetry. The nipples are inspected for redness and cracking, which makes breastfeeding more painful and is a port for entry of microorganisms. Flat or inverted nipples make it more difficult for the infant to grasp the nipple and suckle.

Both nursing and nonnursing mothers should wear a bra to support the heavier breasts. The bra should firmly support the nursing mother's breasts but not be so tight that it impedes circulation. Some nonnursing mothers may prefer to wear an elastic binder to suppress lactation.

The nonnursing mother should avoid stimulating her nipples which stimulates lactation. She should wear a bra at all times to avoid having her clothing brush back and forth over her breasts and should stand facing away from the water spray in the shower.

The nipples should be washed with plain water to avoid the drying effects of soap, which can lead to cracking. The nonnursing woman should minimize stimulation when washing her breasts. Breastfeeding is discussed on pp. 224 to 232.

CARDIOVASCULAR SYSTEM
Cardiac Output and Blood Volume

Because of a 50% increase in blood volume during pregnancy, the woman tolerates normal blood loss at delivery, as follows:

- 500 ml in vaginal birth
- 1000 ml in cesarean birth

Despite the blood loss there is a temporary increase in blood volume and cardiac output because blood that was directed to the uterus and the placenta returns to the main circulation. Added fluid also moves from the tissues into the circulation, further adding to her blood volume. The heart pumps more blood with each contraction (increased stroke volume), leading to bradycardia. After the initial postbirth excitement wanes, the pulse rate may be as low as 50 to 60 beats/min for about 48 hours after birth.

To reestablish normal fluid balance, the body rids itself of excess fluid in the following two ways:

- Diuresis (increased excretion of urine), which may reach 3000 ml/day
- Diaphoresis (profuse perspiration)

Coagulation

Blood clotting factors are higher during pregnancy and the puerperium, yet the woman's ability to lyse (break down and eliminate) clots is not increased. Therefore she is prone to blood clot formation, especially if there is stasis of blood in the venous system. This situation is more likely to occur if the woman has varicose veins, has had a cesarean birth, or must delay ambulation.

Blood Values

The massive fluid shifts just described affect blood values such as hemoglobin and hematocrit, making them difficult to interpret during the early puerperium. Fluid that shifts into the bloodstream dilutes the blood cells, which lowers the hematocrit count. As the fluid balance returns to normal, the values are more accurately interpreted, usually by 8 weeks postpartum.

White blood cells (leukocytes) may increase to as high as 12,000 to 20,000/mm^3, a level that would ordinarily suggest infection. The increase is in response to inflammation, pain, and stress, and it protects the mother from infection as her tissues heal. The white blood cell count returns to normal by 12 days postpartum.

Chills

Many mothers experience tremors that resemble shivering or "chills" immediately after birth. This tremor is thought to be related to a sudden release of pressure on the pelvic nerves and a vasomotor response involving epinephrine (adrenaline) during the birth process. Most women will deny feeling cold. These tremors or "chills" stop spontaneously within 20 minutes. The nurse should reassure the woman and cover her with a warm blanket to provide comfort. Chills accompanied by fever after the first 24 hours suggest infection and should be reported.

Orthostatic Hypotension

Resistance to blood flow in the vessels of the pelvis drops after childbirth. As a result, the woman's blood pressure falls when she sits or stands, and she may feel dizzy, lightheaded, or even faint. Guidance and assistance are needed during early ambulation to prevent injury.

Nursing Care

After the fourth stage, vital signs are taken every 4 hours for the first 24 hours. The temperature may rise to 38° C (100.4° F) in the first 24 hours. A higher temperature or persistence of a temperature elevation for more than 24 hours suggests infection.

The pulse rate helps to interpret temperature and blood pressure values. Because of the normal postpartum bradycardia, a high pulse rate often indicates infection or hypovolemia.

If diaphoresis bothers the woman, she should be reminded that it is temporary. The nurse should help her shower or take a sponge bath and provide dry clothes and bedding.

The nurse checks for the presence of edema in the lower extremities, hands, and face. Edema in the lower extremities is common, as it is during pregnancy. Edema above the waist is more likely to be associated with pregnancy-induced hypertension, which can continue during the early postpartum period.

The woman's legs should be checked for evidence of thrombosis at each assessment, looking for a reddened, tender area (superficial vein) or edema, pain and, sometimes, pallor (deep vein). Homan's sign (calf pain when the foot is dorsiflexed) is of limited value in identifying thrombosis in the postpartum phase. Early and regular ambulation reduces the venous stasis that promotes blood clots.

URINARY SYSTEM

Kidney function returns to normal within a month after birth. A decrease in the tone of the bladder and ureters as a result of pregnancy combined with intravenous fluids administered during labor may cause the woman's bladder to fill quickly but empty incompletely during the postpartum period. This can lead to postpartum hemorrhage when the full bladder displaces the uterus or the potential for urinary tract infection because of stasis of the urine in the bladder.

> **NURSING TIP**
> The woman who voids frequent, small amounts of urine may have increased residual urine because her bladder does not fully empty. Residual urine in the bladder may promote the growth of microorganisms.

Nursing care. The nurse should regularly assess the woman's bladder for distention. The bladder may not feel full to her, yet the uterus is high and deviated to one side. If she can ambulate, the mother should go to the bathroom and urinate. The first two to three voidings after birth or after catheter removal are measured. Women who receive intravenous infusions or have an indwelling catheter continue to have their urine output measured until the infusion and/or catheter are discontinued.

The following measures may help a woman to urinate:
- Provide as much privacy as possible.
- Remain near the woman, but do not rush her by constantly asking her if she has urinated.
- Run water in the sink.
- Have the woman place her hands in warm water.
- Have the woman use the peribottle to squirt warm water over her perineal area to relax the urethral sphincter. Be sure to measure the amount of water in the peribottle when it is filled so the amount used can be deducted from the amount of urine voided.

Some discomfort with early urination is expected because of the edema and trauma in the area. However, continued burning or urgency of urination suggests bladder infection. High fever and chills may occur with kidney infection.

GASTROINTESTINAL SYSTEM

The gastrointestinal system resumes normal activity shortly after birth when progesterone decreases. The mother is usually hungry after the hard work and food deprivation of labor. The nurse should expect to feed and water a new mother often!

Constipation may occur during the postpartum period because of the following:
- Medications may slow peristalsis.
- Abdominal muscles are stretched, making it more difficult for the woman to bear down to expel stool. A cesarean incision adds to this difficulty.
- Soreness and swelling of the perineum or hemorrhoids may make the woman fear her first bowel movement.
- Slight dehydration and little food intake during labor make the feces harder.

The mother is encouraged to drink lots of fluids, add fiber to her diet, and ambulate. A stool softener such as docusate calcium (Surfak) or docusate sodium (Colace) is usually ordered. These measures are generally sufficient to correct the problem. Because constipation is a common problem during pregnancy, measures she has used to relieve it are discussed at that time and efforts are made to build on her knowledge. A common laxative is bisacodyl (Dulcolax), given orally or as a suppository when a laxative is indicated.

INTEGUMENTARY SYSTEM

Hyperpigmentation of the skin ("mask of pregnancy," or chloasma, and the linea nigra) disappears as hormone levels decrease. Striae ("stretch marks") do not disappear but fade from reddish purple to silver.

MUSCULOSKELETAL SYSTEM

The abdominal wall has been greatly stretched during pregnancy and may now have a "doughy" appearance. Many women are dismayed to discover that they still look pregnant after they give birth. They should be reassured that time and exercise can tighten their lax muscles. Also, some women have diastasis recti, in which the longitudinal abdominal muscles that extend from the chest to the symphysis pubis are separated. Abdominal wall weakness may remain for 6 to 8 weeks and contribute to constipation. Hypermobility of the joints usually stabilizes within 6 weeks, but the joints of the feet may remain separated and the new mother may notice an increase in shoe size. The center of gravity of the body returns to normal when the enlarged uterus returns to its prepregnant size.

A woman can usually begin light exercises as soon as the first day after vaginal birth. Women who have undergone a cesarean birth may wait longer. The woman should consult her health care provider for specific instructions about exercise. Common postpartum exercises include the following:
- *Abdominal tightening.* In the supine or erect position, the woman inhales slowly and then exhales slowly while contracting her abdominal muscles.

After a count of 10, she relaxes the muscles. She should begin with three repetitions and increase the number to five, then 10. This may be done three times and then five times daily, up to 10 times each day.

- *Head lift.* The woman lies flat on her bed with her knees bent and inhales. While exhaling, she lifts her head, chin to chest, and looks at her thighs. She holds this position to a count of three, then relaxes. This is repeated several times. After the third week (or when the health care provider permits), the head lift may progress to include the head and shoulders. This may be done five to 10 times daily.
- *Pelvic tilt.* While lying supine with her knees bent and feet flat, the woman inhales and exhales, flattening her lower back to the bed or exercise surface and contracting her abdominal muscles. She holds the position to a count of three. She begins with five repetitions and works up to 10 repetitions daily.
- *Kegel exercises.* Perineal exercises may be resumed immediately after birth to promote circulation and healing. The mother tightens the muscles of the perineal area, as if to stop the flow of urine, and then relaxes them. She should inhale, tighten for a count of 10, exhale, and relax. She may do the exercise five times each hour for the first few days. Then she may increase the number of repetitions. She should not actually stop her urine flow when urinating, however, because this could lead to urine stasis and urinary tract infection.

IMMUNE SYSTEM

Prevention of blood incompatibility and infection are done in the postpartum period according to each woman's specific needs.

Rh$_o$(D) Immune Globulin

The woman's blood type and Rh factor and antibody status are determined on an early prenatal visit or on admission if she did not have prenatal care.

The Rh-negative mother should receive a dose of Rh$_o$(D) immune globulin within 72 hours after giving birth to an Rh-positive infant. This prevents sensitization to Rh-positive erythrocytes that may have entered her bloodstream when the infant was born. *RhoGAM is given to the mother, not the infant,* by intramuscular injection into the deltoid muscle. The woman receives an identification card stating that she is Rh negative and has received RhoGAM on that date.

Rubella (German Measles) Immunization

Rubella titers are done early in pregnancy to determine if a woman is immune to rubella. A titer of 1:8 or greater indicates immunity to the rubella virus. The mother who is not immune is given the vaccine in the immediate postpartum period. The vaccine prevents infection with the rubella virus during subsequent pregnancies, which could cause birth defects. A signed informed consent is usually required to administer the rubella vaccine.

The rubella vaccine is given subcutaneously in the upper arm. The woman should not get pregnant for the next 3 months. The vaccine should not be administered if she is sensitive to neomycin. Women vaccinated during the postpartum period may breastfeed without adverse affects on the newborn (MMWR, July 13, 2001).

CHANGES AFTER CESAREAN BIRTH AND ADAPTATION OF NURSING CARE

The woman who has a cesarean birth has had surgery as well as given birth. Many of her reactions to the surgical birth depend on whether she expected it. The woman who had an unexpected emergency cesarean often has many questions about what happened to her and why because there was no time to answer these questions at the time of birth. In addition, her anxiety may have limited her ability to comprehend any explanations given. Occasionally a woman may feel that she failed if she was unable to give birth after laboring. Terms such as *failed induction* and *failure to progress* imply that the woman herself was not competent in some way.

Some variations of normal postpartum care are needed for the woman who has a cesarean birth (Nursing Care Plan 9-1).

Uterus

The nurse should check the woman's fundus as on any new mother; it descends at a similar rate. Checking her fundus when she has a transverse skin incision is not much different from checking the woman having vaginal birth. If she has a vertical skin incision, the nurse should gently "walk" the fingers toward the fundus from the side to her abdominal midline. If the fundus is firm and at its expected level, no massage is necessary.

Lochia

Lochia is checked at routine assessment intervals, which vary with the time since birth. The quantity of lochia is generally less immediately after cesarean birth because surgical sponges have removed the contents of the uterus.

The Woman Having a Cesarean Birth

PATIENT DATA: A 32-year-old woman is admitted to the postpartum unit after delivering a healthy 8-pound boy via cesarean section. The woman is lying still in bed and refuses to move because she states she fears postoperative pain.

SELECTED NURSING DIAGNOSIS   *Acute pain related to surgical incision and afterpains*

Outcomes	Nursing Interventions	Rationales
The woman will state that pain relief is adequate with pharmacological and nonpharmacological measures.	1. Use a 0-to-10 scale to evaluate pain level before and after interventions.	1. Provides a more objective way for the nurse to evaluate the woman's subjective experience of pain. Evaluates adequacy of pain relief.
	2. Encourage the woman to change positions regularly, (about every 2 hours). Support her body and extremities with pillows as needed.	2. Reduces discomfort from constant pressure and having body in one position too long. Also helps to mobilize respiratory secretions.
	3. Teach the woman to use a small pillow pressed to her incision when moving or coughing.	3. Supports the incision, reducing pain. Increases the likelihood that she will cough adequately, which expels respiratory secretions.
	4. Provide ordered analgesia: a. Patient-controlled anesthesia pump b. Intermittent injections c. Oral analgesia	4. Reduces the perception of pain, which facilitates moving, coughing, and ambulating. Reduces anxiety and fatigue.

SELECTED NURSING DIAGNOSIS   *Impaired skin integrity related to abdominal incision*

Outcomes	Nursing Interventions	Rationales
The woman will have no excessive redness or tenderness and no separation or discharge from incision. The woman will demonstrate knowledge of self-care measures related to her incision by discharge.	1. Observe dressing for drainage with each assessment.	1. Red drainage indicates bleeding, which should not increase. Foul-odored drainage indicates infection.
	2. When dressing is removed, assess incision using REEDA criteria. Assess amount of tenderness.	2. Identifies proper healing of incision. A separating suture line, excessive redness or tenderness, or discharge indicates probable infection.
	3. Determine temperature every 4 hours.	3. A temperature higher than 38° C (100.4° F) after 24 hours is associated with infection.
	4. Teach woman self-care measures: a. Expected progress of healing and how the incision should look b. How to bathe (plastic over incision, if ordered) c. What to report (signs of bleeding or infection) d. When her staples or sutures should be removed if not done before discharge e. Follow-up appointment	4. Women must assume their own care because of short hospital stays. These guidelines give the woman a framework to know what is and is not normal and how to care for herself to prevent infection. Follow-up appointments allow her physician to assess how healing is progressing and to identify complications early.

?CRITICAL THINKING QUESTION

How will your discharge teaching for a patient who delivered by cesarean section differ from that for a patient who delivered vaginally?

Dressing

The dressing should be checked for drainage as in any surgical patient. When the dressing is removed, the incision is assessed for signs of infection. The wound should be clean and dry, and the staples should be intact. The REEDA acronym previously described is a good way to remember key items to check on an incision: *redness, edema, ecchymosis, drainage, approximation*. Staples may be removed and Steri-Strips applied shortly before hospital discharge on the third day. If a woman leaves earlier, the staples may be removed in her health care provider's office.

The woman can shower as soon as she can ambulate reliably. A shower chair reduces the risk for fainting. The dressing or incision can be covered with a plastic wrap, securing the edges with tape. The woman should be told to position herself with her back to the water stream. The dressing is changed after the woman finishes her shower. A similar technique can be used to cover an intravenous infusion site. A glove can cover the infusion site if it is in her hand.

Urinary Catheter

An indwelling urinary catheter is generally removed within 24 hours of delivery. Urine is observed for blood, which may indicate trauma to the bladder during labor or surgery. The blood should quickly clear from the urine as diuresis occurs. Intake and output are measured until both the intravenous infusion and the catheter are discontinued. The first two to three voidings are measured, or until the woman urinates at least 150 ml. The nurse should observe and teach the woman to observe for the following signs of urinary tract infection because the catheter's use increases this risk:

- Fever
- Burning pain on urination
- Urgency of urination

Frequency of urination is hard to assess in any postpartum woman because of normal postpartum diuresis. However, frequent voidings of small quantities of urine, especially if associated with the described signs and symptoms, suggest a urinary tract infection.

Respiratory Care

Lung sounds should be auscultated each shift for clarity. Diminished breath sounds, crackles, or wheezes indicate that lung secretions are being retained. When she is confined to bed, the woman should take deep breaths and turn from side to side every 2 hours. She should be encouraged to cough to move secretions out of her lungs. To reduce incisional pain from coughing or other movement, the nurse can have the woman hold a small pillow or folded blanket firmly against her incision. An incentive spirometer may be used to give the woman a "target" for deep breaths. The woman should begin ambulating as early as possible to mobilize lung secretions.

Preventing Thrombophlebitis

The woman who has undergone a cesarean birth has a greater risk for thrombophlebitis. She should do simple leg exercises, such as alternately flexing and extending her feet or moving her legs from a flexed to an extended position when turning. The nurse should assess for signs of thrombosis as previously described. Early and frequent ambulation also reduces the risk for thrombophlebitis.

Pain Management

Pain control is essential to reduce the woman's distress and facilitate movement that can prevent several complications. The severity, frequency, character, and location of discomfort are assessed. Using a 0-to-10 scale helps to quantify the subjective experience of pain better. Zero would be no pain at all, and 10 would be the worst pain ever. The scale helps the nurse to choose the most appropriate relief methods and provides a method to evaluate the amount of relief the woman receives from the pain interventions.

Some women receive epidural narcotics for long-lasting pain relief. These drugs can cause respiratory depression many hours after they are given, sometimes up to 24 hours. Therefore hourly respiratory monitoring and a pulse oximeter are usual until the drug's effects have worn off. Naloxone (Narcan) should be readily available to reverse the respiratory depression. If the woman has pain not controlled by the epidural narcotic, the health care provider must be consulted for specific orders.

Many women have a patient-controlled analgesia (PCA) pump to provide them with analgesia. The pump has a syringe of a narcotic analgesic inside. It is programmed to deliver a specific dose of the drug when the woman pushes a button. To prevent overdose, there is a lockout interval during which pushing the button has no effect. As with any narcotic, the drug inside the PCA pump is counted at shift change, and the facility's protocol for record keeping is followed to account for all drug doses received, remaining, or wasted when the PCA drug is discontinued.

Most women change to one of the oral analgesics on the day after surgery. The woman should be instructed to call for pain medication when she first becomes uncomfortable. Pain is much harder to relieve if it becomes severe.

The breastfeeding mother should be reassured that timing the administration of analgesia immediately after breastfeeding minimizes passage via breast milk to the infant. It can be explained that adequate pain control helps her to relax so she can breastfeed better and have the energy to become acquainted with her infant.

EMOTIONAL CARE

The birth of an infant brings about physical changes in the mother but also causes many emotional and relationship changes in all family members.

MOTHERS

The transition to motherhood brings many hormonal changes, changes in body image, and intrapsychic reorganization. Fluctuating hormones in pregnancy and the puerperium have an effect on mood, causing early elation at delivery that can be followed by mild depression with tearfulness, irritability, and fatigue peaking on the fifth day postpartum. Most women recover in a few days. However, the physiological factors that affect mood can interact with minor anxieties and stresses to result in a clinical depression. Rubin has described three phases of postpartum change that have been a framework for nursing care for 35 years (Box 9-3). More recent studies have found that women progress through the same three phases, although at a more rapid pace than originally described. The nurse can refer to the three phases when providing postpartum care.

---

box 9-3 *Rubin's Psychological Changes of the Puerperium*

Phase 1: Taking in. Mother is passive and willing to let others do for her. Conversation centers on her birth experience. Mother has great interest in her infant but is willing to let others handle the care and has little interest in learning. Primary focus is on recovery from birth and her need for food, fluids, and deep restorative sleep.

Phase 2: Taking hold. Mother begins to initiate action and becomes interested in caring for infant. Becomes critical of her "performance." She has increased concern about her body's functions and assumes responsibility for self-care needs. This phase is ideal for teaching.

Phase 3: Letting go. Mothers, and often fathers, work through giving up their previous lifestyle and family arrangements to incorporate the new infant. Many mothers must give up their ideal of their birth experience and reconcile it with what really occurred. They give up the fantasy child so they can accept the real child.

New mothers often experience conflicting feelings of joy and emotional letdown during the first few weeks after birth, often called the postpartum blues, or baby blues. She may feel let down, but overall she finds pleasure in life. The symptoms are self-limiting. When providing discharge teaching, the nurse should prepare the woman for these feelings and reassure her that they are normal and temporary.

Postpartum depression is a persistent mood of unhappiness and is discussed on p. 248. When teaching about the postpartum blues, the nurse should explain that persistent depression is *not* expected and should be reported to her health care provider.

FATHERS

New fathers typically display intense interest in their new child (*engrossment*) (Figure 9-5). Their behaviors with their infant parallel those of the new mother. A man's relationship with his own parents, previous experiences with children, and relationship to the mother are important influences on how he will relate to his infant.

Fathers should be included when the nurse is giving instructions about infant care and handling. The nurse must be tactful and supportive of a new father who is trying to assume his new role.

SIBLINGS

The influence of a new child's birth on siblings depends on their age and developmental level. Toddlers may respond by regression and anger when the mother's attention turns to the infant. Preschool children typically

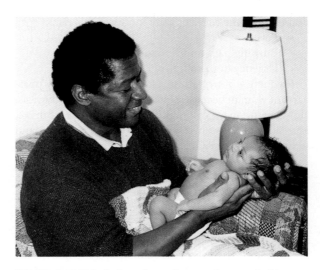

FIGURE **9-5** This father shows intense interest in his new infant (engrossment). The father's reaction to the newborn parallels the mother's. Eye-to-eye contact (en face position) helps the bonding process. (Photo courtesy of Pat Spier, RN-C.)

look at and discuss the newborn but may hesitate to actively touch or hold the infant. Older children often enjoy helping with care of the infant and are very curious about the newcomer.

GRANDPARENTS

The grandparents' involvement with a new child is often dictated by how near they live to the younger family. Grandparents who live a long distance from them cannot have the close, regular contact that they may desire.

Grandparents also differ in what they expect their role to be, and culture sometimes determines their expected role. Some feel that their child rearing days are over and want minimal day-to-day involvement in raising the children. Others expect regular involvement in the grandchild's life, second only to the parents (Figure 9-6). If parents and grandparents agree on their role, little conflict is likely.

GRIEVING PARENTS

The postpartum area is usually a happy area, but nurses occasionally care for grieving parents. With most of these parents, the nurse should simply listen to them and support them. Therapeutic communication techniques such as open-ended questions or reflection of feelings help the parents express their grief—an early step in resolving it.

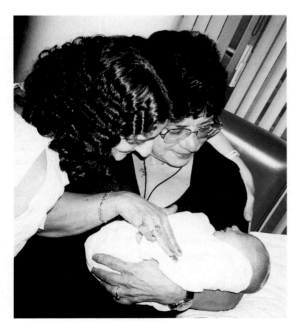

FIGURE **9-6** The daughter's arm around her mother shows how proud she is to introduce her newborn to Grandma. Grandmothers can reinforce cultural customs, help with infant care, and assist with household tasks.

It seems strange to talk of grief when a healthy infant is born, but even a healthy child may be much different in size, sex, or appearance from what parents expected. Most parents eventually come to accept their unique infant and his or her characteristics. Their feelings about their child are not right or wrong—feelings simply exist. The nurse should accept and encourage their expressions of grief to allow them to move forward and accept the infant they have.

A woman who has experienced the loss of a newborn may experience regret, remorse, and sorrow. This can be one of the most difficult kinds of grief. The woman may question what she could have done differently to prevent the loss. The anniversaries of these events are painful, and these feelings often last for many years, if not forever. The birth of a new child may awaken grief that parents thought they had resolved ("We have one child, but we almost had two").

If the condition of a newborn is poor, the parents may wish to have a baptism performed. The minister or priest is notified. In an emergency, the nurse may perform the baptism by pouring water on the infant's forehead while saying, "I baptize you in the name of the Father, and of the Son, and of the Holy Spirit." If there is any doubt as to whether the infant is alive, the baptism is given conditionally: "If you are capable of receiving baptism, I baptize you in the name of the Father, and of the Son, and of the Holy Spirit."

If the infant dies, is stillborn, or has a birth defect, the parents' reactions depend on whether the event was expected. If they have known for some time that the fetus is not living, they may have already begun the grief process and will not display all the typical behaviors. If the death was not expected, the nurse is likely to encounter the following reactions typical of any grieving:

- Shock and disbelief
- Anger (often directed at the physician or staff but rarely at the infant)
- Guilt about what they could have done differently
- Sadness and depression
- Gradual resolution of the sadness

The nurse may encounter grieving families at any point in their grieving process and in many settings. Grieving is often chronic if the infant has a birth defect because of constant reminders of what might have been.

If a newborn dies or is stillborn, nursing units have a protocol to help parents to accept and resolve the event. The parents should be allowed to progress at their individual pace about when they want to see and hold the infant. The parents should be prepared for the infant's appearance. For instance, a stillborn infant may have blue skin that is often peeling. The nurse should try to keep the infant warm so he or she feels more natural to the parents. If this is not possible, they should be prepared for the coolness of the infant's skin and the limp body. The infant should be wrapped in a blanket and the parents allowed to unwrap the infant when and if they want to do so. If an anomaly is present, the infant should be wrapped so the most normal part is showing.

The nurse should listen to the parent's responses to determine the level of support needed; answer questions; and understand the grief behaviors individual to the family or culture. Providing privacy and planning for an interdisciplinary grief conference before discharge are important in the overall plan of care. Parents should be provided with private time with the infant if possible and given mementos to take home. The support system of the parents (and grandparents) should be examined, and some information concerning the expected grief process, its influence on behavior and the ability to perform activities of daily living, coping mechanisms, and resources for follow-up care should be discussed.

Most nursing units make a memory packet containing items such as a lock of hair, footprints on a hospital birth certificate, identification band, a photograph, and clothing or blankets. Some type of code, such as a flower or ribbon on the mother's door, alerts personnel from other departments that a grieving family is inside. This reduces the chance of well-intentioned but painful remarks or questions such as, "What did you have, a boy or girl?"

PARENTHOOD

Whether the parents have one or several children, becoming a parent requires learning new roles and making adjustments. Parents having their first child find themselves in a triangular relationship (the "we" has become an "us"). Many parents say that parenthood, not marriage, made the greatest change in their lives. Adjustments are even greater for women who have professions or who are in the work force because the changes are more extensive.

The demands of parenthood affect communication between the partners, and there is little doubt that children detract from the relationship at times. It is not unusual for one member to feel left out. The division of responsibility can be a source of conflict, particularly when both parents work. Parents often feel inept, which may cause lower self-esteem, depression, and anger. These feelings can be overwhelming.

Fatigue triggers irritability. Even in the ideal situation, waking up two or three times every night is wearing on anyone. For the new mother, physiological changes

continue to play a part in her emotional lability (instability). Both parents are concerned with increased economic responsibilities. Loss of freedom and a decrease in socialization may give the couple a sense of loneliness.

Preparing parents for the lifestyle changes that occur with a new child ideally begins before conception. Parenting courses, group discussions, and support from relatives or friends can be explored. Social service agencies, public health nurses, and other professional resources should be suggested as appropriate. Encouraging parents to share their concerns and worries with one another and to keep communication lines open is foremost. Reestablishing a relationship into which the newborn fits with a minimum of disruption can be accomplished when the parents identify their own needs, set priorities, maintain their sense of humor, and relax their standards.

These tools can make the transition to parenthood, although sometimes difficult, a rewarding experience—one in which the stable family can grow and become stronger. Parents who find themselves at an impasse should seek early intervention with a professional counselor.

THE FAMILY CARE PLAN

The family care plan is similar to the traditional nursing care plan except that the "patient" is the entire family rather than the woman in the hospital. It is most appropriate to use a family care plan in obstetrics when dealing with the birth of a child who will have a profound impact on the family processes. Studying the family as the patient can offer insight to community-based care and help the nurse integrate knowledge of family structure, culture, and composition into a plan of care that will meet some of the goals of *Healthy People 2010*. The data required in a family care plan is listed in Nursing Care Plan 9-2. The nurse should use information concerning cultural practices (see Chapter 6) and family processes presented in general psychology to recognize the implications of specific nursing diagnoses to the delivery of nursing care to families.

Data collection includes the following:

- Demographic information
- Family composition
- Occupation
- Cultural group
- Religious/spiritual affiliation
- Community description
- Developmental tasks
- Health concerns
- Communication pattern

NURSING CARE PLAN 9-2

The Family Care Plan

PATIENT DATA: A woman is admitted to the postpartum unit after delivering a healthy baby girl. The husband, two sons (ages 14 and 10), and the woman's mother are present in the room. The woman tells the nurse she would like to stay in the hospital as long as she can because she has forgotten everything about baby care.

SELECTED NURSING DIAGNOSIS   *Compromised family coping related to new family member (newborn)*

Outcomes	Nursing Interventions	Rationales
Family members will express satisfaction with adaptation to newborn and confident in their roles.	1. Determine relationship of family members to one another.	1. Can help provide a positive experience to prepare the family for new developmental tasks.
	2. Provide unlimited visiting privileges for family and siblings.	2. Facilitates the attachment and bonding process.
	3. Initiate support group concerning breastfeeding and child care.	3. Verbalization of family culture, roles, and perceived responsibilities enables the appropriate person to be included in instruction concerning breastfeeding and child care.
	4. Provide anticipatory guidance concerning changes to expect and family adaptation options.	4. Needs concerning housing, equipment, and community resources available for assisting will help family adapt to changes.
	5. Discuss sexuality needs and plans for contraception.	5. Clarification of contraception options acceptable to the cultural group will enhance learning and enable family to make informed decisions.
	6. Provide written information and suggested books for siblings concerning the new child. Encourage sibling verbalization.	6. Including the needs of each family member will promote family coping and adaptation.

?CRITICAL THINKING QUESTION

How does family care differ from the care of an individual patient?

- Decision making
- Family values
- Socialization
- Coping patterns
- Housing
- Cognitive abilities
- Support system
- Response to care

CARE OF THE NEWBORN

This section presents the Phase 2 care of the newborn after transport to the postpartum unit. Care immediately after birth (Phase 1) was discussed in Chapter 6. Newborn assessments and ongoing care (Phase 3) are presented in Chapter 12. Care of the preterm and post-term infant is presented in Chapter 13.

ADMISSION CARE OF THE NEWBORN TO THE POSTPARTUM OR NURSERY UNIT

If the infant has adequate cardiorespiratory and heat-regulating functions, he or she usually remains undisturbed while the parents and infant become acquainted. The nurse can usually assess temperature, heart rate, and respirations while the parents continue to hold their infant. Within an hour, the admitting nurse does a complete physical and gestational age assessment of the infant and gives prophylactic medications. Chapter 12 offers the expected characteristics, deviations, and related nursing care of the normal newborn.

table 9-1	*Nursing Interventions to Prevent Heat Loss in Newborns*		
MECHANISM OF HEAT LOSS	**SOURCES OF HEAT LOSS**	**INTERVENTIONS**
Evaporation (conversion from liquid to vapor)	Wet skin from amniotic fluid at birth evaporates from skin	Dry infant quickly. Dry and cover head of infant.
Conduction (transfer of heat to a cooler surface)	Cool surface of bed, scale, stethoscope	Prewarm radiant warmer and stethoscope before use. Place scale paper on scale, and place warm blanket on other surfaces.
Convection (loss of heat to the surrounding cooler air)	Drafts from window, air conditioning, oxygen vents	Place crib away from windows and vents.
Radiation (loss of heat to surrounding cold environment)	Cold environment of walls, windows	Place crib away from cold walls. Wrap infant warmly.

The "intensive care concept" has been introduced to the care of all newborns for the immediate neonatal period until they have evidenced a normal transition to extrauterine life (Thureen et al, 1999). The three phases of this transition are as follows:

- *First phase:* 0 to 30 minutes (period of reactivity; see Chapter 6)
  Tachycardia, gradually lowering to normal rate
  Irregular respirations
  Rales present on auscultation
  Infant is alert; frequent Moro (startle reaction) reflex, tremors, crying, increased motor activity (because of sudden release from confines of uterus, response to light)
  Absent bowel sounds
- *Second phase:* 30 minutes to 2 hours (decreased responsiveness)
  Decreased motor activity
  Rapid respirations (up to 60 breaths/min)
  Normal heart rate for term newborn
  Audible bowel sounds
- *Third phase:* 2 to 8 hours (second period of reactivity; see Chapter 12)
  Abrupt, brief changes in color and muscle tone
  Presence of oral mucus (can cause gagging)
  Responsiveness to external stimuli
  Infant stabilizes, begins suck-swallow coordination, and is ready for regular feedings

Supporting Thermoregulation

The temperature of the term newborn is 36° to 36.5° C (96.8° to 97.7° F; skin) or 36.5° to 37° C (97.7° to 98.6° F; axillary). Maintenance of body temperature is very important to the newborn infant, who has a less efficient means of generating heat than an older infant.

Hypothermia (low body temperature) can cause other problems, such as the following:

- Hypoglycemia (low blood sugar) as the infant uses glucose to generate heat
- Respiratory distress, because the higher metabolic rate consumes more oxygen, sometimes beyond the infant's ability to supply it

Hypoglycemia can be both the cause and the result of hypothermia; therefore the nurse must evaluate both factors. Respiratory distress can also require more glucose for the increased work of breathing, causing hypoglycemia.

Heat is lost by any of the following four means:

- *Evaporation* of liquids from the skin
- *Conduction* caused by direct skin contact with a cold surface
- *Convection* of heat away from the body by drafts
- *Radiation* caused by being near a cold surface, although not in direct contact with it

Conduction, convection, and radiation can also be used to add heat to the body. Newborns lose heat quickly after birth because amniotic fluid evaporates from their body, drafts move heat away, and they may contact cold surfaces (Table 9-1).

The infant remains monitored in a radiant warmer until temperature is stabilized and can be cared for in an open crib, clothed, and wrapped in a blanket. The first bath is delayed until the body temperature is stabilized at 36.5° to 37° C (97.7° to 98.6° F). The temperature should be recorded 30 minutes after the bath and 1 hour after transfer to an open crib.

Observing Bowel and Urinary Function

Newborns may not urinate for as long as 24 hours, and occasionally an infant may not void for 48 hours. If an infant urinates in the birthing or operating room, the staff nurse should be informed and the voiding documented on the delivery record. If a long period of time elapses before the second voiding, it will have been established that the urinary tract is open. Seventy percent of term newborns pass meconium in the first 12 hours. Meconium should be passed before discharge to assure a patent gastrointestinal tract.

Identifying the Infant

Wristbands with preprinted numbers are placed on mother, infant, and often the father or other support person in the birthing room as the primary means of identifying the infant. The nurse should check to be sure that all numbers in the set are identical (Figure 9-7). Other identifying information, such as mother's name, birth attendant's name, date and time of birth, sex of the infant, and usually the mother's hospital identification number, should be completed. The bands are applied relatively snugly on the infant and have only a finger's width of slack because infants lose weight after birth.

Each time the infant returns to the mother after a separation, the nurse must check the preprinted band numbers to see that they match. The nurse should either look at the numbers to see that they are identical or have the mother read her own band number while the nurse reads the infant's band.

Some identification bands or umbilical clamps have an alarm that alerts the staff if the infant is removed from the hospital unit. These alarm chips are removed at the time of discharge to the home.

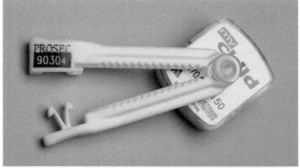
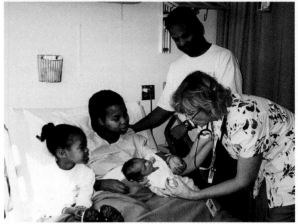

FIGURE **9-7 A,** This umbilical clamp can be used as identification (with an identical numbered wristband for the mother) and also as protection from abduction because it has a lightweight transponder attached to the clamp. When the transponder passes out of the unit, an alarm sounds unless neutralized by a coded signal inputted by the hospital staff. The umbilical clamp is removed before discharge. **B,** The nurse compares the identification bracelet of the newborn with the bracelet on the mother's wrist as the father and sibling look on. (**B** courtesy Pat Spier, RN-C.)

> ### NURSING **TIP**
> Do not check bands in this manner: "Is your band number [state number]?" The mother who is sleepy, sedated, or simply distracted may answer affirmatively and receive the wrong infant.

Observing for Gestational Age and Birth Injuries or Anomalies

Gestational age evaluation. A thorough gestational age assessment is done using a scale such as the new Ballard or Dubowitz form (see Chapter 13). However, the birthing room nurse does a quick assessment to evaluate whether the infant seems to be of the appropriate gestational age. The infant who seems to be preterm may be admitted to the nursery more rapidly than one who is of the expected term gestation. Characteristics to assess include the following:

- *Skin.* Is the skin thin and somewhat transparent (preterm) or peeling (postterm, or possible intrauterine growth retardation [IUGR])?
- *Vernix.* Is this cheesy substance covering most of the skin surface (preterm), is it present only in creases (term), or is it absent (postterm)? Greenish vernix indicates that meconium was passed before birth, which may indicate that the infant is postterm or had poor placental support.
- *Hair.* Is the skin heavily covered with fine lanugo hair (preterm), or is hair only in a few places (term)? Dark-skinned infants often have more lanugo than light-skinned ones.

- *Ears.* When folded toward the lobe, do the ears spring back slowly (preterm) or quickly (term or postterm)? Abundant vernix can stick the ear in place, so that possibility should be considered if the ear does not quickly return to its erect position.
- *Breast tissue.* Is there no or minimal breast tissue under the nipple (preterm), or is there a palpable mass of tissue 5 mm or more (term)? (A millimeter is about the thickness of a dime.)
- *Genitalia.* For males, is the scrotum smooth and small (preterm) or pendulous and covered with rugae or ridges (term)? For females, are the labia majora and labia minora of nearly equal size (preterm) or do the labia majora cover the labia minora (term)?
- *Sole creases.* Are the sole creases on the anterior third of the foot only (preterm), over the anterior two thirds (term), or over the full foot (term or postterm)? Peeling skin may be obvious on the feet in postterm or IUGR infants.

Observing for injuries or anomalies. The nurse notes signs of injury or anomalies while performing other assessments and care. The infant's movements and facial expression during crying are observed for symmetry and equality of movement. The head and face should be assessed for trauma, especially if forceps were used. A small puncture wound is usually apparent on the scalp if an internal spiral electrode was used for fetal monitoring (see Chapter 6). If the infant was born vaginally in a breech presentation, the buttocks may be bruised.

Many anomalies, such as spina bifida (open spine) or a cleft lip, are immediately obvious. The fingers and toes should be counted to identify abnormal numbers or webbing. The feet should be observed for straightness or to determine if deviated feet can be returned to the straight position. The length equality of arms and legs should also be checked. Urination or meconium passage, which confirm patency, must also be noted.

Obtaining Vital Signs

Vital signs begin while parents and infant are bonding. They are measured at 15- to 30-minute intervals at first, then hourly, and every 4 to 8 hours after the infant is stable.

Respiratory rate. For best accuracy, the respiratory and heart rates are assessed before disturbing the infant. The respirations are counted for 1 full minute. Newborn respirations are difficult to count because they are shallow and irregular. The rate can be auscultated by listening with a stethoscope. Placing a hand lightly over the abdomen or watching the abdomen rise and fall also helps to identify each breath. If the infant is crying, a pacifier or gloved finger to suck may quiet him or her so the respiratory rate can be counted.

Heart rate. The newborn's heart rate is assessed apically. A small pediatric head is used on the stethoscope if possible to limit extraneous noise. The nurse should count for 1 minute. The rate is 110 to 160 beats/min. A consistently low or high heart rate can indicate a pathological condition.

NURSING **TIP**
In the past, newborns were placed in a prone position to facilitate the drainage of mucus. Because the prone position has been associated with sudden infant death syndrome (SIDS), it is now recommended that newborns be placed on their side or on their back to sleep. Teach all parents this newer information because they may have been taught to keep a previous infant in a prone position.

Temperature. Some facilities require an initial rectal temperature for newborns, but many have discontinued this practice. To avoid perforating the rectum, the nurse should insert a lubricated thermometer no more than 0.5 inch into the rectum. The thermometer is held securely near the buttocks while it is in place. The nurse must not force the thermometer into the rectum because the infant could have an imperforate anus.

An axillary temperature is most commonly used. The thermometer is placed in the axilla, keeping it parallel to the chest wall. The infant's arm is folded down firmly against the thermometer for the required time. Tympanic temperatures are less accurate in newborns and not generally used during the neonatal period.

Blood pressure. A newborn's blood pressure is measured with an electronic instrument. When blood pressure is assessed on a newborn, all four extremities or one arm and one leg are assessed to identify substantial pressure differences between the upper and lower extremities, which can be a sign of coarctation of the aorta. The normal range of blood pressure is between 65 and 95 mm Hg systolic over 30 to 60 mm Hg diastolic in term infants.

NURSING **TIP**
Remember that the artery runs on the *posterior* aspect of the leg when measuring blood pressure in that extremity.

Weighing and Measuring

Weight. The infant is weighed in the birthing room or when admitted to the nursery. Disposable paper is put on the scale, and the scale is balanced to zero according to its model. The unclothed infant is then placed on the scale. The nurse's hand should not touch the infant but should be kept just above him or her to prevent falls. The weight must be converted to grams for gestational age assessment (see Figure 12-11).

Measurements. Three typical measurements are length, head circumference, and chest circumference. A disposable tape measure is used. The tape should not be pulled out from under the infant to avoid giving a paper cut. Measurements must also be noted in centimeters for gestational age assessment.

Length. There are several ways to measure length. Some facilities have a tape measure applied to the clear wall of a bassinet. The nurse places the infant's head at one end, extends the leg, and notes where the heel ends. Another method is to bring the infant to the bassinet or warmer with the scale paper. The paper is marked at the top of the head, the body and leg are extended, and the paper is marked where the foot is located. Length is measured between the marks. Still another method involves placing the zero end of the tape at the infant's head, extending the body and leg, and stretching the tape to the heel.

Head circumference. The fullest part of the infant's head is measured just above the eyebrows. Molding of the head may affect the accuracy of the initial measurement (see Figure 12-5, A).

Chest circumference. Chest circumference is measured at the nipple line.

Providing Umbilical Cord Care

The health care provider may leave a long length of umbilical cord. If so, the nurse applies a plastic clamp near the skin and cuts the cord just above the clamp.

The cord is assessed for the number and type of blood vessels soon after it is cut. The normal umbilical cord has three vessels: two arteries and one vein. The woman's name "AVA" for "artery-vein-artery" helps the nurse remember the normal number of vessels. A two-vessel cord is associated with other internal anomalies, often of the genitourinary tract. To distinguish the arteries from the vein, the nurse should look at the freshly cut end of the cord. The arteries project slightly from the surface, and the vein looks like a flattened cylinder that does not project from the cut surface.

Umbilical cord care is aimed at preventing infection. It usually includes an initial application of triple-dye solution or antibiotic ointment. Some facilities apply alcohol applications at each diaper change to promote drying of the cord. However, the value of this

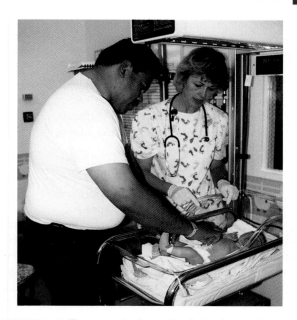

FIGURE **9-8** The nurse includes the father in teaching the care of the newborn's umbilical cord. (Photo courtesy of Pat Spier, RN-C.)

practice is controversial. The diaper should be fastened low to allow air circulation to the cord. The cord should become dry and brownish black as it dries. The clamp is removed when the end of the cord is dry and crisp, usually in about 24 hours. The parents are taught to report redness of the area or a moist, foul-smelling umbilical cord. Tub baths are usually delayed until the cord falls off—about 10 to 14 days after birth (Figure 9-8).

Bleeding from the cord during the first few hours usually indicates that the cord clamp has become loose. Because of the newborn's small blood volume, even a small amount of bleeding can be a significant percentage of the blood volume. The clamp should be checked for closure and another applied if needed.

HYPOGLYCEMIA

The brain is totally dependent on a steady supply of glucose for its metabolism. Until infants begin regular feedings, they must use the glucose stored in their bodies. A blood glucose level below 40 mg/dl in the term infant indicates hypoglycemia.

If the screening test indicates hypoglycemia, a venous blood sample is drawn for a more accurate evaluation. The infant is fed formula or is breastfed as soon as the sample is obtained to prevent a further drop in blood glucose.

Some infants have an increased risk for low blood glucose after birth. Infants at higher risk include the following:

- Preterm/postterm infants
- Infants of diabetic mothers, if maternal glucose is poorly controlled
- Large-for-gestational age (LGA) infants
- Small-for-gestational age (SGA) infants
- Infants with IUGR
- Asphyxiated infants
- Infants who are cold stressed
- Infants whose mothers took ritodrine or terbutaline to stop preterm labor

These infants undergo a blood glucose evaluation within 1 hour after birth and at intervals until their glucose level is stable. They are usually nursed or given formula soon after birth to prevent a fall in their blood glucose level.

Although some infants have a higher risk to develop hypoglycemia, any infant can have a fall in blood glucose levels. Signs of hypoglycemia in the newborn include the following:

- Jitteriness
- Poor muscle tone
- Sweating
- Respiratory difficulty
- Low temperature (which can also cause hypoglycemia)
- Poor suck
- High-pitched cry
- Lethargy
- Seizures

A heel stick is performed when obtaining capillary blood for the glucose screening test. The heel stick should avoid the center of the heel where the bone, nerves, and blood vessels are near the surface.

SCREENING TESTS

Several tests are done to screen for abnormalities that are known to cause physical or mental disability. The mandatory tests vary according to the state. Most of the disorders have therapy that can prevent many, if not all, of the disabilities that would result if left untreated. A test for phenylketonuria (PKU) is mandatory in all states. If the infant has this disorder, a special formula begun in the first 2 months of life can reduce disability and prevent severe mental retardation in most cases. The PKU test is done on the day of discharge for better accuracy and is repeated during early clinic visits. Other tests may include those for hypothyroidism, galactosemia, sickle cell disease, thalassemia, maple syrup urine disease, and homocystinuria.

SKIN CARE

Initial skin care after the infant's condition is stable involves washing off the blood and amniotic fluid that may be present on the infant's skin. Vigorous removal of all remnants of vernix is not advised, because vernix has a protective function on the skin. There should be little vernix present on the skin of the term infant. Until the infant's first sponge bath and shampoo, the nurse must wear gloves while handling the infant. Care of the skin of the newborn is discussed in Chapter 12.

SECURITY

The possibility of abduction must be addressed in any facility that cares for infants and children. In the maternal-newborn setting, security begins with identification bands that the nurse matches every time the infant is reunited with the parent (see Figure 9-7).

Recognition of Employees

Parents should be able to recognize employees who are authorized to take the infant from the mother's room. Employees wear photo identification badges, and maternal-newborn nurses may have an additional badge. They may wear distinctive uniforms. Some units use a code word that changes on a regular basis. The family is taught very early how to recognize an employee who is allowed to take the infant and to refuse to release their infant to any other person. Security measures should be reinforced when providing later care.

Other Security Measures

The mother is taught to keep the infant away from the door to the room. In a semiprivate room the two bassinets are often placed between the mothers. The mother should not leave her infant alone in the room for any reason. If she is alone in her room, she should leave the bathroom door ajar while she toilets or return the infant to the nursery if she showers or naps. These measures also reduce the risk that the infant would aspirate mucus because no one was present for suctioning.

BONDING AND ATTACHMENT

Bonding and *attachment* are terms often used interchangeably, although they differ slightly. Bonding refers to a strong emotional tie that forms soon after birth between parents and the newborn. Attachment is an affectionate tie that occurs over time as infant and caregivers interact. It is important for nurses to promote these processes to help parents claim their infant as their own. Bonding actually begins during pregnancy as the fetus moves and shows individual characteristics on sonogram.

Both partners should view, hold and, most important, *touch* the infant as soon as possible after birth. They must do this to reconcile the fantasy child of pregnancy with the real child they now have. Many parents are not surprised to know the gender of their infant at birth if the sonogram revealed it earlier. However, some do not want to know the infant's gender before birth and some are surprised when the predicted gender differs from the real gender. Most parents count all fingers and toes.

To prevent infant hypothermia, the unclothed infant is kept near the parent's skin. Parents soon identify individual characteristics, such as a nose that looks like Grandpa's, long fingers like the father's, or a cry just like an older sibling. All of these parental behaviors help to identify the infant as a separate individual.

For some, parental feelings do not come naturally. Difficulty in bonding or rejection or indifference in one or both parents should be recorded, and a referral to social services should be considered. Mothers who have little social support may have difficulty forming attachments with their newborns.

> **NURSING TIP**
> Observe the interaction between parents and infant to evaluate the attachment process.

Nursing Care to Promote Bonding and Attachment

The nurse observes parenting behaviors, such as amount of affection and interest shown to the infant. The amount of physical contact, stimulation, eye-to-eye contact (*en face* position; see Figure 9-5), and time spent interacting with the infant are significant. Adults tend to talk with infants in high-pitched voices. The extent to which the parents encourage involvement of siblings and grandparents with the newborn should be noted. This information provides a basis for nursing interventions that may encourage bonding and foster positive family relationships (Figure 9-9).

Parents must learn what their infant's communication cues mean. Soon after birth, most parents begin to recognize when an infant is signaling discomfort from hunger as opposed to discomfort from other causes, such as a wet diaper or boredom. In addition, the parents should quickly be able to distinguish their infant's cry from the cries of other infants. Although this process is just beginning when the mother and infant leave the birth facility, the nurse should note its early signs.

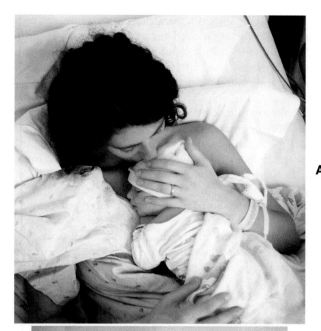

A

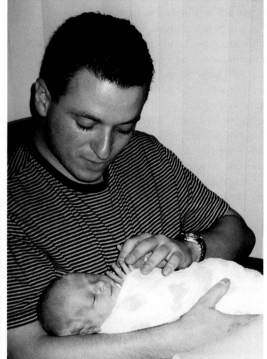

B

FIGURE 9-9 **A,** Mother-infant bonding is obvious in this picture of a mother and her newborn infant. **B,** An uncle bonds with the newborn as he examines features and fingers.

The nurse should observe for parent-infant interactions that dictate a need for additional interventions. Some of these include indifference to the infant's signals of hunger or discomfort, failure to identify their infant's communication, avoidance of eye contact with the infant, or discussing the infant in negative terms. However, the family's culture should also be considered.

Nursing interventions to facilitate parent-infant attachment vary. Calling the infant by name, holding the infant en face, and talking in gentle, high-pitched tones help the nurse to model appropriate behavior for the parent. Role modeling is especially important to adolescent mothers who may feel self-conscious when interacting with their child. Expected infant behaviors should be discussed and unique characteristics pointed out to enhance the bonding process. This is especially important if the parents' "fantasy child" differs from the "real" child in gender, physical attributes, or health.

DAILY CARE

A newborn infant stays in the mother's room most of the time unless either mother or infant has a problem that requires separation. Routine assessments and care provide an opportunity for the nurse to teach the parents normal newborn characteristics, signs of problems that should be reported, and how to provide care for the infant. Involving the parents in care of their infant helps them to learn most successfully. First-time parents may be sensitive to critical remarks, and therefore the nurse should praise their efforts while tactfully giving suggestions for needed improvement.

Feeding and elimination patterns are assessed by discussing them with the mother as well as observing at diaper changes. The mother should be asked how many wet and soiled diapers the infant has had since the last assessment. Voidings are usually totaled for the shift. Stools are also tallied and are described. Meconium stools are expected during the birth facility stay, although they may change to transitional stools before discharge.

If the infant is breastfed, the nurse should discuss with the mother how well the infant is nursing, the frequency and duration of nursing sessions, and any difficulty she is having. Her breasts are checked for engorgement, and her nipples are checked for flatness, inversion, trauma, or tenderness; these problems can impede successful breastfeeding. If the infant is fed formula, the mother should be asked how many ounces the infant has taken since the previous assessment. This is also a good time to remind the mother that bacteria multiply rapidly in formula, so she should discard any leftovers.

The infant's skin should be observed for jaundice at each assessment. Infants have a large number of erythrocytes because they live in a low-oxygen environment in utero. Excess erythrocytes are broken down after birth, which releases bilirubin into the bloodstream. High levels of bilirubin cause yellow skin color, starting at the head and progressing downward on the body. Extremely high levels of bilirubin can cause bilirubin encephalopathy (see Chapter 14).

The infant needs only a shirt and diaper for clothing. A light receiving blanket is used to swaddle the infant and another receiving blanket is placed over the child. A cap is used because the infant's head is the largest body surface area and can be the source of significant heat loss.

Teaching is an important part of mother-infant care. Parent teaching of infant care includes the following:
- Maintenance of an open airway by positioning and use of the bulb syringe
- Temperature maintenance and assessment after discharge
- Expected increase in the number of voidings
- Changes in the stools
- Feeding
- Signs of illness to report
- Follow-up appointments for well-baby care

The first feeding should be observed carefully since anomalies that cause choking could be present.

> ### NURSING **TIP**
> If a pacifier is used to provide extra sucking, teach parents to use a one-piece type to prevent choking. They should use a clip to secure the pacifier to the infant's clothing and not place it on a string around the infant's neck, which can cause an active infant to hang himself or herself.

BREASTFEEDING

Nutrition is especially important in the first few months of life because the brain grows rapidly. Energy use is high because of the newborn's rapid growth. More in-depth discussions of the nutritional needs of the infant are found in Chapters 15 and 16. The mother may choose to nurse her infant or bottle feed. The nurse should support the mother in either decision.

CHOOSING WHETHER TO BREASTFEED

Breastfeeding has many advantages for the newborn, including the following:
- Breast milk contains the full range of nutrients that the infant needs and in the right propor-

tions. No commercial formula has the exact nutritional composition of breast milk.

- Breast milk is easily digested by the infant's maturing digestive system.
- Breast milk does not cause infant allergies.
- Breastfeeding provides natural immunity because the mother transfers antibodies through the milk. Colostrum is particularly high in antibodies.
- Breast milk promotes elimination of meconium. Breastfed infants are rarely constipated.
- Suckling at the breast promotes mouth development.
- Breastfeeding is convenient and economical.
- Breastfeeding eliminates the risks of a contaminated water supply or improper dilution.
- Infant suckling promotes a return of the uterus to its prepregnant state.
- Breastfeeding may play a significant role in improving brain development of the infant.
- Breast milk production uses maternal fat stores, which facilitates maternal weight loss.
- Breastfeeding enhances a close mother-child relationship.
- Breastfeeding may decrease the occurrence of childhood respiratory disorders.

There are also some disadvantages and contraindications to breastfeeding:

- There is a potential for most maternal medications to enter breast milk. Use of antimetabolites, antineoplastic drugs, or chloramphenicol is an absolute contraindication to breastfeeding.
- Working mothers may have more difficulty continuing to nurse after they return to work.
- Women who have untreated active tuberculosis, hepatitis B or C, or infection with the human immunodeficiency virus (HIV) should not breastfeed. Cancer may become worse with the hormonal changes of lactation.
- Women who abuse drugs or alcohol should not breastfeed.

PHYSIOLOGY OF LACTATION
Infectious Diseases and Breastfeeding

The only absolute contraindication to breastfeeding is infection with HIV and human T cell lymphotrophic virus (HTLV 1 and 2) (Schanlen, 2001). HIV infection is an absolute contraindication to breastfeeding because it can be transmitted to the infant via breast milk. The HTLV 1 and 2 viruses are retroviruses that can also be passed to the newborn via breast milk, and breastfeed-

ing is contraindicated. Maternal hepatitis A infection is *not* a contraindication to breastfeeding. The infant can receive immunoglobulin and hepatitis A vaccine therapy. Infants of hepatitis B virus–positive (HBV[+]) mothers should receive HBV vaccine therapy before discharge and can breastfeed. In mothers who are infected with the hepatitis C virus, breastfeeding is contraindicated in the presence of liver failure. In mothers infected with the herpes simplex virus or the varicella zoster virus, breastfeeding is contraindicated when lesions on the breast are present.

Mothers who have active tuberculosis (TB) must be isolated from their newborn infants but infants can be fed breast milk that is pumped because the breast milk does not contain the tubercle bacilli (Schanlen, 2001).

Certain drugs decrease the breast milk volume, such as levodopa, barbiturates, antihistamines, pyridoxine, estrogens, androgens and bromocriptine.

Hormonal Stimulation

To better support the nursing mother the nurse must understand how breast milk production occurs and how the milk changes over time. The following two hormones have a major role in the production and expulsion of breast milk:

- *Prolactin* from the anterior pituitary gland causes the production of breast milk.
- *Oxytocin* from the posterior pituitary gland causes the milk to be delivered from the alveoli (milk-producing sacs) through the duct system to the nipple (*milk ejection,* or let-down reflex). The mother usually feels a tingling in her breasts and sometimes abdominal cramping as her uterus contracts (Figure 9-10).

During pregnancy the glandular tissue of the breasts grows under the influence of several hormones. The woman also secretes high levels of prolactin, the hormone that causes milk production. However, other hormones from the placenta inhibit the breasts' response to prolactin. The influence of prolactin is unopposed after birth and the expulsion of the placenta and milk production begins. If milk is not removed from the breast, prolactin secretion abates and the breasts return to their prepregnant state.

Infant suckling at the breast stimulates the release of oxytocin so that milk is delivered to the nipple where it is ingested by the newborn. Prolactin secretion increases as milk is removed from the breasts, thus stimulating further milk production. Therefore feedings that are infrequent or too short can reduce the amount of milk produced. The opposite is also true, which explains why a mother can produce enough milk for twins.

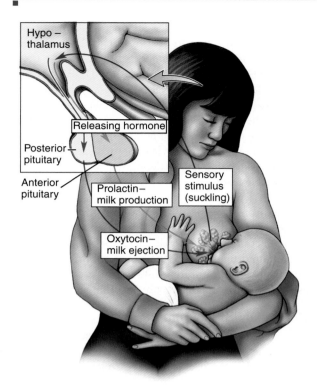

FIGURE **9-10** Lactation reflex arc. The infant suckling on the breast stimulates nerve fibers in the areola of the nipple that travel to the hypothalamus. The hypothalamus stimulates the anterior pituitary to secrete prolactin; this stimulates milk production and stimulates the posterior pituitary to release oxytocin, which causes a "let-down reflex," contracting the lobules in the breast and squeezing milk out into the nipple and to the infant.

Very little milk is stored between feedings. Most is manufactured as the infant nurses. The composition of milk changes slightly from the beginning of a feeding until the end of that feeding, as follows:

- *Foremilk* is the first milk the infant obtains. It is more watery and quenches the infant's thirst.
- *Hindmilk* is the later milk that has a higher fat content. It helps satisfy the infant's hunger. Feedings that are too short do not allow the infant to obtain the hunger-satisfying hindmilk.

✦NURSING **TIP**_____

Anticipatory guidance concerning possible problems associated with breastfeeding helps the mother to see them as common occurrences and not as complications.

Phases of Milk Production

Milk production changes in three phases after birth, as follows:

- Colostrum
- Transitional milk
- Mature milk

Late in pregnancy and for the first few days after birth, colostrum is secreted by the breasts. This yellowish fluid is rich in protective antibodies. It provides protein, vitamins A and E, and essential minerals, but it is lower in calories than milk. It has a laxative effect, which aids in eliminating meconium.

Approximately 7 to 10 days after birth the *transitional milk* emerges as the breasts gradually shift from production of colostrum to production of mature milk. Transitional milk has fewer immunoglobulins and proteins but has increased lactose (milk sugar), fat, and calorie content.

Mature milk is secreted by 14 days after birth. Mature human breast milk has a bluish color, which leads women to think that it is not "rich" enough to nourish the infant. The nurse should explain that the apparent "thinness" of the milk is normal and that the milk has 20 kcal/ounce and all the nutrients the infant needs.

ASSISTING THE MOTHER TO BREASTFEED

Ideally the infant is nursed soon after birth. Although the infant may obtain little colostrum, this first nursing session has the following other advantages:

- Promotes mother-infant bonding
- Maintains infant temperature
- Infant suckling stimulates oxytocin release to contract the mother's uterus and control bleeding

The newborn should be put to breast immediately after delivery—within the first hours when the alert state allows for suckling and bonding. Breastfeeding should not be delayed beyond 6 hours after delivery. The focus of the nurse in the early hours of breastfeeding should be to help the mother position the infant correctly and help the infant have an open, gaping mouth in preparation for suckling. Frequent reassurance and praise of the mother's efforts are essential.

Mothers from many cultures use galactagogues (breast milk stimulators), and nurses should be aware of these practices. Beer, brewer's yeast, rice, gruel, fenugreek tea, and sesame tea are commonly used postpartum. The mother eating garlic to prevent newborn illness will flavor her breast milk but will not harm the newborn. Cultural practices should be respected.

If the mother is too tired or uncomfortable to nurse at this time or if the infant seems disinterested, she should be reassured that she can still breastfeed success-

table 9-2 | *Teaching the New Mother How to Breastfeed*

INSTRUCTION	RATIONALE
Wash hands before feeding; wash nipples with warm water, no soap.	Prevents infection of the newborn and breast; use of plain water avoids nipple cracking and irritation.
Position self (sitting or side-lying).	Alternating positions facilitates breast emptying and reduces nipple trauma.
Sit comfortably in chair or raised bed with back and arm support; hold infant with cradle hold or football hold, supported by pillows.	Pillow support of mother's back and arm and the infant's body in any position reduces fatigue; infant is more likely to remain in correct position for nursing.
Side-lying with pillow beneath head, arm above head; support infant in side-lying position.	Side-lying position reduces fatigue and pressure on abdominal incision.
Turn body of infant to face mother's breast.	Prevents pulling on nipple or poor position of mouth on nipple.
Stroke infant's cheek with nipple.	Elicits rooting reflex to cause infant to turn toward nipple and open mouth wide.
Infant's mouth should cover entire areola.	Compresses ducts and lessens tension on nipples; suction is more even.
Avoid strict time limits for nursing; nurse at least 10 minutes before changing to other breast, or longer if infant is nursing vigorously.	Let-down reflex may take 5 minutes; a too-short feeding will give infant foremilk only, not the hunger-satisfying hindmilk. Strict time limits do not prevent sore nipples.
Use safety pin on the bra as a reminder about which breast to start with the next feeding.	Alternating breasts increases milk production.
Lift infant or breast slightly if breast tissue blocks nose.	Provides a small breathing space.
Break suction by placing finger in corner of infant's mouth or indenting breast tissue.	Removing infant in this way prevents nipple trauma.
Nurse infant after birth and every 2 to 3 hours thereafter.	Early suckling stimulates oxytocin from mother's pituitary to contract her uterus and control bleeding. Breast milk is quickly digested. Early, regular, and frequent nursing reduces breast engorgement.
Burp infant halfway through and following feeding.	Rids stomach of air bubbles and reduces regurgitation.

fully. Table 9-2 reviews techniques the nurse can teach a new mother who wants to breastfeed.

Positions for Nursing

Any of several positions may be used for nursing. The mother may sit in bed or in a chair and hold the infant in a cradle hold, with the head in her antecubital area. To prevent arm fatigue, the infant's body should be supported with pillows or folded blankets. She may prefer the football hold (Figure 9-11), supporting the infant's head with her hand while the infant's body rests on pillows alongside her hip. The football hold is good for mothers who have a cesarean incision.

The mother may prefer to lie on her side with the infant's body parallel to hers. Pillows or folded blankets can be used to support the infant in the proper position. Mothers often use the side-lying position when feeding the infant during the night. It is also good for mothers who have a cesarean birth.

Regardless of the position selected for breastfeeding, the infant's body should be in "chest-to-chest" position with the mother, with the head and neck in alignment. If the infant's chest faces the ceiling of the room, then the infant will have to turn his or her head away from midline to grasp the breast nipple. This position makes swallowing difficult for the infant. The infant should be at the level of the breast nipple to allow easy flow of milk. Holding the infant above the level of the nipple works against gravity flow; holding the infant below the level of the nipple exerts a pressure on the nipple that

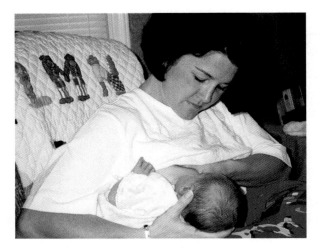

FIGURE **9-11** Football hold. The mother supports the infant's head with her hand while the infant's body rests on pillows alongside her hip. The mother has control of the infant's head and can see the position of the infant's mouth on the breast. The football hold avoids pressure on a cesarean incision and is comfortable for mothers with large breasts.

can cause soreness and bruising. The nipple should be centered to the nose of the infant with the nipple aimed to the roof of the infant's mouth so that the lower jaw latches on first. When the infant's mouth is wide open before latch-on, a more effective latch-on will occur as the mother moves her arm to bring the infant closer to the breast (Box 9-4).

Feeding Technique

The mother is taught to wash her hands before each nursing session. She should wash her breasts gently with plain water.

Position of the mother's hands. The mother should hold her breast in a C position, with the thumb above the nipple and the fingers below it. The thumb and fingers should be well back from the nipple and the nipple should not tip upward. She can also use the scissors hold to grasp the breast between her index and middle fingers, but her fingers are more likely to slip downward over the nipple. Most infants do not need to have the breast indented for breathing room. The mother can lift the infant's hips higher if her breasts are very large or if the infant buries the nose in her breast.

Latch-on. The mother is taught to allow the infant to become alert and hungry but not frantic. To elicit latch-on, the mother should hold her breast so the nipple brushes against the infant's lower lip. A hungry infant usually opens the mouth wide with this stimulation. As soon as the infant's mouth opens wide, the mother should bring the infant close to her breast so

Essential Factors in Breastfeeding

- Proper body alignment of infant
- Infant's mouth is wide open for areola grasp
- Proper hand position of mother on breast
- Infant's mouth moves in rhythmic motion to compress areola
- Audible swallow is heard
- Mother in relaxed, supported position
- Room is warm and private
- Infant ends feeding relaxed and appears satiated
- Mother has soft, nonengorged breasts at end of feeding

that her areola is well into the mouth. The infant's lips should flare outward. The infant's tongue position can be checked to be sure it is under the nipple by gently pulling down on the lower lip.

Suckling patterns. Suckling is the term that specifically relates to giving or taking nourishment at the breast. Infants have different suckling patterns when they breastfeed. Some suck several times before swallowing, and others swallow with each suck. After 4 days the infant generally swallows with every suck at the beginning of breastfeeding, taking in approximately 0.14 ml, and has about two sucks per swallow near the end of the feeding, taking in 0.01 ml with each suck. A soft "ka" or "ah" sound indicates that the infant is swallowing colostrum or milk (nutritive sucking). Noisy sucking or smacking sounds or dimpling of the cheeks usually indicates improper mouth position. "Fluttering" sucking motions indicate nonnutritive suckling.

Removing the infant from the breast. When the infant needs to be repositioned or changed to the other breast, the mother should break the suction and remove the infant quickly. She can break the suction by inserting a finger in the corner of the infant's mouth or indenting her breast near the mouth (Figure 9-12). Pulling the infant away from the breast can cause sore nipples.

Evaluating Intake of Infant

Often the mother must be reassured that she is providing adequate milk for her infant because she cannot see the milk consumed as she can with bottle feeding. Signs that breastfeeding is successful include the following:

- Breast feels full before feedings and softens after.
- "Let-down" reflex occurs—a tingling sensation with milk dripping from breasts when a feeding is due.
- Infant nurses at the breast for 10 to 15 minutes per breast eight to 10 times a day.

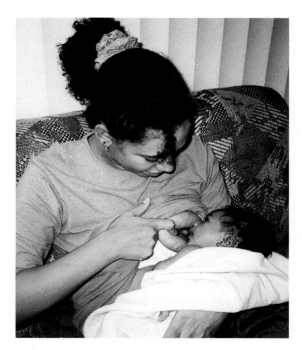

FIGURE **9-12** The mother should break the suction before removing the infant from the breast. She can break the suction by inserting a finger in the corner of the infant's mouth, or indenting the breast near the infant's mouth. The infant should never be pulled away from the breast without first breaking the suction. (Photo courtesy of Pat Spier, RN-C.)

- An audible swallow is heard as infant sucks.
- Infant demands feeding and appears relaxed after feeding.
- Infant has six to eight wet diapers per day.
- Infant passes stools several times a day.

PREVENTING PROBLEMS

Teaching can help new mothers prevent many problems with breastfeeding. If the mother can avoid problems, she is less likely to become discouraged and stop nursing early. Lactation consultants are available in many birth settings to help with breastfeeding problems. Local chapters of the La Leche League may be available to the mother for ongoing support after discharge. Most birth centers have "warm lines" to help with breastfeeding or other problems that occur in mothers and infants after birth.

Frequency and Duration of Feedings

Breastfed infants usually nurse every 2 to 3 hours during the early weeks because their stomach capacity is small and because breast milk is easily digested.

| box 9-5 | *Recognizing Hunger in Newborns* |

- Hand-to-mouth movements
- Mouth and tongue movements
- Sucking motions
- Rooting movements
- Clenched fists
- Kicking of legs
- Crying (a late sign of hunger; may result in shut-down and poor feeding if needs are not met)

Some infants cluster several feedings at frequent intervals and then wait a longer time before nursing again. It is best to maintain flexibility during the early weeks. However, if the infant has not nursed for 3 hours, tell the mother to gently waken the infant and try to breastfeed.

If feedings are too short, the infant may get little milk or only the foremilk. It may take as long as 5 minutes for the woman's let-down reflex to occur. The infant will soon be hungry again if he or she does not receive the richer hindmilk. This can frustrate the mother because her infant wants to "eat all the time." Engorgement will occur if milk is not removed from the breasts, and milk production will decrease or stop. Mothers should be taught how to recognize signs of early hunger in their infant. Crying is usually a late sign of hunger (Box 9-5).

The infant should nurse at least 10 minutes on the first breast, or longer if still nursing vigorously. The mother should then remove the infant from the first breast and have the infant nurse at the second breast until he or she is satisfied. The total duration of early feedings should be at least 15 minutes per breast. The mother should not switch back and forth between breasts several times during a feeding session.

Infants who breastfeed usually do not swallow much air. To burp the infant, the mother can hold the infant in a sitting position in her lap and pat or rub the back to assist (Figure 9-13). Alternately, the infant can be placed against the mother's shoulder for burping. A soft cloth protects the adult's clothing from any "spit-ups."

The mother should begin the next nursing session using the breast that was used last in the previous session. A safety pin attached to her bra helps her to remember which breast to use each time.

The Sleepy Infant

Some newborns are sleepy and need to be awakened for feedings until a routine of feeding on demand is established. To bring the infant to an alert state in prepara-

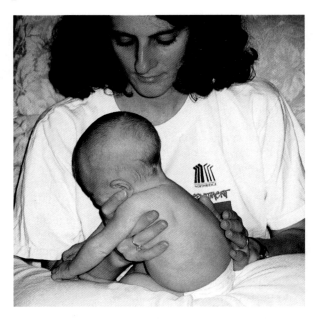

FIGURE **9-13** The mother can burp the infant by holding the infant in a sitting position on her lap, supporting the chin and chest, and gently patting or rubbing the back. In this position the mother can see the infant's face in case of spit-ups.

tion for feeding, the infant should be unwrapped, the diaper can be changed, the mother should hold the infant upright and talk softly to him or her, or she may provide a gentle massage of the back, palms, or soles of the feet. When the infant is awake, feeding will be more successful.

The Fussy Infant

Some infants awaken from sleep crying lustily, eliminating the opportunity to observe for early cues of hunger (see Box 9-5). These infants must be calmed before successful feeding can be attempted. The infant is wrapped snugly (swaddled) and held close. The mother should talk calmly to the infant. When the infant calms, feeding can begin.

Stiffening and crying after feeding starts can indicate a sore mouth from thrush, gas, cramps, or some illness that requires a health care provider's intervention. Collaboration with a lactation consultant is advisable.

Flat or Inverted Nipples

To help the nipples become erect for feedings, the mother can gently roll them between her thumb and forefinger.

Supplemental Feedings and Nipple Confusion

Supplemental feedings of formula or water should not be offered to the healthy newborn who is breastfeeding.

Successful breastfeeding is based on supply and demand. The hungry infant will nurse and stimulate maternal milk production to meet physiological needs. A form of "imprinting" may occur if a newborn is given a bottle of formula and finds it easy to obtain fluid from the nipple with minimal effort. When the infant is then placed at the breast, considerably more effort is needed to obtain the breast milk. As a result, the hungry infant may become fretful and irritable, which causes the mother to lose confidence and decide the infant prefers the formula and artificial nipple. This is often called "nipple confusion." When lactation is firmly established, usually after the neonatal period, the use of a pacifier to meet nonnutritional sucking needs will not cause nipple confusion (Biancuzzo, 1999).

Breast Engorgement

Early, regular, and frequent nursing helps to prevent breast engorgement. If engorgement does occur and the breast and areola are very tense and distended, the mother can pump her breasts to get the milk flow started and soften the areola. She may use a breast pump or manual expression of milk. Cold applications between feedings and heat just before feedings may help to reduce discomfort and engorgement.

Manual massage of all segments of the breasts helps to soften them and express milk downward in the duct system. The mother cups her hands around the breast near the chest wall and firmly slides her fingers forward toward the nipple. She rotates her hands to massage all areas of the breast.

Nipple Trauma

Cracks, blisters, redness, and bleeding may occur. Correct positioning of the infant is the best preventive measure. Feeding formula at this time can worsen the trauma and pain because it is likely to cause engorgement as less milk is removed. Warm water compresses applied to the breasts offer some relief. Rubbing a small amount of breast milk into the nipples may aid healing. Ointments are not effective; if used, they should be removed before nursing.

Hygiene

The mother should not use soap on her breasts. She should wear a supportive and not excessively tight bra 24 hours a day.

SPECIAL BREASTFEEDING SITUATIONS
Multiple Births

Twins can be fed one at a time or simultaneously. The mother's body adjusts the milk supply to the greater demand.

The mother may want to use the crisscross hold when nursing simultaneously. She will need help to position two infants at the breast in a cradle hold in each arm. She positions the first infant in a cradle hold, then her helper positions the second infant at the other breast in the crook of her arm. Their bodies cross over each other. The infants and the mother's arm are supported with pillows.

Premature Birth

Breastfeeding is especially good for a preterm infant because of its immunological advantages. If the infant cannot nurse, the mother can pump her breasts and freeze the milk for gavage (tube) feedings. See Chapter 13 for further information on the preterm infant.

When nursing the preterm or small infant, the mother may prefer the cross cradle hold. She holds the infant's head with the hand opposite the breast that she will use to nurse. She uses the same arm to support the infant's body. The hand on the same side as the nursing breast is used to guide the breast toward the infant's mouth.

Delayed Feedings

When breastfeeding must be temporarily delayed, the mother should be taught how to pump her milk in order to resume full breastfeeding (Figure 9-14).

STORING AND FREEZING BREAST MILK

Milk stored at room temperature over 4 hours has an increased potential for bacterial contamination. Various commercial containers are available for the storage of breast milk, each with advantages and disadvantages. The container size should hold about as much milk as the infant will consume at one feeding.

Milk may be safely stored in glass or hard plastic. Leukocytes may stick to the glass but are not destroyed. Several types of plastic bottles are available in stores. Clear hard plastic bottles are made of *polycarbonate* and, although little research is available, they are considered safe for storing and freezing milk. Dull or cloudy hard plastic bottles are *polystyrene* or milky white *polypropylene*. Polystyrene bottles are not designed for frozen milk storage. Polymers become unstable when heating after freezing. When used for freezing, polypropylene bottles alter the lysozyme, lactoferrin, and vitamin C content of breast milk. *Polyethylene* containers are usually clear plastic bags that may be at risk for puncture and invasion by microorganisms; some brands contain a special nylon between the polyethylene layers to reduce the puncture risk. The loss of lysozyme and fat is significant, and some valuable antibodies that adhere to polyethylene are lost to the infant.

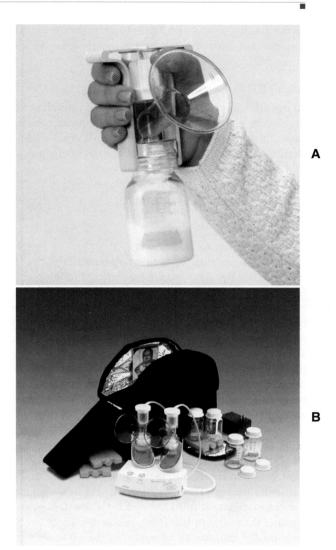

FIGURE **9-14** Breast pumps. Breast pumps can be manual **(A)**, electric **(B)**, or battery operated and pump directly into a bottle or freezer bag. One or both breasts can be pumped, and suction pressure is adjustable. Most hospitals and breastfeeding clinics help new mothers establish breastfeeding and breast pumping schedules to fit their individual needs.

Milk can be thawed in the refrigerator for 24 hours (best to preserve immunoglobulins) or by holding the container under running lukewarm water or placing it in a container of lukewarm water, rotating (not shaking) the bottle often. Microwaving is not advised because it destroys some immune factors and lysozyme contained in the milk and can develop hot spots because of uneven heating.

Milk can be stored in the refrigerator (4° C [39° F]) up to 24 hours without significant changes occurring or in the freezer ($-4°$ C [$-20°$ F]) for up to 3 months. Freezing can destroy some antimicrobial factors in the breast milk.

MATERNAL NUTRITION

To maintain her own nutrient stores while providing for the infant, the mother needs 500 additional calories each day over her nonpregnant diet (see Table 4-4). She should choose foods from each of the following groups in the food guide pyramid:

- Meat, fish, poultry, eggs, beans, and nuts
- Milk and other dairy products
- Vegetables
- Fruits
- Breads, cereals, and grains

She needs to drink fluids to satisfy her thirst (about 8 to 10 glasses per day), excluding those containing caffeine. Women with lactose intolerance may use substitutes such as tofu, soy milk, and canned salmon with bones as a substitute for milk products. A calcium supplement is probably needed to prevent maternal bone loss. The health care provider usually recommends that the nursing mother continue taking prenatal vitamins during lactation, although routine supplementation has been shown to be unnecessary for the well-nourished mother.

Some foods eaten by the mother may change the taste of the milk or cause the infant to have gas. Foods that often cause problems are chocolate, cabbage, beans, and broccoli. If the mother suspects that a particular food is causing fussiness or gas in the infant, she can eliminate it from her diet for a few days to determine if the infant has fewer problems. These problems do not indicate an allergy to breast milk, only irritation with some food by-product contained in the milk.

Many medications taken by the mother are secreted in breast milk but in varying concentrations depending on the drug. In general, timing the drug dose so that it passes its peak of action before the infant's nursing sessions can reduce the amount delivered to the infant.

NURSING **TIP**

Lactation uses fat stores from pregnancy to produce milk, which assists with maternal weight loss.

WEANING

Gradual weaning is preferred to abrupt weaning. Abrupt weaning can cause engorgement and lead to mastitis; it can also be upsetting to the infant.

There is no one best time to wean. Even a short period of breastfeeding provides the infant with many immunological and digestive advantages. As the infant matures, he or she will gradually become less interested in the breast, especially when solid foods are added to the diet around 6 months.

The nurse can teach mothers the following tips when she wants to wean her infant:

- Eliminate one feeding at a time. Wait several days and eliminate another one. The young infant will need formula from a bottle; the older infant may be weaned from the breast to a cup.
- Omit daytime feedings first, starting with the one in which the infant is least interested.
- Eliminate the infant's favorite feeding last. This will often be the early morning or bedtime feeding.
- Expect the infant to need "comfort nursing" if he or she is tired, ill, or uncomfortable.

If the mother must wean abruptly for some reason, breast engorgement is likely to occur. A supportive bra, ice packs, analgesics or cabbage leaves applied to the breasts may relieve discomfort (Schanlen, 2001). Breast pumping is not advised because the breast must remain full enough to decrease the milk supply cycle.

FORMULA FEEDING

Women choose to formula feed for many reasons. Some are embarrassed by breastfeeding or may have little social support. Others are uncomfortable when they cannot see the amount of milk the infant takes at each feeding. Women who have many other commitments and cannot maintain the flexibility needed when lactation is established may find that formula feeding is the only realistic choice. A few women must take medications or have other illnesses that make breastfeeding unwise. Regardless of the reason for choosing to formula feed, the nurse should fully support the mother and reassure her that her infant can receive good nutrition and emotional closeness.

TYPES OF INFANT FORMULAS

Before the first formula feeding, most hospitals have the policy of offering water to the newborn to assure patency of the gastrointestinal tract. If the infant sucks, swallows, and retains the water, formula is then offered. If the infant has an anomaly such as tracheoesophageal fistula (see Chapter 27), aspiration can occur. Management of water aspiration involves less risk than aspiration of formula.

Most formulas are modifications of cow's milk. Similac and Enfamil are examples of *cow's milk-based formulas.* Infants who do not tolerate cow's milk formulas or who come from a family with many allergies may be given soy or protein hydrolysate formulas. *Soy formulas* include ProSobee and Isomil; Nutramigen is a *protein hydrolysate* formula. Other formulas are available to meet special needs, such as those of the preterm infant or the infant with phenylketonuria (PKU).

Common formulas are available in the following three forms:

- Ready-to-feed, either in cans or in glass bottles
- Concentrated liquid
- Powdered

NURSING **TIP**

Overdilution or underdilution of concentrated liquid or powdered formulas can result in serious illness.

PREPARATION

The parent should wash the hands before preparing formula and feeding the infant. Bottles and nipples can be washed in hot soapy water using a nipple brush and rinsed well. Bottles can be washed in a dishwasher, but nipples should be washed by hand to slow their deterioration. Bottles of formula can be prepared one at a time or a 24-hour supply can be prepared. Formula should be refrigerated promptly and kept refrigerated until ready to use.

Ready-to-feed formulas require no dilution. Diluting them with water reduces the amount of nutrients the infant receives and can be dangerous. Ready-to-feed formula for home use comes in cans. The mother should wash the can's lid and open it with a freshly washed can opener. She then pours the approximate amount the infant will take at a feeding into a bottle and caps the bottle.

Concentrated liquid formula also comes in a can. After washing the can and opening it, the mother pours recommended proportions of concentrated liquid formula and tap water into the bottles and caps them. The usual proportions are one part concentrated liquid formula plus one part tap water. Water for formula dilution does not need to be boiled unless its safety is questionable.

Powdered formula is a popular choice for nursing mothers who want to feed their infant an occasional bottle of formula. The parent measures the amount of tap water into the bottle and adds the number of scoops recommended for that quantity.

Sterilization is not required unless the quality of the water is in doubt. Bottled cow's milk or evaporated milk for infant formula are nutritionally inadequate and stress the kidneys of the newborn and young infant.

FEEDING THE INFANT

Formula is digested more slowly than breast milk. Most formula-fed infants initially feed about every 3 to 4 hours. The formula-feeding mother should also be encouraged to avoid rigid scheduling.

Many mothers prefer to warm the formula somewhat, but this is not necessary. Placing the bottle in a container of hot water takes the chill off the milk. Microwave heating of infant formula is *not* recommended, because uneven heating causes hot spots that can cause mouth burns in the infant.

The mother should hold the infant in a semi-upright position in a cradle hold. The nipple should be kept full of formula to reduce the amount of air the infant swallows (Figure 9-15). The infant is initially burped about every ½ to 1 ounce at first, with the amount between burps gradually increased as the stomach capacity enlarges. The infant is also burped at the end of a feeding. Slightly elevating the upper body at the end of the feeding reduces regurgitation.

If milk runs out of the infant's mouth during sucking, the nipple holes may be too large. The nipple should be discarded and replaced with a new one. Leftover

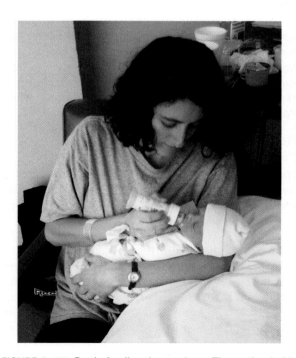

FIGURE **9-15** Bottle feeding the newborn. The mother holds the infant in a semi-upright position in a cradle hold. The nipple should be kept full of formula to reduce the amount of air the infant swallows. Holding the infant close encourages bonding just as breastfeeding does.

formula should be discarded because microorganisms from the mouth grow rapidly in warm formula.

The nurse should caution parents not to prop the bottle, even when the infant is older. Propping the bottle may cause the infant to aspirate formula and is associated with dental caries (cavities) and ear infections.

Fathers or significant others are encouraged to assist with feedings. When teaching new parents about infant care, the father or other support person should be involved to aid his or her involvement and attachment to the infant as well as enhance support for the mother.

DISCHARGE PLANNING

Discharge planning begins on admission or even earlier, when parents attend childbirth classes. Because mothers and infants are discharged quickly after birth, self-care and infant care teaching must often begin before the mother is psychologically ready to learn. Some birth facilities use *clinical pathways* (also called care maps, care paths, or multidisciplinary action plans [MAPs]) to ensure that important care and teaching are not overlooked (see Chapter 12). These plans guide the nurse to identify areas of special need that require referral as well as a means to keep up with the many facets of routine care needed after birth. The nurse must take every opportunity to teach during the short birth facility stay. Ample written materials for both new mother and infant care should be provided to refresh the memory of parents who may be tired and uncomfortable when teaching occurs.

POSTPARTUM SELF-CARE TEACHING

The nurse teaches the new mothers how to best care for themselves to reduce their risk for complications. The health care provider may prescribe more specific instructions for some patients.

Follow-Up Appointments

Most health care providers want to see postpartum women 2 weeks and 6 weeks after birth. The nurse should emphasize the importance of these follow-up appointments to verify that involution is proceeding normally and to identify any complications as soon as possible. Signs of problems the woman should report have been discussed in previous sections.

At the 2-week appointment the healing of the mother's perineum or cesarean incision is assessed. At the 6-week appointment the mother's general health

and recuperation from birth are assessed. The health care provider does a vaginal examination to check the uterus to ensure that involution is complete. Any incision is assessed for healing. The breasts are carefully examined for any signs of problems. Occasionally a complete blood count is done, and vitamins or iron supplements, or both, are ordered if anemia is present.

The woman has the opportunity to discuss any physical or psychological problems she may be having. The health care provider and the nurse usually inquire about how she is adapting to motherhood. Is she getting enough rest? How is breastfeeding coming along? Does she have help at home? How is the partner adapting to this new role?

Hygiene

A daily shower is refreshing and cleanses the skin of perspiration that may be more profuse in the first days after birth. Perineal care should be continued until the lochia stops. Douches and tampons should not be used for sanitary protection until after the 6-week checkup.

Sexual Intercourse

Coitus should be avoided until the episiotomy is fully healed and the lochia flow has stopped. Having sexual relations earlier can lead to infection, trauma, or another pregnancy. A water-soluble lubricant makes intercourse more comfortable for the woman.

Ovulation, and therefore pregnancy, can occur before the 6-week checkup. The health care provider usually discusses contraception with the woman, but the nurse must often clarify or reinforce any explanations. It is important to emphasize that breastfeeding is *not* a reliable contraceptive.

Diet

A well-balanced diet promotes healing and recovery from birth. Because constipation may be a problem, the mother is taught about high-fiber foods (e.g., whole-grain fruits and vegetables with the skins). Breastfeeding mothers should not try to lose weight while nursing. The formula-feeding mother should delay a strict reducing diet until released by her health care provider to do so. Most health care providers recommend that new mothers continue any prescribed prenatal vitamins until after the 6-week checkup.

Danger Signs

By teaching the mother changes to expect as she returns to the prepregnant state, the nurse gives her a framework to recognize when something is not progressing normally. Hemorrhage, infection, and thrombosis are the most common complications. The mother should report the following:

- Fever higher than 38° C (100.4° F)
- Persistent lochia rubra or lochia that has a foul odor
- Bright red bleeding, particularly if the lochia has changed to serosa or alba
- Prolonged afterpains, pelvic or abdominal pain, or a constant backache
- Signs of a urinary tract infection
- Pain, redness, or tenderness of the calf
- Localized breast tenderness or redness
- Discharge, pain, redness, or separation of any suture line (cesarean, perineal laceration, or episiotomy)
- Prolonged and pervasive feelings of depression or being let down; generally not enjoying life

NEWBORN DISCHARGE CARE

Discharge planning for the infant begins at birth. Because of short stays after birth, the nurse must teach the parents how to care for their newborn at every opportunity. Discharge teaching will then be more of a summary than an attempt to crowd all teaching into a short time.

Most newborns are checked by a health care professional within 48 hours of discharge. The infant is assessed at this early check for jaundice, feeding adequacy, urine and stool output, and behavior.

Infants are usually seen again at 6 to 8 weeks after birth to begin well-baby care. When providing discharge teaching, the nurse should emphasize the value of these visits. It should be explained that immunizations can be given to prevent many illnesses. The health care provider assesses the infant for growth and development, nutrition, and any problems the parents or infant are having. Teaching to prepare them for the infant's upcoming needs (anticipatory guidance) helps them to plan ahead to prevent injuries and promote development.

The nurse should teach parents the importance of using infant car safety seats and their correct use (Figure 9-16). The newborn should be placed in semi-reclining position in the car's back seat (never in the front), facing the rear until age 1 year *and* a weight of 22 pounds. The seat's harness is snugly fastened and the seat is secured to the automobile seat with the seat belt. Parents should consult their car's instruction manual for specific instructions on securing safety seats. The National Highway Traffic Safety Administration also has a toll-free number to help parents solve problems when using car safety seats: 800-424-9393.

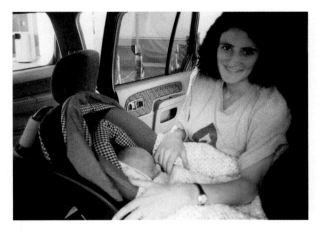

FIGURE **9-16** A new mother prepares to leave the birth facility. The infant is placed in a car seat that will be rear facing and secured by the car's seat belt for the ride home.

NURSING **TIP**

If siblings are waiting on return from the hospital, it is helpful if the father arrives carrying the infant. This leaves the mother's arms free for hugs before turning attention to the new child.

Air bags can prevent serious injuries to older children and adults in motor vehicle accidents. However, the air bag thrusts an infant toward the rear, causing a whiplike motion that can seriously injure the neck or head.

The nurse must emphasize to the parent that even in a low-impact accident, their infant will probably be thrown from their arms and become a "missile" in the car or even be ejected from the car. Death is a likely result.

New parents are often overwhelmed at the volume of information given in such a short time. They should be reassured that the birth facility staff is available 24 hours a day to help them to care for their infant and to refresh their memory if they forget what they have been told.

NURSING **TIP**

Advise parents to limit the newborn's exposure to crowds during the early weeks of life because infants have difficulty forming antibodies against infection until about age 2 months.

key points

- It is essential to consider each patient individually to better incorporate their culture and special needs into the plan of care.

- From its level at the umbilicus, the uterus should descend about one finger's width per day. It should no longer be palpable at 10 days postpartum.
- A slow pulse is common in the early postpartum period. A maternal pulse rate that would be high normal at other times may indicate hemorrhage or infection in the postpartum patient.
- A full bladder interferes with uterine contraction, which can lead to hemorrhage.
- Measures to prevent constipation should be emphasized at each assessment: fluid intake, a high-fiber diet, and activity.
- RhoGAM is given within 72 hours to the Rh-negative mother who delivers a Rh-positive infant.
- The postpartum check should include the status of the fundus, lochia, breasts, perineum, bowel and bladder elimination, vital signs, Homan's sign, pain and evidence of parent-infant attachment.
- Neonatal screening tests such as the phenylketonuria (PKU) test identify disorders that can be treated to reduce or prevent disability.
- The nurse must always keep the possibility of infant abductions in mind when providing care.
- The facility's specific protocol should be maintained during care. Most persons will not be offended by precautions but will be grateful for the security.
- Bonding and attachment require contact between parents and infant. The nurse should promote this contact whenever possible.

- More breast milk removed equals more milk produced. Early, regular, and frequent nursing promotes milk production and lessens engorgement.
- Duration of nursing on the first breast should be at least 10 minutes to stimulate milk production.
- The nursing mother needs 500 extra calories each day plus enough fluid to relieve thirst (about 8 to 10 glasses).
- Weaning from the breast should be gradual, starting with the feeding the infant is least interested in and ending with the one in which he or she has the most interest.
- The three major formula types are modified cow's milk, soy protein, or protein hydrolysate.
- They are available in ready-to-feed, concentrated liquid, or powdered form. Dilution, if required, must be followed exactly according to instructions.
- Discharge planning should take place with every instance of mother or newborn nursing care as the nurse teaches the mother normal findings, significance, and what to report. Written materials should be provided to augment all teaching.

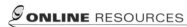 ONLINE RESOURCES

International Lactation Consultant Association: http://www.ilca.org

Breastfeeding Support Consultants Center for Lactation Education: http://www.bsccenter.org

La Leche League International: http://www.lalecheleague.org

REVIEW QUESTIONS *Choose the most appropriate answer.*

1. Which of these assessments is expected 24 hours after birth?
   1. Scant amount of lochia alba on the perineal pad
   2. Fundus firm and in the midline of the abdomen
   3. Breasts distended and hard with flat nipples
   4. Slight separation of a perineal laceration

2. Nursing the infant promotes uterine involution because it:
   1. Uses maternal fat stores accumulated during pregnancy
   2. Stimulates additional secretion of colostrum
   3. Causes the pituitary to secrete oxytocin to contract the uterus
   4. Promotes maternal formation of antibodies

3. The best way to maintain the newborn's temperature immediately after birth is to:
   1. Dry the infant thoroughly, including the hair
   2. Give the infant a bath using warm water
   3. Feed 1 to 2 ounces of warmed formula
   4. Limit the length of time parents hold the infant

4. Eight hours postpartum the woman states she prefers the nurse take care of the infant. The woman talks in detail about her birthing experience on the phone and to anyone who enters her room. She complains of being hungry, thirsty, and sleepy and is unable to focus on the infant care teaching offered to her. The nurse would interpret this behavior as:
   1. Inability to bond with the infant
   2. Development of postpartum psychosis
   3. Inability to assume the parenting role
   4. The normal taking-in phase of the puerperium

5. A new mother asks how often she should nurse her infant. The nurse should tell her to feed the infant:
   1. On a regular schedule, every 2 hours
   2. On demand, about every 2 to 3 hours
   3. At least every 4 hours during the day
   4. Whenever the infant is interested

Nursing Care of Women with Complications Following Birth

objectives

1. Define each key term listed.
2. Describe signs and symptoms for each postpartum complication.
3. Identify factors that increase a woman's risk for developing each complication.
4. Explain nursing measures that reduce a woman's risk for developing specific postpartum complications.
5. Describe additional problems that may result from the original postpartum complication.
6. Describe the medical management of postpartum complications.
7. Explain general and specific nursing care for each complication.

key terms

atony (ĂT-ŏ-nē, p. 240)
curettage (KŪ-rĕ-tăhzh, p. 243)
endometritis (ĕn-dō-mē-TRĪ-tĭs, p. 244)
hematoma (hē-mă-TŌ-mă, p. 242)
hypovolemic shock (hī-pō-vō-LĒ-mĭk shŏk, p. 238)
involution (ĭn-vō-LOO-shŭn, p. 247)
mania (MĀ-nē-ă, p. 249)
mastitis (măs-TĪ-tĭs, p. 246)
mood (p. 248)
psychosis (sī-KŌ-sĭs, p. 248)
puerperal sepsis (pū-ĔR-pĕr-ăl SĔP-sĭs, p. 244)
subinvolution (sŭb-ĭn-vō-LŪ-shŭn, p. 247)

Most women who give birth recover from pregnancy and childbirth uneventfully. However, some experience complications after birth that slow their recovery and may interfere with their ability to assume their new role.

A woman can have any medical problem after a birth, but most complications related to childbirth fall into one of the following six categories:

- Shock
- Hemorrhage

- Thromboembolic disorders
- Puerperal infections
- Subinvolution of the uterus
- Mood disorders

SHOCK

Shock is defined as a condition in which the cardiovascular system fails to provide essential oxygen and nutrients to the cells. Causes of postpartum shock related to childbearing include the following:

- *Cardiogenic shock:* From pulmonary embolism, anemia, hypertension, or cardiac disorders
- *Hypovolemic shock:* Caused by postpartum hemorrhage or blood clotting disorders
- *Anaphylactic shock:* Caused by allergic responses to drugs administered
- *Septic shock:* Caused by puerperal infection

The inherent danger of obstetric shock is that body compensation can mask the signs until the condition becomes life threatening. The vigilance of the nurse can detect early signs and enable prompt intervention.

HEMORRHAGE

Postpartum hemorrhage occurs in about 4% of deliveries (Hacker & Moore, 1998) and is traditionally defined as blood loss greater than 500 ml after vaginal birth or 1000 ml after cesarean birth. Because the average-size woman has 1 to 2 liters of added blood volume from pregnancy, she can tolerate this amount of blood loss better than would otherwise be expected.

Most cases of hemorrhage occur immediately after birth, but some are delayed up to several weeks, as follows:

- *Early postpartum hemorrhage* occurs within 24 hours of birth.
- *Late postpartum hemorrhage* occurs after 24 hours until 6 weeks after birth.

The major risk of hemorrhage is *hypovolemic* (low-volume) *shock,* which interrupts blood flow to body cells. This prevents normal oxygenation, nutrient delivery, and waste removal at the cellular level. Although a less dramatic problem, anemia is likely to occur after hemorrhage.

HYPOVOLEMIC SHOCK

Hypovolemic shock occurs when the volume of blood is depleted and cannot fill the circulatory system. The woman can die if blood loss does not stop and if the blood volume is not corrected.

Body's response to hypovolemia. The body initially responds to reduced blood volume with increased heart and respiratory rates. These reactions increase the oxygen content of each erythrocyte (red blood cell) and more quickly circulate the remaining blood. *Tachycardia (rapid heart rate) is usually the first sign of inadequate blood volume (hypovolemia).* The first blood pressure change is a narrow pulse pressure (a falling systolic pressure and rising diastolic pressure). The blood pressure continues falling and eventually cannot be detected.

Blood flow to nonessential organs gradually stops to make more blood available for vital organs, specifically the heart and brain. This change causes the woman's skin and mucous membranes to become pale, cold, and clammy (moist). As blood loss continues, flow to the brain falls, resulting in mental changes, such as anxiety, confusion, restlessness, and lethargy. As blood flow to the kidneys decreases, they respond by conserving fluid. Urine output decreases and eventually stops.

> ⭐NURSING **TIP**
> Because postpartum women often have a slow pulse, suspect hypovolemic shock or infection if the pulse rate is higher than 100 beats/min.

Medical management. Medical management of hypovolemic shock resulting from hemorrhage may include any of the following actions:

- Stopping the blood loss
- Giving IV fluids to maintain circulating volume and to replace fluids
- Giving blood transfusions to replace lost erythrocytes
- Giving oxygen to increase saturation of remaining blood cells; a pulse oximeter is used to assess oxygen saturation of the blood
- Placing an indwelling (Foley) catheter to assess urine output, which reflects kidney function

Nursing care. Routine postpartum care involves assessing vital signs every 15 minutes until stable so that the signs of postpartum hemorrhage are identified as early as possible. The woman should be observed closely for early signs of shock, such as tachycardia, pallor, cold and clammy hands, and decreased urine output. Decreased blood pressure may be a late sign of hypovolemic shock. Routine frequent assessment of lochia in the fourth stage of labor helps identify early postpartum hemorrhage. When the amount and character of lochia are normal and the uterus is firm but signs of hypovolemia are still evident, the cause may be a large hematoma. Excessive bright red bleeding despite a firm fundus may indicate a cervical or vaginal laceration. The occurrence of petechiae, bleeding from venipuncture sites, or oliguria may indicate a blood clotting problem. In the first hours postpartum the perineal pad should be weighed to determine the output amount, with 1 g equaling 1 ml (see p. 206). Intake and output should be recorded and intravenous (IV) therapy monitored. Oxygen saturation levels are also monitored in early postpartum hemorrhage.

Careful explanations to the mother and family are essential, and providing emotional support and maintaining the integrity of the woman's support system are key nursing roles. Even if the mother is separated from her infant, contact should be maintained concerning the infant's condition. Rooming-in should be established as soon as the woman's condition permits.

Intensive care may be required to allow invasive hemodynamic monitoring of the woman's circulatory status. Nursing Care Plan 10-1 specifies interventions for the woman at high risk for altered tissue perfusion related to hemorrhage.

ANEMIA

Anemia occurs after hemorrhage because of the lost erythrocytes. Anemia resulting from blood loss occurs suddenly, and the woman may be dizzy or lightheaded and is likely to faint. These symptoms are more likely to occur if she changes position quickly, particularly from a lying position to an upright one. Until her hemoglobin and hematocrit counts return to near-normal values, she will probably be exhausted and have difficulty meeting her needs and those of her infant.

Iron supplements are prescribed to provide adequate amounts of this mineral for manufacture of more erythrocytes. Many health care providers have the woman continue taking the remainder of her prenatal vitamins, which usually provide enough iron to correct mild anemia.

EARLY POSTPARTUM HEMORRHAGE

Early postpartum hemorrhage results from one of the following three causes:

NURSING CARE PLAN **10-1**

The Woman with Postpartum Hemorrhage

PATIENT DATA: A woman is admitted to the postpartum unit. She appears anxious and frightened, and her lochia has saturated three perineal pads in the last hour.

SELECTED NURSING DIAGNOSIS   *Risk for ineffective tissue perfusion related to excessive blood loss secondary to uterine atony or birth injury*

Outcomes	Nursing Interventions	Rationales

The woman's blood pressure and pulse will be within 10% of her values when she was admitted.
 The woman will not have signs or symptoms of hypovolemic shock.
	1. Identify whether woman has added risk factors for postpartum hemorrhage.
	 2. Observe the following:
	   a. Fundus for height, firmness, and position
	   b. Lochia for color, quantity, and clots; count pads and degree of saturation (weigh pads for greater accuracy); check blood pressure, pulse, and respiratory rates per hospital protocol
	
	 3. Observe for less obvious signs of bleeding:
	   a. Constant trickle of brighter red blood with a firm fundus
	   b. Severe, poorly relieved pain, especially if accompanied by changes in the vital signs or shock signs and symptoms
	 4. Observe for other signs and symptoms of hypovolemic shock.
	 5. If signs of hemorrhage are noted, take appropriate actions according to the probable cause for hemorrhage:
	   a. Uterine atony: massage uterus until firm—do not overmassage; expel blood from uterine cavity when uterus is firm; have breastfeeding woman nurse infant; notify registered nurse and/or health care provider for orders and medication if uterus does not become firm and stay firm.
	   b. Lacerations: notify registered nurse and/or health care provider to examine woman.
	   c. Hematomas on the vulva: place cold pack on the area.
		1. Women who have risk factors should be assessed more often than those who do not.
		 2. The fundus must be firm to compress bleeding vessels at the placenta site. Bladder distention interferes with uterine contraction and causes the fundus to be high and displaced to one side. A rising pulse rate is often first sign of inadequate blood volume. A rising pulse and falling blood pressure also occur. Most blood lost after birth is visible rather than concealed. Observing lochia provides an estimate of actual blood loss.
		 3. Most postpartum hemorrhage is caused by uterine atony, which often produces dramatic blood loss. However, blood loss from a laceration or hematoma can be significant, even though it is less obvious.
		
		 4. Excessive blood loss can result in hypovolemic shock.
		 5. Hemorrhage can cause death of a new mother if not promptly corrected. Most minor episodes of uterine atony are easily corrected with fundal massage and infant suckling. If the uterus does not remain firm, the health care provider examines the woman to identify and correct cause of bleeding. Oxytocin (Pitocin) infusions are often ordered to contract the uterus. Other drugs, such as methylergonovine (Methergine) or prostaglandin, may be needed. Excessive massage of uterus can tire it, possibly resulting in inability to contract. Trauma such as laceration or hematoma may require repair by

Continued

NURSING CARE PLAN 10-1—cont'd

Outcomes	Nursing Interventions	Rationales
		health care provider. Small hematomas on the vulva can be limited by cold applications because they reduce blood flow to area; cold applications also numb area and make woman more comfortable.

SELECTED NURSING DIAGNOSIS *Fear related to powerlessness*

Outcomes	Nursing Interventions	Rationales
Woman will be able to cope with the unexpected complication. Anxiety will be at a manageable level.	1. Identify woman's reaction to unexpected complication and correct misconceptions and exaggerations of fact or myth. 2. Be calm and reassuring when in contact with the woman. 3. Encourage verbalization of woman concerning her fears and perceptions. 4. Stay with the woman and her partner.	1. Supplying factual information reduces fear. Identifying reaction establishes basis for intervention. 2. Anxiety can be transferred by voice or body language. 3. This helps establish a basis for patient teaching and identification of fears. 4. Having a professional present promotes a feeling of security.

℘CRITICAL THINKING QUESTION

A woman is admitted to the postpartum unit after delivery of a 9-pound, 12-ounce infant. She voids 600 ml. The fundus is difficult to locate and lochia is heavy. What are the priority nursing actions?

- Uterine atony (the most common cause)
- Lacerations (tears) of the reproductive tract
- Hematomas in the reproductive tract

Table 10-1 summarizes the types of postpartum hemorrhage.

Uterine Atony

Atony describes a lack of normal muscle tone. The postpartum uterus is a large, hollow organ with three layers of muscle. The middle layer has interlacing "figure eight" fibers. The uterine blood supply passes through this network of muscle fibers to supply the placenta.

After the placenta detaches, the uterus normally contracts and the muscle fibers compress bleeding vessels. If the uterus is atonic, however, these muscle fibers are flaccid and do not compress the vessels. Uterine atony allows the blood vessels at the placenta site to bleed freely and usually massively.

Normal postpartum changes. After birth, the uterus should easily be felt through the abdominal wall as a firm mass about the size of a grapefruit. After the placenta is expelled, the fundus (top of uterus) is at the

umbilicus level and then begins descending at a rate of about 1 finger's width (1 cm) each day.

Lochia rubra should be dark red. The amount of lochia during the first few hours should be no more than one saturated perineal pad per 1 hour. (Perineal pads containing cold packs absorb less than regular perineal pads.) A few small clots may appear in the drainage, but large clots are not normal.

✹NURSING **TIP**

To determine blood loss most accurately, weigh perineal pads before and after applying them. One gram of weight equals about 1 ml of blood lost.

Characteristics of uterine atony. When uterine atony occurs, the woman's uterus is difficult to feel and, when found, it is boggy (soft). The fundal height is high, often above the umbilicus. If the bladder is full, the uterus is higher and is pushed to one side rather than located in the midline of the abdomen (Figure 10-1). The uterus may or may not be soft if the bladder is full. A

table 10-1 *Types of Early Postpartum Hemorrhage*

	UTERINE ATONY	LACERATIONS	HEMATOMA
Characteristics	Soft, high uterine fundus that is difficult to feel through the woman's abdominal wall Heavy lochia, often with large clots or sometimes a persistent moderate flow Bladder distention that causes uterus to be high and usually displaces it to one side Possible signs of hypovolemic shock	Continuous trickle of blood that is brighter than normal lochia Fundus that is usually firm Onset of hypovolemic shock that may be gradual and easily overlooked	If visible, blue or purplish mass on the vulva Severe and poorly relieved pain and/or pressure in vulva, pelvis, or rectum Large amount of blood lost into tissues, which causes signs and symptoms of hypovolemic shock Lochia that is normal in amount and color
Contributing factors	Bladder distention Abnormal or prolonged labor Overdistended uterus Multiparity (more than 5 births) Use of oxytocin during labor Medications that relax uterus Operative birth Low placental implantation	Rapid labor Use of instruments such as forceps or vacuum extractor during birth	Prolonged or rapid labor Large infant Use of forceps or vacuum extractor

full bladder interferes with the ability of the uterus to contract and, if not corrected, eventually leads to uterine atony.

Lochia is increased and may contain large clots. The bleeding may be dramatic but may also be just above normal for a long time. Some lochia will be retained in the relaxed uterus because the cavity is enlarged. Thus the true amount of blood loss may not be immediately apparent. Collection of blood within the uterus further interferes with contraction and worsens uterine atony and postpartum hemorrhage.

A woman who has risk factors for postpartum hemorrhage (see Table 10-1) should have more frequent postpartum assessments of the uterus, lochia, and vital signs.

Medical management and nursing care. Care of the woman with uterine atony combines nursing and medical measures. When the uterus is boggy, it should be massaged until firm (see Box 9-2). It should not be overly massaged. Because the uterus is a muscle, excessive stimulation to contract it will tire it and can actually worsen uterine atony. If the uterus is firmly contracted, it should be left alone.

Bladder distention is an easily corrected cause of uterine atony. The nurse should catheterize the woman if she cannot urinate in the bathroom or in a bedpan. Any clots or blood pooled in the vagina should be expelled by pressing toward the vagina *after the uterus is firm.* Most health care providers include an order for catheterization to avoid delaying this corrective measure. First the uterus is massaged to firmness, and then the bladder is emptied to keep the uterus firm.

The infant suckling at the breast stimulates the woman's posterior pituitary gland to secrete oxytocin, which causes uterine contraction. A dilute oxytocin (Pitocin) IV infusion is the most common drug ordered to control uterine atony. Other drugs to increase uterine tone include methylergonovine (Methergine) or prostaglandin such as carboprost. Methylergonovine increases blood pressure and should not be given to a woman with hypertension.

The health care provider may examine the woman in the delivery or operating room to determine the source of her bleeding and correct it. Rarely, a hysterectomy is needed to remove the bleeding uterus that does not re-

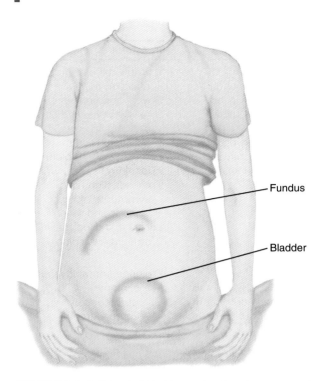

FIGURE **10-1** A distended bladder pushes the uterus upward and usually to one side of the abdomen. The fundus may be boggy or firm. If not emptied, a distended bladder can result in uterine atony and hemorrhage because it interferes with normal contraction of the uterus.

spond to other measures. The woman should have nothing by mouth until her bleeding is controlled.

★ NURSING **TIP**

The woman who develops a hemorrhagic complication should be kept NPO until the health care provider evaluates her in case she needs a general anesthesia for correction of the problem.

Genital Trauma

Lacerations of the reproductive tract. Lacerations of the perineum, vagina, cervix, or area around the urethra (periurethral lacerations) can cause postpartum bleeding. The vascular beds are engorged during pregnancy, and bleeding can be profuse. Trauma is more likely to occur if the woman has a rapid labor or if forceps or a vacuum extractor are used. Blood lost in lacerations is usually a brighter red than lochia and flows in a continuous trickle. Typically, the uterus is firm.

Treatment. The health care provider should be notified if the woman has signs of a laceration—bleeding with a firmly contracted uterus. The injury is usually sutured in the delivery or operating room.

Nursing care. Signs and symptoms of a bleeding laceration should be reported. A continuous trickle of blood can result in as much or more blood loss than the dramatic bleeding associated with uterine atony. The woman should be given nothing by mouth (kept NPO) until further orders are received because she may need a general anesthetic for repair of the laceration. Genital trauma can cause long-term effects such as cystocele, prolapsed uterus, or urinary incontinence (see Chapter 11).

Hematomas of the reproductive tract. A hematoma is a collection of blood within the tissues. Hematomas resulting from birth trauma are usually on the vulva or inside the vagina. They may be easily seen as a bulging bluish or purplish mass. Hematomas deep within the vagina are not visible from the outside.

Discomfort after childbirth is normally minimal and easily relieved with mild analgesics. The woman with a hematoma usually has severe, unrelenting pain that analgesics do not relieve. Depending on the amount of blood in the tissues, she also may describe pressure in the vulva, pelvis, or rectum. She may be unable to urinate because of the pressure.

The woman does not have unusual amounts of lochia, but she may develop signs of concealed blood loss if the hematoma is large. Her pulse and respiratory rates rise, and her blood pressure falls. She may develop other signs of hypovolemic shock if blood loss into the tissues is substantial.

Risk factors for the development of a hematoma are listed in Table 10-1.

Treatment. Small hematomas usually resolve without treatment. Larger ones may require incision and drainage of the clots. The bleeding vessel is ligated or the area packed with a hemostatic material to stop bleeding.

Nursing care. An ice pack to the perineum is sufficient for most small perineal hematomas and requires no physician prescription. The nurse should observe and report for the classic symptom: excessive, poorly relieved pain. Signs of concealed blood loss accompanied by maternal complaints of severe pain, perineal or vaginal pressure, or the inability to void should be reported. The woman is kept NPO until the health care provider examines her and prescribes treatment.

LATE POSTPARTUM HEMORRHAGE

Late postpartum hemorrhage (after 24 hours to 6 weeks after birth) usually occurs after discharge from the hospital and usually results from the following:
- Retention of placental fragments
- Subinvolution of the uterus (discussed on pp. 247 and 248)

table 10-2	*Observation of Venous Thrombosis*	
LOCATION	**MANIFESTATIONS**	**PULMONARY EMBOLISM**
Superficial vein thrombosis	Tender, painful, hard, reddened area along warm vein; easily visible	Rare
Deep vein thrombosis	Increased pain and calf tenderness; leg edema; color and temperature changes; positive Homan's sign (may be present but is unreliable during the postpartum); occasional fever rarely over 38.3° C (101° F)	Possible

Placental fragments are more likely to be retained if the placenta does not separate cleanly from its implantation site after birth. Clots form around these retained fragments and slough several days later, sometimes carrying the retained fragments with them. Retained placental fragments are more likely to occur if the placenta is manually removed (removed by hand rather than being pushed away from the uterine wall spontaneously as the uterus contracts). It is also more likely to occur if the placenta grows more deeply into the uterine muscle than is normal.

Treatment. Treatment consists of drugs such as oxytocin, methylergonovine, or prostaglandins such as carboprost to contract the uterus. Firm uterine contraction often expels the retained fragments and no other treatment is needed. Ultrasonography may be used to identify remaining fragments. If bleeding continues, curettage (scraping or vacuuming the inner surface of the uterus) is done to remove small blood clots and placental fragments. Antibiotics are prescribed if infection is suspected.

Nursing care. The nurse should teach each postpartum woman what to expect about changes in the lochia (see p. 206). She should be taught to report signs of late postpartum hemorrhage to her health care provider:

- Persistent bright red bleeding
- Return of red bleeding after it has changed to pinkish or white

If a late postpartum hemorrhage occurs, the nurse assists in implementing drug and surgical treatment.

THROMBOEMBOLIC DISORDERS

A venous thrombosis is a blood clot within a vein. The size of the clot can increase as circulating blood passes over it and deposits more platelets, fibrin, and cells. It often causes an inflammation of the vessel wall. The pregnant woman is at increased risk for venous thrombosis because of the venous stasis that can occur from compression of the blood vessels by the heavy uterus or by pressure behind the knee when the legs are placed in stirrup leg supports for episiotomy repair. Blood vessel injury during cesarean section can also cause a thrombus. The levels of fibrinogen and other clotting factors normally increase during pregnancy, whereas clot-dissolving factors (such as the plasminogen activator and antithrombin III) are normally decreased, resulting in a state of hypercoagulability (increased susceptibility to develop blood clots). If the woman has varicose veins or remains on bed rest, her state of hypercoagulability places her at increased risk for thrombus formation.

There are three types of thromboembolic disorders:

- *Superficial vein thrombosis (SVT)* involves the saphenous vein of the lower leg and is characterized by a painful, hard, reddened, warm vein that is easily seen.
- *Deep vein thrombosis (DVT)* can involve veins from foot to femoral area and is characterized by pain, calf tenderness, leg edema, color changes, pain when walking, and sometimes a positive Homan's sign (pain when the foot is dorsiflexed), although the Homan's sign is not always reliable during the postpartum period.
- *Pulmonary embolism (PE)* occurs when the pulmonary artery is obstructed by a blood clot that breaks off (embolizes) and lodges in the lungs. It may have dramatic signs and symptoms, such as sudden chest pain, cough, dyspnea (difficulty breathing), decreased level of consciousness, and signs of heart failure. A small pulmonary embolism may have nonspecific signs and symptoms, such as shortness of breath, palpitations, hemoptysis (bloody sputum), faintness, and low-grade fever. Table 10-2 compares the manifestations and likelihood of pulmonary embolism of superficial vein thrombosis with those of deep vein thrombosis.

Treatment. Superficial vein thrombosis is treated with analgesics, local application of heat, and elevation of the legs to promote venous drainage. Deep vein thrombosis is treated similarly, with the addition of subcutaneous or IV heparin anticoagulation. Anticoagulant therapy is continued with heparin or warfarin (Coumadin) for 6 weeks after birth to minimize the risk of embolism.

Antibiotics are prescribed if infection is a factor. The woman with a pulmonary embolism is usually transferred to the intensive care unit.

Nursing care. The woman should be observed for signs and symptoms that suggest venous thrombosis before and after birth. Dyspnea, coughing, and chest pain suggest pulmonary embolism and must be reported immediately.

Prevention of thrombi is most important. Pregnant women should not cross their legs because it impedes venous blood flow. When the legs are elevated, there should not be sharp flexion at the groin or pressure in the popliteal space behind the knee, which would restrict venous flow. Measures to promote venous flow should be continued during and after birth because levels of clotting factors remain high for several weeks.

Early ambulation or range-of-motion exercises are valuable aids to preventing thrombus formation in the postpartum woman. Antiembolic stockings may be used if varicose veins are present. The nurse should teach the woman how to put on the stockings properly, because rolling or kinking of the stocking can further impede blood flow. If stirrups are used during birth or episiotomy repair, they should be padded to prevent pressure to the popliteal angle.

The woman who will be undergoing anticoagulant therapy at home should be taught how to give herself the drug and about signs of excess anticoagulation (prolonged bleeding from minor injuries, bleeding gums, nosebleeds, unexplained bruising). She should use a soft toothbrush and avoid minor trauma that can cause prolonged bleeding or a large hematoma. Home nursing visits are often prescribed to obtain blood for laboratory clotting studies and to help the woman cope with therapy. The antidote for a warfarin overdose is vitamin K.

PUERPERAL INFECTION

Puerperal sepsis is infection or septicemia after childbirth. Tissue trauma during labor, the open wound of the placental site, surgical incisions, cracks in the nipples of the breasts, and the increased pH of the vagina after birth are all risk factors for the postpartum woman. About 7% of women develop a fever of 38° C (100.4° F) or higher after the first postpartum day. Fever after cesarean section occurs in about 14% of patients (Hacker & Moore, 1998). The fever is most often caused by endometritis, an inflammation of the inner lining of the uterus. Blockage of the lochial flow because of retained placenta or clots increases susceptibility to infection. The danger of postpartum infection is that a local-

ized infection of the perineum, vagina, or cervix can ascend the reproductive tract and spread to the uterus, fallopian tubes, and peritoneum, causing peritonitis, a life-threatening condition. Table 10-3 lists characteristics, medical treatment, and nursing care for these infections. Regardless of their location or the causative organism, postpartum infections have several common features.

Manifestations. Puerperal (postpartum) fever is defined as a temperature of 38° C (100.4° F) or higher after the first 24 hours and on at least 2 days during the first 10 days after birth. Slight temperature elevations with no other signs of infection often occur during the first 24 hours because of dehydration. The nurse should look for other signs of infection if the woman's temperature is elevated, regardless of the time since birth. A pulse that is higher than expected and an elevated temperature often occur when the woman has an infection.

Other signs and symptoms of infection may be localized (in a small area of the body) or systemic (throughout the body).

White blood cells (leukocytes) are normally elevated during the early postpartum period to about 20,000 to 30,000 cells/dl, which limits the usefulness of the blood count to identify infection. Leukocyte counts in the upper limits are more likely to be associated with infection than lower counts.

> ⮞NURSING **TIP**
> Proper handwashing is the primary method to avoid the spread of infectious organisms. Gloves should be worn when in contact with any body secretion.

Treatment. The goals of medical treatment are to limit the spread of infection to other organs and eliminate the infection.

A culture and sensitivity sample from the site of the suspected infection is taken to determine what antibiotics will be most effective. A culture and sensitivity test requires 2 or 3 days to complete. In the meantime, antibiotics that are effective against typical organisms that cause the infection are given to limit the spread of infection to nearby structures.

Nursing care. Nursing care objectives focus on preventing infection and, if one occurs, on facilitating medical treatment. To achieve these goals, the nurse should do the following:

- Use and teach hygienic measures to reduce the number of organisms that can cause infection (e.g., handwashing, perineal care)
- Promote adequate rest and nutrition for healing
- Observe for signs of infection

table 10-3 *Postpartum Infections*

	WOUND INFECTIONS	ENDOMETRITIS (UTERUS)	URINARY TRACT	MASTITIS (BREAST)
Characteristics	Signs of inflammation (redness, edema, heat, pain) Separation of suture line Purulent drainage	Tender, enlarged uterus Prolonged, severe cramping Foul-smelling lochia Fever and other systemic signs of infection Signs of uterine sub-involution	Cystitis (bladder) Low temperature Burning, urgency, and frequency of urination Pyelonephritis (kidneys) High fever with a pattern of spikes Chills Pain in the costovertebral angle or flank Nausea and vomiting	Reddened, tender, hot area of the breast Edema and a feeling of heaviness in the breast Purulent drainage (may occur if an abscess forms)
Medical management	Culture and sensitivity of wound exudate Antibiotics	Culture and sensitivity test of uterine cavity Antibiotics by IV route initially	Clean-catch or catheterized urine specimen for culture and sensitivity testing Antibiotics (initially by IV route for pyelonephritis)	Antibiotics (usually oral, although may be IV initially if woman has an abscess) Incision and drainage of abscess
Nursing care	Aseptic/sterile technique for all wound care as indicated Teaching proper perineal hygiene to reduce fecal contamination Sitz baths for perineal wound infections	Teaching woman usual progression of lochia, because infection often occurs after discharge Fowler's position to facilitate drainage of infected lochia Analgesics Observation for absent bowel sounds, abdominal distention, and nausea or vomiting, which suggest spread of infection	Teaching perineal hygiene Encouraging fluid intake of 3 L/day Teaching which foods increase acidity of urine, such as apricots, cranberry juice, plums, and prunes	Teaching effective breastfeeding techniques Moist heat applications with a warm pack Warm shower before nursing to start milk flow Massaging of affected area to reduce congestion and start milk flow Regular and frequent nursing or pumping to keep breasts empty

- Teach signs of infection that the woman should report after discharge
- Teach the woman to take all of the antibiotics prescribed rather than stopping them after her symptoms go away
- Teach the woman how to apply perineal pads (front to back)

Women should be taught to wash their hands before and after performing self-care that may involve contact with secretions. The nurse should explore ways to help the woman get enough rest. Nursing Care Plan 10-2 details interventions for the woman at high risk for infection.

Ultimately, a woman's own body must overcome infection and heal any wound. Nutrition is an essential component of her body defenses. The nurse, and sometimes a dietitian, teaches her about foods that are high in protein (meats, cheese, milk, legumes) and vitamin C (citrus fruits and juices, strawberries, cantaloupe), because these nutrients are especially important for

---

NURSING CARE PLAN 10-2

The Woman with Postpartum Infection

PATIENT DATA: A woman is admitted to the postpartum unit after delivering a baby boy via cesarean section. Her husband is at her bedside, and she is resting in bed.

SELECTED NURSING DIAGNOSIS   *Risk for infection related to loss of skin integrity (cesarean incision) and increased risk factors (blood loss, invasive procedures)*

Outcomes	Nursing Interventions	Rationales
The woman will not have signs of infection as evidenced by an oral temperature below 38° C (100.4° F) and normal progression of lochia that does not have a foul odor. The woman will not self-contaminate.	1. Use handwashing when providing care. Teach woman personal hygiene measures, such as handwashing, perineal care, and regular changes of perineal pads.	1. Limits the transfer of infectious organisms between patients and from one area of the body to another. Regular pad changes also reduce the amount of time organisms have to multiply in its warm, dark, and moist environment.
	2. Determine vital signs every 4 hours or more frequently if signs of infection are present.	2. An elevated temperature and rising pulse are signs of infection. If they occur, woman should be assessed for other signs and symptoms of infection.
	3. Observe lochia for amount, color, and odor with vital signs.	3. Infection is evidenced by foul-smelling lochia that may be increased or decreased; it is sometimes brown.
	4. Observe the wound each shift for redness, edema, ecchymosis, discharge, and approximation (REEDA).	4. A wound infection is characterized by signs of inflammation. The suture line may separate if there is infection in the area.
	5. Maintain medical and surgical asepsis when in contact with the woman.	5. Reduces the potential for infection for the woman at risk because of complications postpartum.
	6. Teach woman wound care protocols and general hygiene.	6. Decreases the spread of infection by self-contamination.
	7. Promote fluid and nutritional intake. Record intake and output.	7. Adequate nutrition is essential for healing. Decreased output can indicate kidney shutdown.

?CRITICAL THINKING QUESTION

You are caring for a woman who had an emergency cesarean delivery and is 1 day postpartum. She is sleepy and asks the nurse to care for the infant. Her temperature at 8 AM was 38° C (100.4° F) and at 10 AM was 38.3° C (100.8° F). What nursing intervention should you provide?

---

healing. Foods high in iron to correct anemia include meats, enriched cereals and breads, and dark green, leafy vegetables.

MASTITIS AND BREASTFEEDING

Mastitis is an infection of the breast. It usually occurs about 2 or 3 weeks after giving birth (Figure 10-2). Mastitis occurs when organisms from the skin or the infant's mouth enter small cracks in the nipples or areolae. These cracks may be microscopic. Breast engorgement and inadequate emptying of milk are associated with mastitis.

Signs and symptoms of mastitis include the following:
- Redness and heat in the breast
- Tenderness
- Edema and a heaviness in the breast
- Purulent drainage (may or may not be present)

The woman usually has fever, chills, and other systemic signs and symptoms. If not treated, the infected

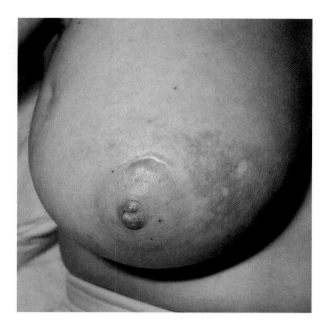

FIGURE **10-2** Mastitis. Mastitis typically occurs several weeks after birth in the woman who is breastfeeding. Bacteria usually enter the breast through small cracks in the nipples. Breast engorgement and milk stasis increase the risk for mastitis.

area becomes walled off and an abscess forms. The infection is usually outside the ducts of the breast, and the milk is not contaminated. However, if an abscess develops, it may rupture into the ducts and contaminate the milk.

Treatment. Antibiotics and continued removal of milk from the breast are the primary treatment for mastitis. Mild analgesics make the woman more comfortable. The woman may need an incision and drainage of the infected area if an abscess forms. IV antibiotics are usually needed to treat a breast abscess.

The mother can usually continue to breastfeed unless an abscess forms. If she should not nurse for any reason, she should pump her breasts and discard the milk. She should not wean her infant when she has mastitis because weaning leads to engorgement and stasis of milk, which worsens the mastitis.

Nursing care. The nursing mother should be taught proper breastfeeding techniques to reduce the risk for mastitis (see Chapter 9). Nursing care for mastitis centers on relieving pain and on maintaining lactation. Heat promotes blood flow to the area, comfort, and complete emptying of the breast. Moist heat can be applied with chemical packs. An inexpensive warm pack can be made by placing a warm wet cloth in a plastic bag and applying it to the breasts. A warm shower provides warmth and cleanliness and stimulates the flow of milk if done just before nursing.

Both breasts should be emptied regularly to reduce milk stasis, which increases the risk for abscess formation. If the affected breast is too painful for the mother to breastfeed, she can use a pump to empty it. She can massage the area of inflammation to improve milk flow and reduce stasis. Nursing first on the unaffected side starts the milk flow in both breasts and can improve emptying with less pain.

Other nursing measures include the following:
- Encouraging fluid intake, about 3 liters a day
- Wearing a good support bra to support the breasts and limit movement of the painful breast; the bra should not be too tight or it will actually cause milk stasis
- Supporting the woman emotionally and reassuring her that she can continue to breastfeed

SUBINVOLUTION OF THE UTERUS

Involution is the return of the uterus to its nonpregnant condition after birth. The muscles of the uterus contract and constrict the blood vessels at the placental site stopping the bleeding. Normally the uterus descends at the rate of 1 cm (one finger's width) per day and is no longer palpable by 12 days postpartum. The placental site heals by 6 weeks postpartum. *Subinvolution* is a slower-than-expected return of the uterus to its nonpregnant condition. Infection and retained fragments of the placenta are the most common causes. Typical signs of subinvolution are as following:
- Fundal height greater than expected for the amount of time since birth
- Persistence of lochia rubra or a slowed progression through the three phases
- Pelvic pain, heaviness, fatigue

Treatment. Medical treatment is selected to correct the cause of the subinvolution. It may include any or all of the following measures:
- Methylergonovine (Methergine) to maintain firm uterine contraction
- Antibiotics for infection
- Dilation of the cervix and curettage to remove fragments of the placenta from the uterine wall

Nursing care. The mother has almost always been discharged when subinvolution of the uterus occurs. All new mothers should be taught about the normal changes to expect so they can recognize a departure from the normal pattern. Women should report fever, persistent pain, persistent red lochia (or return of bleeding after it has changed), or foul-smelling vaginal discharge. The woman should be taught how to palpate the fundus and what normal changes to expect.

The woman may be admitted to the hospital on the gynecology unit. Nursing care involves assisting with medical therapy and providing analgesics and other comfort measures. Specific nursing care depends on whether the subinvolution results from infection or another cause.

DISORDERS OF MOOD

A mood is a pervasive and sustained emotion that can color one's view of life. "Postpartum blues," or "baby blues," are common after birth. The woman has periods when she feels let down, but overall she finds pleasure in life and in her new role as mother. Her roller-coaster emotions are usually self-limiting as she adapts to the changes in her life.

A psychosis involves serious impairment of one's perception of reality. Postpartum depression and postpartum psychosis are disorders that are more serious than postpartum blues.

POSTPARTUM DEPRESSION

Postpartum depression is a nonpsychotic depressive illness that is usually manifested within 2 weeks after delivery and affects 15% of postpartum women (Stables, 1999). The depression is noted by those having close contact with the woman. Signs and symptoms may include the following:

- Lack of enjoyment in life
- Disinterest in others; loss of normal give-and-take in relationships
- Intense feelings of inadequacy, unworthiness, guilt, inability to cope
- Loss of mental concentration
- Disturbed sleep
- Constant fatigue and feelings of ill health

Postpartum depression strains the coping mechanisms of the entire family at a time when all are adapting to the birth of a child. As a result of the strained relationships, communication is often impaired and the depressed woman may withdraw further, which places her further away from her support system. The woman usually remains in touch with reality.

✴ NURSING TIP

If a postpartum woman seems depressed, the nurse should not assume that she has the common "baby blues" or that she will "snap out of it." Explore her feelings to determine if they are persistent and pervasive.

Treatment. Treatment of postpartum depression includes psychotherapy and increased social support and may include antidepressant medications. The influence of hormones on mood changes before, during, and after menstruation supports the theory that fluctuating hormones postpartum may also have an effect on the woman's mood. Falling estrogen levels affect the dopamine levels in the blood, which are thought to be responsible for emotion and thought. Therefore hormonal skin patches are sometimes used in the treatment of postpartum depression (Stables, 1999). Referral to follow-up with a case manager and counseling that includes the woman's partner and family is essential treatment.

Nursing care. The nurse is more likely to encounter the woman with postpartum depression in the health care provider's office or an outpatient clinic. The nurse may help the mother by being a sympathetic listener. Women may be reluctant to express dissatisfaction with their new role, especially if they have waited a long time for a child.

The nurse should elicit the new mother's feelings about motherhood and her infant. She must observe for complaints of sleeplessness or chronic fatigue. The mother's expressions of feeling should be pursued to help her better express them. The nurse must help her see that there is hope for her problem yet not minimize her feelings by saying things such as, "You'll get over it."

Isolation can be both a cause and a result of depression. The new mother should be helped to identify sources of emotional support among her family and friends. Many of her friends may have stopped including her in activities because she has withdrawn from them. She may not have the emotional energy to reach out to them again.

The woman who is physically depleted often has an exaggerated feeling of let-down and depression. The nurse should determine whether she is getting enough exercise, sleep, and proper nutrition to improve her physical health and sense of well-being. The mother should be helped to identify ways to meet her own needs and be reassured that she is not being selfish.

A new mother may feel guilty because she is not happy all the time. The nurse can explain that these feelings are not right or wrong—feelings simply exist. She should be referred to support groups if these are available. Discussing her feelings with others who have similar difficulties can help her realize that she is not alone.

POSTPARTUM PSYCHOSIS

Women experiencing a postpartum psychosis have an impaired sense of reality. Psychosis is much less common than postpartum depression. A woman may have any psychiatric disorder, but the following are more often encountered:

- *Bipolar disorder:* a disorder characterized by episodes of mania (hyperactivity, excitability, euphoria, and a feeling of being invulnerable) and depression
- *Major depression:* a disorder characterized by deep feelings of worthlessness, guilt, serious sleep and appetite disturbance, and sometimes delusions about the infant's being dead

Postpartum psychosis can be fatal for both mother and infant. The mother may endanger herself and her infant during manic episodes because she uses poor judgment and has a sense of being invulnerable. Suicide and infanticide are possible, especially during depressive episodes.

If the woman has resources, such as private health insurance or a health maintenance organization (HMO), case managers, home visits, and outpatient psychiatric counseling may be available. In other cases, social workers within the community may refer the woman for counseling. In some cases an inpatient psychiatric treatment center is the appropriate environment for treatment. Virtually all psychotropic medications prescribed for psychoses pass through the breast milk and will affect the newborn infant. Therefore breastfeeding is contraindicated when psychotropic medications are prescribed for the mother.

THE HOMELESS MOTHER AND NEWBORN

Homelessness is defined as a lack of a permanent home and is not limited to women who must live on the street. Some women live in single-room hotels, and others stay with friends or live in the garage facility of extended family. It is estimated that homeless women are 29% of the current homeless population (Geissler & Braucht, 1999). Homeless women often have difficulty accessing care, receive care from different health care providers at different sites, and have incomplete medical records. Follow-up is difficult. Before discharging a mother with her newborn infant, it is essential to determine that she has a place to go and has a way of accessing help for herself or her newborn. The nurse can be a key link in facilitating referrals to outreach programs, support services, counseling, shelters and follow-up medical care.

key points

- The nurse must be aware of women who are at higher risk for postpartum hemorrhage and assess them more often.
- A constant small trickle of blood can result in significant blood loss, as can a larger one-time hemorrhage.
- Pain that is persistent and more severe than expected is characteristic of a hematoma in the reproductive tract.
- It is essential to identify and limit a local infection before it spreads into the bloodstream.
- The nurse should teach new mothers about normal postpartum changes and indications of problems they should report.
- Early ambulation can prevent thrombosis formation.
- Types of obstetric shock include *cardiogenic* (from anemia or cardiac disorders), *hypovolemic* (from hemorrhage), *anaphylactic* (from a drug response), and *septic* (caused by puerperal infection).
- Careful listening and observation can help the nurse identify a new mother who is suffering from postpartum depression.
- Postpartum psychoses are serious disorders that are potentially life threatening to the woman and others, including her infant.

ONLINE RESOURCES

Behavioral Health Care: http://www.naphs.org

Association of Women's Health, Obstetric, and Neonatal Nurses: http://www.awhonn.org

Child Passenger Safety: www.saferoads.org/issues/fs-child.htm

---

REVIEW QUESTIONS   *Choose the most appropriate answer.*

1. The earliest finding in hypovolemic shock is usually:
   1. Low blood pressure
   2. Rapid pulse
   3. Pale skin color
   4. Soft uterus

2. A bleeding laceration is typically manifested by:
   1. A soft uterus that is difficult to locate
   2. Low pulse and blood pressure
   3. Bright red bleeding and a firm uterus
   4. Profuse dark red bleeding and large clots

3. During the postpartum period, the white blood cell (leukocyte) count is normally:
   1. Higher
   2. Lower
   3. Unchanged
   4. Unimportant

4. A postpartum mother who is breastfeeding has developed mastitis. She states that she does not think it is good for her infant to drink milk from her infected breast. The best response of the nurse would be:
   1. Let the infant nurse only from the unaffected breast until the infection clears up
   2. Suggest she discontinue breastfeeding and start the infant on formula
   3. Encourage breastfeeding the infant to prevent engorgement
   4. Apply a tight breastbinder to the infected breast until the infection subsides

5. A woman is having her checkup with her nurse-midwife 6 weeks after birth. She seems disinterested in others, including her infant. She tells the nurse she does not think she is a very good mother. The nurse should:
   1. Reassure her that almost all new mothers feel let down after birth
   2. Ask her how her partner feels about the infant
   3. Explore her feelings with sensitive questioning
   4. Refer her to a psychiatrist

11 The Nurse's Role in Women's Health Care

objectives

1. Define each key term listed.
2. Explain aspects of preventive health care for women.
3. Describe each menstrual disorder and its care.
4. Explain each gynecological infection in terms of cause, transmission, treatment, and care.
5. Describe the various methods of birth control, including side effects and contraindications of each method.
6. Describe how to use natural family planning methods for contraception or infertility management.
7. Describe possible causes and treatment of infertility.
8. Explain the changes that occur during the perimenopausal period and after menopause.
9. Explain the medical and nursing care of women who are nearing or have completed menopause.
10. Discuss the medical and nursing care of women with pelvic floor dysfunction or problems related to benign growths in the reproductive tract.

key terms

amenorrhea (ă-mĕn-ō-RĒ-ă, p. 254)
climacteric (klī-MĂK-tĕr-ĭk, p. 275)
coitus interruptus (KŌ-ĭ-tŭs ĭn-tĕ-RŬP-tŭs, p. 269)
dysmenorrhea (dĭs-mĕn-ō-RĒ-ă, p. 254)
dyspareunia (dĭs-pă-ROO-nē-ă, p. 255)
endometriosis (ĕn-dō-mē-trē-Ō-sĭs, p. 255)
leiomyoma (lī-ō-mī-Ō-mă, p. 279)
menopause (MĔN-ō-păwz, p. 275)
menorrhagia (mĕn-ō-RĀ-jă, p. 254)
metrorrhagia (mĕ-trō-RĀ-jă, p. 254)
mittelschmerz (MĬT-ĕl-shmārts, p. 254)
myoma (mī-Ō-mă, p. 271)
osteoporosis (ŏs-tē-ō-pă-RŌ-sĭs, p. 276)
retrograde ejaculation (p. 271)

spermicide (p. 266)
spinnbarkeit (SPĬN-băhr-kīt, p. 268)
stress incontinence (p. 279)

GOALS OF *HEALTHY PEOPLE 2010*

Today women from all ethnic backgrounds choose to be active participants in their health care and therefore need information about their bodies, health promotion, self-care techniques, and choices concerning treatment options.

Culturally competent communication is the key to empowering the woman to feel confident about her ability to care for herself and her family. In some cultures, women ask when they want to know; in other cultures, women wait to be told what to do. To be an effective teacher about health behaviors, the nurse must understand the cultural needs, past experiences, and individual goals of the patient. The nurse offers support, knowledge, and caring behaviors that help the woman cope with screening tests or problems.

Some goals of *Healthy People 2010* related to women's health include curbing the rise in breast cancer, increasing the number of women over the age of 40 who have mammograms, reducing the number of deaths from cervical cancer, increasing the number of women over the age of 18 who have Papanicolaou (Pap) tests, reducing the occurrence of vertebral fractures in older women with osteoporosis, and reducing the occurrence of sexually transmitted diseases (STDs). Achievement of these goals requires preventive care, screening, and increasing accessibility to health care.

PREVENTIVE HEALTH CARE FOR WOMEN

The goal of preventive health care, or health maintenance, is the prevention or early identification of disease. The value of preventive health care is that some disabling conditions can be avoided or their severity lessened by specific measures, such as altering the diet or detecting the disorder early and at a more treatable stage. Preventive care for women may include disorders that have the following characteristics:

- Exclusive to women, such as cervical cancer
- Dominant in women, such as breast cancer or osteoporosis
- Prevalent in the general population, such as hypertension or colorectal cancers

This chapter will focus on those disorders that are exclusive or dominant in women. Much of preventive health care involves screening tests. These tests are not diagnostic but can identify whether additional testing is needed. Examples of screening tests that are common in women's health care include mammography to identify breast cancer and Pap tests for cervical cancer.

> ⟩NURSING **TIP**
> Encouraging women to practice preventive health care can help to avoid some disorders or to identify them when they are the most treatable.

BREAST CARE

The following three approaches are needed for early detection of breast cancer:

- Monthly breast self-examination
- Annual professional breast examination
- Mammography as appropriate

The nurse's role is to educate women about the benefit of all three examinations and techniques of self-examination. The reader should consult a medical-surgical text for additional information about the diagnosis and treatment of breast cancer.

Breast Self-Examination

Breast self-examination (BSE) should be performed by all women after age 20 years at about the same time each month. The best time for BSE is 1 week after the beginning of the menstrual period. If she is not menstruating, the woman may choose any day that is easy for her to remember, such as the first day of each month. Box 11-1 describes how to teach a woman BSE.

The chief value of BSE is that a woman learns how her own breasts feel. This is particularly valuable if she has fibrocystic breast changes, in which there are often many lumps that may change with hormonal fluctuations. The woman is more likely to know when something is different about *her* breasts.

Professional Breast Examination

BSE is a supplement to, rather than a substitute for, regular professional examinations. Although the woman who does regular BSE knows what is usual for her own breasts, professionals have the training and experience to identify suspicious breast masses. It is part of every annual gynecological examination and is done more frequently for women who have a high risk for breast cancer. It is recommended at yearly intervals for all women over age 20 years. The professional examination is similar to that for BSE.

Mammography

Mammography uses very-low-dose x-rays to visualize the breast tissue. It can detect breast tumors very early—long before the woman or a professional can feel them. The breast is compressed firmly between two plates, which is briefly uncomfortable. Scheduling the mammogram after a menstrual period reduces the discomfort because the breasts are less tender at that time. The American Cancer Society currently recommends a mammogram every 1 to 2 years for all women age 40 years or over. Women at higher risk for breast cancer may begin mammography earlier.

> ⟩NURSING **TIP**
> Preventive care for breast health involves self-examination, professional examinations, and mammography at the appropriate ages.

VULVAR SELF-EXAMINATION

Women over 18 years of age (or younger, if sexually active) should perform a monthly examination of the external genitalia to identify lesions or masses that may indicate infection or malignancy. The woman should use a hand mirror in a good light to systematically inspect and palpate her vulva and mons pubis for any new growths of any type, any painful or inflamed areas, ulcers, sores, or changes in skin color. She should report any abnormalities to her health care provider.

PELVIC EXAMINATION

The pelvic examination should be scheduled between menstrual periods, and the woman should not douche or have sexual intercourse for at least 48 hours before the examination to avoid altering the Pap test. The purpose of the pelvic examination is to identify conditions such as tumors, abnormal discharge, infections, or unusual pain.

The health care provider first checks the external genitalia to identify signs of problems similar to those noted in vulvar self-examination. Next, a speculum is inserted to visualize the woman's cervix and vagina for inflammation, discharge, or lesions. The speculum is warmed and lubricated with warm water only. A Pap

box 11-1 | *Teaching Women to Perform Breast Self-Examination*

Perform breast self-examination monthly. If you are menstruating, do the examination 1 week after the beginning of your period because your breasts are less tender at this time. If you are not menstruating, choose any day that you can easily remember, such as the first day of each month. Examine your breasts three ways: before a mirror, lying down, and in the shower.

BEFORE A MIRROR

Inspect your breasts in four steps: (1) arms at your sides; (2) arms over your head; (3) with your hands on your hips, pressing them firmly to flex your chest muscles; (4) and bending forward. At each step, note any change in the shape or appearance of your breasts. Note skin or nipple changes such as dimpling of the skin. Squeeze each nipple gently to identify any discharge.

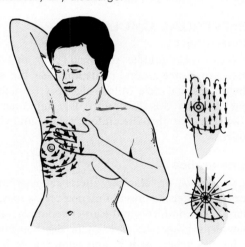

LYING DOWN

Place a small pillow under your right shoulder and put your right hand under your head while you examine your right breast with your left hand. Use the sensitive pads of your fingers to press gently into the breast tissue. Use a systematic pattern to check the entire breast. One pattern is to feel the tissue in a circular pattern, spiraling inward toward the nipple.

Another method is to use an up-and-down pattern. Use the same systematic pattern to examine the underarm area because breast tissue is also present here. Repeat for the other breast.

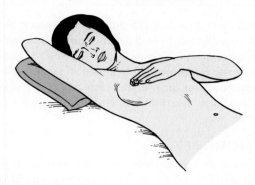

IN THE SHOWER

Raise your right arm. Use your soapy fingers to feel the breast tissue in the same systematic pattern described under Lying Down.

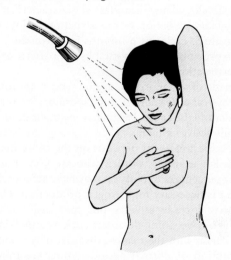

FOR ADDITIONAL INFORMATION

Contact the American Cancer Society at 1-800-ACS-2345 or visit their website at http://www.cancer.org.

test is obtained to screen for changes in the vaginal and cervical tissues that may be precancerous.

The current American Cancer Society recommendations (1999) for the Pap test are as follows:

- Yearly for all women age 18 years or older
- After three or more normal examinations, the Pap test may be performed less frequently at the health care provider's discretion

After the Pap test is obtained, the health care provider will perform an internal, or bimanual, examination to evaluate the internal organs. The index and middle fingers of one hand are inserted into the vagina and the other hand is placed on the abdomen to permit palpation of the cervix, uterus, and ovaries between the fingers.

After the internal examination, a single lubricated finger is inserted into the rectum to identify hemorrhoids or other lesions. A test for fecal occult blood may be done at this time (see a medical-surgical text for details).

MENSTRUAL DISORDERS

Menstrual cycle disorders can cause many women distress. The nursing role in each depends on the disorder's cause and treatment. Common nursing roles involve explaining any recommended treatments (e.g., medications) and caring for the woman before and after procedures. The nurse also provides emotional support to the patient.

AMENORRHEA

Amenorrhea is the absence of menstruation. It is normal before menarche, during pregnancy, and after menopause. Amenorrhea that is not normal may be either of the following:

- *Primary:* failure to menstruate by age 16 years; failure to menstruate by age 14 years if she has not developed any secondary sex characteristics
- *Secondary:* cessation of menstruation for at least three cycles or 6 months in a woman who previously had an established pattern of menstruation

Treatment of amenorrhea begins with a thorough history, physical examination, and laboratory examinations to identify the cause. Pregnancy testing is done for any sexually active woman.

The specific treatment depends on the cause that is identified. For example, women who are very thin or have a low percentage of body fat may have amenorrhea because fat is necessary for estrogen production. These women may include athletes but may also include patients who have eating disorders such as anorexia or bulimia. Therapy for their eating disorder may result in the resumption of normal periods. Other treatments are aimed at correcting the cause, which may be an endocrine imbalance.

ABNORMAL UTERINE BLEEDING

Abnormal uterine bleeding is (1) too frequent, (2) too long in duration, or (3) excessive in amount. Metrorrhagia is uterine bleeding that is usually normal in amount but occurs at irregular intervals. Menorrhagia refers to menstrual bleeding that is excessive in amount. Common causes for any type of abnormal bleeding include the following:

- Pregnancy complications, such as an unidentified pregnancy that is ending in spontaneous abortion

- Lesions of the vagina, cervix, or uterus (benign or malignant)
- Breakthrough bleeding (BTB) that may occur in the woman taking oral contraceptives
- Endocrine disorders such as hypothyroidism
- Failure to ovulate or respond appropriately to hormones secreted with ovulation (dysfunctional uterine bleeding)

Treatment of abnormal uterine bleeding depends on the identified cause. Pregnancy complications and benign or malignant lesions are treated appropriately. BTB may be relieved by a change in the oral contraceptive used. Abnormal hormone secretion is treated with the appropriate medications. Surgical dilation and curettage (D&C) may remove intrauterine growths or aid in diagnosis. Hysterectomy may be done for some disorders if the woman does not want other children. A newer technique, *laser ablation,* can permanently remove the abnormally bleeding uterine lining without a hysterectomy.

MENSTRUAL CYCLE PAIN
Mittelschmerz

Mittelschmerz ("middle pain") is pain that many women experience around ovulation, near the middle of their menstrual cycle. Mild analgesics are usually sufficient to relieve this discomfort. The nurse can teach the woman that this discomfort, while annoying, is harmless.

Dysmenorrhea

Dysmenorrhea, or "cramps," affects many women. It occurs soon after the onset of menses and is spasmodic in nature. Discomfort is in the lower abdomen and may radiate to the lower back or down the legs. Some women also have diarrhea, nausea, and vomiting. It is most common in young women who have not been pregnant (nulliparas).

There are two types of dysmenorrhea: *primary,* in which there is no evidence of pelvic pathology, and *secondary,* in which a known pathology is identifiable. Primary dysmenorrhea affects 50% of menstruating females. Characteristics include the following:

- Onset is shortly after menarche.
- Pain starts no more than a few hours before menstruation starts and lasts no more than 72 hours.
- Pelvic examination is normal.

Secondary dysmenorrhea most commonly results from endometriosis, the use of an intrauterine device (IUD) to prevent pregnancy, pelvic inflammatory disease, uterine polyps, or ovarian cysts. Treatment involves identifying and treating the cause.

Prostaglandins from the endometrium (uterine lining) play an important role in dysmenorrhea. Some women produce excessive amounts of prostaglandins from the endometrium, and these substances are potent stimulants of painful uterine contractions. The following three treatments may provide relief:

- Prostaglandin inhibitor drugs, such as ibuprofen (Motrin, Advil) or naproxen (Naprosyn, Anaprox) (Prostaglandin inhibitors are most effective if taken before the onset of menstruation and cramps.)
- Heat application to the lower abdomen or back
- Oral contraceptives, which reduce the amount of endometrium built up each month and therefore reduce prostaglandin secretion

Low fat and vegetarian diets reduce serum estrogen levels and can relieve menstrual pain in some women. The high-level omega-3 fatty acids in vegetarian diets influence prostaglandin metabolism and may have effects similar to antiinflammatory agents (Barnard et al, 2000).

ENDOMETRIOSIS

Endometriosis is the presence of tissue that resembles endometrium outside the uterus. This tissue responds to hormonal stimulation just as the uterine lining does. The lesions may cause pain, pressure, and inflammation to adjacent organs as they build up and slough during menstrual cycles.

Endometriosis causes pain in many women that is either sharp or dull. It is more constant than the spasmodic pain of dysmenorrhea. Dyspareunia (painful sexual intercourse) may be present. Endometriosis appears to cause infertility in some women.

Treatment of endometriosis may be either medical or surgical. Medications such as danazol and agonists of gonadotropin-releasing hormone (GnRH) may be given via nasal spray to reduce the buildup of tissue by inducing an artificial menopause. The woman may have hot flashes and vaginal dryness, similar to symptoms occurring at natural menopause. She is also at increased risk for other problems that occur after menopause, such as osteoporosis and serum lipid changes.

Surgical treatment includes the following:

- Hysterectomy with removal of the ovaries and all lesions if the woman does not want another pregnancy
- Laser ablation (destruction) of the lesions if she wants to maintain fertility

PREMENSTRUAL DYSPHORIC DISORDER

Formerly called premenstrual syndrome (PMS), premenstrual dysphoric disorder (PMDD) is associated with abnormal serotonin response to normal changes in the estrogen levels during the menstrual cycle.

The following symptom criteria (which are used to diagnose PMDD) occur between ovulation and the onset of menstruation, begin to improve between the menstruation and ovulation phase, and are not present in the week after the menstrual period. Five or more of the following symptoms usually occur regularly:

- Depressed mood
- Anxiety, tension, feeling "on edge"
- Increased sensitivity to rejection
- Irritability
- Decreased interest in usual activities
- Difficulty in concentrating
- Lethargy
- Change in appetite—food cravings
- Change in sleep habits
- Feeling overwhelmed
- Physical symptoms such as breast tenderness, bloating, weight gain, headaches

Treatment includes prescribing calcium, magnesium, and vitamin B_6 (helps convert tryptophan to serotonin) and a diet rich in complex carbohydrates and fiber (to lengthen effects of the carbohydrate meal). Stress management and exercise are also advised. Medical management includes oral contraceptives (low estrogen, progestin dominant), diuretics during the luteal phase of the menstrual cycle (between ovulation and onset of menstruation), and nonsteroidal antiinflammatory drugs (NSAIDs) to prevent headaches.

Serotonin reuptake inhibitors such as fluoxetine (Sarafem) may also be prescribed for negative behavior. Medroxyprogesterone (Depo-Provera) may be indicated to inhibit ovulation and therefore control estrogen levels. Patient education concerning maintenance of a monthly calendar of symptoms, stress management, and dietary guidance are important nursing responsibilities. Although chocolates have been shown to elevate depressed moods, excessive consumption of chocolate should be avoided.

GYNECOLOGICAL INFECTIONS

Vaginal infections are the most common reason for women to seek health care. Nurses play a key role in educating women concerning vaginal health and the prevention of sexually transmitted diseases. Identifying high-risk behavior and providing nonjudgmental, sensitive counseling and education should be part of every physical checkup. Safe sex practices, the reduction of the number of partners, and avoiding the exchange of body fluids are part of primary prevention of STDs. Community-based education in schools and churches are also important in primary prevention.

THE NORMAL VAGINA

At birth the infant's vaginal epithelium is controlled by estrogen from the mother and is rich in glycogen, with a low pH of 3.7 to 6.3. When the maternal estrogen effect decreases, the vaginal epithelium atrophies and contains little glycogen. The pH rises to 7. Estrogen influence returns at puberty and glycogen increases. The interaction of glycogen and estrogen in the vaginal epithelium results in the growth of lactobacilli, which is a bacteriostatic. The pH falls to 3.5 to 4.5. The types of bacteria found in the vagina vary with the pH of the vagina. Factors that change the normal flora of the vagina and predispose to vaginal infection include the following:

- Antibiotics: encourage yeast overgrowth
- Douching: changes pH
- Sexual intercourse: raises pH to 7 or higher for 8 hours after coitus
- Uncontrolled diabetes mellitus: increases glucose that promotes organism growth

The normal acidic pH for the vagina is the first line of defense against vaginal infections. Normal vaginal secretions are made up of creamy white epithelial cells and mucus from the cervix, Skene's glands, and Bartholin's glands. The secretions prevent dryness and prevent infection. Immediately after menstruation the mucus is thin but, as ovulation approaches, the estrogen level increases; at ovulation, the mucus is clear, slippery, and can be stretched without breaking (spinnbarkeit) (see Figure 11-5). After ovulation the mucus is cloudy and sticky. At menopause, lowered estrogen causes vaginal dryness and the pH may change, predisposing the woman to vaginal discomfort and infections.

Other factors can alter the pH of the vagina temporarily and include the following (American College of Obstetricians and Gynecologists, 1996) (Box 11-2):

- Deodorant soap
- Perfumed toilet tissue

---

box 11-2 | *Preventing Vaginal Infections*

By promoting vaginal health, nurses can enhance the quality of life for the women they counsel. The promotion of vaginal health includes wearing cotton underwear, avoiding tight-fitting nylon or spandex pants, wiping front to back after toileting, and frequent handwashing. A healthy lifestyle with a high-fiber, low-fat diet and exercise strengthens the immune system and can prevent many infections. Douching increases the risk for vaginal infections. Women should not douche or use internal feminine hygiene products without first consulting with their health care provider.

- Spermicides
- Tampons
- Hot tubs and swimming pools
- Tight synthetic clothing

Three classes of gynecological infections are covered in the following sections:

- Toxic shock syndrome
- Sexually transmitted diseases
- Pelvic inflammatory disease

TOXIC SHOCK SYNDROME

Toxic shock syndrome (TSS) is a rare and potentially fatal disorder. It is caused by strains of *Staphylococcus aureus* that produce toxins that can cause shock, coagulation defects, and tissue damage if they enter the bloodstream. TSS is associated with the trapping of bacteria within the reproductive tract for a prolonged time. Factors that increase the risk of TSS include the use of high-absorbency tampons and the use of a diaphragm or cervical cap for contraception.

Signs and symptoms of TSS include the following:

- Sudden spiking fever
- Flulike symptoms
- Hypotension
- Generalized rash that resembles sunburn
- Skin peeling from the palms and soles 1 to 2 weeks after the illness

The incidence of TSS has decreased, but the nurse continues to play a role in prevention. The nurse's role is primarily one of education. The following should be included:

- *Tampon use*
  Wash hands before and after inserting a tampon.
  Change tampons at least every 4 hours.
  Do not use superabsorbent tampons.
  Use pads rather than tampons when sleeping because tampons will likely remain in the vagina longer than 4 hours.
- *Diaphragm or cervical cap use*
  Wash hands before and after inserting the diaphragm or cervical cap.
  Do not use a diaphragm or cervical cap during the menstrual period.
  Remove the diaphragm or cervical cap at the time recommended by the health care provider.

NURSING **TIP**

To prevent toxic shock syndrome, the woman should be taught to wash her hands well when using tampons or a diaphragm. The diaphragm should not be used during menstruation. Tampons should be changed every 4 hours and not used during sleep, which usually lasts longer than 4 hours.

SEXUALLY TRANSMITTED DISEASES

Sexually transmitted diseases (STDs) are those that can be spread by sexual contact, although several of these have other modes of transmission as well. It is important that all sexual contacts, even those who are asymptomatic, be completely treated to eradicate the infection. Table 11-1 gives specific information about STDs that the nurse may encounter. Certain STDs must be reported to the health department.

Nursing care related to STDs primarily focuses on patient education to prevent spread of these infections. Nurses may do the following:

- Teach signs and symptoms that should be reported to the health care provider.
- Explain diagnostic tests.
- Teach measures to prevent spread of infection, such as use of a condom.
- Explain treatment measures.
- Emphasize the importance of completing treatment and follow-up and of treating all partners to eliminate the spread of infection.

It is estimated that more than 56 million Americans are infected with STDs (Thomas, 2001). Teaching STD prevention to women across the life span is important because some viral STDs remain in the body for life and can have long-term complications. The most common viral STD is *human papillomavirus (HPV),* with more than 100 variations of the virus. HPV types 16 and 18 are associated with serious cervical cancer, and women who are immunocompromised are at the greatest risk. The use of condoms may not protect the woman if the male lesion is on the scrotum or inguinal folds. It may take 3 to 6 months after infection to develop visible warts. Treatment includes cryotherapy, laser vaporization, electrodiathermy, and electrofulguration with a loop electrode excision procedure. Topical agents are used, such as podofilox (Condylox), imiquimod (Aldara), and bichloroacetic acid (BCA). Lidocaine cream may be used 20 minutes before painful treatments. 5-Fluorouracil (5-FU) is no longer used for this condition because of serious side effects.

Herpes simplex virus II (HSV II) is another example of a viral STD that is recurrent and incurable. HSV infection during pregnancy can have serious consequences for the newborn.

Hepatitis B can be sexually transmitted if sexual practices include anal-oral sexual contact, digital rectal sexual intercourse, or group sex. Symptoms are nonspecific and include malaise, anorexia, nausea, and fatigue. Liver failure can develop. Hepatitis B vaccine can prevent the disease and immunoglobulin can be given if known exposure has occurred.

The occurrence of *gonorrhea (GC)* has decreased from 650,000 in 1997 to 300,000 in 2000 (Centers for Disease Control and Prevention). Casual sex in the 15- to 19-year age-group and sex associated with drug use are the highest risk practices for GC infection. Immunoassays of endocervical exudate or urethral discharge can offer more rapid diagnosis than traditional cultures. Several nucleic acid amplification tests are now available to detect chlamydia, GC, and trichomonas with a simple noninvasive urine test, with results available in a few hours.

Chlamydia trachomatis is the most common bacterial STD in the United States, with 3 million new cases per year (Rawlins, 2001). Treatment tends to be delayed because it is often asymptomatic.

Syphilis was diagnosed in more than 70,000 cases in 1997, with more than 90% of cases in the southern United States (Rawlins, 2001). Untreated syphilis is a risk factor in the spread of human immunodeficiency virus (HIV) infection and also leads to central nervous system (CNS), musculoskeletal, and heart complications. Most newborns of mothers infected with syphilis will have congenital syphilis or die. An external chancre is a characteristic first sign and resolves within 6 weeks without treatment; however, the disease spreads internally. A rash also occurs and resolves, and then the latent period of syphilis occurs and progresses to tertiary syphilis. Aortic aneurysms, dementia, and death can occur.

The number of women infected with *HIV* worldwide is staggering. Patient education plays a key role in prevention, quality of life, and compassionate and knowledgeable referral. Early diagnosis, access to care, medications, and safe sex practices are improving outcomes and decreasing occurrence. Universal HIV screening at pregnancy is a goal of the National Academy of Sciences Institute of Medicine, because many women do not realize they are infected in the early stages. Although education for prevention is essential for adolescents, women account for 23% of those diagnosed with HIV over age 50 years (Boehm, 2001). Nurses may be less likely to consider this age-group high risk and miss opportunities for early detection and education for prevention. Sexual contact and intravenous (IV) drug use are the most common risk behaviors for HIV infection.

Prevention of disease is the key role of the nurse. The nurse must develop strategies, use initiatives, and contact adolescents in the community setting, schools, and churches. Teaching all age-groups healthy behaviors such as abstinence, safe sex practices, and discussion of STD prevention is essential. Improving access to care and early detection is also important. The Centers for

table 11-1 *Sexually Transmitted Diseases*

INFECTION (CAUSATIVE ORGANISM)	SIGNS AND SYMPTOMS	DIAGNOSIS	PREGNANCY, FETAL, AND NEONATAL EFFECTS	TREATMENT	COMMENTS
Candidiasis (yeast) (*Candida albicans*)	Itching and burning on urination, inflammation of vulva and vagina, "cottage cheese" appearance to discharge	Signs and symptoms; identification of the spores of the causative fungus	Can infect newborn at birth	Miconazole nitrate (Monistat), clotrimazole (Gyne-Lotrimin), nystatin (Mycostatin), fluconazole (Diflucan).	Medications are available over-the-counter (OTC), but the woman should seek medical attention to diagnose her first infection or if she has persistent or recurrent infections.
Trichomoniasis (*Trichomonas vaginalis*)	Thin, foul-odored, greenish yellow vaginal discharge, vulvar itching, edema, redness	Identification of the organism under microscope in a wet-mount preparation	Does not cross placenta Can cause postpartum infection	Metronidazole (Flagyl) if not pregnant during first trimester; clotrimazole (Gyne-Lotrimin) for symptom relief during first trimester.	Organism thrives in an alkaline environment. Most infections are thought to be transmitted by sexual contact.
Bacterial vaginosis (*Gardnerella vaginalis*)	Thin, grayish white discharge that has a fishy odor	Microscopic evidence of clue cells (epithelial cells with bacteria clinging to their surface)	Associated with preterm delivery	Bacteria is normal inhabitant of vagina but overgrows. Treatment aims to restore normal balance of vaginal bacterial flora. Metronidazole (Flagyl) may relieve symptoms.	Avoid alcohol during treatment with metronidazole and for 24 hours after. Flagyl cannot be used during first trimester of pregnancy.
Chlamydia (*Chlamydia trachomatis*)	Yellowish discharge and painful urination Often asymptomatic in women, which delays treatment	Culture, rapid detection tests, DNA probe using urine specimen is non-invasive	Transmitted via birth canal Causes conjunctivitis and pneumonia in newborn	Azithromycin, doxycycline, erythromycin in pregnancy. All newborns have prophylactic eye care.	Untreated infection can ascend into fallopian tubes, causing scarring. Infertility or ectopic pregnancy may result. Can spread to neonate's eyes by contact with infected vaginal secretions.

Organism	Signs and Symptoms	Diagnosis	Effect on Fetus/Newborn	Treatment	Comments
Gonorrhea (Neisseria gonorrhoeae)	Purulent discharge, painful urination, dyspareunia	Culture of organism or nucleic acid Amplification of a urine specimen	Transmitted to newborn's eyes during birth, causing blindness (ophthalmia neonatorum)	Antibiotics. All newborns have prophylactic eye care.	Can result in pelvic inflammatory disease with tubal scarring.
Syphilis (Treponema pallidum)	3 stages: *Primary:* painless chancre on the genitalia, anus, or lips. *Secondary:* 2 months after primary syphilis; enlargement of spleen and liver, headache, anorexia, generalized skin rash, wartlike growths on the vulva. *Tertiary:* may occur many years after secondary syphilis and cause heart, blood vessel, nervous system damage	*Primary:* examining material scraped from the chancre with darkfield microscopy to identify the spirochete organism; serological tests are not positive this early. *Secondary or tertiary:* serologic test (VDRL [less specific], RPR, and FTA-ABS [more specific])	Transmitted across placenta Causes congenital syphilis, stillbirth, spontaneous abortion	Penicillin; doxycycline, tetracycline, or erythromycin if allergic. Tetracycline is not recommended during pregnancy; desensitization of the woman is recommended.	Primary and secondary stages are the most contagious. Spread is through sexual contact, by inoculation (sharing needles), or through the placenta from an infected mother.
Herpes genitalis (Herpes simplex virus [HSV], types I and II)	Clusters of painful vesicles (blisters) on the vulva, perineum, and anal areas Vesicles rupture in 1 to 7 days and heal in 12 days	By signs and symptoms; confirmed by viral culture	Can cause spontaneous abortion, stillbirth Active genital infection requires cesarean delivery Causes neonatal CNS problems	No cure exists; acyclovir (Zovirax) or valacyclovir (Valtrex) reduces symptoms. Treated with hygiene, sitz baths during pregnancy.	HSV II usually causes genital lesions. The first episode is usually most uncomfortable. The virus "hides" in the nerve cells and can reemerge in later outbreaks that are as contagious as the first.

Continued

table 11-1 *Sexually Transmitted Diseases—cont'd*

INFECTION (CAUSATIVE ORGANISM)	SIGNS AND SYMPTOMS	DIAGNOSIS	PREGNANCY, FETAL, AND NEONATAL EFFECTS	TREATMENT	COMMENTS
Condylomata acuminata (Human papillomavirus [HPV])	Dry, wartlike growths on the vagina, labia, cervix, and perineum	By typical appearance and location	Growth may obstruct birth canal Infant may have laryngeal papillomas	Removal with cryotherapy (cold), electrocautery, laser, or podophyllin applications are alternatives.	Also known as venereal or genital warts; associated with higher rates of cervical cancer. Women should have more frequent Pap tests.
Acquired immunodeficiency syndrome (AIDS) (Human immunodeficiency virus [HIV])	Initially, no symptoms; later symptoms include weight loss, night sweats, fever and chills, fatigue, enlarged lymph nodes, skin rashes, diarrhea Late symptoms include immune suppression, opportunistic infections, and malignancies	Serology tests: positive ELISA, followed by positive Western blot test	Avoid breaks in skin to mother/fetus during birth process Trasmitted antepartum to newborn Drug therapy advised Infant should be bottle fed	No cure available yet. Zidovudine (AZT, Retrovir) and didanosine (Videx) may slow progression. Lamivudine and nelfinaver are given during pregnancy.	Transmitted through contact of nonintact skin or mucous membranes with infectious secretions, exposure to blood, and transmission from mother to fetus. Standard precautions reduce risk for caregivers. Condom use reduces risk for sexual transmission.

ELISA, Enzyme-linked immunosorbent assay; *CNS,* central nervous system.

Disease Control and Prevention (CDC) offer various free programs that are available over the Internet and can be used by nurses and teachers in the community to teach STD prevention.

PELVIC INFLAMMATORY DISEASE

Pelvic inflammatory disease (PID) is an infection of the upper reproductive tract. Asymptomatic STDs are a common cause of PID. The cervix, uterine cavity, fallopian tubes, and pelvic cavity are often involved. Infertility may be the result.

The woman's symptoms vary according to the area affected. Fever, pelvic pain, abnormal vaginal discharge, nausea and anorexia, and irregular vaginal bleeding are common. When examined, the abdomen and pelvic organs are often very tender. Laboratory tests identify common general signs of infection, such as elevated leukocytes and an elevated sedimentation rate. Cultures of the cervical canal are done to identify the infecting organism. Urinalysis is usually done to identify infection of the urinary tract.

Treatment may be administered on an inpatient or outpatient basis depending on the severity of the infection. Antibiotics are begun promptly to treat the infection. A change in antibiotic(s) is made if culture and sensitivity testing indicates that another one would be more effective.

Douching results in changes in the vaginal flora and predisposes the woman to the development of PID, bacterial vaginosis, and ectopic pregnancies. However, many women practice regular douching in the belief that it is cleansing. The nurse can play an important role in educating the woman to prevent PID.

FAMILY PLANNING

Family planning (birth control) may be part of the nurse's responsibility in family-planning clinics, in physician or nurse-midwife practices, or on the postpartum or gynecology units of an acute care hospital. In addition, family members and friends may turn to the nurse as a resource person who can answer their questions about contraception. The nurse's role in family planning includes the following:

- Answering general questions about contraceptive methods
- Explaining different methods that are available, including accurate information about their advantages and disadvantages
- Teaching the correct use of the method or methods of contraception that the patient chooses

Factors that influence one's choice of a contraceptive include the following:

- Age
- Health status, including risk for STD
- Religion
- Culture
- Impact of an unplanned pregnancy on the woman or family
- Desire for future children
- Frequency of intercourse
- Convenience and degree of spontaneity that is important to the couple
- Expense
- Degree of comfort the partners have with touching their bodies
- Number of sexual partners

A couple's choice of contraception often changes as needs change.

Contraception does not always prevent pregnancy. An important consideration for patients is how likely the method is to fail. A contraceptive technique may fail because the method is ineffective or the user is using the method inappropriately.

The following two *Healthy People 2010* goals are relevant to the provision of family planning services:

- Reduce the percentage of unintended pregnancies to no more than 30%
- Reduce the percentage of women who have an unintended pregnancy despite the use of a contraceptive method to no more than 7%

The nurse can play a part in helping couples choose and correctly use contraceptive methods that enable them to have children that are both wanted and well timed.

TEMPORARY CONTRACEPTION

Reversible contraception is defined as the temporary prevention of fertility.

Abstinence

Abstinence is 100% effective in preventing pregnancy and STDs, including infection with HIV. However, most couples believe that their sexual relationship adds to the quality of life. Therefore abstinence is rarely an option the couple will consider. Most religious groups support abstinence among unmarried people and adolescents.

Hormonal Contraceptives

Hormonal contraceptives have one or more of the following contraceptive effects:

- Prevent ovulation
- Make the cervical mucus thick and resistant to sperm penetration

- Make the uterine endometrium less hospitable if a fertilized ovum does arrive

Hormonal contraceptives do not protect either partner from STDs, including HIV infection.

Oral Contraceptives ("The Pill")

Oral contraceptives (OCs) are a popular, highly effective, and reversible method of birth control (Figure 11-1). They contain either combined hormones (estrogen and progestin) or progestin alone ("minipill"). Combination OCs are highly effective in preventing ovulation. Minipills are slightly less effective in preventing ovulation; their main contraceptive effect is to thicken the cervical mucus and make the endometrium unfavorable for implantation. Minipills are useful for the woman who cannot take estrogen.

Oral contraceptives require a prescription. The woman's history is obtained, and she will have a physical examination, including breast and pelvic examinations and a Pap test. She should have a yearly physical examination, Pap test, breast examination, and blood pressure check. See Hormone Replacement Therapy, pp. 274 and 275, for the use of oral contraceptives for menopause and menstrual irregularities.

Dosing regimens. Combination OCs are available in 21- or 28-pill packs. If the woman has a 21-pill pack, she takes one pill each day at the same time for 21 days, then stops for 7 days. The woman who has a 28-day pack takes a pill each day; the last seven pills of the pack are inert but maintain the habit of taking the pill each day. Menstruation occurs during the 7-day period when either no pills or inert pills are ingested.

Some pills are multiphasic in that their estrogen and progestin content changes during the cycle to mimic natural hormonal activity. If the woman takes multiphasic pills, it is very important that she take each pill in order. Taking the pills at the same time each day is important to maintain a stable blood level of the hormones, regardless of the type of OC.

It is most important that the medication-free interval not be extended beyond 7 days. Taking the first pill of the cycle on time is most important in preventing accidental pregnancies.

Benefits. OCs have a failure rate of 0.2% for combined pills and 0.5% for minipills. They reduce the risk for ovarian and endometrial cancer. Their effect on the risk for breast and cervical cancer risks is not yet definitive. Women tend to have less cramping and lighter periods (and therefore less anemia) when taking OCs. OCs may improve premenstrual symptoms for some women.

Side effects and contraindications. Common side effects of OCs include nausea, headache, breast tenderness, weight gain, and spotting between periods or amenorrhea. These effects generally decrease within a few months and are seen less frequently with low-dose OCs.

Some women should not take OCs or should take them with caution. These women include those who have the following:

- Thromboembolic disorders (blood clots)
- Cerebrovascular accident or heart disease
- Estrogen-dependent cancer or breast cancer
- A smoking pattern of more than 15 cigarettes a day for women older than age 35 years (the pill is safe for women over age 35 years if they do not smoke)
- Impaired liver function
- A confirmed pregnancy or who may be pregnant
- Undiagnosed vaginal bleeding

The first episode of menstrual bleeding after an abortion is usually preceded by ovulation, and therefore contraception should begin immediately to prevent pregnancy. However, after a term delivery the first menstrual cycle is usually anovulatory and there is a higher risk of thromboembolism; therefore the contraceptive is usually started 4 weeks postpartum.

The use of combination OCs also decreases breast milk production, and OCs are therefore contraindicated in the breastfeeding woman until lactation is well established. Women who breastfeed at least 10 times per day usually do not ovulate for 10 weeks postpartum and do not need contraception before that time (Yen, Jaffe, & Barbieri, 1999). Progestin-only OCs (minipill) may be used until menstruation returns in women who breastfeed regularly.

Combination OCs decrease milk supply and should be given postpartum only after lactation is well established; the minipill does not have this drawback. Women should be taught to inform the health care provider of any preexisting health condition or any

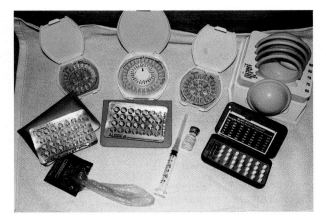

FIGURE **11-1** Contraceptives. This photo shows common types of contraceptives: condoms, diaphragm, oral contraceptives, and parenteral contraceptives.

change in their condition that may affect their use of OCs. The following *ACHES* acronym can help a woman recall the warning signs to report:

- *Abdominal pain* (severe)
- *Chest pain,* dyspnea, bloody sputum
- *Headache* (severe), weakness, or numbness of the extremities
- *Eye problems* (blurring, double vision, vision loss)
- *Severe leg pain* or swelling, speech disturbance

Some medications decrease the effectiveness of OCs. These include the following:

- Some antibiotics, such as ampicillin and tetracycline
- Anticonvulsants
- Rifampin, barbiturates

> ⮞ NURSING **TIP**_____
> Smoking increases the chance of experiencing complications related to oral contraceptives, particularly in women over age 35 years.

Nursing care. The woman needs thorough teaching if the pill is to be a satisfactory contraceptive for her. Teaching should be done in her own language and supplemented by generous written materials if she can read. Teaching points should include the following:

- How to take the specific drug
- What to do if a dose is missed or if she decides to stop using it and does not want to become pregnant
- Common side effects and signs and symptoms that should be promptly reported
- Backup contraceptive methods, such as barrier methods (discussed later in this chapter)
- Supplemental barrier methods of contraception to use in addition to OCs, which also reduce the risk of STDs (including HIV infection)

> ⮞ NURSING **TIP**_____
> The more birth control pills a woman misses, the greater is her risk that pregnancy will occur.

Hormone Implants (Levonorgestrel [Norplant])

Hormone implants involve the placement of six matchstick-size capsules that release progestin under the skin of the upper arm (Figure 11-2). Progestin is released slowly and in small amounts to provide contraception for 5 years. Like the minipill, the hormone implant inhibits ovulation, impairs development of the endometrium, and causes the cervical mucus to impede sperm passage. Its effectiveness is almost 100%. Its advantages are that it does not need to be taken daily and is unrelated to intercourse. It can be removed at any time with a prompt return of fertility. The initial cost of hormone implants is high, but if the woman keeps them for 5 years, they cost about the same as 5 years of OCs.

Side effects and contraindications. The benefits, side effects, and contraindications of the hormone implant are essentially the same as for OCs. A common side effect of the hormone implant is menstrual irregularity. Other side effects include headaches, weight gain, acne, dizziness, and mood changes. Infection may occasionally occur.

Nursing care. The woman should be taught about the side effects of hormone implants. Menstruation is likely to be very irregular or absent when the implants are first inserted. This makes many women anxious because they associate a missed period with pregnancy. Intradermal implants can be removed in the outpatient clinic with the use of a local anesthetic and small incision.

Hormonal Injection (Medroxyprogesterone [Depo-Provera])

Medroxyprogesterone (Depo-Provera) is an injectable form of slow-release progestin. Its contraceptive action is similar to that of the minipill and hormone implant. It provides 3 months of highly effective contraception. Fertility returns about 1 year after stopping the medication (Yen, Jaffe, & Barbieri, 1999). The injection is given deep intramuscularly within 5 days of the menstrual period. If given later than 5 days after the menstrual period, the woman should use another form of contraception because ovulation may have already occurred. The breastfeeding woman usually starts hormone injections 6 weeks after birth, and the nonlactating woman may start 5 days after delivery.

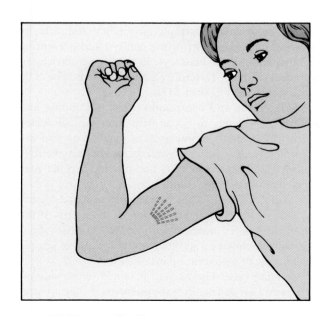

FIGURE **11-2** The Norplant contraceptive system.

Side effects and contraindications. The side effects and contraindications of hormone injections are similar to those of OCs and hormone implants. Menstrual irregularities, breakthrough bleeding, and amenorrhea are common complaints and are often the reason why women stop taking the drug.

Nursing care. The woman should be taught about the side effects and problems to report. It should be emphasized that she return every 3 months for another injection if she wants to maintain a constant level of hormone and thus prevent pregnancy. A backup contraceptive method should be taught if she decides to stop the injections or is delayed in returning for subsequent injections.

Intrauterine Devices

Intrauterine devices (IUDs) are a reversible method of birth control that requires a prescription. They are effective (98% effectiveness or greater), reversible, and unrelated to intercourse.

The ParaGard is a small, T-shaped plastic device containing copper that is effective for 10 years. Other devices carry a sleeve on one segment that contains a reservoir of progesterone or levonorgestrel that is diffused into the uterus each day. The action is local in the uterine cavity and blood levels do not increase. The levonorgestrel type of IUD must be replaced every 5 years, and the progesterone-releasing device must be replaced every year. The main mechanism of contraceptive action of a copper IUD is the production of a sterile inflammatory reaction that is spermicidal and toxic to the blastocyte. Copper impedes sperm transport and viability in the cervical mucus. The progesterone-releasing IUD is associated with a higher incidence of ectopic pregnancy and acts by slowing tubal transport of the embryo and preventing implantation of the blastocyte in the uterine cavity. On removal of the IUD, fertility rapidly returns. The IUD does not protect against STDs.

Side effects and contraindications. Cramping and bleeding are likely to occur with insertion. Increased menstruation and dysmenorrhea may occur and are common reasons why a woman decides to have the IUD removed. The woman who has heavier periods may need iron supplementation.

Possible complications besides infection include expulsion of the IUD or perforation of the uterus. If the woman becomes pregnant with an IUD in place, she is more likely to have a spontaneous abortion, an ectopic pregnancy, or a preterm infant.

Nursing care. The woman is taught about side effects and how to take iron supplements if they are prescribed. The woman will need to feel for the fine plastic strings (tail) that are connected to the IUD to verify that it is in place. She should check the tail weekly for the first 4 weeks after insertion, then monthly. The woman is taught to report if she cannot feel the tail that protrudes into the vagina or if it is longer or shorter than previously. The nurse can teach her signs of infection (fever, pain, change in vaginal discharge) and signs of ectopic pregnancy (see p. 86) that should be promptly reported.

> ### NURSING **TIP**
> An intrauterine device should be used only by women who have no current pelvic infection and are in a mutually monogamous relationship.

Transdermal Patch

Ortho Evra is a transdermal patch used as one patch per week for 3 weeks, followed by a 1-week patch-free interval. It provides effective contraception similar to oral contraceptives (Alexander, 2002).

Vaginal Ring

A flexible, one-size vaginal ring (NuvaRing) that releases estrogen and progestin locally instead of systemically has been approved for contraceptive use in the United States. The ring is worn in the vagina for 3 weeks and removed for 1 week to allow for withdrawal bleeding (Alexander, 2002).

Barrier Methods

Barrier methods work by blocking the entrance of semen into the woman's cervix. Spermicides (sperm-killing chemicals) are part of some of these methods. They avoid the use of systemic hormones. Some barrier methods offer some protection against STDs by providing a barrier to contact.

Some barrier methods must be used just before intercourse (condoms, spermicidal foams, and suppositories), whereas others can be inserted several hours earlier (diaphragm, cervical cap). Spermicidal foams and suppositories are messy and may drip from the vagina. These methods are not suitable for people who are uncomfortable touching their bodies. They are often used as a backup method of contraception.

Barrier methods are inexpensive per use. The diaphragm and cervical cap require a fitting and prescription, which adds to their initial cost. Other barrier methods are over-the-counter purchases. These methods are often chosen as backup methods or when the woman is lactating or if she cannot tolerate OCs or an IUD.

Diaphragm and cervical cap. Diaphragms and cervical caps are rubber domes that fit over the cervix and are used with spermicides to kill sperm that pass the mechanical barrier.

The diaphragm and cervical cap are fitted by a nurse practitioner, nurse-midwife, or physician. The woman must learn how to insert and remove the diaphragm or cervical cap and to verify proper placement. User misplacement, especially of the small cervical cap, is a common reason for unintended pregnancy.

The woman should check either device for weak spots or pinholes before insertion by holding it up to the light. Spermicidal jelly or cream is applied to the ring and center of the diaphragm before inserting it and positioning it over the cervix. It may be inserted several hours before intercourse and should remain in place for at least 6 hours after intercourse but not more than 24 hours to prevent pressure on local tissue. More spermicidal jelly or cream must be inserted into the vagina if the couple repeats coitus within 6 hours.

The diaphragm must be refitted after each birth or a weight change of 10 pounds or more. The cap must be refitted yearly and after birth, abortion, or surgery.

Side effects and contraindications. Women who have an allergy to rubber or spermicides are not good candidates for the diaphragm or cervical cap. Pressure on the bladder may increase the risk of urinary tract infection.

Nursing care. The health care provider who fits the device will provide much of the teaching on insertion, verification of placement, and removal. The nurse often reinforces the teaching, especially about the use and reapplication of spermicide for repeat intercourse. The nurse should teach the woman about signs of uterine infection (pain, foul-odored drainage, or fever) and of sensitivity to the product (irritation or itching). The woman also should be taught to report signs and symptoms of urinary tract infection: fever, pain or burning with urination, urgency, or urinary frequency.

Male condom. Male condoms are sheaths of thin latex, polyurethane, or natural membrane ("skins") worn on the penis during intercourse. Condoms collect semen before, during, and after ejaculation. They come in various styles, such as ribbed, lubricated, and colored, and with or without spermicide. They are single-use, low-cost items that are widely available from vending machines, drugstores, and family planning clinics. Latex condoms provide some protection from STDs, including HIV. Natural membrane condoms do not prevent the passage of viruses, including HIV. See Box 11-3 for the correct use of the condom.

Water-soluble lubricants should be used if the condom or vagina is dry to avoid condom breakage. Unlike other oil-based lubricants, water-soluble lubricants do not damage the latex or cause breakage. The penis should be withdrawn immediately if the man feels that the condom is breaking or becoming dislodged. The condom is removed and a new one applied. Condoms are not reused because even a pinhole can lead to pregnancy or permit the entry of viruses, including HIV. The condom package should be checked for expiration date.

The nurse should educate patients to prevent common condom mistakes, which include the following:
- Allowing the penis to lose erection while still in the vagina
- Opening the condom package with the teeth or a sharp object, which can tear the condom
- Unrolling the condom before applying it to the penis
- Using of out-of-date condoms (condoms with spermicide last 2 years; others, 5 years)
- Using baby oil, cold cream, vegetable oil, or petroleum jelly to lubricate the condom
- Reusing the condom
- Storing condoms in the wallet (heat destroys spermicide)
- Not leaving space between the tip of the penis and the condom to provide a reservoir for ejaculate

Side effects and contraindications. Side effects of and contraindications to condom use are rare. Either of the partners may be allergic to latex. A polyurethane condom can often be used successfully for those who are sensitive to latex.

Female condom. Female condoms are essentially used for the same purpose as male condoms—to prevent pregnancy and to protect the woman from HIV and other STDs (Figure 11-3). Two styles of female condoms are currently available:
- Two flexible rings, one that fits into the vagina and one that remains outside, connected by a polyurethane sheath
- A bikini-panty style that has a pouch that fits inside the vagina

Female condoms are prelubricated, single-use items available over-the-counter. They give the woman control over her exposure to infections without having to rely on the cooperation of her partner. Its failure rate in pregnancy prevention is 5%. Many women find it unattractive.

Side effects and contraindications. There are few problems with the use of the female condom. Few people are sensitive to polyurethane.

>‖ NURSING **TIP**_____
Adolescents must be educated about contraception, reproductive health, and the dangers of unprotected sex.

Spermicides

Spermicidal foam, cream, jelly, film, and suppository capsules are over-the-counter contraceptives. They are inserted into the vagina before intercourse to neutralize vaginal secretions, destroy sperm, and block entrance to the uterus. Each product has specific directions for use. Vaginal films and suppositories must melt before they are effective, which takes about 15 minutes. Most spermi-cides are effective for no more than 1 hour. Reapplication is needed for repeated coitus. The woman should not douche for at least 6 to 8 hours after intercourse.

Adolescents often choose this type of contraception because it is inexpensive and easy to obtain. Teenagers should be taught that products labeled "for personal hygiene use" do not have contraceptive action. Spermicides have an actual failure rate of 21%. The use of a

---

box 11-3 | *Teaching Use of the Male Condom*

Use a new condom each time. Check the expiration date on packages, because condoms deteriorate over time.

Apply the condom before you have any contact with the woman's vagina, because there are sperm in the secretions before you ejaculate.

1. Squeeze the air from the tip when placing the condom over the end of your penis. Leave a half inch of space at the tip to allow sperm to collect and to prevent breakage.

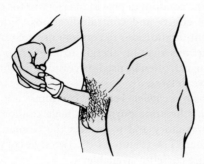

2. Hold the tip while you unroll the condom over the erect penis.

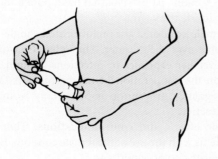

3. Do not use petroleum jelly, grease, or oil as lubricants because they can cause the condom to burst. Instead, use a water-soluble lubricant such as K-Y Jelly.

4. Hold on to the condom at the base of the penis to prevent spillage as you withdraw from the vagina.

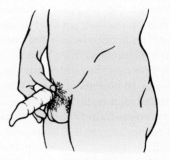

5. Remove the condom carefully to be sure that no semen spills from it.

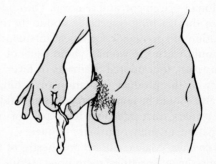

6. Place the condom in the trash or in some safe disposal.

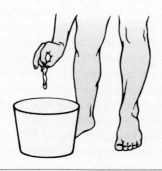

condom with the spermicide increases the contraceptive effectiveness.

Side effects and contraindications. Spermicides can cause local irritation in the vagina or on the penis. The irritation can cause tiny cracks that provide a portal of entry for infection, including HIV.

Natural Family Planning

Natural family planning, also called fertility awareness, involves learning to identify the signs and symptoms associated with ovulation. The couple either abstains from intercourse or uses a barrier method during the presumed fertile period. The ovum is viable up to 24 hours after ovulation, and sperm are viable for 48 to 72 hours in the fallopian tube, although most die within 24 hours (Keye et al, 1995).

Natural family planning methods are acceptable to most religions. They require no systemic hormones or insertion of devices. They are not only reversible but also can actually be used to increase the odds of achieving pregnancy when the couple desires a child.

Natural family planning requires extensive assessment and charting of all the changes in the menstrual cycle. The woman must be highly motivated to track the many factors that identify ovulation. Both partners must be willing to abstain from intercourse for much of the woman's cycle if the method is used to avoid pregnancy. They must also be willing to accept the high failure rate of 20%. There are three ways for a woman to predict when she is fertile. A woman may select only one method, but most women use a combination of the three to increase the predictive value of the methods.

Basal Body Temperature

The basal body temperature (BBT) is taken upon awakening and before any activity (Figure 11-4). This technique is based on the fact that the basal temperature rises very slightly at ovulation (about 0.2° C [0.4° F]) and remains higher in the last half of the cycle. Unfortunately, BBT is better at identifying that ovulation has *already* occurred rather than predicting when it is *about* to occur.

A *basal thermometer* is calibrated in tenths of a degree or is in an electronic digital format to detect these tiny changes. The woman charts each day's temperature to identify her temperature pattern. A rise in the BBT for the last 14 days of the cycle means that ovulation has probably occurred. Some electronic models have a memory to retain each day's temperature and display the pattern on a small screen.

Many factors can interfere with the accuracy of the BBT in predicting ovulation. Poor sleep, illness, jet lag,

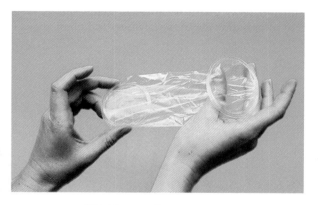

FIGURE **11-3** Female condom.

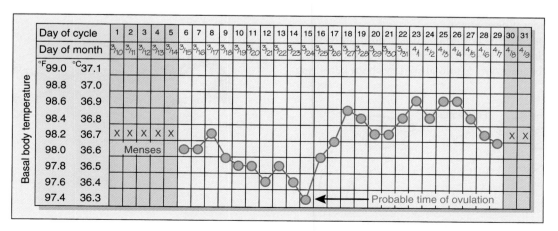

FIGURE **11-4** Basal body temperature chart. By taking and recording her temperature, the woman can determine the probable time of ovulation.

sleeping late, alcohol intake the evening before, or sleeping under an electric blanket or on a heated waterbed can make the BBT unreliable.

Cervical Mucus

The cervical mucus method is also called the *Billings method* to predict ovulation. The character of cervical mucus changes during the menstrual cycle as estrogen and progesterone influence the mucus-secreting glands of the cervix. Immediately after menstruation, the cervical mucus is sticky, thick, and white. As ovulation nears, the mucus becomes thin, slippery, and clear to aid the passage of sperm into the cervix. The slippery mucus can be stretched 6 cm or more and has the consistency of egg white (Figure 11-5). The stretching of the mucus is called spinnbarkeit. After ovulation, the mucus again becomes thicker. Factors that interfere with the accuracy of cervical mucus assessment include the use of antihistamines, vaginal infections, contraceptive foams or jellies, sexual arousal, and recent coitus.

Calendar, or Rhythm, Method

The woman charts her menstrual cycles on a calendar for several months. If they are regular, she may be able to predict ovulation. The rhythm method is based on the fact that ovulation usually occurs about 14 days *before* the next menstrual period. This would be about halfway through a 28-day cycle, but would be on day 16 of a 30-day cycle.

PERMANENT CONTRACEPTION
Sterilization

Sterilization is a permanent method of birth control that is almost 100% effective in preventing pregnancy. Although the procedure may be reversed in some cases, reversal is expensive and not always successful. Therefore patients should carefully think about this decision and consider it permanent.

Advantages. The advantages of sterilization relate to the fact that the person can consider the risk of pregnancy to be near zero. Minimal anxiety about becoming

pregnant may help the individual to enjoy the sexual relationship more.

Disadvantages. A major disadvantage of sterilization is the same as its primary advantage: permanence. Divorce, marriage, death of a child, or a change in attitude toward having children may make the person regret his or her decision. The procedures require surgery, and although the risks are small, they are the same as for other surgical procedures: hemorrhage, infection, injury to other organs, and anesthesia complications.

Male Sterilization

Male sterilization, or *vasectomy,* is performed by making a cut in each side of the scrotum and cutting each vas deferens, the tube through which the sperm travel (Figure 11-6, *A*). Because sperm are already in the system distal to the area of ligation, sterility is not immediate. Another method of birth control must be used until all sperm have left the system, usually about 1 month. The man should return to his physician for analysis of his semen to verify that it no longer contains sperm. Men need information about the anatomy and physiology of

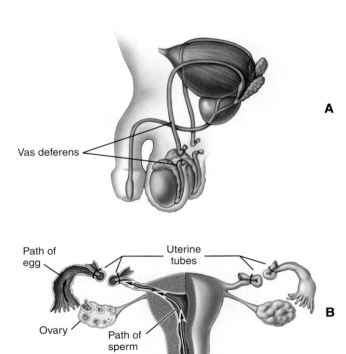

FIGURE **11-6** Surgical methods of birth control. **A,** Vasectomy, the cutting and ligation (tying off) of the vas deferens. **B,** Tubal ligation, the ligation of the fallopian tubes.

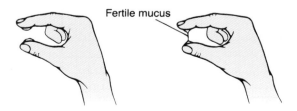

FIGURE **11-5** Spinnbarkeit. The woman tests the ability of her cervical mucus to stretch. This helps to determine the time of ovulation.

their sex organs. They need reassurance that they will still have erections and ejaculations and that intercourse will remain pleasurable.

The surgery takes about 20 minutes and is performed on an outpatient basis with a local anesthetic. There is some pain, bruising, and swelling after the surgery. Rest, a mild analgesic, and the application of an ice pack are comfort measures. As in other surgeries, the man should report the following:

- Bleeding or substantial bruising
- Separation of the suture line, drainage, or increasing pain

Female Sterilization

Female sterilization, called *tubal ligation,* involves blocking or ligating the fallopian tubes. It can be accomplished by using electrocautery or clips. Tubal ligation is easy to perform during the immediate postpartum period because the fundus, to which the tubes are attached, is large and near the surface. Any of the following three methods may be used:

- A *minilaparotomy,* nicknamed "Band-Aid surgery," uses an incision near the umbilicus in the immediate postpartum period or just above the symphysis at other times. The surgeon makes a tiny incision, brings each tube through it, and ligates and cuts the tube.
- *Laparoscopic surgery* is similar, but the tubes are identified and ligated through a lighted tube called a laparoscope (Figure 11-6, *B*).
- The traditional approach is performed during other abdominal surgery, usually a cesarean birth.

The discomfort after the minilaparotomy or laparoscopy is usually easily relieved with oral analgesia. Some women experience nausea from the anesthesia. Even though this is not considered major surgery, the woman requires 1 or 2 days to recuperate. She should report signs of bleeding or infection, as in the male vasectomy.

> ✹NURSING **TIP**_____
> When discussing sexual issues with a couple, the nurse should use the word partner until the couple indicates a preference for an alternative term.

EMERGENCY CONTRACEPTION

The "morning after" pill is a method of preventing pregnancy after unprotected sexual intercourse. It can be used if contraceptives fail (such as a torn condom), in cases of rape, or in other situations as needed.

A larger than normal dose of oral contraceptive can be taken no later than 72 hours after unprotected sex and a second dose is repeated 12 hours later. A kit (Preven)

is available with a prescription. Antiemetics may be needed to treat the side effects of nausea and vomiting.

Levonorgestrel or a combination levonorgestrel and ethinyl estradiol can be administered within 72 hours of unprotected sex in two doses and is considered effective. Inserting a copper 380-A IUD within 5 to 7 days after unprotected sex is also effective in preventing pregnancy and provides long-term protection.

RU486 (mifepristone) in combination with the administration of prostaglandin analogs (misoprostol) 36 to 48 hours later is also considered to be an effective postcoital contraceptive regimen. Side effects include nausea, vomiting and abdominal pain. Counseling the woman concerning birth control and STD prevention is essential.

UNRELIABLE CONTRACEPTIVE METHODS
Withdrawal

Withdrawal, or **coitus interruptus,** is withdrawal of the penis before ejaculation. It demands more self-control than most men can achieve. Preejaculatory secretions often contain sperm that can fertilize an ovum.

Douching

Douching after intercourse is not a form of birth control and may actually transport sperm farther into the birth canal.

Breastfeeding

Breastfeeding inhibits ovulation in many women as long as the infant receives at least 10 feedings in 24 hours. The prolactin secreted to stimulate milk production also inhibits ovulation. If the woman supplements with formula or when the infant begins taking solids, milk intake (and thus prolactin secretion) falls. Ovulation is then likely. Remember that ovulation *precedes* menstruation—pregnancy can occur before the first menstrual period after birth.

> ✹NURSING **TIP**_____
> A woman can become pregnant while breastfeeding.

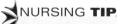
INFERTILITY CARE

Infertility is the inability to conceive when desired. The strict definition of infertility is that a couple who has regular, unprotected sexual intercourse for 1 year cannot conceive. Infertility is *primary* if conception has never occurred and *secondary* when there have been one or more pregnancies before the infertility. The definition is usually expanded to couples who conceive but repeatedly lose a pregnancy.

More couples are seeking help for infertility for many reasons, including the following:

- Couples are delaying childbearing until the mid- to late 30s, when a natural decline in fertility occurs.
- New treatments may cause couples to reconsider their acceptance of childlessness and initiate or resume infertility therapy.

SOCIAL AND PSYCHOLOGICAL IMPLICATIONS

Becoming a parent is a role that most people expect to assume at some time. Because parenting is such an expected and necessary part of society, infertility has implications that go far beyond its physical implications.

Assumption of Fertility

Most couples assume they are fertile and work hard to avoid pregnancy as they pursue educational or career goals. They expect to conceive in a few months at the most when they do decide to have a child. They enjoy being with parents and expectant parents because they foresee joining their ranks shortly. They often begin making preparations for living space and supplies that an infant will need.

As the months pass and the woman's period comes each month, they become less certain that they will join the ranks of other parents. Once-joyful occasions, such as baby showers, become melancholy or anxiety-provoking events. The potential grandparents may think their children are waiting too long to start a family or may even believe they are selfish if they do not realize that the younger couple is trying to conceive.

Psychological Reactions

Shock is often a couple's first reaction to infertility. Their reactions vary based on how easily the infertility is alleviated, their personality and self-images, and their relationship.

Guilt. The partner who has the identified problem may feel guilty because he or she is depriving the other one of children. Either partner may regret past choices that now affect their fertility, such as sexual practices that resulted in infections that scarred the fallopian tubes.

Isolation. Infertile couples often feel different from those who have no problem conceiving. They may isolate themselves from these people to avoid emotional pain. In doing so, they may also isolate themselves from sources of support.

Depression. Infertility challenges one's sense of control and self-image. The couple may experience a roller coaster of hope alternating with despair as the woman has her period each month. They may become judgmental and angry with others.

Stress on the relationship. Either or both partners may feel unlovable because their self-esteem has been shaken by the problem. A man often finds it difficult to perform sexually "on demand" for semen specimens or at specific times each month. Their sexual relationship may take on a clinical air rather than one of love and support.

Cultural and Religious Considerations

In many cultures, fertility (or the lack thereof) is considered strictly a female problem. It may be closely linked to the woman's social status. The stigma of infertility can lead to divorce and rejection from family and society. To choose treatment for infertility may go against the couple's societal norms, particularly if the male must be treated to achieve pregnancy.

Religious norms influence what tests and treatments a couple is willing to pursue. Surrogate parenting, in vitro fertilization, or other techniques may not be acceptable in terms of the couple's personal or religious beliefs. Conflict can arise if a potentially successful therapy is acceptable to one member of the couple but not to the other.

> ⚡NURSING **TIP**_____
> Avoid using the word *fault* when discussing which member of the infertile couple has the identified problem. Although a problem may be identified in only one person, many unknown factors impact fertility.

FACTORS AFFECTING INFERTILITY

Many factors that cause infertility are unknown. Some couples may have a problem that makes it unlikely that they would conceive, yet they have several children. Others have no identified problem but still cannot conceive.

Male Factors

To produce a pregnancy, the man must deposit a sufficient number of normal sperm near the cervix, and the sperm must be protected from the acidic vaginal secretions until they enter the cervix. The sperm must be able to swim purposefully to the waiting ovum. Male factors in infertility can be divided into abnormalities of the sperm, erections, ejaculation, or seminal fluid.

Abnormal sperm. A man may have a sperm count that is too low to achieve fertilization. He may have a sufficient number of sperm, but too many of these are dead or abnormally formed. Sperm are continuously formed, and many factors can affect their formation.

Some factors that can interfere with normal sperm formation and function include the following:

- High scrotal temperature from hot tubs, saunas, or fever
- Abnormal hormone stimulation
- Infections
- Anatomic abnormalities such as a varicocele (enlarged veins in the testicles)
- Medications, illicit drugs, excessive alcohol intake
- Exposure to toxins

Abnormal erections. Anything that impairs nervous system function or blood flow to the penis can interfere with erections. Some drugs, notably antihypertensives, reduce or shorten erections.

Abnormal ejaculation. Some drugs and nervous system disorders may cause retrograde ejaculation, in which semen is released into the bladder rather than from the penis. *Hypospadias* (urethral opening on the underside of the penis rather than the tip) causes semen to be deposited closer to the vaginal outlet rather than near the cervix.

Abnormal seminal fluid. Seminal fluid carries the sperm into the vagina, but only sperm enter the cervix to fertilize the ovum. Semen coagulates immediately after ejaculation, then liquefies within 30 minutes to allow sperm to swim toward the cervix. Sperm will be trapped or will not survive if the seminal fluid remains thick or if its composition does not protect the sperm from the vaginal secretions.

Female Factors

A woman's fertility depends on regular production of normal ova, having an open path from the ovary to the uterus, and having a uterine endometrium that supports the pregnancy.

Disorders of ovulation. Normal ovulation depends on a balanced and precisely timed interaction between the hypothalamus, pituitary, and ovary (see Chapter 2). If the hypothalamus and/or pituitary do not properly stimulate the ovary, ovulation will not occur. Conversely, the ovary may not respond despite normal hormonal stimulation. Chemotherapeutic drugs for cancer, excessive alcohol intake, and smoking can interfere with ovulation. Sometimes ovulation does not occur because the woman is entering the climacteric early.

Abnormalities of the fallopian tubes. Infections such as chlamydia and gonorrhea can cause scarring and adhesions of the fallopian tubes that block them. Adhesions may also occur because of endometriosis, pelvic surgery, appendicitis, peritonitis, or ovarian cysts. If the tubal obstruction allows the smaller sperm to pass but is too narrow for the resulting fertilized ovum, ectopic tubal pregnancy may occur (see p. 86). The same conditions may cause abnormal transport of the ovum through the tube.

Abnormalities of the uterus, cervix, or ovaries. Congenital abnormalities of the reproductive tract or uterine myomas (benign uterine muscle tumors) may interfere with normal implantation of the ovum or may result in repeated spontaneous abortion or early preterm labor. Women with polycystic ovaries have abnormalities of ovulation and menstruation that accompany the hormonal dysfunction associated with this disorder.

Hormone abnormalities. In addition to interfering with ovulation, abnormal hormone stimulation can interfere with proper development of the uterine lining, resulting in an inability to conceive or in repeated spontaneous abortions. Abnormalities in the amount or timing of any hormone necessary for endometrial buildup, ovum development and release, or support of the conceptus can result in infertility.

FACTORS INFLUENCING FERTILITY

Coital frequency. Intercourse more than three times per week is best for conception. The window of opportunity to conceive opens 2 days before ovulation and closes 1 day after ovulation.

Age. Women over 35 years of age have a somewhat decreased (but not absent) chance of conceiving.

Cigarette smoking. Cigarette smoking of more than 15 cigarettes per day suppresses the function of the immune system, leading to an early loss of reproductive function. Nicotine has an effect on tubal motility, resulting in an increased risk of ectopic pregnancies.

Exercise, diet, and weight. Excessive exercise and weight loss may be linked to an increase in infertility. A low-calorie vegetarian diet is associated with a short luteal phase, and excessive weight loss may influence the release of gonadotropins. Ovarian dysfunction is common in obese women, especially those who gain weight rapidly. However, weight is thought to be a cofactor of infertility rather than a direct cause (Keye et al, 1995).

Emotional factors. Emotional factors do not cause infertility, but many infertile couples experience stress and anxiety and require emotional understanding. A strong support system is helpful in the decision to start or stop fertility treatments.

Medical problems. Pelvic adhesions can obstruct the fallopian tube and cause infertility. Adhesions can result from abdominal and/or pelvic surgery, Crohn's disease, ulcerative colitis, or celiac disease. PID and STDs are also associated with infertility.

Drugs and chemicals. Pollutants in the environment and medications or chemicals ingested may influence fertility. Chemotherapeutic agents used in the treatment of cancer are related to infertility. Research is ongoing concerning the protective effect of suppressing ovarian function or storing ova during chemotherapeutic treatments. Recreational drugs such as marijuana and cocaine have an increased risk for infertility. Cocaine use in men has been shown to affect the motility of sperm and contribute to infertility of the couple. Antihistamines can decrease vaginal lubrication, antihypertensives can decrease erectile ability, barbiturates can inhibit the release of gonadotropin, and NSAIDs can block egg release. The use of cimetidine, monoamine oxidase (MAO) antidepressants, and lithium are also thought to alter male reproduction (Keye et al, 1995). Reprotox is a center that maintains a database of reproductive effects of industrial chemicals.

EVALUATION OF INFERTILITY

Both members of a couple are evaluated for infertility. The evaluation begins with a thorough history and physical examination to identify evidence of other conditions that may also be affecting their fertility.

Testing proceeds from the simple to the complex. However, testing may be accelerated if the woman is older because of her natural decline in fertility with age.

Male Testing

A semen analysis is the first male test performed. Semen is best collected by masturbation; if this is unacceptable, semen can be collected in a condom. Endocrine tests identify the hormonal stimulation that is necessary for sperm formation. Ultrasonography can identify anatomical abnormalities. Testicular biopsy is an invasive test to obtain a sample of testicular tissue for analysis.

Female Testing

The methods for predicting ovulation discussed in natural family planning can also be used to evaluate infertility. Ultrasonography is used to assess the structure of reproductive organs, to identify the maturation and release of the ovum, and to ensure proper timing for other tests, such as the postcoital test. Ultrasonography is also used to identify multifetal pregnancies. The postcoital test is done 6 to 12 hours after intercourse to evaluate the action of sperm within the woman's cervical mucus at the time of ovulation. Endocrine tests evaluate the hormone stimulation of ovulation and the buildup of the uterine lining to prepare for pregnancy. More invasive tests are sometimes required. The hysterosalpingogram is an x-ray using contrast medium to evaluate the structure of the reproductive organs. An endometrial biopsy is done to obtain a sample of uterine lining to assess its response to hormones. Hysteroscopy and laparoscopy use an endoscope (instrument that allows visual inspection of internal organs) to examine the uterine interior and the pelvic organs.

THERAPY FOR INFERTILITY

The specific therapy depends on what cause, if any, was identified by testing. Possible therapies are discussed in the following sections.

Medications

Medications may be given to either the man or the woman to improve semen quality, induce ovulation, prepare the uterine endometrium for pregnancy, or support the pregnancy once it is established. Several of the drugs are given with another drug to mimic natural function. Medications are continued for six to nine cycles for optimum outcome. Some of the drugs that may be prescribed include the following:

- Bromocriptine (Parlodel) (Pergolide mesylate and dopamine agonists CV205-502 are newer drugs showing promise.): Corrects excess prolactin secretion by the pituitary, which would interfere with implantation of the fertilized ovum
- Clomiphene (Clomid): Induces ovulation; may be used with hCG
- Gonadotropin-releasing hormone (GnRH, Lutrepulse): Stimulates production of other hormones that, in turn, stimulate ovulation in the female and production of testosterone and sperm in the male (may be administered via IV pump worn on the waist)
- Leuprolide (Lupron): Reduces endometriosis
- Menotropins (Pergonal): Stimulates ovulation and sperm production
- Nafarelin (Synarel): Reduces endometriosis
- Progesterone: Promotes implantation of the fertilized ovum
- Urofollitropin (Fertinex): Stimulates ovulation
- Sildenafil (Viagra): Increases erectile function
- hCG (Pregnyl): Stimulates ovulation and sperm production

Medications given to induce ovulation also increase the risk of multifetal gestations. Although most of these multiple gestations are twins, higher multiples present a much higher risk for maternal, fetal, and neonatal complications. The parents of high multiples may need to make a decision about which, if any, of their fetuses to abort so that the others have a better chance of achieving maturity. This situation presents a difficult ethical situation for both parents and professionals.

Surgical Procedures

Surgery may be used to correct anatomic abnormalities such as varicocele, adhesions, or tubal obstruction.

Therapeutic Insemination

Once called "artificial insemination," therapeutic insemination may use the male partner's sperm or sperm from an anonymous donor. Therapeutic insemination may be used by a woman who wants a biological child without a relationship with a man. If sperm are placed directly in the uterus, they are washed and concentrated to improve their chances of fertilizing an ovum. Donors are screened for genetic defects, infections, and high-risk behaviors. Donor sperm is held frozen for 6 months to reduce the risk of transmitting a disease that was not apparent at the initial screening. Reputable centers limit the number of times a man may donate his sperm to reduce the chance of inadvertent consanguinity (blood relationship) between his offspring when they grow up.

Surrogate Parenting

A surrogate mother may donate the use of her uterus only, with the sperm and ovum coming from the infertile couple who have a problem carrying a pregnancy. Or she may be inseminated with the male partner's sperm, thus supplying both her genetic and her gestational components. Surrogate mothering cannot be anonymous, and the birth mother inevitably forms bonds with the fetus during the months of pregnancy.

Advanced Reproductive Techniques

The field of advanced reproductive technologies gives new hope to couples who may have once considered their infertility to be irreversible (Table 11-2). However, some of the newest techniques are still considered experimental and are thus not covered by insurance.

Bypassing obstacles to conception. The following techniques place intact sperm and ova together to allow fertilization. Each begins with ovulation induction by medications to obtain several ova and thus improve the likelihood of a successful pregnancy.

- *In vitro fertilization (IVF).* Several ova are obtained and mixed with the partner's or a donor's semen. Up to four resulting embryos are then returned to the uterus 2 days later.
- *Gamete intrafallopian transfer (GIFT).* Ova are obtained and mixed with sperm. The gametes are placed in the fallopian tubes where fertilization and entry into the uterus occur normally.
- *Tubal embryo transfer (TET)*, also called zygote intrafallopian transfer (ZIFT). The ova are fertilized outside the woman's body and returned to the fallopian tube at an earlier stage than with IVF.

In general, GIFT and TET have a higher pregnancy rate than IVF. These techniques can result in a multifetal

---

table 11-2 | *Summary of Assisted Reproductive Therapies (ARTs)*

THERAPY	DESCRIPTION
Therapeutic insemination	Donor sperm are placed in the uterus or fallopian tube; sperm may be the partner's or a donor's.
In vitro fertilization (IVF)	After inducing ovulation, ova are recovered by laparoscopy or transvaginal aspiration under sonography; they are then fertilized with sperm from the partner or a donor in the laboratory and transferred to the uterus 2 days later.
Gamete intrafallopian transfer (GIFT)	Oocytes are retrieved into a catheter that contains prepared sperm; up to two ova are injected into each fallopian tube, where fertilization occurs. The woman must have at least one open tube.
Tubal embryo transfer (TET), also called zygote intrafallopian transfer (ZIFT)	Ova are fertilized as in IVF but are transferred to the fallopian tube as soon as fertilization occurs. The resulting embryos enter the uterus normally for implantation.
Donor oocyte	Multiple ova are retrieved from a woman. They are fertilized and placed in the prepared uterus of the infertile woman.
Surrogate mother	A woman allows her ova to be inseminated by the partner or another donor. She then carries the fetus and agrees to relinquish the infant after birth.
Gestational surrogate	The infertile couple undergoes IVF, but the resulting embryos are placed in the prepared uterus of a woman who has agreed to carry the fetus for them. The woman does not donate any of her genetic components.
ICSI (intra-cytoplasmic sperm injection)	Sperm are inserted directly into ova.

pregnancy. Rarely do all ova or embryos returned to the uterus actually implant.

Microsurgical techniques. In these techniques, the surgeon "operates" on the ovum itself to inject a sperm into it (intra-cytoplasmic sperm injection [ICSI]). The fertilized ovum is placed into the uterus, as with IVF. The surgical care of the infertile woman has been revolutionized by the development of laser and microsurgical techniques for male and female infertility.

OUTCOMES OF INFERTILITY THERAPY

The following three outcomes are possible after infertility therapy:

- Achievement of a "take home" infant
- Unsuccessful therapy resulting in a decision about adoption
- Pregnancy loss after treatment

Becoming pregnant changes the couple's anxiety but does not eliminate it. Because of past disappointments, they may be reluctant to invest emotionally in the pregnancy. They may delay preparations for birth because they expect to be disappointed again or fear that something will go wrong at the last minute. Even when their infant is born, they may have unrealistic expectations of themselves as parents after all their hard work in achieving pregnancy.

Couples who decide to pursue adoption must consider their preferences and the realities of the adoption "market." Most couples prefer to adopt an infant of the same race, but that child may not be available. Some couples fear that they will have a biological child after adoption and wonder if they can love the two children equally. When a pregnancy is lost after treatment, the couple may feel optimism mixed with sadness. On one hand, they proved that they could conceive. On the other hand, they did not get an infant.

LEGAL AND ETHICAL FACTORS IN ASSISTED REPRODUCTION

Noncoital reproduction brings with it many legal and ethical problems that must be dealt with. In most cases, assisted reproductive techniques (ARTs) are used to assist infertile couples. However, this technique can also be used by a married couple to avoid known genetic anomalies carried by one partner. Donors and surrogates involve third parties, and their emotional bonds and legal rights must be considered. Homosexual couples or single parents can create a child through surrogacy, and a changed family structure evolves.

Parental rights are a legal challenge. It is now possible for a child to have five parents: a sperm donor, an egg donor, a gestational surrogate, and the two parents who will rear the child. The right to bear a child is protected by the United States Constitution; the government cannot usually interfere. The nontraditional family is therefore entitled to constitutional protection.

Cloning one's lost child is now a possibility. The fate of a frozen embryo when the parents divorce has been challenged in court. The sale of frozen embryos has a growing impact on our legal system. However, federally funded research on fetal tissue can control future research and development. State laws can also prevent funding of private research. The problems of insurance coverage and access to care are also highly debated issues.

NURSING CARE RELATED TO INFERTILITY TREATMENT

Much of the nursing role involves supporting the couple as they undergo diagnosis and make decisions concerning treatment. The nurse must use tactful therapeutic communication to help each member of the couple discuss their feelings. Partners are encouraged to accept their feelings. The normality of feelings that seem out of place (such as ambivalence about a pregnancy after working so hard to achieve it) is reinforced. The couple is helped to identify ways to communicate with each other and to discuss available options that empower them with control.

The couple's sense of control should be increased as much as possible. Their positive coping skills are reinforced, and more constructive alternatives to poor coping are explored. They may benefit from relaxation techniques, support groups, and other stress-management methods. Support groups can also reduce their sense of isolation. The couple should be helped to explore their options at each decision point. Only the person(s) involved can make the decision, but the nurse can help them to explore their feelings.

HORMONE REPLACEMENT THERAPY

When symptoms of menopause interfere with activities of daily living, hormone therapy may help restore quality of life. Hormone replacement therapy (HRT) may be prescribed to relieve many of the uncomfortable symptoms of menopause. In addition, HRT prolongs the protective effects of estrogen on the woman's cardiovascular and skeletal systems. Estrogen cannot prevent osteoporosis, but it can slow bone loss if the woman also takes in adequate calcium.

Estrogen may be administered in various forms depending on the woman's needs. Estrogen comes in tablets, transdermal skin patches, vaginal creams, injections, and pellets. The goal of therapy has a bearing on the dosage and form prescribed (e.g., whether for temporary relief of hot flashes or for osteoporosis). Vaginal changes can be treated locally with vaginal creams or systemically.

Unless a woman had a hysterectomy (removal of the uterus) a combination of progesterone and estrogen is used in HRT. In *cyclic therapy,* estrogen is taken for 13 days and progesterone and estrogen are taken together for the last 12 days. Estrogen may also be administered in a patch. A transdermal patch is applied one to two times a week to a hairless area of the skin. Minor skin irritation can occur. Patches should not be applied to the breast area. Combination estrogen-progestin patches are also available.

Oral progestin can either be taken continuously or 12 days per month to trigger monthly menses. Progesterone is thought to offer some protection against endometrial cancer and is used to manage heavy menstrual bleeding. Low-dose birth control pills may be used to offer contraception. HRT can be prescribed as cyclic or continuous. HRT has the side effect of increasing breast density, which is associated with decreased mammogram accuracy (Archer & Utian, 2001). Therefore women using HRT must be carefully counseled on techniques for breast self-examinations and the need for follow-up visits. Some women use HRT to control the timing of their menstrual periods in relation to business activities or events.

SIDE EFFECTS AND CONTRAINDICATIONS

Side effects of and adverse reactions to estrogen include nausea, vomiting, headache, dizziness, and breast tenderness. The most common side effect of progesterone is irregular bleeding when therapy begins. The less frequent side effects of progesterone include symptoms similar to those of premenstrual syndrome, fluid retention, and depression.

Contraindications for HRT include estrogen-dependent breast cancer, endometrial cancer, thromboembolic disease, a history of malignant melanoma, chronic liver disease, severe hypertriglyceridemia, gallbladder disease, and seizure disorders (Archer & Utian, 2001). Annual breast examinations and regular self-breast assessments are advised for women undergoing HRT.

COMPLEMENTARY REGIMENS

The use of over-the-counter complementary therapy during menopause has become very popular. Some examples include the following:

- Yam root contains natural progesterone in the form of diosgenin and has an oral or topical form but not a proven progesterone effect.
- Soy products are thought to reduce problems such as hot flashes.
- Vitamin E is thought to stabilize estrogen levels.
- Black cohosh, marketed as Remifemin, is thought to reduce luteinizing hormone.
- Calcium and vitamin D supplements are recommended for women who cannot spend at least 30 minutes a day in the sun.

See Chapter 33 for more information concerning complementary and alternative medicine (CAM) therapies. Estrogen helps convert vitamin D into calcitonin, which is essential for the absorption of calcium. Calcitonin is available as a supplement (Calcimar, Miacalcin) to menopausal women. Raloxifene is also approved by the Food and Drug Administration for treatment of osteoporosis in menopausal women. Excessive caffeine intake and alcohol ingestion increases calcium excretion, and smoking further decreases estrogen utilization and so should be avoided.

THERAPY FOR OSTEOPOROSIS

Osteoporosis occurs when the loss of calcium from the bones is faster than its deposition in the bones. Signs of osteoporosis include a loss of height, the development of a "dowager's hump" (a dorsal kyphoses and cervical lordosis), curvature of the upper spine, and increased susceptibility to hip and spinal fractures. Estrogen replacement can slow bone loss if the woman's calcium intake is adequate, particularly if given in the first few years after menopause. Calcium intake from food sources such as dairy products, dark green leafy vegetables, soybeans, and wheat bread and/or calcium supplements can prevent complications of osteoporosis. Exercise such as walking, hiking, stair climbing, and dancing are advisable. High-impact exercises should be avoided. Alendronate (Fosamax) may be prescribed. Esophageal and gastric irritation are common side effects of alendronate, and the woman should be instructed to drink 8 ounces of plain water and sit upright for 30 minutes after taking the drug and before eating a meal.

MENOPAUSE

The definition of menopause according to the World Health Organization (WHO) is the cessation of menstrual periods for a 12-month period because of changes in estrogen production. The climacteric (change of life) is also known as the perimenopausal period, which extends for 2 to 8 years before menstruation ceases. The last menstrual period occurs at approximately 51 years of age (Boston Women's Health Book Collective, 1998). In the 2- to 8-year period before this time, the ova slowly degenerate and menstrual cycles are often anovulatory and irregular. Estrogen production by the ovaries decreases. Pregnancy can occur during the climacteric, and the woman should be encouraged to continue any birth control that she has used in the past. Decreasing estrogen in the woman increases her risk for osteoporosis, arteriosclerosis, and increases in cholesterol levels in the blood. Menopause may be induced at any age by surgery, pelvic irradiation, or extreme stress.

PHYSICAL CHANGES

The decrease in estrogen specifically causes the following:
- Changes in the menstrual cycle
- Vasomotor instability (hot flashes)
- Decreased moisture and elasticity of vagina that can cause dyspareunia (painful intercourse)

Other symptoms such as mood swings and irritability are also experienced. Hot flashes are a well-known phenomenon. The woman suddenly feels a burning or hot sensation of her skin followed by perspiration. Hot flashes often occur during the night, and some women have several sleep interruptions because of them. They are more likely to occur when menopause is artificial, such as through oophorectomy (removal of the ovaries), rather than when it occurs naturally. The woman may also notice chills, palpitations, dizziness, and tingling of the skin as part of the vasomotor instability.

The reproductive organs are estrogen dependent, leading to changes as the estrogen level declines. The uterus shrinks and the ovaries atrophy. The sacral ligaments relax and pelvic muscles weaken, which can result in pelvic floor dysfunction. The cervix becomes pale and shrinks. The vagina becomes shorter, narrower, and less elastic. There is less lubrication. Some women notice a change in *libido* (sexual desire) at this time. Coitus may be uncomfortable because of vaginal dryness. Urinary incontinence may be a problem as the muscles controlling urine flow atrophy. The breasts atrophy.

Loss of estrogen secretion also means an end to its protective effect on the woman's cardiovascular and skeletal systems. Estrogen increases the amount of high-density lipoproteins, which carry cholesterol from body cells to the liver for excretion. The incidence of heart disease rises dramatically after menopause because low-density lipoproteins, which carry cholesterol into body cells (including blood vessels), increase.

Estrogen assists the deposition of calcium in the bones to strengthen them. Loss of bone mass accelerates as estrogen levels fall, resulting in osteoporosis. Osteoporosis is a leading cause of vertebral, hip, and other fractures in postmenopausal women because the bones become very fragile. Both males and females lose bone

mass as they age. Females, who have a lower bone mass to begin with because they are smaller, lose more in proportion to the total amount as they age. In addition, they live longer than males, and the loss continues longer. Therefore problems such as hip fractures related to age affect many more women than men. The bones may be so fragile that a fracture occurs and causes a fall, rather than the fracture being the result of a fall.

PSYCHOLOGICAL AND CULTURAL VARIATIONS

Women from different cultures have different experiences of menopause. How the society views aging, the role of the female, and femininity itself has a bearing. In countries in which age is revered, menopause is practically a "nonevent." In the United States, with its emphasis on youth, sex appeal, and physical beauty, menopause can threaten the woman's feelings of health and self-worth. A positive aspect of menopause is that it is a time of liberation from monthly periods, cramps, and the fear of unwanted pregnancy. It can be the beginning of a satisfying postreproductive life.

TREATMENT OPTIONS

Culture, finances, and access to health care are factors that must be considered. Partnership-building communication with the health care team can help the woman cope with lifestyle changes that may be necessary to maintain health. Exercise, an increase in the dietary intake of calcium and magnesium, and a high-fiber, low-fat diet rich in antioxidants are essential. Stress reduction, daily exposure to sunlight, and annual checkups are also advised as part of self-help care. CAM techniques involved in women's health care are discussed in Chapter 33.

NURSING CARE OF THE MENOPAUSAL WOMAN

Nursing Care Plan 11-1 offers nursing interventions in addition to those discussed here. The woman's knowledge of the changes surrounding menopause is assessed. If she is near the age for the climacteric to begin, any symptoms are identified. Treatments or tests that the woman will have, such as bone density studies, are clarified. The nurse must determine the woman's understanding of the risks and benefits of HRT when helping her to decide about the therapy, with written information given to reinforce verbal teaching.

The woman is taught what signs and symptoms she should report, such as vaginal bleeding that recurs after the cessation of menstrual periods. She should also report signs of vaginal irritation or signs of urinary tract infection because these are more common with atrophy of vaginal tissues.

NURSING CARE PLAN 11-1

The Woman Experiencing Perimenopausal Symptoms

PATIENT DATA: A 49-year-old woman tells the nurse that she is experiencing a lot of discomfort relating to her beginning menopause. She states she is having hot flashes and does not enjoy having sex anymore, among other "embarrassing" symptoms.

SELECTED NURSING DIAGNOSIS   *Impaired comfort related to vasomotor symptoms (hot flashes)*

Outcomes	Nursing Interventions	Rationales
The woman will verbalize measures to increase her comfort during vasomotor symptoms.	1. Suggest that she wear layered cotton clothes.	1. This allows the woman to take off or put on clothes during hot flashes or chills; cotton allows easier passage of air than synthetic fabric.
	2. Advise her to avoid caffeine (coffee, tea, colas, chocolate).	2. Hot flashes often occur at night; caffeine is a stimulant and will contribute to insomnia and perspiration.
	3. Explain that stress exacerbates the condition; explore activities that she finds relaxing.	3. Stress affects virtually every system of the body, including the endocrine and cardiovascular systems, worsening the hot flashes.
	4. Suggest she discuss hormone replacement therapy (HRT) with her physician.	4. HRT is effective at relieving vasomotor symptoms, but its benefits and risks must be evaluated by the individual patient.
	5. Vitamin E, ginseng, and other herbs may reduce vasomotor symptoms.	5. Some women should not take or choose not to take HRT, and these measures provide an alternative.

SELECTED NURSING DIAGNOSIS   *Ineffective sexuality patterns related to painful intercourse*

Outcomes	Nursing Interventions	Rationales
The woman will state measures to reduce vaginal dryness. The woman will express no discomfort with coitus.	1. Teach the woman to use water-soluble lubricant before intercourse.	1. Thinning of vaginal walls and drying of secretions can lead to discomfort during intercourse unless additional lubrication is used; oil-based lubricants can promote bacterial growth.
	2. Teach that products, such as Replens and Lubrin, are available without a prescription to provide relief of vaginal dryness for several days.	2. These products lubricate the vagina for a longer period of time, reducing tissue trauma.
	3. If estrogen vaginal cream is prescribed, teach that it should be inserted at bedtime.	3. Topical applications of estrogen reduce vaginal atrophy; applying at bedtime reduces loss and increases absorption.

SELECTED NURSING DIAGNOSIS   *Risk for stress urinary incontinence and infection related to genital atrophy*

Outcomes	Nursing Interventions	Rationales
The woman will restate measures to promote urinary tract health.	1. Teach Kegel exercises: Contract muscles as if to stop urine flow. Repeat 10 times. Do the cycle of 10 Kegel exercises five times each day. Do not actually stop urine flow while urinating.	1. Kegel exercises increase muscle tone around the urinary meatus and the vagina. Repeatedly stopping the stream of urine could cause retention that could lead to infection.

Continued

NURSING CARE PLAN 11-1—cont'd

2. Drink at least eight glasses of water each day. Caffeine-containing drinks should not be included in the target amount of fluid.

2. Adequate intake of liquid dilutes urine and promotes regular emptying, both of which discourage bacterial growth. Caffeine acts as a diuretic, which reverses some of the benefits of the fluid taken in.

3. Urinate regularly; do not allow the bladder to become overly distended.

3. Prevents stasis of urine, which promotes the growth of bacteria.

4. Wipe from front to back after toileting.

4. Avoids bringing anal organisms to the urinary meatus or vagina, where they could cause infection.

?CRITICAL THINKING QUESTION

A woman, age 49 years, requests help in controlling her anxiety level. She reports hot flashes, night sweats, sleep pattern disturbances, and mood swings. She is afraid her husband will leave her and wants medication to "calm her down." Based on her age and history, what is the best response of the nurse?

The woman is also taught how to take prescribed medications properly. For example, the nurse must teach her that calcium is best used if she also takes vitamin D. Taking foods or other medications before allowing at least 30 minutes (preferably 1 hour) for alendronate to be absorbed will negate the benefit of that dose. Lying down after taking alendronate can cause severe esophageal irritation.

The woman should be informed of medication-related side effects to report. She should contact her health care provider if she has headaches, visual disturbances, signs of thrombophlebitis, heaviness in her legs, chest pain, or breast lumps, because these symptoms may indicate adverse side effects associated with HRT. She should contact her health care provider for the best plan if she decides to stop HRT to reduce the distress associated with abrupt cessation of therapy. Basic education concerning the use of CAM therapy and their side effects (see Chapter 33) and interactions should be included in the teaching plan.

The woman should be taught about the value of weight-bearing exercise in slowing bone loss. She must be helped to identify suitable exercises that she enjoys and cautioned about the high-impact ones that she should avoid. Because even minor falls can result in disabling fractures in women who have osteoporosis, the nurse should teach the woman ways to make her environment safer. Safety needs may be as simple as making sure there are adequate lights with handy switches and that loose cords and obstructions are secured outside of walking paths. Nonskid bath and shower floors and convenient grab bars reduce the risk of falls when bathing.

The nurse should identify the woman's perception of her menopausal status with consideration of cultural factors, sexuality concerns, access to care, and use of self-medication. Teaching the woman about available support groups in the community and the physiology of menopause can increase compliance with preventive health measures.

PELVIC FLOOR DYSFUNCTION

Pelvic floor dysfunction occurs when the muscles, ligaments, and fascia that support the pelvic organs are damaged or weakened. The dysfunction may occur as a result of childbirth injury but often does not become obvious until the perimenopausal period. There are two classifications of pelvic floor dysfunction, and they often occur together:

- Vaginal wall prolapse, which includes cystocele and rectocele
- Uterine prolapse

VAGINAL WALL PROLAPSE

The vaginal wall may prolapse in either the anterior or posterior wall or in both walls.

Cystocele

A *cystocele* occurs when the anterior vaginal wall becomes too weak to support the bladder that contains urine. Stress incontinence may result when the woman loses urine with a sudden increase in intraabdominal pressure, such as with laughing, coughing, or sneezing.

Rectocele

A *rectocele* occurs when the posterior vaginal wall becomes weakened. When the woman strains to defecate, feces are pushed against the weakened wall rather than being directed toward the rectal sphincter for elimination. The woman may use digital pressure against her posterior vaginal wall to facilitate defecation.

UTERINE PROLAPSE

A *uterine prolapse* occurs when the ligaments that support the uterus and vagina are weakened. The uterus sags downward in the vagina. It is more likely to occur in the woman who has had several vaginal births or one who had large infants. Symptoms of uterine prolapse include pelvic fullness, a dragging sensation, pelvic pressure, fatigue, and a low backache. In addition, the woman will often have symptoms characteristic of vaginal wall prolapse.

MANAGEMENT OF PELVIC FLOOR DYSFUNCTION

Medical management of pelvic floor dysfunction depends on several factors, such as age, physical condition, sexual activity, and extent of the problem. Surgical correction gives the most definitive relief. The vaginal wall(s) may be repaired, and a vaginal hysterectomy is often done for uterine prolapse. The two surgeries are often combined. If the woman cannot have surgery, a *pessary* (a device to support the pelvic structures) may be inserted into her vagina. Contraindications to the use of a pessary include pelvic infections, PID, and latex allergy. Careful hygiene and follow-up care are essential when a pessary is inserted to avoid complications such as ulcerations or infections.

NURSING CARE OF THE WOMAN WITH PELVIC FLOOR DYSFUNCTION

Kegel exercises can help to strengthen the pubococcygeal muscle, a major support for the urethra, vagina, and rectum. The woman should contract her muscles as if stopping the flow of urine. She should not actually do the exercise while urinating. She should repeat the contraction 10 times and perform this cycle five times each day. The woman should continue Kegel exercises for the rest of her life to maintain pelvic muscle tone.

To reduce some of the low back and pelvic discomforts associated with pelvic relaxation, the woman can be taught to lie down with her feet elevated. Assuming the knee-chest position for a few minutes may also help.

Measures to prevent constipation, such as adequate fluid and fiber intake, reduce hard feces that would put further pressure on a rectocele.

URINARY INCONTINENCE

Urinary incontinence is an uncontrollable leakage of urine from the bladder. *Stress incontinence* is leakage caused by a sudden increase in intraabdominal pressure (occurs with sneezing or coughing). *Urge incontinence* is the inability to control the urge to urinate because of an overactive bladder. Urinary incontinence in women is often related to genital trauma during birth and is most common in multiparous women. It can be worsened by drugs such as antidepressants, diuretics, caffeine, anticholinergics, alcohol, beta-blockers, and angiotensin-converting enzyme (ACE) inhibitors (Culligan & Heit, 2000).

Treatment and Nursing Care

The nurse can teach the woman how to do Kegel exercises, which can be enhanced by the use of vaginal weights to strengthen the pelvic floor muscles. Electrical muscle stimulation (TENS) may also be prescribed. Medications used for an overactive bladder include oxybutynin (Ditropan XL), tolterodine (Detrol), imipramine (Tofranil), dicyclomine (Bentyl), and hyoscyamine (Cystospaz).

Surgical procedures for stress incontinence include injection of collagen into periurethral tissue. Extracorporeal magnetic innervation is a noninvasive stimulation of muscles that has shown promise in both stress incontinence and overactive bladder. Intraurethral occlusive plugs, valved catheters that act as an artificial urinary sphincter control, are rapidly replacing absorbent pads and surgical intervention (Choe, 2000).

OTHER FEMALE REPRODUCTIVE TRACT DISORDERS

A woman may have other reproductive tract disorders during her life. An overview of some common benign ones is presented in the following sections. A medical-surgical nursing text should be consulted for more information about these and information about malignant female reproductive tract disorders.

UTERINE FIBROIDS

Uterine fibroids are also known as leiomyomas, myomas, and myofibromas. Uterine fibroids are benign growths of uterine muscle cells and are a very common gynecological condition. They grow under the influence of estrogen and are thus most prominent during the childbearing years and often atrophy after menopause. The growths may be within the uterine muscle mass, near the inside or outside uterine surface, or on a pedicle. They may be evident in the pregnant woman as a knotty growth felt on her uterus.

Many women have no problems with fibroids, but they sometimes cause irregular bleeding, pressure on the bladder, or pelvic pressure and dysmenorrhea.

Treatment

Uterine fibroids that are asymptomatic are observed and periodically reevaluated. If the woman is symptomatic, there are surgical and nonsurgical options.

Gonadotropin-releasing hormone agonists (GnRHa) such as leuprolide (Lupron) or nafarelin (Synarel) produce a menopause-like state and can decrease the fibroid size up to 60% (Davidson, 2001). However, changes in bone mass and lipid levels take place, and regrowth of the fibroids can occur when the medication is stopped. The use of hormones such as medroxyprogesterone acetate and danazol requires 3 months to take effect, and regrowth of fibroids often occurs when medication is stopped. Mifepristone and other drugs are being researched.

Surgical interventions include hysteroscopic myomectomy, where the fibroid is removed with a hysteroscope rather than a surgical incision, but this is not an option for large or multiple lesions. A hysterectomy (removal of the entire uterus) can be performed if the woman is past her childbearing years.

A laparoscopic myomectomy is the surgical removal of fibroids and preserves fertility. Myolysis is the laser or electrosurgical destruction of fibroids and also preserves fertility.

Uterine fibroid embolization is a nonsurgical technique of treating uterine fibroids that involves less physiological effect than drug therapy, less psychological effect than surgery, and a faster recovery time. A small catheter is placed into the uterine arteries and a substance is injected that decreases blood supply to the fibroids. This procedure does not require a general anesthetic, and no regrowths have been reported. The nurse should help the woman understand her options in relation to her childbearing goals. Some women feel sexual functioning is related to having a uterus, and the nurse can help clarify misconceptions and reduce anxieties. The preoperative and postoperative care is similar to that for any abdominal surgery (a medical-surgical text should be consulted).

OVARIAN CYSTS

A follicular ovarian cyst may develop if the follicle fails to rupture and release its ovum during the menstrual cycle. This type of cyst usually regresses with the next menstrual cycle. A lutein cyst may occur when the corpus luteum that develops after ovulation fails to regress. The lutein cyst is more likely to cause pain. An ovarian cyst that ruptures or becomes twisted and infarcted as its blood supply is cut off can cause pelvic pain and tenderness.

Diagnosis is by transvaginal ultrasound examination. A laparoscopy may aid in diagnosing and differentiating the ovarian cyst pain from that caused by endometriosis. Laparotomy may be required to remove the cyst.

CULTURAL ASPECTS OF PAIN CONTROL

Pain is considered the fifth vital sign for nurses to assess on a regular basis. Culture and ethnicity may impact the accuracy of pain assessment. Asian women may understand a vertical pain score because they read downward rather than left to right (see Chapter 22 for pain scores). Descriptive words for pain can imply intensity, such as "aches" versus "hurt." In general, any pain score above 5 on a scale of 0 to 10 can interfere with activities of daily living and requires nursing intervention.

Ethnicity can affect drug metabolism so that a dose that is effective for one ethnic group may not be the same in others (Connelly, 1999). Research concerning drugs is often accomplished using white males as subjects.

Diet can affect drug absorption. For example, griseofulvin requires fat in the diet for adequate absorption. Malnutrition can interfere with the absorption and excretion of medications. Smoking is known to impact the metabolism of some drugs.

CAM therapy can affect the action of prescribed drugs. For example, ginseng alters metabolism and therefore affects the absorption and elimination of drugs (see Chapter 33 for details of CAM therapy). Patients should be asked what type of self-care they use for chronic pain. Twenty-one percent of patients report using CAM therapy in addition to prescribed drugs (Benjamin, Gallagher, & Helms, 2001).

Some women suffer in silence with pain that is not relieved by prescribed medication, believing nothing more can be done. These women need guidance and counseling. Pain clinics may be available in some hospitals. Some cultural groups will not report embarrassing side effects, such as diarrhea, and may stop taking the medication because of these side effects. Careful, sensitive questioning by the nurse is essential because this information may not be volunteered.

Understanding pain, its symptoms, and its causes as well as the influence of culture, ethnicity, diet, and CAM therapy on pain relief is essential if nurses are to provide comprehensive care to their patients.

key points

- Preventive care is cost-effective and reduces distress.
- Teaching a woman breast care can reduce her risk of death from breast cancer.
- Several self-help measures can relieve some symptoms of premenstrual syndrome.
- Prevention of toxic shock syndrome involves not allowing microorganisms the time to grow in the woman's reproductive tract.
- Sexually transmitted diseases (STDs) must be adequately treated in all sexual contacts to stop the transmission and to avoid resistance to antibiotics.
- Contraception is an individual choice. The nurse must avoid incorporating personal preferences when educating patients about contraceptive methods.
- Fertility awareness methods can be used both to avoid pregnancy and to increase the chance of achieving it.
- Except for abstinence, condoms (male and female) offer the best protection from STDs, including the human immunodeficiency virus (HIV).
- Nursing care of infertile couples includes helping them to evaluate their options at different phases during evaluation and treatment.
- Common menopausal symptoms, such as hot flashes and vaginal dryness, stem from the cessation of ovulation and decrease in hormonal activity, particularly that of estrogen and progesterone.
- Prevention of disabling osteoporosis begins with adequate calcium and vitamin D intake during youth to achieve maximum bone mass. Reducing osteoporosis after menopause is best accomplished by adequate calcium and vitamin D coupled with supplemental estrogen.
- Alternative drugs are available for women who cannot take estrogen.
- Pain is considered a fifth vital sign and should be assessed with cultural sensitivity.

ONLINE RESOURCES

The National Women's Health Information Center: http://www.4women.gov

Planned Parenthood Federation of America: http://www.plannedparenthood.org

Patient Care: http://www.patientcareonline.com

New Mexico AIDS InfoNet: http://www.aidsinfonet.org

Reproductive Toxicology Database: http://www.reprotox.org

REVIEW QUESTIONS   *Choose the most appropriate answer.*

1. Choose the correct teaching for breast self-examination (BSE).
   1. Monthly BSE eliminates the need for a professional examination until after age 40 years
   2. BSE should be done 1 week after the beginning of each menstrual period
   3. Dry fingers make it easier to feel very small lumps that are just under the skin
   4. Use the palm of the hand to palpate the breast

2. The women's health nurse practitioner recommends ibuprofen to relieve Jenny's menstrual cramps. The nurse should teach her to take the drug:
   1. With a full glass of water and wait 30 minutes before taking any food
   2. On a full stomach, but only if her cramps seem to be getting more severe
   3. Three times per day for 1 week before she expects her period to begin
   4. With food, just before her period begins or soon after it begins

3. Choose the sexually transmitted disease that may cause infertility.
   1. *Chlamydia*
   2. Syphilis
   3. Herpes genitalis
   4. *Candida*

4. To relieve or reduce symptoms of premenstrual dysphoric syndrome, the nurse should recommend that the woman:
   1. Avoid simple sugars and caffeine consumption
   2. Use oral contraceptive medication
   3. Avoid physical exercise
   4. Limit water intake to 1000 ml/day

5. Patient teaching to prevent osteoporosis in the menopausal woman should include:
   1. Limiting total calcium intake to 1000 mg/day
   2. Using pillows to maintain good body alignment when sleeping
   3. Taking alendronate (Fosamax) with the evening meal
   4. Doing low-impact weight-bearing exercise several times each week

1. Define each key term listed.
2. Briefly describe three normal reflexes of the neonate, including the approximate age of their disappearance.
3. State four methods of maintaining the body temperature of a newborn.
4. State the cause and appearance of physiological jaundice in the newborn.
5. Define the following skin manifestations in the newborn: lanugo, vernix caseosa, mongolian spots, milia, acrocyanosis, desquamation.
6. State the methods of preventing infection in newborns.

key terms

acrocyanosis (ăk-rō-sī-ă-NŌ-sĭs, p. 289)
caput succedaneum (KĂP-ĕt sŭk-sĕ-DĀ-nē-ĕm, p. 284)
cephalohematoma (sĕf-ă-lō-hē-mă-TŌ-mă, p. 284)
circumcision (sĭr-kŭm-SĬZH-ŭn, p. 291)
dancing reflex (p. 283)
Epstein's pearls (p. 292)
fontanel (fŏn-tă-NĚL, p. 284)
head lag (p. 283)
icterus neonatorum (ĬK-tĕr-ŭs nē-ō-nă-TŎR-ŭm, p. 295)
lanugo (lă-NOO-gō, p. 292)
meconium (mĕ-KŌ-nē-ĕm, p. 295)
milia (MĬL-ē-ă, p. 292)
molding (p. 283)
mongolian spots (p. 292)
Moro reflex (p. 283)
rooting reflex (p. 283)
scarf sign (p. 290)
tissue turgor (p. 292)
tonic neck reflex (p. 283)
vernix caseosa (VĚR-nĭks kăs-ē-Ō-să, p. 292)

The arrival of the newborn, or *neonate,* begins a highly vulnerable period during which many psychological and physiological adjustments to life outside the uterus must be made. The fetus that remains in the uterus until maturity has reached a major goal. The infant's genetic background, the health of the recent uter-ine environment, a safe delivery, and the care during the first month of life contribute to this adjustment.

The *infant mortality rate* is the ratio between the number of deaths of infants younger than age 1 year during any given year and the number of live births occurring in the same year. The rate is usually expressed as the number of deaths per thousand live births. The infant death rate is highest in the first month and is referred to as the *neonatal mortality rate.* The first 24 hours of life are the most dangerous ones. The infant mortality rate is considered to be one of the best means of determining the health of a country. To obtain accurate figures, all births and deaths must be registered. In the United States this registration is required by law. Each birth certificate is permanently filed with the state bureau of vital statistics. In 1997 the neonatal death rate in the United States was 4.8 deaths per 1000 live births, and the infant death rate was approximately 7 deaths per 1000 live births (National Center for Health Statistics, 1999).

Morbidity (*morbidus,* "sick") refers to the state of being diseased or sick. Morbidity rates show the incidence of disease in a specific population during a certain time frame. *Perinatology* is the study and support of the fetus and neonate. The term *perinatal mortality* designates fetal and neonatal deaths related to prenatal conditions and delivery circumstances. See Chapter 1 for details concerning statistics in the United States.

Low-birth-weight newborns and limited access to health care are major causes of infant morbidity. Reducing infant morbidity rates can reduce the resulting disability, which can impact the growth and development of children. The nurse can play a vital role in educating new parents about health care and the developmental needs of their newborn.

ADJUSTMENT TO EXTRAUTERINE LIFE

When a child is born, an orderly, continuous adaptation from fetal life to extrauterine life takes place. All the body systems undergo some change. Respirations are stimulated by chilling and by chemical changes within the blood. Sensory and physical stimuli also appear to play a role in respiratory function. The first breath opens the alveoli. The infant then enters the world of air exchange, at which time an independent existence begins. This process also initiates cardiopulmonary interdependence. The newborn's ability to metabolize food is hampered by the immaturity of the digestive system, particularly deficiencies in enzymes from the pancreas and liver. The kidneys are structurally developed, but their ability to concentrate urine and maintain fluid balance is limited because of a decreased rate of glomerular flow and limited renal tubular reabsorption. Most neurological functions are primitive (see the discussion of the individual body systems in this chapter).

PHYSICAL CHARACTERISTICS AND PHASE 3 CARE OF THE NEWBORN

Phase 3 care of the newborn covers the physical characteristics and nursing assessment of the normal term newborn, by body system. Refer to Chapter 6 for phase 1 care of the newborn immediately after birth, and refer to Chapter 9 for Phase 2 care of the newborn on admission to the nursery or postpartum unit.

NERVOUS SYSTEM: REFLEXES

The nervous system directs most of the body's activity. Newborns can move their arms and legs vigorously but cannot control them. When the infant is lifted from the bed, the head will fall back because the newborn cannot maintain neutral position of the head. This is called a head lag (Figure 12-1). The reflexes full-term infants are born with, such as blinking, sneezing, gagging, sucking, and grasping (Figure 12-2), help to keep them alive. They can cry, swallow, and lift their heads slightly when lying on their abdomen. If the crib is jarred, they draw their legs up and the arms fan out and then come toward midline in an embrace position. This is normal and is called the Moro reflex (Figure 12-3). Its absence may indicate abnormalities of the nervous system. The rooting reflex causes the infant's head to turn in the direction of anything that touches the cheek, in anticipation of food. The nurse uses this when helping a mother to breastfeed her infant. A breast touching the cheek causes the infant to turn toward it to find the nipple.

The tonic neck reflex is a postural reflex that is sometimes assumed by sleeping infants. The head is turned to one side, the arm and leg are extended on the same side, and the opposite arm and leg are flexed in a "fencing" position. This reflex disappears about the seventh month of life (Figure 12-4). Prancing movements of the legs, seen

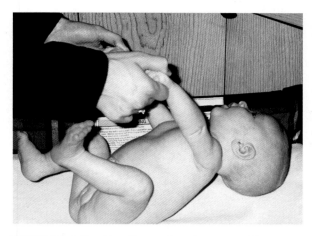

FIGURE **12-1** Head lag. The newborn has some ability to control the head in some positions. When placed on the abdomen the newborn may be able to raise the chin from the bed briefly. However, head lag and hyperextension normally occur when raised from the bed in a supine position. Significant head lag after age 6 months indicates a need for follow-up care.

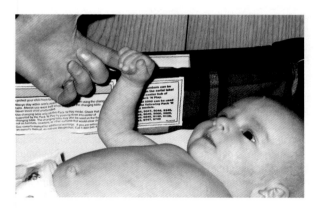

FIGURE **12-2** Grasp reflex. Touching the hands near the base of the fingers causes a reflex flexion of the hands. This grasp reflex is replaced after age 3 months by a voluntary grasp.

when an infant is held upright on the examining table, are termed the dancing reflex. Table 12-1 lists ages at which the neurological signs of infancy appear and disappear.

HEAD

The brain grows rapidly before birth, and therefore the newborn's head is large in comparison with the rest of the body. The normal limits of head circumference range from 12.5 to 14.1 inches (32 to 36 cm) (Figure 12-5, *A*). The head may be out of shape from molding (the shaping of the fetal head to conform to the size and

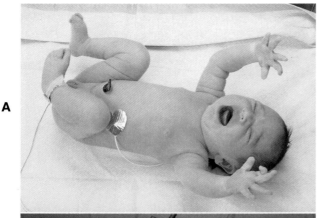

A

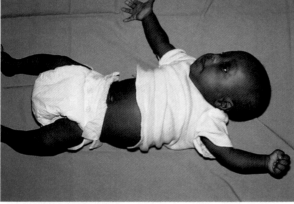

B

FIGURE **12-3** **A,** Moro reflex. Sudden jarring causes extension and abduction (an embracing motion) of the extremities and spreading of the fingers, with the index finger and the thumb forming a C shape. A unilateral (one-sided) Moro reflex may indicate a fractured clavicle. Absence of the Moro reflex may indicate a pathological condition of the central nervous system. **B,** Abnormal Moro reflex. Note the clenched fist of one hand that does not follow a symmetrical embracing motion. This infant requires follow-up care.

table 12-1	*Ages of Appearance and Disappearance of Neurological Signs Peculiar to Infancy*	
RESPONSE	**AGE AT TIME OF APPEARANCE**	**AGE AT TIME OF DISAPPEARANCE**
REFLEXES OF POSITION AND MOVEMENT		
Moro reflex	Birth	1-3 months
Tonic neck reflex (unsustained)*	Birth	5-7 months
Palmar grasp reflex	Birth	4 months
Babinski reflex	Birth	Variable†
RESPONSES TO SOUND		
Blinking response	Birth	
Turning response	Birth	
REFLEXES OF VISION‡		
Blinking to threat	6-7 months	
Horizontal following	4-6 weeks	
Vertical following	2-3 months	
Postrotational nystagmus	Birth	
FOOD REFLEXES		
Rooting response (awake)	Birth	3-4 months
Rooting response (asleep)	Birth	7-8 months
Sucking response	Birth	12 months
OTHER SIGNS		
Handedness	2-3 years	
Spontaneous stepping	Birth	4-5 months
Straight line walking	5-6 years	

Modified from Ross Laboratories. (1986). *Children are different.* Columbus, Ohio: Author.
*Arm and leg posturing can be broken by child despite continued neck stimulus.
†Usually of no diagnostic significance until after age 2 years.
‡Holding the newborn infant upright under the arms will induce eye opening.

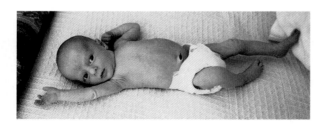

FIGURE **12-4** Spontaneous tonic neck reflex. The infant turns the head to one side and the arm and leg are extended on that side. The opposite arm and leg flexes. Often called the "fencing" reflex, it disappears by age 4 months as the central nervous system matures.

shape of the birth canal) (Figure 12-5, *B*). There may also be swelling of the soft tissues of the scalp, which is termed caput succedaneum. It gradually subsides without treatment. Occasionally, a cephalohematoma (*cephal,* "head," *hemato,* "blood," *toma,* "tumor") protrudes from beneath the scalp (Figure 12-5, *C,D*). This condition is caused by a collection of blood beneath the periosteum of the cranial bone. It may be seen on one or both sides of the head but *does not cross the suture line.* This condition usually recedes within a few weeks without treatment.

The fontanels are unossified spaces or soft spots on the cranium of a young infant. They protect the head

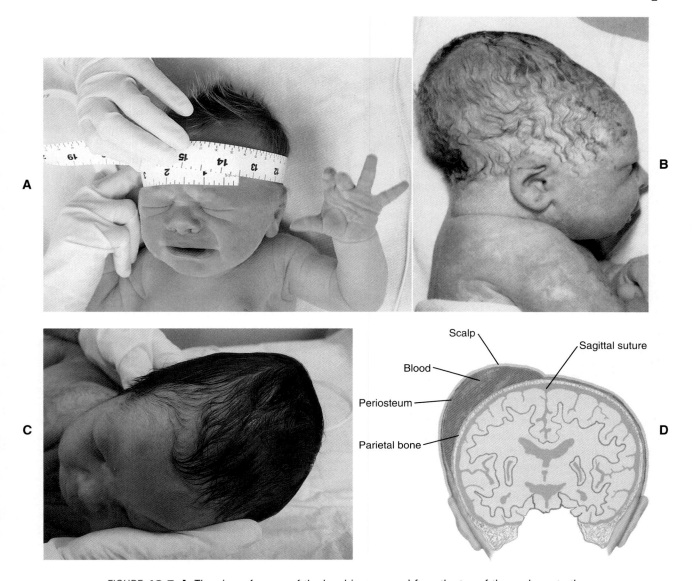

FIGURE **12-5 A,** The circumference of the head is measured from the top of the eyebrow to the widest part of the occiput. **B,** Molding of the head occurs as a result of overriding of the parietal bones as the head passes through the birth canal. Often a collection of fluid under the scalp caused by edema of the presenting part (caput succedaneum) causes the head to appear longer than normal and soft to the touch. This condition disappears without treatment within a few weeks. **C,** Cephalohematoma appears as a lump on one side of the head. **D,** With a cephalohematoma, the blood collects between the surface of the cranial bone and the periosteal membrane. The swelling does not cross the suture lines.

during delivery by the process of molding and allow for further brain growth during the next 1½ years. The *anterior fontanel* is diamond shaped and is located at the junction of the two parietal and two frontal bones. It usually closes by age 12 to 18 months. The *posterior fontanel* is triangular and is located between the occipital and parietal bones. It is smaller than the anterior fontanel and is usually ossified by the end of the second month. These areas are covered by a tough membrane, and there is little chance of their being injured

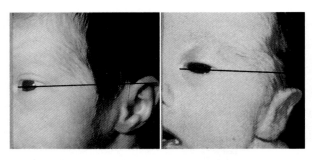

FIGURE **12-6** Ear position. The ears are assessed for placement because low-set ears may indicate a congenital abnormality. An imaginary line drawn from the outer canthus of the eye should be even with the upper tip of the pinna of the ear.

during ordinary care. The features of the newborn's face are small. The mouth and lips are well developed because they are necessary to obtain food. The newborn can both taste and smell. In fact, the newborn can recognize the scent of the mother's milk on the breast pad.

VISUAL STIMULI AND SENSORY OVERLOAD

The healthy newborn can see and can fixate on points of contrast. The newborn shows a preference for observing a human face and follows moving objects. Visual stimulation is thus an important ingredient in newborn care. Toys that make sounds and have contrasting colors attract the newborn. Tears are absent in the newborn and may first appear when the infant cries after 1 to 3 months of age. Sensory overload can occur if there is too much detrimental stimulation. This overload can happen in the hospital environment, where lights are bright and voices carry. The nurse can help to modify this situation by responding quickly to alarms and by speaking quietly when working near the infant.

HEARING

The ears are well developed at birth but are small. The ears are assessed for placement because low-set ears may indicate a congenital abnormality in another part of the body. An imaginary line is drawn from the outer canthus of the eye that should be even with the upper tip of the ear lobe (Figure 12-6). The hearing ability of the newborn is well developed at birth, but the sick or premature newborn may not respond to sounds that are heard. The presence of amniotic fluid in the ear canal can diminish hearing, but normal drainage and sneezing that occurs shortly after birth help clear the ear canal.

The newborn will react to sudden sound by an increase in pulse and respiration or a display of the startle reflex. Newborn infants who do not respond should be referred for a hearing test. Increased responses to vocal stimulation, particularly higher-pitched female voices, have been documented. The ability to discriminate between the mother's voice and the voices of others may occur as early as age 3 days. Hearing is important to the development of normal speech. The nurse observes and records how the newborn reacts to sound, such as a rattle or the voice of the caretaker. The infant will respond to voices by decreasing motor activity and sucking activity and turning the head toward the sound. One test used to measure infant hearing is the Algo hearing screening test. It analyzes hearing by sending a series of soft clicks into the sleeping infant's ear. The infant's brain responds with a specific brain wave that is referred to as an auditory brainstem response (ABR). The response is compared by computer to normal responses, and a pass/fail score is recorded. In some hospitals a hearing test is routine for all newborns.

The ears and nose need no special attention except for cleansing with a soft cloth during the bath. Occasionally they may be *externally* cleansed with a cotton ball moistened slightly with water. The bony canal of the external ear is not well developed, and the tympanic membrane is vulnerable to injury. The nurse should *not* insert applicators. They may cause serious injury to the tympanic membrane if inserted too far into the ear canal or if the infant moves suddenly.

SLEEP

The neonate sleeps approximately 15 to 20 hours a day. There is a gradual change in the quantity and quality of sleep as the newborn matures. At birth the newborn passes through the following phases of sleep-wake states as part of the adjustment to life outside of the uterus:

- *First reactive phase:* During the first 30 minutes of life the newborn is alert, and this is the best time to initiate bonding between the parent and newborn.
- *Sleep phase:* During the next few hours of life the infant gradually becomes more sleepy and less responsive.
- *Second reactive phase:* After a deep sleep the infant again becomes responsive and alert.
- *Stability phase:* After age 24 hours the sleep-wake pattern becomes more stabilized. The pattern of sleep gradually develops into one in which the newborn is awake during the day and asleep during the night.

The environment plays a large role in the infant's sleep behavior. The nurse can help the parent to understand that normal conversational tones can quiet a newborn, whereas high noise levels can cause increased crying. Wrapping an infant snugly can maintain temperature and promote sleep, as can gentle *horizontal* rocking. An infant held upright on the shoulder and rocked in a *vertical* fashion is likely to maintain an alert state. Newborns exhibit a specific *pattern of reactivity* that can influence the response to stimuli and bonding, as follows:

- *Quiet sleep:* Infant sleeps, does not move.
- *Rapid eye movement (REM) sleep:* Respirations are more irregular during REM sleep. Eye movements are evident beneath the eyelid, and limb and mouth movement may be seen.
- *Active alert:* The infant displays diffuse motor activity.
- *Quiet alert:* The infant is awake, relaxed, and quiet. In this state the infant is most responsive to testing and to bonding efforts.
- *Crying:* The infant's cry is accompanied by vigorous motor activity of extremities.
- *Transitional:* The infant is moving between one of the above states. The infant may be quiet and relaxed but not very responsive to the environment.

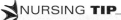

NURSING **TIP**

Advise parents that even the youngest of infants can roll off a changing table or bed when left unattended.

PAIN

In the past it was believed that newborns did not experience pain because of immaturity of the nerve pathways to the brain. It is now thought that fibers that conduct pain stimuli to the spinal cord are in place early in fetal life. These are called *nociceptors* (*noci,* "pain," *ceptus,* "to receive"). The newborn also produces catecholamines and cortisol in response to stress. Heart rate and respiratory rates change. Blood pressure increases, and blood glucose levels rise. Newborns should be medicated for pain when discomfort is anticipated.

Adequate pain relief in newborns who undergo painful procedures (e.g., circumcision) can reduce postoperative morbidity. Evaluation of pain in the neonate can be based on changes in vital signs and behavior of the infant and decreased oxygen saturation rates (Figure 12-7). Swaddling, cuddling, rocking, nonnutritive sucking, and a quiet environment are noninvasive methods of pain relief for newborn infants. Oral sucrose is an effective pain reliever for minor procedures. Morphine, fentanyl, and topical anesthetics can be used safely for severe pain. The nurse must be aware of safe dose ranges and must observe infants closely for side effects or signs

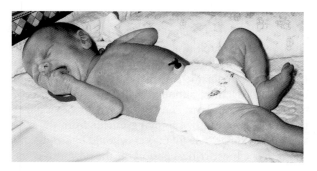

FIGURE **12-7** Pain in the newborn. Note the furrowed brow, clenched fist, irritability or cry, chin quiver, increased muscle tone and activity, tightly closed eyes, and facial grimace. Diaphoresis, a rapid shallow respiration, and increased heart rate and blood pressure also can be observed in the neonate experiencing pain. Pain relief for the neonate during any medical procedure is very important.

of withdrawal when the medication is gradually decreased and then discontinued.

CONDITIONED RESPONSES

A conditioned response or reflex is one that is learned over time. It is an unconscious response to an external stimulus. An example is the hungry infant who stops crying merely at the sound of the caregiver's footsteps, even though food is not yet available. Emotions are particularly subject to this type of conditioning. As an infant matures, the mere sight of an object that once caused pain can precipitate fear.

NEONATAL BEHAVIORAL ASSESSMENT SCALE

The Neonatal Behavioral Assessment Scale, developed by T. B. Brazelton, has increased the understanding of the newborn's capabilities. Among other areas of assessment, this scale measures the inherent neurological capacities of the newborn and responses to selected stimuli. Areas tested include alertness, response to visual and auditory stimuli, motor coordination, level of excitement, and organizational process in response to stress.

RESPIRATORY SYSTEM

The unborn fetus is completely dependent on the mother for all vital functions. The fetus needs oxygen and nourishment to grow. These nutrients are supplied through the bloodstream of the pregnant woman by way of the placenta and umbilical cord. The fetus is relieved of the waste products of metabolism by the same route. The lungs are not inflated and are almost completely inactive. The circulatory system is adapted only to life within the uterus. Little blood flows through the pulmonary artery because of natural openings within the heart and vessels that close at birth or shortly thereafter. When the umbilical cord is clamped and cut, the lungs take on the function of breathing oxygen and removing carbon dioxide. The first breath helps to expand the collapsed lungs, although full expansion does not occur for several days. The health care provider assists the first respiration by removing mucus from the passages to the lungs. The infant's cry should be strong and healthy. The most critical period for the newborn is the first hour of life, when the drastic change from life within the uterus to life outside the uterus takes place.

The nurse can assist newborns to maintain a patent airway by positioning them on their back or side and dressing them in clothing to maintain warmth while allowing full expansion of the lungs. The nurse should record vital signs and suction mucus as needed, first from the mouth and throat and then the nose.

APGAR SCORE

The Apgar score is a standardized method of evaluating the newborn's condition immediately after delivery. Five objective signs are measured: heart rate, respiration, muscle tone, reflexes, and color. The score is obtained at 1 and 5 minutes after birth (see Table 6-4). On admission of the newborn to the nursery, the Apgar score is reviewed to determine any particular difficulties encountered during the birth process. The health care provider's orders are noted. The nurse must observe the newborn *very closely.* Respiratory distress may be evidenced by the rate and character of respirations, color (cyanosis), and general behavior. Sternal retractions are reported immediately (see Chapter 13).

Mucus may be seen draining from the nose or mouth, and it is wiped away with a sterile gauze square. Gently clearing mucus with a bulb syringe may also be indicated. The bulb is depressed, and the tip is inserted into the mouth first and then the nose. The depression is slowly released, which creates the necessary suction (Figure 12-8). When this procedure is done orally, the tip is inserted into the side of the mouth to avoid stimulating the gag reflex. Parents are taught how to use the bulb syringe and are instructed to keep one next to the newborn during the early weeks of life.

CIRCULATORY SYSTEM

The mother's blood has brought essential oxygen to each cell of the fetus in the uterus. The health care provider cuts off this supply by severing the umbilical cord. Thereafter the newborn depends on his or her own systemic circulation and pulmonary circulation.

The newborn has approximately 300 ml of circulatory blood volume. The circulation of blood in the fetus

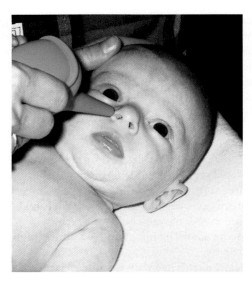

FIGURE **12-8** Bulb suctioning. The bulb is compressed before it is inserted into the nose or mouth; the bulb is then released. If the bulb is depressed after being inserted, the mucus will be forced farther into the respiratory passages. The mouth is suctioned before the nose to avoid causing the infant to gasp and aspirate fluid into the lung.

differs from that in the newborn in that most fetal blood bypasses the lungs (see Chapter 3). Some of the blood goes from the right atrium to the left atrium of the heart through an opening (the foramen ovale) in the septum. Some goes from the pulmonary artery to the thoracic aorta by way of the ductus arteriosus. These normal openings close soon after birth. If they fail to close, the infant may be cyanotic because part of the blood continues to bypass the lungs and does not pick up oxygen.

Murmurs are caused by blood leaking through openings that have not yet closed. Murmurs may be functional (innocent) or organic (caused by improper heart formation). Functional murmurs result from the sound of blood passing through normal valves. Organic murmurs are caused by blood passing through abnormal openings. The majority of heart murmurs are not serious, but they should be checked periodically to rule out other pathological conditions.

◤NURSING **TIP**
Changing Laboratory Values

	Newborn	7 days	3 months
Hemoglobin (Hgb) (g/dL)	18.5	17	11.3
Hematocrit (Hct)	56	44	35
White blood cell count (WBC)	18,000	12,000	10,800
Bilirubin (mg/dL)	6	12	1

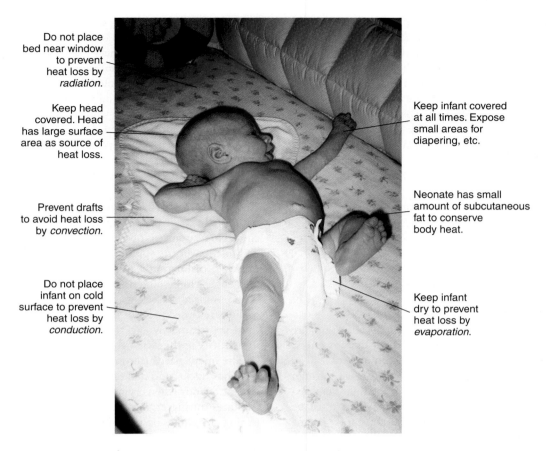

Do not place bed near window to prevent heat loss by *radiation*.

Keep head covered. Head has large surface area as source of heat loss.

Prevent drafts to avoid heat loss by *convection*.

Do not place infant on cold surface to prevent heat loss by *conduction*.

Keep infant covered at all times. Expose small areas for diapering, etc.

Neonate has small amount of subcutaneous fat to conserve body heat.

Keep infant dry to prevent heat loss by *evaporation*.

FIGURE **12-9** Maintaining body temperature of the newborn. Chilling causes "cold stress"—an increased metabolism and oxygen consumption in the neonate—because the infant cannot shiver, as the adult can, to raise body temperature.

PROVIDING WARMTH

The newborn has an unstable heat-regulating system. Body temperature falls immediately after birth to about 35.5° C (96.0° F). Within a few hours, it climbs slowly to a range of 36.6° to 37.2° C (98.0° to 99.0° F). The body temperature is influenced by that of the room and the number of blankets covering the infant. The temperature of the nursery, or of the mother's room in the case of rooming-in, is kept at 69° to 75° F (21° to 24° C). The humidity should be between 45% and 55%. The air in the room must be fresh, but there should be no drafts. The newborn's hands and feet are *not* used as a guide to determine warmth because the infant's extremities are cooler than the rest of the body. Acrocyanosis (*acro,* "extremity" and *cyanosis,* "blue color") is also evident because of sluggish peripheral circulation. The newborn cannot adapt to changes in temperature. The nurse wraps the infant in a blanket whenever the infant leaves the nursery. Because the infant's heat perception is poor, the nurse must be careful when applying any form of external heat.

Because the sweat glands do not function effectively during the neonatal period, the newborn infant is at risk for developing an elevated temperature if overdressed or if placed in an overheated environment. A red skin rash may develop in response to overheating. Maintaining body temperature in the newborn is discussed in Table 9-1 and summarized in Figure 12-9.

OBTAINING TEMPERATURE, PULSE, AND RESPIRATIONS

Some birth facilities recommend that the initial temperature of the newborn be taken by rectum to determine that the rectum is patent. When the temperature is taken rectally, the nurse must be gentle to avoid injuring the rectal mucosa. Daily routine temperatures are taken by axilla. To obtain the axillary temperature, the thermometer is held firmly in the center of the newborn's axilla. During this time, the arm is held against the infant's side. Digital thermometers are read when the indicator sounds.

The newborn's pulse and respirations are counted before the temperature is taken because the infant is apt to cry when disturbed. Figure 12-10 illustrates the apical pulse being obtained from a newborn infant. The newborn's pulse is irregular and rapid and varies from 110 to 160 beats/min. Blood pressure is low and may vary with the size of the cuff used. The average blood pressure at birth is 80/46 mm Hg. The respirations are approximately 30 to 60 breaths/min. The nurse always reports the following changes:

- Temperature elevated to 37.7° C (100° F) or below 36.2° C (97° F)
- Pulse elevated above 160 beats/min or below 110 beats/min
- Respirations elevated above 60 breaths/min or below 30 breaths/min
- Noisy respirations
- Nasal flaring or chest retraction

MUSCULOSKELETAL SYSTEM

The bones of the newborn are soft because they are composed mostly of cartilage, in which there is only a small amount of calcium. The skeleton is flexible. The joints are elastic to accommodate the passage through the birth canal. Because the bones of the infant are easily molded by pressure, the infant's position must be changed frequently. If the infant lies constantly in one position, the bones of the head can become flattened.

The movements of the newborn are random and uncoordinated. The newborn lacks the muscular control to hold the head steady. The development of muscular control proceeds from head to foot and from the center of the body to the periphery (see the discussion of cephalocaudal and proximodistal control in Chapter 15). Therefore the infant holds the head up before sitting erect. In fact, the head and neck muscles are the first ones under control. The newborn's legs are small and short and may appear bowed. There should be no limitation of movement. Fingers clenched in a fist should be separated and observed.

An examination of the newborn for gestational maturity includes checking for the scarf sign (see Figure 13-3). This refers to the full-term infant's resistance to attempts to bring one elbow farther than the midline of the chest. No resistance is observed in the preterm infant.

Most newborns appear cross-eyed because their eye muscle coordination is not fully developed. At first, the eyes appear to be blue or gray; the permanent coloring becomes fixed between ages 6 and 12 months. The eyelids are closed most of the time. Tears do not appear until approximately age 1 to 3 months because of the immaturity of the lacrimal gland ducts.

The infant needs freedom of movement. The infant stretches, sucks, and makes faces and vigorously moves the entire body when crying. Tremors of the lips and extremities during crying are normal. Constant tremors during sleep may be pathological. These are often accompanied by eye movements, are not related to particular stimuli, and should be reported to the health care provider. The morning bath provides excellent opportunities for the newborn to exercise and the nurse to inspect and assess the infant's condition. When handled, the infant should not feel limp. General body proportions are noted. Bathing is also an excellent means of stimulation for the newborn.

LENGTH AND WEIGHT

The length of the average newborn is 19 to 21.5 inches (46 to 56 cm). The weight varies from 6 to 9 pounds (2700 to 4000 g) (Figure 12-11). In general, girls weigh a little less than boys. African-American, Asian-American, and Native-American infants may be somewhat smaller. *In the first 3 to 4 days after birth, the infant loses about 5% to 10% of the birth weight.* This loss may be as high as 15% for preterm infants. This may result from withdrawal from maternal hormones, fluid shifts, and the loss of feces and urine. Mothers should be prepared for this and reassured that the weight will normalize after 3 or 4 days and that the infant will regain his or her birth weight by 10 days of age. Newborns are weighed at the same time each day, when morning care is given. (Instructions for measuring and weighing the infant are provided in Figure 12-11 and Chapter 15.)

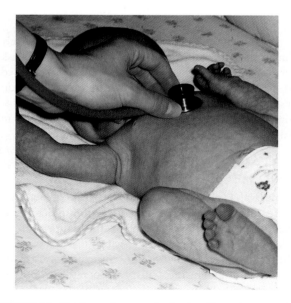

FIGURE **12-10** Assessing an apical pulse. The apical pulse is the most accurate technique of assessing the heart rate in the neonate.

GENITOURINARY SYSTEM

The kidneys function normally at birth but are not fully developed. The glomeruli are small. Renal blood flow is only about one third that of the adult. The ability to handle a water load is reduced, as is the excretion of drugs. The renal tubules are short and have a limited capacity for reabsorbing important substances such as glucose, amino acids, phosphate, and bicarbonate. There is a decrease in the ability to concentrate urine and to cope with fluid imbalances. It is important to note the first voiding of the newborn. This may occur in the delivery room or may not occur for several hours. If voiding does not occur within the first 24 hours, the health care provider is notified. The nurse must keep an accurate record of the frequency of urination. Anuria, changes in color, and any unusual findings are brought to the attention of the health care provider. The newborn should have about six wet diapers per day.

Male Genitalia

The genitalia of the male are developed at birth, although their maturation varies. The testes of the male descend into the scrotum before birth. Occasionally, they remain in the abdomen or inguinal canal. This condition is called *cryptorchidism,* or undescended testes, and is described in Chapter 28. With proper surgical treatment the prognosis is good. The location of the urethral opening should be at the tip of the penis in newborn boys. A white cheesy substance called *smegma* is found under the foreskin.

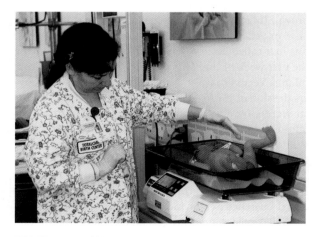

FIGURE **12-11** Weighing the infant. Note the barrier placed under the infant and the nurse's hand held above the infant for safety and protection. The scale used may be a balance scale or digital scale that locks in and displays the weight in pounds and/or kilograms. Gloves should be worn when handling a nude infant. (Photo courtesy of Pat Spier, RN-C.)

Routine retraction of the foreskin of the newborn for cleansing is not recommended. Behrman, Kliegman, and Jenson (2000) state that a lack of retractility is normal in newborns. The foreskin and glans penis gradually separate, and this process is generally completed between age 3 and 5 years. Parents are instructed to test occasionally for retraction during the daily bath. If it has occurred, gentle washing of the glans is begun. The foreskin is then returned to its unretracted position.

Circumcision

Circumcision is the surgical removal of the foreskin on the penis. Circumcision has both advantages and disadvantages. The disadvantages include infection and hemorrhage. Infants with congenital anomalies of the penis, such as *hypospadias* (the opening of the urethra is on the undersurface of the penis), should not be circumcised because the skin may be needed for surgery. The benefits of circumcision include possible prevention of cancer, fewer urinary tract infections, and fewer occurrences of sexually transmitted disease later in life. A discussion of the pros and cons of this procedure is included as part of prenatal and postpartum education. Regardless of whether the male is circumcised, at an appropriate age he is taught daily hygiene of the genitalia. This includes special attention to skin folds, retraction and replacement of the foreskin, cleansing of the penis, and examination for lumps or swelling of the penis or scrotum.

The infant should be physiologically stabilized before circumcision. The newborn is restrained on a circumcision board (Figure 12-12). The Gomco clamp and the Plastibell clamp are two devices commonly used for performing circumcisions. If the Gomco clamp is used, a thin layer of petroleum jelly (Vaseline) or petroleum jelly–impregnated gauze may be applied to the end of the penis to protect it from moisture and from sticking to the diaper. The area is observed for bleeding, infection, and irritation. Voidings are recorded.

When a Plastibell is used, the foreskin is tied over a fitted plastic ring and the excess prepuce cut away. The rim usually drops off 5 to 8 days after circumcision. Parents are instructed not to remove it prematurely. No special dressing is required, and the infant is bathed and diapered as usual. A dark brown or black ring encircling the plastic rim is natural. This disappears when the rim drops off. Parents are instructed to consult their physician if there are any questions, if there is increased swelling, if the ring has not fallen off within 8 days, or immediately if the ring has slipped onto the shaft of the penis. The Jewish religious custom of circumcision, comparable to baptism in the Christian faith, is performed on the eighth day after birth if the newborn's

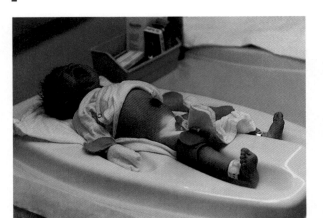

FIGURE **12-12** Circumcision board. A circumcision board is used to restrain the newborn during circumcision. EMLA (eutectic mixture of local anesthetics) is a local skin anesthetic that may be used before the procedure. A sucrose sweetened pacifier may be a helpful pain relief measure during this procedure.

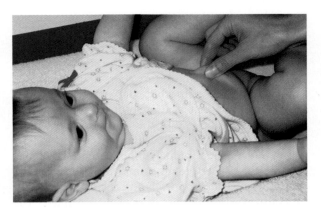

FIGURE **12-13** Testing tissue turgor. The term *turgor* refers to the elasticity of the skin, which is affected by the extent of hydration. The nurse tests skin turgor by gently grasping the skin. When the skin is released, it should instantly spring back into place; if it does not, tissue turgor is considered poor.

condition permits. The infant receives his Hebrew name at that time.

The nurse's role in circumcision includes assessing parental knowledge, checking to see that the surgical consent has been signed, and preparing the newborn. The infant is not fed for 1 to 2 hours before the procedure to prevent possible vomiting and aspiration. A bulb syringe is kept handy in case suctioning is required. A light blanket is placed under the infant on the "circ" board, and the diaper is removed. A heat lamp is positioned to avoid cold stress. The physician may administer a local anesthetic to minimize pain during the procedure and to prevent irritability and sleep disturbances after it. Additional comfort measures include holding and soothing the infant and using a pacifier. If bleeding occurs, gentle pressure is applied to the site with a sterile gauze pad and the physician is notified. The amount and characteristics of the urinary stream are recorded, because edema could cause an obstruction.

Female Genitalia

The female genitalia may be slightly swollen. A thin white or blood-tinged mucus (pseudomenstruation) may be discharged from the vagina. This discharge is caused by hormonal withdrawal from the mother at birth. The nurse cleanses the vulva *from the urethra to the anus,* using a clean cotton ball or different sections of a washcloth for each stroke to prevent fecal matter from infecting the urinary tract. The importance of this is stressed to parents.

INTEGUMENTARY SYSTEM
Skin

Tissue turgor refers to the hydration or dehydration of the skin. To test tissue turgor (elasticity), the nurse gently grasps and releases the skin. It should spring back to place immediately in the well-hydrated infant. When the skin remains distorted ("tented"), tissue turgor is considered poor. Figure 12-13 illustrates the method of testing tissue turgor.

The skin of newborn Caucasian infants is red to dark pink. The skin of African-American infants is reddish brown. Infants of Latin descent may appear to have an olive or yellowish tint. The body is usually covered with fine hair called **lanugo,** which tends to disappear during the first week of life. This is more evident in premature infants. **Vernix caseosa,** a cheeselike substance that covers the skin of the newborn, is made of cells and glandular secretions; it is thought to protect the skin from irritation and the effects of a watery environment in utero. White pinpoint "pimples" caused by the obstruction of sebaceous glands may be seen on the nose and chin. These are called **milia** and disappear within a few weeks. Milia-type lesions on the midline of the hard palate are called **Epstein's pearls** and are caused by a collection of epithelial cells. *Stork bites* (telangiectatic nevi) are flat, red areas seen on the nape of the neck and on the eyelids. They result from the dilation of small vessels. See Table 12-2 for other skin manifestations seen in the newborn.

Mongolian spots, bluish discolorations of the skin, are common in infants of African-American parents, Native-American parents, and parents of Mediter-

table 12-2 | *Common Skin Manifestations in the Newborn*

	APPEARANCE	INTERVENTION
Acrocyanosis 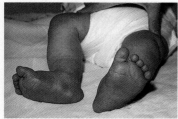	Cyanosis of the hands and feet in the first week of life is caused by a combination of a high hemoglobin level and vasomotor instability.	Parent education concerning this normal phenomenon is helpful.
Cutis marmorata 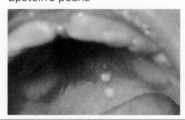	A lacelike red or blue pattern on the skin surface of a newborn's body.	A normal vasomotor response to low environmental temperature. Wrap infant warmly. Intense or persistent appearance should be reported.
Desquamation 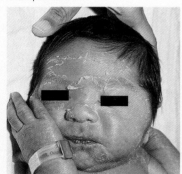	Peeling of the skin at birth may indicate postmaturity. Early removal of vernix can be followed by desquamation in term newborns.	Instruct parents to avoid harsh soaps. Some hospitals do not vigorously remove vernix from the skin of newborns.
Epstein's pearls 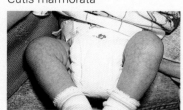	Pearly white pinpoint papules in midline of upper palate.	Distinguish from a thrush lesion (see Chapter 27).
Erythema toxicum 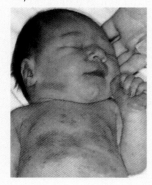	Splotchy erythema with firm yellow-white papules that have a red base.	Can occur at age 2 days; no intervention is required because erythema will spontaneously clear.

Continued

table 12-2 | *Common Skin Manifestations in the Newborn—cont'd*

	APPEARANCE	INTERVENTION
Forceps marks	A bruised area on skin in the shape of forceps or pattern of vacuum extractor.	The bruising and swelling fade within a few days and do not require intervention other than parental support and teaching.
Harlequin color change	An imbalance of autonomic vascular regulatory mechanism. Deep red color over half of body, pallor on the longitudinal half of body. Usually occurs with preterm infants who are placed on their side.	The phenomenon disappears with muscular activity. Changing position of infant is helpful. Condition is temporary and does not usually indicate a problem.
Milia	Pearly white pinpoint papules on face and nose of newborn.	No treatment. Will spontaneously disappear. Educate parents not to attempt to "squeeze out" the white material because infection can occur.
Mongolian spots	Dark blue or slate grey discolorations most commonly found in lumbosacral area. The intensity and hue of color remain until fading occurs.	These lesions are caused by melanin deposits in dark-skinned persons and will gradually disappear in a few years. The nurse must distinguish these lesions from hematoma of child abuse.
Nevi (see Chapter 29)	Known as *stork bites*. These are pink, easily blanched patches that can appear on eyelids, nose, lips, and nape of the neck.	These marks gradually fade and are of no clinical significance.
Port-wine stain	Known as *nevus flammeus*. Is a collection of capillaries in the skin. It is a flat, red-purple lesion that does not blanch on pressure.	This is a permanent skin marking that darkens with age and can become elevated and vulnerable to injury. If a large area of face or neck is involved, laser surgery may be indicated to preserve the child's self-image. Can be associated with genetic disorders.

ranean races. They are usually found over the sacral and gluteal areas (see Table 12-2). They disappear spontaneously during the early years of life. *Acrocyanosis,* or peripheral blueness of the hands and feet, is normal and results from poor peripheral circulation. The hands or feet should not be used to determine general body warmth in the newborn. Central body areas are not cyanotic in normal newborns. Pallor is not normal and should be reported because it may indicate neonatal anemia or another more serious condition.

Desquamation, or peeling of the skin, occurs during the early weeks of life. Skin in areas such as the nose, knees, elbows, and toes may break down because of friction from rubbing against the sheets. The involved area is kept dry, and the infant's position is changed frequently. The buttocks need special attention. A wet diaper should be changed immediately to prevent chafing. The buttocks are washed and dried well.

Physiological jaundice, also called icterus neonatorum, is characterized by a yellow tinge of the skin. It is caused by the rapid destruction of excess red blood cells, which the infant does not need now because he or she is in an atmosphere that contains more oxygen than was available during prenatal life. Plasma levels of bilirubin rise from a normal 1 mg/dl to an average of 5 to 6 mg/dl between the second and fourth days. Physiological jaundice becomes evident between the second and the third days of life and lasts for about 1 week. This is a normal process and is not harmful to the infant. However, genetic and ethnic factors may affect its severity, resulting in pathological hyperbilirubinemia. The skin over the nose or chest is blanched to evaluate for the presence of jaundice. Evidence of jaundice is reported and charted, and the newborn is evaluated frequently to ensure safety.

Table 12-2 discusses nursing interventions for common skin manifestations of the newborn infant.

NURSING **TIP**

Jaundice that appears in the first day of life is not normal and should be recorded and reported.

Bathing the Infant

The bath is an excellent time to provide basic hygiene and to observe the naked newborn for behavior, muscle activity, and general well-being. Special attention must be given to areas of the skin that come in contact with each other because chafing may occur there. These areas are found in the neck, behind the ears, in the axillae, and in the groin. They should be dried well. Powder is seldom used because it can irritate the respiratory tract. Parents are educated about this fact. The use of lotions and oil and the type of soap vary with each institution.

The infant is bathed when his or her temperature is stable; the first bath removes blood and excess vernix. The nurse adheres to standard precautions during the procedure.

The temperature of the bath water should be approximately 38° to 41° C (100° to 105° F) in a warm 24° to 27° C (75° to 80° F) room environment. Special care should be taken to keep the infant covered to prevent chilling. Items such as cotton swabs should *not* be inserted into the nose or ears. Sponge baths using plain tap water should be given to newborns until the cord is well healed. A mild soap can be used for heavily soiled areas. Alkaline soaps and oils and lotions alter the pH of the skin and should be avoided. Parents should be taught to start bathing the face and then proceed in a cephalocaudal (head-to-toe) direction, turning the surface of the washcloth as the bath progresses. The eyes should be cleansed with a moist cotton ball from the inner canthus to the outer, using a clean cotton ball for each eye. The genitalia should be cleansed with a front to back motion to prevent urinary tract infection. The nurse may use a football hold to shampoo the hair (see Chapter 22). The shampoo is given last because the large surface area of the head predisposes the infant to heat loss. The general principles of the infant bath should be explained to parents to foster good techniques at home. Cord care is discussed on p. 221.

GASTROINTESTINAL SYSTEM
Stools

The intestinal tract functions as an outlet for amniotic fluid as early as the fifth month of fetal life. The normal functions of the gastrointestinal tract begin after birth. Food is digested and absorbed into the blood, and waste products are eliminated.

Meconium, the first stool, is a mixture of amniotic fluid and secretions of the intestinal glands. It is dark greenish black, thick, and sticky (tarry) and is passed 8 to 24 hours after birth. The stools gradually change during the first week. They become loose and are greenish yellow with mucus. These are called *transitional stools* (Figure 12-14).

The stools of a breastfed infant are bright yellow, soft, and pasty. There may be three to six stools a day. The number of stools decreases with age. The bowel movements of a bottle-fed infant are more solid than those of the breastfed infant. They vary from yellow to brown and are generally fewer in number. There may be one to four a day at first, but this gradually decreases to one or two a day. The stools are darker when an infant is receiving oral iron supplements and green when an infant is under the phototherapy lamp. Small, puttylike stools or diarrhea and bloody stools are abnormal. When there is a question, the nurse saves the stool specimen for

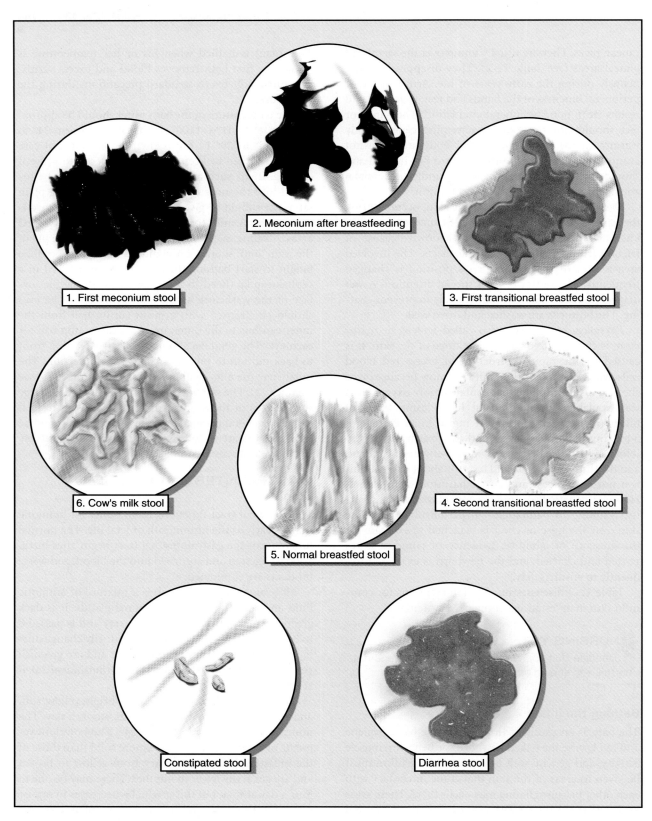

FIGURE **12-14** The normal infant stool cycle. The first meconium is dark, black, and tarry. It gradually changes to a greenish yellow transitional stool. The breastfed infant's "milk" stool is golden yellow, whereas the bottle-fed infant has a pale yellow stool. A green watery stool is indicative of diarrhea and should be reported to the health care provider.

the physician to observe. The nurse keeps an accurate record of the number and character of stools each newborn passes daily.

Constipation

Constipation refers to the passage of hard dry stools. Newborns differ in regularity. Some pass a soft stool every other day. This is not constipation. The nurse explains to parents that straining in the newborn period results from undeveloped abdominal musculature. This is normal and no treatment is required. In the first month of life a breastfed infant will pass at least four stools a day. After the second month of life the infant will increase stool volume and decrease stool frequency. Even if 5 to 6 days pass without a stool, it is not considered constipation if the stool passed is large in volume and soft or pasty in character. Constipation is sometimes seen as the infant grows older and if a formula change is made. Increasing water intake may be all that is necessary to remedy this constipation. If the infant is eating solid foods, an increased intake of fruits, vegetables, and whole-grain cereals is usually sufficient. The nurse encourages mothers to telephone their health care provider's office when questions arise and ask to speak to the nurse. This is particularly emphasized to new mothers, who may be afraid of appearing "ignorant." Very often a simple solution can relieve hours of anxiety.

Hiccoughs

Hiccoughs appear frequently in newborns and are normal. Most disappear spontaneously. Burping the infant and offering warm water may help.

Digestion

Breastfeeding is discussed in Chapter 9. Breastfed infants may be put to the breast in the first hour after delivery for psychological benefits and to help stimulate milk production. Bottle feedings are begun in about 5 hours. An infant's hunger is evidenced by crying, restlessness, fist sucking, and the rooting reflex. The capacity of the stomach is about 90 ml. Emptying time is 2 to 3 hours, and peristalsis is rapid. Feeding the newborn often stimulates the *gastrocolic reflex,* which results in the infant passing a stool.

The immature cardiac sphincter of the stomach causes the young infant to be prone to regurgitation. For this reason parents should be educated to avoid overfeeding their infant and to position the infant on the right side after feeding. Deficiency of pancreatic enzymes such as lipase limits fat absorption. Breast milk contains some lipase enzyme that aids infant digestion. Whole cow's milk does not contain this enzyme and therefore should not be fed undiluted to newborns or young infants.

The salivary glands do not secrete saliva until the infant is age 2 to 3 months. Drooling in the newborn is considered a sign of pathology and should be reported. The liver is immature, especially in its ability to conjugate bilirubin, regulate blood sugar, and coagulate blood.

Vitamins

Infants need extra vitamins C and D. Breast milk contains sufficient vitamin C if the mother's diet is rich in citrus fruits and certain vegetables. Vitamin D may be added to commercial milk (labeled "vitamin D milk") that the mother consumes. Commercial concentrated vitamin preparations may also be prescribed. The fluid is drawn up in the dropper to the prescribed amount (0.3 or 0.6 ml) and is placed directly in the infant's mouth. This is done each morning at approximately the same time to avoid forgetting the vitamins.

PREVENTING INFECTION

Infections that are relatively harmless to an adult may be fatal to the newborn. The newborn's response to inflammation and infection is slow because of the immaturity of the immune system, as follows:

- IgG is an immunoglobulin that crosses the placenta and provides the newborn with passive immunity to infections to which the mother was immune. This type of immunity rarely lasts longer than 3 months.
- IgM is an immunoglobulin produced by the newborn, and an elevated level suggests serious infection.
- IgA is an immunoglobulin produced after the neonatal period (about age 1 month) that is contained in breast milk and provides some resistance to respiratory and gastrointestinal infections. Before age 1 month, infants are at risk for such infections.

An open wound (the umbilical cord) can be a portal of entry for infection. Measures to prevent infections in the newborn nursery includes standard precautions, handwashing, cleansing and replacement of equipment, and proper disposal of soiled diapers and linen.

Nursery standards are developed and enforced by various professional agencies, such as the American Academy of Pediatrics, hospital accreditation boards, and local health agencies. The infection control nurse in each hospital also provides education and surveillance. Provisions governing space, control of temperature and

Text continued on p. 302.

CLINICAL PATHWAY 12-1

CLINICAL PATH DAY	DATE & TIME	EXPECTED PATIENT/ FAMILY OUTCOMES	MULTIDISCIPLINARY ASSESSMENT	TESTS	CONSULT
Immediate Newborn Care		☐ Apgar score >7 at 5 min. [4] ☐ Maintains axillary temp of 36.5C to 37.2C while in radiant warmer or in double blankets [1] ☐ Physiologic parameters WNL [4] ☐ Demonstrates proper latch when breastfeeding [2]	☐ Apgar score 1 & 5 min. ☐ Transitional newborn assessment q 30 min. ☐ Suck reflex	☐ Hypoglycemia protocol when indicated	☐ _____
Newborn Admission		☐ Maintains axillary temp of 36.5C to 37.2C while in radiant warmer or in double blankets [1] ☐ Physiologic parameters WNL [4] ☐ Tolerates initial feeding [2] ☐ Mother's blood type O/Rh- ☐ _____	☐ Weight ☐ V/S q 30 min × 4 ☐ Multisystem admission assessment ☐ Suck reflex ☐ _____	☐ Hypoglycemia protocol when indicated ☐ _____	☐ _____ ☐ _____
Day of Birth		N D E ☐☐☐ Maintains axillary temp of 36.5C to 37.2C independent of external heat source [1] ☐☐☐ Parents/family verbalize understanding of safety & security measures [6] ☐☐☐ Physiologic parameters WNL [4] ☐☐☐ Parent(s)/family & infant demonstrate attachment behaviors [3] ☐☐☐ Feeding [2] ☐☐☐ Latch score is 7 or greater for breastfed newborn [2] ☐☐☐ No jaundice [4] ☐☐☐ Infant seen by physician within 12 hours [6]	N D E ☐☐☐ Temp. apical pulse, neuro, cardiac, resp., GI, GU, integ. q shift ☐☐☐ Parent/infant attachment ☐☐☐ Positioning and LATCH score of breastfed newborn ☐☐☐ Freq. and amount of bottlefeeding ☐☐☐ _____	N D E ☐☐☐ Hypogly-cemia protocol when indi-cated ☐☐☐ _____	N D E ☐☐☐ _____ ☐ Social service consult if indicated

NAME	INITIALS	NAME	INITIALS

An example of a clinical pathway for a newborn from birth to discharge on the second day. This is used by all caregivers to plan and document care. (Courtesy of Women's and Children's Services of the York Health System. York, PA. Modified with permission.)

DOCUMENTATION CODES
Initial = Meets Standard
★ = Exception on pathways identified
C = Chronic problems
N/A = Not applicable

PATIENT/FAMILY PROBLEMS
1. Thermoregulation
2. Nutrition
3. Parent-Infant attachment
4. Potential alteration in newborn metabolism

5. Risk for infection
6. Infant safety
7. _____
8. _____

TREATMENTS	MEDS	NUTR.	EDUC & DC PLANNING
☐ Clamp cord ☐ Dry newborn ☐ Radiant warmer or double blanket while being held until temp stable ☐ ID bands	☐ Neonatal eye prophylaxis & Aquamephylon ☐ HBIG If indicated	☐ Determine if bottlefeeding or breastfeeding ☐ Assist with initial breastfeeding	☐ Initiate safety & security measures with parents/family ☐ Teach breastfeeding mother proper latch
☐ Cord care ☐ Admission bath	☐ _____	Initial feeding: ☐ _____	
N D E ☐☐☐ Cord care ☐☐☐ Circumcision care when indicated ☐☐☐ _____	N D E ☐☐☐ _____	N D E ☐☐☐ Breast/bottle feed on demand (breast: q 2-3 hrs. bottle: q 3-4 hrs)	N D E ☐☐☐ Reinforce safety and security measures w/ parents/family ☐☐☐ Observe & reinforce proper latch and instruct breastfeeding mother/family in alternative positioning ☐☐☐ Give and review new pamphlets: • Message to mothers • Newborn screening • Car seat • Health insurance for newborns • Preparing formula • Breastfeeding. A Guide for Success

NAME	INITIALS	NAME	INITIALS

NOTE: EACH PATIENT REQUIRES AN INDIVIDUAL ASSESSMENT & TREATMENT PLAN, THIS CLINICAL PATH IS A RECOMMENDATION FOR THE AVERAGE PATIENT WHICH REQUIRES MODIFICATION WHEN NECESSARY BY THE PROFESSIONAL STAFF.

Continued

CLINICAL PATH DAY	DATE & TIME	EXPECTED PATIENT/ FAMILY OUTCOMES	MULTIDISCIPLINARY ASSESSMENT	TESTS	CONSULT
Day 1		N D E ☐☐☐ Maintains axillary temp of 36.5C to 37.2C independent of external heat source [1] ☐☐☐ Parent(s)/family & newborn demonstrate attachment behaviors [3] ☐☐☐ Physiologic parameters WNL [4] ☐☐☐ Feeding [2] ☐☐☐ LATCH score 7 or greater for breastfed newborn [2] ☐☐☐ No jaundice [4] ☐☐☐ No signs of Infection [5] ☐☐☐ _____	N D E ☐☐☐ Temp. apical pulse, cardiac, resp., neuro, GI, GU, integ. q 8 hr. N/A/NA Weight ☐☐☐ Parent(s)/family & infant attachment behaviors ☐☐☐ LATCH score of breastfed newborn ☐☐☐ Frequency & amt. of bottlefeeding ☐☐☐ _____	N D E ☐☐☐ _____	N D E ☐☐☐ Referral made to lactation consultant for LATCH score <7 ☐☐☐ _____
Day 2		☐☐☐ Maintains axillary temp of 36.5C to 37.2C independent or external heat source [1] ☐☐☐ Parent(s)/family & newborn demonstrate attachment behaviors [3] ☐☐☐ Physiologic parameters WNL [4] ☐☐☐ Feeding [2] ☐☐☐ LATCH score 7 or greater for breastfed newborn [2] ☐☐☐ No jaundice [4] ☐☐☐ No signs of infection [5] ☐☐☐	☐☐☐ Temp. apical pulse, cardiac, resp., neuro, GI, GU, integ. q 8 hr. N/A/NA Weight ☐☐☐ Parent(s)/family & infant attachment behaviors ☐☐☐ LATCH score of breastfed newborn ☐☐☐ Frequency & amt. of bottlefeeding ☐☐☐	☐☐☐ _____	☐☐☐ Referral made to lactation consultant for LATCH score <7 ☐☐☐ _____
Discharge		☐ Maintains axillary temp of 36.5C to 37.2C independent of external heat source [1] ☐ Parent(s)/family & newborn demonstrate attachment behaviors and appropriate care of newborn [3] ☐ Physiologic parameters WNL [4] ☐ Circumcision w/o bleeding [5] ☐ Voided at least × 1 [4] ☐ Blooded at least × 1 [4] ☐ Feeding [2] ☐ LATCH score 7 or greater for breastfed newborn [2] ☐ Parent(s)/family verbalize newborn D/C instruction [6] ☐ No jaundice [4] ☐ Physician aware of Coombs results ☐ Discharge Day 2 ☐ No signs of infection	☐ Temp. apical pulse, cardiac, resp., neuro, GI, GU, integ. q 8 hr. ☐ Discharge weight ☐ Parent(s)/family & infant attachment behaviors ☐ LATCH score of breastfed newborn ☐ Frequency & amt. of bottlefeeding ☐ _____	☐ Newborn screening tests prior to D/C ☐ _____	☐☐☐ Referral made to lactation consultant for LATCH score <7 ☐ _____

NAME		INITIALS	NAME	INITIALS

NOTE: EACH PATIENT REQUIRES AN INDIVIDUAL ASSESSMENT & TREATMENT PLAN, THIS CLINICAL PATH IS A RECOMMENDATION FOR THE AVERAGE PATIENT WHICH REQUIRES MODIFICATION WHEN NECESSARY BY THE PROFESSIONAL STAFF.

TREATMENTS	MEDS	NUTR.	EDUC & DC PLANNING
N D E [N/A][N/A] Cord care [□□□] Circumcision care when indicated [□□□] _____	N D E [□□□] _____	N D E [□□□] Breast/bottle feed on demand (breast: q 2-3 hrs. bottle: q 3-4 hrs)	N D E [□□□] Observe return demonst. of breast-feeding mother's use of - alternative positioning - infant's suck, swallow [□□□] Observe parent(s) providing appropriate newborn care; reinforce. [□□□] _____
[N/A][N/A] Cord care [□□□] Circumcision care when indicated [□□□] _____	[□□□] _____	[□□□] Breast/bottle feed on demand (breast: q 2-3 hrs. bottle: q 3-4 hrs)	[□□□] Observe return demonst. of breast-feeding mother's use of - alternative positioning - infant's suck, swallow [□□□] Observe parent(s) providing appropriate newborn care; reinforce. [□□□] _____
□ Cord care □ Circumcision care when indicated □ Cord clamp removed prior to D/C □ _____	□ Hepatitis B vaccine per order □ _____	□ NPO for circumcision when indicated □ Breast/bottle feed on demand (breast: q 2-3 hrs. bottle: q 3-4 hrs)	□ Review D/C instructions with parent(s)/family □ Discuss plan for follow-up care □ D/C to mother's care

NAME	INITIALS	NAME	INITIALS

humidity, lighting, and safety from fire and other hazards are considered. Each newborn has an individual crib, bath equipment, and linen supply.

Handwashing is the most reliable precaution available. The nursery nurse washes the hands between handling different babies. The nurse stresses to parents the need for proper handwashing in the home. In many hospitals, nursery personnel wear clean scrub gowns while in the nursery for the purpose of infection control and/or security. Health care providers, technicians, and other nonnursery personnel wear cover gowns when entering the nursery and handling infants.

Health examination of personnel before employment minimizes the spread of infection by unhealthy persons. The nurse who has signs of a cold, earache, skin infection, or intestinal upset should not work in the nursery or care for ill children. Visitors are instructed not to come to the hospital or be around hospital patients if they are not feeling well.

> ⭐NURSING **TIP**_____
> The nurse must adhere to standard precautions while working in the delivery room and/or nursery. These guidelines are of particular importance during the initial care of the newborn, when exposure to secretions, blood, and amniotic fluid is high.

DISCHARGE PLANNING

Discharge teaching ideally begins with the admission of the woman to the hospital or birthing center. Many hospitals have flowsheets, which are helpful in ensuring that all topics have been addressed and that patients understand what has been explained to them. Areas of teaching include the following:

- Basic care of the infant, including bathing, cord care, feeding, and elimination
- Safety measures
- Immunizations
- Support groups, such as La Leche League
- Return appointments for well-baby care
- Telephone number of nursery (note 24-hour availability)
- Proper use of car safety seats
- Signs and symptoms of problems and who to contact; for example, temperature above 38° C (100.4° F) by axilla, refusal of two feedings in a row, two green watery stools, frequent or forceful vomiting, lack of voiding or stooling

The nurse should guide the parents in assessing, bathing, and feeding the newborn so that questions can be answered early and parents can demonstrate understanding of skills and behaviors. The clinical pathway for the newborn (pp. 298 to 301) specifies nursing interventions for assisting the mother, parents, or other caregivers in caring for the infant before and after discharge from the hospital.

HOME CARE

Feeding the newborn is discussed in Chapter 9.

FURNISHINGS

It helps if the newborn has a separate room or a separate area within a room. Simple, durable, easy-to-clean furnishings are necessary. A crib with a firm mattress is a suitable place for the infant to sleep. Crib slats should adhere to safety standards. Mattress covers are usually waterproof. Fitted sheets are convenient, and blankets of lightweight cotton are warm and easy to launder. A pillow should not be placed in the crib of the newborn for safety reasons.

Pictures are attached securely to the wall with wall tapes. Thumbtacks may be swallowed by the growing child. A chest of drawers for clothing, an adult chair (preferably a rocker), and a flat-topped table for changing clothes are necessary. A plastic basin may be used for the first few months to bathe the infant. A tray containing frequently used articles saves time and energy. These items might include a digital thermometer, hairbrush and comb, baby wipes, and baby lotion. A separate linen hamper for the infant's clothes and a closed receptacle for soiled diapers is also necessary.

CLOTHING

Clothing must be soft, washable, of the proper size, and easy to put on and take off. Parents are instructed to launder new clothing and sheets before using them to prevent skin irritation. Nightgowns with drawstring necks are avoided because they may lead to strangulation. Buttons must be sewn on tightly. Snaps or Velcro fasteners are safer. If the mother does not have a clothes dryer, she needs a clothes rack to dry the infant's garments during inclement weather.

Disposable diapers are most commonly used in hospitals and homes. They have an outer waterproof layer. Diapers made of gauze, knitted cotton, or bird's-eye or cotton flannel are available in contoured shapes or prefolded styles. However, they take longer to dry when laundered at home and are more costly. *Diaper liners* are specially treated tissues placed within the diaper. When diapers are soiled, the stool is rinsed into the toilet. The diapers are soaked in cold water, washed with a mild laundry soap, rinsed thoroughly, and dried

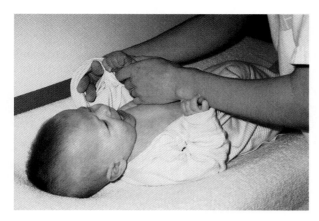

FIGURE **12-15** Dressing the newborn. The simplest technique of dressing the newborn is to place the hand through the sleeve, grasp the infant's hand, and gently pull it through the sleeve.

by clothes dryer or outdoors in the sun. Diapers that have been improperly washed and rinsed may aggravate rashes.

If a rash is present, the buttocks are kept exposed to the air as often as possible. Diapers are changed as soon as they are wet. If a rash becomes increasingly worse, the health care provider is consulted.

The quantity of items that the mother needs is determined by her washing facilities and the climate of the area in which she lives. Figure 12-15 illustrates the simplest way to dress the newborn.

key points

- Assessment of the newborn includes gestational age, weight and measurement, reflexes, system assessment, and bonding with parents.
- Heat loss occurs in the newborn via conduction, convection, evaporation, and radiation.
- The newborn is born with certain reflexes. Three of these are the Moro reflex, the rooting reflex, and the tonic neck reflex.
- The Apgar score is a standardized method of evaluating the newborn's condition at 1 and 5 minutes after delivery. Five objective signs are measured: heart rate, respiration, muscle tone, reflexes, and color.
- The most critical period for the newborn is the first hour of life, when drastic change from life within the uterus to life outside it takes place.
- Physiological jaundice becomes evident after the second and third day of life and lasts for about 1 week.

- The newborn has an unstable heat-regulating system and must be kept warm.
- Although the kidneys function at birth, they are not fully developed. Likewise, the immune system is not fully activated.
- Vernix caseosa is a cheeselike substance that covers the skin of the newborn at birth.
- Meconium, the first stool of the newborn, is a mixture of amniotic fluid and secretions of the intestinal glands. They change in color from tarry greenish black, to greenish yellow (transitional stools), to yellow-gold (milk stools).
- Proper handwashing is essential for preventing infection in newborn infants.
- Nursery standards are developed and enforced by various professional agencies.
- The hydration status of newborns can be evaluated by determining the number and consistency of stools, frequency of voiding, appearance of sunken fontanels, and status of tissue turgor.
- The normal newborn infant will lose about 10% of the birth weight in the first few days of life but will regain the birth weight by age 10 days.
- Discharge teaching begins before birth and continues to discharge date. It includes infant care, follow-up visits, evaluation of support systems, and use of car safety seats.
- The fontanels are spaces between the skull bones of the newborn that allow for molding and provide space for the brain to grow. They are known as "soft spots" on the infant's head.
- Caput succedaneum is edema of the infant's scalp that occurs during the birth process.
- Cephalohematoma is a collection of blood under the periosteum of a cranial bone. The swelling does *not* cross the suture line of the skull bone.

ONLINE RESOURCES

Newborn Care: http://www.parenthood.com

Tips for Parents: http://www.healthology.com

CRITICAL THINKING QUESTION

A new mother brings her 5-day-old infant to the clinic and states she wants to stop breastfeeding and start formula because her infant weighs less now than he did at birth. She states that her breasts are small anyway so she probably is not providing enough milk to help him gain weight. What is the best response of the nurse?

REVIEW QUESTIONS *Choose the most appropriate answer.*

1. The mother of a newborn reports to the nurse that her infant has had a black tarry stool. The nurse would tell the mother that:
   1. This is most likely caused by blood the infant may have swallowed during the birth process
   2. The health care provider will be promptly notified
   3. The infant will be given nothing by mouth (remain NPO) until a stool culture is taken
   4. This is a normal stool in newborn infants

2. The soft spots on a newborn's head are termed:
   1. Hematomas
   2. Fontanels
   3. Sutures
   4. Petechiae

3. Infections in the newborn require prompt intervention because:
   1. They spread more quickly
   2. Infections that are relatively harmless to an adult can be fatal to the newborn
   3. The portals of entry and exit are more numerous
   4. The newborn has no defenses against infection

4. White pinpoint "pimples" caused by obstruction of sebaceous glands seen on the nose and chin of the newborn are termed:
   1. Vernix caseosa
   2. Acrocyanosis
   3. Milia
   4. Mongolian spots

5. The normal respiratory rate of a newborn is:
   1. 12 to 16 breaths/min
   2. 16 to 20 breaths/min
   3. 20 to 30 breaths/min
   4. 30 to 60 breaths/min

objectives

1. Define each key term listed.
2. Differentiate between the preterm and the low-birth-weight newborn.
3. List three causes of preterm birth.
4. Describe selected problems of preterm birth and the nursing goals associated with each problem.
5. Contrast the techniques for feeding preterm and full-term newborns.
6. Describe the symptoms of cold stress and methods of maintaining thermoregulation.
7. Discuss two ways to help facilitate maternal-infant bonding for a preterm newborn.
8. Describe the family reaction to preterm infants and nursing interventions.
9. List three characteristics of the postterm infant.

key terms

apnea (ĂP-nē-ă, p. 309)
Ballard scoring system (p. 306)
bradycardia (brăd-ē-KĂR-dē-ă, p. 310)
bronchopulmonary dysplasia (brŏng-kō-PŬL-mă-năr-ē dĭs-PLĀ-zhă, p. 309)
cold stress (p. 310)
gestational age (p. 306)
hyperbilirubinemia (hī-pĕr-bĭl-ĭ-roo-bĭ-NĒ-mē-ă, p. 312)
hypocalcemia (hī-pō-kăl-SĒ-mē-ă, p. 310)
hypoglycemia (hī-pō-glī-SĒ-mē-ă, p. 310)
icterus (ĬK-tĕr-ŭs, p. 312)
kangaroo care (p. 314)
lanugo (lă-NOO-gō, p. 306)
necrotizing enterocolitis (NEC) (NĔK-rō-tīz-ĭng ĕn-tăr-ō-kō-LĪ-tĭs, p. 312)
neutral thermal environment (p. 313)
postterm (p. 306)
preterm (p. 306)
previability (p. 306)
pulse oximeter (p. 311)
respiratory distress syndrome (RDS) (p. 308)
retinopathy of prematurity (ROP) (p. 311)
sepsis (SĔP-sĭs, p. 310)

surfactant (sŭr-FĂK-tănt, p. 308)
thermoregulation (p. 313)
total parenteral nutrition (TPN) (TŌT-ăl pă-RĔN-tĕr-ăl noo-TRĬ-shĕn, p. 314)

THE PRETERM NEWBORN

The preterm (also known as premature) newborn is the most common admission to the intensive care nursery. With increased specialization and sophisticated monitoring techniques, many infants who in the past would have died are now surviving. The nurse's role continues to be increasingly complex, with greater emphasis placed on subtle clinical observations and technology. This chapter acquaints the student with the preterm infant to encourage an appreciation of his or her struggle for survival and the intense responsibility placed on those entrusted with care. The words *preterm* and *premature* are used synonymously, although the former is now considered more accurate.

Any newborn whose life or quality of existence is threatened is considered to be in a high-risk category and requires close supervision by professionals in a special neonatal intensive care unit (NICU). Preterm newborns constitute a majority of these patients and account for the largest number of admissions to the NICU. Preterm birth is responsible for more deaths during the first year of life than any other single factor. Preterm infants also have a higher percentage of birth defects. Prematurity and low birth weight are often concomitant, and both factors are associated with increased neonatal morbidity and mortality. The less an infant weighs at birth, the greater are the risks to life during delivery and immediately thereafter.

In the past a newborn was classified solely by birth weight. The emphasis is now on gestational age and level of maturation. Figure 13-1 shows two term infants of the same gestational age. One newborn would be classified as small-for-gestational-age (SGA), which may be the result of intrauterine growth restriction (IUGR) because of its weight and size. Term infants

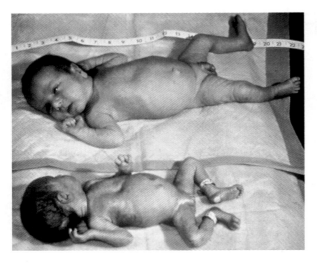

FIGURE **13-1** Two term infants of the same gestational age. These infants are discordant twins. The variation in size and weight resulted from a malformation of the placenta.

over 8.8 pounds (4000 g) may be classified as large-for-gestational-age (LGA). Current data also indicate that intrauterine growth rates are not the same for all infants and that individual factors must be considered. Gestational age refers to the actual time, from conception to birth, that the fetus remains in the uterus. For the preterm infant this is less than 38 weeks, for the *term* infant it is 38 to 42 weeks, and for the postterm infant it is beyond 42 weeks. One standardized method used to estimate gestational age is the Ballard scoring system, which is based on the infant's external characteristics and neurological development (Figures 13-2 and 13-3).

Level of maturation refers to how well developed the infant is at birth and the ability of the organs to function outside the uterus. The physician can determine much about the maturity of the newborn by careful physical examination, observation of behavior, and family history. An infant who is born at 34 weeks' gestation, weighs 3½ pounds at birth, has not been damaged by multifactorial birth defects, and has had a good placenta may be healthier than a full-term, "small for date" infant whose placenta was insufficient for any of a number of reasons. It is also probably in better condition than the heavy but immature infant of a diabetic mother. Each infant has different and distinct needs.

CAUSES

The predisposing causes of preterm birth are numerous; in many instances the cause is unknown. Prematurity may be caused by multiple births, illness of the mother (e.g., malnutrition, heart disease, diabetes mellitus, or infectious conditions), or the hazards of pregnancy itself, such as pregnancy-induced hypertension, placental abnormalities that may result in premature rupture of the membranes, placenta previa (the placenta lies over the cervix instead of higher in the uterus), and premature separation of the placenta. Studies also indicate the relationships between prematurity and poverty, smoking, alcohol consumption, and cocaine and other drug abuses.

Adequate prenatal care to prevent preterm birth is extremely important. Some preterm infants are born into families with numerous other problems. The parents may not be prepared to handle the additional financial and emotional strain imposed by a preterm infant. After delivery, early parental interaction with the infant is recognized as essential to the bonding (attachment) process. The presence of parents in special care nurseries is commonplace. Multidisciplinary care (including parent aides and other types of home support and assistance) is vital, particularly because current studies indicate a correlation between high-risk births and child abuse and neglect.

PHYSICAL CHARACTERISTICS

Preterm birth deprives the newborn of the complete benefits of intrauterine life. The infant the nurse sees in the incubator may resemble a fetus of 7 months' gestation. The skin is transparent and loose. Superficial veins may be seen beneath the abdomen and scalp. There is a lack of subcutaneous fat, and fine hair (lanugo) covers the forehead, shoulders, and arms. The cheeselike vernix caseosa is abundant. The extremities appear short. The soles of the feet have few creases, and the abdomen protrudes. The nails are short. The genitalia are small. In girls the labia majora may be open (Figure 13-3, *A*).

RELATED PROBLEMS
Inadequate Respiratory Function

Important structural changes occur in the fetal lungs during the second half of the pregnancy. The alveoli, or air sacs, enlarge, which brings them closer to the capillaries in the lungs. The failure of this phenomenon leads to many deaths attributed to previability (*pre,* "before" and *vita,* "life"). In addition, the muscles that move the chest are not fully developed; the abdomen is distended, causing pressure on the diaphragm; the stimulation of the respiratory center in the brain is immature; and the gag and cough reflexes are weak because of immature nerve supply. Oxygen may be required and can be administered via nasal catheter, incubator, or oxygen hood (see Figure 13-5). The oxygen must be warmed and humidified to prevent drying of the mucous membranes. Mechanical ventilation may be required. Oxygen saturation levels should be monitored.

MATURATIONAL ASSESSMENT OF GESTATIONAL AGE (New Ballard Score)

NEUROMUSCULAR MATURITY

A

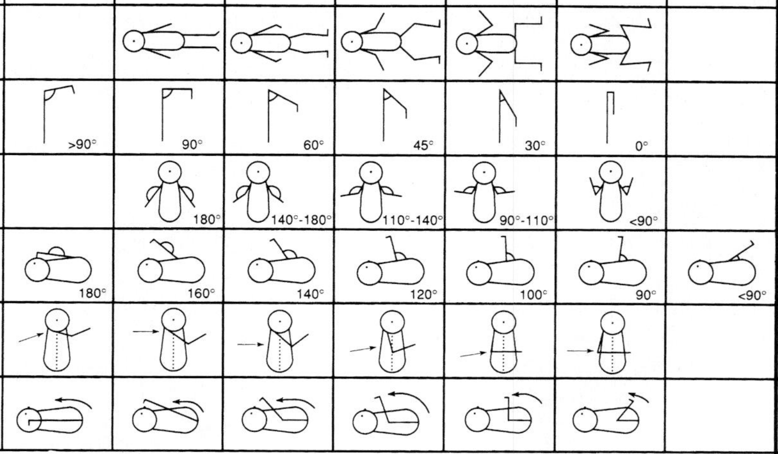

NEUROMUSCULAR MATURITY SIGN	SCORE							RECORD SCORE HERE
	-1	0	1	2	3	4	5	
POSTURE								
SQUARE WINDOW (Wrist)	>90°	90°	60°	45°	30°	0°		
ARM RECOIL		180°	140°-180°	110°-140°	90°-110°	<90°		
POPLITEAL ANGLE	180°	160°	140°	120°	100°	90°	<90°	
SCARF SIGN								
HEEL TO EAR								

TOTAL NEUROMUSCULAR MATURITY SCORE

PHYSICAL MATURITY

B

PHYSICAL MATURITY SIGN	SCORE							RECORD SCORE HERE
	-1	0	1	2	3	4	5	
SKIN	sticky friable transparent	gelatinous red translucent	smooth pink visible veins	superficial peeling &/or rash, few veins	cracking pale areas rare veins	parchment deep cracking no vessels	leathery cracked wrinkled	
LANUGO	none	sparse	abundant	thinning	bald areas	mostly bald		
PLANTAR SURFACE	heel-toe 40-50 mm:-1 <40 mm:-2	>50 mm no crease	faint red marks	anterior transverse crease only	creases ant. 2/3	creases over entire sole		
BREAST	imperceptible	barely perceptible	flat areola no bud	stippled areola 1-2 mm bud	raised areola 3-4 mm bud	full areola 5-10 mm bud		
EYE/EAR	lids fused loosely: -1 tightly: -2	lids open pinna flat stays folded	sl. curved pinna; soft; slow recoil	well-curved pinna; soft but ready recoil	formed & firm instant recoil	thick cartilage ear stiff		
GENITALS (Male)	scrotum flat, smooth	scrotum empty faint rugae	testes in upper canal rare rugae	testes descending few rugae	testes down good rugae	testes pendulous deep rugae		
GENITALS (Female)	clitoris prominent & labia flat	prominent clitoris & small labia minora	prominent clitoris & enlarging minora	majora & minora equally prominent	majora large minora small	majora cover clitoris & minora		

Reference
Ballard JL. Khoury JC. Wedig K. et al: New Ballard Score. expanded to include extremely premature infants. *J Pediatr* 1991: 119:417-423.   Reprinted by permission of Dr Ballard and Mosby-Year Book, Inc.

TOTAL PHYSICAL MATURITY SCORE

SCORE

Neuromuscular_____
Physical _____
Total_____

MATURITY RATING

score	weeks
-10	20
-5	22
0	24
5	26
10	28
15	30
20	32
25	34
30	36
35	38
40	40
45	42
50	44

C

GESTATIONAL AGE (weeks)

By dates_____
By ultrasound_____
By exam_____

FIGURE **13-2** The new Ballard scale estimates gestational age based on the neonate's neuromuscular maturity **(A)** and physical maturity **(B)**. A newborn will score 45 for a 42-week gestation, or only 20 for a 32-week gestation **(C)**.

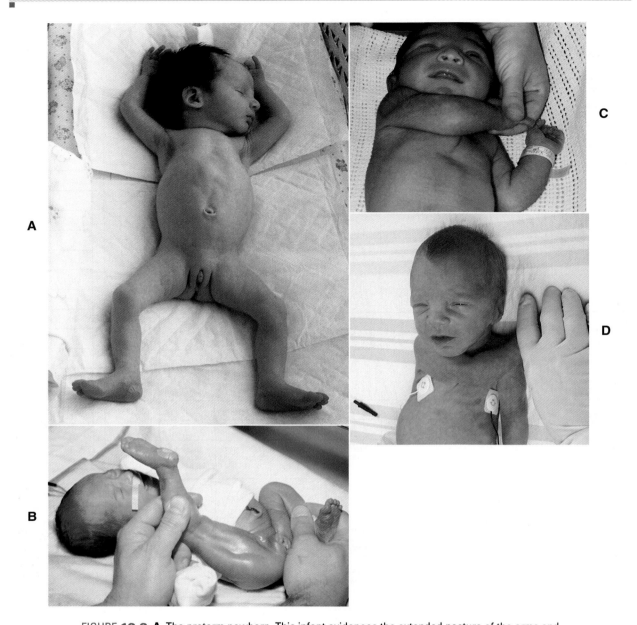

FIGURE **13-3 A,** The preterm newborn. This infant evidences the extended posture of the arms and legs characteristic of the preterm infant. The skin is thin and transparent, and the labia are open and gaping. (See Ballard scale, Figure 13-2.) **B,** Popliteal angle. This heel-to-ear maneuver demonstrates the easy extension of the leg consistent with a 30-week gestation. A full-term infant would show muscle resistance to this maneuver. (See Ballard scale, Figure 13-2.) **C,** When the arm is pulled across the chest of the full-term infant, the elbow goes only as far as the chin in the midline. This is called the *scarf sign.* **D,** When the arm is pulled across the chest of the preterm infant, it can be pulled into a straight line, with the elbow passing the chin at the midline.

Respiratory distress syndrome. Respiratory distress syndrome (RDS), also called hyaline membrane disease, is a result of immaturity of the lungs, which leads to decreased gas exchange. An estimated 30% of all neonatal deaths result from RDS or its complications (Behrman, Kliegman, & Jenson, 2000). In this disease, there is a deficient synthesis or release of surfactant, a chemical in the lungs. Surfactant is high in lecithin, a fatty protein necessary for the absorption of oxygen by the lungs. A test to determine the amount of surfactant in amniotic fluid is the lecithin/sphingomyelin (L/S) ratio.

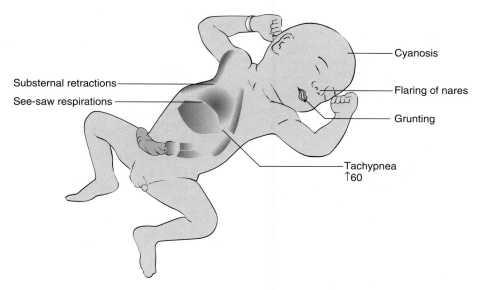

Cyanosis

Flaring of nares

Grunting

Substernal retractions

See-saw respirations

Tachypnea
↑60

FIGURE **13-4** Signs of respiratory distress in a preterm infant.

Manifestations. In general, the symptoms of respiratory distress are apparent after delivery but may not be manifested for several hours (Figure 13-4). Respirations increase to 60 breaths/min or more. Rapid respirations (tachypnea) are accompanied by gruntlike sounds, nasal flaring, cyanosis, and intercostal and sternal retractions. Edema, lassitude, and apnea occur as the condition becomes more severe. Mechanical ventilation may be necessary. The treatment of these infants is ideally carried out in the NICU.

Treatment. Surfactant begins to appear in the fetus alveoli at approximately 24 weeks' gestation and is at a level to enable the infant to breathe adequately at birth by 34 weeks' gestation. If insufficient amounts of surfactant are detected through amniocentesis, it is possible to increase its production by giving the mother injections of corticosteroids such as betamethasone. Administration 1 or 2 days before delivery may reduce the chances of RDS. In preterm newborns, surfactant can be administered via endotracheal (ET) tube at birth or when symptoms of RDS occur, with improvement of lung function seen within 72 hours. Surfactant production is altered during cold stress, hypoxia, and poor tissue perfusion, and such conditions are often present in the preterm infant.

Vital signs are monitored closely, arterial blood gases are analyzed, and the infant is placed in a warm incubator with gentle and minimal handling to conserve energy. Intravenous fluids are prescribed, and the nurse observes for signs of overhydration or dehydration. Oxygen therapy may be given via hood (Figure 13-5) or ventilator in concentrations necessary to maintain ade-

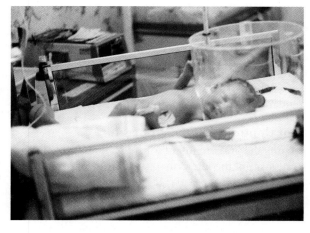

FIGURE **13-5** Oxygen administration via an oxygen hood. Oxygen is administered to this infant by means of a plastic hood. The infant is accessible for treatments without interrupting the oxygen supply.

quate tissue perfusion. Oxygen toxicity is a high risk for infants receiving prolonged treatment with high concentrations of oxygen. Bronchopulmonary dysplasia is the toxic response of the lung to oxygen therapy. Atelectasis, edema, and thickening of the membranes of the lung interfere with ventilation. This often results in prolonged dependence on supplemental oxygen and ventilators that have long-term complications.

Apnea. Apnea is defined as the cessation of breathing for 20 seconds or longer. It is not uncommon in the preterm newborn and is believed to be related to immaturity of the nervous system. An apneic episode may be accompanied by bradycardia (fewer than 100 beats/min) and cyanosis. Apnea monitors alert nurses to this complication. Gentle rubbing of the infant's feet, ankles, and back may stimulate breathing after this occurrence. When these measures fail, suctioning of the nose and mouth and raising of the infant's head to a semi-Fowler's position usually facilitates breathing. If breathing does not begin, an Ambu bag is used.

Sepsis

Sepsis is a generalized infection of the bloodstream. Preterm newborns are at risk for developing this complication because of the immaturity of many body systems. The liver of the preterm infant is immature and forms antibodies poorly. Body enzymes are inefficient. There is little or no immunity received from the mother, and stores of nutrients, vitamins, and iron are insufficient. There may be no local signs of infection, which also hinders diagnosis. Some signs of sepsis include a low temperature, lethargy or irritability, poor feeding, and respiratory distress. Maternal infection and complications during labor can also predispose the preterm infant to sepsis.

Treatment involves administration of intravenous antibiotics, maintenance of warmth and nutrition, and close monitoring of vital signs, including blood pressure. Organization of care will conserve energy. An incubator separates the infant from other infants in the unit and facilitates close observation. Maintenance of strict standard precautions is essential (see Appendix A).

Poor Control of Body Temperature

Keeping the preterm infant warm is a nursing challenge. Heat loss in the preterm results from the following factors:

- The preterm infant has a lack of brown fat, which is the body's insulation.
- There is excessive heat loss by radiation from a surface area that is large in proportion to body weight. The large surface area of the head predisposes the infant to heat loss.
- The heat-regulating center of the brain is immature.
- The sweat glands are not functioning to capacity.
- The preterm infant is inactive, has muscles that are weak and less resistant to cold, and cannot shiver.
- The posture of the preterm infant's extremities is one of leg extension. This increases the surface area exposed to the environment and increases heat loss.
- Metabolism is high, and the preterm infant is prone to low blood glucose levels (hypoglycemia).

These and other factors make the preterm newborn vulnerable to cold stress, which increases the need

> ### ⭐ NURSING **TIP**
> Signs and symptoms of cold stress include the following:
> - Decreased skin temperature
> - Increased respiratory rate with periods of apnea
> - Bradycardia
> - Mottling of skin
> - Lethargy

for oxygen and glucose. Early detection can prevent complications.

Nursing care. The infant's skin temperature will fall before the core temperature falls. Therefore a skin probe is used to monitor the temperature of preterm infants. The skin probe is placed in the right upper quadrant of the abdomen. Care should be taken to ensure that the probe is not directly over a bony prominence, in the line of cool oxygen input, or under a diaper.

The infant is placed under a radiant warmer or in an incubator to maintain a warm environment. The temperature of the incubator is adjusted so that the infant's body temperature is at an optimal level (36° to 37° C [97° to 98° F]).

Hypoglycemia and Hypocalcemia

Hypoglycemia (*hypo,* "less than" and *glycemia,* "sugar in the blood") is common among preterm infants. They have not remained in the uterus long enough to acquire sufficient stores of glycogen and fat. This condition is aggravated by the need for increased glycogen in the brain, heart, and other tissues as a result of asphyxia, sepsis, RDS, unstable body temperature, and similar conditions. Any condition that increases energy requirements places more stress on these already deficient stores. Plasma glucose levels less than 40 mg/dl indicate hypoglycemia.

The brain needs a steady supply of glucose, and hypoglycemia must be anticipated and treated promptly. Any condition that increases metabolism increases glucose needs. The preterm infant may be too weak to suck and swallow formula and often requires gavage or parenteral feedings to supply their 120- to 150-kcal/kg/day needs.

Hypocalcemia (*hypo,* "below" and *calcemia,* "calcium in the blood") is also seen in preterm and sick newborns. Calcium is transported across the placenta throughout pregnancy, but particularly during the third trimester. Early birth can result in infants with lower serum calcium levels.

In *early* hypocalcemia the parathyroid fails to respond to low calcium levels in the preterm infant. Infants stressed by hypoxia, birth trauma, or receiving sodium bicarbonate are at high risk. Infants born to mothers who are diabetic or who have had low vitamin D intake are also at risk for developing early hypocalcemia.

Late hypocalcemia usually occurs about age 1 week in newborn or preterm infants who are fed cow's milk. Cow's milk increases serum phosphate levels, which cause calcium levels to fall.

Hypocalcemia is treated by administering intravenous calcium gluconate. During intravenous therapy the nurse should monitor the infant for bradycardia. Adding calcium lactate powder to the formula also lowers phosphate levels. (Calcium lactate tablets are insoluble in milk and must not be used.) When calcium lactate powder is slowly discontinued from the formula, the nurse should again monitor the infant for signs of neonatal tetany.

> ⭐ NURSING **TIP**_____
> Signs of hypoglycemia in the preterm infant include the following:
> - Tremors
> - Weak cry
> - Lethargy
> - Convulsions
> - Plasma glucose level lower than 40 mg/dl (term) or 30 mg/dl (preterm)

> ⭐ NURSING **TIP**_____
> When an infant is given intravenous calcium gluconate, the nurse should monitor the heart rate closely and report bradycardia.

Increased Tendency to Bleed

Preterm infants are more prone to bleeding than full-term infants because their blood is deficient in prothrombin, a factor of the clotting mechanism. Fragile capillaries of the head are particularly susceptible to injury during delivery, causing intracranial hemorrhage. Ultrasonography is helpful in detecting this problem. The nurse should monitor the neurological status of the infant and report bulging fontanels, lethargy, poor feeding, and seizures. The bed should be in a slight Fowler's position, and unnecessary stimulation that can cause increased intracerebral pressure should be avoided.

Retinopathy of Prematurity

Retinopathy of prematurity (ROP) is a condition in which there is separation and fibrosis of the retina, which can lead to blindness. The damage to immature retinal blood vessels is thought to be caused by high oxygen levels of arterial blood. The condition was formerly termed *retrolental fibroplasia,* but the term ROP is currently used because it is more precise. It is the leading cause of blindness in newborns weighing less than 1500 g. At first it was believed to be caused by oxygen toxicity alone, but now many other problems common to the

preterm infant are thought to contribute to the risk. The disorder is classified into several stages, and preterm infants who have milder forms of the disorder may have no residual effects or visual disabilities (Behrman, Kliegman, & Jenson, 2000). Prevention of preterm births and the problems that beset preterm infants are the key to preventing ROP. Careful monitoring of oxygen saturation in high-risk infants with a pulse oximeter continues to be a priority in the nursery (Figure 13-6). It is the level of oxygen in the blood, rather than the amount of oxygen received, that is of importance in oxygen therapy. There is no "safe level" of oxygen. Infants must be provided with the level of oxygen required to sustain life and prevent neurological damage. Maintaining a sufficient level of vitamin E and avoiding excessively high concen-

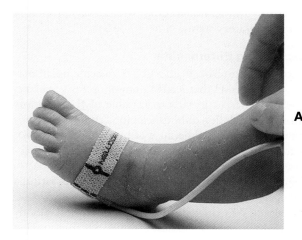
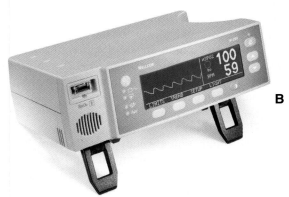

FIGURE **13-6** Pulse oximeter. **A,** A lead with two sensors opposite each other is placed on the toe or foot of the newborn. A red light passes from one sensor, through the vascular bed of the toe or foot, and registers on the sensor on the opposite side. **B,** The determination of oxygen saturation in the blood is shown on the monitor, which displays the heart rate as well as the oxygen saturation level in place. The circle on the foot band indicates the location of the sensor.

trations of oxygen may help to prevent this condition. Cryosurgery may reduce long-term complications of ROP. Consultation with an experienced ophthalmologist is necessary when pathological signs appear.

Poor Nutrition

The stomach capacity of the preterm infant is small. The sphincter muscles at both ends of the stomach are immature, which contributes to regurgitation and vomiting, particularly after overfeeding. Sucking and swallowing reflexes are immature. The infant's ability to absorb fats is poor (this includes fat-soluble vitamins). The inadequate store of nutrients in the preterm infant and the need for glucose and nutrients to promote growth and prevent brain damage contribute to the nutritional problems of the preterm infant. Parenteral or gavage feedings are usually required until the infant is strong enough to tolerate oral feedings without compromising cardiorespiratory status.

Necrotizing Enterocolitis

Necrotizing enterocolitis (NEC) is an acute inflammation of the bowel that leads to bowel *necrosis.* Preterm newborns are particularly susceptible to NEC. Factors implicated include a diminished blood supply to the lining of the bowel wall because of hypoxia or sepsis that causes a decrease in protective mucus and results in bacterial invasion of the delicate tissues. A source for bacterial growth occurs when the infant is fed a milk formula or hypertonic gavage feeding.

Signs of NEC include abdominal distention, bloody stools, diarrhea, and bilious vomitus. Specific nursing responsibilities include observing vital signs, maintaining infection control techniques, and carefully resuming oral fluids as ordered. Measuring the abdomen and listening for bowel sounds are also important. Treatment includes antibiotics and the use of parenteral nutrition to rest the bowels. Surgical removal of the necrosed bowel may be indicated.

Immature Kidneys

Improper elimination of body wastes contributes to electrolyte imbalance and disturbed acid-base relationships. Dehydration occurs easily. Tolerance to salt is limited, and susceptibility to edema is increased.

The nurse should document the intake and output for all preterm infants. The nurse should weigh the dry diaper and subtract its weight from the infant's wet diaper to determine the urine output. The urine output should be between 1 and 3 ml/kg/hr. The infant should be observed closely for signs of dehydration or overhydration. The nurse should document the status of the fontanels, tissue turgor, weight, and urine output.

Jaundice

The liver of the newborn is immature, which contributes to a condition called icterus or jaundice (Table 13-1). Jaundice causes the skin and whites of the eyes to assume a yellow-orange cast. The liver is unable to clear the blood of bile pigments that result from the normal postnatal destruction of red blood cells. The amount of bile pigment in the blood serum is expressed as milligrams of bilirubin per deciliter. The higher the bilirubin level, the deeper is the jaundice and the greater the risk for neurological damage. An increase of more than 5 mg/dl in 24 hours requires careful investigation. Physiological jaundice is normal and is discussed on p. 295. Pathological jaundice is more serious. It occurs within 24 hours of birth and is secondary to an abnormal condition such as ABO-Rh incompatibility (see pp. 338 to 340). In preterm infants the normal rise in bilirubin levels (icterus neonatorum) is slower than in full-term infants and lasts longer, which predisposes the infant to hyperbilirubinemia (*hyper* "excessive," *bilirubin* "bile," and *emia* "blood"), or excessive bilirubin levels in the blood.

There is more evidence of jaundice in infants who are breastfed. Breast milk jaundice begins to be seen about the fourth day, when the mother's milk supply develops. The newborn usually does well but is carefully monitored to rule out problems. In early breast milk jaundice, the lack of infant suckling causes jaundice and requires an increase in breastfeeding. In late breast milk jaundice, the breast milk itself lacks substances that help conjugate bilirubin, and therefore formula may be substituted for 24 to 48 hours to reduce bilirubin levels.

The goals of treatment for hyperbilirubinemia are to prevent *kernicterus* (a serious neurological complication that can cause brain damage) and to reverse the hemolytic process that causes the bilirubin level to rise. The nursing care and treatment for hyperbilirubinemia consists of observing the infant's skin, sclera, and mucous membranes for jaundice. (Blanching the skin over bony prominences enhances the evaluation for jaundice.) Observing and reporting the progression of jaundice from the face to the abdomen and feet is important because it

table 13-1 | *Neonatal Jaundice*

TYPE	APPEARS	PEAK BILIRUBIN CONCENTRATION	DURATION
Physiological			
Full-term	2-3 days	10-12 mg/dl	4-5 days
Preterm	3-4 days	15 mg/dl	7-9 days
Breast milk	4-7 days	15-20 mg/dl	10 weeks
Pathological	First day	Unlimited	Varies

may indicate increasing bilirubin levels. Monitoring and reporting bilirubin laboratory values and response phototherapy should be documented (see p. 340).

SPECIAL NEEDS

The physician appraises the physical status of the preterm newborn at delivery. The immediate needs are to clear the infant's airway and provide warmth. The infant is given care for the umbilical cord and eye care and is then properly identified. Weighing is sometimes omitted until later if the infant's condition is poor. The infant is placed naked in an incubator and taken to the nursery. The nurse in charge is given a report on the general condition of the newborn, the type of delivery, and any complications that have occurred. Many hospitals transfer their preterm infants to special medical centers geared to care for them. The transport team is briefed by the neonatologist and is dispatched to the referring hospital. A life-support infant-transport incubator that can be carried by ambulance (and sometimes helicopter) is used. Box 13-1 lists some nursing goals for care of the preterm newborn.

Thermoregulation (Warmth)

Thermoregulation (*thermo* "heat" and *regulation* "maintenance of") involves maintaining a stable body temperature and preventing hypothermia (low temperature) and hyperthermia (high temperature). A stable body temperature is essential in the survival and management of preterm infants.

Incubator. The preterm newborn is placed in an incubator designed to provide a neutral thermal environment wherein temperature, air, radiating surface temperatures, and humidity are controlled to maintain the infant's temperature within a normal range with minimal oxygen consumption required. The incubator also provides isolation and protection from infection. The top of the incubator is transparent to enable personnel to view the newborn clearly at all times. Models include alarms to indicate overheating or a lack of circulating air, facilities for positioning, and a scale to weigh the infant without removal from the warm environment. Nurses must understand how to use the incubators available in the nurseries to which they are assigned (Figure 13-7). They should request assistance if needed.

The temperature of the incubator is adjusted to a level that will maintain an optimal body temperature in the infant. Smaller infants may require higher incubator temperatures. The nurse records the temperature of the infant and the incubator every 2 hours. The infant's temperature is monitored with a heat-sensitive probe, which is taped to the abdomen. Axillary temperatures may also be taken. A relative humidity of 60% or higher is desirable. Overheating should be avoided because it increases the infant's oxygen and caloric requirements.

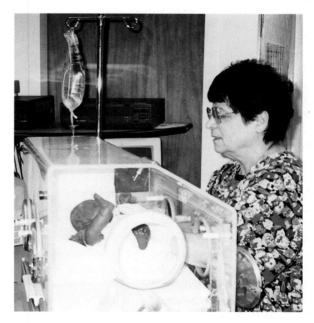

FIGURE **13-7** The incubator. The infant is dressed only in a diaper. Portholes facilitate routine infant care without disturbing the atmospheric conditions in the incubator. The infant can be assessed through Plexiglas windows. Levers under the mattress can place the bed in the Fowler's or Trendelenburg position. Openings at the head and foot of the incubator can be used to remove soiled linen using the principles of aseptic technique. The door of the incubator can be lowered to form a platform that makes the infant accessible for special treatments or tests. The nurse must make sure the door is *locked* in the closed position when the incubator is in use. To promote circadian rhythms, a blanket may be placed over the top of the incubator to shield the infant from environmental lights.

| box 13-1 | *Nursing Goals for the Preterm Newborn* |

The nursing goals in caring for the preterm newborn are as follows:

- Improve respiration
- Maintain body heat (keep the "preemie" warm)
- Conserve energy
- Prevent infection
- Provide proper nutrition and hydration
- Give good skin care
- Observe the infant carefully and record observations
- Support and encourage the parents

Radiant heat. Radiant heat cribs that supply overhead heat have the advantage of providing easier access to the patient while maintaining a neutral thermal environment. Nursing Care Plan 13-1 lists nursing interventions for selected nursing diagnoses pertinent to care of the preterm newborn.

Kangaroo care. Kangaroo care is a method of care for preterm infants that uses skin-to-skin contact. This method of holding the infant is similar to the way a kangaroo keeps its offspring warm in its pouch (Figure 13-8). The practice began in 1979 in Bogota, Colombia, in response to a shortage of incubators and staff and is currently a popular practice in the United States. The infant, wearing only a diaper and a small cap, rests on the mother or father's naked breast. The skin warms and calms the child and promotes bonding.

Nutrition

Feeding of the preterm newborn varies with gestational age and health status. The ability to coordinate breathing, sucking, and swallowing does not develop before 34 weeks' gestation. Therefore a very preterm infant may require gavage feedings (via a tube placed through the nose or mouth into the stomach). Infants weighing more than 1500 g may be able to bottle feed if a small, soft nipple with a large hole is used to minimize the energy and effort required for sucking. Human milk is ideal because the fat is absorbed readily. Breast milk may be manually expressed by the mother and placed in the bottle for her preterm infant. If the infant is gavage fed, the tube is replaced every 3 to 7 days. Intravenous fluids may be provided to meet fluid, caloric, and electrolyte needs in small, weak preterm infants. Often the infants are fed while still in the incubator. Early initiation of feedings reduces the risk of hypoglycemia, hyperbilirubinemia, and dehydration.

The nurse should observe and record bowel sounds and the passage of meconium, which indicate intestinal readiness for oral feedings. When the infant is gavage fed, the contents of the stomach should be aspirated before the feeding is started. If only mucus or air is aspirated, the feeding can be given as planned. If a residual of liquid contents is aspirated, the physician should be notified before proceeding to feed the infant. Infants older than 28 weeks' gestation usually have the digestive enzymes required for the digestion of breast milk. Formulas designed for the term infant are not well tolerated by the preterm infant because they are a burden to their kidneys and can cause central nervous system problems. Formulas designed for preterm infants are not well tolerated by infants older than 34 weeks' gestation or term infants because hypercalcemia may develop. Supplemental vitamins are usually prescribed for the preterm infant. If the infant is too premature or too ill to tolerate oral feedings, total parenteral nutrition (TPN)—the intravenous infusion of lipids and nutrients—may be prescribed to meet the infant's nutritional and growth needs.

Close Observation

The physician examines the preterm newborn and writes specific orders for treatment and nursing care. When the physician leaves the nursery, the nurse is responsible for reporting any significant changes in the infant's condition. The experienced nurse in the preterm nursery observes and charts care and treatment in great detail. Table 13-2 lists the *general* observations to guide care of the preterm newborn. Sudden changes are reported immediately.

Positioning and Skin Care

The preterm newborn is positioned on the back or prone with the head of the mattress slightly elevated unless contraindicated. In this position the abdominal contents do not press against the diaphragm and impede breathing.

Positioning the preterm infant should be compatible with the drainage of secretions and prevention of aspiration. Propping the infant on the side or placing the infant prone can decrease respiratory effort and improve oxygenation. An enclosed space, or *nesting,* can provide a calming, supportive environment for the preterm infant (Figure 13-9). The infant should not be left in one position for long periods because it is uncomfortable and may harm the lungs. Changing the position also prevents breakdown from pressure on the infant's delicate skin. If such a breakdown should occur, the area is exposed to the air, and a suitable ointment is applied as prescribed by the physician (see Chapter 12 for a more extended discussion on the skin of the newborn).

PROGNOSIS

In the absence of severe birth defects and complications, the growth rate of the preterm newborn nears that of the term infant by about the second year. Very low-birth-weight infants may not catch up, especially if there has been chronic illness, insufficient nutritional intake, or inadequate care taking (Behrman, Kliegman, & Jenson, 2000). Additional studies are needed to determine the effects of these factors at various age levels. Parents must be prepared for relatives' comments on the infant's small size and slower development. In general, growth and development of the preterm infant are based on current age minus the number of weeks before term the infant was born; for example, if born at 36 weeks' gestation, a 1-month-old infant would be at a newborn's

NURSING CARE PLAN 13-1

The Preterm Newborn

PATIENT DATA: A newborn infant of 30 weeks' gestation is admitted to the neonatal intensive care unit (NICU). The infant is placed in a prewarmed incubator, and cardiorespiratory sensors are applied.

SELECTED NURSING DIAGNOSIS   *Risk for hypothermia related to decreased subcutaneous tissue, immature body temperature control*

Outcomes	Nursing Interventions	Rationales
Infant's temperature will remain at 36.5° to 37° C (97.6° to 98.6° F).	1. Monitor temperature with skin probe or by axillary method.	1. These methods provide the best indication of the infant's core temperature and are less invasive.
	2. Adjust incubator or radiant warmer to maintain skin temperature.	2. A neutral thermal environment permits the infant to maintain a normal core temperature with minimum oxygen consumption and caloric expenditure.
	3. Observe for signs of cold stress, such as decreased temperature, pallor, and lethargy.	3. Preterm infants have little or no muscular activity; they remain in an extended posture because of lack of muscle tone; they cannot shiver.
	4. Use discretion in bathing.	4. The temperature of a wet infant drops quickly as a result of evaporation.
	5. Avoid cold surfaces.	5. Conductive heat loss occurs when an infant is weighed on a cold scale; prewarm surfaces or use a receiving blanket for protection.

SELECTED NURSING DIAGNOSIS   *Risk for impaired skin integrity related to immature skin, poor nutrition, and immobility*

Outcomes	Nursing Interventions	Rationales
Skin will remain intact.	1. Change position regularly.	1. This prevents pressure sores and aids respiration and circulation.
	2. Be gentle when removing dressings, tape, and electrodes.	2. The preterm infant's skin is fragile and bruises easily; use as little tape as possible.
	3. Cleanse skin with clear water or approved cleansers.	3. Avoid hexachlorophene cleaners because of their toxic effect; all products must be carefully assessed before use because permeability of the preterm infant's skin fosters absorption of ingredients.
	4. Observe skin for signs of infection while recognizing that there may be no local inflammatory response, only vague signs and symptoms.	4. Heel pricks and other invasive procedures are often necessary; the preterm infant's immune system is immature and healing becomes difficult.

?CRITICAL THINKING QUESTION

A mother comes to visit her preterm son in the NICU. She states she wants to see her infant, but she is afraid to touch anything and fears she will hurt her fragile newborn. What is the best response of the nurse?

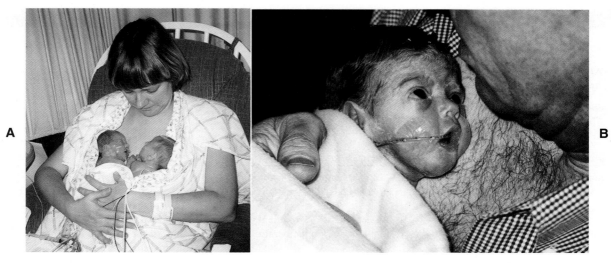

FIGURE **13-8** Kangaroo care. **A,** The mother provides kangaroo care for her preterm infants. Skin-to-skin contact is provided, with warmth maintained by the outer covering. **B,** The father can provide effective kangaroo care. The infant shows a positive response to this contact.

table **13-2** | *Nursing Observations in Care of the Preterm Infant*

OBSERVATION	SIGNS TO LOOK FOR
General activity	Increase or decrease in movements, lethargy, twitching, frequency and quality of cry, hyperactivity
Fontanels	Sunken, flat, or bulging
Eyes	Discharge
Respirations	Regularity, apnea, sternal retractions, labored breathing
Pulse	Rate and regularity
Abdomen	Distention
Cord	Discharge; odor
Feeding	Sucking ability, vomiting or regurgitation, degree of satisfaction
Voiding	Initial, frequency
Stools	Frequency, color, consistency
Mucous membranes	Dryness of lips and mouth, signs of thrush
Color	Paleness, cyanosis, jaundice
Skin	Rashes, irritations, pustules, edema

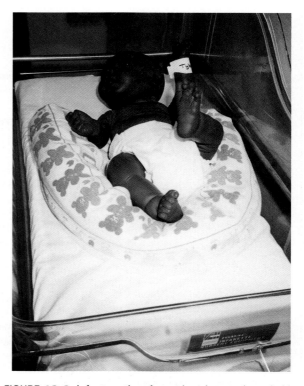

FIGURE **13-9** Infant nesting. An enclosed space bounded by small blanket rolls encircling the preterm infant provides a calming supportive environment.

achievement level. This calculation ensures that no one has unrealistic expectations for the infant.

FAMILY REACTION

The nurse should assist the parents to cope with their responses to having a small, preterm infant. Parents need guidance throughout the infant's hospitalization to help to prepare them for this new experience. They may be disheartened by the unattractive appearance of the preterm newborn. They may believe they are to blame for the infant's condition. They may fear that the infant will die but may be unable to express their feelings. They need time to look at and touch the infant and begin to see the child as uniquely their own (Figure 13-10). This touch and immediate human contact are vital for the infant as well. The mother is usually concerned with her ability to care for such a small and helpless creature. When she feels ready, she may assist the nurse in diapering, bathing, feeding, and other activities. Other aspects of infant care are also stressed during this time.

Nursing care of the preterm infant includes measures to provide short periods of stimulation during the alert phase of activity. The parents can be taught to provide stimulation by using a black-and-white mobile, stroking gently, talking to the infant, rocking, or providing range-of-motion activity or kangaroo care. A pacifier

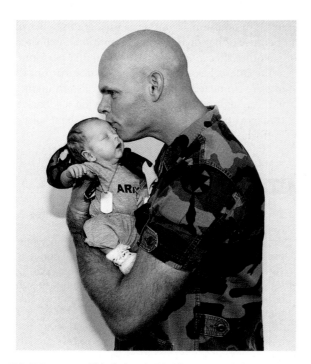

FIGURE **13-10** This father holds his preterm infant in a moment of bonding.

may be used during gavage feeding to provide nonnutritive sucking. Care should be taken not to overly stimulate or tire the infant.

Special effort is required in the NICU environment to reduce noise and light in order to provide rest and preserve the circadian rhythm (sleep pattern). Covering the incubator with a light blanket at intervals can reduce exposure to external stimuli. There should be minimal stimulation *during* feeding in order to enable the infant to concentrate energy on the sucking and swallowing process. Stimulation and interaction with parents should be provided *between* feedings (Medoff-Cooper, McGrath, & Bilker, 2000).

The nurse should collaborate with pediatricians, social workers, nutritionists, psychologists, and staff from other disciplines to plan and coordinate follow-up care of the preterm infant after discharge. Often a mother is discharged without her infant. This is difficult for the entire family and makes attachment and bonding more complicated. The nurse encourages the family to keep in touch by telephone and by visits. Parents can help siblings to accept the infant by addressing the child by name, sharing news of progress, taking pictures of the infant, and encouraging communication by drawings and cards. Listening to what siblings are saying provides information for discussion.

Discharge planning begins at birth. The parents will need to demonstrate and practice routine and/or specialized care. Visits by the nurse to assess home care and provide additional support are valuable. Continued medical supervision is important. The nurse stresses the importance of well-baby examinations, immunizations, and prevention of infection. Good prenatal care for subsequent pregnancies is emphasized because the mother is at high risk for future preterm births.

> **NURSING TIP**
> Encourage parents to talk about their feelings and fears concerning the preterm infant. Answer questions about home care.

THE POSTTERM NEWBORN

The newborn is considered *postterm* if the pregnancy goes beyond 42 weeks. *Postmaturity* refers to the infant showing characteristics of the postmature syndrome. Identification of infants who are not tolerating the extra time in the uterus is the major goal of treatment. Death of the postterm infant is uncommon today because of early detection and intervention. The cause of postmaturity is not yet clear; however, it is known that the placenta does not function adequately as it ages, which could result in fetal distress. The mortality rate of late infants is higher than that of newborns delivered at term. Morbidity rates are also higher. Once the infant makes it through delivery, the risks are fewer.

The late birth is a psychological strain on the mother, father, and other members of the family, who are eagerly awaiting the arrival of the child. The nurse encourages parents to verbalize their feelings and concerns about the delay. Very large newborns, such as those of diabetic mothers, are not necessarily postmature but are larger than normal because of rapid abnormal growth before delivery.

The following problems are associated with postmaturity:

- Asphyxia caused by chronic hypoxia while in the uterus because of a deteriorated placenta
- Meconium aspiration; hypoxia and distress may cause relaxation of the anal sphincter; meconium can be aspirated into the fetal lungs
- Poor nutritional status; depleted glycogen reserves cause hypoglycemia
- Increase in red blood cell production (polycythemia) because of intrauterine hypoxia
- Difficult delivery because of increased size of the infant
- Birth defects
- Seizures as a result of the hypoxic state

PHYSICAL CHARACTERISTICS

The postterm infant is long and thin and looks as though weight has been lost. The skin is loose, especially about the thighs and buttocks. There is little lanugo (downy hair) or vernix caseosa. The loss of the cheeselike vernix caseosa leaves the skin dry; it cracks, peels, and is almost like parchment in texture. The nails are long and may be stained with meconium. The infant has a thick head of hair and looks alert.

NURSING CARE

Labor induction or cesarean deliveries are commonly performed if testing determines that the pregnancy is past 42 weeks or if there are signs of fetal distress or maternal risk. Many postterm infants suffer few adverse effects from the delay, but they still require careful observation in the nursery. Nursing care involves observing for respiratory distress (usually because of aspiration of meconium-stained amniotic fluid), hypoglycemia (caused by depleted glycogen stores), and hyperbilirubinemia (as a result of polycythemia). The infant may be placed in an incubator because fat stores have been used in utero for nourishment and the infant is vulnerable to cold stress.

TRANSPORTING THE HIGH-RISK NEWBORN

Transportation of the high-risk newborn to a regional neonatal center requires the organization and expertise of a special team. A nurse and sometimes a physician accompany the infant unless specialists in emergency medical transport are part of the transport team. Stabilization of the infant before discharge is important. Baseline data, such as vital signs and blood work (blood gases and glucose levels), are obtained. The infant is weighed if this is not contraindicated. Copies of all records are made, including the infant's record, the mother's prenatal history and delivery, and pertinent admission data. A transport incubator is provided for warmth, and the batteries are kept fully charged.

The nurse is responsible for placing an identification band on the infant before transport and for verifying the identification name and number with the mother's identification band. The mother should be reassured that the identification will stay with the infant. The parents should be given the name and location of the receiving hospital and the name and telephone number of a physician to contact for follow-up information and visits.

Parents are shown the newborn before departure. If the mother is unable to hold the infant because of his or her condition, the incubator is wheeled to her bedside for her observation. A picture is taken and given to the parents. On occasion, a mother is unable to see her infant because of her own unstable condition. Such situations require special empathy from nursing personnel. Once the infant has safely reached its destination, the parents are contacted by telephone. It is also thoughtful if the receiving hospital personnel provide feedback to the transport team so that they may enjoy the results of their efforts.

key points

- Early identification of the high-risk fetus facilitates treatment and nursing care.
- Studies indicate that there is a relationship between prematurity and poverty, smoking, alcohol consumption, narcotics use, and lack of prenatal care.
- Preterm infants have poor muscle tone and less subcutaneous fat but more vernix and lanugo than full-term infants.
- The preterm infant is observed for jaundice, low oxygen saturation levels, and unstable vital signs. The intake and output of all preterm infants is monitored.
- The care of preterm infants is organized to minimize handling and stimulation.

- Blanket rolls are used to provide an enclosed space for preterm infants.
- Nurses support parents and encourage participation in care.
- Respiratory distress syndrome has a high mortality rate, and it may precipitate long-term effects.
- Problems associated with prematurity include asphyxia, meconium aspiration, hypoglycemia, hypocalcemia, hemorrhage from fragile vessels, poor resistance to infection, and inadequate nutrition.
- Heat or thermoregulation is essential for the preterm newborn's survival. Cold stress is to be avoided.
- Nursing goals in caring for the preterm newborn are improving respirations, maintaining body heat, conserving the infant's energy, preventing infection, providing nutrition and hydration, providing good skin care, and supporting and encouraging the parents.

- Oxygen is administered very carefully to preterm newborns to prevent eye complications such as retinopathy of prematurity.
- The postterm newborn is born after 42 weeks' gestation and shows certain characteristics that place the infant at risk, such as hypoxia, poor nutritional stores, and polycythemia.
- The postterm newborn has little lanugo and vernix, and the skin is dry and peeling.

ONLINE RESOURCES

March of Dimes 2000 Annual Report: http://www. modimes.org

REVIEW QUESTIONS   *Choose the most appropriate answer.*

1. A standardized method of determining gestational age based on appearance and neuromuscular criteria is the:
   1. Gesell graph
   2. Ballard score
   3. Washington guide
   4. Friedman curve

2. Some preterm infants are fed by gavage because of:
   1. Poor digestion
   2. Overdeveloped gag and cough reflexes
   3. Refusal of formula
   4. Weak sucking and swallowing reflexes

3. A characteristic sign of necrotizing enterocolitis (NEC) in the newborn is:
   1. Bloody diarrhea
   2. Necrosis of the abdomen
   3. Projectile vomiting
   4. High fever

4. The actual time that the fetus remains in the uterus is termed:
   1. Gestational age
   2. Intrauterine growth rate
   3. Neurological age
   4. Level of maturation

5. Providing high oxygen concentrations to a preterm newborn may cause:
   1. Rupture of the alveoli
   2. Cyanosis
   3. Retinopathy of prematurity
   4. Primary atelectasis

14 The Newborn with a Congenital Malformation

CHAPTER

objectives

1. Define each key term listed.
2. List and define the more common disorders of the newborn.
3. Describe the classifications of birth defects.
4. Outline the nursing care for the infant with hydrocephalus.
5. Discuss the prevention of neural tube anomalies.
6. Outline the preoperative and postoperative nursing care of a newborn with spina bifida cystica.
7. Discuss the dietary needs of an infant with phenylketonuria.
8. Describe the symptoms of increased intracranial pressure.
9. Differentiate between cleft lip and cleft palate.
10. Discuss the early signs of dislocation of the hip.
11. Discuss the care of the newborn with Down syndrome.
12. Outline the causes and treatment of hemolytic disease of the newborn (erythroblastosis fetalis).
13. Devise a plan of care for an infant receiving phototherapy.
14. Describe home phototherapy.

key terms

birth defect (p. 320)
cheiloplasty (KĪ-lō-plăs-tē, p. 327)
clubfoot (p. 329)
congenital malformation (p. 321)
erythroblastosis fetalis (ē-rĭth-rō-blăs-TŌ-sĭs fē-TĂL-ĭs, p. 338)
habilitation (p. 325)
hydrocephalus (hī-drō-SĚF-ă-lăs, p. 321)
hyperbilirubinemia (hī-pĕr-bĭl-ĭ-roo-bĭ-NĒ-mē-ă, p. 340)
macrosomia (măk-rō-SŌ-mē-ă, p. 344)
meningocele (mă-NĬNG-gō-sēl, p. 324)
meningomyelocele (mă-nĭng-gō-MĪ-ĕ-lō-sēl, p. 324)
myelodysplasia (mī-ă-lō-dĭs-PLĀ-sē-ă, p. 324)
Ortolani's sign (p. 331)
Pavlik harness (p. 331)

phototherapy (p. 340)
RhoGAM (p. 339)
shunt (p. 322)
spica cast (p. 331)
spina bifida (SPĪ-nă BĬF-ĭ-dă, p. 324)
transillumination (p. 321)

Birth defects, abnormalities that are apparent at birth, occur in 3% to 4% of all live births. The rate is even higher if the defects that become evident later in life are counted. An abnormality of structure, function, or metabolism may result in a physical or mental disability, may shorten life, or may be fatal. Box 14-1 shows the system of classification of birth defects. Because these disorders include so many conditions, it is necessary to limit the number discussed in this chapter and to place others in relevant areas of the text (see the index for specific conditions). Fetal alcohol syndrome and environmental influences on fetal growth are discussed in Chapter 5. Congenital heart is discussed in Chapter 25.

Defects present at birth often involve the skeletal system; limbs may be missing, malformed, or duplicated. Some abnormalities (e.g., congenital hip dysplasia) are more subtle, and the nurse must be alert to detect them. *Inborn errors of metabolism* include a number of inherited diseases that affect body chemistry. There may be an absence or a deficiency of a substance necessary for cell metabolism. The deficient substance is usually an enzyme. Almost any organ of the body may be damaged. Examples of inborn errors of metabolism include cystic fibrosis and phenylketonuria (PKU). In *disorders of the blood*, there is a reduced or missing blood component or an inability of a component to function adequately. Sickle cell disease, thalassemia, and hemophilia fall into this category. *Chromosomal abnormalities* number in the thousands. Most involve some type of mental retardation, and others are incompatible with life. The newborn with Turner's syndrome or Klinefelter's syndrome may have impaired physical growth and sexual development. *Perinatal damage* has many causes and is seen in various forms, the most common of which is premature birth.

| box 14-1 | *Classification of Birth Defects* |

MALFORMATIONS PRESENT AT BIRTH

Structural defects, such as hydrocephalus,* spina bifida,* congenital heart malformations, cleft lip and palate,* clubfoot,* and developmental hip dysplasia*

METABOLIC DEFECTS (BODY CHEMISTRY)

Cystic fibrosis, phenylketonuria,* Tay-Sachs disease, family hypercholesterolemia or high cholesterol that often causes early heart attack, and others

BLOOD DISORDERS

Sickle cell disease, hemophilia, thalassemia, defects of white blood cells and immune defense, and others

CHROMOSOMAL ABNORMALITIES

Down syndrome,* Klinefelter's syndrome, Turner's syndrome, trisomies 13 and 18, and many others; most involve some combination of mental retardation and physical malformations that range from mild to fatal

PERINATAL DAMAGE

Infections, drugs, maternal disorders, abnormalities unique to pregnancy (Rh disease,* difficult labor or delivery, premature birth)

*Topics discussed in this chapter.

As the March of Dimes Birth Defect Foundation (1997) points out, "Few birth defects can be attributed to a single cause. The majority are thought to result from an interplay between environment and heredity, depending on inherited susceptibility, stage of pregnancy, and degree of environmental hazard." Newborns with birth defects may need to remain in the neonatal unit for an extended period of time for intensive care and treatment.

MALFORMATIONS PRESENT AT BIRTH

The following sections discuss congenital malformations, or those defects present at birth, according to body systems.

NERVOUS SYSTEM
Hydrocephalus

Pathophysiology. Hydrocephalus (*hydro*, "water" and *cephalo*, "head") in the newborn is a condition characterized by an increase of cerebrospinal fluid (CSF) within the ventricles of the brain, which causes pressure changes in the brain and an increase in head size. It results from an imbalance between the production and absorption of CSF or improper formation of the ventricles. Hydrocephalus may be congenital or acquired. It is most commonly acquired by an obstruction, such as a tumor, or as a sequela of infections (encephalitis or meningitis) or perinatal hemorrhage. The symptoms depend on the site of obstruction and the age at which it develops.

Hydrocephalus is classified as noncommunicating (obstructive) or communicating. *Noncommunicating hydrocephalus* results from the obstruction of CSF flow from the ventricles of the brain to the subarachnoid space. *Communicating hydrocephalus* results when CSF is not obstructed in the ventricles but is inadequately reabsorbed in the subarachnoid space (Figure 14-1).

Manifestations. The signs and symptoms of hydrocephalus depend on the time of onset and the severity of the imbalance. The classic sign is an increase in head size. If hydrocephalus occurs in utero, the enlarged head will necessitate a cesarean section delivery. At birth the head enlarges rapidly and the fontanels bulge. The cranial sutures separate to accommodate the enlarging mass. The scalp is shiny, and the veins are dilated. In advanced cases the pupil of the eyes may appear to be looking downward and the sclera may be seen above the pupil, much like the look of a *setting sun* (Figure 14-2). A foreshortened occiput suggests pathology of the fourth ventricle, with the brain stem protruding through the cervical canal. This is called the *Chiari* malformation (Behrman, Kliegman, & Jenson, 2000). When the enlarged head involves a prominent occiput, the condition usually involves an atresia of the foramen of Lushka and Magendie and is known as the *Dandy-Walker syndrome*. The infant is helpless and lethargic. The body becomes thin, and the muscle tone of the extremities is often poor. The cry is shrill and high pitched. Irritability, vomiting, and anorexia are present, and convulsions may occur.

When hydrocephalus occurs in the older child, the head cannot enlarge because the cranial sutures are fused; therefore headache is the predominant symptom, with cognitive slowing, personality changes, spasticity, and other neurological signs.

Diagnosis. Transillumination (*trans*, "across" and *illuminare*, "to enlighten"), the inspection of a cavity or organ by passing a light through its walls, is a simple diagnostic procedure useful in visualizing fluid. A flashlight with a sponge-rubber collar is held tightly against the infant's head in a dark room. The examiner observes for areas of increased luminosity. A small ring of light is normal, but a large halo effect is not. The child's head is measured daily. Echoencephalography, computed tomography (CT) scan, and magnetic resonance imaging

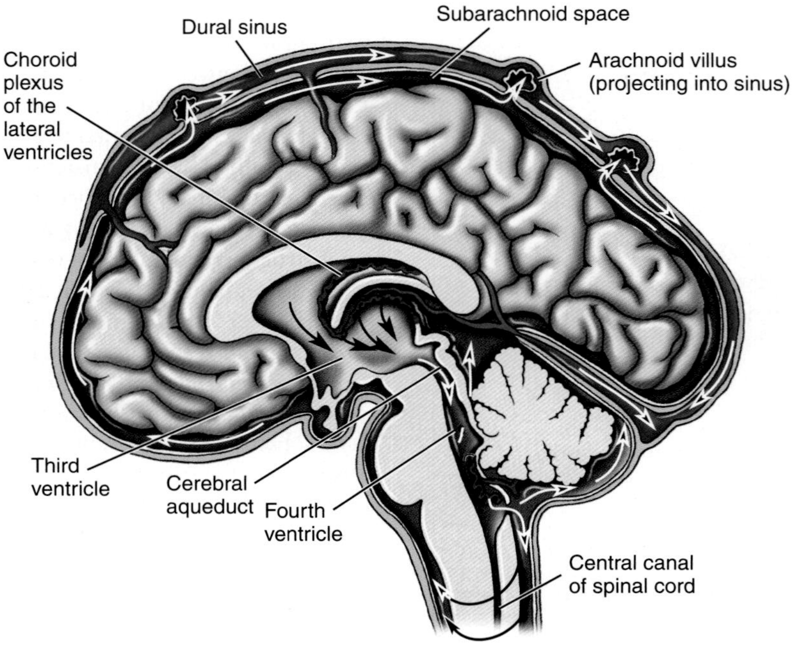

FIGURE **14-1** Cerebrospinal fluid circulation. Cerebrospinal fluid (CSF) is formed in the choroid plexus. The total volume of CSF is approximately 50 ml in the infant and 150 ml in the adult. It flows from the lateral ventricles through the foramen of Monro to the third ventricle. From the third ventricle, the CSF fluid flows through the aqueduct of Sylvius to the fourth ventricle, then through the foramen of Luschka and the foramen of Magendie, and into the cisterns at the base of the brain. Flow continues to the spinal canal. The CSF is then absorbed by the arachnoid villi (which are also known as pacchionian cells). Communicating or nonobstructive hydrocephalus occurs when the arachnoid villi are malformed or malfunction. Noncommunicating or obstructive hydrocephalus results when the tiny aqueduct of Sylvius is obstructed within the ventricles. When hydrocephalus occurs, excessive CSF causes the ventricles to enlarge and press the brain tissue against the bony skull.

(MRI) are used to visualize the enlarged ventricles and to identify the area of obstruction. A ventricular tap or puncture may be performed using sterile technique to determine pressure and drain CSF. The equipment needed is the same as for a lumbar puncture. A specimen is labeled and sent to the laboratory for analysis.

Treatment. The use of acetazolamide and furosemide reduces the production of CSF and may provide some relief, but most often surgery is indicated (Behrman, Kliegman, & Jenson, 2000). The surgeon attempts to bypass, or shunt, the point of obstruction. The CSF may thus be carried to another area of the body, where it is absorbed and finally excreted. This is accomplished by inserting special tubing, which is replaced at intervals as the child grows. The procedure, known as a *ventriculoperitoneal shunt* (Figure 14-3), allows the excess fluid to drain into the peritoneal cavity, where it is absorbed.

The prognosis for the child with hydrocephalus has improved with modern drugs and surgical techniques. If the brain is not seriously damaged before the operation,

mental function may be preserved. Motor development is sometimes slower if the child cannot lift the head, normally because of its weight. Complications of shunts are usually mechanical (kinking or plugging of tubing) or infectious. The shunt acts as a focal spot for infection and may need to be removed if infection persists.

Preoperative nursing care. The general nursing care of an infant with hydrocephalus who has not undergone surgery presents several challenges. The child may be barely able to raise the head. Mental development is delayed. Lack of appetite, a tendency to vomit easily, and poor resistance to infections present challenging problems.

The position of the infant must be changed frequently to prevent hypostatic pneumonia and pressure sores. Hypostatic pneumonia occurs when the circulation of the blood in the lungs is poor and the infant remains in one position too long. It is particularly prevalent in infants who are poorly nourished or weak or who have a debilitating disease. When the nurse turns an

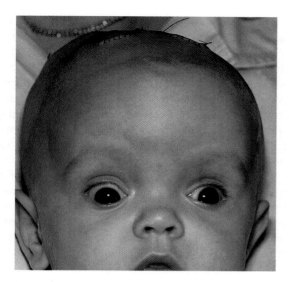

FIGURE **14-2** Marked hydrocephalus with "setting sun" sign of the eyes. Note the characteristic large head, distended scalp veins, and full fontanel.

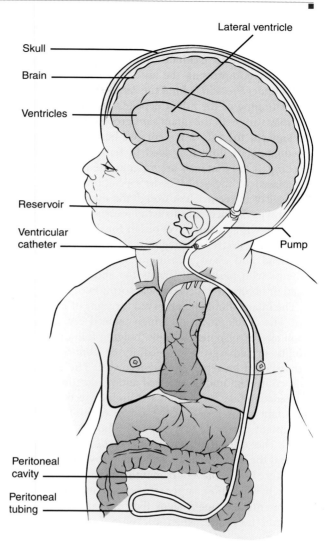

FIGURE **14-3** Shunting procedure for hydrocephalus, in which a catheter drains the ventricular system into the peritoneal cavity. Note the pump behind the ear, which can be depressed intermittently to clear obstructions.

infant who has hydrocephalus, the head must always be supported. To turn the infant in bed, the weight of the head is borne in the palm of one hand, and the head and body are rotated together to prevent a strain on the neck. When the infant is lifted from the crib, the head must be supported by the nurse's arm and chest.

The tissues of the head, ears, and bony prominences tend to break down. A pad of lamb's wool or sponge rubber placed under the head may help to prevent these lesions. If the skin becomes broken, it is given immediate attention to prevent infection. The infant must be kept dry, especially around the creases of the neck, where perspiration may collect.

In most cases the nurse may hold the infant for feedings. The nurse sits with the arm supported because the infant's head is heavy. A calm, unhurried manner is necessary. The room should be as quiet as possible. After the feeding the infant is placed in a side-lying position. The infant is not disturbed once settled, because vomiting occurs easily. The nurse must organize daily care so it does not interfere with meals.

Observations to be recorded and reported include the type and amounts of food taken, vomiting, the condition of the skin, motor abilities, restlessness, irritability, and changes in vital signs. Fontanels are inspected for size and signs of bulging. Head circumference is measured around the occipitofrontal area and is recorded on the chart.

Symptoms of increased pressure within the head are an increase in blood pressure and a decrease in pulse and respiration. Signs of a cold or other infection are immediately reported to the nurse in charge and are recorded.

Postoperative nursing care. In addition to routine postoperative care and observations, the nurse observes the patient for signs of increased intracranial pressure (ICP) and of infection at the operative site or along the shunt line. As with any postoperative care, pain control management is essential.

Bacterial infection is a life-threatening complication that sometimes necessitates shunt removal. Signs of infection include an increase in vital signs, poor feeding, vomiting, pupil dilation, decreased levels of consciousness, and seizures. The operative area is observed for signs of inflammation. An internal flushing device may be used to ensure patency of the shunt tube when increased ICP is suspected. The surgeon may order the pump to be routinely depressed a certain number of times each day to facilitate drainage. This is accomplished by compressing the antechamber or reservoir that is under the skin behind the ear (see Figure 14-3).

Positioning of the infant depends on several factors and may vary with the infant's progress. If the fontanels are sunken, the infant is kept flat because too rapid a reduction of fluid may lead to seizures or cortical bleeding. If the fontanels are bulging, the infant is usually placed in the semi-Fowler's position to promote drainage of the ventricles through the shunt. The infant is always positioned so as to avoid pressure on the operative site. The surgeon leaves orders for the patient's position and activity. Assessment of skin remains a priority. Head and chest measurements are recorded. In patients with peritoneal shunts the abdomen is measured or observed to detect malabsorption of fluid.

The infant should be observed for signs of increased ICP. The development of a high-pitched cry, unequal pupil size or response to light, bulging fontanels, irritability or lethargy, poor feeding, or abnormal vital signs should be reported and recorded. The need for pain control should be assessed and medications given as needed. Intake and output are carefully recorded, and the infant is observed closely for signs of fluid overload. The infant is usually fed after active bowel sounds are heard. The surgical suture lines should be kept clean and dry and the infant's diaper kept well below the abdominal suture line to prevent contamination.

Parent education, support, and guidance are essential. Parents are taught signs that indicate shunt malfunction, how and when to "pump" the shunt by pressing against the valve behind the ear, and the need for multidisciplinary follow-up care. Community resources, such as the National Hydrocephalus Foundation and information concerning special car seats for children with special needs, should be made known to the parents. There is approximately an 80% survival rate for infants treated early, and approximately one third of the cases result in normal physical and neurological functioning. Other survivors may have varying degrees of developmental disabilities.

Myelodysplasia and Spina Bifida

Myelodysplasia refers to a group of central nervous system disorders characterized by malformation of the spinal cord, one of which is spina bifida.

Pathophysiology. Spina bifida (divided spine) is a congenital embryonic neural tube defect in which there is an imperfect closure of the spinal vertebrae. There are two forms: occulta (hidden) and cystica (sac or cyst) (Figure 14-4).

Spina bifida occulta is a relatively minor variation of the disorder in which the opening is small and there is no associated protrusion of structures. It is often undetected and occurs most commonly at the L5 and S1 levels. There may be a tuft of hair (Figure 14-5), dimple, lipoma, or discoloration at the site. In general, treatment is not necessary unless neuromuscular symptoms appear. These symptoms consist of progressive disturbances of gait, footdrop, or disturbances of bowel and bladder sphincter function.

Spina bifida cystica consists of the development of a cystic mass in the midline of the opening in the spine. Meningocele and meningomyelocele are two types of spina bifida cystica. A meningocele (*meningo,* "membrane" and *cele,* "tumor") contains portions of the membranes and CSF. The size varies from that of a walnut to that of a newborn's head.

More serious is a protrusion of the membranes and spinal cord through this opening, or a meningomyelocele. Although it resembles a meningocele, there may be associated paralysis of the legs and poor control of bowel and bladder functions. Hydrocephalus is a common complication. Prenatal detection is possible through ultrasonography and testing for increased alpha$_1$-fetoprotein (AFP) in the amniotic fluid of the mother. (See Chapter 5.)

Prevention. The specific cause of meningomyelocele is unknown. The use of drugs during early pregnancy and poor nutrition may contribute to the development of a neural tube defect. The American Academy of Pediatrics recommends that all women of childbearing age take a daily multivitamin that contains 0.4 mg of folic acid and continue the intake of folic acid until the twelfth week of pregnancy, when basic neural tube development is completed. Studies have shown that the intake of folic acid before conception dramatically decreases the occurrence of neural tube defects such as spina bifida.

> ⚡ NURSING **TIP**
> The intake of a daily multivitamin containing 0.4 mg of folic acid before conception can reduce the risk of neural tube defects such as spina bifida.

Treatment. The treatment for spina bifida is surgical closure. The prognosis for patients with these conditions depends on the extent of involvement. In a meningocele patient with no weakness of the legs or sphincter involvement, surgical correction is performed with excellent results. Surgery is also indicated in a meningomyelocele patient for cosmetic purposes and to help prevent infection. A multidisciplinary approach is necessary because, depending on the extent of the defect, the child may have difficulties associated with

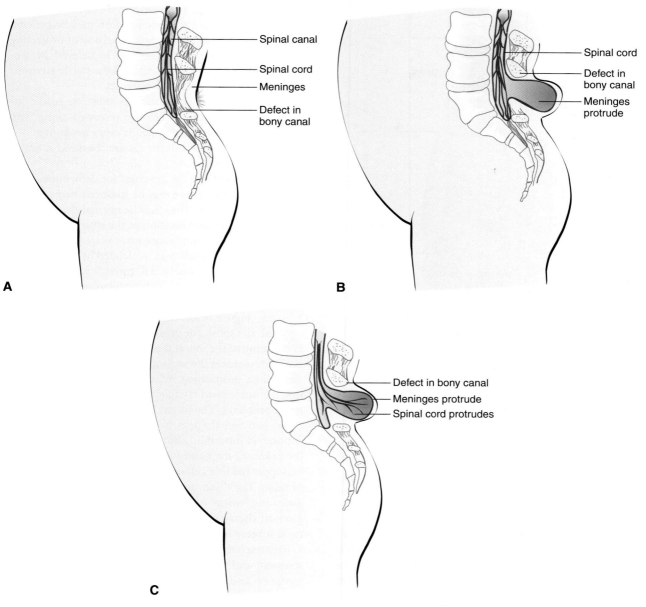

A

B

C

FIGURE **14-4** Types of spina bifida. **A,** Spina bifida occulta. There is a defect in the bony canal. The meninges and spinal cord are normal. **B,** Spina bifida cystica meningocele. The spinal cord is normal, but there is a defect in the bony canal. The meninges protrude through this defect. **C,** Spina bifida cystica meningomyelocele. There is a defect in the bony canal. The meninges protrude and the spinal cord protrudes through the defect.

hydrocephalus, orthopedic problems, and problems relating to urinary and bowel function.

Habilitation is necessary after the operation because the legs remain paralyzed and the patient is incontinent of urine and feces. Habilitation, rather than rehabilitation, is the term used to describe this treatment because the patient is disabled from birth and therefore is learn-ing, not relearning. The aim of habilitation is to mini-mize the child's disability and put to constructive use the unaffected parts of the body. Every effort is made to help the child develop a healthy personality so that he or she may experience a happy and productive life.

Eventually the child can be taught to use a wheelchair and possibly to walk with braces, crutches, or other

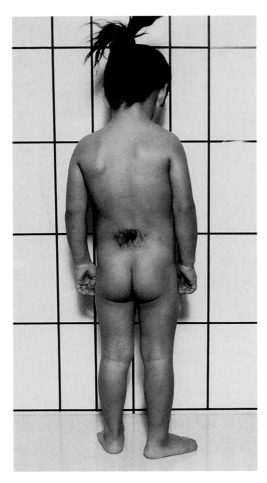

FIGURE **14-5** A child with a hairy patch in the lumbosacral region indicating the site of a spina bifida occulta.

walking devices. The implantation of an artificial urinary sphincter in early childhood can help some children to become continent and prevent the complications associated with constant urinary dribble. Medications such as oxybutynin chloride (Ditropan) are available to increase bladder storage. Children can also be "bowel trained" with the use of suppositories that promote timed bowel movements and avoid the social rejection that can be caused by bowel incontinence.

Nursing care. The main objectives of nursing care include prevention of infection of or injury to the sac, correct positioning to prevent pressure on the sac and development of contractures, good skin care (particularly if the infant is incontinent of urine and feces), adequate nutrition, accurate observations and charting, education of the parents, continued medical supervision, and habilitation.

Immediate care of the sac is essentially the same regardless of whether the cord is involved. On delivery the

newborn is placed in an incubator. Moist, sterile dressings of saline or an antibiotic solution may be ordered to prevent drying of the sac. Some method of protecting the mass is necessary if surgery is to be delayed. Protection from injury and maintenance of a sterile environment for the open lesion are essential.

Pertinent nursing observations must be made, including the following, which are recorded along with the routine observations made for every newborn:

- The size and area of the sac are checked for any tears or leakage.
- The extremities are observed for deformities and movement. (There may be spasticity or paralysis of the limbs, or they may be normal depending on the type and location of the cyst.)
- The head circumference is measured to determine the possibility of associated hydrocephalus.
- Fontanels are observed to provide baseline data.
- The lack of anal sphincter control and dribbling of urine are significant in the differential diagnosis (Figure 14-6). In general, the higher the defect on the spine, the greater the neurological deficit.

Positioning of the infant is of importance. The goal is to avoid pressure on the sac and prevent postural deformities. When positioning infants with multiple deformities, the nurse must try to guard against aggravating existing problems. The infant is usually placed prone with a pad between the legs to maintain abduction and to counteract hip subluxation. A small roll is placed under the ankles to maintain foot position. Some infants may be supported in a side-lying posture to provide periods of relief. The disadvantage of this position is that it reduces movement of the arms and flexes the hips. The physical therapy staff may provide a helpful consultation. Surgery is generally done early.

Postoperative nursing care involves neurological assessment and prevention of infection. The status of the fontanels and any signs of increased ICP, such as irritability or vomiting, are significant. Sometimes a shunt is performed shortly after closure of the spine, if hydrocephalus is present. Complications that can be life threatening include meningitis, pneumonia, and urinary tract infection.

Urological monitoring is essential, because many of these infants have urinary incontinence (see Figure 14-6). Medication to prevent urinary tract infections is routinely given. The Credé method of bladder emptying (applying pressure above the symphasis pubis) may be used for infants. Older children may be taught intermittent, clean self-catheterization. This technique can be performed by parents and learned by children.

Skin care is a challenge. Constant dribbling of feces and urine irritates the perineal area and can infect the

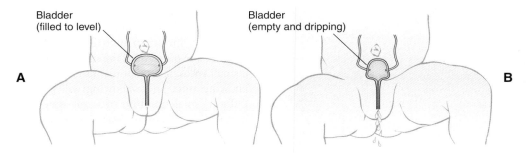

FIGURE **14-6** Incontinence in the newborn. **A,** Normally when the bladder fills to a certain level, a sensor stimulates contraction of the bladder, and expulsion of a volume of urine into the diaper occurs. A normal newborn has about six wet diapers a day. **B,** A newborn is considered *incontinent* when the sensor does not function and the bladder does not fill to its capacity before emptying. There is a constant dribble of urine into the diaper. The diaper is *always* wet.

sac or the incision. Meticulous cleanliness is necessary. The bedding must be dry and free of wrinkles. Frequent cleansing, application of a prescribed ointment or lotion, and light massage help to maintain skin integrity. If range-of-motion exercises are ordered, they are performed gently.

Feeding is facilitated by early closure of the defect. In delayed cases, gavage may be used. These patients need cuddling and sensory stimulation. An infant who cannot be held can be soothed by touch. The nurse talks to the infant and, when possible, provides face-to-face (en face) communication. Mobiles are placed appropriately. Periodically moving the incubator or crib provides diversity of view. Soft music is also soothing.

Many infants with spina bifida develop a latex allergy. A latex-free environment should be initiated whenever possible. Parents should be informed that latex products such as balloons, "koosh" balls, tennis balls, and adhesive strips can cause allergic reactions that may include rashes and wheezing. The parents should be informed about food sensitivities that are common to children with latex allergies. Foods to avoid include bananas, avocados, and kiwi. Other commonly used items to avoid include latex-based pacifiers, feeding nipples, and water toys. The child should wear a medical identification tag indicating the latex allergy. In some cases, antihistamines and steroids may be prescribed before and after surgery. Nurses should wear vinyl gloves instead of latex gloves while caring for these patients.

Special consideration must be given to the establishment of parent-infant relationships. This problem is complicated if the infant is transferred to a large medical center. Understanding and support are given to the parents, who may be overwhelmed. It is not unusual for them to be repulsed by the cyst. Most experience a sense of loss for what was to have been their "perfect baby." Steps of the

grieving process may be recognized by the astute nurse. Information and education about this disorder can be obtained from the Spina Bifida Association of America.

GASTROINTESTINAL SYSTEM
Cleft Lip

Pathophysiology. A *cleft lip* is characterized by a fissure or opening in the upper lip (Figure 14-7). It is a result of the failure of the maxillary and median nasal processes to unite during embryonic development, usually between the seventh and eighth weeks of gestation. In many cases it seems to be caused by hereditary predisposition, but occasionally it can be caused by environmental influences during the stage of oral development. This disorder appears more frequently in boys than in girls and may occur on one or both sides of the lip. The extent of the defect may vary from slight to severe. Sometimes it is accompanied by a *cleft palate,* a fissure in the midline of the roof of the mouth. Cleft lip and cleft palate are common congenital anomalies and occur in about one in 750 births. Transculturally, they occur more often in Asian Americans and Native Americans and less commonly in African Americans (Behrman, Kliegman, & Jenson, 2000).

Treatment and nursing care. The initial treatment for cleft lip is a surgical repair known as cheiloplasty. The cleft lip is repaired by age 3 months when weight gain is established and the infant is free of infection. Surgery not only improves the infant's sucking ability but also greatly improves appearance. Indirectly, this influences bonding and the amount of affection the infant receives because some parents refrain from cuddling an infant who is obviously disfigured.

A complete physical examination is done and routine blood tests are ordered before surgery. Photographs may also be taken. Any signs of oral respiratory or systemic

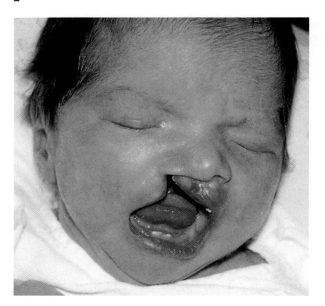

FIGURE **14-7** An infant with a unilateral cleft lip and palate.

infection are reported to the registered nurse. The physician may order elbow restraints to prevent the infant from scratching the lip and to acquaint the infant with them because they are necessary postoperatively. An Asepto syringe with a rubber tip, a long nipple with a large hole attached to a squeeze bottle, or a medicine dropper can be used to feed the infant before and after surgery, because sucking motions must be avoided to decrease tension on the suture line.

Postoperative nursing care. Postoperative nursing goals for the infant undergoing a cheiloplasty include the following:

- Preventing the infant from sucking and crying, which could cause tension on the suture line.
- Careful positioning (never on the abdomen) to avoid injury to the operative site.
- Preventing infection and scarring by gentle cleansing of the suture line to prevent crusts from forming.
- Preventing injury to the operative site by using elbow restraints. A Logan bow (a device used to immobilize the upper lip) may be applied for a short time postoperatively.
- Providing for the infant's emotional needs by cuddling and other forms of affection. This is of particular importance because the infant cannot obtain the usual satisfactions from sucking.
- Providing appropriate pain relief and sedation, which may be required for active infants.

Feeding. The infant receives feedings by dropper until the wound is completely healed (1 to 2 weeks). The infant is usually fed as soon as clear liquids are tolerated postoperatively. Care should be taken to avoid touching the suture line when inserting the medicine dropper. Sucking is avoided until the suture line is healed. Placing a small amount of formula into the infant's mouth and allowing time for swallowing will prevent aspiration. Offering small amounts of sterile water will cleanse the mouth after feeding. Formula or drainage is gently cleaned from the suture line with saline solution, and an ointment may be applied to the skin as prescribed. Holding the infant during feedings, burping frequently, and placing the infant in an infant seat after feeding or on the right side propped with a rolled blanket will aid in a positive outcome for this infant. The mother who has fed her infant preoperatively and has been allowed to assist with feedings during hospitalization will feel more confident after discharge. The immediate improvement as a result of surgery is encouraging to the parents, particularly if the child must have further surgery for cleft palate repair.

Cleft Palate

Pathophysiology. A cleft palate is a failure of the hard palate to fuse at the midline during the seventh to twelfth weeks of gestation. This separation forms a passageway between the nasopharynx and the nose, which not only complicates feeding but also easily leads to infections of the respiratory tract and middle ear that can result in hearing loss. It is generally responsible for the speech difficulties that occur in later life. The cleft may not be readily apparent at birth, and for this reason careful examination of the oral cavity and upper palate at birth is essential. Feeding is a problem because the cleft prevents negative pressure from being formed within the mouth, which is necessary for successful sucking.

Treatment. The goals of therapy are union of the cleft, improved feeding, improved speech, improved dental development, and the nurturing of a positive self-image. Some surgeons prefer to operate between 1 year and 18 months of age if at all possible so that speech patterns are minimally affected. If surgery has been deferred, a dental speech appliance may be used to facilitate communication. This appliance must be changed periodically as the child grows.

Treatment of the child with a cleft lip and palate requires multidisciplinary teamwork with a psychologist, speech therapist, pediatric dentist, orthodontist, social worker, and pediatrician. The public health nurse should be responsible for coordinating parental counseling and referral as needed. The emotional problems that sometimes occur with this condition require more extensive attention than does the repair itself. A child born with a facial deformity encounters many problems. Feedings are difficult and are not relaxed in the initial period. As the child grows, irregular tooth eruptions, drooling, delayed speech, and the need for intermittent hospitalization and frequent clinic appointments can be frustrating. High-resolution ultrasound can detect cleft palate by 13 weeks' gestation, and therefore its correction (without scarring) by fetal surgery appears promising for the near future.

> ## NURSING **TIP**
> Suctioning the mouth should be avoided in infants who have a cleft palate repair.

Psychosocial adjustment of the family. A mother's first reaction to a disfigured newborn is one of shock, hurt, disappointment, and guilt. Some parents regard the deformity as a result of their inadequacies. They may desire to hide the child from relatives and friends. The developing child senses the parents' feelings and acquires either a positive or a negative self-image. The patient and family need understanding, a concrete basis for hope, and practical advice. Family stress often occurs because of the multiple surgeries that may be required throughout childhood.

Follow-up care and home care. In large cities, special cleft palate clinics are available in which several specialists can work together in convenient consultation. The parents are instructed about the resources available in the state in which they live. The American Cleft Palate Association, the Cleft Palate Foundation, the March of Dimes Birth Defect Foundation, and state programs for children with special needs are examples of community referrals that should be offered to parents.

Postoperative treatment and nursing care

Nutrition. Fluids are taken by a cup, although a gravity feeder may be desirable in some cases. The method varies with the plastic surgeon. The diet is progressive, at first consisting of clear fluids and then full fluids. By the time of discharge, a soft diet can generally be taken. Hot foods and liquids are avoided to prevent injury to the operative site. The patient must not suck on a straw. When feeding with a spoon, the nurse should place the spoon into the side of the mouth. The spoon must not touch the roof of the mouth. The nurse teaches parents to keep objects such as the child's thumb, tongue blades, toast, cookies, forks, and pacifiers out of the mouth. Elbow restraints are used to prevent the child from placing his or her fingers or objects in the mouth. The diet is advanced only on consultation with the physician.

Oral hygiene. The mouth is kept clean at all times. Feedings are followed by a little water. The physician may prescribe a mild antiseptic mouthwash.

Speech. It is helpful to speak slowly and distinctly to the child. The child is encouraged to pronounce words correctly. Children who have undergone extensive repairs or have associated deafness need the help of a speech therapist. The speech therapist evaluates the child and assists the parents in specific activities that facilitate speech development.

Diversion. Crying is to be avoided as much as possible. Play should be quiet, particularly in the immediate postoperative period. The nurse reads, draws, or colors with the child.

Complications. Ear infections and dental decay may accompany cleft palate. Parents are instructed to take the child to the health care provider at the first sign of earache. Regular visits to the dentist are scheduled. Throughout the long-term care, a stable goal in the care of this infant is to promote optimum growth and development and to establish positive self-esteem.

MUSCULOSKELETAL SYSTEM
Clubfoot

Pathophysiology. Clubfoot, one of the most common deformities of the skeletal system, is a congenital anomaly characterized by a foot that has been twisted inward or outward. The incidence is about one in 1000 live births. Many mild forms are caused by improper position in the uterus, and these clear up with manipulative exercises. In contrast, true clubfoot does not respond to simple exercise. Several types are recognized. Talipes (*talus,* "heel" and *pes,* "foot") equinovarus (*equinus,* "extension" and *varus,* "bent inward") is seen in 95% of patients. The feet are turned inward, and the child walks on the toes and the outer borders of the feet. It generally involves both feet (Figure 14-8).

Treatment and nursing care. The treatment of clubfoot is started as early as possible or the bones and muscles will continue to develop abnormally. Conservative treatment that consists of splinting or casting to hold the foot in the right position is carried out during infancy. Passive stretching exercises may also be recommended. If these methods are not effective by age 3 months, surgery may be indicated. The infant with a clubfoot is under medical supervision for a long time. Parents must be instructed in developmental behaviors of the infant as well as the clinical aspects of care. Ongoing support is paramount.

Cast care. Casts are made of plaster or synthetic materials such as fiberglass or polyurethane. The plaster cast consists of crinoline that has powdered plaster in its meshwork. It is placed in warm water before being applied over cotton wadding or a stockinet. The wet plaster of Paris hardens as it dries. This type of cast dries from the inside out and takes 24 to 48 hours to dry.

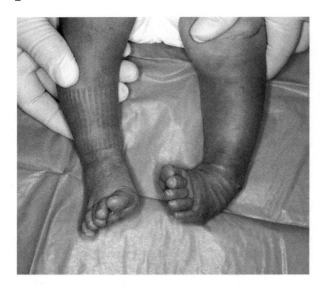

FIGURE **14-8** Clubfoot. A child with a clubfoot showing a flexed ankle, turned heel, and adducted forefoot.

If the patient returns to the unit before the cast is dry, the cast must be left uncovered and protected from pressures that could cause a depression in it. If the physician orders that the leg and foot be elevated on pillows to prevent swelling, the nurse who assists must use the palms of the hands, not the fingers, to lift the cast. Indentations made in a wet cast by fingers can press on the underlying skin and cause damage. This precaution is also explained to parents. Lighter synthetic casts dry in less than 30 minutes; however, they are more expensive and not as strong.

The toes are left exposed for observation. The nurse checks them for capillary refill and signs of poor circulation, pallor, cyanosis, swelling, coldness, numbness, pain, or burning. If circulation is impaired, the physician may split the cast to relieve the pressure, or the cast may need to be removed and reapplied. The nurse also reports irritation of the skin around the edges of the cast and lack of movement of the toes. Adhesive petals may be placed around the edges of the cast to prevent skin irritation.

As the infant grows the cast may need to be removed and reapplied. Because an infant grows rapidly, parents should be taught how to check for circulation impairments, which could be caused by a tight cast.

If surgery on tendons and bones has been performed, the nurse also observes the cast for evidence of bleeding. If a discolored area appears on the cast, it is circled and the time is recorded. Further bleeding can then be estimated. If bleeding is noted, the patient's vital signs are also checked and compared with preoperative

readings. After surgery the cast is changed about every 3 weeks to bring the foot gradually into position. When the cast is removed for the final time, exercise and special shoes may be indicated.

Emotional support. The nurse is an important figure in the care of the long-term patient with clubfoot. Nurses review the normal growth and development of children in the patient's age range to anticipate problems and to educate caretakers in parenting.

Children in a cast may be slow in developing certain motor abilities. Education concerning the therapy and referral for follow-up care is an important nursing responsibility. The financial burdens of hospitalization, surgery, special shoes, and continued medical supervision may pose a serious problem. If the nurse suspects that the parents need financial help, a social service referral is made.

NURSING TIP

In the long-term care of orthopedic patients, educating the parents about orthopedic devices, cast care, exercise, hygiene, and treatment goals is necessary. The nurse explains the importance of frequent clinic visits, reinforces physicians' information, and clarifies directions as necessary.

Developmental Hip Dysplasia

Pathophysiology. Developmental hip dysplasia, formerly known as congenital hip dysplasia, is a common orthopedic deformity. The incidence is about 1 in 1000 births. The term *hip dysplasia* is a broad description applied to various degrees of deformity: subluxation or dislocation, either partial or complete. The head of the femur is partly or completely displaced due to a shallow hip socket (acetabulum). Hereditary and environmental factors appear to be causal factors. Hip malformation, joint laxity, breech position, and maternal hormones may all contribute. Developmental hip dysplasia is seven times more common in girls than in boys. Newborn infants seldom have complete dislocation. However, the child beginning to walk exerts pressure on the hip, which can cause complete dislocation. Therefore early detection and treatment are of particular importance.

There is a high risk for developmental hip dysplasia in cultures in which the newborn is wrapped snugly with the hips in adduction and extension. There is a lower risk for developmental hip dysplasia in cultures in which the infant is carried straddled on the mother's waist with the infant's hips flexed and widely abducted.

Manifestations. A dislocation of the hip is commonly discovered at the periodic health examination of the infant during the first or second month of life. One of the most reliable signs is a limited abduction of the

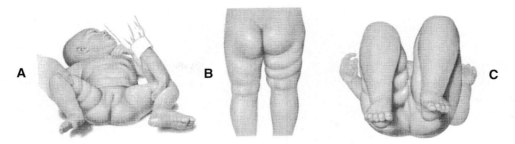

FIGURE **14-9** Early signs of dislocation of the right hip. **A,** Limitation of abduction. **B,** Asymmetry of skin folds. **C,** Shortening of femur.

leg on the affected side. When the infant is placed on the back with knees and hips flexed, the physician can press the thigh of the normal hip backward until it almost touches the examining table. This can be accomplished only partially on the affected side. The knee on the side of the dislocation is lower, and the skin folds of the thigh are deeper and often asymmetrical (Figure 14-9). When the infant is in a prone position, one buttock appears higher than the other.

Barlow's test is performed by a physician to detect an unstable hip in the newborn. The physician adducts and extends the hips while stabilizing the pelvis and may "feel" the dislocation occur as the femur leaves the acetabulum.

In infants age 1 to 2 months with developmental dislocation of the hip, the physician can actually feel and hear the femoral head slip back into the acetabulum under gentle pressure. This is called Ortolani's sign or Ortolani's click and is also considered diagnostic of the disorder. The child who is walking and has had no treatment displays a characteristic limp. Bilateral (*bi,* "two" and *latus,* "side") dislocation may occur; however, unilateral (*uni,* "one" and *latus,* "side") dislocation is more common. X-ray studies confirm the diagnosis.

Treatment. Treatment begins immediately on detection of the dislocation. The hips are maintained in constant flexion and abduction for 4 to 8 weeks to keep the head of the femur within the hip socket. This constant pressure enlarges and deepens the acetabulum; thus it can correct the dislocation.

A triple-thick diaper may be used in the newborn to maintain a "froglike" abduction of the legs. In infants more than 2 months of age, soft tissue contractures prevent stabilization of the hip, and longer term immobilization with a Pavlik harness may be required (Figure 14-10). Traction may be necessary if the dislocation is severe or is not detected until the child begins to walk. This pulls the head of the femur down to the correct

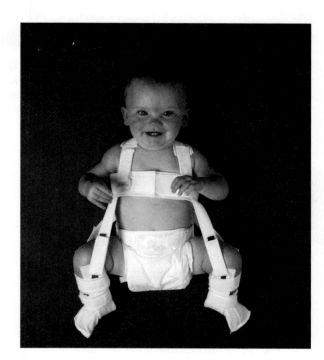

FIGURE **14-10** The Pavlik harness is used in infants age 1 to 6 months to maintain hips in a position of flexion and abduction.

position opposite the acetabulum and helps to overcome muscle spasm. Casting in a froglike position is then done. This type of cast, known as a body spica cast, is shown in Figure 14-11. (See Chapter 24 for care of the orthopedic patient.)

The length of time spent in a cast varies according to the patient's progress and growth and the condition of the cast; however, it is usually 5 to 9 months. During this time the cast may be changed about every 6 weeks. Surgery may be required in infants more than 18 months of age. In such cases, open reduction of the

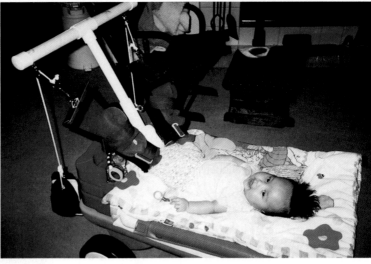

FIGURE **14-11 A**, Infant in a spica body cast. This cast maintains the legs in a froglike position and is used to treat developmental hip dysplasia. Note that the infant is able to move her toes freely. A diaper tucked inside prevents the cast from becoming soiled with urine or feces. **B**, Traction is sometimes necessary before surgery or casting. Home care enables the child to be in familiar surroundings that will nurture growth and development.

dislocation or repair of the shelf of the hip bone are performed. After surgery a cast is applied to keep the femur in the correct position.

Nursing care. The nursery nurse carefully observes each infant during the morning bath to detect signs of a hip dysplasia, as follows:

- When the infant is prone, the nurse observes the buttocks for variation in size.
- The legs of the infant should be equal in length.
- The infant should be kicking both legs, not just one leg.
- The depth and number of the skin folds of the infant's upper thighs should be symmetrical.
- In the well-baby clinic the nurse notes the posture and gait of older children and records observations.

Infants who progress well with the Pavlik harness or Frejka splint (or a similar brace) remain at home. The mother and infant visit the physician regularly. The parents need assurance that the infant may be held and may sit in a chair. They should be encouraged to ask questions of the clinic nurse and physician.

The child who is admitted to the hospital with a diagnosis of developmental hip dysplasia is given as much personal attention as possible. The first admission sets the pattern for future hospitalization; therefore the child must make a satisfactory adjustment. The nurse becomes familiar with the child's habit and plan

of care. Every effort is made to provide a homelike environment for children who are hospitalized for many weeks.

The spica cast. The body spica cast encircles the waist and extends to the ankles or toes. Neurovascular assessment, discussed in Chapter 24, should be reviewed at this point. Nursing Care Plan 14-1 gives selected nursing diagnoses and interventions for the patient with a spica cast.

Firm, plastic-covered pillows are required. These are placed beneath the curvatures of the cast for support. Older children may benefit from an overhead bar and trapeze. The room should be adequately ventilated. A fracture pan should be available at the bedside for toileting as developmentally appropriate.

The head of the patient's bed is slightly elevated so that urine or feces drain away from the body of the cast. One should not use pillows to elevate the head or shoulders of a child in a body cast, because this thrusts the patient's chest against the cast and causes discomfort or respiratory difficulty. The child who is not toilet trained may be placed on a Bradford frame to facilitate nursing care. Frequent changes of position are important; immobilized patients must be turned often. Infants may be held in the nurse's lap after the cast has dried. A ride on a wagon or gurney to the playroom or around the hospital provides changes of position and scenery.

NURSING CARE PLAN 14-1

The Infant/Child with a Spica Cast

PATIENT DATA: An infant returns from the cast room after having a spica cast applied. The infant is scheduled for discharge after the cast is dry.

SELECTED NURSING DIAGNOSIS   *Risk for ineffective tissue perfusion due to cast constriction*

Outcomes	Nursing Interventions	Rationales
Tissues and circulation will appear adequate as evidenced by pink, warm skin, good capillary refill, and lack of numbness or swelling. Parents will understand signs of inadequate circulation and explain importance of seeking immediate assistance if these signs appear.	1. Observe exposed extremities and skin distal to the cast every 30 minutes for the first few hours of a new cast and every 1 to 4 hours thereafter; watch for signs of pallor, cyanosis, swelling, coldness, numbness, pain, or burning. 2. Circle any drainage on cast with date and time; monitor and record findings. 3. Observe nonverbal communication for signs of pain; ask older child if pain is experienced. 4. Educate parents and patient, if old enough, in all of above. 5. Provide written instructions.	1. Circulation can be impaired, leading to ischemia. Peripheral nerves in contrast to muscles do not degenerate with disuse, but loss of *innervation* can take place if nerves are damaged by pressure or if the blood supply is disrupted. 2. An increase in size of circle indicates further bleeding or possibly a draining infection. 3. Unrelieved pain, especially after a few days, may indicate *compartment syndrome;* compartment syndrome appears in a group of muscles and fascia where an increase in pressure within this closed space may disrupt circulation within the space. 4. Education reduces stress of parents and patient. 5. Written instructions provide reinforcement and help to ensure the success of other interventions.

SELECTED NURSING DIAGNOSIS   *Risk for injury related to awkwardness and weight of cast*

Outcomes	Nursing Interventions	Rationales
Patient will remain safe and as independent as possible.	1. Inform older child when turning as to how and when you are going to proceed (e.g., "ready, set, go"). 2. Leave articles and toys within reach. 3. Some car seats are adapted to accommodate a small child in a spica cast.	1. Involving child in procedure as age appropriate gives him or her a sense of control; procedure will go more smoothly. 2. Child will not need to strain or move awkwardly to reach articles; patient will feel greater mastery if articles can be obtained independently. 3. These children need protection in a car.

❓CRITICAL THINKING QUESTION

A mother brings her 2-year-old child to the clinic complaining that the spica cast has a strong, unpleasant odor. The child has a temperature of 100° F. He appears to be in no acute distress and is playing with a small toy car in one hand and has a half-eaten cracker in the other hand. What nursing intervention is indicated?

The supporting bar between the legs should not be used as a lever when turning the child (Box 14-2). All body curvatures are supported with pillows or sheet rolls. Whenever possible, the older child should be on the abdomen during mealtime to facilitate swallowing and self-feeding. When placing a child in a body cast on a fracture pan, the upper back and legs are supported with pillows so that body alignment is maintained.

Itching is a problem for the patient in a body cast. If at all possible, a strip of gauze is placed beneath the cast before it is applied; this gauze extends through the opened area required for toilet needs. It is gently moved back and forth to relieve itching. When the strip becomes soiled, a clean one is tied to one end of the soiled gauze and pulled through the cast; this soiled portion is then removed. Other methods that might cause injury to the skin beneath the cast are discouraged because any break in the skin under a cast is difficult to heal.

Toys small enough to be "hidden" inside the cast should not be given to the child. Toys that can be used when the child is in a prone position are best.

The child with this long-term disability requires help in meeting his or her everyday needs. This child is growing and developing rapidly, and therefore frequent adjustments in home and clinic care are necessary. Dressing and clothing are a problem. The child cannot fit into regular furniture and much of the play equipment enjoyed by other children. Transportation is difficult. A special wagon built up with pillows may be used (see Figure 14-11). The child should be included in everyday family and play activities to encourage normal growth and development. A referral for home health care should be made on discharge.

box 14-2 | *Technique for Turning the Child in a Body Cast*

Two people, one on each side of the bed, are needed to turn a child in a body cast, as follows:

1. Move the child to the edge of the bed as far as possible so that the nurse who receives the child is farther away from him or her.
2. The nurse nearer to the child places one hand under the head and back and one hand under the leg part of the cast and turns the child to the midway point on the side.
3. The nurse farther away then accepts the support of the child and cast as turning is completed.

METABOLIC DEFECTS

The infant with an inborn error of metabolism has a genetic defect that is not apparent before birth. As the infant adjusts to the birth process and begins to ingest nourishment, symptoms can rapidly emerge that quickly become life threatening. Symptoms such as lethargy, poor feeding, hypotonia, a unique odor to the body or urine, tachypnea, and vomiting must be reported by the nurse in the newborn nursery to avoid long-term or life-threatening sequelae. The nurse must also be prepared to offer psychological support and help parents deal with the impact of having an infant with a genetic problem.

PHENYLKETONURIA

Pathophysiology. Classic phenylketonuria (PKU) is a genetic disorder caused by the faulty metabolism of phenylalanine, an amino acid that is essential to life and is found in all protein foods. This inborn error of metabolism, which is transmitted by an autosomal recessive gene, is termed *classic PKU* and is associated with blood phenylalanine levels above 20 mg/dl. The hepatic enzyme phenylalanine hydrolase, which is normally needed to convert phenylalanine into tyrosine, is missing. When the infant is fed formula, phenylalanine begins to accumulate in the blood. It can rise to as high as 20 times the normal amount. Its by-product, phenylpyruvic acid, appears in the urine within the first weeks of life.

Classic PKU results in severe retardation that is evidenced in infancy. Early detection and treatment are paramount. By the time the urine test is positive, brain damage has already occurred. The infant appears normal at birth but begins to show delayed development at about 4 to 6 months of age. The child may show evidence of failure to thrive, have eczema or other skin conditions, have a peculiar musty odor, or have personality disorders. About one third of the children have seizures. PKU occurs mainly in blond and blue-eyed children; these features result from a lack of tyrosine, a necessary component of the pigment melanin. Less severe forms of the disorder are now recognized. They are designated as "atypical PKU" and "mild hyperphenylalaninemia."

Diagnosis. The *Guthrie blood test* is widely used and is currently considered the most reliable test for PKU. Blood is obtained from a simple heel stick. A few drops of capillary blood are placed on a filter paper and mailed to the laboratory for screening. It is recommended that the blood be obtained after 48 to 72 hours of life, preferably after the ingestion of proteins, to reduce the possibility of false-negative results. Many states require that the test be done on all newborns before they leave the nursery, but because of early discharge the test may be repeated within 2 weeks. The infant can be tested at home by a public health nurse or at the clinic or physician's office. Confirmation of the diagnosis requires quantitative elevations of phenylalanine compound in the blood (Behrman, Kliegman, & Jenson, 2000). Screening programs for pregnant women have also been advocated to detect elevated phenylalanine levels that could have an effect on the newborn.

Treatment and nursing care. Treatment of PKU consists of close dietary management and frequent evaluation of blood phenylalanine levels. Because phenylalanine is found in all natural protein foods, a synthetic food that provides enough protein for growth and tissue repair but little phenylalanine must be substituted. The most commonly used formulas are Lofenalac for infants, Phenyl-Free for children, and Phenex-2 for adolescents. The goals of the diet are to provide enough essential proteins to support growth and development while maintaining phenylalanine blood levels between 2 and 10 mg/dl. A phenylalanine level below 2 mg/dl may result in growth retardation, whereas levels above 10 mg/dl can result in significant brain damage.

There is a low phenylalanine content in breast milk, and infants can be partially breastfed and supplemented with Lofenalac while phenylalanine blood levels are monitored. Solid foods that are low in phenylalanine are added at the same age that solid foods are added for infants without PKU. Phenyl-Free is introduced between ages 3 and 8 years. Cookbooks and family recipes provide variety. Eventually the child learns to assume full management of the diet.

A dietitian may be consulted concerning parental guidance and support in maintaining the dietary regimen, especially for the school-aged child and adolescent. Many foods that contain a high level of phenylalanine are clearly labeled and provide easier choices for parents at the supermarket. A single 12-ounce can of diet cola containing NutraSweet or Equal (aspartame) will not significantly raise blood levels of phenylalanine, but the intake of most meat, dairy products, and diet drinks must be restricted. An exchange list for food selection can aid the child in participating in and monitoring his or her progress. Flavoring the milk substitute with a fruit-flavored powder or chocolate flavoring can increase the child's compliance.

Genetic counseling is important for the affected child for future family planning. Women of childbearing age who have PKU must follow a low-phenylalanine diet before conception to avoid brain damage of the fetus during development.

> ★ **NURSING TIP**
>
> Children with PKU must avoid the sweetener aspartame (NutraSweet) because it is converted to phenylalanine in the body.

MAPLE SYRUP URINE DISEASE

Pathophysiology. Maple syrup urine disease is caused by a defect in the metabolism of branched-chain amino acids. It causes marked serum elevations of leucine, isoleucine, and valine. This results in acidosis, cerebral degeneration, and death within 2 weeks if left untreated.

Manifestations. The infant with maple syrup urine disease appears healthy at birth but soon develops feeding difficulties, loss of the Moro reflex, hypotonia, irregular respirations, and convulsions. The urine, sweat, and cerumen (ear wax) have a characteristic sweet or maple syrup odor. This is caused by ketoacidosis, a process similar to that which may occur in diabetic children, and causes a fruity odor of the breath. However, the condition does not resolve with the correction of blood glucose levels. The urine contains high levels of leucine, isoleucine, and valine. Diagnosis is confirmed by blood and urine tests.

Treatment and nursing care. Early detection in the newborn period is extremely important. The nursery nurse should report any newborn whose urine has a sweet aroma. Initial treatment consists of removing these amino acids and their metabolites from the tissues of the body. This is accomplished by hydration and peritoneal dialysis to decrease serum levels. The patient is placed on a lifelong diet low in the amino acids leucine, isoleucine, and valine. Several formulas specifically for this disease are available. Exacerbations are most often related to the degree of abnormality of the leucine level. These exacerbations are frequently related to infection and can be life threatening. The nurse must frequently assess the patient and instruct parents about the need to prevent infections.

GALACTOSEMIA

Pathophysiology. In galactosemia the body is unable to use the carbohydrates galactose and lactose. In the healthy person the liver converts galactose to glucose. In the patient with galactosemia, an enzyme is defective or missing and therefore there is a disturbance in a normally occurring chemical reaction. The result is an increase in the amount of galactose in the blood (galactosemia) and in the urine (galactosuria). This can cause cirrhosis of the liver, cataracts, and mental retardation if left untreated. Because galactose is present in milk sugar, early diagnosis is necessary so that a milk substitute can be used.

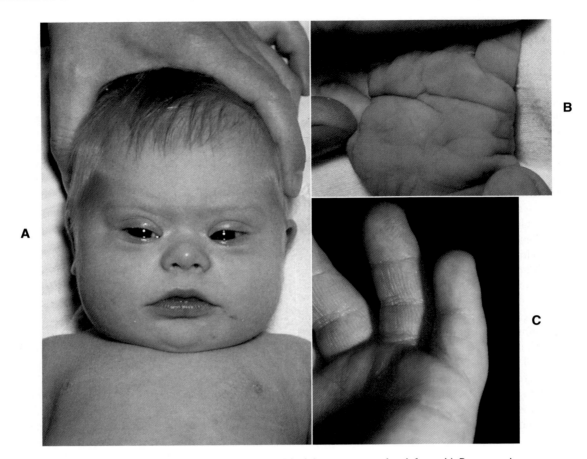

FIGURE **14-12** Down syndrome. **A,** The typical facial appearance of an infant with Down syndrome shows the upward slant of the canthal folds of the eyes, protruding tongue, and short, thick neck. **B,** The straight simian crease in the palm of the hand is a typical finding in children with Down syndrome. **C,** The short fifth finger is a typical finding in children with Down syndrome. The tip of the fifth finger does not extend to the distal joint of the adjoining finger.

Manifestations. The symptoms of galactosemia begin abruptly and worsen gradually. Early signs consist of lethargy, vomiting, hypotonia, diarrhea, and failure to thrive. These commence as the newborn begins breastfeeding or ingesting formula. Jaundice may be present. Diagnosis is made by observing galactosuria, galactosemia, and evidence of decreased enzyme activity in the red blood cells. Screening tests are available.

Treatment and nursing care. Milk and lactose-containing products are eliminated from the diet of the patient with galactosemia. The nursing mother must discontinue breastfeeding. Lactose-free formulas and those with a soy-protein base are often substituted. The nurse must realize the frustration and anxiety that this diagnosis creates. Parents experience periods of feeling overwhelmed and inadequate. They can also become totally absorbed in the dietary program. A rare disease creates feelings of isolation and uncertainty. Because

surveillance is ongoing, some of the emotional characteristics of the family with a child who has a chronic disease are pertinent.

CHROMOSOMAL ABNORMALITIES

DOWN SYNDROME

Pathophysiology. Down syndrome is one of the most common chromosomal abnormalities. Its incidence is approximately nine in 10,000 live births. It may increase to one in 365 live births among children of mothers age 35 years or older (Behrman, Kliegman, & Jenson, 2000). Paternal age is also a factor, particularly when the father is age 55 years or over. Sometimes the first infant of a young mother has Down syndrome, but subsequent children are usually born free of the defect. Children born with this birth defect have mild to severe mental

| table 14-1 | *Time of Occurrence of Developmental Milestones in Normal Children and Those with Down Syndrome (in Months)* | | | |

MILESTONE	CHILDREN WITH DOWN SYNDROME		NORMAL CHILDREN	
	AVERAGE	RANGE	AVERAGE	RANGE
Smiling	2	1.5-4	1	0.5-3
Rolling over	8	4-22	5	2-10
Sitting alone	10	6-28	7	5-9
Crawling	12	7-21	8	6-11
Creeping	15	9-27	10	7-13
Standing	20	11-42	11	8-16
Walking	24	12-65	13	8-18
Talking, words	16	9-31	10	6-14
Talking, sentences	28	18-96	21	14-32

From Levine, M.D., Carey, W.B., & Crocker, A.C. (1999). *Developmental-behavioral pediatrics* (3rd ed.). Philadelphia: W.B. Saunders.

| table 14-2 | *Time of Occurrence of Self-Help Skills in Normal Children and Those with Down Syndrome (in Months)* | | | |

MILESTONE	CHILDREN WITH DOWN SYNDROME		NORMAL CHILDREN	
	AVERAGE	RANGE	AVERAGE	RANGE
EATING				
Finger feeding	12	8-28	8	6-16
Using spoon and fork	20	12-40	13	8-20
TOILET TRAINING				
Bladder	48	20-95	32	18-60
Bowel	42	28-90	29	16-48
DRESSING				
Undressing	40	29-72	32	22-42
Putting on clothes	58	38-98	47	34-58

From Levine, M.D., Carey, W.B., & Crocker, A.C. (1999). *Developmental-behavioral pediatrics* (3rd ed.). Philadelphia: W.B. Saunders.

retardation and generally some physical abnormalities. In the past, children with this condition were called "mongoloid" because of the Oriental ("Mongolian") appearance of their faces, but this term is now considered inappropriate.

There are three phenotypes (genetic makeups) of Down syndrome: trisomy 21, mosaicism, and translocation of a chromosome. The most common type, trisomy 21 syndrome, accounts for 95% of patients. In this instance there are three number 21 chromosomes rather than the normal two. This is a result of *nondisjunction,* the failure of a chromosome to follow the normal separation process into daughter cells. The earlier in the embryo's development this occurs, the greater the number of cells affected. When nondisjunction occurs late in development, both normal and abnormal cells are present in the newborn. This condition is *mosaicism,* and patients tend to be less severely affected in physical appearance and intelligence. The third condition is *translocation.* In translocation, a piece of chromosome in pair 21 breaks away and attaches itself to another chromosome.

Screening for Down syndrome is offered during prenatal care at 15 weeks' gestation to allow parents the choice of terminating the pregnancy or continuing the pregnancy with preparation for the care the infant will require. Alpha$_1$-fetoprotein (AFP), unconjugated estriol, and human chorionic gonadotropin (hCG) levels are used for prenatal diagnosis (see Chapter 5), and this is known as the "triple test." Amniocentesis and chorionic

villus sampling are the most accurate methods of prenatal screening but are invasive tests and carry a risk for pregnancy loss. An increased nuchal fold thickness can be detected on abdominal ultrasound, and the clinician must be alert to the possibility of this condition.

Manifestations. Down syndrome can be diagnosed by the clinical manifestations, but a chromosomal analysis will confirm the specific type. The signs of Down syndrome, which are apparent at birth, are close-set and upward-slanting eyes, small head, round face, flat nose, protruding tongue that interferes with sucking, and mouth breathing (Figure 14-12, *A*). The hands of the infant are short and thick, and the little finger is curved (Figure 14-12, *C*). There is a deep straight line across the palm, which is called the *simian crease* (Figure 14-12, *B*). There is also a wide space between the first and the second toes. The undeveloped muscles and loose joints enable the child to assume unusual positions. Physical growth and development may be slower than normal (Tables 14-1 and 14-2). The child is limited intellectually. Some children have been found to have intelligence quotients (IQs) in the borderline to low-average range. Congenital heart deformities are also associated with this condition.

Children with Down syndrome are very lovable. They may be restless and somewhat more difficult to train than the normal youngster. Their resistance to infection is poor, and they are prone to respiratory and ear infections as well as speech and hearing problems. The life span of children with Down syndrome has increased with the widespread use of antibiotics. The incidence of acute leukemia is higher in these children than in the normal population, and Alzheimer's disease is common to those who reach middle adult life (Jackson & Vessey, 2000).

The limp, flaccid posture of the infant is caused by hypotonicity of the muscles, makes positioning and holding more difficult, and contributes to heat loss from the exposed surface areas. The infant should be warmly wrapped to prevent chilling. The hypotonicity of muscles also causes respiratory problems and excess mucus accumulation. Bulb suctioning may be necessary before feedings. The hypotonicity of muscles also contributes to the development of constipation, which can be controlled by dietary intervention.

Nursing care

Counseling parents. The counseling of families of Down syndrome children is ongoing. Maternity nurses must be aware of their own feelings before they can effectively support parents. They, too, will feel saddened at the birth of an imperfect child. They may identify with the parents. It is appropriate to express one's feelings of initial helplessness, and it may encourage the parents to verbalize their concerns. The nurse must listen and provide honest, tactful, and compassionate support.

Empathy from the nurse is particularly important. Involving parents in the care and planning for the infant from the start facilitates bonding. The need for the staff's warm concern cannot be overestimated. Pampering the infant by putting a little curl in the hair, for example, shows that others care.

Counseling family. Siblings of the patient must be informed and included in discussions about the newborn. Even very young children are aware of parental distress, and their imaginations can be more frightening than the reality. Open communications early on will prevent isolation, avoid misconceptions, and promote an easier transition period. The nurse should connect the family with a Down syndrome support group in their area if there is one. Other parents with a Down syndrome child are an important resource. The National Association for Down Syndrome is one organization that provides education and support to families. (See Chapter 23 for further discussion of nursing care of the cognitively impaired child.)

PERINATAL DAMAGE

HEMOLYTIC DISEASE OF THE NEWBORN: ERYTHROBLASTOSIS FETALIS

Pathophysiology. Erythroblastosis fetalis (*erythro,* "red," *blast,* "a formative cell," and *osis,* "disease condition") is a disorder that becomes apparent in fetal life or soon after birth. It is one of many congenital hemolytic diseases found in the newborn. It is caused when an Rh-negative mother and an Rh-positive father produce an Rh-positive fetus. Although fetal and maternal blood do not mix during pregnancy, small leaks may allow fetal blood to enter the maternal circulation and sensitize the mother. The mother's body responds by producing antibodies that cross the placenta and destroy the blood cells of the fetus, causing anemia and possible heart failure (see Chapter 5). The terms *isoimmunization* and *sensitization* refer to this process (Box 14-3). The incidence of erythroblastosis fetalis has greatly decreased as a result of the protective administration of an Rh immune globulin (RhoGAM) to women at risk. Incompatibility of ABO factors is now more common and generally less severe than Rh incompatibility (Box 14-4).

The process of maternal sensitization is depicted in Figure 14-13. The mother accumulates antibodies with each pregnancy; therefore the chance that complications may occur increases with each gestation. If large numbers of antibodies are present, the infant may be severely anemic. In the gravest form, *hydrops fetalis,* the progressive hemolysis causes anemia, heart failure, fetal *hypoxia,* and *anasarca* (generalized edema). This is rare today because of early detection methods.

Diagnosis and prevention. An extensive maternal health history is obtained. Of particular interest are pre-

---

| box 14-3 | *Terms Helpful in Understanding Rh Sensitization* |

antigen (*anti,* "against" and *gen,* "to produce") A substance that induces the formation of antibodies; the antigen-antibody reaction is the basis of immunity.

Coombs' test *Indirectly* measures Rh-positive antibodies in the *mother's* blood; *directly* measures antibody-coated Rh-positive red blood cells in the *infant's* blood.

erythroblastosis fetalis The severe form of this disease produces anemia in the *fetus* as a result of the incompatibility of the red blood cells of the mother and those of the fetus.

Rh$_o$(D) immune globulin (RhoGAM) Immunoglobulin given after delivery of an Rh-positive fetus to an Rh-negative mother to prevent the maternal Rh immune response.

sensitization (isoimmunization) The phenomenon in which an Rh-negative mother develops antibodies against an Rh-positive fetus.

vious Rh sensitizations, an ectopic pregnancy, abortion, blood transfusions, or children who developed jaundice or anemia during the neonatal period. The mother's blood titer is carefully monitored. An *indirect Coombs'* test on the mother's blood will indicate previous exposure to Rh-positive antigens.

Diagnosis of the disease in the prenatal period is confirmed by amniocentesis and monitoring of bilirubin levels in the amniotic fluid. Information gained from these tests helps to determine early interventions such as

induction of labor or intrauterine fetal transfusions that allow the fetus to remain in utero until the lungs mature. Repeated transfusions may be required (Behrman, Kliegman, & Jenson, 2000).

Prevention of erythroblastosis by the use of $Rh_o(D)$ immune globulin (RhoGAM) is now routine. An intramuscular injection is given to the mother within 72 hours of delivery of an Rh-positive infant. RhoGAM may also be given to the pregnant woman at 28 weeks' gestation. It is also administered, when appropriate, after a spontaneous or therapeutic abortion, after amniocentesis, and to women who have bleeding during pregnancy because fetal blood may leak into the mother's circulation at these times.

---

box 14-4 | *ABO Incompatibility*

Hemolytic disease with symptoms similar to those of erythroblastosis can occur with ABO incompatibility. A mother who has an "O" blood type and who gives birth to an infant with an A or B blood group constitutes the most commonly seen ABO incompatibility. Treatment and nursing care are the same as for erythroblastosis.

⚡NURSING TIP

RhoGAM is administered to Rh-negative mothers by the intramuscular route after a normal delivery, after an ectopic pregnancy, or after an abortion to prevent the development of Rh-positive antibodies. RhoGAM has no effect on existing Rh-positive antibodies.

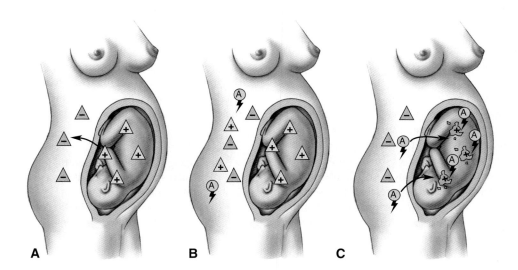

△ Rh– Red blood cell (RBC) of mother

⊕ Rh+ RBC of fetus with Rh antigen on surface

Ⓐ⚡ Anti–Rh antibody made against Rh+ RBC

Hemolysis of Rh+ RBC

FIGURE **14-13** Maternal sensitization producing erythroblastosis in the newborn. **A,** During the first pregnancy the mother is sensitized to the Rh-positive antigen from the fetus. **B,** The mother produces Rh antibodies to the Rh antigen to which she was exposed. **C,** During a second pregnancy, these Rh antibodies cross the placenta to the fetus and destroy the fetal Rh-positive blood cells.

Manifestations. At the time of delivery, a sample of the infant's cord blood is sent to the laboratory. The *direct Coombs' test* detects damaging antibodies. The symptoms of erythroblastosis fetalis vary with the intensity of the disease. Anemia and jaundice are present. The anemia is caused by hemolysis of large numbers of erythrocytes. This *pathological jaundice* differs from *physiological jaundice* in that it becomes evident within 24 hours after delivery. The liver is unable to handle the massive hemolysis, and bilirubin levels rise rapidly, causing hyperbilirubinemia (*hyper,* "excess," *bilis,* "bile," *rubor,* "red," and *emia,* "blood"). Early jaundice is immediately reported to the physician.

Enlargement of the liver and spleen and extensive edema may develop. The circulating blood usually contains an excess of immature nucleated red blood cells (erythroblasts) caused by the infant's attempts to compensate for the destruction of cells. The oxygen-carrying power of the blood is diminished, as is the blood volume, and therefore shock or heart failure may result. Severe jaundice may cause *kernicterus* (accumulation of bilirubin in the brain tissues). This may cause serious brain damage, may leave the newborn mentally retarded, and often results in death.

> ⭐NURSING **TIP**_____
> Jaundice that occurs on the first day of life is always pathological and requires prompt intervention.

Treatment and nursing care. Treatment includes prompt identification, laboratory tests, drug therapy, phototherapy, and exchange transfusion if indicated. Phototherapy may be used to reduce serum bilirubin levels. It may be used alone or in conjunction with an exchange transfusion. The newborn is placed in an incubator under a bank of fluorescent lights (Figure 14-14). The eyes and gonads are protected from the lights, and specific protocols are carried out. Although this procedure may prevent the rise of bilirubin, it has no effect on the underlying cause of jaundice. The nursing care of the infant receiving phototherapy is presented in Nursing Care Plan 14-2.

During an exchange transfusion, a plastic catheter is inserted into the umbilical vein of the newborn, small amounts of blood (10 to 20 ml) are withdrawn, and equal amounts of Rh-negative blood are injected. The amount of donor blood used is about twice the infant blood volume to a limit of 500 ml. In this way, healthy cells are added to the infant's blood, and antibodies are removed. Additional small transfusions may be necessary later. After a second exchange transfusion, approximately 85% of the infant's blood will have been replaced. Antibiotics may be given to prevent infection.

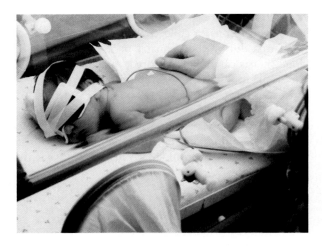

FIGURE **14-14** Phototherapy. The infant is in an incubator with phototherapy lights. When an infant receives phototherapy in an incubator, the eyes are protected from the fluorescent lights. The infant is turned frequently so that all skin surfaces are exposed to the lights.

The nurse is usually responsible for the following: observing the newborn's color and reporting any evidence of jaundice during the first and second days; applying wet, sterile compresses to the umbilicus, if ordered, until an exchange transfusion is completed; stressing to mothers the importance of good prenatal care for subsequent pregnancies; helping to interpret the treatment to parents by giving reassurance as needed; and observing and assisting the physician with the exchange transfusion.

> ⭐NURSING **TIP**_____
> Assessing jaundice involves the following:
> - The skin and the whites of the eyes assume a yellow-orange cast.
> - Blanching the skin over the bony prominences enhances the evaluation of jaundice.

> ⭐NURSING **TIP**_____
> An infant born with cardiac failure and edema as a result of hemolytic disease is a candidate for immediate exchange transfusion with fresh whole blood.

Home phototherapy. Home phototherapy programs are being used for newborns with mild to moderate physiological (normal) jaundice. These programs are advocated because bilirubin levels generally begin to rise on the third day after birth, when the mother and newborn are discharged. A rise in bilirubin levels may necessitate the newborn's return to the hospital and possible separation of mother and infant. Home

NURSING CARE PLAN 14-2

The Infant Receiving Phototherapy

PATIENT DATA: A newborn, 12 hours of age, is diagnosed with hyperbilirubinemia and placed in an incubator for phototherapy.

SELECTED NURSING DIAGNOSIS   *Risk for injury to eyes and gonads related to phototherapy*

Outcomes	Nursing Interventions	Rationales
Infant does not have eye drainage or irritation. Genitals are protected.	1. Apply eye patches over infant's closed eyes before placing infant under lights. 2. Remove patches at least once per shift to assess eyes for conjunctivitis. 3. Remove patches to allow eye contact during feeding. 4. Cover ovaries or testes with diaper.	1. Closing eyes prevents corneal abrasion and protects retina from damage by high-intensity light. 2. Facilitates early detection of inflammation and jaundice (sclera may yellow). 3. Provides for visual stimulation and bonding. 4. Protects gonads from damage by heat.

SELECTED NURSING DIAGNOSIS   *Impaired skin integrity related to immature structure and function, immobility*

Outcomes	Nursing Interventions	Rationales
Skin will remain intact as evidenced by absence of skin rash, excoriation, or redness.	1. Observe for maculopapular rash. 2. Cleanse rectal area gently, because stools are often green and liquid. 3. Reposition at least every 2 hours. 4. Observe for jaundice or bronzing (NOTE: Serum bilirubin may be high even though infant may not appear jaundiced under lights.) 5. Observe for pressure areas.	1. Rashes and burns have been known to occur as a result of phototherapy. 2. Frequent stools may cause breakdown of skin; loose stools are a result of increased bilirubin excretion. 3. Repositioning provides exposure of all skin areas. 4. Observation of jaundice may be initial sign of hyperbilirubinemia. Bronze baby syndrome appears in preterms who do not excrete the photo-oxidation products adequately. 5. Early intervention prevents skin breakdown.

SELECTED NURSING DIAGNOSIS   *Risk for deficient fluid volume related to increased water loss through skin and loose stools*

Outcomes	Nursing Interventions	Rationales
Infant will not become dehydrated as evidenced by good skin turgor, normal fontanels, and moist tongue and mucous membranes. Weight maintenance, urine output satisfactory.	1. Monitor intravenous fluids. 2. Check skin turgor. 3. Observe for depressed fontanel. 4. Anticipate the need for additional water between feedings. 5. Daily weights unless contra-indicated.	1. IV fluids are sometimes used to prevent dehydration or in anticipation of exchange transfusion. 2. Helps to determine extent of dehydration. 3. Sign of dehydration. 4. Adequate hydration facilitates elimination and excretion of bilirubin. 5. Assess progress; helps to determine extent of dehydration.

Continued

NURSING CARE PLAN 14-2—cont'd

SELECTED NURSING DIAGNOSIS *Risk for hyperthermia or hypothermia*

Outcomes	Nursing Interventions	Rationales
Infant will not become overheated or chilled; temperature will be maintained between 36.3° and 37.4° C (97.4° and 99.4° F).	1. Monitor infant's temperature. 2. Adjust incubator to maintain neutral thermal environment.	1. Hyperthermia and hypothermia are common complications of phototherapy. 2. Avoid overheating incubator or warming unit.

SELECTED NURSING DIAGNOSIS *Risk for injury (neurological) related to nature of hyperbilirubinemia*

Outcomes	Nursing Interventions	Rationales
Infant will show no signs of neurological involvement (lethargy twitching).	1. Anticipate daily bilirubin blood levels. 2. Turn off phototherapy lights when blood is being drawn to avoid false readings. 3. Observe parameters for neurological deficit (e.g., twitching, lethargy).	1. Phototherapy success determined by frequently measuring serum bilirubin levels. 2. Promotes accuracy of blood test. 3. Kernicterus (brain damage) is rare but is evidenced by neurological sequela such as hypotonia, diminished reflexes, twitching, lethargy.

SELECTED NURSING DIAGNOSIS *Imbalanced nutrition: less than body requirements*

Outcomes	Nursing Interventions	Rationales
Infant will receive adequate nutrients as evidenced by stabilization of weight, laboratory reports.	1. Provide feedings as ordered. 2. Assist mother to reestablish breastfeeding if temporarily halted.	1. Early feedings within 4 to 6 hours after delivery tend to decrease high bilirubin levels and provide nourishment. 2. Encourages mother, helps her feel more in control, promotes bonding; opinions of physicians vary regarding discontinuance of breastfeeding, because the cause of breast milk jaundice is not known.

SELECTED NURSING DIAGNOSIS *Anxiety (parental) related to deficient knowledge crisis of having an infant with jaundice*

Outcomes	Nursing Interventions	Rationales
Parents express fears concerning infant's welfare.	1. Explain procedures and treatment. 2. Provide reassurance. 3. Provide follow-up.	1. Information decreases parental stress. 2. Parents are in need of support persons. 3. Follow-up care is reassuring to parents and medical personnel that family is progressing nicely without complications.

CRITICAL THINKING QUESTION

The mother of an infant receiving phototherapy states she has other children and always fed them every 4 hours. She states she does not want her infant to become "fat" and therefore does not want to feed more often. What is the appropriate response of the nurse?

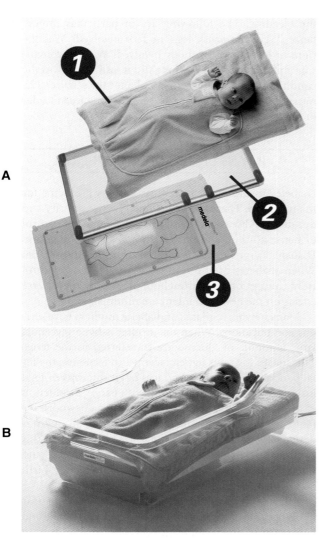

A

B

FIGURE **14-15** Phototherapy Bilibed. **A,** The infant is diapered and placed in the therapy blanket, which fits on a light permeable infant support. This plastic support is placed over the irradiation unit, which fits into the standard bassinet instead of the mattress. **B,** The infant in the Bilibed can room-in with the mother and requires no eye patch protection. The therapeutic light focuses directly on the infant's skin through the underside of the phototherapy blanket.

therapy is less costly. A referral for home care is made by the infant's pediatrician on the basis of the newborn's health, bilirubin levels (generally between 10 and 14 mg/dl), evidence of jaundice, and suitability of the family for complying with the home program.

A phototherapy blanket in a bassinet (Figure 14-15) or a fiberoptic pad (Figure 14-16) can be used. These allow for holding the infant and decrease the risk of eye damage. Written instructions are given to the parents. Parents keep a daily record of their infant's temperature,

---

| box 14-5 | *Phototherapy Tips* |

If the infant is in an incubator:

- Eyes must be covered while the infant is under lights.
- A small diaper should cover the gonad area.
- The infant is turned frequently to expose all skin surfaces.
- The infant should be in an incubator to prevent chilling.
- Loose greenish stools caused by photodegradation products must be distinguished from true diarrhea.

weight, intake and output, stools, and feedings. (See Nursing Care Plan 14-2.) Phototherapy tips are listed in Box 14-5.

INTRACRANIAL HEMORRHAGE

Pathophysiology. Intracranial hemorrhage, the most common type of birth injury, may result from trauma or anoxia. It occurs more often in the preterm infant, whose blood vessels are fragile. Blood vessels within the skull are broken, and bleeding into the brain occurs. When the diagnosis is made, the specific location of the hemorrhage may be noted (i.e., subdural, subarachnoid, or intraventricular). This injury may also occur during precipitate delivery or prolonged labor or when the newborn's head is large in comparison with the mother's pelvis.

Manifestations. The signs of intracranial hemorrhage may occur suddenly or gradually. Some or all signs are present depending on the severity of the hemorrhage and can include poor muscle tone, lethargy, poor sucking reflex, respiratory distress, cyanosis, twitching, forceful vomiting, a high-pitched shrill cry, and convulsions. Opisthotonic posturing may be observed (see Figure 23-8). The fontanel may be tense and under pressure rather than soft and compressible. The pupil of one eye is likely to be small (constricted) and the other large (dilated).

If the symptoms are mild, most patients have a good chance of complete recovery. Death results if there is a massive hemorrhage. The infant who survives an extensive hemorrhage may suffer residual effects such as mental retardation or cerebral palsy. The diagnosis is established by the history of the delivery, computed tomography (CT) scan, MRI, evidence of an increase in cerebrospinal fluid pressure, and the symptoms and course of the disease.

Treatment and nursing care. The newborn is placed in an incubator, which allows proper temperature control,

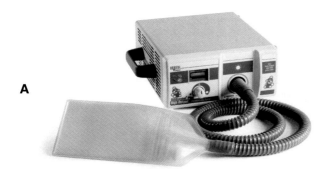

A

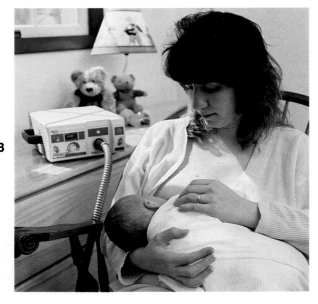

B

FIGURE **14-16** Biliblanket Plus High Output Phototherapy System. **A,** A pad of woven fibers is used to transport light from a light source to the infant. This fiberoptic pad is wrapped directly on the infant's skin to bathe the skin in light. **B,** The infant can then be diapered, clothed, held, and nursed during treatment at home.

ease in administering oxygen, and continuous observation (p. 313). The infant is handled gently and as little as possible. The head is elevated. The physician may prescribe vitamin K to control bleeding and phenobarbital if twitching or convulsions are apparent. Prophylactic antibiotics and vitamins may be used. The infant is fed carefully because the sucking reflex may be affected. The infant vomits easily. The nurse observes the infant for signs of increased ICP (see Chapter 23) and convulsions and assists the physician with procedures such as lumbar punctures and aspiration of subdural hemorrhage. Performing neurochecks, monitoring vital signs and head circumference, and palpating fontanels are essential.

If a convulsion occurs, observation of its character aids the physician in diagnosing the exact location of the bleeding. The following are of particular importance: Were the arms, legs, or face involved? Was the right or left side of the body involved? Was the convulsion mild or severe? How long did it last? What was the condition of the infant before and after the seizure? The nurse records observations and notifies the team leader or health care provider.

INFANT OF A DIABETIC MOTHER

Diabetes in the mother presents various problems for the newborn. These are determined by the severity and duration of disease in the mother, the degree of control of her condition, and the gestational age of the infant. Diabetes in pregnancy is discussed on pp. 100 to 106. When diabetes of the mother is under good control from conception and throughout pregnancy, the adverse effects on the newborn infant are minimal.

Many newborn infants of diabetic mothers have serious complications. When the mother is hyperglycemic, large amounts of glucose are transferred to the fetus. This makes the fetus hyperglycemic. In response, the fetal pancreas (islet cells) produces large amounts of fetal insulin. Hyperinsulinism, along with excess production of protein and fatty acids, often results in a newborn infant who weighs more than 9 pounds. Such an infant is designated "large for gestational age" (LGA), and this condition is termed macrosomia (*macro,* "large" and *soma,* "body"). This infant is prone to injuries at birth because of his or her size.

After delivery the infant often has low blood sugar levels because of the abrupt loss of maternal glucose and hypertrophy of the pancreatic islet cells, which results in a temporary overproduction of insulin. The infant has a characteristic *cushingoid* appearance because of increased subcutaneous fat. The face is round and appears puffy, and the infant appears lethargic. The size of these newborn infants makes them appear healthy, but this is deceptive because they often have developmental deficits and may suffer complications of respiratory distress syndrome (RDS) or congenital anomalies. In contrast, some infants born to a mother with severe diabetes may be small for gestational age (SGA) because of poor placental perfusion. These infants suffer from hypoglycemia, hypocalcemia, and hyperbilirubinemia.

The nursing care of the infant of a diabetic mother includes close monitoring of vital signs, early feeding, and frequent assessment of blood glucose levels for the first 2 days of life. Hypoglycemia in the first days of life is defined as a blood glucose level that falls below 40 mg/dl. It can result in rapid and permanent brain damage. The infant should be closely watched for signs of irritability, tremors, and respiratory distress.

key points

- The nurse manages communication between parents and the multidisciplinary health care team to meet the needs of the newborn with congenital problems and of their families.
- Measuring head size is important in infants with hydrocephalus.
- Spina bifida is a congenital embryonic neural tube defect in which there is an imperfect closure of the spinal vertebrae.
- Folic acid supplementation during the early weeks of pregnancy can prevent neural tube anomalies.
- Postoperative nursing care of the infant with a cleft lip includes preventing the infant from sucking and crying, which could impair healing of the suture line.
- Newborns feel pain, and adequate pain control after invasive procedures and surgery is essential.
- The body spica cast encircles the waist and extends to the ankles or toes. It is used to treat developmental hip dysplasia.
- A positive Barlow's test and Ortolani's sign are indicative of developmental hip dysplasia.
- Newborn infants are routinely screened for phenylketonuria.

- Lofenalac is a formula used for infants with phenylketonuria.
- RhoGAM is given to an Rh-negative mother after delivering an Rh-positive fetus to prevent maternal Rh sensitization.
- Hyperbilirubinemia results from rapid destruction of red blood cells.
- Jaundice that occurs in the first 24 hours of life is considered pathological.
- Distinguishing pathological jaundice from physiological jaundice can facilitate early intervention and prevent serious complications.
- Macrosomia is a condition in which the infant is large for gestational age (LGA) and usually occurs in infants of diabetic mothers.
- In intracranial hemorrhage, blood vessels within the skull are broken and there is bleeding into the brain.

ONLINE RESOURCES

Spina Bifida Association of America: http://www.sbaa.org

Centers for Disease Control and Prevention: http://www.cdc.gov

March of Dimes: http://www.modimes.org

American Cleft Palate–Craniofacial Association: http://www.cleftline.org

REVIEW QUESTIONS   *Choose the most appropriate answer.*

1. The inspection of a cavity by passing a light through its wall to visualize fluid is called:
   1. Transillumination
   2. Phototherapy
   3. Hydrotherapy
   4. Photosynthesis

2. A congenital defect that results in enlargement of the patient's head and pressure changes within the brain is:
   1. Hydrocephalus
   2. Microcephalus
   3. Hydrocele
   4. Anencephaly

3. Meningomyelocele is:
   1. A protrusion of the meninges through an opening in the spine
   2. Primarily a disorder of the muscular tissue of the body
   3. A protrusion of the membranes and cord through an opening in the spine
   4. A tumor in the meningocele space

4. A Pavlik harness is often used to correct:
   1. Clubfoot
   2. Juvenile arthritis
   3. Developmental hip dysplasia
   4. Fractured femur

5. When bathing an infant, the nurse observes the hips for dislocation. Which of the following observations may indicate developmental hip dysplasia?
   1. Toes turned inward
   2. Limitation of abduction of legs
   3. Asymmetry of epicanthal folds
   4. Shortening of patella

An Overview of Growth, Development, and Nutrition

1. Define each key term listed.
2. Explain the differences between growth, development, and maturation.
3. Recognize and read a growth chart for children.
4. List five factors that influence growth and development.
5. Discuss the nursing implications of growth and development.
6. Describe three developmental theories and their impact on planning the nursing care of children.
7. Discuss the nutritional needs of growing children.
8. Differentiate between permanent and deciduous teeth and list the times of their eruption.
9. Recognize the influence of the family and cultural practices on growth, development, nutrition, and health care.
10. Understand the characteristics of play at various age levels.
11. Describe the relationship of play to physical, cognitive, and emotional development.
12. Understand the role of computers and computer games in play at various ages.
13. Define therapeutic play.
14. Understand the use of play as an assessment tool.
15. Discuss the importance of family-centered care in pediatrics.

adolescent (p. 349)
cephalocaudal (sĕf-ă-lō-KAW-dăl, p. 349)
cognition (kŏg-NĬ-shŭn, p. 363)
community (p. 356)
competitive play (p. 382)
cooperative play (p. 382)
deciduous (dē-SĬD-ū-ŭs, p. 378)
dysfunctional family (p. 355)
Erikson (p. 363)
extended family (p.355)
fluorosis (floo-RŌ-sĭs, p. 380)
growth (p. 349)
height (p. 352)

infant (p. 349)
Kohlberg (p. 363)
length (p. 352)
Maslow (p. 363)
maturation (p. 349)
metabolic rate (p. 350)
neonate (p. 349)
nuclear family (p. 355)
nursing caries (p. 380)
parallel play (p. 382)
personality (p. 356)
Piaget (pē-ă-ZHĀ, p. 363)
proximodistal (prŏk-sī-mō-DĬS-tăl, p. 349)
therapeutic play (p. 383)
toddler (p. 349)

GROWTH AND DEVELOPMENT

The main difference between caring for the adult and caring for the child is that the latter is in a continuous process of growth and development. This process is orderly and proceeds from the simple to the more complex (Box 15-1). Although the process is orderly, it is not steadily paced. Growth spurts are often followed by plateaus. One of the most noticeable growth spurts is at the time of puberty. The rate of growth varies with the individual child. Each infant has an individual timetable that revolves around established norms. Siblings within a family vary in growth rate. Growth is measurable and can be observed and studied. This is done by comparing height, weight, increase in vocabulary, physical skills, and other parameters. There are variations in growth within the systems and subsystems. Not all parts mature at the same time. Skeletal growth approximates whole-body growth, whereas the brain, lymph, and reproductive tissues follow distinct and individual sequences.

THE IMPACT OF GROWTH AND DEVELOPMENT ON NURSING CARE

Pediatrics is a subspecialty of medical-surgical nursing. Adult acute care units in a hospital may contain a separate neurology unit, a separate cardiac unit, a separate medical unit, and a separate surgical unit. On the pedi-

box 15-1 | *Emerging Patterns of Behavior from Age 1 to 5 Years*

12 MONTHS

Motor: Walks with one hand held; rises independently; takes several steps

Adaptive: Picks up pellet with pincer action of thumb and forefinger; releases object to another person on request

Language: Says "mama," "dada," and a few similar words

Social: Plays simple ball game; makes postural adjustment to dressing

15 MONTHS

Motor: Walks alone; crawls up stairs

Adaptive: Makes tower of three cubes; makes a line with crayons; inserts pellet in bottle

Language: Jargon; follows simple commands; may name a familiar object (ball)

Social: Indicates some desires or needs by pointing; hugs caregivers

18 MONTHS

Motor: Runs stiffly; sits on small chair; walks up stairs with one hand held; explores drawers and wastebaskets

Adaptive: Makes tower of four cubes; imitates vertical stroke; imitates scribbling; dumps pellet from bottle

Language: 10 words (average); names pictures; identifies one or more parts of body

Social: Feeds self; seeks help when in trouble; may complain when wet or soiled; kisses caregivers with pucker

2 YEARS

Motor: Runs well; walks up and down stairs, one step at a time; opens doors; climbs on furniture; jumps

Adaptive: Tower of seven cubes (6 at 21 months); circular scribbling; imitates horizontal stroke; folds paper once imitatively

Language: Puts three words together (subject, verb, object)

Social: Handles spoon well; often tells immediate experiences; helps to undress; listens to stories with pictures

2 ½ YEARS

Motor: Goes up stairs alternating feet

Adaptive: Tower of nine cubes; makes vertical and horizontal strokes but generally will not join them to make a cross; imitates circular stroke, forming a closed figure

Language: Refers to self by pronoun "I"; knows full name

Social: Helps put things away; pretends in play

3 YEARS

Motor: Rides tricycle; stands momentarily on one foot

Adaptive: Tower of 10 cubes; imitates construction of "bridge" of three cubes; copies a circle; imitates a cross

Language: Knows age and sex; counts three objects correctly; repeats three numbers or a sentence of six syllables

Social: Plays simple games (in "parallel" with other children); helps in dressing (unbuttons clothing and puts on shoes); washes hands

4 YEARS

Motor: Hops on one foot; throws ball overhand; uses scissors to cut out pictures; climbs well

Adaptive: Copies bridge from model; imitates construction of "gate" of five cubes; copies cross and square; draws a man with two to four parts besides head; names longer of two lines

Language: Counts four pennies accurately; tells a story

Social: Plays with several children with beginning of social interaction and role playing; goes to toilet alone

5 YEARS

Motor: Skips

Adaptive: Draws triangle from copy; names heavier of two weights

Language: Names four colors; repeats sentence of 10 syllables; counts 10 pennies correctly

Social: Dresses and undresses; asks questions about meaning of words; domestic role playing

Modified from Behrman, R., Kliegman, R., & Jenson, H. (2000). *Nelson's textbook of pediatrics* (16th ed.). Philadelphia: W.B. Saunders. Data are derived from those of Gesell (as revised by Knobloch), Shirley, Provence, Wolf, Bailey, and others.

After 5 years the Stanford-Binet, Wechsler-Bellevue, and other scales offer the most precise estimates of developmental level. To have the greatest value, they should be administered only by an experienced and qualified person.

atric acute care unit in the general hospital, all medical-surgical specialties are usually housed on one unit—for patients from newborn to adolescent. The developmental needs of the child have an impact on his or her response to illness and on the approach required by the nurse in developing a plan of care. Choosing the right words to explain to a child what will happen to him or her is essential. For example, if the nurse states that the child will be "put to sleep" before the operation, will the child relate that to a pet at home being "put to sleep" and never heard from again? The fractured jaw of an 8-month-old after a motor vehicle accident may affect his developmental process more seriously than the same injury in a 4-year-old because the 8-month-old is in the oral phase of development.

Because the child differs from the adult both anatomically and physiologically, differences in response to therapy as well as manifestations of illness can be anticipated. The nurse must understand the normal to recognize deviations within any age-group and to plan care that considers these developmental differences (Box 15-2).

An understanding of growth and development, including its predictable nature and individual variation, has value in the nursing process. Such knowledge is the basis of the nurse's anticipatory guidance of parents. For example, the nurse who knows when the infant is likely to crawl can, at the appropriate age, expand teaching on

safety precautions. The nurse also incorporates these precautions into nursing care plans in the hospital. *Age-appropriate care cannot be administered without an understanding of growth and development.*

While explaining various aspects of child care to families, the nurse stresses the importance of individual differences. Parents tend to compare their children's development and behavior with those of other children and with information in popular magazine articles. This may relieve their anxiety or cause them to impose impossible expectations and standards. In addition, many parents had poor role models who influenced their own experiences as children. Lack of knowledge about parenting can be recognized by the nurse and suitable interventions begun.

The nurse who understands that each child is born with an individual temperament and "style of behavior" can help frustrated parents cope with a newborn who has difficulty settling into the new environment. Specific parameters can be used to determine whether an infant is merely on an individual timetable or whether the infant varies from normal.

The nurse must also recognize when to intervene to prevent disease and/or accidents. For example, a brief visit with a caregiver may reveal that the child's immunizations are not up-to-date. A review of the characteristics of a 2-year-old with a teenage mother may prevent the ingestion of poisons. Complications of the newborn can be avoided by advising the expectant mother to avoid alcohol and cigarettes. Other threats to health may likewise be anticipated. Knowing that specific diseases are prevalent in certain age-groups, the nurse maintains a high level of suspicion when interacting with these patients. This approach, based on developmental knowledge, experience, and effective communication, helps to ensure a higher level of family care. Finally, the nurse must understand how to provide nursing care to children of various ages to enhance their physical, mental, emotional, and spiritual development according to their specific needs and comprehension.

| box 15-2 | *The Nursing Process Applied to Growth and Development*

DATA COLLECTION

Obtain height and weight and plot a standard growth chart.
Record developmental milestones achieved related to age.
Observe infant; interview parents.

ANALYSIS/NURSING DIAGNOSIS

Determine appropriate nursing diagnoses related to parenting, coping skills, and unmet developmental needs.

PLANNING

Offer guidance and teaching to family, school personnel, and child to meet child's developmental needs. For example, the toddler and preschooler may have specific needs related to safety or the use of age-appropriate toys.

IMPLEMENTATION

Interventions that foster growth and development in the hospital setting can include encouraging age-appropriate self-care. In the home, the school-age child with diabetes may be taught to participate in performing blood sugar tests and administering insulin.
Anticipatory guidance may be given to parents so they understand changes in behavior, eating habits, and play of the growing child.

EVALUATION

Ongoing evaluation of growth and development of the child and follow-up of teaching and guidance offered at prior clinic/home visits are essential.

>NURSING **TIP**_____
The nursing approach should be governed by the developmental level of the child and family values, with choices and active participation offered when appropriate.

>NURSING **TIP**_____
Arnold Gesell, founder of the Clinic for Child Development at Yale University, was the first to study children scientifically over a period of time. He coined the term *child development*.

TERMINOLOGY

The following stages of growth and development are referred to throughout this text:

- Fetus: Ninth gestational week to birth
- Neonate: Birth to 4 weeks
- Infant: 4 weeks to 1 year
- Toddler: 1 to 3 years
- Preschool: 3 to 6 years
- School age: 6 to 12 years
- Adolescent: 12 to 18 years

Growth refers to an increase in physical size and is measured in inches and pounds. *Development* refers to a progressive increase in the function of the body. These two terms are inseparable. Maturation (*maturus,* "ripe") refers to the total way in which a person grows and develops, as dictated by inheritance (Box 15-3). Although maturation is independent of environment, its timing may be affected by environment.

DIRECTIONAL PATTERNS

Directional patterns are fundamental to all humans. Cephalocaudal development proceeds from head to toe. The infant is able to raise the head before being able to sit, and he or she gains control of the trunk before walking. The second pattern is proximodistal, or from midline to the periphery. Development proceeds from the center of the body to the periphery (Figure 15-1). These patterns occur bilaterally. Development also proceeds from the general to the specific. The infant grasps with the hands before pinching with the fingers.

SOME DEVELOPMENTAL DIFFERENCES BETWEEN CHILDREN AND ADULTS
Height

Height refers to standing measurement, whereas length refers to measurement while the infant is in a recumbent position. At birth the newborn has an average length of about 20 inches (50 cm). Linear growth is caused mainly by skeletal growth. Growth fluctuates until maturity is reached. Infancy and puberty are both rapid growth periods. Height is generally a family trait, although there are exceptions. Good nutrition and general good health are instrumental in promoting linear growth. Height is measured during each well-child visit (Figure 15-2). The length of the infant usually increases about 1 inch per month for the first 6 months. By age 1 year, the birth length increases by 50% (mostly in the trunk area).

Weight

Weight is another good index of health. However, the weight of a newborn infant does not always imply gestational maturity (see Chapter 13 and Figure 13-1). The average full-term newborn weighs 6 to 9 pounds (2.72 to 4.09 kg), with a general average of 7.5 pounds. Approximately 5% to 10% of the birth weight is lost by age 3 or 4 days as the result of the passage of stools and a limited fluid intake. The infant usually regains his or her birth weight by age 10 to 12 days. *Birth weight usually doubles by age 5 to 6 months and triples by age 1 year.* After the first year, weight gain levels off to approximately 4 to 6 pounds (1.81 to 2.72 kg) per year until the pubertal growth spurt begins.

Weight is determined at each office visit. A marked increase or decrease requires further investigation. The body weight of a newborn is composed of a higher percentage of water than in the adult. This extracellular

| box 15-3 | *Key Terms in Child Development* |

development A progressive increase in the function of the body (e.g., infant's increasing ability to digest solids).

growth An increase in physical size, measured in feet or meters and pounds or kilograms.

maturation The total way in which a person grows and develops, as dictated by inheritance.

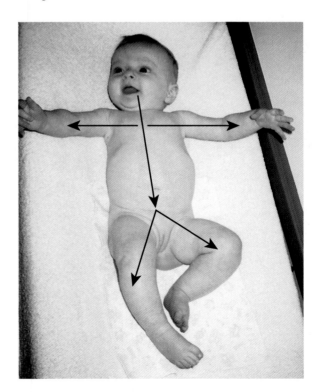

FIGURE **15-1** The development of muscular control proceeds from head to foot (cephalocaudally) and from the center of the body to its periphery (proximodistally).

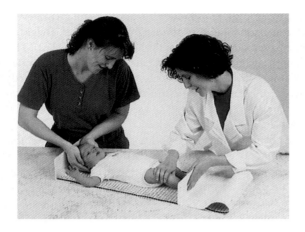

A

Head in
midline

Line of
vision
parallel
to floor

Shoulders
touching

Buttocks
touching

Heels
touching
and
together

B

fluid falls from 40% in the newborn to 20% in the adult. The high proportion of extracellular fluid in the infant can cause a more rapid loss of total body fluid, and therefore every infant must be closely monitored for dehydration. (See technique of weighing infants, Chapter 12 and Figure 12-11.)

Body Proportions

Body proportions of the child differ greatly from those of the adult (Figure 15-3). The head is the fastest growing portion of the body during fetal life. During infancy the trunk grows rapidly, whereas during childhood growth of the legs becomes the predominant feature. At adolescence, characteristic male and female proportions develop as childhood fat disappears. Alterations in proportions in the size of head, trunk, and extremities are characteristic of certain disturbances. Routine measurements of head and chest circumference are important indices of health.

Metabolic Rate

The metabolic rate (energy utilization and oxygen consumption) in children is higher than in adults. Infants require more calories, minerals, vitamins, and fluid in proportion to weight and height than do adults. Higher metabolic rates are accompanied by an increased production of heat and waste products. The body surface area of young children is far greater in relation to body weight than that of adults. The young child loses relatively more fluid from the pulmonary and integumentary systems.

Respirations

The respirations of infants are irregular and abdominal. Small airways can become easily blocked with mucus. The short, straight eustachian tube connects with the ear and predisposes the infant to middle ear infections. The chest wall is thin and the muscles are immature, and therefore pressure on the chest can interfere with respiratory efforts.

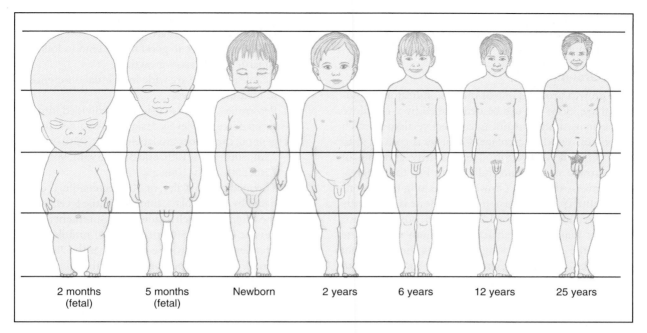

FIGURE **15-3** Changes in body proportions. Approximate changes in body proportions from fetal life through adulthood are shown. These changes in body proportions affect body surface areas that are used to determine the percentages of body burns in burn injuries. (See the "rule of nines," Figure 29-15.)

Cardiovascular System

In neonates, the muscle mass of the right and left ventricles of the heart is almost equal. An increased need for cardiac output is often met by an increase in *heart rate.* Newborns have a high oxygen consumption and require a high cardiac output in the first few months of life. The presence of fetal (immature) hemoglobin in the first months of life also contributes to the need for a high cardiac output. The disappearance of fetal hemoglobin along with the loss of maternal iron stores contributes to the development of *physiological anemia* in infants after 3 or 4 months of age.

Immunity

For the first 3 months of life, the newborn is protected from illnesses to which the mother was exposed. The infant gradually produces his or her own immunoglobulin until adult levels are reached by puberty. Therefore the infant and child must be protected from nosocomial infections in the hospital and from unnecessary exposure to pathogens. Immunizations against common childhood communicable diseases is discussed in Chapter 31.

Kidney Function

Kidney function is not mature until the end of the second year of life. Therefore drugs that are eliminated via the kidney can accumulate in the body to dangerous levels before age 2 years. Immature kidney function also predisposes the infant to dehydration. Nursing responsibilities for children under age 2 years include monitoring for dehydration and observing closely for toxic effects of drug therapy.

Nervous System

Maturation of the brain is evidenced by increased coordination, skills, and behaviors in the first years of life. Primitive reflexes, such as the grasp reflex, are replaced by purposeful, controlled movement. Head circumference increases 1.5 cm per month to an approximate total of 43 cm at age 6 months. During the second 6 months of life, head circumference increases 0.5 cm per month to an approximate total of 46 cm at 1 year of age. The age-appropriate toy is correlated with nervous system maturation. When selecting play activities, the nurse should consider the diagnosis and the child's developmental level and abilities to be sure the toy is safe.

Sleep Patterns

Sleep patterns vary with age. The neonate sleeps 8 to 9 hours per night and naps an equal amount of time during the day. The 2-year-old may sleep 10 hours during the night and have only one short daytime nap. The 7-year-old usually requires 8 to 8½ hours of sleep and rarely has a daytime nap. These patterns may be altered by cultural practices. For example, Israeli Kibbutzim often have *all* family members nap after work or school, before dinner.

Bone Growth

Bone growth provides one of the best indicators of biological age. Bone age can be determined by x-ray films. In the fetus, bones begin as connective tissue, which later is converted to cartilage. Cartilage is converted to bone through ossification. The maturity and rate of bone growth vary within individuals, but the progression remains the same. Growth of the long bones continues until *epiphyseal* fusion occurs. Bone is constantly synthesized and reabsorbed. In children, bone synthesis is greater than bone destruction. Calcium reserves are stored in the ends of the long bones. Vitamin A, vitamin D, sunlight, and fluorine are necessary for the growth and development of skeletal and soft tissue.

Critical Periods

There appear to be certain periods when environmental events or stimuli have their maximum impact on the child's development. The embryo, for example, can be adversely affected during times of rapid cell division. Certain viruses, drugs, and other agents are known to cause congenital anomalies during the first 3 months after conception. It is believed that these sensitive periods also apply to factors such as developing a sense of trust during the first year of life and learning readiness.

Integration of Skills

As the child learns new skills, they are combined with ones previously mastered. The child who is learning to walk may sit, pull the body up to a table by grasping it, balance, and take a cautious step. Tomorrow the child may take three steps! Children connect and perfect each skill in preparation for learning a more complex one.

GROWTH STANDARDS

Growth is measured in dimensions such as height, weight, volume, and thickness of tissues. Measurement alone, without any standard of comparison, limits the interpretation of the data. A number of standards have been developed to make it possible to (1) compare the measurement of a child to others of the same age and sex (and ideally race), and (2) compare that child's present measurements with the former rate of growth and pattern of progress. These standards, available as *growth charts,* are among the tools that have been used to assess the child's overall development (Figure 15-4).

Length refers to horizontal measurement; it is used before a child can stand, usually between birth to 2 years. Height is measured with the child standing, usually

between 2 and 18 years. Some pointers in reading and interpreting growth charts are as follows:

- Children who are in good health tend to follow a consistent pattern of growth.
- At any age, there are wide individual differences in measured values.
- Percentile charts are customarily divided into seven percentile levels designated by lines. In general, these lines are labeled 97th, 95th, 90th, 75th, 50th, 25th, 10th, and 3rd, or 95th, 90th, 75th, 50th, 25th, 10th, and 5th.
- The median (middle), or 50th percentile, is designated by a solid black line. Percentile levels show the extent to which a child's measurements deviate from the 50th percentile or middle measurement. A child whose weight is at the 75th percentile line is *one percentile above* the median. A child whose height is at the 25th percentile is *one percentile below* the median.
- A difference of two or more percentile levels between height and weight may suggest an underweight or overweight condition and prompts further investigation.
- Deviations of two or more percentile levels from an established growth pattern require further evaluation.

DEVELOPMENTAL SCREENING

Developmental screening is a vital component of child health assessment. One widely used tool is the Denver II, a revision of the Denver Developmental Screening test. This tool assesses the developmental status of children during the first 6 years of life in four categories: personal-social, fine motor-adaptive, language, and gross motor. It is *not* an intelligence test. Its purpose is to identify children who are unable to perform at a level comparable to their age-mates. A low score merely indicates a need for further evaluation. It is designed for use by both professionals and paraprofessionals. Proper administration and interpretation will aid in developing an individualized plan of care for the child.

> ⟩NURSING **TIP**_____
> "Catch-up" growth refers to the process by which a child who has been sick or malnourished and whose growth has slowed or stopped experiences a more rapid period of recovery as the body attempts to compensate.

INFLUENCING FACTORS

Growth and development are influenced by many factors, such as heredity, nationality, race, ordinal position in the family, gender, and environment. These factors

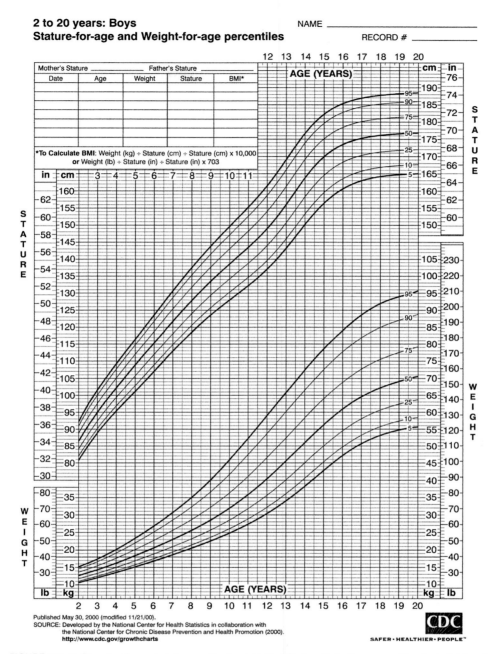

2 to 20 years: Boys
Stature-for-age and Weight-for-age percentiles

FIGURE **15-4** Sample of a complete growth chart, United States. Note the percentiles for height and weight. *Continued*

are closely related and dependent on one another in their effect on growth and development. They make each person unique. If a child is ill, physically or emotionally, the developmental processes may be delayed.

Hereditary Traits

Characteristics derived from our ancestors are determined at the time of conception by countless genes within each chromosome. Each gene is made of a chemi-

cal substance called deoxyribonucleic acid (DNA), which plays an important part in determining inherited characteristics. Examples of inherited traits are eye color, hair color, and physical resemblances within families.

Nationality and Race

Many physical differences among people of various nationalities and races, who were formerly distinguished with ease, have become less apparent in our age of com-

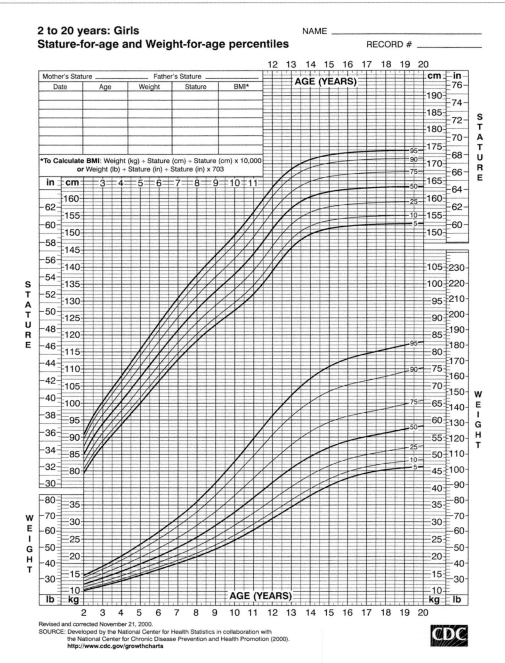

2 to 20 years: Girls
Stature-for-age and Weight-for-age percentiles

NAME _____

RECORD # _____

Revised and corrected November 21, 2000.
SOURCE: Developed by the National Center for Health Statistics in collaboration with the National Center for Chronic Disease Prevention and Health Promotion (2000).
http://www.cdc.gov/growthcharts

FIGURE **15-4, cont'd** For legend, see p. 353.

mon environment and customs. For instance, a person of Japanese origin might be thought of as being of short stature. However, Japanese children living in the United States are comparable in height to other children in this country. Nevertheless, ethnic differences extend into many areas, including speech, food preferences, family structure, religious orientation, and code of conduct. The nurse should ascertain cultural beliefs and practices when collecting data for nursing assessment (see Table 15-2).

Ordinal Position in the Family

Whether the child is the youngest, middle, or oldest in the family has some bearing on growth and development. The youngest and middle children learn from their older sisters and brothers. However, motor development of the youngest may be prolonged if the child is babied by the others in the family. The only child or the oldest child may excel in language development because his or her conversations are mainly with adults.

These children are often subject to greater parental expectations.

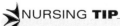NURSING **TIP**
Acceptance of the child's value system and cultural beliefs will assist in positive nurse-child interactions.

Gender

The male infant often weighs more and is slightly longer than the female. He grows and develops at a slightly different rate. Parents and relatives may treat boys differently from girls by providing "gender-appropriate" toys and play and by having different expectations of them. Current trends promote unisex activities in play and career development.

Environment

The physical condition of the newborn is influenced by the prenatal environment. The health of the mother at the time of conception and the amount and quality of her diet during pregnancy are important for proper fetal development. Infections or diseases may lead to malformations of the fetus. A healthy and strong newborn can easily adapt to its surroundings.

The home greatly influences the infant's physical and emotional growth and development. If a family is financially strained by an added member and the parents are unable to provide nourishing foods and suitable housing, the infant is directly affected. An uneducated mother may not know how to properly cook foods to preserve their nutritional value. Immunizations and other medical attention may be neglected. The infant senses tension within the family and is affected by it.

In contrast, energies can be directed toward positive development when the surroundings are secure and stable and the infant feels secure, wanted, and loved. Most environments are neither completely positive nor completely negative but fall somewhere between the two extremes. Intelligence plays an important role in social and mental development. Potential intelligence is believed to be inherited but greatly affected by the environment.

NURSING **TIP**
"Different" does not mean "inferior."

The Family

The *family* has been defined in many different ways and fulfills many different purposes. Traditionally, the **nuclear family,** or biological family, has been the basic unit of structure in American society (mother, father, siblings). Today many nuclear families do not share the same household because of single parenthood, divorce,

table 15-1	*Variations of Family Living*
TYPE OF FAMILY*	**COMMENT**
Nuclear	Traditional—husband, wife, children (natural or adopted)
Extended	Grandparents, parents, children, relatives
Single parent	Women or men establishing separate households through individual preference, divorce, death, illegitimacy, or desertion
Foster parent	Parents who care for children who require parenting because of dysfunctional family, no family, or individual problems
Alternative	Communal family
Dual career	Both parents work because of desire or need
Blended	Remarriage of persons with children
Polygamous	More than one spouse
Homosexual	Two persons of the same sex who have adopted children or who have had children from a previous marriage
Cohabitation	Heterosexual or homosexual couples who live together but remain unmarried

*Not all family types may be legally sanctioned.

and remarriage. Kinship lines have become blurred, and fundamental changes from what was once perceived are occurring in the family. The **extended family** refers to three generations: grandparents, parents, and children. Because of an increasing life span, however, there are a greater number of living grandparents and great-grandparents, and the proportion of them living in the family home may increase. Table 15-1 lists the various types of families and a description of each.

By far, the *interactions* of family unit members is most influential in the growth and development of the child. The nurse must understand the interaction of the family unit to affect a positive change that may be necessary to prevent or treat childhood illnesses. Some families have solid support systems and use available community resources to maintain health. Other families may lack support systems and require closer follow-up care and encouragement by the health team. Parenting is a learned behavior, often modeled by past experience and modified by the acceptance of specific roles and responsibilities. A family that does not provide for the optimum physical, psychological, and emotional health of the children is called a **dysfunctional family.** A dysfunctional family does not necessarily imply that its members are not loving and caring. A dysfunctional family does not know how to be successful in its efforts and interactions and requires intervention.

Historically, in middle-class families the father was the breadwinner and the mother managed the home and raised the children. This trend has shifted. Because of changing economic conditions, both parents' earnings may be necessary to maintain the family's standard of living. In dual-career families both the father and the mother are often absent for most of the day because of long commutes or the demands of the working environment. Both parents may share child care and domestic chores. The parents may need to transfer to different locations to maintain their careers. This decreases extended family support and makes it necessary for children to change schools frequently.

Divorce, separation, death, and pregnancy outside marriage create many one-parent families. The percentage of children living in single-parent families has more than doubled since the 1970s. Most single-wage families have an economic disadvantage, but families with women as the single-wage earner often have considerably lower incomes than those in which men are the single-wage earner. The problem of providing good, affordable child care is a serious one for both dual-career families and single parents. Relatives and the noncustodial parent may assist in raising the child. Many single parents remarry, creating the *blended* family. The addition may be merely a stepfather or stepmother, or two families may unite. These family units must make many adjustments. To succeed, parents and children have to learn problem-solving techniques, communication skills, and flexibility.

A *family APGAR* first described by Smilkstein (1984) is a tool that can be used as a guide today to assess family functioning. This assessment is valuable in determining the approach to home care needs:

- *Adaptation:* How the family helps and shares resources
- *Partnership:* Lines of communication and partnership in the family
- *Growth:* How responsibilities for growth and development of child are shared
- *Affection:* Overt and covert emotional interactions among family members
- *Resolve:* How time, money, and space are allocated to prevent and solve problems

Questions concerning each of these areas should be posed and evaluated. The goal in family assessment is to enable the nurse to develop interventions that aid the family to achieve a healthier adaptation to the child's health needs or problems.

NURSING TIP

Special care may be required to assist in the growth and development of infants who are blind or whose parents are chronically depressed.

NURSING TIP

An infant who is hypersensitive to noise or touch needs the parent to understand the need for quiet surroundings. A chronically depressed parent may interpret fussiness or lack of smiling as rejection. Therefore an assessment of parent-child interaction is essential in the home, clinic, or hospital setting.

The family as part of a community. The term community is defined in many ways, but here it is used to refer to the immediate geographical area in which the family lives and interacts (e.g., "I come from the South Side"). Families are greatly influenced by the communities in which they reside. Nurses must understand the culture of the community in which they work or to which the patient will return (Table 15-2). Assessment of the community is particularly important in creating discharge plans for families from various cultures. Their lives may be broadened or restricted depending on the facilities within the community. A few factors to consider are housing, access to public transportation, city services, safety, and health care delivery systems. The nurse has immediate access to the patient and therefore becomes an important liaison between various agencies that address specific needs.

The homeless family. The homeless family with children is a modern-day problem that impacts the growth, development, and health of the child. Support systems and financial resources are often lacking, and the school nurse or emergency department nurse may be the first to identify this family. Community referrals to provide shelter, food, education, and financial aid are primary needs that must be met before health teaching can be effective.

It is imperative that nurses take advantage of the strengths of the family while attending to its weaknesses. Nurses are in an excellent position to help the health profession move toward truly contemporary models of family-centered care. The nuclear family of the past is no longer dominant. Pediatric nursing research and care must reflect this phenomenon.

PERSONALITY DEVELOPMENT

Most people tend to equate personality with social attractiveness: "She has a lot of personality, and he has no personality" or "There's an example of personality plus." The term personality is more broadly defined by psychologists. One definition states that personality is a

Text continued on p. 363

table 15-2 *Cultural Influences on the Family*

CULTURAL GROUP	FAMILY AND KINSHIP STRUCTURE	COMMUNICATION	HEALTH BELIEFS AND PRACTICES	FAMILY AND CHILD CARE PRACTICES
HISPANIC				
Mexican American	Family is an extensive network composed of nuclear and extended family members. Father is provider and decision maker; mother is family caregiver. Decisions are made by father after discussion with older or extended family members. Divorce is uncommon. Out-of-wedlock relationships are common. Children are the center of family life.	Eye contact may be considered rude. Looking at or admiring an infant without touching the child can bring about *mal ojo* (evil eye).	Health represents an equilibrium between hot and cold, wet and dry. An imbalance in these forces causes disease. Cold remedies are used to treat hot diseases, and hot remedies are used to treat cold diseases. Balance and harmony are accomplished through avoiding some foods and consuming others. Seek curandero, a folk healer, for treatment remedies and spiritual healing ceremonies. May combine advice from curandero with the antibiotics or other therapies from a physician. Resort to prayer or home remedies (remedias caseras) before seeking help from folk practitioner or health care provider. Often delay seeking medical attention and obtaining screening examinations and immunizations. Higher incidence of jobs with no health insurance. Mother is unlikely to sign consent for child's health care without discussion with the father.	Delay breastfeeding until milk comes in. Believe that stress and anger make milk bad and infant can become ill. Neutralize infant bowel when weaning from breast to bottle by feeding only anise tea for 24 hours. More likely to have children without prenatal or postnatal care. *Mal ojo*, or "evil eye," is an illness that affects children and occurs when someone with special powers looks at or admires a child but does not touch or hold the child. A curandero can treat the child through massage and prayer. Wearing special amulets or charms can protect child from the evil eye. The practice of binding the umbilicus of the newborn is done to prevent bad air from entering the infant. Parent-child relationship is warm and nurturing. Parents are often quite permissive in respect to their child's behavior.
Puerto Rican	Extended and patriarchal family.	Bilingual—Spanish and English.	Avoid iron supplements because they are considered "hot" medications. Classify foods and medications as hot, cold, and cool. Classify foods as hot and cold.	Children are viewed as a gift from God. Children are taught to obey and respect their parents. Male-female roles are taught.
Cuban	Family ties are strong, and this continues as children grow into adulthood.	Bilingual—Spanish and English.	Health promotion is important. Believe in the biomedical model, although supernatural forces (evil eye) are thought to cause some illnesses that can be cured by ethnic treatments or magic spells.	Mother is the primary child caregiver. Plump infants and young children are idealized. School system assumes much of the childrearing responsibilities.

Continued

Modified from Bowden, V., Dickey, S., & Greenberg, C. (1998). *Children and their families: The continuum of care.* Philadelphia: W.B. Saunders; and Lipson, J. Dibble, S., & Minarek, P. (1998). *Culture and nursing care;* San Francisco: University of California—San Francisco Nursing Press.

table 15-2 *Cultural Influences on the Family—cont'd*

CULTURAL GROUP	FAMILY AND KINSHIP STRUCTURE	COMMUNICATION	HEALTH BELIEFS AND PRACTICES	FAMILY AND CHILD CARE PRACTICES
Cuban—cont'd	Several generations live together.		Amulets on a bracelet or necklace may be worn to ward off the evil eye. Diet is high in fat, cholesterol, sugar, and fried foods.	Fathers make the decisions.
HAITIAN	Extended family is important as the support system. Matriarchal society with male as figurehead.	Rely on native language.	Believe that God's will must prevail. Rely on folk foods and treatments for illness management. Believe in hot-cold theory. Avoid eggplant, okra, tomatoes, black pepper, cold drinks, milk, rice, bananas, and fish during pregnancy. White foods are believed to cause increased vaginal discharge in pregnancy.	Usually breastfeed and believe strong emotions affect quality of milk. Folk medicine is the first line of treatment.
AFRICAN-AMERICAN	Family is of great importance. Many are headed by mother in absence of a father. In two-parent families, egalitarian structure is most prominent. It is not uncommon to have extended family living together and older members assisting with child care.	English	Wife or mother is the source of advice on medical ailments and when to seek medical treatment. Many believe that illness comes from germs. Others believe that illness can result from natural causes (e.g., exposure to wind, rain) or unnatural causes (witchcraft, voodoo, punishment for sin). Poverty and lack of health insurance lead to inadequate health care. Many rely on folk remedies passed from one generation to next before seeking care from physician. "Granny" or "old lady" is woman in community with knowledge of herbs to treat common illnesses. Spiritualist is someone with a special gift from God to heal certain diseases. Prayer is commonly used in response to illness.	Begin cereal consumption in infancy at early age. This culture is least likely to breastfeed. Religious orientation is strong (Baptist predominant). Use belly band or binder to protect newborn's umbilicus from dirt, injury, or hernias. Strict parenting practices are encouraged and are meant to develop effective coping abilities in children to prepare them for the racial discrimination they are likely to encounter in society. There is a high respect for authority figures, a strong work ethic, and an emphasis on achievement. Expression of emotions by males and females is encouraged. Children are expected to use their time wisely, assume responsibilities at an

ASIAN

Group	Family Organization	Communication	Nutrition	Health Beliefs	Child-Rearing/Health Practices
Vietnamese	Patriarchal in structure. Extended families are predominant. Primogeniture (first son inherits family's worth).	Avoid confrontations with health care professionals, perhaps answering questions with what they believe the other person wants to hear. May consider health practitioners to be loud and boisterous. Do not touch children on the head. The head is considered sacred because it is where one's consciousness lies. Eye contact may be considered rude. Beckoning with one's hand or finger is the gesture used to beckon dogs and is considered insulting when used with people.	A diet high in fat and sodium is considered an indication of well-being. Many individuals have lactose intolerance; therefore milk may be inadequate in the diets of pregnant women and children.	Forces of yang (light, heat, or dryness) and yin (darkness, cold, and wetness) influence the balance and harmony of a person's state of health. Seek a shaman (a physician-priest) for treatment remedies and spiritual healing ceremonies. Evil spirits enter the body through open orifices such as the ears, nose, and mouth, causing infection. If the opening is covered, the bad spirits cannot enter and the illness is cured. Health represents an equilibrium between hot and cold, wet and dry. An imbalance in these forces causes disease.	early age, and participate in decision making. Physical forms of discipline are often used. Breastfeeding may be delayed for 3 days because the colostrum is considered "dirty." Breastfeeding is low among immigrant Southeast Asians. Boys are breastfed longer than girls. Delay the introduction of solid foods up to 18 months. Diet may consist of breast milk and rice water; the diet is low in calcium and iron. Excessive consumption of cow's milk (up to eight bottles a day) in the second year of life is common, as is the continual use of the bottle instead of the cup into the third year of life. Avoid praising an infant for fear that a spirit may overhear the praise and be tempted to steal the infant. Parents have an approach to childrearing that is more controlling, achievement oriented, and more encouraging of independence than that of other parents. Balance and harmony are accomplished.
Chinese	Needs of the family come before the needs of the individual.	Silence does not necessarily indicate the end of a conversation; it		Forces of yang (light, heat, or dryness) and yin (darkness, cold, and wetness) influence the balance and harmony of person's state of health.	Primary responsibility for child care belongs to mother. Grandparents may be asked to assist in child care.

Continued

Modified from Bowden, V., Dickey, S., & Greenberg, C. (1998). *Children and their families: The continuum of care.* Philadelphia: W.B. Saunders; and Lipson, J. Dibble, S., & Minarek, P. (1998). *Culture and nursing care;* San Francisco: University of California—San Francisco Nursing Press.

table 15-2 *Cultural Influences on the Family—cont'd*

CULTURAL GROUP	FAMILY AND KINSHIP STRUCTURE	COMMUNICATION	HEALTH BELIEFS AND PRACTICES	FAMILY AND CHILD CARE PRACTICES
Chinese— cont'd	Children repay their parents' love and care by providing for them in their old age. Extended family important, with older adults respected and cared for in the homes of the adult children. Interracial marriages are frowned upon.	may mean the speaker wishes the listener to consider the content before the speaker continues.	Health is a state of physical and spiritual harmony with nature. Prevention is key to healthy living. Traditional Chinese medicine is sought before Western medical services. Use acupuncture, herbal medicines, massage, cupping, skin scraping, and moxibustion as therapies to restore yin and yang. Avoid eating soy sauce during pregnancy because it is believed to darken the infant's skin; shellfish is believed to cause allergies in the infant, and iron supplements are believed to harden bones and lead to difficult delivery.	Cultural healing practices can cause visible bruising or injury to child's skin. It is important for children to exhibit self-control. Children are socialized not to challenge authority. Pregnancy means woman has "happiness in her body." Many children are breastfed until they are 4 to 5 years of age. Jade is often worn in the form of a charm to keep the child safe. Believe physical illness is caused by an imbalance of ying and yang in body.
Japanese	Value social group harmony over individual needs and autonomy. Family structure is extended and patriarchal. Women are traditionally passive.	Silence does not necessarily indicate the end of a conversation; it may mean the speaker wishes the listener to consider the content before the speaker continues. Handshakes are acceptable; a pat on the back is not acceptable. Direct eye contact considered a lack of respect.	When in pain, patients stoically withstand comfort. Women labor in silence. After delivery, long periods of rest and recuperation are encouraged. Use natural herbs—Kampō medicine. Use both Western and traditional Oriental healing methods.	Mother has primary responsibility for childrearing and ensuring the child's success in school. Mother may sleep with her child. Colostrum is not fed to infants. Only half of all breastfed infants continue to be breastfed after age 1 month.
Hmong	Extended family structure.	Do not touch children on the head. The head is considered sacred because it is where one's consciousness lies.	Seek shaman (a physician-priest) for treatment remedies and spiritual healing ceremonies.	Avoid praising an infant for fear that a spirit may overhear the praise and be tempted to steal the infant. Infants may wear colorful hats so they are disguised as "flowers" and the spirits will not notice them.

EUROPEAN

	Family	Communication	Health Beliefs	
Caucasian American	Nuclear family is highly valued. Divorce and remarriage are a common practice. Goal of individual often seen as more important than goal of the family. Success is measured in terms of financial wealth and status in society.	Pat children on head to show affection or approval. Uncomfortable with periods of silence. Expect people to look you in the eye when they are speaking to you. Avoiding eye contact can be considered an indication that a person is lying.	Rely on modern medicine and health care professionals to treat illness.	Style of parenting is authoritative. Children are encouraged to value individual differences, the future rather than the present, material well-being, and competition and to consider many options when making decisions. Adults readily praise the infant's and child's behavior and appearance. Self-reliance is highly valued.
Irish American	Strong family bonds. Emphasis is placed on the well-being of family, not individual members.	May communicate with flowery and sometimes exaggerated words. May be overly verbose in descriptions of their condition.	Health comes when person is goal oriented and nurtures a strong religious faith. Health is maintained with a great deal of sleep combined with fresh air, exercise, and balanced diet. Home remedies or treatments are first resort to treat illness. Medical assistance should be sought only in cases of emergency.	Strict followers of the church—typically Protestant or Catholic.
Italian American	Family roles are traditional. Father is head of household, and mother is heart of the household, although mother has powerful sway over internal family matters. Children are valued members and are showered with love and affection.	Complaining loudly and making demands are often rewarded with attention.	Health is maintained by strong religious influence (primarily Catholic). Faith in God and saints will see them through illness. Beliefs about the cause of illness have been found to include winds and currents that bear diseases, contagion or contamination, heredity, supernatural or human causes, and psychosomatic explanations.	It is important to keep child warm in cold weather, stay out of drafts, and not go outside with wet hair. Maintain health with a nutritious diet of fruit, vegetables, pasta, hard cheese, and wine. Children are introduced to water-wine mixture at a young age.

Continued

Modified from Bowden, V., Dickey, S., & Greenberg, C. (1998). *Children and their families: The continuum of care.* Philadelphia: W.B. Saunders; and Lipson, J. Dibble, S., & Minarek, P. (1998). *Culture and nursing care;* San Francisco: University of California—San Francisco Nursing Press.

table 15-2 *Cultural Influences on the Family—cont'd*

CULTURAL GROUP	FAMILY AND KINSHIP STRUCTURE	COMMUNICATION	HEALTH BELIEFS AND PRACTICES	FAMILY AND CHILD CARE PRACTICES
Italian American—cont'd	Family is a source of comfort and pride for individual members. Members maintain close contact or close proximity with nuclear and extended family. Divorce is uncommon in traditional families. Large family size is attributed to adherence to Catholic beliefs and traditions.			
NATIVE AMERICAN	Grandparents retain important role in parenting their grandchildren. Extended family network is valued. Many Native Americans have married into other tribes and other ethnic groups. Children respect elders.	Silence is critical during interactions. Strong need to sit quietly and think before responding to questions. Eye contact may be considered rude. May consider health practitioners to be loud and boisterous. Spokesperson may not be decision maker.	Wellness exists when there is harmony in body, mind, and spirit. Seek shaman (a physician-priest) for treatment remedies and spiritual healing ceremonies. High incidence of lactose intolerance. Eat nonperishable food items because of lack of refrigeration. Beans are the main source of protein. Frequent problems with obesity and alcoholism. Often feel that Western medicine places too much emphasis on medications. A holistic approach to healing is valued. Alcoholism is a major problem for many families.	High rate of breastfeeding. Mothers retain primary responsibility for childrearing and discipline. Medicine bag is often worn by ill person and must not be handled by caregivers.

Modified from Bowden, V., Dickey, S., & Greenberg, C. (1998). *Children and their families: The continuum of care.* Philadelphia: W.B. Saunders; and Lipson, J. Dibble, S., & Minarek, P. (1998). *Culture and nursing care;* San Francisco: University of California—San Francisco Nursing Press.

"unique organization of characteristics that determine the individual's typical or recurrent pattern of behavior." No two persons are exactly alike. An individual's personality is the result of interaction between biological and environmental heritages.

Although no one group of theories can explain all human behavior, each can make a useful contribution to it. Many experts have devoted their lives to understanding why children and families behave as they do. Some experts, called *systems theorists,* believe that everyone in the family or system is affected by each of its members. This theory focuses on the interrelatedness of the various persons as opposed to an analysis of an individual in the group. Nurses using systems theory focus on caring for the child by caring for the whole family. They see the family as protector, educator, resource, and health provider for the child. In turn, they see the child's health as having an impact on each member of the family as a whole.

Many experts see human development as a composite of various theories. The hierarchy of needs developed by Abraham Maslow is depicted in Figure 15-5, and the developmental theories of Erik Erikson, Sigmund Freud, Lawrence Kohlberg, Harry Stack Sullivan, and Jean Piaget are presented in Table 15-3. Other theorists are briefly contrasted within appropriate chapters devoted to specific age-groups. Theories provide a framework for the practitioner; however, humans are not a gathering of isolated parts, even though these parts must be dissected for investigative purposes.

Cognitive Development

Cognition (*cognoscere,* "to know") refers to intellectual ability. Children are born with inherited potential, but the potential must be developed. "It requires opportunities for exploration that are neither too easy nor too hard" (Levine, Carey, & Crocker, 1999). The development of logical thinking and conceptual understanding is a complex process. One outstanding authority on cognitive development was Piaget, a Swiss psychologist. He proposed that intellectual maturity is attained through four orderly and distinct stages of development, all of which are interrelated: *sensorimotor* (up to 2 years), *preoperational* (2 to 7 years), *concrete operations* (7 to 11 years), and *formal operations* (11 to 16 years). The ages for each stage are approximate, and each stage builds on the preceding one.

Piaget believed that intelligence consists of interaction and coping with the environment. Infants begin their interaction by reflex response. As they grow older, their use of symbolism (particularly language) increases. Gradually they acquire a here-and-now orientation (concrete operations) and finally a fully abstract comprehension of the world (formal operations). Table 15-4 relates Piaget's theory to feeding and nutrition. It is a good example of how a knowledge of development can help in understanding the behavior of a child at a particular time.

Moral Development

Lawrence Kohlberg, a childhood theorist, suggests that moral development in children is sequential. His theories on moral development are based on Piaget's cognitive development investigations. He describes three levels: *preconventional, conventional,* and *postconventional.* Each level contains two stages. In the preconventional stage (4 to 7 years), children try to be obedient to their parents for fear of punishment. During the conventional phase (7 to 11 years), children show conformity and loyalty, and they focus on obeying rules. In the postconventional level (12 years and older), *moral values* are developed to solve complex problems. There is an emphasis on the conscience of the individual within the society. Although rules are still important, changing them to meet the needs of a culture is considered.

THE GROWTH AND DEVELOPMENT OF A PARENT

Table 15-5 shows the task of the parent that relates to the child's developmental task of Erikson's stages, as well as some suggestions for nursing interventions that can assist in the growth and development of a parent and a child.

Erikson's stages of child development demonstrate the various tasks that must be mastered at each age to achieve optimum maturity. Each stage builds on the successful completion of the previous stage. Achievement of the tasks of childhood do not occur in isolation. Parents must *interact* appropriately to assist the child to

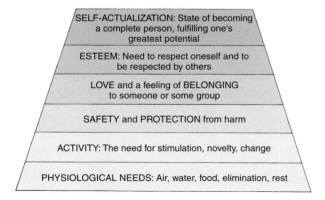

FIGURE **15-5** Maslow's hierarchy of basic needs. The needs at the bottom of the pyramid must be met before one can fulfill needs at the next higher level.

table 15-3 | *Comparison of the Developmental Theories of Erikson, Freud, Kohlberg, Sullivan, and Piaget*

DEVELOPMENTAL PERIOD	ERIKSON	FREUD	KOHLBERG	SULLIVAN	PIAGET
Infancy	*Trust/mistrust* Getting Tolerating frustration in small doses Recognizing mother as distinct from others and self	*Orality*—understanding the world by exploring with the mouth	*Preconventional/ premoral*—cannot distinguish right from wrong	Security Patterns of emotional response Organization of sensation	*Sensorimotor stage* (birth to 2 years)—at birth, responses are limited to reflexes; begins to relate to outside events; concerned by sensations and actions that affect self directly
Toddler	*Autonomy/shame and doubt* Trying out own powers of speech Beginning acceptance of reality versus pleasure principle	*Anality*—learning to give and take	*Punishment/ obedience*—performance based on fear of punishment	Mastery of space and objects	*Preoperational* (2 to 7 years)—child is still egocentric; thinks everyone sees world as self does
Preschool	*Initiative/guilt* Questioning Exploring own body and environment Differentiation of sexes	*Phallic/oedipal phase*—becoming aware of self as sexual being	*Morality*—rules are absolute; breaking rules results in punishment; behavior based on rewards	Speech and conscious need for playmates, interpersonal communication	*Perceptual* (4 to 7 years)—capable of some reasoning but can concentrate on only one aspect of a situation at a time
School age	*Industry/inferiority* Learning to win recognition by producing things Exploring, collecting Learning to relate to own sex	*Latency*—focusing on peer relations; learning to live in groups and to achieve	*Conventional morality*—rules are created for the benefit of all; adhering to rules is the right thing to do (7 to 11 years)	Chumship, one-to-one relationship, self-esteem, compassion (homosexuality)	*Concrete operations* (7 to 11 years)—reasoning is logical but limited to own experience; understands cause and effect
Adolescence	*Identity/role diffusion* Moving toward heterosexuality Selecting vocation Beginning separation from family Integrating personality (e.g., altruism)	*Genitality*	*Principled morality* (autonomous stage) (12 years on)—acceptance of right or wrong on basis of own perceptions of world and personal conscience	Capacity to love, empathy, partnership (heterosexuality)	*Formal operational stage* (11 to 16 years)—acquires ability to develop abstract concepts for self; oriented to problem solving

table 15-4 | *Piaget's Theory of Cognitive Development in Relation to Feeding and Nutrition*

DEVELOPMENTAL PERIOD	COGNITIVE CHARACTERISTICS	RELATIONSHIPS TO FEEDING AND NUTRITION
Sensorimotor (birth to 2 years)	Progression is from newborn with automatic reflexes to intentional interaction with the environment and the beginning use of symbols.	Progression is made from sucking and rooting reflexes to the acquisition of self-feeding skills. Food is used primarily to satisfy hunger, as a medium to explore the environment, and to practice fine motor skills.
Preoperational (2 to 7 years)	Thought processes become internalized; they are unsystematic and intuitive. Use of symbols increases. Reasoning is based on appearances and happenstance. Approach to classification is functional and unsystematic. Child's world is viewed egocentrically.	Eating becomes less the center of attention than social, language, and cognitive growth. Food is described by color, shape, and quantity, but there is limited ability to classify food into "groups." Foods tend to be classed as "like" and "don't like." Child can identify food as "good for you," but reasons are unknown or mistaken.
Concrete operations (7 to 11 years)	Child can focus on several aspects of a situation simultaneously. Cause-effect reasoning becomes more rational and systematic. Ability to classify, reclassify, and generalize emerges. Decrease in egocentrism permits child to take another's view.	Child begins to realize that nutritious food has a positive effect on growth and health but has limited understanding of how or why this occurs. Mealtimes take on a social significance. Expanding environment increases the opportunities for, and influences on, food selection (peer influence rises).
Formal operations (11 to 16 years)	Hypothetic and abstract thought expand. Understanding of scientific and theoretic processes deepens.	The concept of nutrients from food functioning at physiological and biochemical levels can be understood. Conflicts in making food choices may be realized (knowledge of nutritious food versus preferences and nonnutritive influences).

From Mahan, L. K., & Escott-Stump, S. (2000). *Krause's food, nutrition and diet therapy* (10th ed.). Philadelphia: W.B. Saunders.

table 15-5 | *The Growth and Development of a Parent*

CHILD'S TASKS (ERIKSON'S STAGES)	PARENT'S TASK	NURSING INTERVENTION
FIRST PRENATAL TRIMESTER		
Growth	Develop attitude toward newborn: Happy about child? Parent of one disabled child? Unwed mother? These factors and others will affect the developing attitude of the mother.	Develop positive attitude in both parents concerning expected birth of child. Use referrals and agencies as needed.
SECOND PRENATAL TRIMESTER		
Growth	Mother focuses on infant because of fetal movements felt. Parents picture what infant will look like, what future he or she will have, and other ideas.	Parents' focus is on child care and needs and providing physical environment for expected infant. Therefore information concerning care of the newborn should be given at this time.

Continued

| table 15-5 | *The Growth and Development of a Parent—cont'd* |

CHILD'S TASKS (ERIKSON'S STAGES)	PARENT'S TASK	NURSING INTERVENTION
THIRD PRENATAL TRIMESTER		
Growth	Mother feels large. Attention focuses on how fetus is going to get out.	Detailed information should be presented at this time concerning the birth processes, preparation for birth, breastfeeding, and care of sibling at home.
BIRTH		
Adjust to external environment	Elicit positive responses from child and respond by meeting child's need for food and closeness. If parents receive only negative responses (e.g., sleepy infant, crying infant, difficult feeder, congenital anomaly), development of the parent will be inhibited.	Encourage early touch, feeding, and other practices. Explain behavior and appearance of newborn to allay fears. Help parents to identify positive responses. (Use infant's reflexes, such as grasp reflex, to identify a positive response by placing mother's finger into infant's hand.)
INFANT		
Develop trust	Learn "cues" presented by infant to determine individual needs of infant.	Help parents assess and interpret needs of infant (avoid feelings of helplessness or incompetence). Do not let in-laws take over parental tasks. Help parents cope with problems such as colic.
TODDLER		
Autonomy	Try to accept the pattern of growth and development. Accept some loss of control but maintain some limits for safety.	Help parents cope with transient independence of child (e.g., allow child to go on tricycle but don't yell "Don't fall" or anxiety will be radiated).
PRESCHOOL		
Initiative	Learn to separate from child.	Help parents show standards but "let go" so child can develop some independence. A preschool experience may be helpful.
SCHOOL AGE		
Industry	Accept importance of child's peers. Parents must learn to accept some rejection from child at times. Patience is needed to allow children to do for themselves, even if it takes longer. Do not *do* the school project *for* the child. Provide chores for child appropriate to his age level.	Help parents to understand that child is developing his or her own limits and self-discipline. Be there to guide child, but do not constantly intrude. Help child get results from his or her own efforts at performance.
ADOLESCENT		
Establishing identity Accepting pubertal changes Developing abstract reasoning Deciding on career Investigating lifestyles Controlling feelings	Parents must learn to let child live his or her own life and not expect total control over the child. Expect, at times, to be discredited by teenager. Expect differences in opinion and respect them. Guide but do not push.	Help parents adjust to changing role and relationship with adolescent (e.g., as child develops his or her own identify, he may become a Democrat if parents are Republican). Expose child to varied career fields and life experiences. Help child to understand emerging emotions and feelings brought about by puberty.

achieve successfully at his or her developmental level. For example, if the parent constructs a school project for a child, the child will not achieve a sense of industry. If the parent does not accept a positive attitude toward the pregnancy and attempts to abort unsuccessfully, the parent may become overly protective or abusive to the newborn infant, and bonding will not occur.

Parents should be guided not to attempt to prevent frustration in the lives of their children. Experiences in dealing with challenges and disappointments prepare the child to function independently in adulthood. Parents should encourage a child to deal with successes and failures, provide socially acceptable outlets, and intervene only if the frustrations become overwhelming. The parent's task is to provide the child with the skills and tools appropriate at each age level to deal with events. Current tips concerning parenting skills can be accessed at http://www.iamyourchild.org.

NUTRITION

NUTRITIONAL HERITAGE

Good nutrition begins before conception. Nutritional needs during pregnancy are discussed in Chapter 4. The dependent child is fed for many years by adults whose eating habits may be based on misinformation, income level, folklore, fads, or religious, cultural, and ethnic preferences. Table 15-6 describes some common and selected food patterns of various cultures found in the United States. Many families are poor, others have inadequate knowledge of how to prepare foods, and many rely on convenience foods to save time.

Some families do not consider food a priority in the home. However, optimum nutrition is essential for the child to reach his or her growth potential. A lack of adequate nutrition can lead to mental retardation. The obese child may be subject to decreased motor skills and peer rejection, leading to low self-esteem.

The nurse is in a position to identify children at risk and to help families modify eating habits to ensure proper nutrition. An important resource for the nurse is the nutritionist in the community or on the staff of the health agency where the nurse is employed. Formula feeding and breastfeeding are discussed in Chapter 9.

FAMILY NUTRITION

The U.S. Departments of Agriculture and Health and Human Services guidelines for good eating are illustrated by a food pyramid (see Figure 15-6, *A*). The food pyramid is intended to help Americans make informed decisions about what they eat. Families who practice such principles are educating their children by good

example. Many families are vegetarian, and the use of teaching tools that respect the dietary limitations will encourage compliance. Figure 15-6, *B*, demonstrates a modification of the standard food pyramid. This food pyramid is directed toward vegetarian families and applies to children as young as age 2 years. The nurse should assess restricted foods in the vegetarian diet and ensure that the diet is adequate in protein, vitamins, and minerals to promote growth and development in children. Children on vegetarian diets often consume large amounts of high-fiber foods. High-fiber foods cause increased losses of calcium, zinc, magnesium, and iron in the stool and may require supplements. A diet containing meat, poultry, or fortified foods lessens this nutrient deficiency.

Different types of fiber are contained in foods (Table 15-7). The water-soluble fiber found in oats, apples, and citrus fruits delays intestinal transit and decreases serum cholesterol levels. The water-insoluble fiber found in whole-grain breads, wheat bran, and some cereals accelerates intestinal transit and slows starch digestion.

A well-balanced diet supplies all essential nutrients in the necessary amounts. Food provides heat and energy, builds and repairs tissues, and regulates body processes. A given food is a mixture of elements such as minerals (e.g., calcium, phosphorus, sodium, iron), compounds (carbohydrates, fats, proteins, some vitamins), and water. The body needs approximately 50 nutrients, which it absorbs at various sites (Figure 15-7). Table 15-8 specifies the new recommended dietary allowances (RDA) and recommended dietary intakes (RDI) for children.

Children are susceptible to nutritional deficiencies because they are growing and developing. Infants require more calories, protein, minerals, and vitamins in proportion to their weight than do adults. Fluid requirements are also higher for infants. Eating a *variety* of foods selected from the basic food groups ensures good health for children. The *amount* and *size* of portions are important in maintaining a reasonable weight. *There are no known advantages to consuming excessive amounts of any nutrients, and there are risks for overdoses.*

> ⭐NURSING **TIP**
>
> The American Academy of Pediatrics recommends 0.5 g of fiber/kg of body weight in childhood, gradually increasing to adult levels of 20 to 35 g/day by the end of adolescence. High-fiber foods can fill the small stomach capacity and provide few of the nutrients and calories needed by the active, growing child.

table 15-6 | *Culturally Diverse Food Patterns of Americans*

CULTURE	HISTORICAL DIETARY PATTERN*
African American	All meats, fish, and chicken; pork is often consumed (spareribs, bacon, and sausage). Vegetables are cooked in salt pork for long periods of time; grits and cornbread muffins. There is some lactose intolerance. Popular vegetables include collard greens, beet greens, and sweet potatoes.
Chinese American	Rich in vegetables (bean sprouts, broccoli, bamboo shoots, and mushrooms). Vegetables are cooked until crisp; meat is consumed in small portions with other food. Soy sauce, tofu, peanut butter; limited milk and cheese; fish baked with native spices; soups with egg, meat, and vegetables. Tea is China's national beverage. Rice is staple of diet.
Jewish American	Diet varies according to whether family is Orthodox, Reformed, or Conservative. For an Orthodox family, food must be kosher (clean); meat is soaked in salt water to remove blood; only meat eaten is that of divided-hoofed animals that chew a cud; fish without scales (shellfish) and pork are prohibited; milk and meat cannot be combined. Favorites are gefilte fish, lox (smoked salmon), herring, eggs, bagels, cream cheese, and matzo.
Laotian American	Numerous varieties of freshwater fish and shellfish (eaten fresh, dried, or salted); pork, beef, chicken, rabbit, often mixed with vegetables and spices; eggs, peanuts, black-eyed peas; vegetables eaten raw, as juice, or cooked with meat or fish and preserved by drying or pickling; sticky rice, rice or bean thread noodles, and legumes often used in desserts; soybean drink, sugar cane drink, tea, and coconut juice. Popular seasonings include padek, chilies, curry, tamarind, and red and black pepper.
Italian American	All meats, fish, and chicken, including cold cuts (salami, mortadella) and Italian pork sausage; pasta (staple of diet), breads, olive oil, wine, cheese, and all varieties of fruits and vegetables.
Japanese American	Fish and seafood (fresh, smoked, and raw) and beef. Food is cut into small portions. Principal fruit is nasi, which tastes much like a pear. Many vegetables are eaten, such as seaweed, bamboo shoots, onions, beans, and dried mushrooms (shitake); enjoy pickled vegetables. Rice is national staple. Beverages include tea and sake. Little cheese, milk, butter, or cream is consumed. Chief cooking fat is soybean oil or rice oil.
Mexican American	Chicken, pork chops, wieners, cold cuts, hamburger, eggs (used frequently), beans (eaten mashed or refried with lard), potatoes (basic item, usually fried), chilies, fresh tomatoes, corn (maize—often used as basic grain), tortillas, packaged cereals; little milk because of lactose intolerance.
Native American	Acorn flour, a staple food made into mush or bread; salmon, fresh or dried; other varieties of fish, deer, duck, geese, and other small game; nuts such as buckeye and hazel; wild berries, seeds, and roots.
Puerto Rican American	Meat cooked in stews; poultry, pork, fish, dried beans or peas mixed with rice; milk in combination with coffee (cafe con leche), variety of fruits, starchy vegetables (plantains, cassava, sweet potatoes), salad, soft drinks.
Vietnamese American	Pork—most common meat; meats cut into small pieces and fried, boiled, or steamed; fish—all types of freshwater and saltwater fish and shellfish, often fried and dipped in fish sauce; eggs, soybeans, legumes, and wide variety of fruits and vegetables; rice often eaten with every meal; seasonings including oyster sauce, soy sauce, monosodium glutamate, ginger, garlic, nuoc mam sauce; tea, coffee, soft drinks, soybean milk.

Data from Mahan, L. K., & Escott-Stump, S. (2000). *Krause's food, nutrition and diet therapy* (10th ed.). Philadelphia: W.B. Saunders; Wetter, A., et al. (2001). How and why do individuals make food and activity choices? *Nutrition Review, 59*(3), 11-21; and Booth, S., et al. (2001). Environmental and societal factors affect food choice and physical activity: Rationale, influences, and leverage points, *Nutrition Review, 59*(3), 21-40.
*More diverse eating patterns occur as future generations of a culture become assimilated.

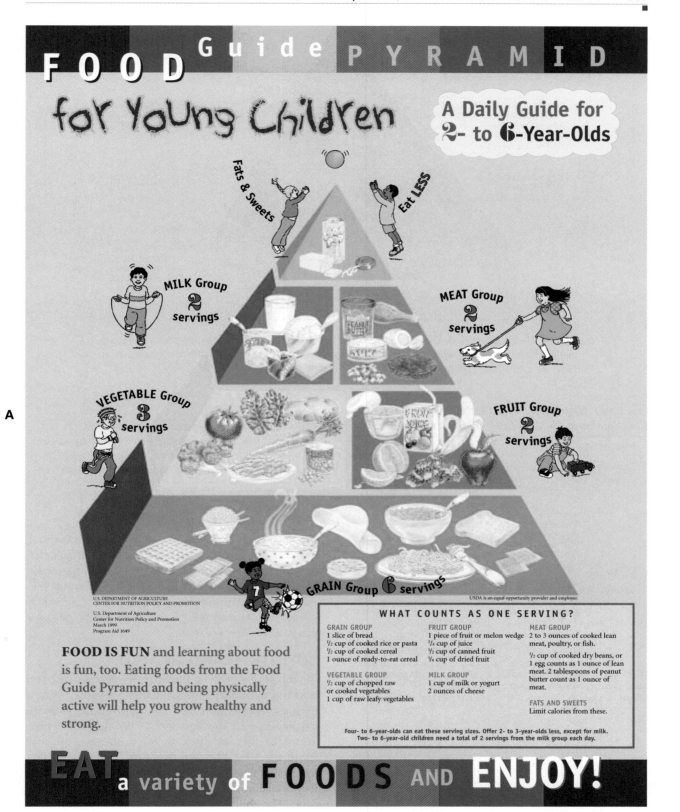

FIGURE **15-6, A,** The Children's Food Pyramid. This food pyramid can be used to teach children about a balanced diet that will promote growth and development. *Continued*

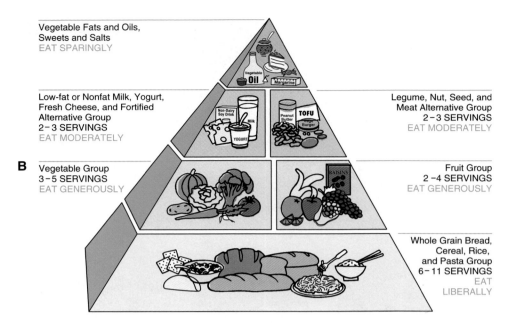

B

Vegetable Fats and Oils,
Sweets and Salts
EAT SPARINGLY

Low-fat or Nonfat Milk, Yogurt,
Fresh Cheese, and Fortified
Alternative Group
2–3 SERVINGS
EAT MODERATELY

Legume, Nut, Seed, and
Meat Alternative Group
2–3 SERVINGS
EAT MODERATELY

Vegetable Group
3–5 SERVINGS
EAT GENEROUSLY

Fruit Group
2–4 SERVINGS
EAT GENEROUSLY

Whole Grain Bread,
Cereal, Rice,
and Pasta Group
6–11 SERVINGS
EAT
LIBERALLY

FIGURE **15-6, cont'd B,** The Vegetarian Food Pyramid. A food pyramid designed for vegetarians will promote compliance when teaching parents and children concerning recommended dietary intakes for a balanced diet that will promote growth and development.

---

table 15-7	High-Fiber Foods for Relief of Mild Constipation in Children Over 12 Months of Age	
TYPE OF FOOD	**SERVING SIZE**	**EXAMPLE***
Cereals, bread	1 ounce	Raisin Bran, Grapenuts, Shredded Wheat, Bran Chex
	1 slice	Whole-grain bread
	1 medium	Bran muffin
	2½-inch square	Corn bread
Fruits	½ cup	Cooked prunes
Vegetables	½ cup	Spinach
	1 medium	Corn on the cob
Meat substitute	½ cup	Beans (baked, black, garbanzo, kidney, lima, pinto, lentil)

Modified from Baker, S. (1994). Introduce fruits, vegetables, and grains but don't overdo high-fiber foods. *Pediatric Basics,* 69, Summer, 2-4.
*All products indicated are registered trademarks of their respective companies.

NURSING TIP

Raw fruits that contain seeds or some raw vegetables and nuts may not be appropriate foods for infants and young children because of the risk of choking. Beans and vegetables should be well cooked.

NURSING TIP

Foods containing essential minerals such as iron, zinc, and calcium should be combined with citrus, fish, or poultry to enhance absorption of the minerals. Vitamin D and lactose sugars also enhance mineral absorption in the body.

NUTRITIONAL CARE PLAN

The nutritional care plan can be used in the hospital, home, or outpatient department. Parts of the care plan may already have been collected by other professionals, and the nurse should refer to the patient's chart for pertinent data. The nutritional care plan provides information and stores it in one place. It can also be put on a computer for easy retrieval.

NUTRITION AND HEALTH

The digestive system of the newborn is immature and functions minimally during the first 3 months. Saliva is minimal; hydrochloric acid and renin in the stomach and trypsin aid in the digestion of milk. Amylase (a pancreatic enzyme) and lipase are not in adequate quantity before age 4 months, and therefore complex carbohydrates and fats cannot be digested effectively. Excess fiber intake in the young infant results in loose, bulky stools. The ability of the liver to function is limited in the first year of life. The teeth are not present for chewing before 6 to 8 months of age.

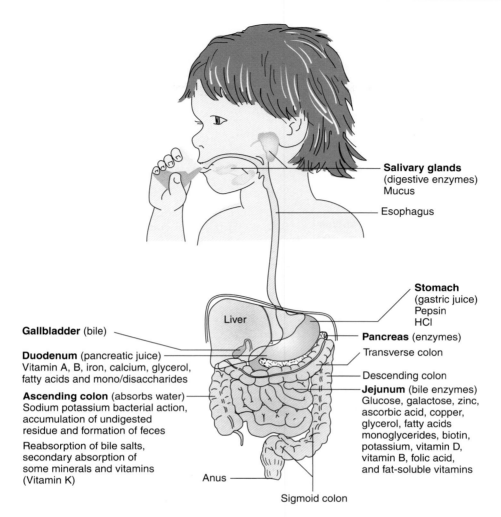

Salivary glands
(digestive enzymes)
Mucus

Esophagus

Stomach
(gastric juice)
Pepsin
HCl

Pancreas (enzymes)

Transverse colon

Liver

Gallbladder (bile)

Descending colon

Duodenum (pancreatic juice)
Vitamin A, B, iron, calcium, glycerol,
fatty acids and mono/disaccharides

Jejunum (bile enzymes)
Glucose, galactose, zinc,
ascorbic acid, copper,
glycerol, fatty acids
monoglycerides, biotin,
potassium, vitamin D,
vitamin B, folic acid,
and fat-soluble vitamins

Ascending colon (absorbs water)
Sodium potassium bacterial action,
accumulation of undigested
residue and formation of feces

Reabsorption of bile salts,
secondary absorption of
some minerals and vitamins
(Vitamin K)

Anus

Sigmoid colon

FIGURE **15-7** Nutrient digestion. The sites of absorption of major nutrients are shown in this illustration. Most nutrient absorption occurs in the duodenum and jejunum of the small intestine. Most water absorption occurs in the large intestine. Absorption of nutrients depends on adequate secretion of digestive enzymes, normal motility, and normal villi on the mucosal surface of the intestines. Portal circulation, lymphatic circulation, and hormones also play a role in the digestion and absorption of nutrients.

The physiology of digestion is the basis for food introduction in the first year of life. Breast milk or iron-fortified formula are the foods of choice for the first 6 months to 1 year of life. Introducing baby food before age 5 to 6 months is not for the purpose of nutritional gain. Overnutrition and its link to obesity in adults have been explored. The effects of childhood nutrition on adult health and illness patterns, such as heart disease, have been established.

NUTRITION AND ILLNESS

Therapeutic diets, such as the diabetic diet, are well established in medical care. Some foods can promote dental caries, and others contain protective fiber that are known to prevent some diseases. Atherosclerosis can be prevented by starting healthy dietary patterns in childhood. However, restrictive diets are not advised for infants and young children. Fat and cholesterol are needed for calories and the development of the central nervous system. The sodium content of baby foods has been decreased because the average diet contains adequate sodium. Some food additives, such as aspartame (an artificial sweetener), may be harmful to children with phenylketonuria. Food additives that prolong the shelf life of foods and food dyes that make food look more attractive should be minimized in the child's diet. Fast-food chains, often depended on by working parents and preferred by adolescents, make available to the con-

table 15-8 | *Recommended Dietary Allowances—RDI and RDA*

1997-1998 DIETARY REFERENCE INTAKES (DRI)

AGE (YR)	RECOMMENDED DIETARY ALLOWANCES (RDA)							ADEQUATE INTAKE (AI)						
	THIAMINE (mg)	RIBOFLAVIN (mg)	NIACIN (mg)	VITAMIN B6 (mg)	FOLATE (µg)	VITAMIN B12 (µg)	PHOSPHORUS (mg)	MAGNESIUM (mg)	VITAMIN D	PANTOTHENIC ACID (mg)	BIOTIN (µg)	CHOLINE (mg)	CALCIUM (mg)	FLUORIDE (mg)
INFANTS[a]														
0.0-0.5	0.2	0.3	2[b]	0.1	65	0.4	100	30	5	1.7	5	125	210	0.01
0.5-1.0	0.3	0.4	4	0.3	80	0.5	275	75	5	1.8	6	150	270	0.5
CHILDREN														
1-3	0.5	0.5	6	0.6	150	0.9	460	80	5	2.0	8	200	500	0.7
4-8	0.6	0.6	8	0.6	200	1.2	500	130	5	3.0	12	250	800	1.1
MALES														
9-13	0.9	0.9	12	1.0	300	1.8	1250	240	5	4.0	20	375	1300	2.0
14-18	1.2	1.3	16	1.3	400	2.4	1250	410	5	5.0	25	550	1300	3.2
FEMALES														
9-13	0.9	0.9	12	1.0	300	1.8	1250	240	5	4.0	20	375	1300	2.0
14-18	1.0	1.0	14	1.2	400	2.4	1250	360	5	5.0	25	400	1300	2.9

1989 RECOMMENDED DIETARY ALLOWANCES (RDA)

AGE (YR)	ENERGY (kcal)	PROTEIN (g)	VITAMIN A (µg)	VITAMIN E (mg)	VITAMIN K (µg)	VITAMIN C (mg)	IRON (mg)	ZINC (mg)	IODINE (µg)	SELENIUM (µg)
INFANTS										
0.0-0.5	650	13	375	3	5	30	6	5	40	10
0.5-1.0	850	14	375	4	10	35	10	5	50	15
CHILDREN										
1-3	1300	16	400	6	15	40	10	10	70	20
4-6	1800	24	500	7	20	45	10	10	90	20
7-10	2000	28	700	7	30	45	10	10	120	30
MALES										
11-14	2500	45	1000	10	45	50	12	15	150	40
15-18	3000	59	1000	10	65	60	12	15	150	50
FEMALES										
11-14	2200	46	800	8	45	50	15	12	150	45
15-18	2200	44	800	8	55	60	15	12	150	50

Modified from *Dietary Recommended Allowances*, 10th edition, and the first two of the *Dietary Reference Intakes* series, National Academy Press. Copyright 1989, 1997, and 1998, respectively, by the National Academy of Sciences. Courtesy of the National Academy Press, Washington, D.C.

[a]For all nutrients, an AI was established instead of an RDA as the goal for infants; for the B vitamins and choline, the age groupings are 0 through 5 months and 6 through 11 months.

[b]The AI for niacin for this age-group only is stated as milligrams of preformed niacin instead of niacin equivalents.

sumer the nutrient content of their foods served. The caloric content of the menu often depends on the foods selected and the toppings added. Therefore a "salad bar" is not necessarily synonymous with a low-calorie meal.

Height and weight should be plotted on a growth chart at each clinic visit to enable early identification of health problems related to dietary intake. The weight or triceps skinfold thickness greater than the 85th percentile or below the 3rd percentile indicates a need for further evaluation. The role of the grandparents in providing a diet that may lead to obesity must often be addressed, because the principles of good nutrition that were adhered to 20 or 30 years ago may no longer be valid. Concern is expressed over the level of cholesterol in children. Methods to reduce cholesterol in families are listed in Box 15-4. The National Cholesterol Education Program's recommendations are cited in Box 15-5.

Dietary supplements, formulas, and nutritional support techniques for preterm infants, children with cancer, and those with long-term disorders (e.g., cystic fi-

brosis) have become sophisticated and are used successfully. Total parenteral nutrition allows the physician to choose preparations ranging from amino acids and intravenous fats to complete multivitamins. Total

---

box 15-4 | ***Methods to Reduce Cholesterol in School-Age Children***

- Exercise more with your children.
- Provide fresh fruits and vegetables rather than empty calories such as those found in doughnuts and store-bought pastries.
- Decrease trips to fast-food restaurants.
- Switch to low-fat foods; use vegetable oil cooking sprays in place of butter; bake or broil foods instead of frying them.
- Seek the advice of a nutritionist.
- If you have a family history of heart disease, have your child's as well as your levels of cholesterol tested.

---

box 15-5 | ***National Cholesterol Evaluation Program (NCEP) Recommendations for Detecting and Managing Hypercholesterolemia in Children and Adolescents***

The NCEP has made recommendations for managing hypercholesterolemia to be applied to adolescents and children over 2 years of age.

For the general population of children and adolescents in the United States, NCEP recommends that eating patterns be adopted to meet the following criteria:

- Nutritionally adequate, varied diet
- Adequate energy intake to support growth and development and maintain appropriate body weight
- Saturated fat—less than 10% of total calories
- Total fat—an average of no more than 30% of total calories
- Dietary cholesterol—less than 300 mg/day

To implement these patterns means involving the entire community—parents (in the selection and preparation of food), schools (by modification of school food service), health care clinics (by providing health education), government (by mandating improvement of food labeling), and the food industry (by developing low-saturated-fat, low-fat foods that are appealing to children).

NCEP also aims to identify and treat individual children and adolescents who have hypercholesterolemia and a family history of premature cardiovascular disease or whose parents have hypercholesterolemia. For this group, NCEP recommends the following:

- Blood cholesterol screening of children and adolescents whose parents or grandparents (at age 55 years or younger) were found to have coronary atherosclerosis; suffered myocardial infarction, peripheral vascular disease, cerebrovascular disease, or sudden death; or underwent invasive cardiac therapy (balloon angioplasty or coronary artery bypass surgery)
- Blood cholesterol screening of offspring of a parent with a blood cholesterol of 240 mg/dl or greater
- Appropriate levels for total cholesterol and low-density-lipoprotein (LDL) cholesterol. For children with levels above these, dietary change is recommended:

Category	Total Cholesterol	LDL Cholesterol
Acceptable	<170 mg/dl	<110 mg/dl
Borderline	170-199 mg/dl	110-129 mg/dl
High	≥200 mg/dl	≥130 mg/dl

A family history of high cholesterol is indication for screening of the child.

If there is insufficient blood lipid lowering after 6 months to 1 year of dietary therapy, drug therapy can be considered in children over 10 years of age.

Modified from Mahan, L.K., & Escott-Stump, S. (2000). *Krause's food, nutrition, and diet therapy* (10th ed.). Philadelphia: W.B. Saunders.

parenteral nutrition and enteral feedings allow children who need nutritional support to be cared for at home, thus greatly enhancing the quality of life.

In the 1990s an oral rehydration solution (ORS) used by third world populations for treating acute diarrhea in children gained acceptance and is now produced and distributed by the World Health Organization. It is composed mainly of electrolytes, glucose, and water. Health care workers are able to teach parents how to save the lives of their infants by using this simple solution. Medicine women, the respected leaders of some tribes, are being incorporated into the educational process. One example of a commercial preparation available in the United States is Pedialyte.

A cereal-based oral rehydrating solution can be made by mixing $\frac{1}{2}$ to 1 cup of infant rice cereal, 2 cups water, and $\frac{1}{4}$ teaspoon of table salt (Bartholmey, 1994). Often the older child who refuses the oral rehydrating solution can be offered a saltine cracker with half-strength apple juice.

FEEDING THE HEALTHY CHILD

Table 15-9 specifies the nursing interventions that help to meet the nutritional needs of children from infancy to adolescence.

The Infant

Infants require more calories, protein, minerals, and vitamins in proportion to their weight than do adults. Their fluid requirements are also high. Breast milk is excellent, and a nursing mother may continue this even when her infant is hospitalized. The nurse stresses that the mother should avoid fatigue because it affects milk production. Breast milk can be manually expressed and refrigerated at the hospital and then given in the mother's absence.

Some infants cannot tolerate milk because of intestinal bleeding, allergy, or other negative reactions. Many milk substitutes are available for therapeutic use. Among these are soybean mixtures (such as ProSobee and Isomil) for infants with milk-protein sensitivity. Most products come in dry and liquid forms, and parents must be made aware of what concentrations the physician recommends. Rice cereal is the first solid food introduced at age 6 months (Figure 15-8).

The nurse must be aware of the problems of underfeeding and overfeeding infants. Underfeeding is suggested by restlessness, crying, and failure to gain weight. Overfeeding is manifested by symptoms such as regurgitation, mild diarrhea, and too rapid a weight gain. Diets high in fat delay gastric emptying and cause abdominal distention. Diets too high in carbohydrates may cause distention, flatus, and excessive weight gain.

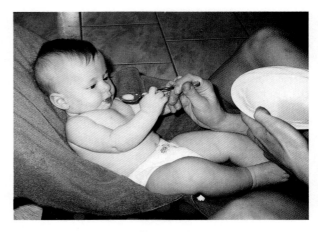

FIGURE **15-8** Spoon feeding. Solid foods should be introduced at age 6 months and fed by spoon to the infant. Cereal should not be mixed into the formula bottle when feeding the healthy infant.

Constipation may be the result of too much fat or protein or a deficiency in bulk. Increased amounts of cereals, vegetables, and fruits can often correct this problem.

Most infants naturally adapt to a schedule of three meals a day by the first year of life. At this time the appetite fluctuates as the growth rate slows somewhat. The child may not be interested in eating. Spills are frequent. At age 1 year, children cannot manipulate a spoon, but hand-to-mouth coordination is good enough that they enjoy holding a piece of toast while the nurse assists. In the hospital, children in highchairs are secured with safety belts. The nurse remains in constant attendance. Developmental advancements that change eating patterns are explained to parents to prevent feeding difficulties.

NURSING **TIP**

Whole milk should not be introduced before 1 year of age. Low-fat milk should not be introduced before 2 years of age.

The Toddler

Toddlers can feed themselves by the end of the second year. This is important in developing a sense of independence. The toddler may be rebellious at times, and food may be pushed away or completely refused. Toddlers benefit most from the caregivers' presence at mealtime. Feeding difficulties may result from the anxieties of parents and a lack of time planned for meals.

table 15-9 *Nursing Interventions for Meeting the Nutritional Needs of Children*

COMMENT	NURSING INTERVENTIONS
NEWBORNS AND INFANTS	
High energy maintenance because of immature systems (e.g., heat loss)	Assist mother with breastfeeding. Assist family with bottle feeding. Teach formula preparation.
Immature digestive system	Burp infant frequently. Place infant on right side after feeding.
Nutrient requirements related to body size	Observe infant for tolerance to formula. Consider vitamin C and D supplementation. Anticipate iron deficiencies (particularly in preterm newborns).
Need for additional nutrients, satiety	Introduce solids when age-appropriate, at about 6 months, starting with rice cereal, which is the least allergenic. Fruits and then vegetables may be added one at a time in 1-week intervals to allow time to observe for adverse responses (consider variety, portions, texture). Instruct parents not to add salt or sugar to baby foods to avoid high sodium and calorie intake.
Danger of choking decreases as swallowing matures	Anticipate allergies; as teething progresses, junior or chopped foods can be substituted for strained food. Explain selection and makeup of soy-based formulas if prescribed.
Prevention of dental decay	Encourage use of fluorides (after age 6 months) if fluoride content of community water supply is less than 0.6 ppm. Encourage weaning as appropriate to prevent bottle-mouth caries. Rinse infant's mouth after feedings.
Continued requirements for basic food groups	Assess the educational and financial needs of family. Use supplemental food programs (e.g., Women, Infants, and Children [WIC] program).
TODDLERS AND PRESCHOOLERS	
Slower rate of growth; although body needs are still high, energy requirements decrease	Emphasize that from a nutritional viewpoint, child can regulate intake if appropriate foods are offered.
Picky eater	Provide nutritional snacks. Respect need for independence; do not force child to eat. Use colored straws; if milk is refused, offer cheese, yogurt (not fortified with vitamin D); add milk to potatoes. Offer meat in bite-sized portions. Add fruit to cereal. Reduce sweets. Invite playmate to lunch. Relax at meals. Promote harmony.
CHILDREN OF SCHOOL AGE	
Growth rate that continues to be slow but steady until puberty, some spurts and plateaus	Maintain education in nutrition. Introduce new foods when eating out. Assist child in preparing nutritious lunches. Provide fruits and raw vegetables for snacks. Encourage parents to include children in meal planning, preparation, and food shopping.

Continued

table 15-9	*Nursing Interventions for Meeting the Nutritional Needs of Children—cont'd*
COMMENT	**NURSING INTERVENTIONS**
ADOLESCENT GIRLS	
Girls' caloric requirements less than those of boys	Emphasize that skipping meals can lead to decrease in essential nutrients.
	Encourage physical exercise to maintain body weight.
Concern with body image may lead to anorexia or bulimia	Educate regarding proper nutrients to maintain body weight (e.g., skim milk, fruits).
	Avoid high-calorie fast foods.
	Consider emotional components related to foods (e.g., difficulty with peers, need for love and approval).
Athletic activities	See interventions for adolescent boys.
Oral contraceptives	Explain that oral contraceptives increase requirements for several nutrients (folic acid, vitamin B_6, ascorbic acid).
Adolescent pregnancy	Educate concerning increased nutritional needs to complete growth and nourish fetus.
ADOLESCENT BOYS	
Concern with body image, bodybuilding	Instruct regarding proper nutrition for sports.
	Avoid quack claims.
	Promote proper conditioning, well-balanced diet (increased calories), proper hydration without supplements—salt tablets unnecessary.
Overnutrition	Explain that this can lead to adult obesity.
	Teach that in order to lose weight the following are advised:
	Eat a variety of foods low in calories and high in nutrients
	Eat less fat and fewer fatty foods
	Eat less sugar and fewer sweets
	Drink less alcohol
	Eat more fruits, vegetables, whole grains
	Increase physical activity

The Preschool Child

Preschoolers and toddlers like finger foods. Dawdling and regression are common in this age-group. In general, preschoolers are more vulnerable to protein-calorie deficiencies; their younger siblings receive priority at home, and older brothers and sisters may receive the benefits of school lunch programs.

The School-Age Child

School-age children need food from the basic food groups but in increased quantities to meet energy requirements. Their attitudes toward food are unpredictable. Intake of protein, calcium, vitamin A, and ascorbic acid tends to be low. The intake of sweets decreases the appetite and provides empty calories.

The Adolescent

Nutrition is particularly important during the adolescent years. Teenagers grow rapidly and expend large amounts of energy. Their food needs are great. The nurse attempts to involve the teenager in selecting foods that are nutritious and appetizing. This may be done by reviewing choices made on the daily menu. Sometimes it helps to stress how important good nutrition is to physical appearance and fitness. The need for peer approval is at its height during adolescence, and food fads and skipped meals may result in malnutrition, even in families of means. Fatigue is a common complaint at this age. If it is accompanied by a lack of appetite and irritability, anemia should be suspected. Some adolescents consult computer chat rooms for weight loss information, and this can lead to anorexic behavior. Parental guidance of computer use is necessary.

Table 15-10 reviews some nutritional services in the community that are available to children.

FEEDING THE ILL CHILD

Children in the hospital are in the process of growing. Well-nourished children can be characterized as follows:

- Nearly always show steady gains in weight and height

table 15-10 | *Nutrition Resources Within the Community*

PROGRAM	ELIGIBILITY	PROGRAM CONTENT
Maternal and child health	Pregnant women and children of low-income families	Free or reduced price Improved health care services for mothers and children at a clinic affiliated with a specific hospital Free vitamins, immunizations
Special Supplemental Food Program for Women, Infants, and Children (WIC) Aid to Families with Dependent Children (AFDC)	Individuals at nutritional risk: Pregnant women up to 6 months postpartum Nursing mothers up to 1 year Infants and children up to age 5 years identified as being at nutritional risk: must live in geographically determined low-income area and be eligible for reduced price or free medical care; must be certified by WIC staff member Periodic assessment of risk status	Provision of supplemental foods Over 1 year: iron-fortified formula and infant cereals, fruit juice high in vitamin C Women and children: whole fluid milk or cheese, eggs, iron-fortified hot or cold cereal, fruit or vegetable high in vitamin C Food distribution: directly from participating agency, via voucher system, or by home delivery Nutrition education is an integral part of program
Program for Children with Special Health Needs (formerly Crippled Children's Services)	Children with developmental disabilities	Under Title V Free nutrition counseling Funds available for equipment or supplies
Child Care Food Program (CCFP)	Preschool children in nonprofit facilities, Head Start, day care, after-school facilities	Year-round program Cash in lieu of commodities available
School Breakfast Program	All public and nonprofit private schools Public and licensed nonprofit residential child care institutions For needy children or those who travel great distances to school	As set by U.S. Department of Agriculture Nonprofit breakfasts meeting nutritional standards Served free or at a reduced price to children from low-income families Costs to schools reimbursed by federal funds
National School Lunch Program	All public and nonprofit private school pupils of high-school grade or under, some residential institutions and temporary shelters	As set by U.S. Department of Agriculture Nonprofit nutritious lunches offered free or at a reduced price to those who cannot pay Lunch follows specified guidelines and meets one third or more of daily dietary allowance Schools reimbursed by federal and state funds
Summer Food Service Programs for children	Public agency–sponsored preschool and school-age recreation programs, summer camps	Free lunch to children in summer programs Federal monetary support
Special Milk Program	Schools, child care centers, summer camps	Federal reimbursement for all or part of the milk served
Food Distribution (donated foods)	Supplemental programs for mothers and infants	Distribution of surplus food to eligible persons, schools, institutions
Food Stamps	Eligibility based on total income, expenses, number being fed in household Each applicant is considered on an individual basis	Patient should apply at local Food Stamp Office within the community, presenting wage slips, sources of income, rent receipts, utility bills Food Stamps are given free of charge depending on eligibility needs Used like cash to purchase food at authorized food stores (nonfood items and alcoholic beverages not allowed)

- Are alert
- Have shiny hair
- Have no fatigue circles beneath the eyes
- Have a skin color within normal limits
- Have a flat abdomen
- Have an erect posture
- Have well-developed muscles
- Have mouth and gum mucous membranes that are firm and pink, not swollen or bleeding
- Have no mouth or tongue lesions
- Have teeth that are erupting on schedule
- Have a generally good appetite and eliminate regularly
- Sleep well at night, have energy and vitality, and are not irritable

This picture changes somewhat during illness, but the child who is basically well nourished can easily be distinguished from one who is malnourished.

Many hospitalized children have poor appetites. This may be due to age, the nature of the illness, the type of diet, sudden exposure to strange foods and a strange environment, a reaction to hospitalization, or the degree of satisfaction obtained during mealtimes. The child may also refuse to eat in an attempt to manipulate the parents, particularly if lack of appetite was a concern in the past.

The nurse observes the patient's tray to determine if the food is of the right consistency. Does the child have any teeth? Do lesions in the mouth prevent chewing? Can the child use a knife and fork? Children with bandaged limbs or those receiving intravenous fluids require assistance. The size of servings is important.

One should serve less than one hopes will be eaten. A tablespoonful of food (not heaping) for each year of age is a good guide to follow. More is given if the patient appears hungry. One item at a time is placed before small children who feed themselves so they do not become overwhelmed. The nurse avoids showing personal dislikes because negative attitudes are easily transmitted. The nurse proceeds slowly with unfamiliar children to determine their level of mastery. Food is served warm, and sufficient time is allotted. Sweet drinks and snacks should not be served just before meals. Treatments such as chest physiotherapy should not be scheduled immediately after a meal.

Infants who are placed on "nothing by mouth" (NPO) status should be provided with a pacifier to meet their sucking needs. Some children prefer to use their thumb for nonnutritive sucking (Figure 15-9).

FOOD-DRUG INTERACTIONS

Whenever a child is ill and treated with prescription medications, the nurse is responsible for monitoring

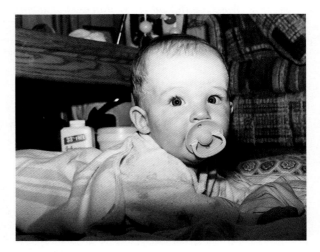

FIGURE **15-9** Nonnutritive sucking. Nonnutritive sucking involving the finger or a pacifier is common in infants under age 1 year and fulfills the needs of the oral phase of development. In general, malocclusion from nonnutritive sucking will not be a problem if the habit is discontinued before age 3 years. *Frequency, duration,* and *intensity* of sucking influence the occurrence of malocclusion associated with finger or pacifier use. Behavior modification can help to decrease thumb sucking (e.g., a dental appliance or substances placed on the finger). The child must be physically and emotionally "ready" to discontinue thumb sucking, and appropriate rewards should be predetermined.

drug-drug interactions, drug-food interactions, and drug-environment interactions. Drug-drug interactions involve a knowledge of the side effects of each drug prescribed. Drug-environment interactions involve the effects of a drug on the response of the patient to his or her environment. For example, certain antibiotics have photosensitivity as a side effect. Nurses armed with this knowledge advise the patient or parent to avoid prolonged exposure to sunlight. Drug-food interactions are often overlooked but can impact treatment and/or the growth and development of the child. The nurse should remain alert to food-drug interactions while dealing with the sick child.

THE TEETH
Deciduous Teeth

The development of the 20 deciduous, or baby, teeth begins at about the fifth month of intrauterine life. The health and diet of the expectant mother affect their soundness. Primary teeth erupt during the first 2½ years of life. It is a normal process and is generally accompanied by little or no discomfort. Wide individual differences in tooth eruption occur in normal, healthy infants. Occasionally an infant is born with teeth; neonatal teeth are removed to prevent the possibility of choking

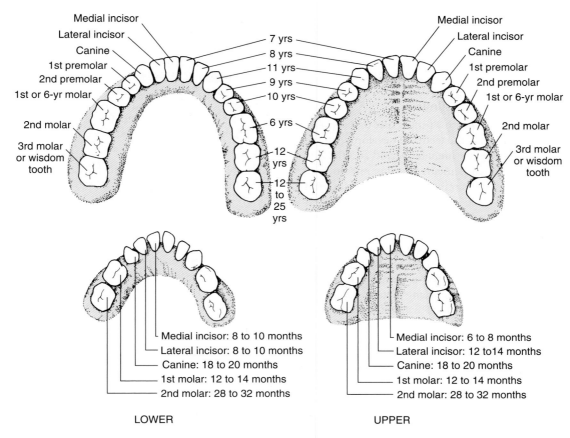

FIGURE **15-10** Permanent and deciduous teeth and age of eruption.

should they fall out. A delay in teething is significant if other forms of immaturity or illness are present. The physician evaluates the process of teething during the infant's regular health checkups.

The first tooth generally appears at about the sixth or seventh month. The 1-year-old has about six teeth, four above and two below. The order in which the teeth appear is almost always the same (Figure 15-10). They are shed in about the same order in which they appear (i.e., lower central incisors first, and so forth). Although the Academy of Pediatric Dentistry recommends that the first dental visit occur by 1 year, the majority of children begin seeing a dentist between age 2 and 3 years. Tetracycline antibiotics stain developing teeth a yellowish brown and therefore are to be avoided during pregnancy and in the first 8 years of life.

Parents and nurses must not neglect baby teeth, thinking that they will eventually be lost. A 2-year-old who wants to brush his teeth when Mommy does is encouraged to do so. The deciduous teeth serve not only in the digestive process but also in the development of the jaw. When the deciduous teeth are lost early because of neglect, the permanent teeth become poorly aligned. The nurse checks that all patients age 1 year and older have toothbrushes. Children sometimes must be reminded of oral hygiene at bedtime. Parental supervision of toothbrushing is necessary until age 7 years.

Permanent Teeth

The 32 permanent teeth develop just before birth and during the first year of life. They do not erupt through the gums, however, until the sixth year. Nutrition and general health during the first year of life affect the formation of permanent teeth. This process is not completed until the wisdom teeth appear at about age 18 to 25 years. The first permanent teeth do not replace any of the deciduous teeth but appear behind the deciduous molars. Cavities in them are often neglected because they are mistaken for baby teeth. The most common site of decay in children is the fissures of the molar teeth. These areas can be protected by the professional application of plastic sealants.

✦NURSING **TIP**_____
To assess the number of teeth a child under age 2 years is expected to have, use the following formula: Age in months - 6.

Oral Care in Health and Illness

Good dental care begins with a proper diet that supplies adequate nutrients while the teeth are developing in the jaws, especially during the prenatal period and the first year. The many essential elements found in milk include calcium, phosphorus, vitamins A and B complex, and protein. Vitamin D (the sunshine vitamin) and vitamin C (found in citrus fruits) are also valuable. Dietary practices influence the development of cavities (Box 15-6), and parents are encouraged to limit the *frequency* of fermentable carbohydrate intake.

In the past, total carbohydrate consumption was thought to be the most important dietary consideration for dental health. Today more attention is given to the frequency with which sweets are eaten and how long they stick to the teeth. Sticky retentive foods have more caries (cavity) potential than do sugared drinks that are quickly cleared from the mouth. Oral care after eating sticky foods is recommended. Recommended snack foods include cheese, peanuts, milk, sugarless gum, and raw vegetables. Items to be avoided include sugared gum, dried fruits, sugared soft drinks, cakes, and candy.

Of most importance in preventing caries is the administration of fluoride by mouth after age 6 months. Ideally, fluorides are present naturally in the water supply or are added to it. The fluoride content of city water or prepared formula may decrease the need for fluoride supplements. When necessary, systemic fluorides can be offered until the last permanent tooth erupts at about age 13 years. Many fluoride preparations are available and are often incorporated with vitamins. These tablets are obtained by prescription and should not be interchanged among children of various ages, because too much fluoride may cause the teeth to become "mottled" (fluorosis). Fluoride may also be applied directly to the teeth by the dentist.

Another aspect of tooth care is the prevention of *bottle-mouth caries* (nursing caries). (Figure 15-11). This condition occurs when an infant is falls asleep while breastfeeding or put to bed with a bottle of milk or sweetened juice. Sugar pools within the oral cavity, causing severe decay. It is seen most often in children between 18 months and 3 years of age. Eliminating the bedtime bottle or substituting water is recommended.

| box 15-6 | *Developmental Dental Hygiene* |

FIRST YEAR OF LIFE

Gentle brushing each night with soft, small toothbrush; no toothpaste necessary (infant may not like foaming action or taste and the fluoride in the toothpaste should not be swallowed).

Child is not put to bed with bottle of milk or juices. If infant must have a bottle, water is used.

2 TO 3 YEARS

Parents introduce soft brush and toothpaste. Only a pea-sized amount of toothpaste is used to minimize fluoride ingestion.

3 TO 6 YEARS

Deciduous teeth erupt, and baby teeth start to exfoliate (fall out) toward the end of this period.

Parents assist children and remind them to brush and floss until at least age 8 years. A small, soft toothbrush is used.

Bedtime routine of brushing is established, as salivary flow rates slow during sleep, reducing natural protective mechanisms.

Parents are advised to brush for the child at least once a day and to clean teeth that are in contact with each other with dental floss.

Sweets are limited to daytime meals, when saliva content is high.

6 TO 12 YEARS

First permanent molars appear. The pits and fissures of molars make them primary site for caries. Sealants (plastic coating) professionally applied to molars provide a mechanical barrier against bacteria.

Parents continue with fluorides, flossing, reducing *frequency* of exposure to fermentable carbohydrates. Adolescent gingivitis (*gingi*, "gum" and *itis*, "inflammation of") characterized by redness, swelling, and bleeding is common in children and adolescents and may be aggravated by hormonal changes at puberty.

Motivating the adolescent to assume responsibility for dental care may be complicated by rebellion against authority and some incapacity to appreciate long-term consequences.

Topical fluorides and fluoride toothpastes are available.

Orthodontic treatments place adolescent at high risk for gingivitis and caries around appliances or braces.

Mouth protectors should be used to prevent dental injuries from contact sports.

Data from Griffen, A. (2000). Pediatric oral health, *Pediatric Clinics of North America*. Philadelphia: W.B. Saunders.

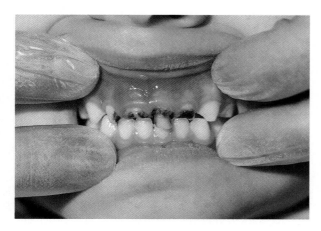

FIGURE **15-11** Nursing caries. During sleep, saliva decreases and the teeth become more vulnerable to decay. When the infant is put to sleep with a bottle containing milk or sweetened juice, the sugar combines with the bacterial flora in the mouth to cause tooth decay. This is known as "milk caries." Parents should be taught to use unsweetened water as the only liquid in a bottle at bedtime.

The maintenance of good oral health is an integral portion of comprehensive care for a sick or disabled pediatric patient. Education, prevention, and referral in the home, school, or hospital setting must be part of the child's plan of care. Untreated dental caries or malposition of the erupting teeth can cause periodontal disease in later years if not treated promptly. Delayed or early eruption of teeth can be indicative of certain endocrine disorders or other pathological condition and should be recorded and reported. Parents and caregivers should avoid "tasting" baby food fed to infants and young children because the transmission of acid-producing bacteria from their mouths can be passed on to the food or feeding utensils and contribute to tooth decay in the infant. Regular toothbrushing can start with tooth eruption. Children should brush before bedtime because the protective bacteriocidal effects of saliva decrease during sleep, and bacterial growth can cause tooth decay.

Parents and children should be educated concerning the care of the toothbrush to provide maximum effectiveness of the toothbrushing activity:
- Replace toothbrush every 3 months.
- Replace toothbrush after a viral illness.
- Avoid rinsing bristles in hot water.
- Do not use a closed container for toothbrush storage.
- Avoid sharing toothbrushes among children.

A properly sized toothbrush will aid in developing good toothbrushing technique. Dental flossing should be done with an up-and-down motion. A back-and-forth "sawing" motion can cause injury to gingival tissues. Children need assistance and supervision with flossing until at least age 7 years.

Trauma to the teeth often occurs in school-age children. Appropriate protective devices can prevent injury during sports activities. If a primary tooth is knocked out (avulsed) because of trauma, the child should be referred to a dentist for a "spacer" that will maintain tooth alignment until the permanent tooth erupts. If a permanent tooth is avulsed because of trauma, the tooth should be immersed in milk and brought with the child to the dentist for immediate care. Open wounds to oral tissues may require tetanus prophylaxis or antibiotics. All tooth fractures should be referred to a dentist for evaluation and treatment.

Dental problems that occur often with adolescents include puberty gingivitis; gingivitis associated with oral contraceptive use; drug-related gingivitis, and hyperplastic gingivitis associated with orthodontic therapy. Temporomandibular joint problems (TMJ) and malocclusion caused by missing teeth require a dental referral. Orthodontic appliances such as fixed braces can trap plaque and food and increase tooth decay. Meticulous oral hygiene, brushing, flossing, and fluoride applications are part of comprehensive orthodontic care.

A team approach to dental care for the child receiving chemotherapy or radiation therapy includes the dentist, physician, nurse, parent, and patient. Brushing and flossing when the platelet count is more than $20,000/mm^3$ or using moist gauze when platelet count is under $20,000/mm^3$ is advised to prevent infection and bleeding. The use of chlorhexidine may be prescribed to reduce oral lesions. Table 15-11 reviews medical problems that have an effect on dental health.

Disabled children can master independent toothbrushing by modifying the toothbrush. Using padded tongue depressors to visualize the oral cavity and an aspirating catheter attached to the toothbrush and connected to a suction machine can assist in providing dental care for a severely disabled child. Battery-operated toothbrushes can help to achieve optimum brushing technique.

In March 2000 the U.S. Surgeon General convened a meeting to discuss the accessibility of oral care for all children. Preventive oral health was considered to be vital to the maintenance of general health. The principal goals established were to urge health care providers to integrate oral health concepts into education and general health care and to increase the accessibility of oral care for children.

table 15-11 *Medical Problems and Dental Health*

HEALTH PROBLEM	EFFECT ON TEETH
Asthma	Sucrose content of medication can cause decay
Hemophilia Cancer	Can cause oral bleeding, impaired healing
Seizure disorders	Causes decreased saliva; gingival overgrowth (use of diphenylhydantoin)
Medications that depress the central nervous system	Decrease salivary flow, increasing susceptibility to dental caries
Juvenile rheumatoid arthritis	Sucrose-containing medications increase risk of cavities
Bulimia	Erosion of teeth caused by acid contact during vomiting episodes
Chemotherapy	Oral ulcerations
Fluoride ingestion	Excess fluoride can cause fluorosis (mottling of teeth)

NURSING TIP

When a tooth is "knocked out" or avulsed traumatically, the tooth should be gently cleansed of obvious dirt and placed in milk until dental care is obtained.

PLAY

Play is the business of children. Observing the child at play can assist in assessing growth and development and understanding the child's relationship with family members. Any plan of care for a hospitalized child of any age should include a play activity that either encourages growth and development or encourages the expression of thoughts and feelings. Playrooms in the hospital pediatric unit can be used for children who have conditions that are not communicable. Medications and treatments should not be carried out in the playroom setting. Play can also be therapeutic and assist in the recovery process. An example of therapeutic play is the game of having the child "blow out" the light of a flashlight as if it were a candle to promote deep breathing. Table 15-12 reviews age-appropriate play behaviors.

Art is an appropriate play activity at almost any age and provides an avenue of experimentation as well as

table 15-12 *Development of Play*

AGE-GROUP	TYPE OF PLAY	SUGGESTED PLAY ACTIVITY
Infants	Explore, imitate	Provide visual stimuli for newborns; touch stimuli for infants, and toys involving manipulation for 1-year-olds.
1 to 2 years	Parallel play	Children play next to each other but not with each other. Provide each child with toys that reflect activities of daily living.
3 to 5 years	Cooperative play	Children play with each other, each taking a specific role. "You be the mommy and I'll be the daddy."
	Creative play	A simple box can become a train to a 3-year-old.
5 to 8 years	Symbolic group play; secret clubs	Secret codes, "knock knock" jokes, and rhymes are popular at this age.
8 to 10 years	Competitive play	Children at this age can accept competition with structured rules and highly interactive physical activity.
13 to 19 years	Fantasy play; cliques	Leadership activities such as baby-sitting or tutoring are popular. Daydreaming occurs. Board games are popular. Interactive social activities in "cliques" occur at and after school.

creative expression and feeling of accomplishment in the child. Computer programs are popular with all age-groups, providing problem-solving games, manipulative skills, and opportunities for new learning. Both of these activities must be balanced with active play experiences.

Nursing interventions should focus on encouraging optimal play activities and experiences that are age appropriate. Parents need guidance concerning the value of play that may not always be a neat and clean activity. Helping parents to select appropriate toys that are safe as well as appropriate to the age and illness is essential. For example, a stuffed animal may not be the toy of choice for an asthmatic child. In the health care setting a blood pressure cuff can give the child a "hug." Children can play with the equipment they see in their environment to provide stress relief.

key points

- Growth and development are orderly and sequential, although there are spurts and plateaus.
- Cephalocaudal development proceeds from head to toe.
- Children are susceptible to nutritional deficiencies because they are in the process of growth and development.
- Maslow depicted human development on the basis of a hierarchy of needs.
- Freud's theories view personality development as phases of psychosexual development.
- Piaget describes phases of cognitive development.
- Erikson described eight stages of psychosocial development from birth to adulthood.
- Developmental theories can serve as guides to nursing intervention; however, each child grows and develops at an individual pace.
- A family is two or more persons that interact together.
- Parent-child interactions affect positive growth and development.

- Deciduous teeth are baby teeth. The proper care of the teeth depends on caregiver supervision and the child's physical level of development and mastery.
- Optimal nutrition is essential to physical and neurological growth and development.
- Motor development follows a predictable sequence.
- Nutritional practices of early childhood persist through adulthood.
- The nurse is responsible for counseling and teaching positive nutritional practices that are acceptable to the family's culture, religion, and lifestyle.
- The availability of age-appropriate toys enhances physical, emotional, and mental development in infants, children, and adolescents.
- Computer games can foster problem solving, cognitive development, and motor coordination but should be balanced with active play activities.
- Many hospitals have playrooms, which must be kept safe from painful or invasive experiences.
- A nurse is an advocate, educator, and collaborator in a family-centered care environment.

ONLINE RESOURCES

Cholesterol Guidelines: http://www.nhlbi.nih.gov/chd

Inheritance and Development:
http://www.ncbi.nlm.nih.gov/omim

Gerber: http://www.gerber.com

2000 CDC Growth Charts: http://cdc.gov/growthcharts

CRITICAL THINKING QUESTION

The parents discuss oral hygiene for their 15-month-old child with the nurse at the clinic. The father states he is not sure the child has enough teeth to warrant toothbrushing at this time, but the child does seem to enjoy it. The mother states the child enjoys brushing his teeth and says, "He likes me to put a lot of toothpaste on the toothbrush because he loves the taste of it. He is so cute when he has a mouthful of toothpaste." What nursing intervention and teaching would be appropriate?

REVIEW QUESTIONS *Choose the most appropriate answer.*

1. How many erupted teeth would an 8-month-old infant be expected to have?
   1. 2
   2. 4
   3. 6
   4. 8

2. During the first week of life, the newborn's weight:
   1. Increases about 5% to 10%
   2. Decreases about 5% to 10%
   3. Stabilizes
   4. Fluctuates widely

3. The nurse should encourage the parent to introduce toothbrushing to her child by:
   1. Age 6 months
   2. Age 1 year
   3. Age 3 years
   4. Age 7 years

4. To meet the needs (as described by Erikson) of a school-aged child diagnosed with diabetes, the nurse should:
   1. Explain carefully to the mother the need to rigidly adhere to dietary modifications
   2. Allow the child to eat whatever he or she wants and administer insulin to maintain optimum glucose levels
   3. Allow the child to perform his own Accuchecks and administer his own insulin
   4. Perform Accuchecks four times a day and at bedtime

5. It is most appropriate to first introduce competitive games at:
   1. Age 3 to 5 years
   2. Age 7 to 8 years
   3. Age 9 to 10 years
   4. Age 12 to 15 years

objectives

1. Define each key term listed.
2. Describe the physical and psychosocial development of infants from age 1 to 12 months, listing age-specific events and guidance when appropriate.
3. Discuss the major aspects of cognitive development in the first year of life.
4. Discuss the nutritional needs of growing infants.
5. Describe how to select and prepare solid foods for the infant.
6. List four common concerns of parents about the feeding of infants.
7. Discuss the development of feeding skills in the infant.
8. Identify the approximate age for each of the following: posterior fontanel has closed; central incisors appear; birth weight has tripled; child can sit steadily alone; child shows fear of strangers.
9. Describe normal vital signs for a 1-year-old infant.
10. Discuss safety issues in the care of infants.
11. Discuss the approach and care of an infant with colic.
12. Identify age-appropriate toys and their developmental or therapeutic value.
13. Discuss principles of safety during infancy.
14. Discuss the development of positive sleep patterns.

key terms

colic (p. 395)
extrusion reflex (ĕk-STROO-zhŭn RĒ-flĕks, p. 398)
grasp reflex (p. 386)
milestones (p. 385)
norms (p. 385)
object permanence (p. 403)
oral stage (p. 386)
parachute reflex (p. 386)
pincer grasp (p. 386)
prehension (p. 386)
satiety (să-TĪ-ĕ-tē, p. 399)
separation anxiety (sĕp-ă-RĀ-shăn ăng-ZĪ-ĭ-tē, p. 385)
weaning (p. 402)

Physical, emotional, and cognitive growth and the development of motor abilities occur rapidly during the first year of life. Milestones of growth and development describe general patterns of achievements at various stages of infancy. These milestones, or patterns, are referred to as norms. Norms can vary greatly for the individual child, but the nurse must understand the normal range for milestone achievement to assess the progress of growth and development of the infant and initiate early referral for follow-up care.

During the neonatal phase of development, the chief tasks mastered were the establishment of effective feeding patterns and a predictable sleep-wake cycle. Infants who have unmet hunger needs can become irritable, may not perceive feeding as pleasurable, and may fail to develop trust in the caregiver. Parental bonding and social interaction begin in the neonatal phase but heighten when the infant begins to respond with a social smile, making the caregiver feel "loved."

By the time the infant is age 4 to 6 months, the positive parental interaction with the infant should be obvious during clinic visits. If the parent does not appear to enjoy the developmental changes in the infant at this age or does not appear relaxed during interactions with the infant, further follow-up of possible family dysfunction or social or mental stresses should be initiated.

By age 9 months, control of feeding may become an issue of conflict between parent and infant. The parent needs to "let go" and introduce the infant to finger foods and initiate drinking from a cup. Offering limited choices can reduce conflict as the infant reaches toward autonomy. If the nurse notices an overly neat and orderly approach during feeding, parental guidance may be necessary. Separation anxiety (see Chapter 21) can be expected by the ninth-month clinic visit, and the nurse should expect to spend some time playing with and getting to know the infant to establish the rapport necessary for a successful physical assessment. Repetition is the key to successful parent teaching and counseling by the nurse.

Children, unlike adults, are in the process of growing while they are hospitalized. To provide total patient care

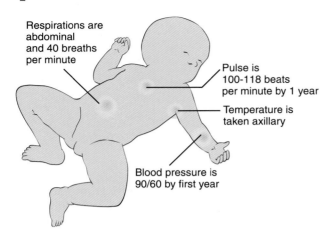

FIGURE **16-1** Average vital signs of the infant.

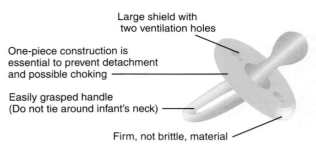

FIGURE **16-2** Pacifier. Pacifiers provide nonnutritive sucking to meet the needs of the oral phase of infancy. A safe pacifier is illustrated. Note that it is constructed in one piece.

the nurse must be able to recognize a patient's needs at various stages of growth and development. The pulse rate, respiration, and blood pressure that are normal for an infant are not normal for the adult patient (Figure 16-1). The nurse must try to meet individual needs effectively and to administer the specialized nursing care required for the particular patient. *The most common cause for concern about a child is a sudden slowing, not typical for age, of any aspect of development.*

GENERAL CHARACTERISTICS

ORAL STAGE

Sucking brings the infant comfort and relief from tension. This oral stage of personality development is important for the infant's physical and psychological development. The nurse, knowing the importance of sucking to the infant, holds the infant during feedings and allows sufficient time to suck. Infants who are warm and comfortable associate food with love. The infant who is fed intravenous fluids is given added attention and a pacifier to ensure the necessary satisfaction of sucking (Figure 16-2). When the teeth appear, the infant learns to bite and enjoys objects that can be chewed. Gradually, the infant begins to put fingers into the mouth. When infants can use their hands more skillfully, they will not suck their fingers as often and will be able to derive pleasure from other sources.

MOTOR DEVELOPMENT

The grasp reflex is seen when one touches the palms of the infant's hands and flexion occurs. This reflex disappears at about 3 months. Prehension, the ability to grasp objects between the fingers and the opposing thumb, occurs slightly later (age 5 to 6 months) and follows an orderly sequence of development (Figure 16-3).

The parachute reflex appears by age 7 to 9 months. This is a protective arm extension that occurs when an infant is suddenly thrust downward when prone. By age 1 year the pincer grasp coordination of index finger and thumb is well established.

EMOTIONAL DEVELOPMENT

Love and security are vital needs of infants. They require the continuous affection of their parents. If trust is to develop, consistency must be established. Parents are assured that they need not be afraid of spoiling their infants by attending promptly to their needs. Infants who are consistently picked up in response to crying show fewer crying episodes when they are toddlers and less aggressive behavior at age 2 years. Loving adults affirm that the world is a good place in which to live. Each day the infant becomes impressed by parental actions and learns to imitate and trust caregivers. A sense of trust is vital to the development of a healthy personality. Many consider it to be the foundation of emotional growth. The child who does not develop a sense of trust learns to mistrust people, which could have a permanently negative effect on personality development.

Parents are taught to talk, sing, and touch their infants while providing care. They should not expect too much or too little from them. Infants will easily accomplish various activities if they are not forced before they reach maturity. When an infant shows readiness to learn a task, parents should provide encouragement.

NEED FOR CONSTANT CARE AND GUIDANCE

The full-time caregiver needs and deserves the understanding of and kind support from relatives at home and from the nurse in the hospital. Pediatrics involves family-centered care. A short break from pressures provides renewed energy with which to enjoy the infant. A

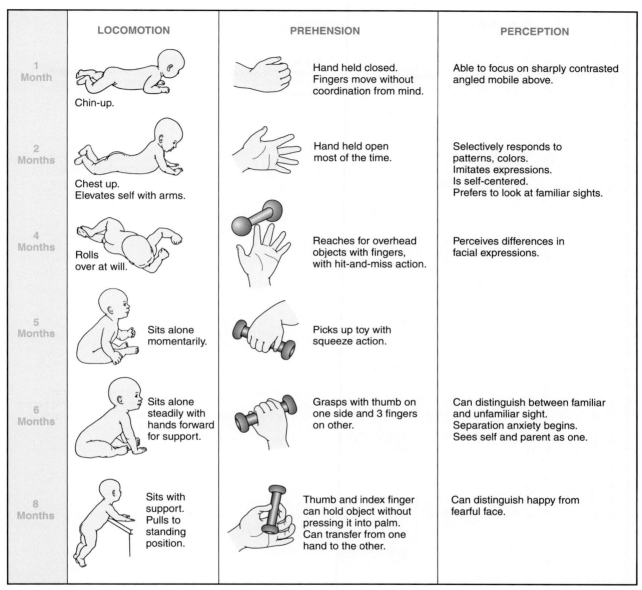

	LOCOMOTION	PREHENSION	PERCEPTION
1 Month	Chin-up.	Hand held closed. Fingers move without coordination from mind.	Able to focus on sharply contrasted angled mobile above.
2 Months	Chest up. Elevates self with arms.	Hand held open most of the time.	Selectively responds to patterns, colors. Imitates expressions. Is self-centered. Prefers to look at familiar sights.
4 Months	Rolls over at will.	Reaches for overhead objects with fingers, with hit-and-miss action.	Perceives differences in facial expressions.
5 Months	Sits alone momentarily.	Picks up toy with squeeze action.	
6 Months	Sits alone steadily with hands forward for support.	Grasps with thumb on one side and 3 fingers on other.	Can distinguish between familiar and unfamiliar sight. Separation anxiety begins. Sees self and parent as one.
8 Months	Sits with support. Pulls to standing position.	Thumb and index finger can hold object without pressing it into palm. Can transfer from one hand to the other.	Can distinguish happy from fearful face.

Continued

FIGURE **16-3** The development of locomotion, prehension, and perception.

trip to the store or a stroll with the infant in the carriage affords stimulation and a change of environment for the infant and the caregiver. The infant who is constantly left in a crib or playpen and is not introduced to a variety of learning experiences may become shy and withdrawn. *Sensory stimulation is essential for the development of the infant's thought processes and perceptual abilities.*

If a mother is unable to room-in with her hospitalized infant, personnel should try to imitate her care by promptly fulfilling the infant's physical and emotional needs. In the nursery the nurse first feeds the infant who appears hungry, rather than delaying feeding to adhere to

a specific routine. Wet diapers are changed as soon as possible. The crying child is soothed. The exactness of time or method of bathing or feeding the infant is less important than the care with which it is done. The infant easily recognizes warmth and affection or the lack thereof.

DEVELOPMENT AND CARE

Table 16-1 is a guide to infant care from the first month to the first year. Some of the aspects of care (e.g., safety measures) are important throughout the entire year.

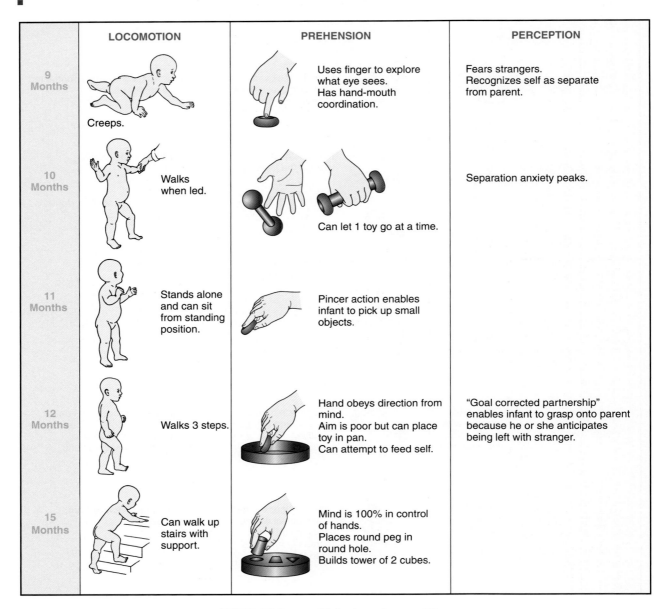

	LOCOMOTION	PREHENSION	PERCEPTION
9 Months	Creeps.	Uses finger to explore what eye sees. Has hand-mouth coordination.	Fears strangers. Recognizes self as separate from parent.
10 Months	Walks when led.	Can let 1 toy go at a time.	Separation anxiety peaks.
11 Months	Stands alone and can sit from standing position.	Pincer action enables infant to pick up small objects.	
12 Months	Walks 3 steps.	Hand obeys direction from mind. Aim is poor but can place toy in pan. Can attempt to feed self.	"Goal corrected partnership" enables infant to grasp onto parent because he or she anticipates being left with stranger.
15 Months	Can walk up stairs with support.	Mind is 100% in control of hands. Places round peg in round hole. Builds tower of 2 cubes.	

FIGURE **16-3 cont'd** For legend, see p. 387.

The nurse explains to parents that physical patterns cannot be separated from social patterns and that abrupt changes do not take place with each new month. Human development cannot be separated into specific areas any more than the body's structure can be separated from its function.

No two infants are just alike at a certain age. Table 16-1 is just a guide! However, individual variations fall in a range about central norms that serve as guidelines in the evaluation of an infant's or child's progress. The addition of the various solid foods to the diet and the time of immunizations vary slightly, depending on the in-

fant's health and the physician's protocol. Table 15-5 outlines the parental tasks involved in guiding the infant through the stages of growth and development.

COMMUNITY-BASED CARE: A MULTIDISCIPLINARY TEAM

The prevention of disease during infancy is of the utmost importance and includes all measures that improve the physical health and psychosocial adjustment of the child. The concept of periodic health appraisal is

Text continued on p. 395

1 MONTH

Physical Development

Weighs approximately 8 lb. Has regained weight lost after birth. Gains about 1 inch in length per month for the first 6 months. Lifts head slightly when placed on stomach. Pushes with toes. Turns head to side when prone. Head wobbles. Head lags when infant pulled from lying to sitting position. Clenches fists. Stares at surroundings.

Vaginal discharge in girls and breast enlargement in boys and girls from maternal hormones received in utero are not unusual and disappear without treatment.

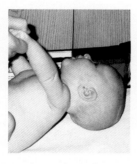

Note head lag of 1-month old.

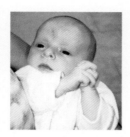

Infant keeps hands at midline.

Social Behavior

Makes small throaty noises. Cries when hungry or uncomfortable. Sleeps 20 out of 24 hr. Awakens for 2 AM feeding.

Care and Guidance

Sleep. Back; if side-lying position, support back with blanket roll. Use a firm, tight-fitting mattress in a crib with bars properly spaced so that the infant's head cannot be caught between them. Raise crib rails. Do not use a pillow.

Diet. Breast milk every 2 to 3 hours or iron-fortified formula every 4 hours as infant indicates need. Vitamin D (400 IU/day) in dark-skinned infants, breast-fed infants, or infants who are not regularly exposed to sunlight. Burp infant well.

Exercise. Allow freedom from the restraints of clothing before bath. Provide fresh air and sunshine whenever possible. (Protect the infant from sun and insects with sunscreen or protective clothing.) Support head and shoulders when holding infant. Attend promptly to physical needs. Provide colorful hanging toys for sensory stimulation out of infant's reach.

2 MONTHS

Physical Development

Posterior fontanel closes. Tears appear. Can hold head erect in midposition. Follows moving light with eyes. Holds a rattle briefly. Legs are active.

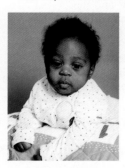

The 2-month-old can hold head erect in midline for brief periods of time.

Social Behavior

Smiles in response to mother's voice. Knows crying brings attention. Awakens for 2 AM feeding.

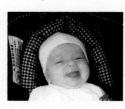

The smile of the 2-month-old delights parents.

Care and Guidance

Sleep. Develops own pattern; may sleep from feeding to feeding.

Diet. Breast milk or formula.

Exercise. Provide a safe, flat place to kick and be active. Do not leave infant alone, particularly on any raised surface. Physical examination by the family doctor or pediatrician.

Immunization. First diphtheria, whooping cough, and tetanus (DPT). Oral polio vaccine (OPV), *Haemophilus influenzae* type b (Hib), and second hepatitis B virus (HBV) vaccine. Still completely depends on adults for physical care. Needs a flexible routine throughout infancy and childhood.

Pacifier. If used, select for safety. Choose one-piece construction and loop handle to prevent aspiration (see Figure 16-2).

Hiccups. Are normal and subside without treatment. Small amounts of water may help.

Colic. Consists of paroxysmal abdominal pain, irritable crying. Usually disappears after 3 months. Place infant prone over arms (see Figure 16-4). Use pacifier. Massage back. Relieve caregiver periodically.

Continued

| table 16-1 | *Physical Development, Social Behavior, and Care and Guidance of Infants—cont'd* |

3 MONTHS

Physical Development

Weighs 12 to 13 lb. Stares at hands. Reaches for objects but misses them. Carries hand to mouth. Can follow an object from right to left and up and down when it is placed in front of face. Supports head steadily. Holds rattle.

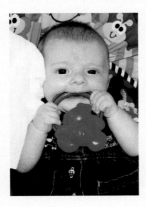

The 3-month-old carries hands to mouth.

Social Behavior

Cries less. Can wait a few minutes for attention. Enjoys having people talk to him. Takes impromptu naps.

Care and Guidance

Sleep. Yawns, stretches, naps in mother's arms.
Diet. Mother's milk or formula.
Exercise. May have short play period. Enjoys playing with hands.

4 MONTHS

Physical Development

Weighs about 13 to 14 lb. Drooling indicates appearance of saliva and beginning of teething. Lifts head and shoulders when on abdomen and looks around. Turns from back to side. Sits with support. Begins to reach for objects he or she sees. Coordination between eye and body movements. Moves head, arms, and shoulders when excited. Extends legs and partly sustains weight when held upright. Rooting, Moro, extrusion, and tonic neck reflexes are no longer present.

Social Behavior

Coos, chuckles, and gurgles. Laughs aloud. Responds to others. Likes an audience. Sleeps through the night.

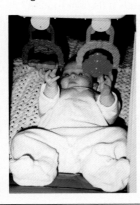

Visual stimulation is important to the growing infant

Care and Guidance

Sleep. Stirs about in crib. Sleeps through ordinary household noises.
Diet. Mother's milk or formula.
Exercise. Plays with hand rattles and dangling toys. Start acquainting with a playpen, where infant can roll with safety.
Immunization. Second DPT, OPV, and Hib.
Elimination. One or two bowel movements per day. May skip a day.

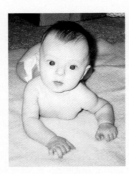

While on the abdomen the 4-month-old can lift the head and shoulders and look around.

table 16-1 | *Physical Development, Social Behavior, and Care and Guidance of Infants—cont'd*

5 MONTHS

Physical Development

Sits with support. Holds head well. Grasps objects offered. Puts everything into mouth. Plays with toes.

Social Behavior

Talks to himself. Seems to know whether persons are familiar or unfamiliar. May sleep through 10 AM feeding. Tries to hold bottle at feeding time.

Care and Guidance

Sleep. Takes two or three naps daily in crib.
Diet. Mother's milk or formula.
Exercise. Provide space to pivot around. Makes jumping motions when held upright in lap.
Safety. Check toys for loose buttons and rough edges before placing them in playpen.

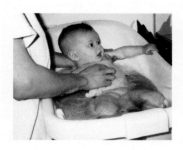

At 5 months the infant enjoys the bath. Firm head and shoulder support is essential for safety.

6 MONTHS

Physical Development

Doubles birth weight. Gains about 3 to 5 ounces per week during the next 6 months. Grows about a half inch per month. Sits alone momentarily. Springs up and down when sitting. Turns completely over. Hitches (moves backward when sitting). Bangs table with rattle. Pulls to a sitting position. Chewing more mature. Approximates lips to rim of cup.

Social Behavior

Cries loudly when interrupted from play. Increased interest in world. Babbles and squeals. Sucks food from spoon. Awakens happy.

Care and Guidance

Sleep. Needs own room. Should be moved from parents' room if not previously done. Otherwise, as infant becomes older, may become unwilling to sleep away from them.
Diet. Introduce first solid foods, usually rice cereal fortified with iron. See Figure 16-5 for progression.
Exercise. Grasps feet and pulls toward mouth.
Immunization. DPT, Hib, and HBV.
Safety. Remove toxic plants. Provide a chewable object, such as a teething ring, for enjoyment.

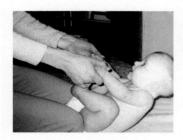

The infant can pull to sitting position without head lag at 6 months.

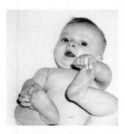

A 6-month-old discovers and plays with the feet.

Continued

table 16-1 | *Physical Development, Social Behavior, and Care and Guidance of Infants—cont'd*

7 MONTHS

Physical Development

Two lower teeth appear. These are the first of the deciduous teeth, the central incisors. Begins to crawl. Moves forward, using chest, head, and arms; legs drag. Can grasp objects more easily. Transfers objects from one hand to the other. Appears interested in standing. Holds an adult's hands and bounces actively while standing. Struggles when being dressed.

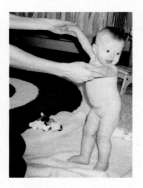

The infant enjoys standing position with assistance.

Social Behavior

Shifts moods easily—crying one minute, laughing the next. Shows fear of strangers. Anticipates spoon feeding. Sleeps 11 to 13 hours at night.

Care and Guidance

Sleep. Fretfulness caused by teething may appear. This is generally evidenced by lack of appetite and wakefulness during the night. In most cases, merely soothing and offering a cup of water are sufficient.

Diet. Add fruit. Add finger foods, such as toast or zwieback.

Exercise. Primitive locomotion.

8 MONTHS

Physical Development

Sits steadily alone. Uses index finger and thumb as pincers. Pokes at object. Enjoys dropping article into a cup and emptying it.

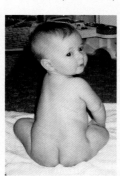

At 8 months, the infant is able to sit steady with back straight.

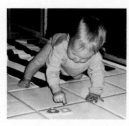

The pincer action is developed and the infant can pick up small objects between the two fingers.

Social Behavior

Plays pat-a-cake. Enjoys family life. Amuses self longer. Reserved with strangers. Indicates need for sleep by fussing and sucking thumb. Impatient especially when food is being prepared.

Care and Guidance

Sleep. Takes two naps a day.

Diet. Add vegetables. Continue to add new foods slowly, observing for reactions.

Exercise. Enjoys jump chair. Rides in stroller. Stuffed toys or those that squeak or rattle are appropriate.

Safety. Remain with infant at all times during bath in tub. Protect from chewing paint from windowsills or old furniture. Paint containing lead can be poisonous. Safety-lock doors to ovens, dishwashers, washing machines, dryers, and refrigerators.

| table 16-1 | *Physical Development, Social Behavior, and Care and Guidance of Infants—cont'd* |

9 MONTHS

Physical Development

Shows preference for use of one hand. Can raise self to a sitting position. Holds bottle. Creeps. (Carries trunk of body above floor but parallel to it. More advanced than crawling.)

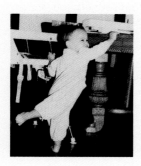

Infant cruises on furniture. Be sure it is stable!

Social Behavior

Tries to imitate sounds (e.g., says "ba-ba" for bye-bye). Cries if scolded. Drops food from highchair at mealtime. May fall asleep after 6 PM feeding.

Care and Guidance

Sleep. Has generally begun to sleep later in the morning.

Diet. Add meat, beans. Introduce chopped and mashed foods. Place newspaper beneath feeding table. Use unbreakable dishes. Allow infant to pick up pieces of food by hand and put them into mouth.

Safety. Keep a supply of syrup of ipecac on hand. Know phone number of nearest poison control center. Avoid tablecloths with overhangs infant could reach.

Exercise. Is busy most of the day exploring surroundings. Provide sufficient room and materials for safe play. Help infant to learn. Distract curious child from danger. In this way punishment is limited—avoid excessive spankings and "no's."

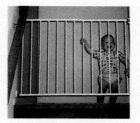

Stairway gates prevents falls. (Photo courtesy of Pat Spier, RN-C.)

10 MONTHS

Physical Development

Pulls to a standing position in the playpen. Throws toys to floor for parent to pick up. Cries when they are not returned. Walks around furniture while holding on to it.

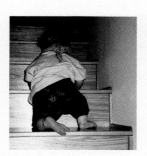

Infant is able to climb steps but needs supervision. (Photo courtesy of Pat Spier, RN-C.)

Social Behavior

Knows name. Plays simple games such as peek-a-boo. Feeds self a cookie. May cry out in sleep without waking.

Care and Guidance

Sleep. Avoid strenuous play before bedtime. A night light is convenient for parent and makes infant's surroundings more familiar. Pajamas with feet are warm, because infant becomes uncovered easily.

Diet. Takes juice and water from cup. Solid foods in general are taken well.

Exercise. Tours around room holding adult's hands. Daytime clothing should be loose so as not to interfere with movement.

Continued

table 16-1 *Physical Development, Social Behavior, and Care and Guidance of Infants—cont'd*

11 MONTHS

Physical Development

Stands upright holding on to an adult's hand.

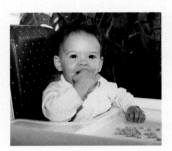

The 11-month-old can feed self finger foods and drink from a "sippy cup."

Social Behavior

Understands simple directions. Impatient when held. Enjoys playing with empty dish and spoon after meals.

Care and Guidance

Sleep. Greets parents in morning with excited jargon.

Diet. Still spills from cup. Enjoys blowing bubbles.

Exercise. Plays with toys in tub. Enjoys gross motor activity. Kicks, pulls self up.

Safety. Cover electrical outlets. Put household cleaners and medicines out of reach if not previously done. Needs to be sat down in playpen at times, because tends to stand until becomes exhausted.

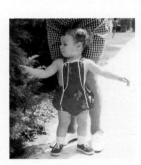

The 11-month-old is alert to surroundings and touches the leaves.

12 MONTHS

Physical Development

Pulse 100 to 140 beats/min. Respirations 20 to 40 breaths/min. Triples birth weight. Height is about 29 inches. Stands alone for short periods. May walk. Puts arm through sleeve as an aid to being dressed. Six teeth (four above and two below). Drinks from a cup, eats with a spoon with supervision. Pincer grasp is well established. Handedness (the preference for the use of one hand), although not fully established, may be evidenced.

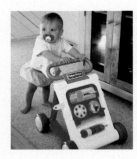

At 12 months, the infant can stand alone and walk with assistance.

Social Behavior

Friendly. Repeats acts that elicit a response. Recognizes "no-no." Verbalization slows because of concentration on getting about. Enjoys rhythmic music. Shows emotions such as fear, anger, and jealousy. Reacts to these emotions from adults. Plays with food and removes it from mouth.

Care and Guidance

Sleep. May take one long nap daily.

Diet. Gradually add egg white and fish (baked, steamed, or boiled). Add orange juice. Add well-cooked table foods. Interest in eating dwindles.

Exercise. Enjoys putting objects in a basket and then removing them. Places objects on head. Distraction is an effective way to deal with determination to do what infant wants regardless of outcome.

not new. In the late 1800s, "milk stations" were established at various locations throughout the United States to provide safe water and milk for infants in an effort to reduce the number of deaths from infant diarrhea.

HEALTH MAINTENANCE
The Infant

Parenting skills can be impaired by several socioeconomic factors, as well as by physical and mental problems. A prime responsibility of the nurse in the community-based clinic is to guide the parent and assist in the development of the skills necessary to ensure the proper growth and development of their child. The nurse can provide encouragement and explanations of strategies that will enable parents to be successful in coping with various infant behaviors.

The nurse is the important link in the initiation of referral to the multidisciplinary health care team, follow-up of progress, and maintenance of communication between the family and members of the health care team. A home-based infant stimulation program can use a teacher, nurse, occupational or speech therapist, or physical therapist (depending on the specific need of the infant) to directly stimulate the infant and teach the parents how to provide the care.

Coping with the irritable infant. One of the goals of early parent-infant interaction is to promote a calm, alert infant who can respond to parents and the environment. Success in this area promotes a feeling of competence in the parent. Some infants cannot tolerate environmental stimulation and handling and start to cry during diaper changes, feeding, and rocking. Lights, sound, and movement cause some infants to become irritable. Techniques to cope with these problems include the following:

- Shield the infant's eyes from bright light.
- Sit quietly with the infant. Do not talk or sing.
- Eliminate noise from radio, television, and computer.
- Talk in a soft voice.
- Change the infant's position slowly.
- If the infant turns away, squirms, grimaces, or puts the hands in front of the face, stop the interaction and reduce environmental stimuli.
- Swaddle the infant snugly in a light blanket with extremities flexed and hands near the face.
- Provide nonnutritive sucking.
- Rock the infant slowly and gently. Avoid sudden movements.
- Cradle the infant firmly in lap during feeding and remain still during sucking efforts.

Repetitious banging of toys on a table by an infant may be perceived by the parent as an irritating type of behavior. Counseling may be required to help the parent to understand that this is a developmental phase of motor activity and should be encouraged!

Colic. Colic is characterized by periods of unexplained irritability and crying in a healthy, well-fed infant. Although the exact cause is unknown, it is thought to be a combination of infant, parental, and environmental factors. Colic can interfere with parent-infant interactions if the infant is not soothed by holding or carrying and parental fatigue and guilt grow. Providing periods of rest and "breaks" to parents of colicky infants can prevent a cycle that may lead to child abuse. Figure 16-4 illustrates the "colic carry." Holding the infant close to the body while supporting the abdomen and providing a gentle rocking motion often soothes the colicky infant. See Nursing Care Plan 16-1 for care of the infant with colic.

Coping with the lethargic infant. Stimulation, interaction, and nourishment are essential for optimum infant growth and development. Some infants respond to an excessively stimulating environment by "shutting down" and sleeping. Coping strategies for dealing with this infant include the following:

- Avoid bright lights.
- Move and handle the infant slowly and gently.

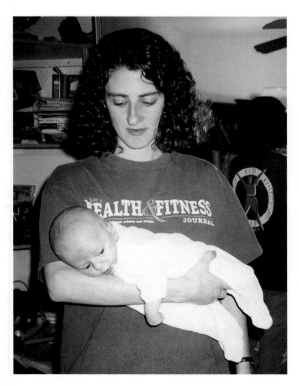

FIGURE **16-4** The colic carry. The infant is carried face down and is fully supported. Gentle motion may be soothing.

NURSING CARE PLAN 16-1

The Infant with Colic

PATIENT DATA: The parents of a 3-week-old infant state they feel inadequate as parents because their infant is often fussy and irritable and does not respond to their efforts to calm him. They ask what they are doing wrong.

SELECTED NURSING DIAGNOSIS *Interrupted family processes related to fussiness of infant*

Outcomes	Nursing Interventions	Rationales
Parents will demonstrate increased coping behaviors by 1 week. Parents will verbalize feelings of increased confidence in caring for the infant.	1. Educate parents about common manifestations of colic.	1. No single cause has been established for colic. Infant appears otherwise healthy but demonstrates cramplike pain, drawing legs to abdomen and demonstrating irritable cry. It is time-limited to about 3 months.
	2. Determine whether other causes have been ruled out by physician.	2. Intestinal obstruction and infection may mimic symptoms of colic. Bowel movements are not abnormal with colic.
	3. Review caregiver's history and usual day with infant.	3. This helps to determine if colic is related to type of feedings, diet of breastfeeding mother, passive smoking, milk allergy, activities of family members while infant is being fed, or other factors.
	4. Identify soothing measures used by parents and their effectiveness.	4. Environment may be overstimulating infant; parents may not know how to soothe the infant.
	5. Suggest abdominal massage, wind-up swing, and car rides.	5. These measures may help to relieve symptoms; burping before and after feedings and placing in an upright position after feedings may also decrease distress.
	6. Demonstrate "colic carry" (see Figure 16-4).	6. This may comfort infant by applying a little extra pressure on abdomen.
	7. Suggest periods of free time for parents.	7. Constant crying by infants produces a great deal of frustration in family members; caution against shaking infant, which can be harmful to the head and neck.
	8. Emphasize that colic is not a reflection on parenting skills.	8. First-time parents may feel anxious and incompetent. Nurse provides reassurance and support and builds on their strengths.

?CRITICAL THINKING QUESTION

A mother brings her 8-week-old infant to the clinic and complains that the infant is fussy and acting like he has colic. What information does the nurse need to obtain from the parent to develop a teaching plan?

- Talk in a calm voice.
- Sit the infant upright at intervals.
- *Slowly* dress and undress the infant.

Developing positive sleep patterns. Most newborns sleep at 4-hour intervals and increase their sleep intervals to 8 hours by age 4 to 6 months. Synchronizing the circadian rhythm of the infant to the family routine is a learned behavior. Parents must be alert to the infant's individual rhythm and promote activities that foster a stable synchronized pattern. Infants should be positioned for sleep on their backs and on a firm mattress, both for their safety and to prevent SIDS.

Until age 6 months, infants rely on parents to soothe them back to sleep when they awaken during the night. If the parent resorts to midnight pacing or car rides, the infant will learn to rely on the parent to get them back to sleep after age 6 months. The mother should assist the infant to develop "self-soothing" behaviors so the infant can roll over, grasp the pacifier, and return to sleep on his or her own. Helping the infant to achieve this ability will also make parents feel more confident in their parenting skills and less fatigued and frustrated.

> ⟫NURSING **TIP**_____
> The American Academy of Pediatrics recommends a supine or side-lying position for infants to avoid sudden infant death syndrome (SIDS). Care should be taken to use a sturdy mattress and avoid soft pillows that inhibit breathing.

Special Needs

A day care nursery school can be used, and the public school system offers special classes and tutoring for children in need. Counseling, behavior management techniques, and cognitive therapy can be provided by a psychologist. Neurodevelopmental therapy (NDT) can be provided by a professional or occupational or physical therapist. Speech therapy and auditory testing are also available within the community. The social worker can assist with social and environmental problems (see Chapter 18).

ILLNESS PREVENTION

Skilled health services today encompass periodic health appraisal; immunizations; assessment of parent-child interaction; counseling in the developmental processes; identification of families at risk (e.g., for child abuse); health education and anticipatory guidance; referrals to various agencies; follow-up services; appropriate record-keeping; and evaluation and audit by peers. These services are provided in a variety of health care facilities. Ideally the infant is seen in the clinic at least five times during the first year at specific intervals (2 months, 4 months, 6 months, 9 months, and 1 year). Private group practice, hospital-based clinics, and neighborhood health centers are examples of health care settings.

These visits are as important for parents as they are for the infant. They provide caregiver support and reassurance as well as information and anticipatory guidance for the many developmental changes and health issues of the infant's first year. A common concern is diaper rash, which can cause discomfort to the infant. The mother should be taught the importance of frequent diaper changes, how to wipe from front to back, and the importance of exposing the skin in the diaper area to the air for periods of time. Some commercial diaper wipes may contain fragrance or other ingredients that can further irritate a diaper rash. Soiled areas can be washed with water and mild soap if needed. To avoid skin breakdown, A and D or another protective ointment such as Desitin can be applied when the skin in the diaper area appears pink and irritated.

A careful health history is obtained during routine clinic visits. Growth grids during infancy include measures of weight, length, and head circumference. The reading and recording of growth charts are described in Chapter 15. There are numerous developmental screening tests. In the 1986 Amendment to the Education of All Handicapped Children Act (PL99-457), all states are required to assess for developmental disabilities before age 5 years. Most pediatricians initiate their assessment at birth to enable early intervention. General screening tools are available to identify children in need of referral and further care. Some of the tests include the following:

- Denver Developmental Screening Test (DDST): widely used and tests social, fine-motor adaptive, language, and gross motor abilities from birth to age 6 years
- Denver Home Screening Questionnaire: provides information concerning the child-rearing environment
- Early Language Milestone Scale (ELM): because language is necessary for cognitive development, this test assesses expressive, receptive, and visual language from birth to age 3 years
- Clinical Linguistic and Auditory Milestone scale (CLAMS): assesses language milestones from birth to age 3 years
- Ages and Stages Questionnaire (ASQ): administered between ages 4 and 48 months
- Brazelton Neonatal Behavioral Assessment Scale: is of particular value during the newborn period, helping to describe the infant's emerging personality and evaluating infant reflexes, general activity, alertness, orientation to spoken voice, and response to visual stimuli (see p. 287).

The physical examination is adapted to the infant's needs. Routine assessments of hearing and vision are an integral part of the examination. In the newborn period, loud noises should precipitate the *startle,* or *Moro, reflex.* Localization of sound during infancy can be roughly ascertained by standing behind the child seated on the mother's lap and ringing a bell or repeating voice sounds. The infant's response is compared with the average for that age level. Vision is mainly assessed by light perception. The examiner shines a penlight into the eyes and notes blinking, following to midline, and other responses. Laboratory tests may include a hemoglobin or hematocrit to detect anemia and urinalysis. Screening tests for various asymptomatic diseases are assuming greater importance; examples of these are the phenylketonuria (PKU) test, tuberculin test, and sickle cell test.

Immunizations

Health personnel must repeatedly stress to parents the importance of immunizations. A delay can lead to undue risks of serious illness, sometimes with fatal complications.

The nurse can stress to working parents that an unprotected child may become sick, making it necessary for them to lose valuable working hours. Immunization also prevents numerous physician and hospital expenses and is required before school entry. A delay or interruption in a series does not interfere with final immunity. It is not necessary to restart any series, regardless of the length of delay. Accurate records prevent confusion. A detailed discussion of immunizations and common childhood communicable diseases is in Chapter 31.

Nutrition Counseling

The nutritional needs of infants reflect rates of growth, energy expended in activity, basal metabolic needs, and the interaction of the nutrients consumed (Mahan & Escott-Stump, 2000). The infant is born with a rooting reflex, which assists in finding the nipple. The sucking reflex is present at birth. There is a forward and backward movement of the tongue. As the infant grows, neuromaturation of the cheeks and tongue enables advancement to a more mature sucking pattern that uses negative pressure to obtain milk. At about the third to fourth month, the extrusion reflex (protrusion), which pushes food out of the mouth to prevent intake of inappropriate food, disappears.

The digestive system continues to mature. By 6 months, it can handle more complex nutrients and is less susceptible to food allergens. The stomach capacity expands from 10 to 20 ml at birth to 200 ml by 12 months. This expansion enables the infant to consume more food at less frequent intervals. As the pincer grasp becomes more developed, the infant can pick up food with tiny fingers and place it in the mouth. By age 2 years the child masters spoon feeding.

Parental concerns. Parents have many concerns about feeding their infant during the first year of life. This is a period when readiness to receive nutritional education is usually high; therefore the nurse looks for opportunities to provide accurate information. Assessment of parental knowledge; infant development, behavior, and readiness; parent-child interaction; and cultural and ethnic practices is important. Nutritional care plans based on developmental levels assist parents in recognizing changes in feeding patterns. The components of a nutritional assessment are discussed in Chapter 15.

A suggested parental guide to determining the adequacy of the diet includes the following:
- The infant has gained 4 to 7 ounces/week for the first 6 months.
- The infant has at least six wet diapers per day.
- The infant sleeps peacefully for several hours after feedings.

Monitoring of weight, height, head circumference, and skin fold thickness determines if the diet is adequate; therefore the value of periodic well-baby examinations is stressed. Bottle-fed infants are usually fed at 3- to 4-hour intervals. Breastfed infants may require feedings at 2- to 3-hour intervals because breast milk is more easily digested. A flexible but regular schedule that provides a rest period between feedings is best for the parent and infant. The nurse reassures parents that most children eat enough to grow normally, although intake is seldom constant and varies in quantity and quality. Forced feedings are not appropriate.

> **NURSING TIP**_____
> Human milk and properly prepared formula supply adequate fluid for the infant under normal conditions. The infant may require additional water during illness or hot, humid weather.

Breastfeeding and bottle feeding. Infants, in proportion to their weight, require more calories, protein, minerals, and vitamins than do adults. Their fluid requirements are also high. Human milk is the best food for infants under age 6 months. It contains the ideal balance of nutrients in a readily digestible form. Breastfeeding soon after birth helps to promote bonding and stimulates milk production. It protects the infant from certain bacteria, and allergic reactions are minimal.

Nutritious infant formulas are also available. Many pediatricians recommend iron-fortified formulas because maternal iron stores decrease by age 6 months. An

table 16-2 *Common Milk Preparations for the First Year*

	ADVANTAGES	DISADVANTAGES
Human breast milk	No preparation needed; nonallergenic; provides antibodies	Lifestyle or illness of mother may influence availability
Prepared, ready-to-feed formula	No preparation needed; no refrigeration needed before opening the bottle	Expensive
Formula concentrate	Easy to prepare; can prepare one bottle at a time or a maximum of one day's feeding at a time	Must be refrigerated after preparation. Must use accurate proportions; safe water supply must be used to dilute the concentrate (water from a natural well may have a high mineral concentrate)
Formula powder	Least expensive formula; lasts up to 1 month once opened	Needs accurate measurement; needs safe water supply and must be shaken thoroughly to dissolve powder

infant who cannot tolerate milk-based formulas may be placed on a soy-based formula. These formulas are nutritionally sound. Whole cow's milk is not recommended for infants under age 1 year because the tough, hard curd is difficult to digest. This type of milk may also contribute to iron-deficiency anemia by causing gastrointestinal blood loss. Formula preparation and breast milk storage is discussed in Chapter 9. Table 16-2 reviews the advantages of the various types of milk available. Box 16-1 reviews how to heat formula in a microwave oven.

It is suggested that infants remain on human milk or iron-fortified formula for the first year of life. Parents are sometimes unsure of when their infant has had enough formula. It is important to explain satiety (hunger satisfaction) behavior at the various ages (Table 16-3). Coaxing infants to finish the last drop in a bottle is unnecessary. Infants who are breastfed longer than 6 months gain less weight by age 1 year than bottle-fed infants.

Taste cells develop during the eighth week of gestation and the fetus begins to respond to flavors when swallowing amniotic fluid. At birth the infant demonstrates a preference for certain tastes, preferring sweet and rejecting sour. Breast milk may supply flavor experiences based on the mother's diet. Infants should be given an opportunity to develop their own personal tastes by being offered various foods when solid foods are introduced. Figure 16-5 illustrates how feeding skills develop in infants and toddlers.

NURSING TIP
Whole milk and "imitation milk" should not be given to infants until after age 1 year.

box 16-1 *Heating Refrigerated Formula in a Microwave Oven*

Most formula can be fed at room temperature. If a formula has been refrigerated, it can be warmed by running warm water over the bottle. Microwave warming is not recommended because it can produce "hot spots" within the formula. Microwaving frozen breast milk may destroy some immune properties and is not advisable. However, because microwaving is a popular current practice, the nurse should explain the proper technique:
- Heat only one portion at a time.
- Keep the bottle in upright position and uncovered.
- Heat a 4-ounce bottle for a *maximum* of 30 seconds.
- Heat an 8-ounce bottle for a *maximum* of 45 seconds.
- Replace nipple and invert bottle several times.
- Test formula temperature before feeding by placing a few drops on your wrist.

Modified from Bush, G., & Anentheswaran, R. (1992). Microwave heating of infant formula: A dilemma resolved. *Pediatrics, 90*(3), 414.

Adding solid foods. Parents often wonder when to begin adding solid foods. The addition of solid food at about 6 months is recommended because this is when the tongue extrusion reflex has completely disappeared and the gastrointestinal tract is mature enough to digest the foods. There are a number of commercially prepared brands of baby foods. Parents should be instructed to read the labels on the jars to obtain nutrition information. Home-prepared foods may also be used (Box 16-2).

table 16-3 | *Growth and Development of Mealtime Behavior*

AGE	HUNGER BEHAVIOR	COMMUNICATION	FEEDING BEHAVIOR	SATIETY	PARENTAL GUIDANCE
Birth to 3 months	Cries; hands fisted; body tense	Roots in search of nipple	Strong suck reflex; needs to be burped	Falls asleep when full; hands relaxed; body relaxed; withdraws head from nipple	Burp frequently. Avoid overfeeding or underfeeding. Recognize signs of satiety.
3 to 5 months	Grasps and draws bottle to mouth; tongue protrudes in anticipation of nipple; fusses; mouths hands	Reaches with open mouth to receive nipple	Strong suck; holds nipple firmly; preference for tastes; pats bottle	Tosses head back; ejects nipple; distracted easily by surroundings; plays with nipple	Provide predictable routine. Allow infant to gain experience with varied textures of fingers/toys.
6 to 9 months	Reacts to food preparation; reaches for bottle	Vocalizes hunger; pulls spoon to mouth; holds bottle	Picks up small food with raking, then pincer action; draws food from spoon with lips; chewing begins	Changes posture; closes mouth; plays with utensils; shakes head "no"	Offer one new food at a time at spaced intervals to assess responses. Include familiar favorites.
10 to 12 months	Vocalizes; grasps utensils; fussy	Attempts to feed self; purses lips to cup's edge	Skilled pincer action to pick up pieces of food and place in mouth; drinks from cup; chews food	Shakes head "no"; sputters food; throws food to floor	Allow infant to assist with feeding. Introduce foods with varied textures. Avoid foods that can be aspirated.

NOTE: Parents who are alert to infant's communication of hunger and satiety help the infant develop self-regulation and communication skills.

Between 4 and 6 months of age, sucking becomes more mature, and munching (up-and-down chopping motions) commences. Rice cereal is often recommended as the first solid food because it is less allergenic.

Only small amounts are offered at first (1 teaspoonful). A small amount of food is placed on the back of the tongue. Cereal may be diluted with formula or water. The consistency is thickened and amounts of solid foods are gradually increased as the infant becomes more familiar with them. A small bowl and a spoon with a long, straight handle is suggested. Single-ingredient foods are introduced (green beans rather than mixed vegetables), because it is easier to determine food allergies this way. Only one new food is offered in a 4-day to 1-week period to determine tolerance.

If the infant refuses a certain food, it is temporarily omitted. Mealtime is kept pleasant. The infant is allowed to try new foods, even ones that the parents dislike. New foods should not be introduced when the infant is ill because adverse responses may not be effectively assessed. The amount of food consumed varies with the child. Fruit juices are generally offered at about 5 to 6 months of age, when the infant begins to drink from a cup. An exception is the addition of orange juice, which is withheld until the infant is 1 year old, especially when family members have known allergies. Other highly allergenic foods that may be delayed include fish, nuts, strawberries, chocolate, and egg whites.

A children's "sipper" plastic cup is helpful at first. The juice is initially diluted. The National Research Council (NRC) recommends a daily liquid intake of 140 to 160 ml/kg/day for a 3-month-old; 130 to 155 ml/kg/day for a 6-month-old; 120 to 135 ml/kg/day for a 1-year-old, and 90 to 100 ml/kg/day for a 6-year-old (Behrman, Kliegman, & Jenson, 2000). Baby food can be prepared

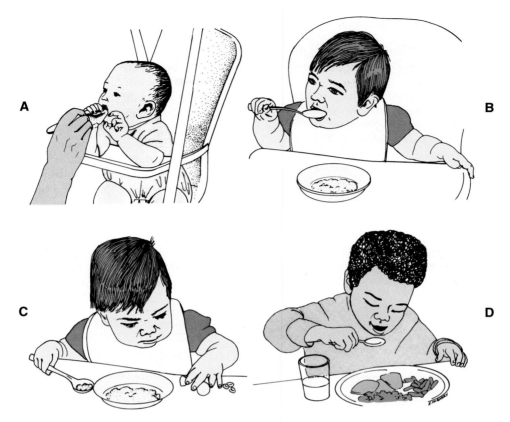

FIGURE **16-5** Development of feeding skills in infants and toddlers. **A,** At 7 months, this child begins to reach for the spoon. **B,** At 9 months, this little girl begins to use her spoon independently, although she is not yet able to keep food on it. **C,** The 9-month-old shows a refined pincer grasp to pick up food. **D,** The 2-year-old is much more skillful at self-feeding and has the ability both to rotate the wrist and to elevate the elbow to keep food on the spoon.

in a food grinder, electric blender, or food mill or by mashing the food to the desired texture.

>NURSING **TIP**_____
Cereal and baby food should *not* be mixed in a bottle with formula.

>NURSING **TIP**_____
To prevent the development of botulism, honey should not be included in the diet of infants under age 2 years.

>NURSING **TIP**_____
New solid foods should be introduced *before* the milk feedings to encourage the infant to try the new experience. As solid food intake increases, the amount of formula or milk should decrease to avoid overfeeding.

Recommended fat intake during infancy. Fat contains more calories than carbohydrates and proteins. Because infants have a limited stomach capacity and a high caloric need, fats in easily digestible forms are needed for meeting their caloric needs for growth and development and for brain development. Infants have a high basal metabolic rate (BMR) and require almost three times more calories per kilogram of weight than adults do to maintain their rapid growth and development in the first year of life. In the young infant, breast milk and infant formulas provide the necessary fats that the infant is able to digest. *Feeding a low-fat diet to infants under age 2 years will compromise their growth and development.*

The fat and cholesterol content may not be designated on the label of many baby foods. By age 6 months, amylase and lipase are present in the digestive tract to aid in digesting fat content present in solid foods. A well-balanced diet provides appropriate fat and choles-

box 16-2 *Directions for Home Preparation of Infant Foods*

1. Select fresh, high-quality fruits, vegetables, or meats.
2. Be sure all utensils, including cutting boards, grinder, and knives, are thoroughly clean.
3. Wash hands before preparing the food.
4. Clean, wash, and trim the food in as little water as possible.
5. Cook the foods until tender in as little water as possible. Avoid overcooking, which may destroy heat-sensitive nutrients.
6. Do not add salt. Add sugar sparingly. Do not add honey to food for infants less than age 2 years. (Botulism spores have been reported in honey, and young infants do not have the immune capacity to resist this infection.)
7. Add enough water so the food can be easily pureed.
8. Strain or puree the food with an electric blender, food mill, baby food grinder, or kitchen strainer.
9. Pour the pureed food into an ice cube tray and freeze.
10. When food is frozen hard, remove the cubes and store in freezer bags.
11. Unfreeze and heat (in water bath or microwave oven) in serving container the amount of food that will be consumed at a single feeding.

From Mahan, L.K., & Escott-Stump, S. (2000). *Krause's food, nutrition and diet therapy* (10th ed.). Philadelphia: W.B. Saunders.

terol intake. Evaluating the height and weight of infants on a growth chart during clinic visits is an essential assessment of growth and development. Whole cow's milk can be introduced after age 1 year, and low-fat milk can be introduced after age 2 years.

Buying, storing, and serving foods. Baby foods stored in jars are vacuum-packed. Parents are taught to check safety seals before purchase. Directions are generally indicated on the jar (e.g., to reject product if safety button is up). The expiration date of the product should be checked. Dates are usually found on the caps of jars and on the sides of cereal and bakery items. Unopened jars of baby food and juices are stored in a dry, cool place. Jars are rotated, and those on hand the longest are used first.

When a jar is opened, a definite "pop" is heard as the vacuum seal is broken. Food is transferred to a serving dish. The infant should not be fed out of the jar, and leftovers should not be returned to the jar because saliva may turn certain foods to liquid by digesting them in the jar. Unused portions may be stored in the refrigerator in the original jar. Special precautions are taken when food is heated in the microwave, because food sometimes heats unevenly.

Weaning. Weaning is defined as substituting a cup for a bottle or breastfeeding. Because sucking is a major source of pleasure in the first year of life, weaning is a major step in growth and development. Signs of readiness to wean can be seen in the infant who eagerly looks forward to new tastes and textures found on the spoon. The infant may not want to be held close during feedings and may start to "bite" the nipple as teeth erupt. The approaching stage of autonomy provides the child with motivation to manipulate the cup. Imitation of older siblings or parents also contributes to readiness. Weaning should be very gradual and start with daytime feedings. Weaning is usually completed by age 2 years but may continue longer in some cultures.

INFANT SAFETY

CAR SAFETY

Infant seats should be used for all infants traveling in automobiles. A rear-facing infant seat should be used for infants under age 1 year and 22 pounds, and it should be located in the center of the rear seat of the automobile. Cars with passenger-side safety air bags pose a danger to infants in infant seats who are placed in the front seat. The infant seat should be firmly anchored to the vehicle by the car seat belt (see Chapter 17).

FALL PREVENTION

An infant should never be left unattended on a flat surface, such as a changing table. Newborn infants have crawling reflexes that can cause them to fall off a changing table. Infants under age 4 months have rounded backs and can accidentally roll off a flat surface. Infants over age 4 months can voluntarily roll over. Crib rails should be raised and securely locked. Infants should be secured in high chairs or swings. An infant seat should not be placed on a table or high surface. Crawling infants should be protected from stairways, and heavy or unsturdy furniture should not be available for use in pulling themselves to a standing position.

A safe environment for a crawling infant includes storage of poisonous items out of the sight and reach of the infant. Cabinet locks are available for purchase. Plants, batteries, pool areas, plugs, loose hanging wires, and pets can be hazardous to an infant. Close supervision at all times is essential to the safety of any environment. Resource consultants are available in most communities for information concerning "childproofing" the home.

| table 16-4 | *Toys for the First Year* |

AGE	VISUAL STIMULATION	AUDITORY STIMULATION	SENSORIMOTOR STIMULATION
0 to 2 months	Black-and-white contrasting mobiles placed at midline of infant's vision	Talk Music Ticking clock	Cuddle, rock
3 to 5 months	Unbreakable mirrors Infant seat positioned to view the room	Talk to infant, provide rattles	Cradle gym, infant swing
6 to 9 months	Peek-a-boo (teaches object permanence) Encouraging imitation of facial expression	Use appropriate names for objects Speak clearly	Introduce various textures for infant to touch Use teething toys
10 to 12 months	Large picture books Shopping trips Soft blocks Nested boxes	Reading, singing nursery rhymes Imitating sounds of animals	Push-pull toys Activity boxes

NOTE: Toys for each age-group should be varied to stimulate sight, touch, sound, and movement. Safety for age and diagnosis is of utmost importance in selection of a play activity or toy.

TOY SAFETY

Toys should be appropriate for the age and diagnosis, but safety is the most important feature involved in toy selection. Infants put everything into their mouths, and therefore choking is a major problem if a toy has small or removable parts. When the pincer skill is developed, infants will be able to pick up small objects such as pins and put them in their mouths. Toys appropriate for older siblings can be dangerous to infants. For example, if an infant drinks the glue from a model airplane set an older sibling is playing with, the results can be deadly. Constant supervision is essential. Toys should nurture growth and development (Table 16-4). A child's response to a toy can indicate readiness to learn new skills. An infant who is able to reach for and pick up a toy shows readiness for communication.

SUMMARY OF MAJOR DEVELOPMENTAL CHANGES IN THE FIRST YEAR

- Weight doubles by age 6 months and triples by age 1 year.
- Height increases by 1 inch per month for first 6 months to 29 inches (74 cm) by age 1 year (increase is mainly in the trunk of the body).
- Head circumference increases 0.6 inches (1.5 cm) each month for the first 6 months and is 18 inches (46 cm) by age 12 months.
- Head circumference and chest circumference are equal by the first year of life.

- Closure of the posterior fontanel occurs by age 2 months.
- Closure of the anterior fontanel occurs by age 18 months.
- Primitive reflexes are replaced by voluntary movements.
- Maternal iron stores decrease by age 6 months.
- Digestive processes increase functioning at age 3 months. Amylase and lipase are deficient until age 4 to 6 months, which decreases the ability to digest the fats found in solid foods.
- Tooth eruption begins at age 6 months, when "biting" activities start.
- Binocular vision is established by age 4 months.
- Depth perception begins to develop at age 9 months.
- Infants over age 4 months can voluntarily roll over.
- By age 1 year, infants can take some independent steps.
- *Separation* (of self from others), object permanence (objects exist even if they are out of visual field), and *symbols* (saying bye-bye means someone is leaving) are major aspects of cognitive development in the first year of life.

key points

- A development of a sense of trust begins in infancy and is vital to a healthy personality.
- Breast milk or formula is the most desirable food for the first 6 months of the infant's life, followed by gradual introduction of a variety of solid foods.

- Sensory stimulation is essential for the development of the infant's thought processes and perceptual abilities.
- Health maintenance visits are essential during the first year to detect variations from normal growth patterns, to provide immunizations, and to educate and support parents.
- Infants should be positioned for sleep on their backs, on a firm mattress, for safety and to prevent sudden infant death syndrome (SIDS). The infant can be placed on his or her abdomen during playtime.
- The nurse must stress to parents the value of immunizations for infants and children.
- Human milk and properly prepared formula supply an adequate fluid intake for the infant under normal conditions. The infant may require additional water during illness or in very hot, humid weather.
- Feeding an infant a low-fat diet before age 2 years will compromise growth and development.
- The most common cause of concern is an atypical-for-age slowing of any aspect of development.

ONLINE RESOURCES

Recommendations of the ACIP: http://www.cdc.gov/nip/publications/acip-list.htm

Child Health Statistics: http://www.childstats.gov

Immunization Action Coalition: http://www.immunize.org

National Immunization Programs: http://www.cdc.gov/nip

Poison Control Center: http://www.aapcc.org

REVIEW QUESTIONS *Choose the most appropriate answer.*

1. The startle reflex is also known as the:
   1. Moro reflex
   2. Rooting reflex
   3. Pincer reflex
   4. Grasp reflex

2. A car seat for an infant under age 1 year:
   1. Is not needed if the infant is held securely in the lap of an adult
   2. Should be placed close to the driver in the front passenger seat
   3. Should face the rear and be placed in the center of the back seat
   4. Should face forward and be placed on the driver's side of the back seat

3. To detect allergies when feeding new foods:
   1. Introduce single-ingredient foods
   2. Mix the food with one the infant likes
   3. Mix the food with formula
   4. Offer two new foods at a time

4. The nurse is discussing home safety with the mother of a 4-month-old infant. Which of the following is a priority topic?
   1. Placing locks on cabinet doors that contain cleaning supplies
   2. Covering electrical outlets
   3. Raising and securing crib side rails
   4. Encouraging reading and talking to infant

5. A mother expresses concern that her 1-year-old infant is overweight. She states that her family has a tendency to be overweight and wishes to discontinue formula feedings and start the infant on low-fat milk. The nurse assesses that the present weight of the infant is 24 pounds. The infant's birth weight was 8 pounds, 2 ounces. The best response of the nurse would be:
   1. To place the infant on low-fat milk because the infant is slightly overweight at this time
   2. To place the infant on regular whole milk as the infant's weight is appropriate for his age
   3. To indicate that the infant is underweight for his age and needs to have supplemental formula added to the diet
   4. To note that infancy is a period of rapid growth and weight loss will occur as the infant becomes more active

objectives

1. Define each key term listed.
2. Describe the physical, psychosocial, and cognitive development of children from 1 to 3 years of age, listing age-specific events and guidance when appropriate.
3. Describe the task to be mastered by the toddler according to Erikson's stages of growth and development.
4. List two developmental tasks of the toddler period.
5. Discuss speech development in the toddler.
6. Discuss how adults can assist small children in combating their fears.
7. Identify the principles of toilet training (bowel and bladder) that will assist in guiding parents' efforts to provide toilet independence.
8. List two methods of preventing the following: automobile accidents, burns, falls, suffocation and choking, poisoning, drowning, electric shock, and animal bites.
9. Describe the characteristic play and appropriate toys for a toddler.
10. Discuss the principles of guidance and discipline for a toddler.
11. Describe the nutritional needs and self-feeding abilities of a toddler.

key terms

autonomy (p. 411)
cooperative play (p. 420)
egocentric thinking (p. 420)
negativism (p. 405)
object permanence (p. 409)
parallel play (p. 420)
ritualism (p. 405)
separation anxiety (sĕp-ă-RĀ-shăn ăng-ZĪ-ĭ-tē, p. 409)
temper tantrum (p. 411)
time-out (p. 411)
toddler (p. 405)

GENERAL CHARACTERISTICS

Children between 1 and 3 years of age are referred to as toddlers. They are able to get about by using their own powers and are no longer completely dependent persons. By this time, they have generally tripled their birth weight and gained control of their head, hands, and feet. The remarkably rapid growth and development that took place during infancy begins to slow down. The toddler period presents different challenges for the parents and the child.

The toddler is in Erikson's stage of autonomy versus shame and doubt, which is based on a continuum of trust established during infancy (see Chapter 15). The challenging tasks to be mastered by the toddler include increasing independence, toilet training, self-feeding, self-dressing, speech development, and a curiosity to explore the widening environment. One major parental responsibility is to maintain safety while allowing the toddler the opportunity for social and physical independence. Another major parental responsibility is to maintain a positive self-image and body image in the child whose behavior is inconsistent and often frustrating. Toddlers alternate between dependence and independence. They test their power by saying "no" frequently. This is called negativism. Offering limited choices and the use of distraction can be helpful tools in handling toddlers (too many choices can cause confusion). Developing self-control and socially acceptable outlets for aggression and anger are important factors in the formation of personality and behavior. Ritualism is another characteristic of toddler behavior. Toddlers increase their sense of security by making compulsive routines of simple tasks, and therefore their rituals should be respected. Table 17-1 summarizes the toddler's physical development, social behavior, and abilities at various ages.

PHYSICAL DEVELOPMENT

The toddler's body changes proportions (Figure 17-1). The legs and arms lengthen through ossification and growth in the epiphyseal areas of the long bones. The

table 17-1 *Physical Development, Social Behavior, and Abilities of Toddlers*

	SOCIAL	FINE MOTOR	GROSS MOTOR	LANGUAGE	COGNITION
12 to 16 months	Imitates adults' activities Seeks alternate methods of achieving solitary play	Drinks from cup, holds spoon Builds tower of 2 blocks Prefers finger feeding	Begins to walk	Uses words Is activity oriented Follows simple commands	Classifies objects with function Object permanence begins to develop
16 to 18 months	Curious, parallel play Ritualistic behavior	Places objects in appropriately shaped openings Improved self-feeding	Walks alone, can walk backward	Use symbolic language ("bye-bye") Is able to point to familiar objects	Can imitate from memory Begins to realize cause and effect

The toddler uses pincer action of the fingers as well as the spoon to self-feed.

24 months	Increased independence Egocentric—everything is "mine" Increased autonomy, can say "no"	Builds tower of 6 to 7 blocks Turns pages of book Can undress self	Runs, throws ball Climbs steps Imitates oral hygiene Jumps with both feet	Uses plural words Uses words to tell story Names familiar objects	Continuous investigation and exploring Develops likes and dislikes
36 months	Establishes toilet independence Identifies sexual roles Begins to share May have imaginary playmate	Holds cup by handle and spoon with two fingers Copies a circle	Balances (hops) Jumps on one foot Uses tricycle Climbs stairs using alternate feet	Can hold conversation Frequently asks why and how Says full name	Can understand one idea or concept at a time Knows two colors Imitates parental roles

This 2 1/2-year-old has all of her deciduous teeth.

Imitating parental behaviors can help the toddler to prepare for the arrival of a new sibling.

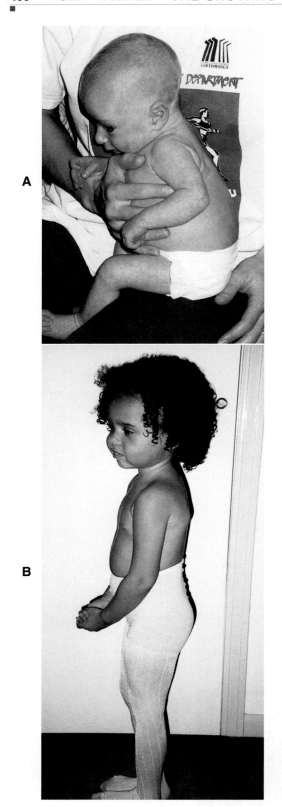

FIGURE **17-1** Change in body contour. **A,** The back of the infant is rounded. **B,** In the toddler, the exaggerated lumbar lordosis makes the abdomen protrude.

trunk and head grow more slowly. The toddler gains 4 to 6 pounds (1.8 to 2.7 kg) per year. The birth weight has quadrupled by 2½ years of age. The toddler grows 4 inches (10 cm) per year in height. The height of a 2-year-old is thought to be one half of the potential adult height of that child. The height and weight are plotted carefully on a growth chart during each clinic visit to reflect the steady pace of growth and development. (See Chapter 15, Figure 15-4.)

The rate of brain growth decelerates. The increase in head circumference during infancy is 10 cm (4 inches), whereas during the second year of life it is only 2.5 cm (1 inch). Chest circumference continues to increase. After the second year the child appears leaner because the chest circumference begins to exceed the abdominal circumference. The protuberant abdomen flattens when the muscle fibers increase in size and strength.

Myelination of the spinal cord is practically complete by 2 years, allowing for control of anal and urethral sphincters. Bowel and bladder control is usually complete by 2½ to 3 years of age.

Respirations are still mainly abdominal but shift to thoracic as the child approaches school age. The toddler is more capable of maintaining a stable body temperature than is the infant. The shivering process, in which the capillaries constrict or dilate in response to body temperature, has matured.

The skin becomes tough as the epidermis and dermis bond more tightly, which protects the child from fluid loss, infection, and irritation. The defense mechanisms of the skin and blood, particularly phagocytosis, work more effectively than they did during infancy. The lymphatic tissues of the adenoids and tonsils enlarge during this period. The eustachian tube continues to be shorter and straighter than in the adult. Tonsillitis, otitis media, and upper respiratory infections are common problems. Eruption of deciduous teeth continues until completion at about 2½ years of age (see Chapter 15).

The blood pressure of a toddler may average 90/56 mm Hg, and the respiratory rate slows to 25 breaths/min and continues to be abdominal breathing. The pulse of a toddler slows to a range of 70 to 110 beats/min. Digestive processes and the volume capacity of the stomach increase to accommodate a three-meal-a-day schedule.

SENSORIMOTOR AND COGNITIVE DEVELOPMENT

The senses and motor abilities of the toddler do not function independently of one another. Two-year-old toddlers reach, grasp, inspect, smell, taste, and study objects with their eyes. Their attention becomes centered on characteristics of their surroundings that capture their interest. Binocular vision is well established by age 15 months. Visual acuity is about 20/40 by 2 years of age.

As memory strengthens, toddlers can compare present events with stored knowledge. They assimilate information through trial and error plus repetition. They try alternative methods of accomplishing a goal. Thought processes advance, preparing the way for more complex mental operations. The sensorimotor and preconceptual phase of development described by Piaget develops rapidly between 1 and 3 years of age and affects the toddler's behavior.

Separation anxiety, which consists of *protest, despair,* and *detachment,* develops in infancy and continues throughout toddlerhood. Toddlers are able to tolerate longer periods of separation from parents to explore their environment. They become aware of cause and effect. Often they correlate a type of object with its function. For example, if their toys are stored in a paper bag, they will gleefully open any paper bag they see, expecting to find toys. If the bag contains garbage or drugs, they can be injured or may be punished. This can be confusing to the toddler and frustrating to the parents.

The concept of spatial relationships develops, and toddlers are able to fit square pegs in a square hole and round pegs in a round hole. Toys should be selected to promote this ability. Object permanence continues to develop, and the toddler becomes aware that there may be fun items behind closed doors and in closed drawers. The toddler's curiosity and ability to explore make it important to educate parents to keep dangerous objects out of their reach. The toddler begins to internalize standards of behavior as evidenced by saying "no-no" when tempted to touch a forbidden object.

The toddler copies the words and the roles of the models seen in the home. The toddler may "help Mommy clean" or "help Daddy shave." By 2 years of age there is a recognition of sexual differences.

Toddlers may confuse essential with nonessential body parts. Expelling feces and flushing it down the toilet can be upsetting to some toddlers because they may feel they expelled a part of themselves that has disappeared. Toddlers' body image and self-esteem may be impaired if they are scolded in a way that makes them feel *they* are bad rather than their *behavior* is bad. The nurse must help the parents develop skills that will enable toddlers to feel they are loved even though the specific behavior is unacceptable.

SPEECH DEVELOPMENT

Language development parallels cognitive growth. The increase in the level of comprehension is particularly striking and exceeds verbalization. By 3 years of age the child has a rather extensive vocabulary of about 900 words. Speech is more than 90% intelligible (Table 17-2).

At about the end of the first year, the infant begins to make noises that sound like "bye-bye," "ma-ma" and "da-da." When toddlers see the happy response to these sounds, they repeat them. This is true throughout the

table 17-2 | *Language Milestones*

EXPRESSIVE LANGUAGE	AGE (MONTHS)	RECEPTIVE LANGUAGE	AGE (MONTHS)
Social smile	2	Alerts	1
Coos	3	Recognizes mother	2
Laughs	4	Orients to voice	4
Razzes	5	Orients to bell	5
"Ah-goo"	5	Looks directly at bell	9
Babbles	6	Understands "no"	9
Dada/Mama		Plays gesture games	9
Nonspecific	8	Follows one-step command	
Specific	10	With gesture	12
First word	11	Without gesture	16
Second word	12	Knows one body part	18
Jargon	15	Points to one picture	18
4 to 6 words	16	Follows two-step command	24
Two-word phrases	21	Points to seven pictures	24
Two-word sentences	24	Follows prepositional commands	36
Pronouns	36		
Plurals	36		

Modified from Montgomery, T. (1994). When not talking is the chief complaint. *Contemporary Pediatrics, 11*(9), 49.
NOTE: This table of language milestones is a guide to assessing normal language development. Although most mentally retarded children are language delayed, not all language-delayed children are mentally retarded. Some normal children also are late talkers.

toddler period. To want to learn to talk, small children must have an appreciative audience.

Children first refer to animals by the sounds the animals make. For example, before saying "dog," the toddler repeats "bow-bow." Soon the child can say short phrases such as "Daddy gone car." Toddlers also respond to tone of voice and facial expression. If an adult sounds threatening, the toddler may answer "no" and then repeat it in a louder voice.

Sometimes adults scold the child merely for being too young to understand what is requested. However, imagine being punished in a foreign country because you could not speak or comprehend the language well enough to defend yourself. Adults who show empathy to the small child can help to minimize their frustrations.

Parents who are concerned about their child's delayed speech can discuss it with their health care provider during a routine physical examination so it can be evaluated in light of total physical growth and development (Table 17-3). Many late talkers are perfectly normal children who prefer listening over active participation. Many common household items, such as vertical window blinds and decorative metal vases, contain lead. Lead poisoning and hearing deficits should be ruled out before screening for other developmental problems (Box 17-1).

GUIDANCE AND DISCIPLINE

Discipline for the toddler involves guidance. The goal is to teach, not to punish. Teaching the toddler self-control with positive self-esteem is desirable rather than encouraging a completely submissive, "obedient" child.

table 17-3	*When a Child with a Communication Disorder Needs Help*	
AGE	**BEHAVIOR INDICATING HELP IS NEEDED**
0 to 11 months	Before 6 months the child does not startle, blink, or change immediate activity in response to sudden loud sounds.
	Before 6 months the child does not attend to the human voice and is not soothed by his or her mother's voice.
	By 6 months the child does not babble strings of consonant + vowel syllables or imitate gurgling or cooing sounds.
	By 10 months the child does not respond to his or her name.
	At 10 months the child's sound making is limited to shrieks, grunts, or sustained vowel production.
12 to 23 months	At 12 months the child's babbling or speech is limited to vowel sounds.
	By 15 months the child does not respond to "no," "bye-bye," or "'bottle.'"
	By 15 months the child will not imitate sounds or words.
	By 18 months the child is not consistently using at least six words with appropriate meaning.
	By 21 months the child does not respond correctly to "Give me . . .," "Sit down," or "Come here" when spoken without gestural cues.
	By 23 months two-word phrases have not emerged that are spoken as single units (e.g., "Whatzit," "Thank you," "Allgone").
24 to 36 months	By 24 months, at least 50% of the child's speech is not understood by familiar listeners.
	By 24 months the child does not point to body parts without gestural cues.
	By 24 months the child is not combining words into phrases ("Go bye-bye," "Go car," "Want cookie").
	By 30 months the child does not demonstrate understanding of on, in, under, front, back.
	By 30 months the child is not using short sentences ("Daddy went bye-bye").
	By 30 months the child has not begun to ask questions, using where, what, why.
	By 36 months the child's speech is not understood by unfamiliar listeners.

At any age the child is consistently dysfluent (not clear) with repetitions, hesitations, blocks, or struggles to say words. Struggle may be accompanied by grimaces, eye blinks, or hand gestures.

From Behrman, R., & Kliegman, R. (1998). *Nelson's essentials of pediatrics* (3rd ed.). Philadelphia: W.B. Saunders.

The toddler who scribbles on the wall must be given the opportunity to scribble on paper, a more socially acceptable outlet.

Temper tantrums (an uncontrolled anger reaction) often occur during the toddler years, and parent responses reinforce to the child either the desirability or the risks involved with such behavior. Expectations must be commensurate with the child's physical and cognitive abilities. Toddlers get into many situations that are over their heads. When adults make firm decisions, the problem is resolved, at least for the time being. The child feels secure.

Limit setting should include praise for desired behavior as well as disapproval for undesired behavior. A time-out period in a safe place helps the child to develop self-regulation. Timing should not begin until the child has settled down. The child is praised once calm. Timing for time-out is usually based on 1 minute per year of age.

Children, like adults, seek approval. It is effective and helps to increase their self-confidence. The positive approach should be taken as often as possible. One assumes that the toddler is going to be good rather than bad. "Thank you, Johnny, for giving me the matches" will make them arrive in your hand more quickly than "Give me those matches right now," said in a threatening tone. The use of fear or physical aggression should not be a part of discipline because it does not foster self-control and can lead to physical or mental abuse.

Fear is a valuable emotion to the child if it does not become too intense. Unfortunately, many children fear situations that are not in themselves dangerous, and this sometimes deprives them of activities that otherwise would be enjoyable. If the parent warns, "Be careful, don't fall," when a toddler begins to ride a tricycle, the toddler may develop a fear of the risk taking that may be involved in experiencing new activities.

The physical and mental health of the child at the time of a fear-provoking experience affects the extent of the reaction. If the child is alone, fear may be greater than if someone such as a parent or nurse is present. Once a fear has been learned, it is more difficult to eliminate. Favorite possessions and repetitive rituals are *self-consoling behaviors* for the toddler, particularly at bedtime and during separation from parents.

Stress increases fear of separation. Adults should attempt to control their own fears in the presence of young children. Respect and understanding should always be accorded to children who are afraid. Making fun of the fear or shaming the child in front of others is detrimental to self-esteem.

Many toddlers who independently explore the clinic examining room while waiting to be examined may cling to the parent when the stranger (the health care provider) enters the room and approaches the child. The toddler who does not seek the parent during stressful situations or turns to a stranger for comfort reflects a need for closer evaluation of the parent-child relationship.

The "terrible two's," during which negativistic behavior is predominant, begin the disciplinary pattern of the family that will carry throughout childhood and affect the child's personality. Corporal punishment, involving spanking, is accepted in many traditional cultures as the mainstay of discipline. However, regular spanking reflects a desperate effort by the parent to gain control over a toddler who is exercising his or her beginning autonomy (independent functioning) and developing negativism. Potential injury, child abuse, and reciprocal aggressive behavior in the child can be avoided with careful parental guidance concerning alternative techniques of discipline. Time-out, limit setting, clear communication, and frequent rewards/approval for positive behavior are effective noncorporal techniques of discipline.

Communicating love and respect to the child with a clear message that it is the *behavior,* not the *child,* that is disapproved by the adult are the keys to effective discipline. Behavior problems that can occur during early childhood are detailed in Table 17-4.

> **NURSING TIP**
>
> Caregivers must provide safe areas for the toddler to explore. They need to watch carefully before saying "no."

box 17-1 | *Screening for Signs of Autism*

No pointing, gesturing (bye-bye) by 12 months
No single words by 16 months
No spontaneous two-word phrases by 24 months
Loss of achieved language or social skills

These are preliminary symptoms. Lead poisoning or hearing deficits should be ruled out.

From Filipek, P., et al. (2000). Practice parameter: Screening and diagnosis of autism. *Neurology* 55:468-479.

DAILY CARE

Nutrition, dentition, and oral care are discussed in Chapter 15. When talking to the toddler, the adult should be at eye level with the child so the adult seems less overwhelming. This is of particular importance when the child is in a fear-provoking environment, such as the hospital. A flexible schedule organized around the needs of the entire household is best for the toddler. The

table 17-4 *Behavior Problems During Early Childhood, Normal Expectations, and Parental Guidance*

BEHAVIOR	NORMAL EXPECTATIONS	CHILD FACTORS CONTRIBUTING TO PROBLEM	PARENTAL GUIDANCE
Sleep disorders	Occasional nightmares begin at about 36 months.	Excessive napping during the day	Provide one nap a day until end of second year, when naps can be eliminated.
	Ritual bedtime routine begins; attempt to delay sleep peaks between 2 and 3 years.	Insufficient adult interaction during the day, leading to the use of bedtime as opportunity to gain adult attention	Use of bedtime rituals, such as a quiet activity or bedtime stories, are helpful.
	Head banging and rocking between 1 and 4 years provide a release of tension.	Unusual fears related to darkness, being left alone	Use of favorite toy or blanket in the bed can ease insecurities involved in separation.
		Discomfort of wet diapers	Provide environment conducive to sleep.
		Illness	Avoid scary television shows.
			Restrict fluids before bedtime.
Temper tantrums	Tantrums peak at age 2 years, decreasing in frequency and intensity until they rarely occur by about 4 years of age.	Used as a manipulative device to gain control of parental behavior	Use simple explanations of behavior expectations.
	Tantrums usually occur in response to the frustrated desires of a child, such as wanting a toy that cannot be purchased.	Insufficient positive interaction with adults, leads to use of tantrums to gain attention	Use "time out" responses (1 minute per year of age). Maintain consistency of expectations from both parents. Reward good behavior.
Toilet training and bed wetting	Child has full physiological capacity for day control by 3 years, night control by 4 years.	Fears and anxiety in response to negative toilet training	Use positive rewards for successful toileting and ignore accidents.
	Daytime and nighttime "accidents" occur throughout early childhood, decreasing in frequency by 4 years.	Used as an attention-getting device if positive means of gaining attention are lacking	Recognize signals of need to use toilet. Restrict fluids before bedtime.
		May use constipation as a control mechanism	

From Chinn, P., Leitch, C. (1979). *Child health maintenance* (2nd ed.). St. Louis: Mosby

toddler needs a consistent routine, but it can differ for special occasions.

The clothing of toddlers should be simple and easy for them to put on and take off. Pants with elastic waists are convenient for them to pull down when they use the toilet. All clothing must be fairly loose to provide freedom of movement for jumping and other strenuous activities. Sunburn protection with clothing or sunscreen is necessary to prevent skin damage.

The toddler wears shoes mainly for protection. They should fit the shape of the foot and be ½ inch longer and ¼ inch wider than the foot. The heels must fit securely. Children should wear their usual shoes at their periodic checkups because these show how the shoes have been worn, which indicates to the health care provider how the children are using their bodies. The toddler may go barefoot whenever it is safe and possible, because this strengthens the foot muscles. Socks must be large enough that they do not flex the toes. The toddler should be taught to pull socks free from the toes before putting on shoes.

Good posture is the result of proper nutrition, plenty of fresh air and exercise, and sufficient rest. The toddler's mattress must be firm. The chair and play table are adapted to size. In some cases this can be easily accomplished by placing a rolled-up blanket or pad in the seat of the chair. A sturdy small stool placed in the bathroom will bring the child to the proper height for brushing the teeth.

table 17-4 *Behavior Problems During Early Childhood, Normal Expectations, and Parental Guidance—cont'd*

BEHAVIOR	NORMAL EXPECTATIONS	CHILD FACTORS CONTRIBUTING TO PROBLEM	PARENTAL GUIDANCE
Toilet training and bed wetting—cont'd	Regression occurs with environmental or social changes, such as arrival of sibling, moving, or divorce.	Excessive fluid intake before bedtime	Use clothing that toddler can easily remove for self-toileting.
Aggressive or quarrelsome behavior, sibling rivalry	Ability to play cooperatively begins to emerge at 3 to 5 years. Before this age, the child is seldom able to share toys and often wants toys that another child has.	Insufficient positive adult attention, leading to deliberate use of aggression to gain adult attention	Prepare toddler for the separation and change involved in the arrival of a new sibling. Provide for any changes involved 1 to 2 months before arrival of sibling (e.g., change to a new bed or room).
	There is a predominant use of physical hitting and shoving to express displeasure; verbal abilities begin to emerge.	May arise from actual or perceived adult preference for sibling or playmate	Provide toddler with doll to imitate parental behaviors. Provide for special individual time with toddler each day.
Inability to separate, excessive shyness	Child can separate easily by 3 years if surroundings are consistent, predictable, and positive. Child continues to protest separation if environment changes or if confronted by total strangers. Child is shy in new and strange surroundings but relaxed and spontaneous in familiar surroundings.	Inadequate establishment of self-concept, leading to lack of confidence, even in familiar surroundings. Uses protest of separation as a manipulative control device. Fear of being abandoned	Prepare toddler for anticipated separation. Refer to time using concrete terms ("I will return after lunch" rather than "I will return at 1 PM"). Avoid radiating parental anxiety at the planned separation. Spend time with toddler and in new environment or with new caregiver before leaving.

As in all areas of learning, the child's posture is greatly influenced by that of other members of the family. The toddler who is happy and is allowed gradually increasing independence develops a sense of security, which is reflected in the posture. Slouching is sometimes seen in children who are insecure and lack self-confidence.

TOILET INDEPENDENCE

There are many approaches to toilet training. Much depends on the temperament of both the individual child and the person guiding the child. Readiness is important. Voluntary control of anal and urethral sphincters occurs at about 18 to 24 months. The child's waking up dry in the morning or from naptime is an indication of maturity. Children must be able to communicate in some fashion that they are wet or need to urinate or defecate. They must be willing to sit on the potty for at least 5 to 10 minutes.

Toddlers seek approval and like to imitate the actions of parents. They wander into the bathroom and are curious about what is taking place there. If a parent feels that the child will respond to training at this time, the child might first be put in training pants or pull-up diapers. These can be removed quickly and easily, and the child becomes more aware of being wet.

The use of a child's potty-chair or a device that attaches to an adult seat is a matter of personal preference.

A potty-chair may make the toddler feel more secure because it is small (Figure 17-2). It should support the back and arms of the child. The feet should touch the floor. If a potty-chair is not available, the child can be placed on the standard-size toilet, facing the toilet tank. This method may increase feelings of security. The toddler can use a regular toilet with a bench to support the child's feet.

Bowel training is generally attempted first; however, some toddlers become bladder trained during the day because they enjoy listening to the "tinkle" in the potty. If toddlers have bowel movements at the same time each day, they may progress fairly rapidly. They should not be left on the potty-chair for more than a few minutes at a time.

Demands and threats do more damage than good. Life is smoother for all if the parent remains patient and keeps this new adventure pleasant. Training should not be undertaken when the family or child is under stress, such as during illness or a move to a new location.

Bladder training is begun when the toddler stays dry for about 2 hours at a time. The parent may discover that the toddler has gone the entire night without wet-ting. It is then logical to put the child on the potty-chair and to praise success. Bladder training varies widely, particularly during the night. Restricting fluids before bedtime may help. Placing the half-asleep child on the potty-chair accomplishes little.

Most children continue to have occasional accidents until age 4 years. If the toddler has a mishap, parents should accept it matter-of-factly and merely change the clothes. Children benefit when adults show continuous affection to them and accept both bad and good days.

The word that toddlers use to signal defecation or urination should be one that is recognized by others besides the immediate family. Sometimes a parent may forget to inform the baby-sitter or nursery school teacher of the word that the child uses. This causes the toddler unnecessary frustration because those about them cannot understand what they are trying to say.

Toddlers who are toilet trained at home should continue to use the potty in the hospital setting. They may be acutely embarrassed by wetting the crib. Although regression of bowel and bladder training is common during hospitalization, personnel often contribute to it by not taking time to investigate the child's needs. Nurses regularly consult the child's nursing care plan to maintain continuity of care as well as promote growth and development of the toddler.

> ⭐ NURSING **TIP**
> Nurses can help parents identify readiness for toilet independence.

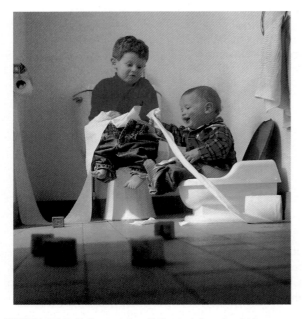

FIGURE **17-2** Toilet training. Toilet training should be a non-stressful experience for the toddler. Nurses can help parents identify readiness for toilet independence. The nurse assesses the parents' expectations, family and cultural preferences, and developmental readiness of the child when instructing parents. Often the younger sibling enjoys imitating the older sibling. Sitting on the potty too long without supervision may result in bathroom playtime! (Photo by Camile Tokerud, New York.)

NUTRITION COUNSELING

Caloric requirements per unit of body weight decline in the toddler from 120 Calories/kg during infancy to 100 Calories/kg. Children need an adequate protein intake to cover maintenance needs and to provide for optimum growth. Milk should be limited to 24 ounces a day. Too few solid foods can lead to dietary deficiencies of iron. Children between 1 and 3 years of age are high-risk candidates for anemia.

The toddler who is well nourished shows steady proportional gains on height and weight charts and has good bone and tooth development. The diet history should be adequate, avoiding excessive calories and large amounts of vitamins.

The toddler is noted for having a fluctuating appetite with strong food preferences. The nurse reminds parents that any nutritious food can be eaten at any meal; for example, soup for breakfast and cereal for dinner are acceptable. Serving size is important (Table 17-5). Too-large servings are discouraged because they may overwhelm the child and can lead to overeating problems. One tablespoon of solid food per year of age serves as a measurement guide. A quiet time before meals provides an opportunity for the child to "wind down." The toddler's refusal to eat may result from fatigue or not being particularly hungry. The toddler may eat one food with vigor one week and refuse it the next. A flexible schedule designed to meet the needs of the toddler and the rest of the family must be worked out by the individual family. Forcing toddlers to eat only creates further difficulties. They are quick to sense parents' frustration and may use mealtime to obtain attention by behaving poorly and refusing to eat. Discipline and arguments during mealtime only upset everyone's digestion.

Toddlers are fond of ritual. This is often seen at mealtime. They want a particular dish, glass, and bib. It is best to go along with their wishes as long as they do not become too pronounced. It gives them a sense of security and, in the long run, saves time and energy for the adult.

Toddlers have a brief attention span. They may try to stand in the high chair or wander away from the table. They may be excused if they have eaten a fair amount of the meal; otherwise distraction of some type is necessary. Toddlers who regularly feed themselves may enjoy being helped by mommy or daddy. Some restaurants that cater to families provide crayons and special place mats to keep the small child occupied until adults finish their dinners. In the hospital the toddler who is fed in a high chair wears an appropriate safety restraint, and the nurse remains with the child.

The toddler's food is chopped into fine pieces. Various foods are offered, and one should try to plan contrasts of colors and textures. A 2-year-old likes finger foods. Foods are served at moderate temperatures. Candy, cake, and soda between meals are to be avoided. (See p. 369 for a nutritional guide.)

Children like colorful dishes, which must be made of an unbreakable substance. Washable plastic bibs, placemats, and protection for the floor around the high chair are advisable. Eating utensils should be small enough that it can be handled easily. Seating equipment should be adjusted so the child is comfortable and maintains good posture. Table 17-1 illustrates the skills of the 18-month-old toddler.

NURSING **TIP**

When determining the size of portions, toddlers and young children should be offered 1 tablespoon of solid food per year of age.

DAY CARE

Family life has changed dramatically since the 1970s. Today many more children are cared for in community settings outside of the home. Since 1992 the fastest growing group of persons in the labor force were women with infants. Not only were more mothers working, but they were also returning to the work force sooner after the child was born. It was clear that alternative methods of child care were necessary. These arrangements must meet families' personal preferences, cultural perspectives, and financial and special needs. Parents must take an active role in ensuring high-quality care. Nurses need to be resource persons and family advocates because finding adequate day care can be stressful.

The decision to place a toddler in the care of others while parents work can be difficult and produce feelings of guilt in the parent. The concept of such care is not new. Many cultures, such as the Israelis', have traditionally placed toddlers in day care while working on a "kibbutz." The hours of care extend from early morning to the dinnertime hour. Successful alternate child care arrangements depend on specific guidelines in selecting the facility (see Chapter 18), frequent visits to the facility, and close communication and conferences with the staff in the facility. Day care for the toddler differs somewhat from the preschool child because of the toddler's shorter attention span, the tendency to engage in *parallel play* rather than group play, and the need for closer supervision to maintain safety (Figure 17-3).

There are various types of child care. Many children today can be cared for by relatives, friends, neighbors, or those who have advertised such services. However, there is little research on these types of home arrangements and few standards of quality control. Most licensed day care centers are private businesses run for profit. They are subject to state regulations about physical layout, number of children per caretaker, education of personnel, and other factors. Parents must plan ahead for times when the child is sick and unable to attend. A few innovative programs for the in-home care of sick children have been

table 17-5	*Approximate Serving Sizes per Meal*	
	AGE 1 YEAR	**AGE 2 TO 3 YEARS**
Bread	1 slice	1 slice
Cereal	1 ounce	1 ounce
Rice/pasta	1 cup	1 cup
Vegetables	2 tbsp	3 tbsp
Fruit	1 cup	1 cup
Milk	1 cup	1 cup
Meat, beans	2 tbsp	3 tbsp

NOTE: Approximate serving sizes per meal for a toddler. For food pyramid, see Figure 15-6.

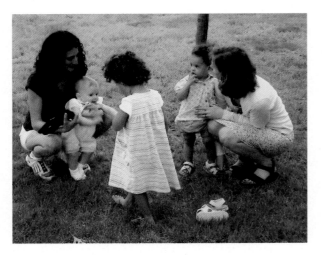

FIGURE **17-3** Beginning social skills, parallel play, and short attention spans of toddlers require them to have close supervision in day care settings.

developed. Employer-supported child care is a rapidly growing area, and these programs are very diverse. Some companies provide family day care (care of the child in the provider's home). Other employers assist parents through reimbursement, referral programs, or support of existing child care programs in the community.

For low-income and some middle-income families, the cost of child care is difficult if not impossible to maintain. Some form of continued or expanded government assistance or private funding is necessary. Inspection and monitoring of child care facilities to ensure compliance with health (physical and mental) and safety standards are paramount. Ideally, all day care programs would include comprehensive health services and health education programs. Criteria for selecting a day care center are similar to those discussed for nursery schools (see Chapter 18).

✴NURSING **TIP**
A major task for parents is to "let go" and allow the toddler to interact with influences outside the family in day care centers or preschools.

INJURY PREVENTION

Accidents kill and cripple more children than any disease known and are *the leading cause of death* in childhood. The best prevention is knowledge of age-appropriate risks and anticipatory guidelines. If parents understand their child's activities at certain ages, they can prevent many serious injuries by taking necessary precautions (Table 17-6).

Nurses have an important responsibility to review injury prevention with parents during each clinic visit. The normal behavior characteristics of a toddler, including curiosity, mobility, and negativity, make the toddler prone to injuries, which often occur in and around the home (Figure 17-4).

Car safety is important. The use of seat belts is effective if they are worn properly. A shoulder strap that extends across the neck or a lap belt that fits high on the abdomen or waist area can be harmful rather then helpful. A child seat placed in the front car seat close to the passenger air bag can be dangerous. Table 17-6 correlates hazards that are often associated with the toddler age-group.

Nurses demonstrate safety measures to their patients and their families. This is most effectively done by good example. Safety measures pertinent to the pediatric unit are discussed in Chapter 22. Nurses in the community can often contribute indirectly to the welfare of others by the example set and by being aware of emergency medical facilities available in the community.

CONSUMER EDUCATION

The federal government and concerned private agencies have attempted to regulate some of the variables that cause injuries. A few examples are ensuring the use of nonflammable material for children's sleepwear, child-proof caps on medicine bottles and certain household products, and establishing maximum temperatures for home hot-water heaters. Smoke detectors in homes and public places are commonplace. The United States Consumer Product Safety Commission has established regulations for crib slats, locks, and latches and crib mattress size and thickness. Safety warnings on the crib's carton advise buyers to use a snug mattress only. The nurse should reinforce this type of information.

Laws have been passed in virtually all states that require infants and small children to be restrained while riding in automobiles (Figure 17-5). These restraints must follow standards established by the Federal Motor Vehicle Safety Department. Rental cars also loan child seat restraints. The use of car seats begins with the first ride home from the hospital.

New homes are required to have smoke detectors. Consumers who live in older homes and apartment complexes are also encouraged to install them. Various other safety codes are mandatory for public buildings, with additional measures required for buildings specifically for the disabled. Nevertheless the problems of surveillance and upkeep are considerable. Many children live in substandard housing with little supervision. The education of parents is of monumental importance in decreasing death and disability.

BEHAVIORAL CHARACTERISTICS	HAZARD AND PREVENTION STRATEGIES
AUTOMOBILE	
Impulsive	Teach child street safety rules.
Unable to delay gratification	Teach child the meaning of red, yellow, and green traffic lights.
Increased mobility	Caution children not to run from behind parked cars or snow banks.
Egocentric	Use car seat restraints appropriately.
	Hold toddler's hand when crossing the street.
	Supervise tricycle riding.
	Do not allow children to play in the car alone.
	Driver must look carefully in front and behind vehicles before accelerating.
	Teach children what areas are safe in and around the house.
	Supervise child under age 3 years at all times.
BURNS	
Fascination for fire	Teach the child the meaning of "hot" (one mother taught this by allowing the
Can reach articles by climbing	child to touch beach sand warmed by the sun).
Pokes fingers in holes and openings	Put matches, cigarettes, candles, and incense out of reach and sight.
	Turn handles of cooking utensils toward the back of the stove.
Can open doors and drawers	Beware of hot liquids; avoid tablecloths with overhang.
Unaware of cause and effect	Keep appliances such as coffee pots, electric frying pans, and food processors and their cords out of reach.
	Test food and fluids heated in microwave ovens to ensure that center is not too hot.
	Beware of hot charcoal grills or gas barbecues.
	Use snug fireplace screens.
	Mark children's rooms to alert firefighters in emergency.
	Keep a pressure-type fire extinguisher available, and teach all family members who are old enough how to use it.
	Practice what to do in case of fire in the home.
	Install smoke detectors.
	Cover electrical outlets with protective caps.
	Check bath water temperature before placing child in water.
	Do not allow child to handle water faucets.
FALLS	
Like to explore different parts of the house	Teach children how to go up and come down stairs when they show a readiness for this task.
Can open doors and lean out open windows	Fasten crib sides securely and leave them up when child is in the crib.
	Use side rails on a large bed when child graduates from crib.
Have immature depth perception	Lock basement doors or use gates at top and bottom of stairs.
	Mop spilled water from floor immediately.
Capabilities change quickly	Use window guards.
May seem quite grown up at times but still require constant supervision at home and on the playground	Use car seat restraints appropriately.
	Keep scissors and other pointed objects away from the toddler's reach.
	Use childproof door knobs and drawer closures.
	Secure child in shopping cart at store.
	Supervise climbing child in playground.
	Clothing and shoelaces should be appropriate to prevent tripping.
SUFFOCATION AND CHOKING	
Explores with senses; likes to bite on and taste things	Do not allow small children to play with deflated balloons; these can be sucked into airway.
Eats on the run	Inspect toys for small or loose parts.
	Remove small objects such as coins, buttons, and pins from reach.
	Avoid popcorn, nuts, small hard candies, chewing gum, or large chunks of meat, such as hot dogs.
	Debone fish and chicken.
	Learn the Heimlich maneuver and CPR.

Continued

BEHAVIORAL CHARACTERISTICS	HAZARD AND PREVENTION STRATEGIES
	Inspect width of crib and playpen slats.
	Keep plastic bags away from small children; do not use as mattress cover.
	If child is vomiting, turn him or her on side.
	Avoid nightclothes with drawstring necks.
	Discard old refrigerators and appliances or remove doors.
POISONING	
Ingenuity increases, can open most containers	Store household detergents and cleaning supplies out of reach and in a locked cabinet.
Increased mobility provides child access to cupboards, medicine cabinets, bedside stands, interior of closets	Do not put chemicals or other potentially harmful substances into food or beverage containers.
	Keep medicines in a locked cabinet; put them away immediately after use.
	Use child-resistant caps and packaging.
Looks at and touches everything	Flush old medicine down toilet.
	Follow health care provider's directions when administering medication.
Learns by trial and error	Do not refer to pills as "candy."
Puts objects in mouth	Educate parents regarding when and how to use ipecac syrup.
	Explain poison symbols to child and to parents not fluent in English.
	Keep telephone number of poison control center available.
	When painting, use paint marked "for indoor use" or one that conforms to standards for use on surfaces that may be chewed on by children.
	Wash fruits and vegetables before eating.
	Obtain and record name of any new plant purchased.
	Alert family of location and appearance of poisonous plants on or around property or frequently encountered when camping.
	Use childproof locks on cabinets.
	Use dishes that do not have high lead content.
DROWNING	
Lacks depth perception	Watch child continuously while at beach or near a pool.
Does not realize danger	Empty wading pools when child has finished playing.
Loves water play	Cover wells securely.
	Wear recommended life jackets in boats.
	Begin teaching water safety and swimming skills early.
	Lock fences surrounding swimming pools.
	Supervise tub baths; be aware that a young child can drown in a very small amount of water.
ELECTRIC SHOCK	
Pokes and probes with fingers	Cover electrical outlets.
	Cap unused sockets with safety plugs.
	Water conducts electricity; teach child not to touch electrical appliances when wet; keep appliances out of reach.
	Keep electrical appliances away from tub and sink area.
ANIMAL BITES	
Has immature judgment	Teach child to avoid stray animals.
	Do not allow toddler to abuse household pets.
	Supervise closely.
SAFETY	
Easily distracted	Teach toddler stranger safety.
Trusting of others	Do not personalize clothes.
Falls frequently	Do not allow toddler to eat or suck lollipops while running or playing.
	Keep sharp-edged objects out of reach.
	Keep sharp-edged furniture out of play area.

Keep first aid chart and emergency numbers handy. Know location of and how to get to nearest emergency facility.

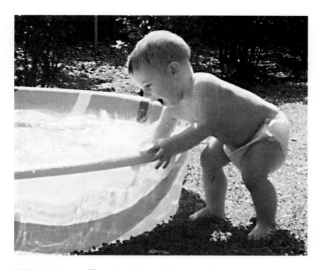

FIGURE **17-4** The playful toddler needs close supervision during water play. Falling into a kiddie pool can result in serious injury.

TOYS AND PLAY

In 1970 the Child Protection and Toy Safety Act was passed in an effort to halt the distribution of unsafe toys. In addition, parents must be taught to inspect toys and to buy toys suitable for the age, skills, and abilities of the individual child. Some labels now give safety information and intended age. Parents are also taught to inspect toys routinely for damage.

In general, notification of recall for a specific toy is announced on radio and television and is published in newspapers and consumer journals. Toy boxes and toy chests are also a potential hazard. The most serious injuries caused by a box or chest are the result of the lid falling on a child or a child being trapped inside. A parent can report a product hazard by writing to the United States Consumer Product Safety Commission, Washington DC 20207.

Play is the work of a toddler. Through play, toddlers learn how to manipulate, understand their environment, socialize, and explore their world. High-priced toys are not necessary. Pots and pans from the kitchen,

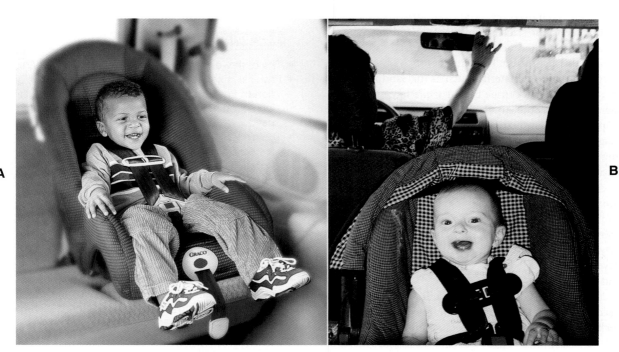

FIGURE **17-5 A,** The toddler's car seat can be front facing in the center of the rear seat of the car and secured by the car's seat belt. **B,** The infant's seat faces the rear of the car to prevent the infant's large and heavy head from falling forward when the car stops suddenly or in case of an accident. The driver can look through the rearview mirror of the car toward a mirror mounted on the rear window or seat back to see the face of the infant in a rear-facing car seat. Note that the metal clip or lock of the car seat belt is not under the chin of the infant but rests firmly on the chest.

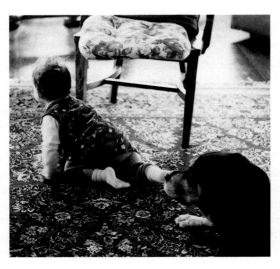

FIGURE **17-6** Close supervision is necessary when a child plays in any home where there is a large or small pet. Both the toddler and the pet have unpredictable behavior.

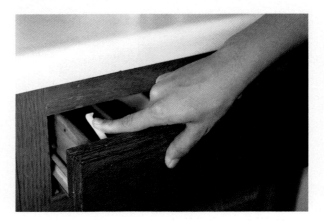

FIGURE **17-7** Childproofing the home. A simple drawer or cabinet latch prevents access to the contents by the young child while still remaining accessible to the adult, who can press and release the latch with one finger.

supervised water play, dancing to music, and crayons or finger paint and paper are preferred by toddlers. A picture book reviewed while on the lap of a family member can often be enjoyed over and over again. Tricycles can be adapted to the size and ability of the toddler. Objects that can be pushed or pulled are preferred to wind-up toys for this age-group. The sense of touch can be stimulated by providing materials such as fur, sandpaper, felt, and nylon. Colors can be taught while having the toddler help to sort the laundry. Memory can be stimulated by pointing to familiar pictures in a book, newspaper, or magazine. Counting can be taught while climbing stairs. Supervision and maintenance of safety are the keys to a positive play experience for the toddler (Figure 17-6).

As toddlers become aware of their expanding environment, their social development takes form. Egocentric thinking, in which children relate everything to themselves, predominates. They engage in parallel play, playing next to, but not with, their peers. They gradually develop cooperative play, which involves imagination and sharing skills.

Nurses must closely assess children with special needs for safety precautions. Children with disabilities such as visual, motor, or intellectual impairments; convulsive disorders; or diabetes require extended instruction according to the child's particular needs. Immobile children must be protected from sunburn and wind or rainy weather. Adults must also guard these children from mosquitoes and other vectors. Injury prevention involves some of the methods mentioned in the discussion of consumer education; the use of items such as electric outlet covers, cabinet locks, drawer locks; and the creation of a hazard free or "childproof" environment for the child (Figure 17-7).

key points

- The birth weight has quadrupled by age 2½ years.
- Physical changes of the toddler include the acquisition of fine and gross motor skills, among which is increased mobility and increased eye-hand coordination.
- The digestive volume and processes of the toddler increase to accommodate a three-meal-a-day schedule.
- Complete bowel and bladder control is usually achieved by age 2½ to 3 years.
- Erikson refers to the toddler stage as one in which the child's task is to acquire a sense of autonomy (self-control) while overcoming shame and doubt.
- The most evident cognitive achievements of the toddler are language and comprehension.
- Some important self-regulatory functions mastered by the toddler include toilet independence, self-feeding, tolerating delayed gratification, separation from parents, and perfecting newfound physical skills and speech.
- Separation anxiety includes the stages of protest, despair, and detachment.
- Parental guidance is needed to deal with the negativism, temper tantrums, and sibling rivalry that is characteristic of this age-group.
- Discipline for the toddler should be designed to teach rather than punish.

- Some methods of dealing with the inconsistencies of the toddler include distraction, ignoring minor infractions, reward and praise, and time-out in a safe place.
- Accidents and poisoning are the leading causes of death in the toddler age-group.
- Infants and young children should ride in a car safety seat for all car trips.

ONLINE RESOURCES

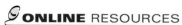

Health Information: http://www.aafp.org

Alliance for Children and Families: http://www.alliance1.org

Resources for Toddler Development: http://www.zerotothree.org

?CRITICAL THINKING QUESTION

The parents of a toddler discuss safety in the home with the nurse. The parents state they will use a car seat as required by law and safety gates on the stairs to prevent accidental falls. However, they believe no other safety "childproofing" is necessary because their child is a good child and they plan to teach him to be obedient so he will learn what not to touch. What is the best response of the nurse?

REVIEW QUESTIONS   *Choose the most appropriate answer.*

1. The term used to denote the toddler's concentration on self is:
   1. Ritualism
   2. Negativism
   3. Egocentric
   4. Egomania

2. The nurse assesses the vital signs of a 2-year-old. A normal respiratory rate (per minute) would be:
   1. 18 to 20
   2. 25 to 30
   3. 35 to 40
   4. 45 to 50

3. Which statement by the parent would indicate *a need for further guidance*?
   1. I use a car seat for my toddler whenever we are in the car, and he is right beside me as I drive so I can keep an eye on him
   2. I use a car seat for my toddler whenever we are in the car and secure it onto the rear seat of the car
   3. I use a car seat for my toddler that is designed to hold children up to 40 pounds
   4. I use a car seat for my toddler that is designed to fasten with the seat belt

4. A mother tells the nurse that her 2-year-old toddler often has temper tantrums at the family dinner table and asks how to handle the behavior. The best response of the nurse would be:
   1. Temper tantrums are normal for a 2-year-old and the child will grow out of it
   2. The toddler should be removed from the family dinner table until he or she is old enough to behave
   3. Strict discipline and corporal punishment are appropriate to help the child to gain self-control
   4. Parents should agree on a method of discipline, such as time-out, and use it when the child misbehaves

5. One of the developmental tasks of the toddler that is most hazardous to safety is:
   1. Brief attention span
   2. Need for ritual
   3. Fluctuating appetite
   4. Need to explore

objectives

1. Define each key term listed.
2. List the major developmental tasks of the preschool-age child.
3. Describe the physical, psychosocial, and spiritual development of children from age 3 to 5 years, listing age-specific events and guidance when appropriate.
4. Describe the development of the preschool child in relation to Piaget's, Erikson's, and Kohlberg's theories of development.
5. Discuss the characteristics of a good preschool.
6. Discuss the value of play in the life of a preschool child.
7. Designate two toys suitable for the preschool child, and provide the rationale for each choice.
8. Describe the speech development of the preschool child.
9. Discuss the value of the following: time-out periods, consistency, role modeling, rewards.
10. Describe the developmental characteristics that predispose the preschool child to certain accidents, and suggest methods of prevention for each type of accident.
11. Discuss the development of positive bedtime habits.
12. Discuss the approach to problems such as enuresis, thumb sucking, and sexual curiosity in the preschool child.
13. Discuss one method of introducing the concept of death to a preschool child.

key terms

animism (p. 423)
art therapy (p. 435)
artificialism (p. 423)
associative play (p. 427)
centering (p. 423)
echolalia (ĕk-ō-LĀ-lē-ă, p. 424)
egocentrism (p. 423)
enuresis (ĕn-ū-RĒ-sĭs, p. 431)
modeling (p. 430)
parallel play (p. 427)
play therapy (p. 435)
preconceptual stage (p. 423)
preoperational phase (p. 423)
separation anxiety (sĕp-ă-RĀ-shăn ăng-ZĪ-ĭ-tē, p. 435)
symbolic functioning (p. 423)
therapeutic play (p. 435)
time-out (p. 429)

GENERAL CHARACTERISTICS

The child from age 3 to 5 years is often referred to as the *preschool child.* This period is marked by slowing of the physical growth process and mastery and refinement of the motor, social, and cognitive abilities that will enable the child to be successful in his or her school years.

The major tasks of the preschool child include preparation to enter school, development of a cooperative-type play, control of body functions, acceptance of separation, and increase in communication skills, memory, and attention span. Dentition and nutrition are discussed in Chapter 15.

PHYSICAL DEVELOPMENT

The infant who tripled his or her birth weight at 1 year has only doubled the 1-year weight by 5 years of age. For instance, the infant who weighs 20 pounds on the first birthday will probably weigh about 40 pounds by the fifth birthday. The child between 3 and 6 years of age grows taller and loses the chubbiness seen during the toddler period. Between 3 and 5 years of age, there will be an increase of 3 inches in height, mostly in the legs, that contributes to the development of an erect, slender appearance. Visual acuity is 20/40 at 3 years of age and 20/30 at 4 years of age. All 20 primary teeth have erupted. Hand preference develops by 3 years of age, and efforts to change a left-handed child to a right-handed child can cause a high level of frustration. Appetite fluctuates widely. The normal pulse rate is 90 to 110 beats/min. The rate of respirations during relaxation is about 20 breaths/min. The systolic blood pressure is about 85 to 90 mm Hg, and the diastolic blood pressure is about 60 mm Hg.

Preschool children have good control of their muscles and participate in vigorous play; they become more adept at using old skills as each year passes. They can swing and jump higher. Their gait resembles that of an adult. They are quicker and have more self-confidence than they did as toddlers.

COGNITIVE DEVELOPMENT

The thinking of the preschool child is unique. Piaget calls this period the preoperational phase. It comprises children from 2 to 7 years of age and is divided into two stages: the preconceptual stage (2 to 4 years of age) and the *intuitive thought stage* (4 to 7 years of age). Of importance in the preconceptual stage is the increasing development of language and symbolic functioning. Symbolic functioning is seen in the play of children who pretend that an empty box is a fort; they create a mental image to stand for something that is not there.

Another characteristic of this period is egocentrism, a type of thinking in which children have difficulty seeing any point of view other than their own. Because children's knowledge and understanding are restricted to their own limited experiences, misconceptions arise. One misconception is animism. This is a tendency to attribute life to inanimate objects. Another is artificialism, the idea that the world and everything in it are created by people.

The intuitive stage is one of prelogical thinking. Experience and logic are based on outside appearance (the child does not understand that a wide glass and a tall glass can both contain 4 ounces of juice). A distinctive characteristic of intuitive thinking is centering, the tendency to concentrate on a single outstanding characteristic of an object while excluding its other features.

More mature conceptual awareness is established with time and experience. This process is highly complex, and the implications for practical application are numerous. Interested students are encouraged to explore these concepts through further study. Table 18-1 summarizes some major theories of personality development for the preschooler.

EFFECTS OF CULTURAL PRACTICES

Cultural practices can influence the development of a sense of initiative in families who practice authoritarian-type parenting styles that put a great value on obedience and conformity. Parents and older siblings are models for language development, and the mastery of sounds proceeds in the same order around the world. Some parents speak both English and a native language in the home. Studies have shown that young children adapt quickly to a bilingual environment (Figure 18-1). Cultural preferences related to dietary practices are discussed in Chapter 15.

LANGUAGE DEVELOPMENT

The development of language as a communication skill is essential for success in school (Figure 18-2). Delays or problems in language expression can be caused by physiological, psychological, or environmental stressors. Typically, in the preschool period between 2 and 5 years

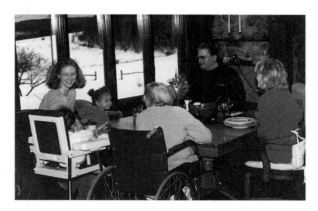

FIGURE **18-1** The family meal. The multigenerational family enjoys a meal together. Cultural traditions and family bonding occur here.

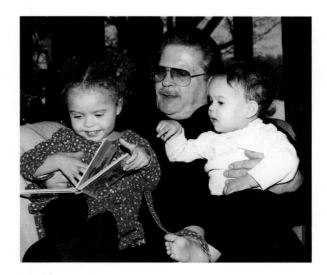

FIGURE **18-2** Grandpa reads to the children. Preschool language development depends on exposure to the written word and picture familiarity. In interactive reading the child is asked questions about the pictures she sees and receives immediate feedback. It is the ideal way to optimize the mastery of language.

■

table 18-1 *Preschool Growth and Development*

	INTELLIGENCE	EMOTIONAL	LANGUAGE	PLAY	PARENTAL GUIDANCE
3 years	Piaget's preoperational phase Understands time in relation to concrete activities Knows own sex Has attention span of approximately 15 minutes, is easily distractible	Freud's phallic stage Oedipus complex may develop in boys Erikson's stage of initiative versus guilt Wishes to please parents Ritualism provides security Egocentric (unable to see viewpoint of others)	Has vocabulary of approximately 300 to 800 words Uses plurals Forms three-word sentences Can repeat three numbers Understanding occurs before expressive ability	Kohlberg: beginning moral development Identifies with same-sex parent Develops understanding of good/bad Explains different emotions in pretend play Starts to engage in group play Is highly imaginative	Child usually wants to please parents. Guidance techniques are based on this principle. Overprotection during this stage of initiative can thwart the development of a coping mechanism in the child. Self-esteem will be enhanced by having the child "help" the parent.
4 years	Can count to 5 Knows simple songs Sexual curiosity is high Has attention span of approximately 20 minutes Adds logic to thinking Understands that feelings are connected to actions	May use tantrums to relieve frustrations and; if successful, they may become a coping mechanism Has mood swings Is highly imaginative Asks many questions Likes to "show off" accomplishments Experiments with masturbation	Has vocabulary of 1500 words Uses four- to five-word sentences Experiments with language and words May use offensive words without understanding the meaning	Engages in rough and tumble play Learns how much he can control Demonstrates sibling rivalry	Minimize passive activity, such as doing puzzles *for* the child. Repetition of words without comprehension (echolalia) should be referred for follow-up care. Teach self-control through limit setting. Guide parent in discipline techniques. Provide nutritious snacks. Answer questions truthfully.

of age, the number of words in the child's sentence should equal the child's age (e.g., two words at 2 years of age). By 2½ years of age, most children evidence possessiveness (*my* doll). By 4 years of age, they can use the past tense, and by 5 years of age they can use the future tense. The development of language skills includes both the understanding of language and the expressing of

oneself in language. Children who have difficulty expressing themselves in words often exhibit tantrums and other acting-out behaviors.

Table 18-2 lists the language, cognitive, and perceptual abilities required for success in school. Problems detected and treated during the preschool years can prevent many school problems in later years. Table 18-3 de-

| table 18-1 | *Preschool Growth and Development—cont'd* | | | | |

	INTELLIGENCE	EMOTIONAL	LANGUAGE	PLAY	PARENTAL GUIDANCE
5 years	Beginning concept of past, present, and future, although time is evidenced in activity rather than hour Knows the days of the week Attention span reaches 30 minutes Can count to 10 Knows name and address Behaviors that result in rewards are considered right, behaviors that result in punishment are considered wrong	Is less egocentric and has beginning awareness of the outside world Enjoys activities with parent of the same sex	Has vocabulary of 2000 words Can name four colors Uses six- to eight-word sentences with pronouns, etc.	Wants to play "by the rules" but cannot accept losing Can copy sample shapes and print first name Establishes preference for hand use	Child can participate in own care. Teach front-to-back wiping after bowel movements. Provide information concerning vision and hearing assessment facilities in community. Review immunization status. Prepare parent for separation and entrance of child to school.

scribes the clinical symptoms of typical language disorders. Evaluation of language development must be done together with an assessment of problem-solving skills.

DEVELOPMENT OF PLAY

Play activities in the preschool child increase in complexity. At 2 to 3 years of age, the child imitates the activities of daily living of the parents (hammering, shaving, feeding the doll). By 4 years of age, the child may develop a broader theme such as a trip to the zoo. By 5 years of age, a trip to the moon demonstrates the child's imaginary abilities. Play enables the child to experience multiple roles and emotional outlets, such as the aggressor, the victim, the superpower, or the acquisition of toys or friends they wish for. Appealing to the child's magical thinking is the best approach to communication.

SPIRITUAL DEVELOPMENT

Preschoolers learn about religious beliefs and practices from what they observe in the home. The preschooler cannot yet understand abstract concepts. Their concept of God is concrete, sometimes treated as an imaginary friend. Preschool children can memorize Bible stories and related rituals, but their understanding of the concepts are limited. Observing religious traditions practiced in the home during a period of hospitalization (e.g., before-meal or bedtime prayers) can help the preschool child deal with stressors.

SEXUAL CURIOSITY

When guiding parents concerning the sexual education of young children, the nurse should use the following principles of teaching and learning common to other patients:

- First assess the knowledge base of the child, then assess what specific information the child is asking for.
- Be honest and accurate in providing information at the child's level. Although the child may not understand completely at first, the child's repeated questions and explanations will form the basis of later learning and understanding.

table 18-2 *Selected Perceptual, Cognitive, and Language Processes Required for Elementary School Success*

PROCESS	DESCRIPTION	ASSOCIATED PROBLEMS
PERCEPTUAL		
Visual analysis	Ability to break a complex figure into components and understand their spatial relationships	Persistent letter confusion (e.g., between *b*, *d*, and *g*); difficulty with basic reading and writing and limited "sight" vocabulary
Proprioception and motor control	Ability to obtain information about body position by feel and unconsciously program complex movements	Poor handwriting, requiring inordinate effort, often with overly tight pencil grasp; special difficulty with timed tasks
Phonological processing	Ability to perceive differences between similar-sounding words and to break down words into constituent sounds	Delayed receptive language skills; attention and behavior problems secondary to not understanding directions; delayed acquisition of letter-sound correlations (phonetics)
COGNITIVE		
Long-term memory, both storage and recall	Ability to acquire skills that are "automatic" (i.e., accessible without conscious thought)	Delayed mastery of the alphabet (reading and writing letters); slow handwriting; inability to progress beyond basic mathematics
Selective attention	Ability to attend to important stimuli and ignore distractions	Difficulty following multistep instructions, completing assignments, and behaving well; peer interaction problems
Sequencing	Ability to remember things in order; facility with time concepts	Difficulty organizing assignments, planning, spelling, and telling time
LANGUAGE		
Receptive language	Ability to comprehend complex constructions, function words (e.g., if, when, only, except), nuances of speech, and extended blocks of language (e.g., paragraphs)	Difficulty following directions; wandering attention during lessons and stories; problems with reading comprehension; problems with peer relationships
Expressive language	Ability to recall required words effortlessly (word finding), control meanings, and vary position and word endings to construct meaningful paragraphs and stories	Difficulty expressing feelings and using words for self-defense, with resulting frustration and physical acting out; struggling during "circle time" and in language-based subjects (e.g., English)

From Behrman, R., Kliegman, R., & Jenson, H. B. (2000). *Nelson's textbook of pediatrics* (16th ed.). Philadelphia: W.B. Saunders.

- Use correct terminology so that misinformation or misinterpretation can be avoided.
- Provide sex education at the time the child asks the question. The asking of the question often indicates readiness to learn.
- Parents must understand that sexual curiosity starts as an inquiry into anatomical differences. Differences in how urination occurs may later become the focus. A general understanding of infants coming from Mommy's tummy precedes the more mature concept of sexual organs and functioning.

Preschool children are as matter-of-fact about sexual investigation as they are about any other learning experience and are easily distracted to other activities. Sexual curiosity displayed in the form of masturbation or "playing doctor" should be approached in a positive manner. The appropriate touch or dress can be taught without generating a "bad" or "dirty" concept of the activity. Teaching socially acceptable behavior must be in the form of guidance rather than discipline.

Masturbation. Masturbation is common in both genders during the preschool years. The child experiences pleasurable sensations, which lead to a repetition of the behavior. It is beneficial to rule out other causes of this activity, such as rashes or penile or vaginal irritation. Masturbation in the preschool child is considered harmless if the child is outgoing, sociable, and not preoccupied with the activity.

Education of the parents consists of assuring them that this behavior is a form of sexual curiosity and is normal and not harmful to the child, who is merely curious about sexuality. The cultural and moral background of the family must be considered in assessing

table 18-3	*Not Talking: A Clinical Classification*

WHEN PARENTS SAY	CLASSIFY THE SYMPTOMS AS
"I'm the only one who understands what she says."	Articulation disorder
"She'll do what I say, but when she wants something, she just points."	Expressive language delay
"He can't play 'show me your nose,' and the only word he says is 'mama.'"	Global language delay
"He never made those funny baby sounds or said 'mama' and 'dada,' and now he just repeats everything I say."	Language disorder
"He used to say things like 'Joey go bye-bye,' but now he doesn't talk at all."	Language loss

From Montgomery, T. (1994). When children do not talk. *Contemporary Pediatrics, 11*(9), 49.

the degree of discomfort about this experience. A history of the time and place of masturbation and the parental response is helpful. Punitive reactions are discouraged. Parents are advised to ignore the behavior and distract the child with some other activity. The child should know that masturbation is not acceptable in public, but this must be explained in a nonthreatening manner. Children who masturbate excessively and who have experienced a great deal of disruption in their lives benefit from ongoing counseling.

BEDTIME HABITS

The development and reinforcement of optimum bedtime habits is important in the preschool years. Parents should be guided to engage the child in quiet activities before bedtime, to maintain specific rituals that signal bedtime readiness such as storytelling, and to verbally state "after this story, it will be bedtime." The use of a night-light, a favorite bedtime toy, or a glass of water at the bedside is an option. Attention-getting behavior that results in taking the child into the parent's bed should be discouraged because it rewards the attention-getting behavior and defeats the objectives of the bedtime ritual. The nurse should be aware that specific cultures encourage "family beds," where children regularly sleep with siblings and parents. Understanding cultural practices is essential before preparing a teaching plan.

PHYSICAL, MENTAL, EMOTIONAL, AND SOCIAL DEVELOPMENT

THE THREE-YEAR-OLD

Three-year-olds are a delight to their parents. They are helpful and can assist in simple household chores. They obtain articles when directed and return them to the proper place. Three-year-olds come very close to the ideal picture that parents have in mind of their child. They are living proof that their parents' guidance during the trying 2-year-old period has been rewarded. Temper tantrums are less frequent, and in general the 3-year-old is less erratic. They are still individuals, but they seem better able to direct their primitive instincts than previously. They can help to dress and undress themselves, use the toilet, and wash their hands. They eat independently, and their table manners have improved.

Three-year-olds talk in longer sentences and can express thoughts and ask questions. They are more company to their parents and other adults because they can talk about their experiences. They are imaginative, talk to their toys, and imitate what they see about them. Soon they begin to make friends outside the immediate family. Parallel play (playing independently within a group) and associative play are both typical of this period. Children play in loosely associated groups. Because they can now converse with playmates, they find satisfaction in joining their activities. Three-year-olds play cooperatively for short periods. They can ask others to "come out and play." If 3-year-olds are placed in a strange situation with children they do not know, they commonly revert to parallel play because it is more comfortable.

Preschoolers begin to find enjoyment away from Mom and Dad, although they want them nearby when needed. They begin to lose some of their interest in their mother, who up to this time has been more or less their total world. The father's prestige begins to increase. Romantic attachment to the parent of the opposite gender is seen during this period. A daughter wants "to marry Daddy" when she grows up. Children also begin to identify themselves with the parent of the same gender.

Preschool children have more fears than the infant or older child because of increased intelligence (which enables them to recognize potential dangers), memory development, and graded independence (which brings them into contact with many new situations). Toddlers are not afraid of walking in the street because they do not understand its danger. Preschool children realize that trucks can injure, and they worry about crossing the street. This fear is well founded, but many others are not.

The fear of bodily harm, particularly the loss of body parts, is unique to this stage. The little boy who discovers that his infant sister is made differently may worry that she has been injured. He wonders if this will happen to him. Masturbation is common during this stage as children attempt to reassure themselves that they are all right. Other common fears include fear of animals, fear of the dark, and fear of strangers. Night wandering is typical of this age-group.

Preschool children become angry when others attempt to take their possessions. They grab, slap, and hang onto them for dear life. They become very distraught if toys do not work the way they should. They resent being disturbed from play. They are sensitive, and their feelings are easily hurt. Much of the unpleasant social behavior seen during this time is normal and necessary to the child's total pattern of development.

THE FOUR-YEAR-OLD

Four-year-olds are more aggressive and like to show off newly refined motor skills. They are eager to let others know they are superior, and they are prone to pick on playmates. Four-year-olds are boisterous, tattle on others, and may begin to swear if they are around children or adults who use profanity. They recount personal family activities with amazing recall but forget where their tricycle has been left. At this age, children become interested in how old they are and want to know the exact age of each playmate. It bolsters their ego to know that they are older than someone else in the group. They also become interested in the relationship of one person to another, such as Timmy is a brother but is also Daddy's son.

Four-year-olds can use scissors with success. They can lace their shoes. The vocabulary has increased to about 1500 words. They run simple errands and can play with others for longer periods. Many feats are done for a purpose. For instance, they no longer run just for the sake of running. Instead, they run to get someplace or see something. They are imaginative and like to pretend they are doctors or firefighters. They begin to prefer playing with friends of the same gender.

The preschool child enjoys simple toys and common objects. Raw materials are more appealing than toys that are ready-made and complete in themselves. An old cardboard box that can be moved about and climbed into is more fun than a doll house with tiny furniture. A box of sand or colored pebbles can be made into roads and mountains. Parents should avoid showering their children with ready-made toys. Instead, they can select materials that are absorbing and that stimulate the child's imagination.

Stories that interest young children depict their daily experiences. If the story has a simple plot, it must be related to what they understand to hold their interest.

They also enjoy music they can march around to, music videos, and simple instruments they can shake or bang. (Make up a song about their daily life, and watch their reaction.)

The concept of death. Children between 3 and 4 years of age begin to wonder about death and dying. They may pretend to be the hero who shoots the intruder dead, or they may actually witness a situation in which an animal is killed. Their questions are direct. "What is 'dead'? Will I die?" The view of the family is important to the interpretation of this complex phenomenon.

Children may become acquainted with death through objects not of particular significance to them. For instance, the flower dies at the end of the summer and does not bloom anymore. It no longer needs sunshine or water because it is not alive. Usually young children realize that others die, but they do not relate death to themselves. If they continue to pursue the question of whether or not they will die, parents should be casual and reassure them that people do not generally die until they have lived a long and happy life. Of course, as they grow older they will discover that sometimes children do die.

The underlying idea is to encourage questions as they appear and gradually help them accept the truth without undue fear. There are many excellent books for children about death. Two that are appropriate for the preschool child are *Geranium Mornings* by S. Powell, and *My Grandpa Died Today* by J. Fassler. The dying child is discussed in Chapter 26.

THE FIVE-YEAR-OLD

Five is a comfortable age. Children are more responsible, enjoy doing what is expected of them, have more patience, and like to finish what they have started. Five-year-olds are serious about what they can and cannot do. They talk constantly and are inquisitive about their environment. They want to do things correctly and seek answers to their questions from those whom they consider to "know" the answers. Five-year-old children can play games governed by rules. They are less fearful because they believe their environment is controlled by authorities. Their worries are less profound than at an earlier age.

The physical growth of 5-year-olds is not outstanding. Their height may increase by 2 to 3 inches, and they may gain 3 to 6 pounds. They may begin to lose their deciduous teeth at this time. They can run and play games simultaneously, jump three or four steps at once, and tell a penny from a nickel or a dime. They can name the days of the week and understand what a week-long vacation is. They usually can print their first name.

Five-year-olds can ride a tricycle around the playground with speed and dexterity. They can use a hammer to pound nails. Adults should encourage them to develop motor skills and not continually remind them to "be careful." The practice children experience will enable them to compete with others during the school-age period and will increase confidence in their own abilities. As at any age, children should not be scorned for failure to meet adult standards. Overdirection by solicitous adults is damaging. Children must learn to do tasks themselves for the experience to be satisfying.

The number and type of television or computer programs that parents allow the preschool child to watch are topics for discussion. Although children enjoyed television at age 3 or 4 years, it was usually for short periods. They could not understand much of what was going on. The 5-year-old, however, has better comprehension and may want to spend a great deal of time watching television or playing computer games. The plan of management differs with each family. Whatever is decided must be discussed with the child. For example, television and computers should not be allowed to interfere with good health habits, sleep, meals, and physical activity. Most parents find that children do not insist on watching television if there is something better to do.

GUIDANCE

DISCIPLINE AND LIMIT SETTING

Much has been written on the subject of discipline, which has changed considerably over time. Today, authorities place much importance on the development of a continuous, warm relationship between children and their parents. They believe this helps to prevent many problems. The following is a brief discussion that may help the nurse in guiding parents.

Children need limits for their behavior. Setting limits makes them feel secure, protects them from danger, and relieves them from making decisions that they may be too young to formulate. Children who are taught acceptable behavior have more friends and develop good self-esteem. They live more enjoyably within the neighborhood and society. The manner in which discipline or limit setting is carried out varies from culture to culture. It also varies among different socioeconomic groups. Individual differences occur among families and between parents and vary according to the characteristics of each child.

The purpose of discipline is to teach and to gradually shift control from parents to the child, that is, self-discipline or self-control. Positive reinforcement for appropriate behavior has been cited as more effective than punishment for poor behavior. Expectations must be appropriate to the age and understanding of the child.

The nurse encourages parents to try to be consistent because mixed messages are confusing for the learner.

Timing the Time-Out

Most researchers agree that to be effective, discipline must be given at the time the incident occurs. It should also be adapted to the seriousness of the infraction. The child's self-worth must always be considered and preserved. Warning the preschool child who appears to be getting into trouble may be helpful. Too many warnings without follow-up, however, lead to ineffectiveness. For the most part, spankings are not productive. The child associates the fury of the parents with the pain rather than with the wrong deed because anger is the predominant factor in the situation. The real value of the spanking is therefore lost. Beatings administered by parents as a release for their own pent-up emotions are totally inappropriate and can lead to child abuse charges. In addition, the parent serves as a role model of aggression. Whether a parent is affectionate, warm, or cold (uncaring) also plays a role in the effectiveness of child rearing.

Time-out periods, *usually lasting 1 minute per year of age,* with the child sitting in a straight chair facing a corner is considered an effective discipline technique. There should be no interaction or eye contact during the time-out period, and a timer with a buzzer should be used. Often a child will attempt interaction during this period by asking, "How much more time is left?" The child should learn that any interaction starts the timer at zero. Using the child's room or a soft comfortable chair for time-out is not effective because the child will either fall asleep or engage in another activity and the objective of time-out is defeated. Time-out should be preceded by a short (no longer than 10-word) explanation of the reason and followed by a short (no more than 10 word) restatement of why it was necessary. Longer explanations are not effective for young children. If the child knows the rules and the behavior that will precipitate a time-out and receives no more than one warning that there will be a time-out if the undesirable behavior continues, he or she will learn self-control. Consistency is the key to helping the child learn acceptable behavior. Parents must be taught to resist using power and authority for their own sake. As the child matures and understands more clearly, privileges can be withheld. The reasons for such actions are carefully explained.

Reward

Rewarding the child for good behavior is a positive and effective method of discipline. This can be done with hugs, smiles, tone of voice, and praise. Praise can always be tied with the act, such as "Thank you, Suzy, for picking up your toys," or "I appreciate your standing quietly like that." The encouragement of positive behavior eliminates many of the undesirable effects of punishment.

Rewards should not be confused with bribes. The parent may offer a child a reward if he or she behaves in a specific situation *before* an incident occurs. For example, the parent may say, "You may pick out one small toy after we are finished shopping if you behave during this trip." If this agreement is not made *prior* to an incident and the child misbehaves and *then* is offered one small toy to behave, this is a bribe that serves to reinforce the bad behavior and is not a desirable technique of behavior management.

Consistency and Modeling

Being consistent is difficult for parents. Realistically, it is only an ideal to strive for—no parent is consistent all the time. Consistency must exist *between* parents as well as within each parent. It is suggested that parents establish a general style for what, when, how, and to what degree punishment is appropriate for misconduct. Parents who are lax or erratic in discipline and who alternate it with punishment have children who experience increased behavioral difficulties.

The influence of modeling or good example has been widely explored. Studies show that adult models significantly influence children's education. Children identify and imitate adult behavior, verbal and nonverbal. Parents who are aggressive and repeatedly lose control demonstrate the power of action over words. Those who communicate, show respect and encouragement, and set appropriate limits are more positive role models. Finally, parents need assistance in reviewing parental discipline during their own childhood to recognize destructive patterns that they may be repeating.

JEALOUSY

Jealousy is a normal response to actual, supposed, or threatened loss of affection. Children or adults may feel insecure in their relationship with the person they love. The closer children are to their parents, the greater is their fear of losing them. Children envy the newborn. They love the sibling but resent his or her presence. They cannot understand the turmoil within themselves (Figure 18-3). Jealousy of a new sibling is strongest in children under 5 years of age and is shown in various ways. Children may be aggressive and may bite or pinch, or they may be rather discreet and may hug and kiss the infant with a determined look on their face. Another common situation is children's attempt to identify with the infant. They revert to wetting the bed or want to be powdered after they urinate. Some 4-year-olds even try the bottle, but it is usually a big disappointment to them.

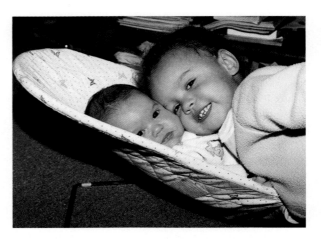

FIGURE **18-3** Child and new sibling. A new sibling is welcomed into the home. Both children need attention to minimize the development of jealousy.

Preschool children may be jealous of the attention that their mother gives to their father. They may also envy the children they play with if they have bigger and better toys. There is less jealousy in an only child, who is the center of attention and has a minimum number of rivals. Siblings of varied ages are apt to feel that the younger ones are "pets" or that the older ones have more special privileges.

Parents can help to reduce jealousy by the early management of individual occurrences. Preparing young children for the arrival of the new brother or sister minimizes the blow. They should not be made to think that they are being crowded. If the newborn is going to occupy their crib, it is best to settle the older child happily in a large bed before the infant is born. Children should feel they are helping with care of the infant. Parents can inflate their ego from time to time by reminding them of the many activities they can do that the infant cannot.

If it is convenient, the newborn is given a bath or a feeding while the older child is asleep. In this way, the older sibling avoids one occasion in which the mother shows the newborn affection for a relatively long time. Some persons think that it helps to give the child a pet to care for. Many hospitals offer sibling courses that assist parents in helping the child to overcome jealousy.

If the child tends to hit the infant or another child, both children must be separated. The child who has caused or is about to cause the injury needs as much attention as the victim, if not more. Similar aggressiveness is seen when the child is made to share toys. It is even more difficult to learn to share Mother, so the child must be given time to adjust to new situations. Children are assured that they are loved but are told that they cannot injure others.

THUMB SUCKING

Thumb sucking is an instinctual behavioral pattern and is considered normal. It is seen by sonogram about the twenty-ninth week of embryonic life. Although the cause is not fully understood, it satisfies and comforts the infant. Nonnutritive sucking in the form of thumb sucking or use of a pacifier has several documented benefits in the first year of life—when the infant is in the oral phase of development. Increased weight gain, decreased crying, the development of self-consoling ability, and increased behavioral organization have been documented in infants who have been allowed to suck unrestrained. If a pacifier is used, safe construction is essential (see Figure 16-2). The pacifier causes fewer dental problems than the rigid finger and is more easily relinquished. Parents need guidance in the safe use of pacifiers. Cleanliness is essential, because the pacifier often falls onto a dirty surface.

Finger- or thumb sucking will not have a detrimental effect on the teeth as long as the habit is discontinued before the second teeth erupt. Most children give up the habit by the time they reach school age, although they may regress during periods of stress or fatigue. Management includes education and support of the parents to relieve their anxiety and prevent secondary emotional problems in their children. The child who is trying to stop thumb sucking is given praise and encouragement.

ENURESIS
Pathophysiology

Enuresis is involuntary urination after the age at which bladder control should have been established. The term *enuresis* is derived from the Greek word *enourein,* "to void urine." Bed-wetting has existed for generations and affects many cultures. There are two types: primary and secondary. Primary enuresis refers to bed-wetting in the child who has never been dry. Secondary enuresis refers to a recurrence in a child who has been dry for a period of 1 year or more. *Diurnal,* or daytime, wetting is less common than *nocturnal,* or nighttime, episodes. It is more common in boys than in girls, and there may be a genetic influence. In many children a specific cause is never determined.

Approximately 92% of children achieve daytime dryness by 5 years of age. By 12 to 14 years of age, approximately 98% of children remain dry during the night. Sometimes enuresis is the result of inappropriate toilet training. Parents who demand early toilet training can cause a child to rebel and defy them by contin-

uing to wet the bed. Parents who are not alert to the needs of the child may not recognize readiness to toilet train and therefore thwart the child's efforts to master this developmental task. Stressful events can precipitate bed-wetting.

In some cases, organic causes of nocturnal enuresis include urinary tract infections, diabetes mellitus, diabetes insipidus, seizure disorders, obstructive uropathy, abnormalities of the urinary tract, and sleep disorders. Maturational delay of the nervous system and small bladder capacity have also been suggested as causes.

Treatment and Nursing Care

A detailed physical and psychological history is obtained. Factors such as the pattern of wetting, number of times per night or week, number of daytime voidings, type of stream, dysuria, amount of fluid taken between dinner and bedtime, family history, stress, and reactions of parents and child are documented. The nurse also determines any medications that the child may be taking and the extent to which his or her social life is inhibited by the problem, such as the inability to spend the night away from home. Developmental landmarks, including toilet training, are reviewed. If there appears to be an organic cause, appropriate blood and urine studies are undertaken. In most cases, the physical findings are negative.

Education of the family is extremely crucial to prevent secondary emotional problems. Parents are reassured that many children experience enuresis and that it is self-limited. Power struggles, shame, and guilt are fruitless and destructive. Reassurance and support by the nurse are of great help.

It is essential that the child be the center of the management program. The positive approach of rewarding dry nights and charting the progress is very helpful. Liquids after dinner should be limited, and the child should routinely void before going to bed.

When the child does not respond to routine management, other techniques include counseling, hypnosis, behavior modification, and pharmacotherapy. Moisture-activated conditioning devices are also commercially available (an alarm rings when the child wets). These have had limited success. Bladder-training exercises in which the child is asked to hold the urine for as long as possible may stretch the bladder and increase its size. The child's bedroom should be as close to the bathroom as possible, and a night-light should be used.

The nurse prepares the parents for relapses, which are common. The response to various therapies is highly individual. Overzealous treatment is to be avoided. A nonpunitive, matter-of-fact attitude is most prudent. Imipramine hydrochloride (Tofranil) has been found to decrease enuresis. It is administered before bedtime. Imipramine has a variety of side effects, including mood and sleep disturbances and gastrointestinal upsets. Overdose can lead to cardiac arrhythmias, which may be life threatening. Dosage and administration should be closely supervised. It is not recommended for children under age 6 years. Desmopressin (DDAVP) nasal spray has been used with some success but is expensive.

NURSERY SCHOOL

The change from home to nursery school or preschool is a big step toward independence. At this age, children are adjusting to the outside world as well as to the family. Some children have the complicating factor of a new brother or sister in the house.

Many parents work outside the home and find it necessary to provide alternate care settings for their children. Some parents who have only one child seek preschool experiences for their child to enhance their growth and development by providing experience with playmates. Nurses can provide guidance to parents in selecting an appropriate preschool to meet their child's needs. A *family day care center* provides child care for small groups of children for 6 or more hours of a 24-hour day Work-based group care may be provided by some employers as a convenience to their employees. *Preschool programs* provide structured activities that foster group cooperation and the development of coping skills. The child can gain self-confidence and a positive self-esteem in a good preschool program. Qualified preschool teachers are objective in their interaction with the child and often can detect problems that can be followed up before the child enters kindergarten. Parents may need guidance in selecting a preschool for their child.

The following is a list of suggestions to guide the nurse in helping parents to select a facility appropriate for their child:

- A state licensing agency should be contacted for a list of local day care centers or preschools.
- The accreditation criteria for preschools can be obtained by writing the National Association for the Education of Young Children, 1834 Connecticut Avenue NW, Washington, DC 20009.
- Teachers prepared in early childhood education should staff the preschool.
- The student-to-staff ratio should be reviewed.
- The philosophies of the facility, including discipline procedures, environmental safety, sanitary provisions, fee schedules, and facilities

for snacks, meals, and rest time should be reviewed.
- Schedules and facilities for active/passive and indoor/outdoor play should be reviewed.
- The school should routinely require a personal and health history of the child before admission to the program.
- The parent should visit the preschool and personally observe the environment. Talking with the parents of other children attending the school is helpful. Children are accepted into nursery schools between ages 2 and 5 years. Most sessions last about 3 hours.

DAILY CARE

The child between ages 3 and 6 years does not require the extensive physical care given to an infant but still needs a bath each day and a shampoo at least twice a week. It is best to keep hairstyles simple. Dental hygiene and nutrition are discussed in Chapter 15.

CLOTHING

Clothes should be loose enough to prevent restriction of movement and allow for active play without stepping on hems. Clothes should be washable. Simple clothes make it easy for preschoolers to dress themselves. A hook nailed to the door within reach is helpful. These children should dress and undress themselves as much as they can. The child's mother or father can assist but should not take over.

Shoes should be sturdy and supportive. Protective gear such as helmets for bicycling should be a natural part of dressing for play activities. Dressing appropriately for the weather encountered is essential. Flame-retardant sleepwear is available in most stores.

ACCIDENT PREVENTION

Accidents are still a major threat during the years from 3 to 5. At this age, children may suffer injuries from a bad fall. Preschool children hurry up and down stairs. They climb trees and stand up on swings. They play hard with their toys, particularly those they can mount. Stairways must be kept free of clutter. Shoes should have rubber soles, and new ones are bought when the tread becomes smooth. When buying toys, parents must be sure they are sturdy and age appropriate. Preschool children should not be asked to do anything that is potentially dangerous, such as carrying a glass container or sharp knife to the kitchen sink.

Automobiles continue to be a threat. Children are taught where they can safely ride their tricycle and where they can play ball, and they should not be allowed to use sleds on streets that are not blocked off for this purpose. They must not play in or around the car or be left alone in the car. The use of *car seats* or *seat belt restraints* continues to be important.

Burns that occur at this age often result from the child's experimentation with matches. Burns from hot coffee are also common. These items are common hazards for this age-group; they should be kept well out of reach, and their dangers should be explained to the child.

Poisoning is still a danger. Children try to imitate adults and are apt to sample pills, especially if they smell good. Their increased freedom brings them into contact with many interesting containers in the garage or basement.

Preschool children are also taught the dangers of talking to or accepting rides from strangers. If they are stopped by a driver, they should run to the house of people they know. Parents should make it clear to children in nursery school that they will never send a stranger to call for them. Children must know the dangers of playing in lonely places and of accepting gifts from strangers. Children should always know where to go if Mother or Father or the baby-sitter cannot be found. Preschool children still require a good deal of indirect supervision to protect them from dangers that arise from their immature judgment or social environment (Figure 18-4).

PLAY IN HEALTH AND ILLNESS

VALUE OF PLAY

Play is important to the physical, mental, emotional, and social development of both healthy and sick children (Figure 18-5). Children climbing on a jungle gym develop muscles coordination and exercise all parts of their bodies. They use energy and develop self-confidence. Their imagination may take them to the jungle, where they swing from limb to limb. They may face imagined fears and solve problems that would be much more trying, if not impossible, in reality. They communicate with other children and take a further step in developing moral values, that is, taking one's turn and considering others. Other types of play help children learn colors, shapes, sizes, and textures and can teach creativity. This natural and readily available outlet must be tapped by nursing and health care personnel. Children may be unfamiliar with every facet of the hospital, but they know how to play, and playing is a good way for the nurse to establish rapport with them.

THE NURSE'S ROLE

Some hospitals have well-established playroom programs supervised by play therapists. *Play therapy* is an important part of every pediatric nursing care plan. It is not necessary to be an expert in manual dexterity, art, or music; rather one must understand the needs of the child. Play is not just the responsibility of those assigned to it, nor is it confined to certain times or shifts.

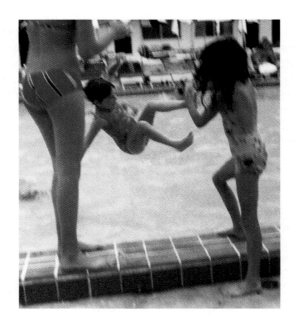

FIGURE **18-4** Unsupervised water play can quickly lead to unexpected injuries.

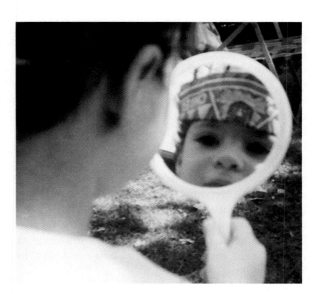

FIGURE **18-5** A self-image begins to develop during the preschool years with imaginative play.

Many factors are involved in providing suitable play for children of various ages in the hospital. The patient's state of health determines the amount of activity in which he or she can participate. The nurse can provide many activities that relieve stress and provide enjoyment for the child on bed rest. Overstimulation would be hazardous for some severely ill children. Nurses are always on guard for signs of fatigue in patients and use their judgment accordingly.

The diagnosis of the hospitalized child should also be considered when choosing an appropriate toy. For example, a friction toy is inappropriate for a child in an oxygen-rich environment. Sparks from the toy can cause an explosion. A stuffed animal may not be an appropriate toy for a child with asthma, who may be allergic to the contents of the stuffing. A washable laundry bag tied to the bed of a hospitalized child can be used to store the child's own toys neatly and safely. Toys may be taken home with the child or discarded after he or she is discharged from the hospital.

Safety must be considered in selecting an appropriate toy. Toys should be safe, durable, and suited to the child's developmental level. Toys should not be sharp or have parts that are easily removed and swallowed. Too many toys at one time are confusing to the child. Complicated toys are frustrating and disappointing. Well-selected toys such as crayons, blocks, and dolls are useful throughout the years. Each child needs sufficient time to complete an activity. In general, quiet play should precede meals and bedtime for both well and sick children. Investigations have shown that the toys enjoyed by boys and those enjoyed by girls are more similar than dissimilar.

During routine procedures the nurse can entertain the child with nursery rhymes, stories, nonsense games, songs, finger play, or puppets. Often the other children on the unit can be included for "I'm thinking of something blue, red, and green," and so forth. Simple crafts are fun. The nurse may find various instructions from children's magazines or the local public library. Scrapbooks are entertaining. Children may even enjoy making a storybook about their hospital experience. The nurse involved in enrichment programs for children can make a definite contribution. Surprise boxes in which a gift is opened every day provide anticipation for the patient. Collections of scraps containing bright ribbons, bits of string, pipe cleaners, paper bags, newspapers, or bits of cotton can be started. Because the turnover of patients is rapid, many projects can be repeated with different children.

Music is provided by radio, tape recorders, video cassette recorders (VCRs), computers, and piano. Older children enjoy sending messages to friends via a computer. Special children's recordings and videotapes are available. The services of a music therapist are available in some institutions. Drawing materials, finger paints, and modeling clay foster expression and creativity. They require only a flat surface, such as the overbed table, and a particular medium. The bedridden child can participate in messy projects, too. The bed is simply protected with newspapers or plastic. Children in cribs require adequate back support for such projects. This is done by elevating the mattress or using pillows. Simple computer games may be available in the hospital setting.

Playmates may be limited in the hospital setting if the child has a condition that is communicable. However, surgical and orthopedic patients can play together in a playroom with appropriate supervision. The nurse should guide the parents to play *for* a child who is fatigued or weakened by illness. The child can maintain the role of observer.

TYPES OF PLAY

Preschool children need playmates to promote social development. The play characteristic of each age-group is shown in Table 15-12. The preschool-age child gradually moves from parallel and associative play to cooperative play with playmates.

The play of preschool children should be noncompetitive. The healthy preschool child requires active play activities that are supervised for safety. Large construction sets, number or alphabet games, crayons, play tools, housekeeping toys, musical toys, pop-up books, large puzzles, and clay are examples of suitable toys for the preschool-age child. Active play can involve simple climbing, sliding, and running activities. Imaginary friends are common to the preschool-age child. They serve many purposes in helping the child adjust to an expanding world and increased independence. Parents can acknowledge the presence of the imaginary friend as part of pretend play, but the responsibilities of reality do not include the pretend friend. Parents should not intervene in play groups. Allowing the child to master frustration and develop social skills is essential to growth and development.

> ➤ NURSING **TIP**_____
> Imaginary playmates are common and normal during the preschool period and serve many purposes, such as relief from loneliness, mastery of feats, and a "scapegoat."

Play and the Handicapped Child

The child who is mentally handicapped needs more stimulation through play than the child who is not. The nurse must consider the mental age of the child rather than the chronological age when guiding parents about the selection of toys. The environment should be as colorful and bright as possible. The child may be introduced to objects of various sizes and textures. Play with other children must be supervised because the poorer judgment of mentally handicapped children may get them into difficulty. They may be aggressive and unaware of their own strength. Adequate space in which to run is necessary. These children should be brought into group play gradually. Materials are presented one at a time.

Mentally handicapped children may need to be taught how to play, because they may not have had the preschool play experience of the nonhandicapped child. Repetition of play experiences is necessary. Equipment and play materials must be altered to accommodate the child's size and yet be suitable for the mental age. The nurse or teacher should improvise games and songs to meet the special needs of this group. (See Chapter 23 for a more complete discussion of the growth and development and care of the mentally handicapped child.)

Therapeutic Play

Play and toys can be of therapeutic value in retraining muscles, improving eye-hand coordination, and helping children crawl and walk (push-pull toys). A musical instrument such as the clarinet promotes flexion and extension of the fingers. Blowing is an excellent prerequisite for speech therapy. Therapists supervise such activities. They leave specific instructions if they wish their work to be reinforced on the unit. Blowing out the light of a flashlight as if it were a candle is therapeutic play for a postoperative preschool child.

Play Therapy

The nurse may also hear the term play therapy. This technique is used for the child under stress. A well-equipped playroom is provided. Children are free to play with whatever articles they choose. A counselor may be in the room observing and talking with the child, or the child may be observed through a one-way glass window. By using these as well as other methods, the therapist obtains a better understanding of the patient's struggles, fears, resentments, and feelings toward self and others. When children act out their feelings through "dramatic play," the feelings are externalized, which relieves tension. The interpretation of child behavior is complex and requires a great deal of time, study, and sensitivity to be fully understood.

Art Therapy

Art therapy is useful in communicating with children and adults. It is becoming more widely used. The art therapist is especially trained to assist children to express their feelings and communicate through drawings, clay, and other media. Some hospitals with inpatient mental health units have art therapy departments.

NURSING IMPLICATIONS OF PRESCHOOL GROWTH AND DEVELOPMENT

The nurse should anticipate parental concern with nutritional problems in the preschool child. Daily appetites may fluctuate widely, but the weekly pattern will probably show stability to meet the child's growth needs. During clinic visits the parents should be guided to provide age-appropriate foods at mealtimes in appropriate portions. The child's developing self-regulatory mechanism will determine how much he or she will eat based on feelings of hunger or satiety. Efforts to control the preschool child's intake may result in power struggles or patterns of overeating or under-eating.

Safety is a high priority in this active age range. "Childproofing" the home and the need for adequate supervision and safety equipment during sports activities should be emphasized. Preschoolers who will be given immunizations via a "shot" can be calmed by giving pretend "shots" to their doll and having a parent present to comfort them. Explanations such as "the shot will hurt just a little but will prevent you from getting sick" are beyond the Piaget preoperational level of understanding of the preschool child. The ability to understand detailed explanations is not yet present in preschool-age children, even if verbal ability is high. The preschool-age child may have unfounded fears that respond best to reassurance and "protection" by parents, rather than reasoning why the fear is unfounded.

The nurse should provide parental guidance concerning the changing behavior patterns of the preschool-age child. The characteristic alternating dependence and independence can be frustrating for parents. Parents who do not volunteer any positive comments about their child during conversations may require further investigation and interview. Problems with day care and discipline must be discussed. The use of corporal punishment (spanking) as a major disciplinary technique can lead to child abuse. The use of time-out and alternative methods of discipline (p. 429) should be stressed.

Hospitalization can be frightening to a preschool child who is egocentric and prone to magical thinking. Because the preschool child cannot fully understand cause and effect, he or she may perceive hospitalization as punishment for his behavior. The preschool child may feel abandoned by the parents and continues to be subject to separation anxiety. Separation anxiety is manifested by the stages of *protest, despair, detachment,* and *regression* to earlier behaviors. Bed-wetting is common in the hospitalized preschool child, and parents should be encouraged to be patient and positive. Assigning a consistent caregiver and providing age-appropriate diversional activities are essential for a hospitalized preschool child.

The nurse who is with children daily can describe their behavior. It is important to describe good and poor behavior, conversations that seem pertinent, and the child's relationships with other children in the hospital. What is the approach to play? Do they join in freely or linger outside the group? Do they prefer active or quiet activities? Do they seem to tolerate frustrations? Can they talk with their playmates and convey their ideas? What type of attention span do they have? These observations and charting are meaningful and promote better understanding and appropriate interventions by nurses and other personnel.

key points

- The child age 3 to 5 years is often referred to as the "preschool child." During this period, the child grows taller and loses the chubbiness of the toddler period.
- The major tasks of the preschool child include preparation to enter school, the development of a cooperative-type play, control of body functions, acceptance of separation, and increase in communication skills, memory, and attention span.
- Gross and fine motor skills become more developed, as evidenced by participation in running, skipping, and drawing pictures.
- Piaget refers to the preschool period as one in which symbolic thought processes and language emerge.
- Erikson's preschool stage involves the development of initiative. Kohlberg's theory concerning preschoolers refers to the moral development and the beginning awareness of needs of others.
- Language ability develops rapidly, and the child is able to construct rather complicated sentences by the end of this period.
- The many questions of the preschool child must be listened to carefully and answered thoughtfully and truthfully.

- Play is the business of children. It contributes to physical and mental well-being by encouraging communication, socialization, and outlets for energy.
- Cooperative and highly imaginative play is characteristic of the preschool child.
- Social issues of the preschool period include learning to share and to control impulses.
- Common concerns of parents during this period include how to set limits, handle jealousy, and respond to thumb sucking and masturbation.
- Corporal punishment of the preschool child can nurture rebellion and aggression. Appropriate discipline techniques can assist the child to develop self-control.
- Careful evaluation of day care and nursery school programs is important to ensure high-quality care.
- Accidents are still a major hazard for preschool children because of their immature judgment and increased locomotive skills.
- During the preschool years the parents need guidance to understand the developmental road map of physical, emotional, and cognitive growth to help the child to meet life's challenges and goals and to enrich family interaction.
- Primary enuresis refers to bed-wetting in a child who has never been dry. Secondary enuresis refers to bed-wetting in a child who has been dry for a period of 1 year or more.

ONLINE RESOURCES

Children's Health Topics: http://www.aap.org

Sexuality Information and Education Council of the U.S.: http://www.siecus.org

CRITICAL THINKING QUESTION

The parents of a preschool child discuss the typical play activities of their child. They express concern that they have seen their child choose to play the role of "the aggressive bad guy" in play scenarios and are concerned that he may be developing aggressive behavior. They ask if they should stop him from assuming roles in play that are not acceptable behaviors. What is the best response of the nurse?

REVIEW QUESTIONS *Choose the most appropriate answer.*

1. When selecting play activities for a healthy 4-year-old, the parent should be guided to understand that the 4-year-old:
   1. Enjoys solitary play, sitting next to a friend
   2. Enjoys cooperative play with friends
   3. Enjoys competitive play with teams
   4. Enjoys observing rather than participating

2. Masturbation is:
   1. Uncommon during preschool years
   2. Common in both sexes during the preschool years
   3. A sign of extreme anxiety in the preschool child
   4. A sign of incompetent parenting

3. The nurse is guiding a parent concerning techniques of dealing with a child with enuresis. The most appropriate suggestion by the nurse would be:
   1. Wake the child in the middle of the night and take him to the bathroom to void
   2. Limit liquids after dinner and have the child void before going to bed
   3. Use a consistent technique of discipline whenever the bed is wet
   4. Keep the child in diapers until bed-wetting is no longer a problem

4. The appropriate amount of time to use in time-out period for a 3-year-old child is:
   1. 1 minute
   2. 3 minutes
   3. 5 minutes
   4. 10 minutes

5. A 4-year-old child is in Erikson's stage of:
   1. Autonomy
   2. Industry
   3. Initiative
   4. Identity

CHAPTER 19

The School-Age Child

objectives

1. Define each key term listed.
2. Describe the physical and psychosocial development of children from 6 to 12 years of age, listing age-specific events and type of guidance where appropriate.
3. Discuss how to assist parents in preparing a child for school.
4. List two ways in which school life influences the growing child.
5. Contrast two major theoretical viewpoints of personality development during the school years.
6. Discuss accident prevention in this age-group.
7. Discuss the value of pet ownership for the healthy school-age child and the family education necessary for the allergic or immunocompromised child.
8. Discuss the role of the school nurse in providing guidance and health supervision for the school-age child.

key terms

androgynous (ăn-DRŎJ-ĭ-năs, p. 440)
concrete operations (p. 438)
latchkey children (p. 443)
preadolescent (prē-ăd-ō-LĔS-ĕnt, p. 446)
Sex Information and Education Council of the United States (SIECUS) (p. 440)
sexual latency (p. 438)
stage of industry (p. 438)

GENERAL CHARACTERISTICS

School-age children (6 to 12 years of age) differ from preschool children in that they are more engrossed in fact than in fantasy and are capable of more sophisticated reasoning. School-age children develop their first close peer relationships outside of the family group and their first affiliation with adults outside of their family who will influence their lives in a significant way (see Table 19-2).

As a result of the increased contact with the world outside and increased cognitive abilities, school-age children begin to understand how others evaluate them. School-age children are often judged by their performance—good grades or athletic feats. Their sense of industry and the development of a positive self-esteem are directly influenced by their ability to become an accepted member of a peer group and meet the challenges in the environment.

The school-age child must be able to pay attention in class (with at least a 45-minute attention span), understand language, and progress from the *skill* of writing or reading to *understanding* what is written or read. To be successful in school, the child must work toward a delayed reward and must risk being unsuccessful in his or her efforts. However, parents must be guided to understand that multiple unsuccessful experiences for their child can lead to the development of a fear of trying in the future. New experiences for the school-age child include the first night sleeping away from home at a friend's house or camp, successes that are formally celebrated, chores that are dependably performed, conflict resolution with peers, and the selection of adult role models.

School-age children have an ardent thirst for knowledge and accomplishment. They tend to admire their teachers and adult companions. They use the skill and knowledge they obtain to attempt to master the activities they enjoy, including music, sports, and art. Thus this phase is referred to by Erikson as the stage of industry. Unsuccessful adaptations at this time can lead to a sense of inferiority. Participation in group activities heightens. Romantic love for the parent of the opposite sex diminishes, and children identify with the parent of the same sex. Freud refers to this period as a time of sexual latency. The type of acceptance school-age children receive at home and at school will affect the attitudes they develop about themselves and their role in life. Piaget refers to the thought processes of this period as concrete operations.

Concrete operations involves logical thinking and an understanding of cause and effect. The egocentric view of the preschool child is replaced by the ability to understand the point of view of another person. The child can understand the origin or consequence of an event he or she is experiencing. By 10 years of age, the child understands that people do not always control events in life, such as death, spirituality, or the origin of the world (Box 19-1).

Between 6 and 12 years of age, children prefer friends of their own sex and usually prefer the company of their friends to that of their brothers and sisters. Outward displays of affection by adults are embarrassing to them. Although they are now too big to cuddle on their parents' laps, they still require much love, support, and guidance.

Between 6 and 12 years of age, self-esteem becomes very important in the developmental process. Children are evaluated according to their social contribution, such as the ability to attain good grades or hit home runs (Figure 19-1). Children's feelings about themselves are very important and should be assessed.

PHYSICAL GROWTH

Growth is slow until the spurt directly before puberty. Weight gains are more rapid than are increases in height. The average gain in weight per year is about 5.5 to 7 pounds (2.5 to 3.2 kg). The average increase in height is approximately 2 inches (5.0 cm). Growth in head circumference is slower than before because myelinization within the brain is complete by 7 years of age. Head circumference increases from 20 to 21 inches between 5 and 12 years of age. At the end of this time, the brain has reached approximately adult size. (Dentition and nutrition are discussed in Chapter 15.)

Muscular coordination is improved, and the lymphatic tissues become highly developed. The skeletal bones continue to ossify, and the body has a lower center of gravity. The body is supple, and sometimes skeletal growth is more rapid than is growth of muscles and ligaments. The child may appear "gangling." There is a noticeable change in facial structures as the jaw lengthens. The sinuses are often sites of infection. The 6-year molars (the first permanent teeth) erupt. The loss of primary teeth begins at about age 6 years, and about four permanent teeth erupt per year. The gastrointestinal tract is more mature, and the stomach is upset less often. Stomach capacity increases and caloric needs are less than in preschool years. The heart grows slowly and

---

box 19-1 | **Features of Major Theories of Development During Later Childhood**

SIGMUND FREUD

The child is in a period of sexual latency.
The child's repression of sexuality makes it possible to form same-sex friendships; the child assumes the role of leader or follower.
The child is heavily influenced by parents and teachers, who can bolster his or her self-image or more deeply repress sexuality.

ERIK ERIKSON

The child's development is heavily influenced by others.
The child's leadership abilities and popularity depend on successfully controlling the environment.
By learning to be productive, self-directing, and accepted at school and in society, the child gains a positive self-concept.

JEAN PIAGET

The child can concentrate on more than one aspect of a situation at a time.
The child becomes capable of abstract reasoning, but thought is still limited to his or her own experience.
The child understands cause and effect.

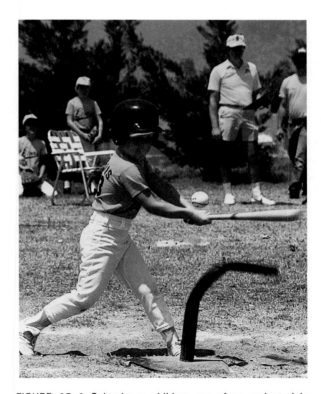

FIGURE **19-1** School-age children are often evaluated by their peers according to their performance, such as the ability to achieve good grades or hit a home run. (Photo courtesy of Pat Spier, RN-C.)

is now smaller in proportion to body size than at any other time of life.

The shape of the eye changes with growth. The exact age at which 20/20 vision occurs, once believed to be about 7 years of age, is now believed to be sometime during the preschool years. The capabilities of the child's sense organs, including hearing, have an important bearing on learning abilities.

The vital signs of the child of school age are near those of the adult. The temperature is 37° C (98.6° F), the pulse is 85 to 100 beats/min, and respirations are 18 to 20 breaths/min. The systolic blood pressure ranges from 90 to 108 mm Hg; the diastolic blood pressure ranges from 60 to 68 mm Hg. Boys are slightly taller and somewhat heavier than girls until changes indicating puberty appear. The differences among children are greater at the end of middle childhood than at the beginning.

The changes in body proportions help the child prepare for activities commonly enjoyed in school. However, size is not correlated with emotional maturity and a problem is created when a child faces higher expectations because he or she is taller and heavier than peers. Sedentary activities and habits in the school-age child are associated with a high risk of developing obesity and cardiovascular problems later in life.

➤ NURSING **TIP**

Emergency Treatment of an Avulsed Tooth. When a permanent tooth is accidentally knocked out of the socket, the tooth should be picked up by the crown to avoid damaging the root area. Place the tooth in milk until the child and tooth arrive at a dentist's office.

GENDER IDENTITY

The sex organs remain immature during the school-age years, but interest in gender differences progresses to puberty. Sex role development is greatly influenced by parents through differential treatment and identification. These two interdependent processes are at work in the family and in society. In infancy, boys and girls are often wrapped in pink or blue blankets. Later their dress, the types of toys and games chosen for them, television, and the attitudes of family members may serve to fortify gender identity, although unisex dress and play are currently popular.

The influence of the school environment is considerable. The teacher can directly foster stereotyping in the assignment of schoolroom tasks, the choice of textbooks, and the disapproval of behavior that deviates from the child's sex role. Aggressive behavior is sometimes overlooked in boys but is discouraged in girls.

Some adults develop a sex role concept that incorporates both masculine and feminine qualities, sometimes

termed androgynous. Because healthy interpersonal relationships depend on both assertiveness and sensitivity, the incorporation of traditionally masculine and feminine positive attributes may lead to fuller human functioning.

SEX EDUCATION

Sex education is a lifelong process. Parents convey their attitudes and feelings about all aspects of life, including sexuality, to the growing child. Sex education is accomplished less by talking or formal instruction than by the whole climate of the home, particularly the respect shown to each family member.

Children's questions about sex should be answered simply and at their level of understanding. Correct names should be used to describe the genitalia. The hospitalized child who complains, "My penis hurts," is understood by all. Private masturbation is normal and is practiced by both males and females at various times throughout their lives. It does not cause acne, blindness, insanity, or impotence. The young boy must be prepared for erections and nocturnal emissions (wet dreams), which are to be expected and are not necessarily the result of masturbation. The young girl is prepared for menarche and is provided with the necessary supplies. This is particularly important to the early maturer because an elementary school may not provide dispensing machines in the restrooms. (See the discussion of menstrual cycle in Chapter 2.)

Both sexes are concerned during the school years with the disproportion of their bodies, and they may be self-conscious when undressing. They may compare themselves with their friends. They need reassurance about their awakening sexuality, which affects their thoughts and behavior.

Factual knowledge concerning sex and drugs is an essential component of sex education both in the home and at school. School nurses can assist in preparing sex education programs, but participation of parents is valuable. Sex education can be taught in the context of the normal process and function of the human body. Facts must be provided. Values clarification can be added and influenced by parents in the home. If children realize that their parents are uncomfortable with discussing the subject, they may turn to peers, who often supply erroneous and distorted information. The Sex Information and Education Council of the United States (SIECUS) (SIECUS, 130 W. 42nd Street, Suite 350, New York, NY 10036; http://www.siecus.org) maintains that every sex education program should present the topic from six aspects: biological, social, health, personal adjustment and attitudes, interpersonal associations, and establishment of values.

Regardless of the practice setting, nurses can help parents and children with sex education through careful listening and anticipatory guidance (Table 19-1). They can teach decision-making skills and responsibility. Nurses should review normal developmental behavior and explain age-specific information. They provide families with useful written information that stresses sexuality as a healthful rather than as an illness-related concept. The nurse should always consider cultural differences when counseling.

AIDS education. Education concerning sexually transmitted diseases and human immunodeficiency virus/acquired immunodeficiency syndrome (HIV/AIDS) prevention should be presented in simple terms. The school nurse is a vital link in the education of the child and the parents. There are audiovisual materials designed for the school-age child. Factual information about AIDS and concrete information on how to say "no" to sexual intercourse and drugs is an essential component in AIDS education of the preadolescent. The nurse can help to implement educational programs in the school, clinic, church, and other community organizations. The facts concerning the harmful effects of drugs and unprotected sex should be communicated to the child without using scare tactics.

✕NURSING **TIP**

When discussing sexuality with school-age children, it is necessary to review slang or street terms. Most children hear the terms but may be confused about their meaning.

INFLUENCES FROM THE WIDER WORLD

SCHOOL-RELATED TASKS

The home, the school, and the neighborhood each have an impact on the growth and development of the child. Schools have a profound influence on the socialization of children, who bring to school what they have learned and experienced in the home. Although some children come from healthy, intact, and financially secure families, many do not. The child may be disabled or abused or may suffer from a chronic illness. Parents may be alcoholics, substance abusers, unemployed, or suffering from numerous other physical or stress-related conditions. Nurses must remember these factors because they surface continually with this age-group.

Children may be unable to verbalize their needs; therefore caretakers must become particularly astute in their observations. Table 19-2 reviews the expected growth and development abilities related to required school tasks. Success in school requires an integration of cognitive, receptive, and expressive (language) skills. Repeating a grade in school can seriously impair self-image, and therefore it is important to identify deficits or health problems that affect learning as early as possible.

A holistic attitude of child care must focus not only on intellectual achievement and test scores but also on such qualities as artistic expression, creativity, joy, cooperation, responsibility, industry, love, and other attributes. The sensitive nurse can assist parents by affirming the individuality of children and by encouraging parents

---

table 19-1 *Using the Nursing Process in Sex Education of the School-Age Child*

INTERVENTION	OBSERVATION
Data collection, history taking	Readiness to learn is indicated by asking questions concerning sex, menstruation, "wet dreams," and pregnancy.
Analysis	Observe parent-child interactions and determine level of communication.
	Observe peer interaction to determine the child's self-image, self-confidence, and ability to communicate.
	Observe parent's knowledge and ability to discuss issues pertaining to sex education.
	Determine child's understanding of sexual development and body changes.
Planning/implementation	Discuss growth and development with the parent and child.
	Reinforce teaching techniques and opportunities with parents.
Evaluation	With each clinic or home visit, evaluate the results of parent-child interaction concerning sex education.

table 19-2 *Growth and Development of the School-Age Child in School-Related Tasks*

CHILD'S TASK	PARENT'S TASK	NURSING INTERVENTIONS
Adapt to differences in expectations of teachers.	Communicate with teacher to maintain consistency in expectations and discipline.	School nurse should be contacted to facilitate parent-teacher-child interaction.
Compete with 30 or more peers for adult attention.	Praise child's accomplishments. Avoid comparisons to other children.	Evaluate parent-teacher interactions, and provide guidance and positive support.
Learn to accept criticism from peers and teachers without losing self-esteem.	Supervise peer activities. Provide constructive activities.	Provide teacher-parent guidance.
Assimilate peer values with family values.	Maintain open communication. Encourage peer activity. Introduce and accept other cultures in community.	Provide anticipatory guidance in dealing with behavior problems. Observe and deal with signs of prejudice.
Find satisfaction in achievements at school.	Allow children to achieve. Do not complete tasks for them.	
Participate in group activities.	Encourage child to join a group or club and actively participate as a member.	Refer to community agencies such as churches, organizations, and club activities as needed.
Learn self-control. Handle prejudice from others in a positive way.	Encourage participation in activities away from home and with peers. Have faith in child's problem-solving abilities. Discuss coping with prejudices of others.	Encourage parents to "let go" and provide guidance while encouraging independence.

to share with their children the pride they are experiencing as the children learn and progress through the elementary grades. Box 19-2 is a summary of parental guidance that the nurse may find useful in preparing children for the beginning of school.

The nurse observes patterns of communication between parents and child and assists with specific behavioral problems. In general, the transition to junior high school or "middle schools" means multiple classrooms, a series of teachers, and a change of buildings. The child is developing adult characteristics and has new feelings about his or her body, parents, teachers, and peers. Anticipatory guidance includes a review of normal physiology and how it changes with puberty. Information concerning sexuality is reviewed, and the child is encouraged to ask questions at the time they arise.

A warm, ongoing relationship between the parents and child helps to provide a safe atmosphere of caring. Adults should develop a heightened awareness for things such as school attendance problems, tardiness, and signs of loneliness or depression. They should continue to encourage children to discuss their school problems, feel-ings, and worries. Parents and children must set realistic goals. A good question for adults to contemplate periodically is, "When was the last time this child had a success?" Homework should be the child's responsibility, with a minimum of assistance from parents. For some children, visits to the nurse's office may be their only continuous contact with a health care worker. The nurse may be instrumental in establishing positive health patterns that may be carried into adulthood.

The school nurse can guide the parents in determining health care requirements for the school-age child. Schools provide some health screening, but the financial resources of the family may prevent adequate follow-up care, clothing, or transportation. School lunch programs are available in most schools for the child identified as being in need.

Safety is an important issue for the school-age child. The rules of the road should be taught before the child walks to school. Car safety and the use of seat belts must be a regular ritual. Caution in play is essential, but a child must not be made to feel afraid to try new activities or skills.

box 19-2	*Parental Guidance for Children Starting School*

Encourage parents to:

- Review normal growth and development of 5- to 6-year-olds.
- Anticipate regression such as thumb sucking, clinging behavior, and occasional soiling.
- Encourage children to express what they think school will be like.
- Arrange for children to meet others who will be entering school with them.
- Tour the school with the child.
- Introduce the child to the school crossing guard and bus driver.
- Teach the child his or her family name and telephone number.
- Teach safety precautions about crossing the street, strangers, and "blue star" homes (community-established "safe homes" for children in an emergency; such houses are designated by a blue star or other symbol).
- Allow sufficient time in the morning to prepare for school.
- Provide a cheerful send-off.
- Instruct the child where to go in case of emergency at home, such as neighbor or relative.
- Walk to school until the child understands the route, or designate a bus stop.
- Listen to the child at the end of the day; become interested in his or her school life.
- Get to know the child's teacher; take an interest in the school.
- Inform the teacher of sudden or unusual stress in the child's life.

Data from Rogers, F., & Head, B. (1983). *Mister Rogers talks with parents.* New York: Berkley Books; and Behrman, R.E., Kliegman, R.M., & Jenson, H.B. (2000). *Nelson's textbook of pediatrics* (16th ed.). Philadelphia: W.B. Saunders.

PLAY

Play activities in the school-age child involve increased physical and intellectual skills and some fantasy. The sense of belonging to a group is very important, and conformity to "be just like my friends" is of vital importance to the child. The culture of the school-age child involves membership in a group of some type. If parents do not provide a club, scout, or church group, the child may find a group of his or her own, which may be a gang.

Teams are important to growth and development, and competition is a new challenge. Rituals such as collecting items and playing board games are enjoyable quiet activities for the school-age child. Television is often considered to be a "baby-sitter" when overused, but

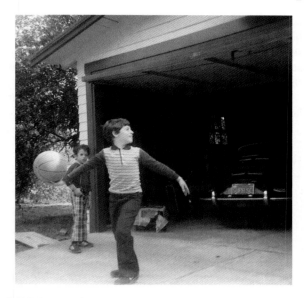

FIGURE **19-2** Developing the skills of a team sport is important to the school-age child.

many educational and exciting programs are offered during prime-time hours. Computer and video games challenge intellect and skill and are healthy outlets as long as they do not completely replace active physical play. Play enables the child to feel powerful and in control. Mastering new skills helps the child to feel a sense of accomplishment, which is necessary to successfully achieve Erikson's phase of industry (Figure 19-2). Participation in organized sports can develop skill, teamwork, and fitness, but excessive pressure and unrealistic expectations can have negative effects. High-stress and high-impact sports such as football are not desirable sports activities for the school-age child because of the risk of injury to the immature skeletal system.

⭐NURSING **TIP**

Caution parents about the safe storage of firearms. Many deaths caused by firearms occur in the home, not on the streets.

LATCHKEY CHILDREN

In the United States, latchkey children are those who are left unsupervised after school because parents are away from home or at work and extended family is not available to care for them. These children are subject to a higher rate of accidents and are at risk of feeling isolated and alone. Some latchkey children, however, enjoy the independence and become skilled in problem solving and self-care. A back-up adult should be available to the child in case of emergencies. Many latchkey children do not participate in after-school social and sports activities and may be slower to identify themselves as belonging to a group. The school nurse can be a key source for providing information about the needs of the school-age child and quality after-school care programs that may be available in the community.

Box 19-3 shows parental and child guidance for latchkey children. Nurses should be aware of local re-sources, such as "Prepared for Today" (a program sponsored by the National Boy Scouts of America) and Young Men's Christian Association (YMCA) and Young Women's Christian Association (YWCA) after-school activities. They can also assist in developing innovative programs such as cooperative baby-sitting, in which parents exchange child care services. The nurse must spend time with parents, lend support, and help them to explore their options.

---

box 19-3 | *Guidance for Latchkey Families*

TEACH CHILD ABOUT SAFETY

Do not enter the house if the door is ajar or if any-thing looks unusual.
Do not leave the house or yard without permission.
Never admit a stranger into the house.
Never agree to meet with someone you met online.
Never respond to messages on the computer that sound weird.
Do not display keys; keep the door locked.
Teach how to answer the telephone (parents are busy, not "out").
Do not take shortcuts to school through alleys or across train tracks.
Walk to and from school with friends.
Never accept rides with strangers.
Know how to reach a trusted adult.
Teach first aid techniques; know how to call 911.
Review fire safety rules and the route of escape; walk through the procedure with the child.
Know and obey basic safety rules.

TEACH PARENTS TO

List emergency numbers and post them near the telephone.
Designate a neighbor who is usually home for help in emergencies.
Teach the child his or her own name, telephone number, address, and parents' name.
Leave work number with the child.
Lock up firearms or remove them from the house.
Prepare a first aid kit and designate its location.
Address street safety with the child when returning from school; include precautions with strangers.
Consider obtaining a pet for the child.
Be home on time or call the child.
Leave a tape-recorded message to decrease the loneliness of the child, recommend specific ac-tivities rather than television.
Help the child to feel successful and appreciated.
Assess the home and neighborhood for hazards specific to their locale.

Data modified from State of California Office of Criminal Justice Planning, Sacramento, California 95814; and McClellan, M. (1984). On their own: Latchkey children. *Pediatric Nursing, 10,* 2000.

PHYSICAL, MENTAL, EMOTIONAL, AND SOCIAL DEVELOPMENT

THE SIX-YEAR-OLD

At 6 years of age, children burst with energy and are on the go constantly. They soon become overtired, and it is necessary to limit their activities. They like to start tasks but do not always finish them because their attention span is fairly brief. They tend to be bossy, are sometimes rude, and experiment with language, but they are very sensitive to criticism. Their conscience is active, and they find it difficult to make decisions.

One of the most obvious physical changes at this age is the loss of the temporary teeth (Figure 19-3). The im-portant 6-year molars also erupt. Children can jump rope, throw and catch a ball, tie shoelaces, and perform

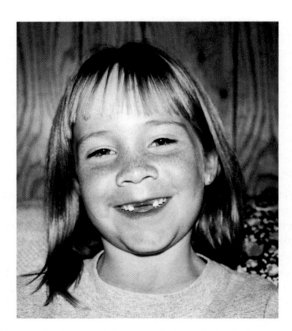

FIGURE **19-3** One of the most obvious physical changes of the 6-year-old is the loss of primary teeth. The loss of primary teeth starts at 6 years of age, and about four permanent teeth erupt each year.

numerous other feats that require muscle coordination. Their language differs from that of the preschool child. They use it for a purpose rather than for the pure joy of talking. Their vocabulary consists of about 2500 words. They require 11 to 13 hours of sleep a night.

Boys and girls play together at this age, although they begin to prefer to associate with children of the same gender. Most children enjoy collecting objects such as shells, leaves, or stones. Play at this time usually reflects events that occur in the immediate environment.

Six-year-old children need time and support to help them adjust to school. The transition may be more comfortable if they have nursery school or kindergarten experience. Most children go to school expecting the same reception they are accustomed to at home. If parents are critical or overly protective, children will assume that the teacher will be also. When the teacher's response differs markedly from the child's expectations, they feel insecure and may even be hostile toward the teacher. Parents must observe children for signs of fatigue and stress. Not all children are ready for school merely because they reach the proper age. Even those who are ready need time and support from parents and teachers before they can settle down to the job at hand. Being in school exposes the child to infection more frequently than being at home. Preschool immunizations and a physical examination are indicated. (See Immunizations in Chapter 31.)

THE SEVEN-YEAR-OLD

The 7-year-old is a quieter child, and some educators have noted that second graders are the easiest children to teach. They set high standards for themselves and for their families. They have a good sense of humor, tend to be somewhat of a "tease" (wiggle loose teeth to annoy adults), and are a little more modest than at an earlier age. They enjoy being active but also appreciate periods of rest. The second grader may have a "crush" on a friend of the opposite sex.

These children know the months and seasons of the year and begin to tell time. They have a beginning concept of arithmetic, can count by twos and fives, and know that money is valuable. Their hands are steadier. Their interest in God or heaven may be heightened.

Active play is still important to both genders. The boys are more apt to tease the girls than to participate in games such as jump rope or tag. Both genders enjoy bike riding and table games. Realistic toys, such as dolls that can be bathed and fed and battery-powered trains or radio-controlled cars, appeal to the 7-year-old. Comic books are also popular. Becoming increasingly independent, the children imagine themselves accomplishing feats more adventurous than those of their parents. They cannot understand how Mom and Dad ever chose to lead such "dull lives."

THE EIGHT-YEAR-OLD

The 8-year-old wants to do everything and can play alone for a longer period than can the 7-year-old. The work of an 8-year-old is usually creative. These children enjoy group activities, such as Brownies and Cub Scouts, and prefer companions of the same gender. They become interested in group fads. Eight-year-olds like to be considered important, particularly by adults. They may behave better for company than for the family. Hero worship is evident.

The arms and hands of the 8-year-old seem to grow faster than the rest of the body. The large and small muscles are better developed, and movements are smoother and more graceful. The child can write rather than print and understands the number of days that must pass before special events such as Christmas, birthdays, and discharge from the hospital.

The 8-year-old enjoys competitive sports but is generally a poor loser. Long, involved arguments often occur. A healthy way to teach a child to express anger is to have the child pound on a pillow (Figure 19-4). Wrestling is common, and dramatic play is popular. Most children like to be the hero or heroine of their favorite program. Neighborhood secret clubs are organized, and all members must strictly adhere to the rules.

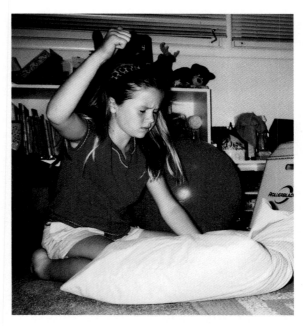

FIGURE **19-4** A healthy outlet for feelings of anger is pounding on a pillow. (Photo courtesy of Pat Spier, RN-C.)

THE NINE-YEAR-OLD

Nine-year-olds are dependable, show more interest in family activities, assume more responsibility for personal belongings and for younger brothers and sisters, and are more likely to complete tasks. They resist adult authority if it does not coincide with the opinions or ideals of the group. However, they are more able to accept criticism for their actions. Individual differences are pronounced.

Worries and mild compulsions are common. Nervous habits, sometimes referred to as tics, may appear and may vary widely. Eye blinking, facial grimacing, and shoulder shrugging are but a few examples. The child cannot help such actions and should not be scolded for them because they are mainly caused by tension; they usually disappear when home and social life become more relaxed.

Hand and eye coordination is well developed, and manual activities are managed with skill. The child works and plays hard and can become overly tired. About 10 hours of sleep a night are needed. The permanent teeth are still erupting.

Competitive sports are still popular, as are reading, listening to the radio, watching television, and playing computer games. Sports programs that take into consideration the limitations of children at various ages should be encouraged. Teaching proper techniques and the use of adequate safety devices is essential (Figure 19-5). Boys develop more muscle mass than girls as puberty approaches; therefore competitive contact sports should have separate teams for boys and girls.

An interest in music is shown, and the child may desire to take lessons. Children know the date, can repeat months of the year in order, can multiply and do simple division, and are ready for more complex math. They take care of their body needs, and by now their table manners have improved considerably.

PREADOLESCENCE
The Ten-Year-Old

Age 10 marks the beginning of the preadolescent years. Girls are more physically mature than boys. The child begins to show self-direction, is courteous to adults, and thinks clearly about social problems and prejudices. The 10-year-old wants to be independent and resents being told what to do but is receptive to suggestions. The ideas of the group are more important than are individual ideas. Interest in sex and sexual curiosity continues.

In general, girls are more poised than boys. Both genders are fairly reliable about household duties (Figure 19-6). Slang terms are used. The 10-year-old can write for a relatively long period of time and maintains good writing speed. The child uses fractions and knows abstract numbers. Boys and girls begin to identify themselves with skills that pertain to their sex role. They are intolerant of the opposite sex. The play enjoyed by the 10-year-old is similar to that enjoyed by the 9-year-old. In addition, the child takes more interest in personal appearance.

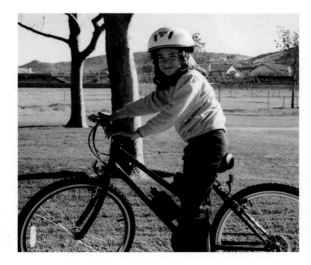

FIGURE **19-5** Protective clothing is necessary for potentially hazardous play. Providing protective equipment appropriate for any sport the child plays is an important parental responsibility (e.g., helmets for bicycling, skateboarding, or ice hockey).

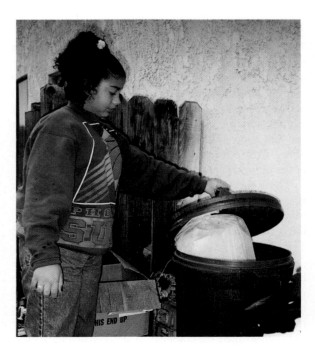

FIGURE **19-6** Household chores. The school-age child contributes to the smooth running of the household by performing household chores. (Reminders may be needed!)

Eleven- and Twelve-Year-Olds

Adjectives that describe 11- and 12-year-olds include intense, observant, all-knowing, energetic, meddlesome, and argumentative. This period before the onset of puberty is one of complete disorganization. It begins earlier in some children; the onset and rate of physical maturity vary greatly. Before the end of this period the hormones of the body begin to influence physical growth. Posture is poor. There are 24 to 26 permanent teeth.

The child has an overabundance of energy and is on the go every minute. Girls become "tomboyish" in their actions. Table manners are a thing of the past, and the refrigerator is constantly emptied. Children at this age are less concerned with their appearance. They often seem to be preoccupied; this, along with physical activities and numerous anxieties, accounts for some of the decline seen in school grades. The ability to concentrate decreases, and parents complain that the child "never hears anything." When asked to do a new task, these children moan and groan.

Group participation is still important. They enjoy being team players. Preadolescent children are not ready to stand alone, but they cannot bear the thought of depending on parents. They must overcome the problems they confront without parental help. Their attitude implies, "Can't you see that I'm not a child anymore?"

During preadolescence, children are interested in their bodies and watch for signs of growing up. Girls look forward to menstruation and wearing their first bra. Boys and girls tend to "ignore" the opposite sex, but really they are very much aware of them. There is a tendency to tease one another. Their descriptions of each other are far from complimentary: "stupid," "crazy," and "nerd." Both sexes enjoy earning money by obtaining odd jobs. The preadolescent often seeks an adult friend of the same sex to idolize.

Guiding preadolescents is not easy. They need freedom within limits and recognition that they are no longer infants. They should know why parents make a decision. They should not be expected to follow household rules blindly. Their conscience enables them to understand and accept reasonable discipline. They ignore constant verbal nagging. They should be provided constructive opportunities to release pent-up emotions and energy. One can more easily accept their irritating behavior by realizing that much of it is indeed "just a phase."

The American Academy of Pediatrics Committee on Sports Medicine and School Health recommends teaching motor skills and fitness exercises in the school setting to promote positive attitudes toward exercise in later life. The focus should be on mastering the skill of the sport and enjoying the exercise rather than winning a game. Selecting students for teams based on athletic prowess is inappropriate for the preadolescent child. Ceremonies should recognize all participants rather than star players. In the physical education or gym class, discipline for misbehavior should not be in the form of assigned extra pushups or extra laps of running on the track. Such discipline measures foster a negative attitude toward healthy exercise.

GUIDANCE AND HEALTH SUPERVISION

HEALTH EXAMINATIONS

The yearly preschool physical examination is given in the spring preceding school admission. This allows time to correct any problems that are found. Booster immunizations are given as needed; the child's teeth are examined and dental work is completed. (See Immunizations in Chapter 31.) Good dental hygiene and regular professional dental care are essential as the permanent set of teeth erupts. Dental health and nutrition are discussed in Chapter 15.

School health programs aimed at maintaining and promoting health are provided in most school systems. Nurses and other professional persons who take part in such programs can play an important role in counseling parents. They also help to meet the needs of disabled children enrolled in their schools. A carefully obtained health history provides the nurse with much-needed information. Table 19-3 reviews the development of the school-age child.

The eating habits of a child of this age should be basically sound, as long as a variety of nutritious foods is offered. Food preferences occur. A nutritious breakfast is important. The federal government has established the school breakfast program in many areas. The National School Lunch Program has been ongoing. Summer lunch programs are also available. These lunches must provide certain nutritional standards (the goal is to provide one third of the recommended daily allowance of foods).

Children who are inattentive at school should be screened for vision or hearing deficits and language or learning disabilities before being diagnosed as having attention deficit disorder (ADD). Increasing structure and decreasing distractions is the first step in helping any child with a school problem. Emphasis should be placed on producing successful experiences and increasing complexity slowly. Realistic demands must be balanced by unconditional support during the successes and failures of the developing child. If the development

table 19-3 *Summary of Growth and Development and Health Maintenance of School-Age Children*

AGE (YEARS)	PHYSICAL COMPETENCY	INTELLECTUAL COMPETENCY	EMOTIONAL-SOCIAL COMPETENCY	NUTRITION	PLAY	SAFETY
General: 6 to 12 years	Gains an average of 2.5 to 3.2 kg/yr (5.0 to 7 lb/yr) Has overall height gains of 5.0 cm/yr (2 in/yr); growth occurs in spurts and mainly in the trunk and extremities Loses deciduous teeth; most permanent teeth erupt Progressively more coordinated in both gross and fine-motor skills Caloric needs increase during growth spurts	Masters concrete operations Moves from egocentrism; learns that he or she is not always right Learns grammar and expression of emotions and thoughts Vocabulary increases to 3000 words or more Handles complex sentences	Central crisis; industry versus inferiority; wants to do and make things Progressive sex education needed Wants to be like friends; competition is important Fears body mutilation, alterations in body image; earlier phobias may recur; nightmares; fears death Nervous habits are common	Fluctuations in appetite because of uneven growth pattern and tendency to get involved in activities Tendency to neglect breakfast in rush of getting to school Although school lunch is provided in most schools, child does not always eat it	Plays in groups, mostly of same sex; gang activities predominate Books for all ages Bicycles important Sports equipment Cards, board and table games Most play is active games requiring little or no equipment	Enforce continued use of seat belts during car travel. Bicycle safety must be taught and enforced. Teach safety related to hobbies, handicrafts, mechanical equipment.
6 to 7 years	Gross motor skill exceeds fine motor coordination Has good balance and rhythm— runs, skips, jumps, climbs, gallops Throws and catches ball Dresses self with little or no help	Has vocabulary of 2500 words Learning to read and print Begins concrete concepts of numbers, general classification of items Knows concepts of right and left; morning, afternoon, and evening; coinage	Boisterous, outgoing, and a know-it-all Whiny; parents should sidestep power struggles, offer choices Becomes quiet and reflective during seventh year; very sensitive Can use telephone	Persistence of preschool food dislikes Tendency for deficiencies in iron, vitamin A, and riboflavin, 100 ml/kg of water per day, 3 g/kg protein daily	Still enjoys dolls, cars, and trucks Plays well alone but enjoys small groups of both sexes; begins to prefer same-sex peers during seventh year Ready to learn how to ride a bicycle	Teach and reinforce traffic safety. Child needs adult supervision of play. Teach child to avoid strangers and never to take anything from strangers. Teach illness prevention and reinforce continued practice of other health habits.

Age						
	Has intuitive thought process Is verbally aggressive, bossy, opinionated, argumentative Likes simple games with basic rules	Likes to make things; starts many projects, finishes few Give some responsibility for household duties		Prefers imaginary, dramatic play with real costumes Begins collecting for quantity, not quality Enjoys active games such as hide-and-seek, tag, jump rope, roller skating, kickball		Restrict bicycle use to home ground and no-traffic areas; teach bicycle safety. Child should wear helmet. Teach and set examples about harmful use of drugs, alcohol, and smoking.
8 to 10 years	Myopia may appear Secondary sex characteristics begin in girls Hand-eye coordination and fine motor skills are well established Movements are graceful, coordinated Cares for own physical needs completely Is constantly on the move; plays and works hard	Learning correct grammar and expression of feelings in words Likes books he or she can read alone; will read funny papers and scan newspaper Enjoys making detailed drawings Mastering classification, seriation, spatial, temporal, and numerical concepts Uses language as a tool; likes riddles, jokes, chants, word games Rules are a guiding force in life now Very interested in how things work and what and how weather, seasons, and the like are made	Strong preference for same-sex peers Antagonizes opposite-sex peers Self-assured and pragmatic at home; questions parental values and ideas Has a strong sense of humor Enjoys clubs, group projects, outings, large groups, camp Modesty about own body increases over time; sex-conscious Works diligently to perfect the skills he or she does best Happy, cooperative, relaxed, and casual in relationships	Needs about 2100 calories/day; nutritious snacks Tends to be too busy to bother to eat Tendency for deficiencies in calcium, iron, and thiamine Problem of obesity may begin now Has good table manners Able to help with food preparation	Ready for lessons in dancing, gymnastics, music Restrict television time to 1 to 2 hour each day. Likes hiking, sports Enjoys cooking, woodworking, crafts Enjoys cards and table games Likes radio and records Begins qualitative collecting	Stress safety with firearms. Keep them out of reach and allow their use only with adult supervision. Know who the child's friends are; parents should still have some control over friend selection. Teach water safety; swimming should be supervised by an adult. Enforce balance in rest and activity.

Continued

From Betz, C., Hunsberger, M., & Wright, S. (1994). *Family-centered nursing care of children* (2nd ed.). Philadelphia: W.B. Saunders.

table 19-3 *Summary of Growth and Development and Health Maintenance of School-Age Children—cont'd*

AGE (YEARS)	PHYSICAL COMPETENCY	INTELLECTUAL COMPETENCY	EMOTIONAL-SOCIAL COMPETENCY	NUTRITION	PLAY	SAFETY
8 to 10 years—cont'd			Increasingly courteous and well mannered with adults Gang stage at a peak; secret codes and rituals prevail Responds better to suggestion than to dictatorial approach			
11 to 12 years	Vital signs approximate adult norms Growth spurt for girls Inequalities between sexes increasingly noticeable, with boys having greater physical strength Eruption of permanent teeth complete except for third molars Secondary sex characteristics begin in boys Menstruation may begin	Able to think about social problems and prejudices; sees others' points of view Enjoys reading mysteries, love stories Begins playing with abstract ideas Interested in whys of health measures and understands human reproduction Very moralistic; religious commitment often made during this time	Intense team loyalty; boys begin teasing girls, and girls flirt with boys for attention Best-friend period Wants unreasonable independence; is rebellious about routines; has wide mood swings; needs some time daily for privacy Very critical of own work Hero worship prevails Facts-of-life chats with friends prevail Masturbation increases Appears under constant tension	Male needs 2500 Calories/day; female needs 2250 (70 Calories/kg/day), both need 75 ml/kg of water/day and 2 g/kg protein daily	Enjoys projects and working with hands Likes to do errands and jobs to earn money Very involved in sports, dancing, talking on phone Enjoys all aspects of acting and drama	Continue monitoring friends. Stress bicycle and roller blade safety on streets and in traffic and the use of helmets and other protective gear.

From Betz, C., Hunsberger, M., & Wright, S. (1994). *Family centered nursing care of children* (2nd ed.), Philadelphia: W.B. Saunders.

of behavior problems is to be averted, the school nurse should be aware of parenting styles that demonstrate difficulty in "letting go" and parenting styles that demonstrate excessive pressure.

Active play with family members is important to the school-age child. Divorce, separation, domestic violence, and neighborhood gangs can negatively affect the progress of development in the school-age child. The school nurse can initiate appropriate referrals to community agencies.

Health supervision should include the assessment of physical activity and school performance. A child who avoids activities that may reveal his physical appearance, such as changing into gym clothes or cooperating in health examinations, may have a negative perception of his or her own physical appearance. Parents need guidance to understand the difference between participation in sports activities that help to develop skill, teamwork, and fitness and participation in high-stress activities that increase the risk of skeletal injury and focus on winning as a central theme. Often a 6-year-old with advanced athletic ability who is guided into early competition and experiences outstanding commendations loses his or her self-esteem on reaching 12 years of age—when the ability of peers reaches or exceeds his or her level and he or she no longer experiences the spotlight. The school-age child can understand simple explanations of his or her illness but sometimes can revert to believing illness is "punishment" for bad behavior or thoughts.

School-age children need time and a place to study. They require a desk in their own room or at least a private area of the house where they can concentrate. Their furniture should be of the proper size; lighting should be adequate. They must learn to take responsibility for their assignments and school supplies. Parents can encourage school children by showing interest in what they are learning, by joining parent-teacher organizations, and by visiting periodically with the teacher. Parents should be encouraged to vote on civic matters that will benefit the school system in their community.

At this age an allowance or at least a means of earning money provides children with opportunities to learn its value. It takes time and encouragement for them to learn to spend money wisely. Such experiences aid in making the school-age child a more responsible person.

NURSING **TIP**

Mutual respect involves accepting the child's feelings. When helping children to identify feelings, start with the terms *mad, glad, sad,* or *scared.*

PET OWNERSHIP

Pet ownership is a common practice in families with children. After 7 years of age, children can be responsible for caring for the needs of a family pet. Pets that have close contact with children have the potential of transmitting disease (Table 19-4). Studies have documented the positive influence of pet ownership on improving the medical and psychological outcome after illness or surgery. Disabled children especially benefit from interacting with pets (increased self-esteem and positive attitudes). Pets allow the ill child who feels separated from other people to feel companionship and acceptance. Shy children often find pet ownership eases the path to socialization with others who initiate contact because of the pet.

The age of the child, the presence of allergies, and an immunocompromised family member are major factors that influence the desirability of pet ownership. Toddlers and young children may not understand the limitations in handling pets that can respond by biting or scratching. Certain breeds of dogs have a greater tendency to bite (e.g., chows, German shepherds, Saint Bernards, pit bulls, bull terriers, Akitas, rottweilers, Doberman pinschers, Chihuahuas, dachshunds); these breeds of dogs should be avoided as pets for young children.

Immunocompromised children are at risk of contracting illness that is spread by some animals. Box 19-4 explains methods advised to minimize risks to immunocompromised children. Birds, rodents, turtles, and reptiles are not recommended as pets because they cannot be screened for potential pathogens, have few vaccines, and are most likely to transmit disease. Infection can occur via contact with saliva, feces, fecal droppings, or urine and/or by inhalation or skin contact with organisms. Risk factors in pet ownership of cats and dogs can be further reduced if children are cautioned not to kiss pets, if pets are not allowed to sleep in bed with the child, if exposure to animal feces is avoided, and if handwashing after handling a pet is encouraged. Families and pets can benefit by taking obedience courses, which are available at low cost in many communities.

Having an allergy to animal dander does not always rule out having a pet. Parent education concerning pet selection and hygiene can assist the family in making a decision that is best for all family members. Toddlers who spend most of their time indoors and infants born in winter months are more likely to have a cumulative exposure to allergens that increases a sensitivity response. Cats are most often the allergen offender because allergens are secreted in the saliva and by sebaceous glands onto the cat hair and skin. Cats shed their hair and dander, and electrostatic properties enable the allergens to adhere to carpets and walls, making allergy-proofing the

table 19-4	*Diseases That Can Be Transmitted by Pets to Humans*
VECTOR	**DISEASE**
Dog bites	Cellulitis, septicemia
Geckos	*Salmonella*
Dogs, cats, birds, farm animals	*Campylobacter pylori* (gastroenteritis, Guillain-Barré syndrome)
Cats, dogs, ferrets, raccoons, skunks, bats, foxes, and wolves	Rabies
Reptiles, rodents, cats, dogs	Cryptosporidiosis (gastroenteritis)
Dogs, cats	Parasites, pneumonia, hypereosinophilia, toxocariasis, fungal skin infections
Dogs, cats, reptiles, turtles	Leptospirosis
Blood contact during birth of animals	Brucellosis, Q fever
Kittens	Cat scratch disease (lymphadenopathy and preauricular adenitis)
Cats	Toxoplasmosis*
Birds, farm animals, cats	Q fever
Birds	Psittacosis, cryptococcosis, histoplasmosis
Fish	Fish tank granuloma (related to *Mycobacterium tuberculosis* organism that causes ulcerated skin lesions after cleaning the fish tank)

*Toxoplasmosis can cause congenital malformations in the fetus. Pregnant females are urged to avoid contact with litter boxes.

| box 19-4 | *Ten Ways to Protect Immunocompromised Children from Pet-Transmitted Disease* |

1. Choose a healthy animal (preferably a dog or cat) older than age 1 year to reduce the likelihood of colonization with human pathogens.
2. Neuter the pet at an early age to minimize roaming activity and interaction with animals in the wild.
3. Feed pets only cooked meat and foods unlikely to be contaminated with animal feces to minimize gastrointestinal colonization with potential pathogens.
4. Keep the animal indoors as much as possible to limit interaction with other animals and reduce exposure to disease.
5. Treat the animal for fleas during flea season to prevent transmission of disease by these ectoparasites.
6. Do not keep birds, reptiles, turtles, or rodents as pets because they are more likely to carry unusual human pathogens, cannot be immunized, and are difficult to screen for transmissible diseases.
7. Make sure a pet dog or cat receives booster immunizations for rabies, distemper, canine hepatitis, leptospirosis, parvovirus, and feline leukemia virus.
8. Have a veterinarian test the pet's stools annually for *Salmonella, Campylobacter, Giardia,* and *Cryptosporidium* species and screen the animal for dermatophytes (which are transmissible to humans).
9. Have cats tested annually for feline leukemia, because cats with this disease are more likely to acquire human infectious agents such as cryptosporidiosis.
10. Avoid exposure to farm animals and petting zoos unless the animals have been carefully screened for human pathogens.

Modified from Steele, R. (1997). Sizing up the risks of pet transmitted diseases. *Contemporary Pediatrics, 14*(9), 65.

house a difficult challenge. The poodle breed of dog does not have a shed cycle and therefore may be the least offensive pet for the allergic child. Shar-peis, terriers, Labrador retrievers, and pit bulls may release more allergens because they are very susceptible to atopic conditions that cause scratching. Young neutered female dogs produce fewer allergens than older, unneutered males.

If an allergenic pet is already part of the family, the risks can be minimized by frequent bathing and by keeping the pet outdoors or at least out of the child's bedroom. A 3% tannic acid spray to carpets and furniture can reduce the allergen potential of cat dander. Desensitization of the child by an allergist is also an option. Except for bite injuries, where secondary infection is common, the benefits of pet ownership often outweigh the risks. Education concerning the approach to and handling of pets is beneficial to children whether or not they own pets, because they are likely to come in contact with pets in their neighborhood or at their friend's house.

key points

- School age (6 to 12 years of age) is a time of increased independence and is a time in which the child begins to incorporate, perfect, and process the skills and information gained in earlier years.
- Erikson calls this stage the *stage of industry* or accomplishment.
- Freud describes this period as the *sexual latency stage,* when the child's energy is directed toward cognitive and physical skills.
- Major changes occur in the child's cognitive-perceptual patterns. Piaget refers to this stage as the *concrete operational stage.*
- Growth is slow until the spurt that occurs directly before puberty.
- School has an important influence on the socialization of children.
- The child acquires a positive self-concept from the ability to be productive, self-directed, and accepted.
- Peers range from same-sex friends in the early years to opposite-sex friends around puberty.
- Group acceptance is important.
- Both sexes need accurate information and reassurance in advance about changes of puberty and reproduction.

- The availability of junk food hampers efforts to provide proper nutrition. Meals may be sporadic because of the child's activities and the parents' working schedules.
- Accident prevention is still extremely important. These children are prone to injuries from motor vehicles, bicycles, skateboards, swimming, and their tendency to be overactive and distracted.
- Language development during the school-age years develops and expands the ability to communicate. The school-age child experiments with words without fully understanding the meaning.
- Moral development includes an understanding of rules, fairness, values, and knowledge of right and wrong.
- After-school day care in relation to developmental needs is a concern of working parents.
- Pet ownership can nurture a sense of responsibility and encourage socialization in a shy child.
- Selection of an appropriate pet for the child and family is essential.
- The school nurse plays an important role in providing anticipatory guidance, health assessment, and community referral.

ONLINE RESOURCES

Alliance for Children and Families: http://www.alliance1.org
National Institute of Child Health and Human Development: http://www.nichd.nih.gov
Parents Without Partners: http://www.parentswithoutpartners.org

CRITICAL THINKING QUESTION

Parents discuss their child's behavior with the nurse. They state they are anxious for their child to succeed in school so he can have all the advantages of a good education. However, the child does not seem to want their help, nor does he appreciate their efforts to help him. They give the example of a science project that was due for school last week. His father, an engineer, built the best-looking project for his child to take to school. "It earned an easy 'A' grade for the boy." However, the boy didn't appreciate the help given him and didn't seem to care about the "A" grade received. They are worried that school may not have the same meaning for the child as it does for them. What is the best response of the nurse?

REVIEW QUESTIONS *Choose the most appropriate answer.*

1. The pulse of the school-age child is approximately:
   1. 100 to 120 beats/min
   2. 95 to 120 beats/min
   3. 85 to 100 beats/min
   4. 60 to 80 beats/min

2. By age 12 years, the brain:
   1. Decreases in circumference
   2. Reaches approximately adult size
   3. Reaches approximately child size
   4. Divides into the cerebrum and cerebellum

3. While playing in school, a 9-year-old child suffers an injury that knocks his tooth out of his mouth. The teacher or school nurse should:
   1. Place the tooth in a cup of clean water and send the child home
   2. Place the tooth in a cup of milk and call the parent to take the child to the dentist
   3. Wrap the tooth in a clean cloth and call the parent to take the child to the dentist
   4. Rinse the child's mouth and place the tooth in an envelope for the child to show his parent

4. The parent of an 8-year-old child seeks advice from the nurse because her child is overweight. The nurse would advise the parent to:
   1. Provide a reward for the child when he avoids between-meal snacks for a full week
   2. Limit privileges when the child eats sweets or junk food
   3. Include the child in meal planning and preparation
   4. Limit party-going activities where sweets will be served

5. Sandra, age 9 years, is practicing the piano. She continues to have difficulty in playing the theme song from a popular movie. She starts to pound on the piano keys in frustration. You would enter the room and say:
   1. "Just what do you think you're doing? That piano cost money!"
   2. "That's not difficult. Pull yourself together or you'll never amount to anything."
   3. "That piece sounds hard. I can see how you could be discouraged."
   4. "Here, let me show you how to play that."

objectives

1. Define each key term listed.
2. Identify two major developmental tasks of adolescence.
3. Discuss three major theoretical viewpoints on the personality development of adolescents.
4. List five life events that contribute to stress during adolescence.
5. Describe menstruation to a 13-year-old girl.
6. Describe Tanner's stages of breast development.
7. Identify two ways in which a person's cultural background might contribute to behavior.
8. List three guidelines of importance for the adolescent participating in sports.
9. Summarize the nutritional requirements of the adolescent.
10. Discuss the importance of peer groups, cliques, and best friends in the developmental process of an adolescent.
11. Discuss two main challenges during the teen years to which the adolescent must adjust.
12. List a source for planning sex education programs for adolescents.

key terms

abstract thinking (p. 463)
adolescence (p. 455)
asynchrony (p. 456)
cliques (p. 463)
epiphyseal closure (ĕp-ĭ-FĬZ-ē-ăl KLŌ-zhĕr, p. 460)
formal operations (p. 463)
gay (p. 467)
gender roles (p. 456)
growth spurt (p. 456)
homosexual (p. 467)
intimacy (p. 455)
lesbian (p. 467)
menarche (mĕ-NĂR-kē, p. 459)
puberty (p. 456)
self-concept (p. 462)
sexual maturity ratings (SMR) (p. 468)

GENERAL CHARACTERISTICS

Adolescence is defined as the period of life beginning with the appearance of secondary sex characteristics and ending with cessation of growth and emotional maturity. The term comes from the word *adolescere,* meaning "to grow up." Adolescence is often divided into early, middle, and late periods because the 13-year-old adolescent differs a great deal from the 18-year-old adolescent. Middle adolescence appears to be the time of greatest turmoil for most families. Perhaps one of the most characteristic features of adolescence is its uncertainty. It is a period of life that in our culture lasts a comparatively long time and involves a great number of adjustments. The major tasks of adolescence include establishing an identity, separating from family, initiating intimacy, and developing career choices for economic independence. Some of the major theories of development are summarized in Box 20-1.

Life is never dull when there are adolescents in the family. The surge toward independence becomes more and more pronounced, making it practically impossible for adolescents to get along with their parents, who represent authority. When adolescents submit to parental wishes, they may feel humiliated and childish. If they revolt, conflicts arise within the family. Parents and teenagers must weather the storm together and try to come up with solutions that are relatively satisfactory to all.

Numerous other factors account for the restlessness of adolescents. Their bodies are rapidly changing, and they experience intense sexual drives. They want to be accepted by society, but they are not sure how to go about it. Adolescents question life and search to find what psychologists call their sense of identity; they ask, "Who am I?" "What do I want?" This is followed by the intimacy stage, in which teenagers must learn to avoid emotional isolation. They must face the fear of rejection in shared activities such as sports, in close friendships, and in sexual experiences. The older adolescent thinks about the future and is generally idealistic. Jean Piaget and other investigators indicate that during this time

box 20-1 *Features of Major Theories of Development During Adolescence*

SIGMUND FREUD

Adolescent is in the genital stage, the final stage of psychosexual development.

Self-love (narcissism) disappears; love for others (altruism) develops.

Peers and parents are less influential than before but still provide love and support.

ERIK ERIKSON

The adolescent's main concerns are self-definition and self-esteem.

The adolescent experiences an identity crisis brought on by physical (including sexual) changes and conflict about future choices and expectations of others.

The adolescent must adapt to these changes and develop a new self-concept and appropriate vocational choices.

The adolescent learns to understand self in relation to others' perceptions and expectations.

JEAN PIAGET

The adolescent is in the stage of formal operations and therefore has the ability to reason logically and abstractly.

The adolescent is oriented toward problem solving.

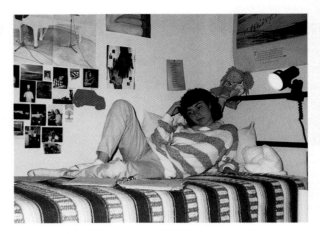

FIGURE **20-1** Adolescents need privacy.

the teen years include adjusting to rapid physical and physiological changes, maintaining privacy, coping with social stresses (Figures 20-1 and 20-2) and pressures, maintaining open communication, and developing positive health care practices and lifestyle choices.

GROWTH AND DEVELOPMENT

PHYSICAL DEVELOPMENT

Preadolescence is a short period immediately preceding adolescence. In girls it comprises the ages of 10 to 13 years and is marked by rapid changes in the structure and function of various parts of the body. It is distinguished by puberty, the stage at which the reproductive organs become functional and secondary sex characteristics develop. Both sexes produce male hormones (*androgens*) and female hormones (*estrogens*) in comparatively equal amounts during childhood. At puberty the hypothalamus of the brain signals the pituitary gland to stimulate other endocrine glands—the adrenals and the ovaries or testes—to secrete their hormones directly into the bloodstream in differing proportions (more androgens in the boy and more estrogens in the girl).

The age of puberty varies and is somewhat earlier for girls than for boys. The final 20% of mature height that is achieved during adolescence is called the growth spurt and usually occurs by 18 years of age. The major cause of weight gain is the increase in skeletal mass. The implications of growth and development for nursing assessments are illustrated in Figure 20-3.

The general appearance of the adolescent tends to be awkward, that is, long-legged and gangling; this growth characteristic is termed asynchrony because different body parts mature at different rates. The sweat glands are very active, and oily skin and acne are common.

adolescents reach the final stages of *abstract reasoning,* logic, and other symbolic forms of thought, which increases sophistication in moral reasoning.

These facts sound complicated in themselves, but they are intensified by a world that is constantly changing. Gender roles are less well defined in many households, and parents may not be traditional role models for their children. Many adolescents live in single-parent homes or with working relatives where little, if any, supervision is available.

Conformity is one of the strongest needs of the adolescent in society. Today, with electronic technology bringing common experiences to people all over the world via radio, television, and computers, the strength of conformity often overrides cultural or traditional practices. Assimilation is beginning to occur via technology.

The needs of the family often compete with the needs of the adolescent when parents try to push him or her into an activity or career that meets the parent's own personal need or dreams. Parents must be guided to enjoy the interests and activities of the adolescent without imposing their personal desires. The main challenges of

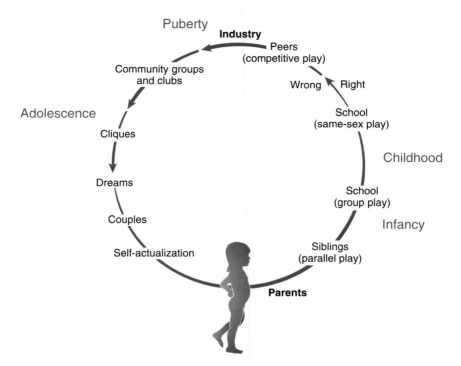

FIGURE **20-2** Roadmap of social interaction. In infancy and early childhood the child's focus is on parents. As the child grows, peers replace parents in importance. When adolescents mature, they return to the family with new respect, independence, and cooperation.

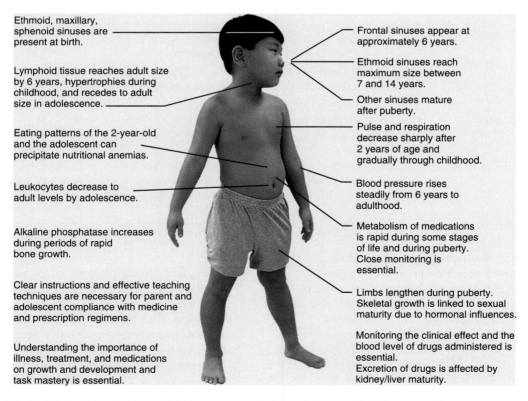

Ethmoid, maxillary, sphenoid sinuses are present at birth.

Lymphoid tissue reaches adult size by 6 years, hypertrophies during childhood, and recedes to adult size in adolescence.

Eating patterns of the 2-year-old and the adolescent can precipitate nutritional anemias.

Leukocytes decrease to adult levels by adolescence.

Alkaline phosphatase increases during periods of rapid bone growth.

Clear instructions and effective teaching techniques are necessary for parent and adolescent compliance with medicine and prescription regimens.

Understanding the importance of illness, treatment, and medications on growth and development and task mastery is essential.

Frontal sinuses appear at approximately 6 years.

Ethmoid sinuses reach maximum size between 7 and 14 years.

Other sinuses mature after puberty.

Pulse and respiration decrease sharply after 2 years of age and gradually through childhood.

Blood pressure rises steadily from 6 years to adulthood.

Metabolism of medications is rapid during some stages of life and during puberty. Close monitoring is essential.

Limbs lengthen during puberty. Skeletal growth is linked to sexual maturity due to hormonal influences.

Monitoring the clinical effect and the blood level of drugs administered is essential. Excretion of drugs is affected by kidney/liver maturity.

FIGURE **20-3** Many developmental changes occur between infancy and adolescence. The nurse must understand the implications of growth and development for nursing assessments.

table 20-1 | *Growth and Development of the Adolescent*

	EARLY (10 TO 13 YEARS)	MIDDLE (14 TO 16 YEARS)	LATE (17 TO 21 YEARS)
Physical growth	Appearance of secondary sex characteristics	Spurt in height growth	Growth slows
Body image	Self-conscious Adjusts to pubertal changes	Experiments with different "images" and "looks"	Accepts body image Personality emerges
Self-concept	Low self-esteem Denial of reality	Impulsive Impatient Identify confusion	Positive self-image Empathetic Independent thinker
Behavior	Behaves for rewards	Behaves to conform	Shows responsible behavior
Sexual development	Sexual interest	Sexual experimentation	Sexual identity emerges Develops caring relationships
Peers	Cliques of unisex friends Has "best friend" Hero worship Has adult "crushes"	Begins dating Has need to please significant peer Develops heterosexual peer group	Values individual relationships Partner selection
Family	Is ambivalent to family Strives for independence	Struggles for autonomy and acceptance Rebels/withdraws Demands privacy	Achieves independence Reestablishes family relationships
Cognitive development	Concrete thinking Here and now is important	Early abstract Daydreams, fantasizes Starts inductive and deductive reasoning	Abstract thinking Idealistic
Goals	Socializing is priority Goals are unrealistic	Identifies skills/interests Becomes a superachiever or dropout	Identifies career goals Enters work or college
Health concerns	Concerned about normalcy	Concerned about experimenting drugs or sex	Idealistic Decision making for lifestyle choice
Nursing interventions	Convey limits Encourage verbalization	Help them solve problems from choices Use peer group sessions Provide privacy	Discuss goals Allow participation in decisions Provide confidentiality

Both sexes mature earlier and grow taller and heavier than in past generations. Because of the gross motor development that occurs during adolescence, teenagers can gain satisfaction from sports. Table 20-1 outlines the growth and development of adolescents.

NURSING TIP

A rapid period of growth in which a body reaches adult height and weight before age 18 years is known as a *growth spurt*.

Boys

During fetal life the placental chorionic gonadotropin stimulates Leydig cells to secrete testosterone. Thus weeks 8 to 12 of fetal life are important in the sexual development of the male (XY) child. Luteinizing hormone (LH) maintains testosterone levels. Serum levels of LH increase during sleep 1 to 2 years before puberty. The secretion of gonadotropins stimulate gonad enlargement and the secretion of sex hormones. The interaction between the hypothalamus, pituitary, and gonads supports the development of puberty.

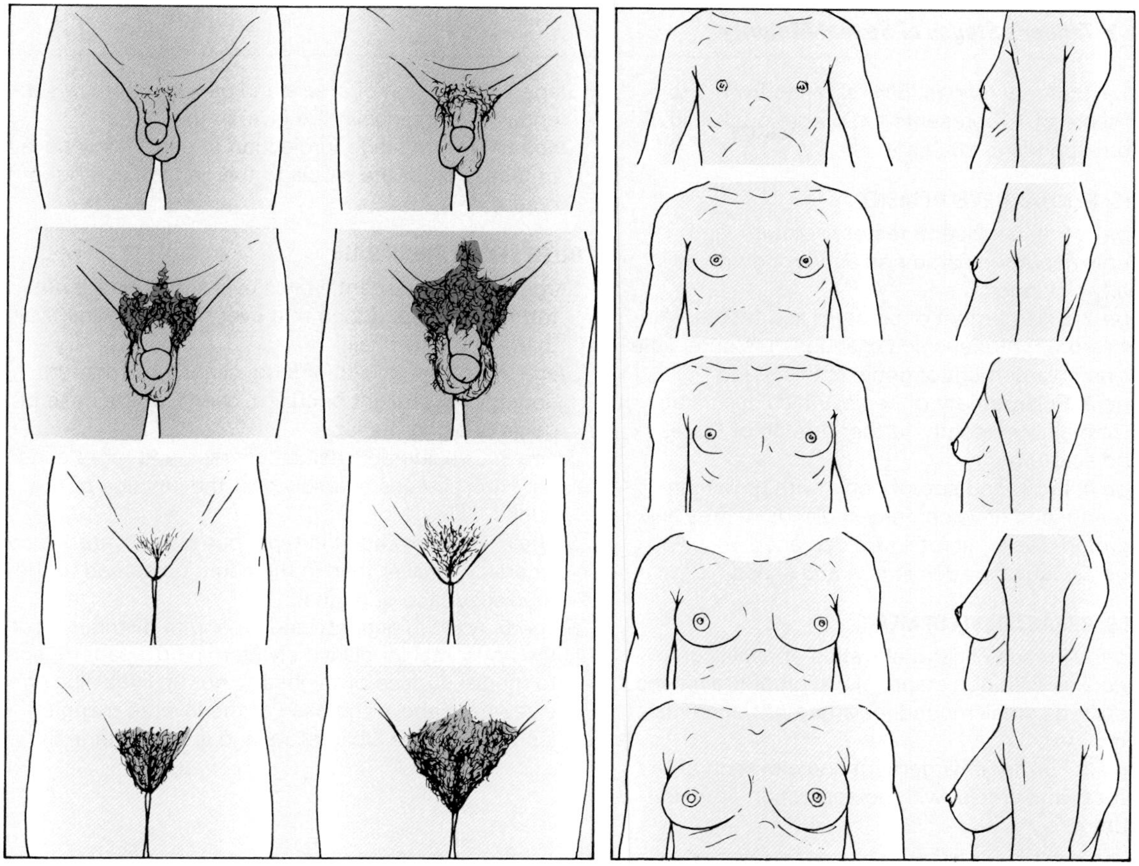

FIGURE **20-4 A,** Sexual maturity ratings (SMRs) of pubic hair changes in adolescent boys and girls.
B, SMR of breast changes in adolescent girls.
Bone growth is closely correlated with SMR because epiphyseal closure is controlled by hormones.

In boys, puberty begins with hormonal changes between 10 and 13 years of age. Enlargement of the testicles and of internal structures and pigmentation of the scrotum are followed by enlargement of the penis. Erections and nocturnal emissions take place. The production of sperm begins between 13 and 14 years of age. The shoulders widen, the pectoral muscles enlarge, and the voice deepens. Hair begins to grow on the face, chest, axillae, and pubic areas (Figure 20-4 and Box 20-2).

An athletic scrotal support (jock strap) is necessary for boys participating in sporting events, for dancers, and the like. It supports and protects the genitalia and also prevents embarrassment from exposure. A support is purchased by size. Good personal hygiene is necessary because heat and friction may lead to jock itch, a fungal infestation of the groin. Sharing athletic supporters is discouraged.

The American Cancer Society recommends that boys examine their testes during or after a hot bath or shower.

Each testicle is examined using the index and middle fingers of both hands on the underside of the testicle and the thumbs on the top of the testicle. The testicles are gently rolled between the thumb and the fingers. Testicular and scrotal self-examinations are performed once a month. If a lump is discovered, it should be reported immediately to a health care provider.

Girls

Pubertal changes in girls occur 6 months to 2 years before boys. Puberty is easily recognized in girls by the onset of menstruation (Figure 20-5). The first menstrual period is called the menarche. It commonly occurs about age 12 or 13 years, but this varies. It may occur as early as age 10 years or as late as age 15 years. Secondary sex characteristics become more apparent before the menarche. Fat is deposited in the hips, thighs, and breasts, causing them to enlarge (see Box 20-2).

At this time the adolescent girl may need to be fitted for a bra. Measurements must be ascertained and vari-

box 20-2   *Tanner's Stages of Sexual Maturity*

Sexual maturity ratings (SMRs) range from 1 to 5. A score of 1 represents the prepubertal child; 5 corresponds to adult status.

BOYS: GENITAL DEVELOPMENT

Stage 1: Preadolescent; testes, scrotum, and penis about the same size and proportion as in early childhood

Stage 2: Enlargement of scrotum and testes; skin of scrotum reddens and changes in texture; little or no enlargement of penis at this stage

Stage 3: Enlargement of penis, which occurs at first mainly in length; further growth of testes and scrotum

Stage 4: Increased size of penis with growth in breadth and development of glands; testes and scrotum larger; scrotal skin darkened

Stage 5: Genitalia adult in size and shape

GIRLS: BREAST DEVELOPMENT

Stage 1: Preadolescent: elevation of papilla only

Stage 2: Breast bud stage: elevation of breast and papilla as small mound; enlargement of areolar diameter

Stage 3: Further enlargement and elevation of breast and areola, with no separation of their contours

Stage 4: Projection of areola and papilla to form a secondary mound above the level of the breast

Stage 5: Mature stage; projection of papilla only because of recession of the areola to the general contour of the breast

BOTH SEXES: PUBIC HAIR

Stage 1: Preadolescent; vellus over the pubes is not further developed than that over the abdominal wall, that is, no pubic hair

Stage 2: Sparse growth of long, slightly pigmented, downy hair, straight or curled, chiefly at the base of the penis or along the labia

Stage 3: Considerably darker, coarser, and more curled hair; hair spreads sparsely over the junction of the pubes

Stage 4: Hair now adult in type, but area covered is considerably smaller than in the adult; no spread to the medial surface of thighs

Stage 5: Adult in quantity and type with distribution of the horizontal (or classically "feminine") pattern; spread to medial surface of thighs but not up linea alba or elsewhere above the base of the inverse triangle (spread up linea alba occurs and is rated stage 6)

Data from Tanner, J.M. (1962). *Growth of adolescence* (2nd ed.). Oxford: Blackwell Scientific.

ous styles tried on for comfort. Straps should fit so that they do not continually fall from the shoulders. Cups need to be large enough to support fullness near the underarms. The garment must fit across the back so that it is not uncomfortably tight. Teenagers generally like attractive undergarments that have some type of lace trim. Sports bras are available for girls who participate in active sports. Puberty is a good time to begin to teach breast self-examination (see Box 11-1). Informational materials are available through the American Cancer Society.

The external genitalia grow. Hair develops in the pubic area (see Figure 20-4 and Box 20-2) and the underarms. It is important to note that in ballet dancers, runners, gymnasts, and adolescents engaged in other athletic activities that involve a lean body and high level of physical activity, the mechanisms affecting puberty can be altered and cause a delay in the onset of menarche. Energy balance, activity, and nutrition are important factors to evaluate when menstruation is delayed. Further growth can no longer take place when the ends of the long bones knit securely to their shafts (epiphyseal closure). See Chapter 2 for a detailed discussion of physiology of reproductive organs.

NURSING TIP

Young women are taught breast self-examination, and young men are instructed in self-examination of the testes.

PSYCHOSOCIAL DEVELOPMENT
Sense of Identity

Physical growth and sexual interest correlate with sexual maturity. Cognitive growth and social changes correlate with chronological age and placement in school. Stresses can increase when physical growth and cognitive growth occur at different rates in the same adolescent. Although the early-maturing male often finds positive social adjustment and acceptance, early-maturing females are often embarrassed and develop low self-esteem. The teenager's desire for freedom and independence is extremely important and necessary for developing individuality. To accomplish this, young persons must reject their childhood self and often the people most closely associated with it. Erikson identifies the major task of this group as *identity versus role confusion.* Emancipation is a critical element in the establishment of identity.

1. The *pituitary gland* is a small gland at the base of the brain. It sends out chemical messengers through the blood to various parts of the body. These messengers, or hormones, are responsible for many steps of growth and change as we develop. When a girl reaches the age of puberty, the pituitary gland sends out a new hormone that affects the functions of a group of organs concerned with menstruation.

3. The *ovaries* are two small female organs that manufacture human egg cells. When a girl reaches the age of puberty, these little cells receive a signal from the pituitary gland and begin to grow. Each month a cell escapes from an ovary and starts to travel along a passageway—one of the fallopian tubes. This movement of the egg cell is called ovulation. If one of these cells becomes fertilized by a male cell, it can develop into a baby.

4. The *fallopian tubes*, into which the egg cells pass, lead toward the uterus.

5. The *uterus* is also called the womb. This is where the egg cell develops if it has been fertilized. Each month a soft, thick lining (the endometrium) of tissue and blood vessels forms inside the uterus.

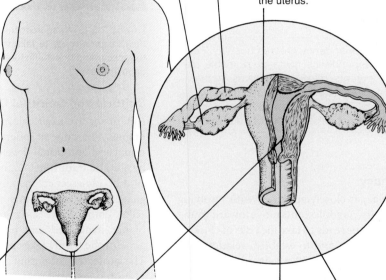

2. The *pelvic area* is located in the lower part of the body in the region of the hips. It is here that the organs associated with menstruation are located.

7. The *cervix* is the lower part of the uterus, which connects it with the vagina.

6. The *endometrium*, or uterus lining, serves as a warm nest to shelter and nourish the unborn child until it has grown enough to be ready to come into the world as a baby. But unless an egg cell has been fertilized and a baby started on its way toward birth, there is no need for the cell or for the blood and tissues of the endometrium. Therefore they are passed from the body.

8. The *vagina*, a passageway leading to the outside of the lower part of the body, carries away these materials in a flow of blood. This is called menstrual flow. When it occurs, it lasts for several days each month and is known as menstruation.

FIGURE **20-5** Menstruation.

Adolescents want to be people in their own right, and they "try on" different roles. Self-concept (one's view of oneself) fluctuates during this time and is molded by the demands of parents, peers, teachers, and others. Interaction with others helps teenagers determine who they are and in what direction they want to proceed. This process is more difficult for low-income minorities and is complicated by many factors, such as illness, broken homes, and the extent of formal education. Young persons who are unable to master confusion and establish an identity may become rigid in their actions, bewildered, or depressed, or they may cling to the conformity of peer groups long after the need should have passed. Some show an inordinate need for something "new and exciting." They may experience low self-esteem and alienation, and they may confront many other difficulties on entering the adult world.

> ◥NURSING **TIP**_____
> In adolescence, dependency creates hostility. Parents who foster dependence invite unavoidable resentment. Wise parents make themselves increasingly dispensable. Their language is sprinkled with such statements as "The choice is yours," "You decide about that," "If you want to," and "It's your decision."

Sense of Intimacy

Developing intimacy is closely entwined with resolving one's sense of identity. As adolescents move toward young adulthood, they become ready to take the risks of close affiliations and friendships and to establish relationships with the opposite sex (Figure 20-6). Avoidance of this may lead to a deep sense of isolation. Adolescence is a period of trying and testing. Disagreements with parents often revolve around dating, the family car, money, chores, school grades, choice of friends, smoking, sex, and the use of illicit drugs. The young person questions parental values and morals and is particularly sensitive to hypocrisy.

Adults who associate with adolescents should try to create an atmosphere of interest and understanding. Adolescents must know that adults care. They need practice in making decisions that must be respected even if they have made a mistake. Parents should set limits and expect them to be challenged but not exceeded. Parents and nurses who see other people's intrinsic worth, feel good about themselves, and do not see the teenager's behavior as a reflection on their parenting or nursing provide a more secure environment for growth. Loving detachment is not easy, but it is an effective tool in dealing with adolescents.

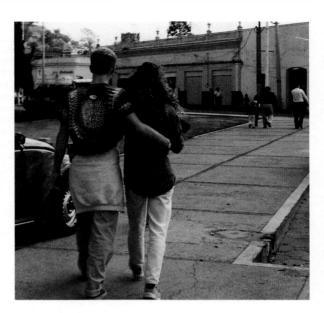

FIGURE **20-6** As adolescents move toward young adulthood, they become ready to take the risks of close affiliations and friendship and to establish relationships with members of the opposite sex.

Cultural and Spiritual Considerations

Americans are multicolored, multicultural, and multilingual. The value of independence as a goal of maturational and emotional development may not be adopted by all. The traditional Chinese do not recognize the period of adolescence; there is no word for it in their language. Many immigrants and Americans of Asian descent come from societies that are patriarchal and highly structured and have distinct social roles. The good of the family takes precedence over personal goals. The protection of family image and neighborhood reputation is essential.

As part of a search for their identity, adolescents focus on the values and ideals of the family and decide either to embrace them or to separate from them. Adolescents often perceive their feelings and thoughts as unique and therefore do not express their feelings freely. Adolescents can understand abstract concepts and symbols, and exposure to religion and religious practices other than those experienced within their own traditional family can help them stabilize their group identity (Figure 20-7). The nurse's awareness of these and other cultural influences on the adolescent's behavior will help to provide holistic care.

> ◥NURSING **TIP**_____
> Every culture is unique. Adolescent behavior problems and expectations differ in other areas of the world and must be respected.

Realistic Body Image

In early adolescence the young person must adjust to the dramatic changes of puberty. Focusing on body development during early and middle adolescence is one factor that contributes to egocentrism, or self-centeredness. Young persons create what has been termed an "imaginary audience." They believe everyone is looking at them. This preoccupation with self is normal and accounts for the constant hair combing and makeup repairing often observed in a group of teenagers. Young adolescents may try to hide their changing body or may advertise it. They may take pride in their abilities or feel frustrated when their actual abilities do not match their perceived abilities.

In early adolescence every effort is made to be just like their peers. A pimple on the skin or a disability is disastrous to the young adolescent. By late adolescence, most have completed their growth and are less self-conscious and enjoy their individual skills, abilities, and interests. Chronic illness or eating disorders (see Chapter 32) may complicate or exacerbate unresolved problems of body image.

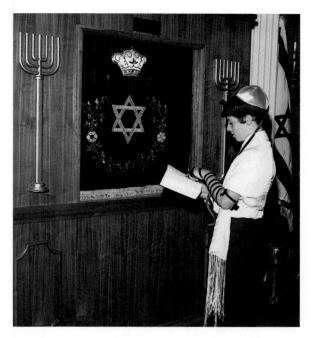

FIGURE **20-7** Adolescents can understand abstract concepts and symbols, and religious traditions can help to stabilize identity. The bar mitzvah is a spiritual rite of passage into adulthood.

> 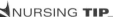NURSING **TIP**
>
> Psychosocial milestones that must be accomplished during adolescence include the five *I's*:
> - Image of self
> - Identity
> - Independence
> - Interpersonal relationships
> - Intellectual maturity
>
> Modified from Cohall, A. (1997). What's normal and what's not. *Patient Care, 31*(11), 84.

COGNITIVE DEVELOPMENT

Piaget's theory of cognitive development states that development is systematic, sequential, and orderly. Young adolescents are still in the *concrete phase* of thinking. They take words literally. A young teenage girl, if asked by the nurse, "Have you ever slept with anyone?" may not connect the question with a vaginal infection or sexual intercourse. By middle adolescence the ability to think abstractly has increased. Piaget calls this the stage of formal operations.

Older adolescents can see a situation from many viewpoints and can imagine or organize unseen or unexperienced possibilities. Abstract thinking emerges. Therefore the nurse must focus on concrete issues and concerns when teaching early adolescents about menstruation. When abstract thinking emerges in later adolescence, the abstract meaning of menstruation relating

to womanhood or motherhood can be discussed. Empowering young adolescent girls by educating them according to their intellectual and emotional developmental level can increase their self-image. Adolescents are able to sympathize and empathize. They can understand their own values and actions and can also understand and accept differing values and actions of people from other cultures.

PEER RELATIONSHIPS

Peer groups help adolescents to feel that they "belong" and make it possible to experiment with social behaviors (Figure 20-8). School assumes an important role in the psychological development of the adolescent by providing the focus for initiating social interaction. Small, exclusive groups called cliques form. These unisex groups are made up of adolescents with similar interests, values, and tastes. Belonging to the group is of utmost importance to the young adolescent.

Within the clique, the adolescent often develops a close personal relationship with one peer of the same sex. This *best friend* interaction supports social development by enabling adolescents to experiment with behaviors together and listen and care about each other (Figure 20-9). Stable "best friend" experiences often precede successful heterosexual relationships in later life.

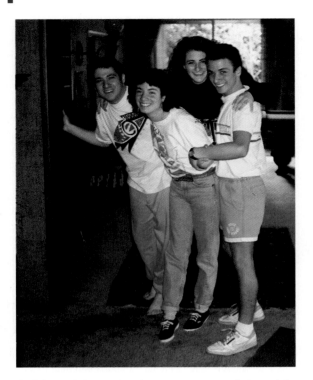

FIGURE **20-8** Immersion into a peer group helps adolescents free themselves from childhood dependence.

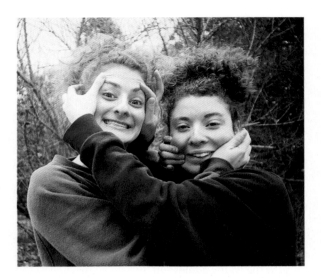

FIGURE **20-9** Adolescents practice facial expressions and try out new hair arrangements. "Best friend" interaction supports social development by enabling the adolescent to experiment with behavior and care about each other.

The peer group serves as a mirror for "normality" and helps to determine where one "fits in." It is vitally important in helping adolescents define themselves. Acceptance by one's friends helps to decrease the loneliness and sense of loss many teenagers experience on the road to adulthood.

The social norms and pressures exerted by the group may cause problems. The selection of friends and allegiance to them may bring about confrontations within the family. Parents need help in understanding that the adolescent's exaggerated conformity is necessary to moving away from dependence and obtaining approval from persons outside the nuclear family. Failure to develop social competence may produce feelings of inadequacy and low self-esteem.

Nurses can assist the family by supporting and educating them in the dynamics of this age-group. Parents can be directed to groups such as peer helpers (for the adolescent) and community educational programs sponsored by various agencies. Organizations such as Parents Without Partners might be another resource.

CAREER PLANS

Some adolescents graduate from high school with a definite idea of what they would like to do. Many, however, are unsure of what they want. To choose a career that is best suited for them, teenagers must first know themselves. What particularly interests them? What are they good at? What are their shortcomings?

By this time, adolescents have already taken some definite steps toward a goal. Choice of high school curriculum and grades determine eligibility for college or preparation for a specific vocation. Parents should observe the interests of their children and encourage them to take advantage of their talents (Figure 20-10). Whenever possible, a teenager should investigate various fields by talking to people who are involved in them.

Valuable information can also be obtained by career exploration, which is available at most colleges, and by pamphlets from professional organizations, the government, Internet sites, and other sources. The school guidance counselor administers aptitude tests as an additional guide and can work with adolescents to expose them to as wide a selection of careers as possible. The teenager must make the final decision. To be happy in a career, the teenager must choose it of his or her own free will and not because parents expect him or her to follow in their footsteps.

The job market today is extremely competitive and almost nonexistent for some people without skills or higher education. Productive employment must fit young people's life framework and offer an opportunity for personal growth. Some positive aspects of employment include helping to build self-esteem, promoting responsibility, testing new skills, constructively channeling energies, providing money for increased independence, engaging the young person in interactions with adults,

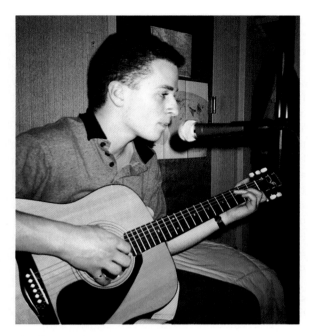

FIGURE **20-10** Parents should encourage adolescents to take advantage of their talents. Singing, playing a musical instrument, or developing mechanical skills is part of adolescent life.

and allowing them to assume an active rather than a passive role. In contrast, when adolescents are forced to take a job because of economic or personal pressures, they may need to drop out of school. With few skills and no experience, they may remain locked into low-level employment. This is often perpetuated from one generation to another.

RESPONSIBILITY

Adolescents look forward to challenges. Parents must encourage their children to take on new responsibilities. The adolescent is often humiliated by being placed in a dependent role, such as when a parent or sibling drives them to school. Driving a car or a bicycle or walking provides a sense of independence and responsibility. Even routine jobs can be made more inspiring if youths are taught to see them in relation to a longer-term objective.

Young adolescents must also be taught the value of money. An allowance helps them to learn financial management. If money is simply handed out as requested, it is more difficult to develop responsibility for finances. Allowances should be increased from time to time to comply with the age and needs of the teenager.

Middle and older adolescents who have jobs can be taught to use a checkbook and a savings account. Many

find satisfaction in purchasing their own clothes. A teenager who buys an old car soon discovers that it takes money to insure, run, and repair it. Such experiences provide valuable lessons in finance. Baby-sitting is a common means of earning money among younger adolescents. Many boys and girls begin to assist with baby-sitting at about 12 or 13 years of age. Baby-sitting courses are valuable because young people need to be prepared for this important responsibility.

DAYDREAMS

Adolescents spend a lot of time daydreaming in the solitude of their rooms or during a class lecture. Most of this behavior is normal and natural for this age-group. Daydreaming is usually considered harmless if the young person continues the usual active pursuits. It also serves several purposes. Adolescence is a lonely, in-between age; daydreaming helps to fill the void. Imaginatively acting out what will be said or done in various situations prepares adolescents to deal with others so they can better cope with real situations. Daydreams are also a valuable safety valve for the expression of strong feelings.

SEXUAL BEHAVIOR

Adolescents must meet and become acquainted with members of the opposite sex. This may begin by admiration from afar, which is accompanied by daydreams as the young person attempts to attract the other's attention.

Group dates for structured school or church functions are followed by double dating and then single-couple dating. Popular dancing provides an opportunity for the symbolic expression of sexual urges without physical contact. Slow dancing provides a mode of close physical contact in public that is socially acceptable. Long telephone conversations or Internet chat rooms link the teen with peers when they are at home or feeling alone. "Crushes" or feelings of attachment to a person of the opposite sex who is popular or possesses qualities important to the adolescent is a common occurrence. Competition and rivalry may be keen, but long-term commitment and deep romantic attachments are not often present.

Sexual experimentation often occurs as a response to peer pressure, as a means for momentary pleasure, as a learning experience to satisfy curiosity, or as a means of gaining a feeling of being loved and cared about. Sexual behavior can affect the growth and development of the adolescent. Unplanned pregnancies or sexually transmitted diseases are two major complications of adolescent sexual interaction, because few adolescents responsibly use protection (Behrman, Kliegman, & Jenson, 2000).

The adolescent's cultural background influences patterns of dating. Conflict often arises when the teenager wants to be independent and quickly adopts American norms of dating while parents insist on strict traditional values. This is particularly noticeable with daughters.

Dating is one of the early social aspects of growing up. Attending the high school prom is a ritual of adolescence. As such, it may become a battleground for the struggle for independence. Parental opposition is often based on their unspoken fears. Parents may also fear sexual experimentation, pregnancy, or acquired immunodeficiency syndrome (AIDS). They may respond by imposing strict restrictions, such as curfews, chaperones, and limitations on use of the car. When these problems are not discussed openly, the adolescent may react by rebelling sexually or by other means to test general parental control, rather than for the prohibited act itself.

Sexual curiosity and masturbation are common among adolescents. There is also a need for the intimacy of close personal friendships. Seeking one person of the opposite sex to share confidences and feelings may lead to sexual intimacies. This may produce guilt feelings and can lead to isolation from friends and family. The breaking up of such romances is often a source of great emotional pain.

Most of our knowledge about the sexual behavior of Americans comes from the pioneering efforts of Alfred Kinsey. Although his studies had flaws, they provided much in-depth information. A wide variety of sexual behavior is freely discussed and depicted in movies, in magazines, and on television. Music directed toward young people often centers on sexual themes. Premarital sexual activity has become much more widespread, and adolescents are initiating their sexual activity at increasingly younger ages. Thirty percent of girls and 45% of boys report having had sexual intercourse by 18 years of age (Behrman et al, 2000).

Sex Education

Sex education for the adolescent is a challenge. Nurses must put aside their own attitudes and biases; understand society, cultural, and moral values; and incorporate a broad understanding of physical and psychological growth and development to prepare an effective school or clinic program. Television, movies, magazines, and computer chat rooms or websites provide a source of sex education for the adolescent that may or may not be accurate and helpful to the young adult.

The incidence of human immunodeficiency virus (HIV) exposure, AIDS, and other sexually transmitted diseases (STDs) was a factor that resulted in the formalized incorporation of sex education in schools. This education focuses on the physiology of sex, the reproductive systems, and STDs as well as personal values concerning sexuality, facts about contraception, safe sex, and peer pressure. Formal structured comprehensive sex education programs are available from the Sexuality Information and Education Council of the United States (SIECUS, 130 W. 42nd Street, Suite 350, New York, NY 10036; http://www.siecus.org) and other community agencies. These types of programs are geared to kindergarten through grade 12 and present information about all aspects of health, such as nutrition, dental care, avoidance of drugs, and STDs. These courses should be presented as age appropriate. The physiology of the reproductive systems can be taught at about grade 5. By grade 8 topics such as coping skills for dating and sexuality, pregnancy, and birth can be reviewed. Abstinence and contraception are also discussed.

Decision making is emphasized. Flowcharts should show the possible consequences of certain actions. The high school units can include how to handle teenage pregnancy, prenatal and postnatal care, and effective parenting techniques. A unit on intimate relationships can be presented as a series of discussions and activities designed to help students think about the nature of love. It can cover ideas such as compromise, problem solving, and communication skills. It should emphasize the many reasons why teenagers should say "no" to casual sex.

Factual and sensitive information provided by concerned parents is, of course, the ideal. However, too often peers provide erroneous material or parents postpone education until a crisis arrives. Children must be told what bodily changes to expect and why these changes occur. *Two years too soon is better than 1 day too late!* Parents who have answered their children's questions truthfully throughout childhood offer a secure and natural foundation on which to build. Studies have shown that adolescents who obtain early sex education information from caring parents or well-informed adults do *not* have a higher rate of sexual activity.

Concerns About Being "Different"

Adolescents have certain concerns that are specific to puberty. The girl who begins to experience physical changes at about 10 years of age may feel self-conscious because she towers over her friends or needs to wear a bra. She may be teased because she is different. The other extreme is the latecomer who feels abnormal and unattractive because her friends look more feminine.

Such problems are not limited to girls. Of particular concern is the boy on a slow schedule of development. Still short at age 15 years, he is unable to compete for placement on school teams because of his size. He sees his male friends being admired for their height and strength, and this is a threat to him. Such fears are natural and usually are alleviated by reassurances that, although boys begin to grow later than girls, their growth spurt lasts longer. During data collection, the nurse has an opportunity to support the adolescent who is concerned about normal growth and development.

Traditional sex stereotypes define being "male" by activity and achievement and being "female" by sensitivity and interpersonal competence. Society's current trends toward equality of the sexes may affect these roles. Nevertheless, few adolescents escape the social pressures that dictate acceptable sexual attitudes and behavior for each gender.

Homosexuality

When a person has an attraction for a person of their own gender, that person is referred to as homosexual. A lesbian is a female who prefers other females as sexual partners. A male is called gay when he prefers another male as his sexual partner. Homosexual behavior in adolescence is not uncommon. *This experimentation is not a positive predictor of adult sexual preference;* rather, it may merely indicate a desire to explore alternative lifestyles. Homosexuality occurs in about 5% of men and women (Behrman et al, 2000) but is no longer listed as a mental disorder by the American Psychiatric Association. It is now believed that a combination of cultural, biological, and psychological factors contribute to sexual orientation and development. The nursing role is not to change homosexual behaviors but to help the child understand how to cope with the reaction of others.

Nurses must be sensitive to these issues when obtaining histories and working with young adolescents. They must also be aware of their personal biases to determine their potential effectiveness with this population. Support groups for parents and friends of gays and lesbians are available. Those who question their sexual orientation are referred to counselors and health agencies that can respond to their needs. Table 20-2 provides an example of the use of the nursing process in planning sex education for the adolescent.

PARENTING

Parenting an adolescent requires major adaptations on the part of the parents. At times it is difficult for parents to cope with adolescents. The shift in parenting philosophies from the rigid rules of discipline to permissiveness, or a current middle-of-the-road position, often leads to confusion. Some parents are unsure of their own opinions and may hesitate to exert authority. Others refuse to "let go" or change any of their beliefs to accommodate today's youth. Issues of privacy and trust abound, and conflict occurs as the adolescent desires more adult liberties. Adolescents may need time alone to separate themselves from family and search for their identity.

Adolescents need to talk about their fears, such as school examinations or how they will look with a certain haircut. They need assistance in sorting out confused feelings. A confidential, accepting atmosphere will promote quality communications (Figure 20-11). Physical symptoms, such as stomachaches, insomnia, and headaches, surface in relation to anxiety. Bizarre behavior may be a call for long-overdue help.

table 20-2 *Using the Nursing Process in Planning Sex Education for the Adolescent*

Data collection	Determine the level of knowledge concerning puberty and body changes. Discuss peer acceptance. Determine sexual practices and outlets such as masturbation. Discuss the use of drugs, alcohol, and cigarettes.
Analysis	Review body image and understanding concerning body changes. Observe for signs of abuse. Determine risk factors involving sexual behavior and substance abuse. Clarify sexual practices, including contraception. Review for sexual variation or deviation.
Planning/implementation	Provide a private area and nonjudgmental environment for teaching. Discuss safe sex practices and personal views and values of the adolescent. Teach techniques and the value of self-breast/testicular examination. Discuss contraceptive choices, if appropriate. Teach the need for regular follow-up health care.
Evaluation	Follow-up during return home or clinic visits concerning problems identified or teaching completed.

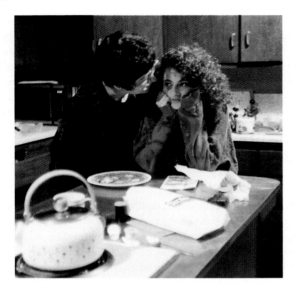

FIGURE **20-11** Listening is an important tool for establishing rapport. A confidential accepting atmosphere will promote quality communications.

Some approaches to such problems are presented in Table 20-3. As adolescents try to separate themselves from their family, they may reject some family traditions such as family outings or dress codes. When parents respond to this behavior negatively, the separation widens and tension grows. Often adolescents search for adults outside of the family as role models and confidants. Coaches or scout leaders can fulfill this role and serve as positive outlets for gaining a sense of "belonging" when there are conflicts at home.

Nurses should help parents keep the lines of communication open, promote respect and trust, and provide confidentiality and a sense of privacy. Despite the problems parents face with their teenagers throughout adolescence, the family continues to play a major role in socialization.

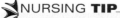

NURSING **TIP**
Privacy and confidentiality are essential when communicating with adolescents.

HEALTH EDUCATION AND GUIDANCE

NUTRITION

Teenagers grow rapidly; therefore they need foods that provide for their increase in height, body cell mass, and maturation. Adolescents appear to be "always hungry" because their stomach capacity is too small to meet the increased caloric and protein requirements of their rapid growth spurt. Frequent meals are needed. Dietary deficiencies are more likely to occur at this age because of this acceleration and because eating patterns become more irregular. Nutritional requirements are more strongly correlated with sexual maturity ratings (SMR) (see Box 20-2) than with age. For example, girls at SMR 2 and boys at SMR 3 are close to their peak growth velocities. They require adequate intake of nutrients and calories, regardless of chronological age.

The most noticeable changes in the adolescent's eating habits are skipped meals, more between-meal snacks, and eating out more often. Breakfast and lunch are often omitted. Part-time jobs, school activities, and socialization may result in the teenager's eating little or nothing during the day and then "catching up" in the evening. Fast-food restaurants are inexpensive and provide food quickly for the busy adolescent. These foods tend to be high in calories, fat, protein, sugar, and sodium and low in fiber. In general, to assess fiber intake in children, add 5 g to the age in years to determine dietary fiber needs (Kolasa, Poehlman, & Peery, 2000). Most food chains have added salads and other, healthier foods, which is applauded. Carbonated drinks often replace milk, resulting in low intakes of calcium, riboflavin, and vitamins A and D.

Foods should be selected from the basic food pyramid (see Figure 15-6, *B*). In estimating calories, variables such as physical activity and gender must also be considered. The elements most likely to be inadequately supplied in the adolescent's diet are calcium, iron, and vitamin B_{12}. Zinc is known to be essential for growth and sexual maturation and is therefore of great importance in adolescence. The recommended dietary allowances (RDAs) for adolescents is listed in Chapter 15.

Vegetarian Diets

Foods and eating fads are often the main conflict between adolescents and their parents. However, teenagers are now a growing segment of the vegetarian population. Ninety percent of teenage vegetarian diets include eggs and milk. Iron-rich foods include fortified grain products. However, a high intake of whole grains, bran, and foods rich in oxalic acid (e.g., spinach) can impair the absorption of iron. Tofu, nuts, wheat germ, and legumes can provide the zinc necessary for cognitive development. If animal products are totally excluded in the diet, a vitamin B_{12} supplement may be necessary. The nursing role is to understand the eating pattern, identify fad diets, understand the reason the diet was selected, and then evaluate and discuss any deficiencies or needs within that diet. Developing a partnership with the adolescent in meeting growth needs and allowing

table 20-3 *Effective Approaches to Problems*

APPROACH	PURPOSE	EXAMPLE
Reflective listening	Showing you understand teenager's feelings. Used when teenager "owns" problem.	"You're very worried about the semester exam." "Sounds like you're feeling discouraged because the job's so difficult."
"I" message	Communicating your feelings about how teenager's behavior affects you. Used when you own problem.	"When I'm ill and the dishes are left for me to do, I feel disrespected because it seems no one cares about me." "When you borrow tools and don't return them, I feel discouraged because I don't have the tools I need when there's a job to do."
Exploring alternatives	Helping teenagers decide how to solve problems they own.	"What are some ways you could solve this problem?" "Which idea appeals to you most?" "Are you willing to do this until . . .?"
	Negotiating agreements with teenager when you own problem.	"What can we do to settle this conflict between us?" "Are we in agreement on that idea?" "What would be a fair consequence if the agreement is broken?"
Natural and logical consequences	Permitting teenagers, within limits, to decide how they will behave and allowing them to experience consequences. Natural consequences apply when teenager owns problem. Logical consequences apply when either parent or teenager owns problem.	*Natural:* Teenager who forgets coat on cold days gets cold; teenager who skips lunch goes hungry. *Logical:* Teenager who spends allowance quickly does not receive any more money until next allowance day; teenager who neglects to study for a test gets low grade.

From *Systematic training for effective parenting of teens: Parenting teenagers,* Circle Pines, Mich.: American Guidance Service. © 1990 by Don Dinkmeyer and Gary D. McKay.

the child to take responsibility for meeting his or her own health needs is the cornerstone for success in nutritional education.

Vegetarians who eat no animal protein, eggs, or dairy products (vegans) are at particular risk of developing deficiencies in protein, vitamin B_{12}, calcium, iron, iodine, and possibly zinc. A total vegetarian diet is adequate only if it is carefully planned.

Sports and Nutrition

The best training diet is one that contains foods from each of the basic food groups in sufficient quantities to meet energy demands and nutrient requirements. What to eat and when to eat it in relation to muscle exercise are vital to successful athletic performance. Athletes exhaust reserves of muscle glycogen. Carbohydrates that can be rapidly converted to blood glucose and transported to muscles will provide the rapid recovery of muscle glycogen necessary for maintaining prolonged intense muscle activity. Eating a slowly absorbed glucose source will prevent the development of chronic low muscle energy stores. To hasten muscle energy recovery, the young athlete should consume at least 50 g of a rapidly used carbohydrate within 4 hours after exercise. Foods high in fat and protein will prolong carbohydrate metabolism.

Carbohydrates that provide both energy and other nutrients are best for athletes. Therefore fruits and fruit juices are a better choice than sugar-rich soft drinks and candy. The fat content in candy will slow carbohydrate absorption. Some foods that provide a rapid supply of carbohydrates to muscles include corn flakes, bagels, raisins, maple syrup, potatoes, and rice. Some foods that supply a slow release of carbohydrates to muscles include apples, pears, green peas, chickpeas, skim milk, and plain yogurt. Fluids lost by sweat must be replaced by drinking small amounts of fluid during a workout. Thirst is one guide for intake.

Caffeine and alcohol deplete body water and are to be avoided. Anabolic steroids, used by some athletes to gain weight and increase strength, are detrimental to bone growth. Iron is particularly necessary for female athletes, who may be borderline or deficient in their intake of this mineral.

Nutrition and School Examinations

The role of diet in the treatment of illness has become traditional practice. The role of nutrition in health is becoming prominent in health education today. Nutritional practices are the focus of weight control programs, and special nutritional supplements are available for athletes, pregnant women, and the elderly. Studies have shown that foods can affect behavior, moods, and alertness.

For the adolescent who is scheduled to take an important school examination, the nurse can offer nutritional guidance as part of the examination preparation. Carbohydrates such as pancakes and syrup, breakfast pastries, or a muffin and jelly increase serotonin in the brain, resulting in a soothing, sleepy response. Bacon and eggs are high in fat and cholesterol and are therefore slow to digest, diverting blood from the brain during the digestion process and causing decreased alertness. Drinking more than 4 cups of a caffeine-containing beverage such as coffee can cause overstimulation and nervousness. However, protein-rich meals increase amino acids and tyrosine, which will break down into norepinephrine in the brain and result in increased alertness. Fish, soy, peanuts, and rice increase choline and acetylcholine in the brain, which results in increased memory. Therefore a "proper" meal before a big school test may help the adolescent's achievement as well as his or her health.

PERSONAL CARE
Hygiene

The adolescent needs personal hygiene information because body changes require more frequent bathing and the use of deodorants. The nurse can help the young person sort out the various claims of reliability for hair removal, menstrual hygiene, and cosmetics products and procedures. The practice of body piercing, a popular teenage fad, should be performed by an experienced person using sterile instruments. The skin around the point of insertion of the body ring should be regularly inspected for signs of infection. Swapping of body rings is discouraged. Teenagers are warned not to use another's razor or toothbrush, particularly in light of the risk for AIDS.

Dental Health

The prevalence of tooth decay has substantially decreased. This is believed to result from the widespread use of fluorides, including community fluoridation, dental sealants, and dental products containing fluorides. Teenagers are nonetheless at risk for dental caries because of inadequate dental maintenance and frequent snacking on sucrose-containing candies and beverages. When dental hygiene is neglected, the period of greatest tooth decay in the permanent teeth is from ages 12 to 18 years. Lack of oral hygiene (inadequate brushing, flossing, and rinsing, particularly after meals) fosters the accumulation of plaque and food debris. Missing, aching, or decayed teeth contribute to poor nutrition. Young people with unattractive teeth may suffer from low self-esteem. Corrective orthodontic appliances are often worn during adolescence, and meticulous oral hygiene is essential to prevent discoloration of tooth enamel and other complications.

According to media hype, healthy, white teeth are synonymous with popularity and sex appeal. Regular dental visits during adolescence must be maintained as a priority in the health care teaching of adolescents and their families. See Chapter 15 for a detailed discussion of dental health.

Sunbathing

Adolescents respond to movie and magazine pictures of the ideal "healthy suntanned body" as an attractive aspect of a body image. The young adult looks forward to sunbathing on the beach or at the pool during summer vacations and often prepares his or her body by trying to obtain a tanned appearance using artificial means. The nurse plays a vital role in educating the adolescent concerning the danger of the sun's rays and the need for skin protection with a sun protective factor (SPF) of at least 15. Protection of the eyes from the sun is also essential. Excessive sunlight and the use of artificial tanning machines can cause serious long-term reactions such as early aging of the skin or skin cancer.

SAFETY

The chief hazard to the adolescent is the automobile (Figure 20-12). Road and off-road vehicle accidents kill and cripple teenagers at alarming rates. Some schools now offer driver training courses as an integral part of the educational program. Students learn how to drive and the accompanying responsibilities; however, this does not ensure compliance. Preventing motor vehicle accidents is of utmost importance to every community. Adolescents who ride motorcycles, motor scooters, or motorbikes should know the rules of the road and wear special safety equipment, such as helmets.

Young people should learn how to swim and practice swimming safety. Accidents result from diving into un-

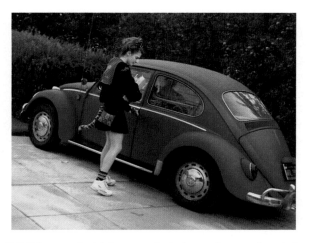

FIGURE **20-12** Adolescents look forward to getting their driver's license. The search for independence also brings responsibilities.

safe areas, from using alcohol or drugs while swimming, and from unsafe use of jet skis. If adolescents are interested in hunting or similar sports that require a gun, they must be instructed in the proper safeguards.

Sports Injuries

Sports involving body contact can be hazardous to the adolescent. Sports teams separated by age only are a special problem, because adolescents of one specific age-group can vary in size, weight, and muscle strength. Protective gear should be worn by all team players in any contact sport. The feeling of strength and the need to show off can motivate the adolescent to participate in risky behavior. Assessment of the female athlete in training should include identification of the "female athlete triad," which includes an eating disorder, amenorrhea, and osteoporosis. Coaches, parents, and health care providers must be vigilant for this condition, which has serious long-term complications.

All student athletes should have comprehensive cardiovascular screening before participating in competitive sports activities. Each year 1 out of every 200,000 high school athletes die in nontraumatic sports-related deaths (Maron et al, 1998). Most result from cardiac problems that are not obvious. The American Academy of Pediatrics Committee on Sports Medicine has established guidelines for medical clearance for sports activities. There may be a future role for genetic testing for cardiac disease in athletes with a family history of cardiac problems. The school nurse can play a key role in safety education by working closely with school coaches and parents.

> **NURSING TIP**
>
> Obtaining a driver's license, graduating from high school, and reaching the legal drinking age are American rites of passage through adolescence. Other cultures offer specific ceremonies to mark phases of development.

COMMON PROBLEMS OF ADOLESCENCE

SUBSTANCE ABUSE

The growing drug trade and the increase in vandalism and crime expose adolescents to unprecedented assaults in their schools and neighborhoods. Gang-related deaths from guns and knife wounds have escalated greatly. This growing menace is a source of great frustration and concern to parents and to all who provide services to children.

When adolescents experiment with different types of behavior in a search for their identity, they may experiment with drugs. The best weapon against drug addiction is education. Drugs are often made available in the schools and in the streets of the neighborhood where adolescents congregate. The need to conform, the need to be accepted, peer pressure, and the emotional depression often occurring in the turmoil of adolescent adjustments are strong influences for drug use. Education concerning the dangers of drug use is essential in the home and in the school.

Adolescents are prone to mood swings as they try to adjust to the many physical and psychological changes occurring in their lives. The present may feel overwhelming, and the future blurs. The following PACE interview (Schwartz, 1997) can assist in distinguishing the drug-free adolescent from one who may be experimenting with drugs and requires a follow-up referral:

P—Parents, peers, and pot. Question the adolescent concerning his or her parents, relationships with peers, and attitude and exposure to marijuana.

A—Alcohol, automobiles. Question the adolescent concerning alcohol use (e.g., beers at parties) and his or her driving record.

C—Cigarettes. Discuss the adolescent's smoking history.

E—Education. Discuss the adolescent's attitude and performance in school.

If two or more of the PACE letters are problem areas, the adolescent may be at high risk for drug abuse and require a professional referral. Follow-up care may involve making a contract with the adolescent to be drug free, educating the adolescent, teaching coping skills, and referring the parents to a support group such as Tough

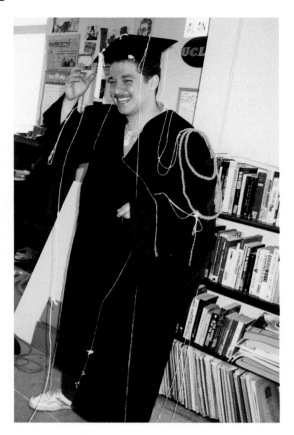

FIGURE **20-13** Graduation from high school is the self-actualization of the adolescent. Peers and family share the joy with the new graduate.

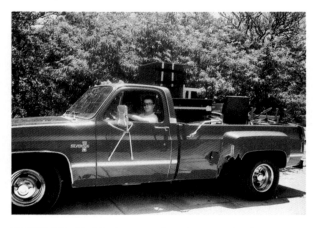

FIGURE **20-14** Moving away from home and going away to college mark the entrance into adulthood.

Love Groups or the National Federation of Parents for Drug Free Youth (Silver Springs, MD).

DEPRESSION

Sometimes an adolescent who appears to be adjusted and performing well in school may become depressed. Drug use can precede the development of depression. Working parents and busy teachers can easily overlook slowly changing behaviors. A change in school performance, in appearance, or in behavior can be a warning sign of depression, which can lead to suicide if left untreated. A threat of suicide is a call for help that must be taken care of without delay. Suicide is the third leading cause of death in the adolescent group age 15 to 19 years (American Academy of Child and Adolescent Psychiatry, 1998). The school nurse can help the adolescent by recognizing the depression, encouraging open communication, posting the numbers of available hotlines, identifying appropriate coping mechanisms, and providing professional referrals.

THE NURSING APPROACH TO ADOLESCENTS

The nurse must open the lines of communication with adolescents and enable them to feel at ease before initiating care or teaching. A sense of humor is helpful. Providing privacy and ensuring confidentiality and respect are basic to adolescent communication. The nurse must be careful not to behave like a teenager, because the adolescent may perceive that behavior as "phoney." Adolescent hostility may be evidence of fear of the unknown, and rebellion may be an effort at grasping independence. The nurse should guide the parents concerning the need to listen, understand, and share with teens. Helping parents distinguish between normal problems of adolescence and problems that require referral and follow-up is essential. For example, demands for privacy are normal, but overall withdrawal requires referral and follow-up care.

Health care teaching should include nutrition, dental care, personal care, body piercing, accident prevention, substance abuse, self-control, risk-taking behavior, money, and time management. Open-ended questions concerning common problems of adolescence may encourage the discussion of a topic that adolescents may not initiate by themselves.

Graduation from high school is self-actualization for the adolescent (Figure 20-13). Getting a job that will provide for self-support or going to college, which may involve leaving home, is the first step of entrance into independent adulthood (Figure 20-14).

key points

- Adolescence is defined as the period of life that begins with the appearance of secondary sex characteristics and ends with emotional maturity and the cessation of growth.
- According to Erikson, the major developmental task of adolescence is to establish a sense of identity. Other major tasks of adolescence include separating from family, initiating intimacy, and making career choices.
- Freud considered adolescence as the last stage of psychosexual development. He termed this the genital stage.
- Jean Piaget suggests that the cognitive development during adolescence reflects abstract reasoning and logic. He calls this stage the period of formal operations.
- The physical development seen during this period is distinguished by puberty, the stage at which the reproductive organs become functional and secondary sex characteristics develop.
- Adolescents vary in their rate of physical and social maturation and their ability to resolve conflicts concerning self-esteem and autonomy.
- A nonjudgmental adult role model who can maintain a confidence can help avoid a crisis for the adolescent.
- The Sexuality Information and Education Council of the United States (SIECUS) is an example of a national organization that assists in the development and implementation of sex education programs.
- Some main challenges of the adolescent years include adjusting to rapid physical changes, maintaining privacy, coping with stresses and pressures, maintaining open communication, and developing positive lifestyle choices.

- Peer groups help the adolescent to separate from the family and experiment with social behaviors.
- A clique affords the adolescent the opportunity to "belong" and to develop close personal relationships with others who have similar interests and values.
- The first menstrual period is called *menarche.*
- The teenager struggles with the development of a realistic body image.
- The epidemic of AIDS creates new demands for accurate, safe, and timely sex education.
- Adolescence is a time of conflict with parental authority and values. The influence of peers and heterosexual relationships increase.
- Motor vehicle accidents, homicide, and drownings are the leading causes of mortality in this age-group.

ONLINE RESOURCES

It's Your Sex Life: http://www.itsyoursexlife.com

Bicycle Helmets: http://www.aap.org/policy/0103.html

Parents Without Partners:

http://www.parentswithoutpartners.org

CRITICAL THINKING QUESTION

A high school senior expresses her concern to the nurse about taking her college entrance examination. The exam is given early in the morning, which is when she often feels sleepy and less alert and has trouble concentrating. She states that she usually studies hard the night before an exam and tries to eat a good breakfast on the day of the exam. The breakfast usually consists of bacon and eggs, a muffin, and chocolate milk. What is the appropriate response of the nurse?

REVIEW QUESTIONS   *Choose the most appropriate answer.*

1. One of the tasks of adolescence as defined by Erikson is:
   1. Finding an identity
   2. Sexual latency
   3. Heterosexuality
   4. Concrete operations

2. When teaching an adolescent concerning safety, which of the following concepts of adolescent behavior should be considered?
   1. The typical adolescent understands teaching and respects and usually follows the advice of adults
   2. Growth and development are complete in the adolescent, and muscle coordination and skills lessen the risks for injury
   3. Safety concerns at this age mostly focus on sports injuries
   4. Adolescents are risk takers and tend to experiment with potentially dangerous outcomes

3. Puberty can most accurately be defined as the period of life characterized by the:
   1. Occurrence of sexual maturity and appearance of secondary sex characteristics
   2. Substitution of adult interests and value systems for child interests
   3. Most rapid rate of physical and mental growth and development
   4. Awakening of sexual feelings and the initiation of sexual experience

4. Pat, age 16 years, towers over her companions. This bothers her, and she confides in you and says, "I just hate school—everyone is always staring at me." Your best response would be:
   1. "Don't pay any attention to it."
   2. "You just don't know how lucky you are to be tall."
   3. "This will resolve itself in time. Don't worry."
   4. "Tell me more about how this embarrasses you."

5. Which of the following actions is most important when planning the management of obesity in adolescents?
   1. Planning a low-calorie diet
   2. Incorporating favorite or fad foods into the diet
   3. Encouraging a positive attitude toward obesity
   4. Offering rewards for self-control

21 The Child's Experience of Hospitalization

objectives

1. Define each key term listed.
2. Describe three phases of separation anxiety.
3. Identify two problems confronting the siblings of the hospitalized child.
4. List two ways in which the nurse can lessen the stress of hospitalization for the child's parents.
5. Discuss the management of pain in infants and children.
6. Describe two milestones in the psychosocial development of the preschool child that contribute either positively or negatively to the adjustment to hospitalization.
7. Contrast the problems of the preschool child and school-age child facing hospitalization.
8. List three strengths of the adolescent that the nurse might use when formulating nursing care plans.
9. Interpret a clinical pathway for a hospitalized child.
10. Organize a nursing care plan for a hospitalized child.
11. Identify various health care delivery settings.

key terms

clinical pathway (p. 484)
emancipated minor (ē-MĂN-sĭ-pā-tăd MĪ-nŏr, p. 491)
narcissistic (năhr-sĭ-SĬS-tĭk, p. 490)
personal space (PŬR-să-năl spās, p. 482)
pictorial pathway (p. 486)
regression (rē-GRĔSH-ăn, p. 479)
respite care (RĔS-pĭt kăr, p. 492)
separation anxiety (sĕp-ă-RĀ-shăn ăng-ZĪ-ĭ-tē, p. 477)
transitional object (trăn-ZĬSH-ăn-ăl ŎB-jĕkt, p. 487)

HEALTH CARE DELIVERY SETTINGS

OUTPATIENT CLINIC

Many hospitals today have well-organized outpatient facilities and satellite clinics for preventive medicine and care of the child who is ill. The advent of Medicaid and other such programs has made these services available to low-income families. Within clinics, there may be specialty areas (particularly at children's facilities) such as well-child clinics, asthma clinics, cardiac clinics, and orthopedic clinics. In some institutions, information is distributed and brief classes are held for waiting parents.

In many offices the pediatricians or their nurses are available at certain hours of each day to answer telephone inquiries. The pediatric nurse practitioner may visit patients in the home, give routine physical examinations at the clinic, and otherwise work with the physician so that a higher quality of individual care may be attained. The nurse practitioner is often the primary contact person for children in the health care system.

Types of Outpatient Clinics

Satellite clinics are convenient and offer families flexible coverage. Some are located in shopping malls. Parents may walk with children and be contacted by a beeper when it is their turn to see the health care provider. This eliminates confining children in a small area and is less frustrating to caregivers. In many cities, a group of pediatricians practice in an office removed from the hospital, which aids in the distribution of health services and provides evening and weekend health coverage.

Another area of outpatient care is the pediatric research center, such as the one at St. Jude's Hospital in Memphis, Tennessee. This type of institution offers highly specialized care for patients with particular disorders, often at little or no expense to the patient. In the outpatient clinic, as in all other settings, documentation and record review are important parts of data collection.

For patients with uncomplicated conditions (e.g., herniorrhaphy or tonsillectomy), elective surgery at an outpatient surgery clinic offers the advantage of lower cost, reduced incidence of nosocomial infection, and recuperation at home in familiar surroundings. These outpatient clinics eliminate the need to separate the child from the family so that the treatment and the emotional impact of the illness are reduced. Careful preparation must be given, and assurance must be obtained that the child's home environment is adequate to meet recovery needs.

Promoting a Positive Experience

The attitude of nurses, receptionists, and other personnel in the clinic, office, or hospital unit is of the utmost importance. It can make the difference between an atmosphere that is warm and friendly and one in which the child is made to feel dehumanized. As more and more medical care is offered in outpatient clinics, there will be an even greater reduction in the number of children who require hospitalization. For many, the only exposure to medical personnel is through brief clinic appointments. Therefore it is very important that these encounters are positive ones for children and their families.

HOME

Because hospitalization is now brief for most children, the choice is not either hospital or home care but a combination of the two. They are becoming interdependent. Dramatic technical improvements and research in specific disease entities are also helping to advance the movement to home care (e.g., cryoprecipitate for hemophiliacs, Broviac catheters for chemotherapy, heparin locks, glucometers). Home care, however, is broader than in years past. It is not merely a matter of supplying appliances and nursing care, but it also includes assessment of the total needs of children and their families. Families need to be linked to a wide variety of network services. This ideally involves a multidisciplinary approach headed by the health care provider.

The hospice concept for children has received accolades from parents who have benefited from its service. Local and national support groups for specific problems afford opportunities for families to share and support one another and to learn from others' successes and failures. Special groups and camps for children with chronic illnesses are also well established. Group therapy for children under stress is equally important in preventing mental health problems (e.g., groups for children whose parents are divorced, Alateen for children of alcoholics). These and other programs not only have the potential for improving life for the child and family but also may help to reduce the high cost of medical care. There have been dramatic changes in the delivery of health care to children and families. These changes impact the role and responsibilities of the nurse working both in wellness centers providing preventive care and in hospitals or homes treating illness.

CHILDREN'S HOSPITAL UNIT

The children's unit differs in many respects from adult divisions. The pediatric unit or hospital is designed to meet the needs of children and their parents. A cheerful, casual atmosphere helps to bridge the gap between home and hospital and is in keeping with the child's emotional, developmental, and physical needs. Nurses wear colorful smocks or pastel uniforms, and colored bedspreads and wagons or strollers for transportation provides a more homelike atmosphere.

The physical structure of the unit includes furniture of the proper height for the child, soundproof ceilings, and color schemes with eye appeal. There is a special treatment room for the health care provider to examine or treat the child. In this way the other children do not become disturbed by the proceedings. Some hospitals have a schoolroom. When this is not available, it is necessary for the home-school teacher to visit each school-age child individually. Today's modern general hospitals have separate waiting rooms for children. This is more relaxing for parents, because they do not need to worry about whether their child is disturbing adult patients, and it is less frightening to the child.

Most pediatric departments include a playroom. It is generally large and light in color. Bulletin boards and whiteboards are within reach of the patients. Mobiles may be suspended from the ceiling. Some playrooms are equipped with an aquarium of fish because children love living things. Various toys suitable for different age-groups are available. This room may be under the supervision of a child life specialist or a play therapist. Parents usually enjoy taking their children to the playroom and observing the various activities. The playroom is considered an "ouch-free" area or a safe haven from painful treatments.

When the child is not able to be taken to the playroom because of the diagnosis or physical condition, bedside play activities appropriate to the developmental level and diagnosis of the child should be provided. The daily routine of the pediatric unit emphasizes parent rooming-in, the provision of consistent caregivers, and flexible schedules designed to meet the needs of growing children.

THE CHILD'S REACTION TO HOSPITALIZATION

The child's reaction to hospitalization depends on many factors such as age, amount of preparation given, security of home life, previous hospitalizations, support of family and medical personnel, and child's emotional health. Many children cannot grasp what is going to happen to them even though they have been well prepared. At a time when children need their parents most, they may be separated from them, placed in the hands of strangers, and even fed different foods. Add to this a totally new environment and physical discomfort, and the result is one frightened and unhappy child.

Each child reacts differently to hospitalization. One may be demanding and exhibits temper tantrums, whereas another may become withdrawn. The "good" child on the unit may be going through greater torment than the one who cries and shows feelings outwardly. The best-prepared nurse cannot replace the child's parents. However, hospitalization can be a period of growth rather than just an unpleasant interlude. Children may see the nurse as someone who cares for them physically, as their parents would, and as a source of security and comfort (Figure 21-1).

The major causes of stress for children of all ages are separation, pain, and fear of body intrusion. This is influenced by the child's developmental age, the maturity of the parents, cultural and economic factors, religious background, past experiences, family size, state of health on admission, and other factors.

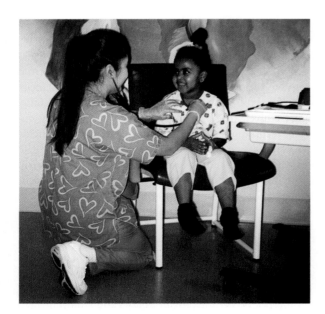

FIGURE **21-1** The nurse greets the child at eye level in a nonthreatening manner. This child views the nurse as a person who cares for her physically and is a source of security and comfort. (Photo courtesy of Pat Spier, RN-C.)

> **NURSING TIP**
> Familiar rituals and routines must be incorporated into the plan of care for a hospitalized child.

SEPARATION ANXIETY

Separation anxiety occurs in infants age 6 months and older and is most pronounced at the toddler age. There are three stages of separation anxiety: *protest, despair,* and *denial* or *detachment.* Unless infants are extremely ill, their sense of abandonment is expressed by a loud *protest.* Toddlers may watch and listen for their parents. Their cry is continuous until they fall asleep in exhaustion. Toddlers may call out "Mommy" repeatedly, and the approach of a stranger only causes increased screaming. The crying gradually stops, and the second stage of *despair* sets in. Children appear sad and depressed. They move about less and withdraw from strangers who approach. They do not play actively with toys. In the third stage, *denial* or *detachment,* children appear to deny their need for the parent and become detached or disinterested in their visits. They become more interested in their surroundings, their toys, and their playmates. On the surface, it appears the child has adjusted to the separation. However, it is important for the nurse to understand that the child is using a coping mechanism to detach and reduce the emotional pain.

If the detachment stage is prolonged, an irreversible disruption of parent-infant bonding may occur. Health care workers who do not understand the stages of separation anxiety may label the crying, protesting child as "bad," the withdrawn depressed child in despair as "adjusting," and the child who is in the detachment phase as a "well-adjusted" child. This misinterpretation can prevent health care workers from providing desperately needed assistance and guidance to the child and family.

The nurse must understand that the child who is in despair reverts back to the protest stage when the parent arrives for a visit. Rather than showing joy, the child cries loudly when the parent appears at the door. This is good! The child who has reached the detached phase appears unmoved and uninterested in the parent's arrival. Nursing interventions are needed in this case to preserve and heal parent-child relationships. The nurse should help the parents to understand they should not deceive the child into believing they will stay and "sneak out" while the child is distracted. This can tear the bond of trust.

> **NURSING TIP**
> The stages of separation anxiety include protest, despair, and detachment or denial.

1. Visual analog scale
   Child points to where the pain falls on the scale.

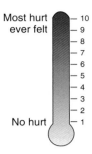

Most hurt ever felt — 10

— 9

— 8

— 7

— 6

— 5

— 4

— 3

— 2

No hurt — 1

2. Descriptive word scale
   Child chooses the word that describes the pain.

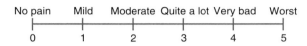

No pain	Mild	Moderate	Quite a lot	Very bad	Worst
0	1	2	3	4	5

3. Faces (Oucher) scale
   Child tells which face represents the pain at that moment.

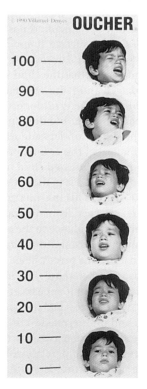

OUCHER

100 —
90 —
80 —
70 —
60 —
50 —
40 —
30 —
20 —
10 —
0 —

4. Poker chip
   a. Use 4 red poker chips (color variations have also been cited).
   b. Place horizontally in front of child.
   c. Say "These are pieces of hurt—one piece is a little, and four pieces are a lot."
   d. Ask "How many pieces of hurt do you have right now?"
   e. Record number on flow sheet (no pain equals zero).

FIGURE **21-2** Four pain assessment tools for children.

PAIN

The accepted definition of pain is that "pain is whatever the experiencing person says it is, existing whenever the experiencing person says it does" (McCaffery & Pasero, 1999). This includes verbal and nonverbal expressions of pain. Freedom from pain is a basic need and right of the infant and child.

The negative physical and psychological consequences of pain are well documented. Patients in pain secrete higher levels of cortisol, have compromised immune systems, experience more infections, and show delayed wound healing. Nurses must maintain a high level of suspicion for pain when caring for children. Infants cannot show the nurse where it hurts, and often a child's report of pain is not given the credibility of an adult's report. In addition, children may not realize they are supposed to report pain to the nurse.

The nurse should ask the child about pain using a pain rating scale. See Figure 21-2 for sample pain assessment tools. Children may sometimes refrain from complaining if they believe they will receive an injection to relieve the pain. In infants, pain may be assessed according to a behavior scale that includes tightly closed eyes, clenched fists, and a furrowed brow (see Figure 12-7.) In toddlers, crying may be caused by anxiety and fear rather than by the degree of pain. On the other hand, chronically ill children may not grimace or cry when in pain, but withdraw from interacting with their surroundings. All factors relating to pain assessment should be considered. Family members also experience emotional pain when they see their child in pain.

Nonpharmacological techniques such as drawing, distraction, imagery, relaxation, and cognitive strategies may enhance analgesia to provide necessary relief from pain symptoms. The child may draw "how the pain feels" and where it is located. Distractions such as storytelling, quiet conversation, and puppet play are effective. Imagery techniques, such as having children imagine themselves in a safe place, relieves anxiety. Slowing down breathing and listening to relaxation tapes is effective in reducing pain in adolescents. Cognitive (thinking) techniques such as "thought stopping" are also helpful in older patients. In this technique, the patient is instructed to repeat the word "stop" in response to negative thoughts and worries. A backrub or hand massage is also relaxing, depending on the child's age and diagnosis. In newborns and infants undergoing brief painful procedures, oral sucrose may provide some analgesia. Pain medications should not be withheld from infants and children when needed.

DRUG PHYSIOLOGY

Infants and children respond to drugs differently than adults. Elimination of the drug from the body may be prolonged because of an immature liver enzyme system. However, the renal clearance of drugs may be greater in toddlers than in adults. A decreased protein-binding capacity in the blood of small newborns may allow a greater proportion of free unbound drug to remain in the body of the small infant. Dosages are influenced by weight and differences in expected absorption, metabolism, and clearance. Every medication must be calculated by the nurse to determine the safety of the dose before the medication is administered. See the dosage calculation technique in Chapter 22.

Drugs Used for Pain Relief in Infants and Children

Acetaminophen is commonly used for the relief of mild to moderate pain in infants and children. The maximum dose is 15 mg/kg/dose for infants and children, with a maximum of 5 doses in 24 hours. Toxicity involves liver failure.

Nonsteroidal antiinflammatory drugs (NSAIDs), such as ibuprofen (Motrin), are given in a maximum dosage of 8 to 10 mg/kg every 6 hours (q6h). Ketorolac is a parenterally administered NSAID given for a maximum of 5 days.

Opioids are used for moderate to severe pain such as postoperative pain, sickle-cell crises, and cancer and should be administered with stool softeners to avoid constipation. If used for long periods of time, tolerance to the pain-relieving effect as well as the respiratory depression effects can develop. The right dose of an opioid drug is the amount that relieves pain with a margin of safety for the child. The dose should be repeated *before* the pain recurs. Addiction is rare in children and adults receiving opioids for pain (Behrman, Kliegman, & Jenson, 2000). Providing adequate pain relief enables patients to focus on their surroundings and other activities, whereas inadequate pain relief causes the patient to focus on the pain and when more medication will be given to stop the pain.

Fentanyl is a potent analgesic given for short surgical procedures. It has a rapid onset with a short duration of action.

Naloxone should be available for use in case of opioid overdose. Flumazenil (Romazicon) should be on hand for a midazolam (Versed) or diazepam (Valium) overdose.

Local anesthetics are used with safety and effectiveness in children. *Topical anesthetics* are used for skin sutures, intravenous (IV) catheter placement, and lumbar punctures. *EMLA Cream* is a mixture of lidocaine and prilocaine that is applied topically to the intact skin (Figure 21-3) and can be used in neonates. Preoperative and postoperative care is discussed in Chapter 22.

Patient-controlled analgesia (PCA) allows the patient to press a button attached to an IV analgesic infusion to administer a bolus of medication. Parents and children as young as 7 years of age can be taught to use PCA. A built-in lockout interval prevents accidental overdosing. Any child receiving opioid analgesic drugs should be observed closely for side effects, such as respiratory depression.

More effective pain relief at lower doses may be achieved when a low-dose analgesic is administered around-the-clock on a regular schedule rather than as needed (PRN). However, "breakthrough pain" can occur, and additional doses of an analgesic may need to be given. This type of pain management is called preventive pain control.

Conscious Sedation

Conscious sedation is the administration of IV drugs to a patient to impair consciousness but retain protective reflexes, the ability to maintain a patent airway, and the ability to respond to physical and verbal stimuli. Conscious sedation is used to perform therapeutic or diagnostic procedures outside the traditional operating room setting. A skilled registered nurse is required to continuously monitor the patient in an area where emergency equipment and drugs are accessible for resuscitation.

A 1:1 nurse-patient ratio is continued until there are stable vital signs, age-appropriate motor and verbal abilities, adequate hydration, and a pre-sedation level of responsiveness and orientation. Parents are instructed concerning diet, home care, and follow-up visits.

FEAR

Intrusive procedures, such as placing IV lines and performing blood tests, are fear provoking. They disrupt the child's trust level and threaten self-esteem and self-control. They may require restriction of activity. Care must be taken to respect the modesty, integrity, and privacy of each child. Hospital personnel can provide an environment that supports the child's need for mastery and control. These interventions are discussed according to age in this chapter and throughout the text. Selected nursing diagnoses for the hospitalized child and family are presented in Nursing Care Plan 21-1.

REGRESSION

Regression of growth and development during hospitalization can be expected. Regression is the loss of an achieved level of functioning to a past level of behavior that was successful during earlier stages of development. Examples of regression include demanding a bottle in a child who usually drinks from a cup, refusal to use a potty chair in a child who has achieved bowel and bladder control, or demanding to be carried by a child who had been walking independently. Regression can be minimized by an accurate nursing assessment of the child's abilities and

INSTRUCTIONS FOR APPLICATION OF EMLA CREME

 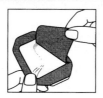 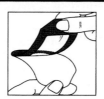 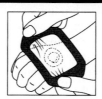 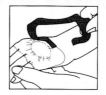 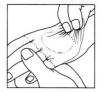

1. In adults, apply 2.5 g of cream (1/2 the 5 g tube) per 20 to 25 cm² (approx. 2 in. by 2 in.) of skin in a thick layer at the site of the procedure. For pediatric patients, apply as prescribed by your physician.

2. Take an occlusive dressing (provided with the 5 g tubes only) and remove the center cut-out piece.

3. Peel the paper liner from the paper framed dressing.

4. Cover the EMLA Cream so that you get a thick layer underneath. Do not spread out the cream. Smooth down the dressing edges carefully and ensure it is secure to avoid leakage. (This is especially important when the patient is a child.)

5. Remove the paper frame. The time of application can easily be marked directly on the occlusive dressing. EMLA must be applied at least 1 hour before the start of a routine procedure and for 2 hours before the start of a painful procedure.

6. Remove the occlusive dressing, wipe off the EMLA Cream, clean the entire area with an antiseptic solution and prepare the patient for the procedure. The duration of effective skin anesthesia will be at least 1 hour after removal of the occlusive dressing.

Manufactured by:
Astra Pharmaceutical Production, AB
Södertälje, Sweden

PRECAUTIONS

1. Do not apply near eyes or on open wounds.
2. Do not use in children under one month of age.
3. Keep out of reach of children.

ASTRA
Astra USA, Inc.
Westborough, MA 01581
021700R01

FIGURE **21-3** EMLA Cream, a topical anesthetic used before an invasive procedure to reduce pain involved in piercing the skin.

the planning of care to support and maintain growth and development. However, regression should not be punished. Nurses can guide parents to praise appropriate behavior and ignore regressions. When the child is free of the stress that caused the regression, praise will motivate the achievement of appropriate behavior.

CULTURAL NEEDS

Showing culturally sensitive attitudes toward families with hospitalized children decreases anxiety. Flexibility and careful listening are necessary to understand cultural needs. Studies of children in many different societies show that American culture is different from childhood environments derived from other traditions. Nurses must also be aware of their own cultural biases and how they might affect the assessment. In some cases a translator may be required.

The nurse must create a bridge between the health care system of the United States and the diverse people that system serves. Effective utilization of health care service and compliance with treatment plans is en-

hanced when the nurse's approach is compatible with cultural needs and beliefs. Teaching will be effective only if the parents or child understand the language used. Interpreters should be used as needed. Nonverbal cues and body language are important in intercultural communication. Nurses should take the time to learn what their gestures and movements mean to the family from another culture.

In some developing countries the energies of parents are focused on survival rather than on promoting growth and development or intellectual skills. These practices become ingrained in the childrearing practices handed down from generation to generation. For example, within these cultures, parents may believe that an ill infant must be near the caregiver's body at all times. Therefore, in the Western hospital, the nurse may find it a challenge to coax parents to allow the infant to remain in the crib, separated from them, and enveloped by an oxygen tent.

Crying may be interpreted by some cultures as a signal of an organic upset or illness. Because diarrhea is a

NURSING CARE PLAN 21-1

The Hospitalized Child and Family

PATIENT DATA: A 5-year-old girl is admitted to the hospital with a diagnosis of a compound fracture of the right tibia. She cries whenever her parents leave or return to her room, and she has had episodes of bedwetting since admission.

SELECTED NURSING DIAGNOSIS   *Anxiety related to hospitalization of the child as evidenced by restlessness, facial tension, insomnia, crying, clinging behavior, regression to previous stage of growth and development, or maladaptive behaviors*

Outcomes	Nursing Interventions	Rationales
Child/family will experience decreased anxiety as demonstrated by ability to relax, present a calm demeanor, and effectively participate in child's care.	1. Determine child's/family's knowledge regarding reason for hospitalization.	1. Provides information to the nurse as to what areas need clarification and reinforcement of correct information.
	2. Explain routines usually followed on unit and orient the child and parent to the unit, including playroom.	2. Helps to decrease level of anxiety for the child and parents.
	3. Suggest that parents or family members bring in a photograph, favorite toy, or favorite music tape/CD for child.	3. These items help to provide a link to home and help to promote a sense of security in the child.
	4. Recognize and teach the parent about age-appropriate separation anxiety.	4. The age of the child is a major factor to consider in adjusting to separation from familiar people and surroundings.
	5. Instruct parents to explain to the child when they will return in an age-appropriate manner (e.g., "After *Rugrats* is over" or "When *Recess* starts" or "before dinner").	5. Establishes a sense of trust that the child has not been abandoned. Also, toddlers and young children do not fully understand the concept of time. By using a favorite show or a mealtime as a marker, helps to lessen the degree of anxiety the child may feel.
	6. Provide for consistency in personnel assigned to child as much as possible.	6. Consistency is necessary to develop a sense of trust. Maladaptive behaviors may be normal in unfamiliar circumstances. However, if consistency and support are not given, coping abilities decrease.
	7. Support parents by showing a willingness to be available to them to listen and/or to answer questions.	7. Nurse's availability to show interest in parents and answer questions shows concern, prevents the potential for misunderstanding of prescribed treatments, and helps to lessen the anxiety of family members.
	8. Maintain child's contact with family; involve family in child's care when appropriate.	8. Increases sense of security in child and provides a sense of purpose for the family.

Continued

NURSING CARE PLAN 21-1—cont'd

?CRITICAL THINKING QUESTION

A 5-year-old child has been hospitalized for 2 days. She is watching the television mounted above her bed. She is expressionless but does not cry or appear to be in distress. Her mother calls on the telephone and states that since her child seems to be adjusted, she may not come in today to visit because she does not want to "upset her." How should the nurse interpret the child's behavior? How should the nurse respond to the mother?

common cause of infant death in developing countries, frequent feeding in response to crying is a survival response. When families from developing countries that use these survival practices move to the United States (where survival threats decrease), it may take generations to change the child care practices and focus on promoting optimum growth and development.

One cultural group may prize autonomy and initiative in their children, whereas another may tolerate only complete obedience. Protective amulets or charms placed on the wrists or clothing of infants must be respected. In the gypsy culture, the color red and the number three are positive symbols. Therefore a red-colored medicine to be given three times a day will receive more compliance than a white-colored medication prescribed two times a day. Respecting cultural and religious beliefs will enhance compliance.

The nurse must be careful to separate survival practices from cultural beliefs. It may be advantageous to change care practices based on survival when the threat to survival is no longer present. If the practice is based on cultural belief, however, then the practice must be respected and no attempt should be made to change. The nurse must assess the family through the eyes of its culture to avoid labeling a family who is "different" as dysfunctional.

FOSTERING INTERCULTURAL COMMUNICATION
Personal Space

Personal space is defined as an imaginary circle that surrounds us. The size of that space is determined by culture. We can observe the space by watching two friends of the same culture talk to each other. Some people stand close to each other. Nurses who invade that "personal space" can be thought of as "pushy" or suspect, and the parent who retreats can be thought of by the nurse as "cold."

Smiling

A smiling nurse may not be received by varying cultures as a "friendly" nurse. In Russia a smile indicates happiness and is inappropriate in a serious or sad situation.

Nurses may interpret a nonsmiling Russian as "unfriendly" if they are unaware of this cultural difference. Some cultures, however, smile in all circumstances. Their smile is a show of respect. When they are reprimanded, they smile to show they did not mind being reprimanded.

Eye Contact

In the United States, eye-to-eye contact with the person with whom one is communicating is considered a show of respect and attention. In some Asian cultures, however, eye-to-eye-contact is seen as disrespect. Native Americans consider it rude to stare at a speaker. Eye contact is acceptable for short periods only. The cultural term the *evil eye* originates from cultures that interpret eye-to-eye contact as disrespectful.

Touch

In the United States, touch is often considered a gesture of friendliness. However, touch can give misleading messages. A pat on the head may infer superiority of the person touching the head. In the Vietnamese culture, touching the head is thought to rob those being touched of their souls.

Focus

Some cultures are receptive to communication or teaching if the focus is on the problem. Some cultures deal with the problem by focusing on its future impact on the family or life of the child. Teaching strategies must be designed to approach the topic from the perspective appropriate to that culture.

When teaching infant and child care, the nurse must always determine the values of the cultural practice of the family before imposing a standardized process. Avoiding cultural conflict is essential to the successful outcome of parent and child teaching. Culture evolves and is not static. However, most families from varying cultures strive to maintain their cultural identities while adapting to Western practices. The nurse should support maintaining the individual cultural identity of that family. Culturally sensitive health care is also discussed in Chapter 15.

THE PARENTS' REACTIONS TO THE CHILD'S HOSPITALIZATION

When children are hospitalized, the entire family is affected. The parents of the hospitalized youngster need others to show interest in their physical and emotional needs. If they are frightened and tense, the child soon senses it.

Parents may believe they are to blame for the child's illness; they may believe they should have recognized the symptoms earlier or could have prevented an accident by closer supervision. Immunizations and other types of preventive care may also have been neglected. These feelings can cause a sense of guilt, helplessness, and anxiety.

Parents seldom are the cause for direct hospital admission of a child. Even in cases of child abuse or neglect, nothing is gained by blaming the parents. The nurse must remain objective and empathetic. The nurse listens carefully to parental concerns and acknowledges the legitimacy of their feelings, for example, "It is understandable that you feel this way; everything happened so fast." Parents also commonly express feelings of helplessness at the loss of the parental role as protector. The nurse encourages and supports parents and other family members, stresses their importance to the child's recovery, and encourages their participation in the care of the child. The admission of a child to the hospital is anxiety producing. The uncertainty of the situation can become overwhelming, causing feelings of panic. However, these feelings are usually temporary. The nurse should remain relaxed, reassure the parents, and reinforce positive parenting. Information about the child's condition and treatment plan is given. Needs are assessed, and interventions are planned to meet specific needs.

Poor communication results in unnecessary fears. The nurse should explain in simple terms some of the equipment being used and facilities available on the unit. The nurse listens attentively and tries to clear up misconceptions. Rooming-in may alleviate some anxieties of parents. However, the nurse must continue to promptly and cheerfully tend to the needs of the child to indicate to the parents that their child is in good hands. Parental involvement in a child's care offers the nurse the opportunity to assess the relationship and to provide guidance and teaching as needed.

Parents may need to take time from work, especially if treatment involves travel to special centers. Ronald McDonald homes offer lodging and other familiar amenities for parents of patients with life-threatening illness. The availability of these facilities is explored with the family. The social service worker may be of help in such instances. The care and welfare of other children at home while one parent is at work and the other is rooming-in with the ill child should be discussed. Parents should be advised that pain control techniques are available and will be used to minimize painful experiences for the ill child.

Parents may ventilate their feelings and stresses through anger, crying, or body language. Behavior is not only a response to the current situation but often involves attitudes resulting from early childhood experiences. The nurse must not pass judgment on individuals whose behavior may seem demanding or unreasonable. An understanding and acceptance of people and their problems is essential for the successful pediatric nurse.

Siblings are also affected when a brother or sister is hospitalized. They may feel left out, guilty, or resentful of the attention focused on the ill child. Suitable interventions by the nurse include directing some attention to the siblings, supporting their efforts to comfort the family member, and engaging them in play or drawing pictures, such as "How it feels to have an ill brother or sister." They may also make cards and pictures for the patient.

NURSING **TIP**

When a child is admitted to the hospital, every family member is affected.

THE NURSE'S ROLE IN HOSPITAL ADMISSION

Nurses are responsible for admitting new patients to the hospital unit. Besides performing the procedure skillfully, they must be prepared to meet the emotional needs of those involved. The impression the nurse gives, whether good or bad, definitely affects the child's adjustment. Empathy in responding to the fears of the child and family members makes the admission procedure stimulating and educational—a positive experience for all.

A child should be prepared for hospitalization when possible. Ideally, the child and parents should tour the pediatric unit before admission. This enables the parents to meet some of the people who will care for their child. Children and their families may be overwhelmed by the size of the institution and the fear of becoming lost.

Between 1 and 3 years of age, children are worried about being separated from their parents. After 3 years of age, children may become more fearful about what is going to happen to them. Parents should try to be as matter-of-fact as possible about this new experience. Unless they have been hospitalized before, children can only try to imagine what will happen to them. It is not necessary to go into much detail; the child's imagination is great, and giving information that is beyond comprehension may create unnecessary fears. It is logical to dwell on the more pleasant aspects, but not to the extent of saying that hospitalization involves no discomforts. For example, one might mention that meals will be served on a tray, that baths will be taken from a basin at the bedside, and that the child will be with other children. The fact that there is a buzzer for calling the nurse may add to the child's sense of security. The parents may plan with the child what favorite toy or book to bring.

Perhaps more important than explaining certain occurrences is listening to how the child feels and encouraging questions. Parents should prepare them a few days, but not weeks, in advance. Parents should never lure children to the hospital by pretending that it is some other place. In emergency situations, there is little time for preparation. In such cases the entire medical team must try to give added emotional support to the child. The initial greeting should show warmth and friendliness—smile and introduce yourself.

Some hospitals allow the patient to be taken to the playroom for a short time before going to the room. When the parent tells the nurse the child's name, associating it with a familiar person who has the same name will help the nurse to remember it. It creates a much warmer feeling to speak of "John" or "Suzy" than "your little boy" or "your daughter."

The parent is encouraged to do as much for the child as possible, for example, remove clothes. The nurse tries not to appear rushed. A matter-of-fact attitude must be maintained regardless of the patient's condition. A soft voice and quiet approach are less frightening to the child. A nurse who looks anxious causes unnecessary worry for everyone concerned. A troubled look may have nothing to do with the child. Taking one step at a time is advised. Calmness is catching. The nurse remains available to answer questions that might arise. When there is a good relationship between the parent and nurse, the child benefits from higher quality care.

When children are hospitalized, the nurse should be aware of the developmental history as well as the medical history. A developmental history includes the following:

- Family relationships and support systems
- Cultural needs that may affect care and hospital routine
- Nicknames, rituals, routines
- Developmental level and abilities
- Communication skills
- Personality, adaptability, coping skills
- Past experiences, divorce, new siblings, extended family
- Previous separation experiences—vacations or hospitalizations

- Impact of current health problem on growth and development
- Preparation given the child
- Previous contact with health care personnel

NURSING TIP

When explaining procedures to children, it is helpful to identify the child's role in the event, for example, "You will be asked to step on the scale."

DEVELOPING A PEDIATRIC NURSING CARE PLAN

Developing the pediatric nursing care plan is similar to developing an adult care plan. The care plan is the result of the nursing process. It states specifically what is to be done for each child and keeps the focus on the child—not on the condition or therapy. An established list of accepted nursing diagnoses is available and in use (see Appendix C). These serve as a standard for organizing data collection. They also serve as a vehicle by which one nurse can communicate with another. A nursing diagnosis for a pediatric patient may require some modification. A survey of the child includes a knowledge of growth and developmental processes. It also includes evaluating the primary caregiver, who has a direct role in the safety and maintenance of the child's health. Nursing care plans are guides that need continual evaluation and reevaluation to determine whether the goals for the individual child are being met. Some hospitals use a Kardex system (Figure 21-4). Figure 21-5 shows a nurse entering data for later retrieval into the unit computer.

NURSING TIP

Play is an important part of a nursing care plan for children.

NURSING TIP

The achievement of developmental tasks should be part of the plan of care for the hospitalized child.

CLINICAL PATHWAYS

Clinical pathways are used in acute care settings as well as in alternate care settings. The clinical pathway is an interdisciplinary plan of care that displays the progress of the entire treatment plan for the patient. The main difference between a clinical pathway and a nursing care

12-1

DIET 1800 calorie
Constant Carbohydrate

Self Select __X__ Evenflo _____ Warm _____
Cup _____ Playtex _____ Cold _____

Intake	✓
doctor's order	12-1
Output	✓
doctor's order	12-1

IV's Heparin lock
for blood draws

Date started 12-1
IV site Ⓛ hand
Needles #20 jelco
Tubing Change _____

Activity
Bedrest _____
Bathroom Priv. _____
May be held _____
Up ad lib __X__ 12-1
Playroom _____
Other Pt to be up and dressed
Interim Summary 12-5

Bath
Complete _____
Partial _____
Tub/Shower 12-1
Shampoo _____
Special Instructions:

Safety Precautions
Crib Net _____
Restraints _____
Seiz. Prec. _____
ID band on 12-1
Name Tag
  on Crib _____
Siderail release _____

Vital Signs 12-1
TPR Routine
BP Routine
Neuro Check ___
Growth Chart ___
OFC _____
Weight daily

Special Equipment
Glucometer

Allergies
none Known

Resp. Therapy

Routine Lab Orders

Therapy Schedule
Exercise 1000 and
1400

STANDING	MEDICATIONS	DATE	TREATMENTS
12-1	Sliding Scale Insulin Sub-q Give the following! 5 units Regular insulin acetone large 3 units Regular insulin acetone moderate 1 unit Regular insulin acetone small	12-1	Blood glucose tests to be done at 0700, 1100, 1600, 2100, 0200 using dextrostix or chemstrips unless patient has own meter. Patient or parent to do testing except at 0200
		12-1	Call resident if blood sugar is less than 50 or greater than 240
		12-1	Acetest all urines until negative or blood sugar below 240
PRN 12-1	Tylenol 325mg q 3°-4° prn headache.	12-1	Oral treatment of insulin reaction 15 grams carbohydrate (6oz of orange juice) Repeat if signs or symptoms persist after rechecking.

Room	Name	Diagnosis	Assoc. Nurse	Primary Nurse	Doctor
364-1	Cory Johnson	Newly diagnosed diabetes mellitus	Peg T	Craig J	Roberts

PEDIATRIC NURSING CARE PLAN

Date	Patient Problems/Teaching Needs	Expected Outcomes	Nursing Orders	Initials
12-2	Deficient Knowledge related to newly diagnosed diabetes mellitus	Patient and patient's family will discuss disease and its treatment.	① Show patient and family new equipment A. Syringes B. Insulin C. Glucometer D. Dextrosticks	CR
			② Allow patient time to begin accepting disease	CR
			③ Discuss resources outside hospital A. ADA B. JDF	CR
			④ Be supportive to patient and family during learning process	CR

Age 13	Birth Date 2-12-89	Hospital # 7391-85	Religion Methodist	Service PEDS	Admission Date 12-1-02	Time 1200

NURS 372 4/80
632034462

FIGURE **21-4** The Kardex serves as a reference to patient problems that require nursing intervention.

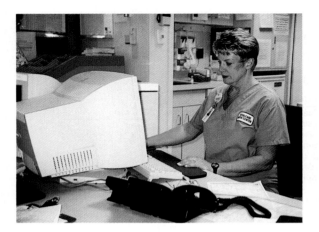

FIGURE **21-5** The nurse enters data and retrieves information about the patient's progress on the unit computer. (Photo courtesy of Pat Spier, RN-C.)

plan is that the nursing care plan focuses on the nurse's role in the care of the patient, and the clinical pathway focuses on the broader view of the entire multidisciplinary health care team and general outcome goals of care with specific timelines. Understanding the nursing process and the nursing care plan is essential to understanding the nurse's role in the clinical pathway. See Chapter 1 for further details concerning the clinical pathway.

Pictorial pathways (Figure 21-6) have been used and are especially valuable in patient education and anticipatory guidance. Clinical pathways for children with specific conditions are presented in various chapters of this text.

NEEDS OF THE HOSPITALIZED CHILD

THE HOSPITALIZED INFANT

Hospitalization is frustrating for infants. During infancy, rapid physical and emotional development takes place. Infants are used to getting what they want when

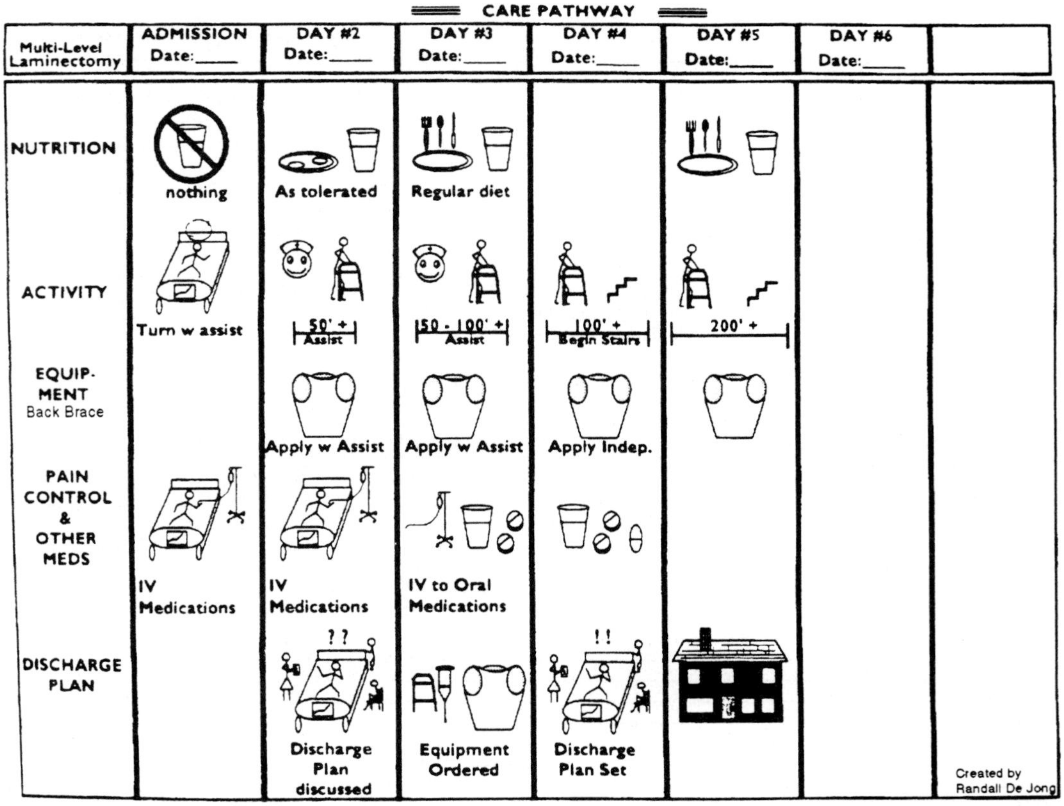

Multi-Level Laminectomy	ADMISSION Date:____	DAY #2 Date:____	DAY #3 Date:____	DAY #4 Date:____	DAY #5 Date:____	DAY #6 Date:____	
NUTRITION	nothing	As tolerated	Regular diet				
ACTIVITY	Turn w assist	50' + Assist	50 - 100' + Assist	100' + Begin Stairs	200' +		
EQUIP- MENT Back Brace		Apply w Assist	Apply w Assist	Apply Indep.			
PAIN CONTROL & OTHER MEDS	IV Medications	IV Medications	IV to Oral Medications				
DISCHARGE PLAN		?? Discharge Plan discussed	Equipment Ordered	!! Discharge Plan Set			Created by Randall De Jong

FIGURE **21-6** Pictorial clinical pathway. Pictorial clinical pathways are especially valuable in patient education and anticipatory guidance.

they want it, and they show their displeasure quickly when illness restricts the satisfaction of their desires. Infants who were breastfed at home may be unable to continue this regimen. They miss the continuous affection of their parents. Their daily schedule is upset. The infant who drinks well from a cup at home may refuse it entirely at the hospital.

Nursing personnel must try to meet the needs of these patients by protecting them from excess frustration. It is not wise to expect them to develop new habits when they need energy to cope with their illness and the strange environment. One of the nurse's major goals during this period is to assist with the parent-infant attachment process and to promote sensorimotor activities. This can be fostered by providing means for the infant and significant other to interact and by attempting to ease the tension of the parents. The nurse can serve as a role model by performing activities with the infant, such as cuddling, rocking, talking, and singing. A swing, a bath with squeeze toys, a pacifier, and a hanging mobile are also appropriate as the infant's condition permits.

Because the infant cannot understand explanations, the nurse administers uncomfortable procedures as gently as possible and returns the infant to the parents for consolation. Liberal visiting hours are essential (Figure 21-7). When parents are not available, soothing support and gentle touch are provided; otherwise the infant may learn to associate only pain with nursing care. Consistency in caregivers is also important at this stage of development.

THE HOSPITALIZED TODDLER

The toddler's world revolves around the parents, particularly the mother (or significant caregiver). Hospitalization is a painful experience for toddlers. They cannot understand why they are separated from their mothers, and they become very distressed. Toddlers who have a continuous, secure relationship with their mothers react more violently to separation because they have more to lose. Nursing goals in the care of the hospitalized toddler are presented in Box 21-1.

The stages of separation anxiety are at their peak in the toddler (see p. 477). The nurse who comprehends the various separation stages sees parental visits as necessary, even though the process of separation and reunion is painful. A cohesive staff is essential to meet the needs of the children and their parents. Education of the parents helps to promote their continued visits and to decrease feelings of inadequacy. Ritualistic patterns of care that involve structure are appropriate for children in this age-group.

Repetitive games that deal with disappearance and return are helpful. Peekaboo and hide-and-seek serve such a purpose. The use of a transitional object, such as a blanket or a favorite toy from home, promotes security. Pictures of the family and tape recordings of favorite stories are other measures that help the child remain connected with the family. When the nurse or parent leaves, he or she explains when he or she will return in terms of the toddler's experience (e.g., after naptime or lunch) and then returns promptly at that time. A loving hug, good-bye, and prompt exit are then necessary. The continued reappearance of the parents as promised is of value in reducing the child's anxiety and reestablishing his or her sense of trust. The parent should not wait until a child falls asleep to depart. This avoids confrontations but disturbs the child's sense of trust. The nurse assures the parents that he or she will remain with the child for comfort.

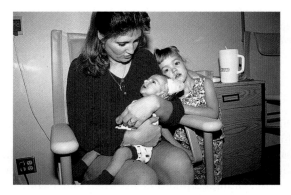

FIGURE **21-7** Liberal visiting hours enable the parent to meet the needs of the hospitalized infant. Family-centered hospital care allows the sibling to maintain contact with the parent while visiting in the hospital.

box 21-1 | *Nursing Goals in the Care of Hospitalized Toddlers*

- Reassure parents, particularly the child's primary caregiver.
- Maintain the toddler's sense of trust.
- Incorporate home habits of the child into nursing care plans, for example, transitional objects.
- Allow the child to work through or master threatening experiences through soothing techniques and play.
- Provide individualized, flexible nursing care plans in accordance with the child's development and diagnosis.

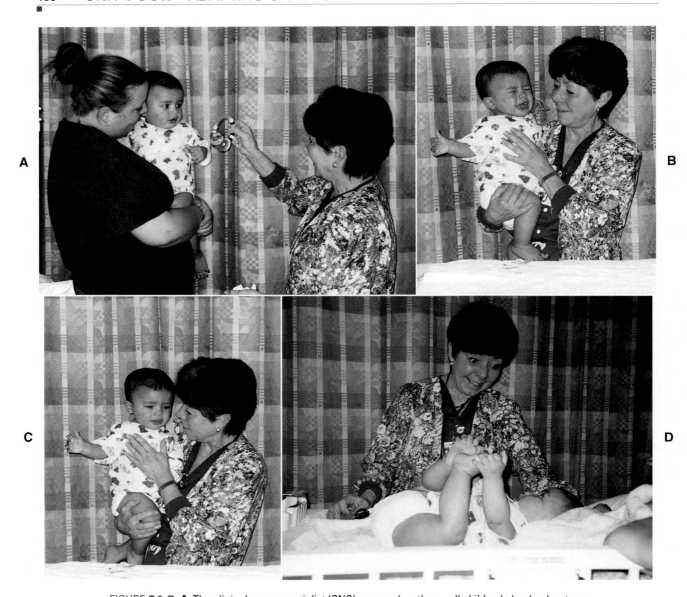

FIGURE **21-8 A,** The clinical nurse specialist (CNS) approaches the small child calmly, slowly, at eye level, and with the parent present. **B,** The infant shows apprehension and anxiety when carried by the CNS. **C,** Beginning trust is established. **D,** After trust is established, general assessment can begin. (Photo Courtesy of Pat Spier, RN-C.)

Rooming-in is highly desirable. When rooming-in is impossible, consistent caregivers should be assigned to care for the child and the parent. The nurse indicates by his or her approach that he or she considers the parent's contributions extremely important to the child's well-being. The nurse interprets the stages of separation anxiety to the parent (Figure 21-8). The nurse must also realize that parents are under stress and should not be asked to assume responsibilities beyond their capabilities. The nurse observes parents for signs of fatigue and suggests appropriate interventions.

Occasionally parents do not choose to care for their child; for example, "We feel that since we are paying for this, we should just be able to entertain him." In such instances, the parents' wishes are respected. Referral to the clinical nurse specialist might also be appropriate to facilitate communication and to better understand the underlying dynamics of the situation.

The home habits of the toddler are recorded and used. A potty chair is provided if the child is trained. Some regression in behavior is to be expected. If the toddler still prefers bottles to cups, there should be no attempt to change this in the hospital. Familiar toys and books are important. A steady, calm voice communicates safety. Toddlers are in the stage of autonomy. Loss of a small amount of the self-control they have achieved usually results in resistance and negativism.

Children are forewarned about any unpleasant or new experience that they may need to undergo while in the hospital. This is done in keeping with their level of understanding. Being truthful about things that may hurt prevents the child from feeling betrayed. Preparation and explanation are done immediately before a procedure so that the child does not worry needlessly for an extended time. Crying and protesting when told about certain procedures are healthy expressions of feelings and relieve tension. Distractions such as blowing bubbles, looking through a kaleidoscope, and pop-up toys may help to reduce anxiety and pain.

Supervised playroom activity contributes to intellectual, social, and motor development. Treatments in the playroom are avoided. Toddlers are encouraged to play with safe equipment used in their care, such as bandages, tongue blades, and stethoscopes. Whenever possible, they are allowed out of their cribs because confinement is frustrating for little ones who have just begun to enjoy walking. Playtime establishes rapport and is an important part of the nursing care of children.

There are indications that restraining the child's mobility by surgical and medical procedures involving splints, IV therapy, burn dressings, and so on may contribute to the development of emotional or personality problems or to speech and learning difficulties (Behrman et al., 2000). Therefore, when restraint is required, it must be accompanied by increased emotional support such as rooming-in, additional attention from nurses, and suitable diversion.

It is common for children to experience changes in behavior on their return home. They may be demanding and may cling to the parent every minute. "He just won't let me out of his sight" is a common description. The parent should give the toddler extra attention and reassurance until trust is regained.

NURSING **TIP**

Toddlers experience some degree of separation anxiety any time they are left by their parent or primary caregiver, such as when they are left with day care personnel, baby-sitters, or relatives.

THE HOSPITALIZED PRESCHOOLER

The experience of hospitalization may be easier for preschool children who have had outside contact (e.g., nursery school and kindergarten) than for those who have never been separated from their parents. Because children of this age operate with concrete thinking, they can understand more and they can be better prepared for hospitalization. Explanations must be made in realistic terms, because preschool children cannot understand abstract explanations. They are made to realize that hospitalization is not a punishment for something they have done wrong. Children may feel guilty, particularly if an accident happens because of some mischief on their part, such as in the case of burns or falls.

Preschool children are distressed when their parents prepare to leave them, but unlike the toddler, they can understand time relationships through activities—at breakfast, after lunch, and the like. The nurse and parents must not tell the child that they will return unless they intend to do so.

At this age the child is afraid of bodily harm, particularly invasive procedures. The surgical patient must be shown the part of the body that requires surgery. The nurse can sketch a body outline and draw a circle around the operative site, giving simple information about the system that will be affected. It is stressed that only this area of the body will be involved. Children in this age-group engage in magical thinking and fantasy. Fantasizing the unknown can be frightening to a young child. The preschooler needs clear, understandable, and truthful explanations. Children who ask questions should be complimented and listened to; any misinterpretations should be corrected. The child is helped to increase self-esteem through praise. The child relieves tension through role playing. Tongue depressors, adhesive bandages, and other materials related to everyday hospital life are relished by the sick child.

Parents are faced with a disrupted home life throughout the child's hospitalization. Parents cannot cope with everyday tasks when they are lonely for and are worried about their child. The frequent trips to the hospital interfere with the daily routine, and other children in the family may resent them. Contact with the physician is needed. Parents have a legal and ethical right to be informed of the benefits and risks of therapy and to be included in the decision-making process. When the child is finally discharged, he or she may be demanding and irritable. Parents need the kind support of hospital personnel to enable them to make informed decisions and deal with these added strains.

THE HOSPITALIZED SCHOOL-AGE CHILD

Children of school age can endure separation from their parents if it is not prolonged. Children who have been cherished from birth can tolerate brief interruptions in their lives more easily than can those who have been denied a secure environment. The school-age child is in a stage of industry and independence. Forced dependency in the hospital (such as immobilization) can result in a feeling of loss of control and loss of security. School-age children need to feel "grown up." They can participate in their care and be offered simple choices to foster their feeling of independence. They can choose their menus within appropriate restrictions, "help the nurse" in various activities, and keep busy with age-appropriate toys.

Knowledge of growth and development in the school-age child assists in anticipatory guidance. Nurses can also enlist parents to determine what, if any, successful approaches they use in guiding the child. Behavioral problems may be addressed by a team conference. Nurses who work with children should keep abreast of current trends and guidance approaches. Positive direction and consistency are tools of particular importance to the pediatric nurse.

The education of the school-age child must continue throughout any illness. This gives the child a sense of continuity with the outside world, provides periods of socialization, reinforces weak academic areas, and reassures the child that he or she can return to his or her peers after discharge. The parents may act as liaisons between school and hospital. The teacher must be informed of the child's physical and emotional health to be effective. The nurse provides children with opportunities to study undisturbed so that they will be prepared for classes. Diagnostic tests and treatments should be scheduled around established school routines whenever possible. Many school districts have individual tutors for homebound or hospitalized school-aged children.

It is common for school-age children to be "brave" and to show little, if any, fear in situations that actually upset them a good deal. Observation of body language may provide some clues to emotional states. The nurse's presence during unfamiliar procedures is comforting. Following treatments the nurse should encourage children to draw and talk about their drawings or to act out their feelings through puppet play.

⮞NURSING **TIP**

Observation of nonverbal clues such as facial grimaces, squirming about, and finger tapping is important in determining the need for pain relief and support for the child.

THE HOSPITALIZED ADOLESCENT

Adolescents, in particular, experience feelings of loss of control during hospitalization. Daily routines are disrupted, and dependence-independence issues come to the foreground. When feelings of independence, self-assertion, and identity are threatened, the adolescent may respond by withdrawal, noncompliance, or anger. Care plans must be designed to incorporate choice, privacy, and understanding.

Early Adolescence

Nursing care plans must be oriented to the adolescent's age. Illness during early adolescence, approximately 10 to 13 years of age, is seen mainly as a threat to body image. There is a narcissistic concern about height, weight, and sexual development. Patients are aware of heightened body sensations and often have numerous physical complaints. Intense relationships with members of one's own sex are prevalent; they precede heterosexual involvement. Patients in this age-group are anxious about how the illness will affect their physical appearance, functioning, and mobility; however, they are not usually overwhelmed by forced dependence. Self-portrait drawings are effective at this time. Maintaining privacy and same-sex room assignments are essential.

Middle Adolescence

During middle adolescence (approximately 14 to 16 years of age), adolescents are anxious about their ability to appeal to the opposite sex and to meet sex role expectations. Physical growth is practically complete. The peer group assumes greater importance in determining acceptability and behavior. During middle adolescence the struggle for emancipation from the family, although erratic, is at its peak. It is disturbing not only to the adolescent but also to parents, who must relinquish much of their control to hospital personnel. Incorporating choice, privacy, appropriate hair and cosmetic appearance, and the opportunity for peer visitors is important during hospitalization.

Late Adolescence

Late adolescents, approximately 17 to 21 years of age, are mainly concerned with the tasks of education, career, marriage, children, community, and style of life. The dating partner becomes the person of primary importance. Hospitalization may pose the threat of postponement of career and future plans. Contact with school personnel, counselors, and teachers is important to prevent long-term impact on the education and development of the adolescent.

Adjustment to Illness

The adolescent has many intellectual strengths, including the ability to think abstractly and to solve problems. Adolescents can understand the implications of their disease both in the present and in the future, and they are capable of participating in decisions related to treatment and care. The nurse who recognizes these skills and encourages their practice helps patients gain confidence in their intellectual abilities, thus increasing their sense of independence and self-esteem.

Roommate Selection

Roommate selection, although often overlooked, is extremely important for this age-group. Adolescents usually do better with one or more roommates than in single rooms. Because few community hospitals have adolescent wings, it is helpful if the patients participate in the decision regarding whether the adolescent is admitted to the pediatric or the adult unit. A few adjoining rooms at the ends of these units will suffice. Placing the teenager next to a senile, dying, or severely debilitated patient in the adult unit or an infant in the pediatric unit should be avoided.

CONFIDENTIALITY AND LEGALITY

Respecting the confidentiality of children is important to establishing trust. In general, information should not be divulged or shared without consent. Many problems can be avoided if the confidentiality of the relationship is clearly defined during initial meetings. Patient records must be carefully monitored to avoid loss or observation by unauthorized personnel. The nurse must avoid giving private information about any patient to telephone callers or visitors. Appointment books and computer screens in an office are kept concealed rather than open to view on the desk.

An emancipated minor generally refers to an adolescent younger than 18 years of age who is no longer under the parent's authority. Married minors or minors in the military are automatically considered emancipated and may give consent for medical treatment for themselves and their children.

In some parts of the United States the young adolescent may receive medical assistance without parental awareness for certain conditions, such as sexually transmitted diseases, contraception, pregnancy, abortion, and drug abuse. These laws are designed to afford the young person immediate medical help without fear of reprisal. However, some laws are being challenged in the courts. In a medical emergency a minor can be treated without the consent of parents if the situation is life-threatening.

Because laws vary from state to state, nurses must keep abreast of policies and legislation within their practice. Such information is available from the local medical or state nursing licensing boards.

DISCHARGE PLANNING

Preparation for the patient's discharge ideally begins on admission, because the goal of hospitalization is to return a healthier and happier child to the parents. An approach directed only toward good physical care of the patient's disease is not sufficient. The nurse must also consider the emotional growth of the child and the education of the patient and family. This will provide a positive learning experience for all involved.

If a patient requires specific home treatment, such as hyperalimentation, colostomy care, crutches, special diet, or insulin therapy, instructions are given to the parents gradually throughout their child's hospitalization. The instructions are written so they can be referred to as needed. If the older child is to administer any self-treatment, careful explanations and supervision are required until both patient and parents are confident they can carry out the procedure safely at home. This may require the home health services.

Parents also must be prepared for behavioral problems that may arise after hospitalization. Severe stress may be obvious during the patient's stay. The services of a children's counselor are helpful if nightmares and regression occur. Guidance suggestions include the following:

- Anticipating behaviors such as clinging, regression in bowel and bladder control, aggression, manipulation, and nightmares
- Allowing the child to become a participating family member as soon as possible
- Taking the focus off the illness; praising accomplishments unrelated to it
- Being kind, firm, and consistent with misbehavior
- Building trust by being truthful
- Providing suitable play materials such as clay, paints, and doctor and nurse kits
- Allowing time for free play
- Listening to and clarifying misconceptions about the illness
- Avoiding long periods of separation until a sense of security is regained
- Allowing the child to visit hospital staff during routine clinic visits if desired

Whenever possible, parents are given at least 1 day's notice of their child's discharge from the hospital so they can make the necessary arrangements. This is particularly important if both parents work or if transportation is a problem. The physician writes the discharge order. The approximate hour of dismissal is relayed to the parents. The child is weighed and dressed, and all personal belongings are collected. Parents are given a written return clinic appointment card when indicated.

Parents sign a release form and visit the hospital business office according to hospital procedure. The nurse may accompany the child and parents to the hospital exit to say good-bye. According to condition, the child is placed in a hospital wagon, wheelchair, or stretcher for transport. The nurse assists the child into the car seat or assists in fastening seat belts. Charting includes when and with whom the child departed, patient's behavior (smiling, alert, crying, and so on), method of transportation from the division, patient's weight, and any instructions or medications given to the child or parents.

NURSING TIP

Discharge charting should include who accompanied the child (and identification given), time of discharge, behavior and condition of the child, method of transportation, vital signs and weight, medications, and instructions given to parents or caregiver.

HOME CARE

Many children with acute and chronic conditions are being cared for in the home. Home health care and other community agencies work together to provide holistic care. Respite care provides trained workers who come into the home for brief periods to relieve parents of the responsibility of caring for the child. This enables the parents to shop, do business transactions, or simply take time for much-needed self-care. The school systems also share in the responsibility for care, which is crucial if a family is to be successful in home care. The health care worker assisting in the home should do the following:

- Observe how the parents interact with the child.
- Observe facial expressions and body language.
- Post signs above the bed denoting special considerations, such as "Never position on left side" and "Do not feed with plastic spoon."
- Listen to the parents and observe how they attend to the physical needs of the youngster.
- Ask questions or discuss apprehensions the parents may have about their ability to care for the child.
- Be attuned to the needs of other children in the home.
- Be creative in exploring avenues for socialization because these children are seldom invited to birthday or slumber parties.

- Explore community facilities or support groups that might benefit the family.

key points

- The care of sick children can take place in a variety of settings.
- Play is an important part of a nursing care plan for children.
- Nursing care plans for hospitalized children should include measures to minimize negative impact on growth and development.
- Three major causes of stress for children of all ages are separation, pain, and fear of bodily harm.
- Separation anxiety is most pronounced in the toddler.
- The three stages of separation anxiety are protest, despair, and detachment.
- When a school-age child requires hospitalization, a school, home, or hospital teacher should be requested by the nurse to prevent loss of grade status.
- Nurses caring for children must maintain a high level of suspicion for pain because children are often unable to verbalize discomfort.
- Techniques such as drawing, distraction, imagery, relaxation, and cognitive strategies, as well as analgesia, provide relief from pain.
- A culturally sensitive attitude toward families with hospitalized children decreases anxiety.
- Treatments in the playroom should be avoided.
- The surgical patient must be shown the part of the body that will be operated on. Children are assured that this is the only area of the body that will be involved.
- Respecting the confidentiality of the adolescent is important to establishing trust.
- The pediatric nursing care plan is the result of the nursing process applied to the child.
- Clinical pathways are a multidisciplinary plan of care with outcome goals that involve timelines.
- The developmental level of the child influences specific needs during the hospitalization experience.
- The age, sex, developmental level, and diagnosis of the child are factors that influence placement on a unit.
- Discharge planning begins on the day of admission.
- Pain is the fifth vital sign and should be assessed and treated in infants and children.

ONLINE RESOURCES

Pain Resource Center—City of Hope: http://mayday.coh.org
Safety Syringe Products: http://www.bd.com

REVIEW QUESTIONS   *Choose the most appropriate answer.*

1. The stages of separation anxiety in the toddler are:
   1. Protest, despair, denial
   2. Denial, dependence, submission
   3. Protest, sadness, despair
   4. Despair, anxiety, regression

2. An object such as a blanket or favorite toy is referred to as:
   1. A transitory item
   2. A transitional object
   3. A transitional task
   4. A cuddly

3. The best way to minimize separation anxiety in a hospitalized infant is to:
   1. Explain routines carefully
   2. Encourage parent to room-in
   3. Provide age-appropriate roommates
   4. Provide an age-appropriate toy

4. Which of the following statements by the parent of a hospitalized 4-year-old child indicates an understanding of the child's needs?
   1. "I am going to buy him a box of new toys to keep him busy while in the hospital"
   2. "I am going to bring some of his favorite toys from home for him to play with while in the hospital"
   3. "I'm glad there is a television in the room for him to watch all day"
   4. "I will stay every day until he falls asleep and then I will go home"

5. A 4-year-old hospitalized child wets his bed. The parents tell the nurse that the child was completely toilet trained. The nurse should understand that:
   1. The parents are denying a problem exists
   2. The child may be developmentally delayed
   3. The child may be experiencing regression
   4. The child is probably "punishing" the parents

objectives

1. Define each key term listed.
2. List five safety measures applicable to the care of the hospitalized child.
3. Devise a nursing care plan for a child with a fever.
4. Position an infant for a lumbar puncture.
5. Contrast the administration of medicines to children and adults.
6. Discuss two nursing responsibilities necessary when a child is receiving parenteral fluids and the rationale for each.
7. Summarize the care of a child receiving oxygen.
8. List the adaptations necessary when preparing a pediatric patient for surgery.
9. Illustrate techniques of transporting infants and children.
10. Plan the basic daily data collection for hospitalized infants and children.
11. Identify the normal vital signs of infants and children at various ages.
12. Discuss the technique of obtaining urine and stool specimens from infants.
13. Demonstrate techniques of administering oral, eye, and ear medications to infants and children.
14. Compare the preferred sites for intramuscular injection for infants and adults.
15. Calculate the dosage of a medicine that is in liquid form.

key terms

auscultation (ăw-skŭl-TĀ-shŭn, p. 499)
body surface area (BSA) (p. 510)
Broviac catheter (BRŌ-vē-ăk KĂTH-ă-tăr, p. 517)
clean-catch specimen (p. 505)
dimensional analysis (p. 511)
dorsogluteal (dŏr-sō-GLŪ-tē-ăl, p. 515)
gastrostomy (găs-TRŎS-tă-mē, p. 519)
heparin lock (HĔP-ă-rĭn lŏk, p. 517)
informed consent (ĭn-FŌRMD kŏn-SĔNT, p. 494)
intramuscular (IM) injection (ĭn-tră-MŬS-kŭ-lăr ĭn-JĔK-shăn, p. 515)

low-flow oxygen (p. 527)
lumbar puncture (LŬM-băhr PŬNGK-chăr, p. 506)
mist tent (p. 527)
mummy restraint (p. 514)
nomogram (NŎM-ō-grăm, p. 510)
O.D. (p. 514)
O.S. (p. 514)
O.U. (p. 514)
parenteral (pĕ-RĔN-tĕr-ăl, p. 518)
phototoxicity (fō-tō-tŏk-SĬS-ĭ-tē, p. 511)
saline lock (SĀ-lēn lŏk, p. 517)
subcutaneous (SC) injection (sŭb-kū-TĀ-nē-ĕs ĭn-JEK-shăn, p. 515)
total parenteral nutrition (TPN) (TŌT-ăl pă-RĔN-tĕr-ăl noo-TRĬ-shĕn, p. 518)
tracheostomy (trā-kē-ŎS-tō-mē, p. 519)
tympanic thermometer (tĭm-PĂN-ĭk thĕr-MŎM-ă-tĕr, p. 503)
vastus lateralis (VĂS-tŭs lăt-ĕr-Ā-lĭs, p. 515)
ventrogluteal (vĕn-trō-GLOO-tē-ăl, p. 515)

ADMISSION TO THE PEDIATRIC UNIT

INFORMED CONSENT

When the child is admitted to the pediatric unit, a written informed consent is obtained for treatments that are given. An informed consent implies that the parent or legal guardian is capable of understanding information given to him or her, including the purpose and risks of the procedure, and voluntarily agrees to that procedure. The consent must be signed by the parent, the health care provider who provides the information, and a witness. The nurse acts as a patient advocate in ensuring that proper consent has been signed *before* a procedure and that the child is also given age-appropriate information concerning what to expect.

IDENTIFICATION

Every child admitted to the pediatric unit must have an identification (ID) bracelet applied. The ID bracelet of the patient should be checked before medications are administered or treatments are carried out. If a bracelet

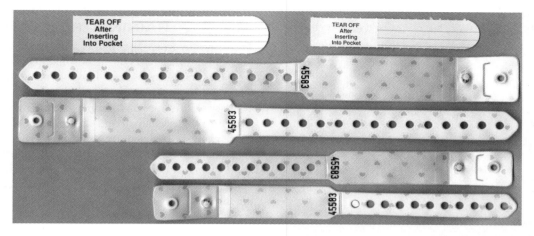

FIGURE **22-1** Identification (ID) bracelet. All hospitalized children must have an identification bracelet that is checked before the nurse administers medications or provides care. Some ID bracelets may have a computer chip attached to alert the staff if the child leaves the unit.

applied on admission is taken off by the child or falls off, identification should be verified and a new bracelet reapplied (Figure 22-1). The bracelet should be snug enough to prevent voluntary removal by the child.

ESSENTIAL SAFETY MEASURES IN THE HOSPITAL SETTING

The nurse must be especially conscious of safety measures on the children's division. Accidents are a major cause of death among infants and children. By demonstrating concern about safety regulations, the nurse not only reduces unnecessary accidents but also sets a good example for parents. Although the physical layout of each institution cannot be altered by personnel, many simple safety measures can be carried out by the entire hospital team. The following is a list of measures applicable to the children's unit:

DOs

- Keep crib sides up at all times when the child is unattended in bed (Figure 22-2).
- Identify child by ID bracelet, not room number.
- Use a bubble-top or plastic-topped crib for infants and children capable of climbing over the crib rails (Figure 22-3).
- Place cribs so that children cannot reach sockets and appliances.
- Inspect toys for sharp edges and removable parts.
- Keep medications and solutions out of reach of the child.
- Identify the child properly before giving medications.
- Keep powder, lotions, tissues, baby wipes, disposable diapers, safety pins, and so on out of the infant's reach.

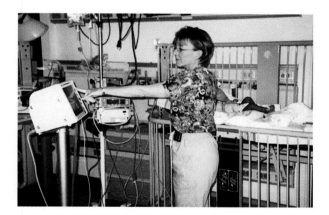

FIGURE **22-2** The nurse should maintain hand contact if it is necessary to turn the back on the infant or toddler. If the nurse needs equipment that is out of reach, the side of the crib should be raised before leaving the infant or child. (Photo courtesy of Pat Spier, RN-C.)

- Prevent cross-infection. Diapers, toys, and materials that belong in one patient's unit should not be borrowed for another patient's use.
- Remain with the child who uses the bathtub.
- Apply safety belt for children in high chairs.
- Take proper precautions when oxygen is in use.
- Locate fire exits and extinguishers on your unit and learn how to use them properly. Become familiar with your hospital's fire procedure.

DON'Ts

- Don't prop nursing bottles or force-feed small children. There is a danger of choking.
- Don't allow ambulatory patients to use wheelchairs or stretchers as toys.

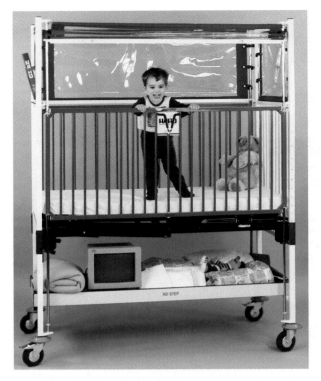

FIGURE **22-3** A hard plastic "bubble-top" or a soft plastic crib extender must be in place on the crib if the child is capable of climbing over the side rails. The extender stays in place when the side rails are lowered.

- Don't leave an active child in a baby swing, feeding table, or high chair unattended.
- Don't leave a small child unattended when out of the crib.
- Don't leave medications at the bedside.

Many other safety measures must be carried out as each nurse becomes more familiar with the hazards of individual units. Nurses must use their eyes to see with, not just to look at, and then must take the necessary precautions.

✱ NURSING **TIP**

Crib Safety
- The mattress must fit securely into the crib.
- Tucked-in blankets should not be used in cribs.
- Soft or contour pillows should not be placed in cribs.
- The distance between crib slats should be no more than 2⅜ inches (6 cm).
- Decorative extensions on the corners of cribs can catch onto clothing and strangle the child.
- A bubble-top or extension should be in place if the child is capable of climbing over the crib side.

TRANSPORTING, POSITIONING, AND RESTRAINING THE INFANT

The means by which the child is transported within the unit and to other parts of the hospital depends on age, level of consciousness, and how far one must travel. Older children are transported in the same way as adults. Younger children are often transported in their cribs, in a wagon or wheelchair, or on a stretcher. The side rails on a stretcher are raised during transport. The nurse ensures that the child's ID band is secured before leaving the division. A notation is made as to where the child is being taken, for what purpose, and who is accompanying the child.

Figure 22-4 depicts three safe methods for holding an infant. Head and back support are necessary for young infants. The movements of small children are often random and uncoordinated; therefore they must be held securely. The football hold is useful when one hand needs to be free, such as for bathing the infant's head. The *mummy restraint* is a short-term restraint that might be necessary for examination or treatments such as a venipuncture or placement of a nasogastric tube. This restraint effectively controls the child's movements and can be modified to expose an arm, a leg, or the chest as needed. *Swaddling* of the newborn infant is accomplished by the same technique. Many young infants respond positively to snug wrapping with a light baby blanket. Box 22-1 lists the principles for swaddling or applying a mummy restraint on infants and children.

VERIFYING THE CHILD ASSESSMENT

Children are different from adults both anatomically and physiologically. Data collection is done to determine the level of wellness, the response to medication or treatment, or the need for referral.

BASIC DATA COLLECTION

Basic data collection involves casual observation without touching. The child's general appearance will indicate if he or she is seriously ill or within normal limits. In general, serious illness may be suspected if the child is not alert and responsive to the environment. If the child is lethargic, prompt intervention by a health care provider is essential. Applying knowledge of basic growth and development will enable the nurse to determine whether the activities and behavior of the child are age appropriate. A child who has not mastered age-appropriate milestones should be referred for follow-up care. The presence of bruises on the body of the child that may be in different stages of healing, the lack of body cleanliness or appropriate dress, and the interac-

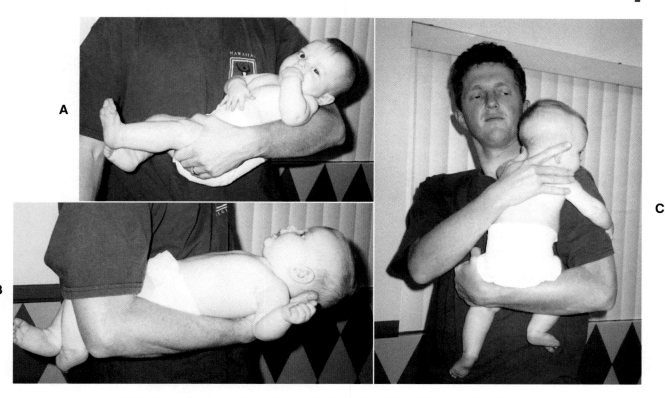

FIGURE **22-4** **A,** The cradle position. **B,** The football position. **C,** The upright position.

tion or lack of interaction between parent and child are also areas that may require prompt referral for follow-up care. Is the child tipping his head? Rubbing the ears? Is the child maintaining a rigid body position to breathe? If stridor or grunting sounds are heard during respiration, prompt referral should be made.

THE HISTORY SURVEY

The *history survey* affords the nurse the opportunity to teach parents about the child's needs and prevention of injury and illness. The immunization record should be reviewed and plans for future immunizations discussed. Encouraging safe environments that include the use of car seats and protective gear for sports activities should be part of every teaching plan.

THE PHYSICAL SURVEY

The *physical survey* includes a head-to-toe review that should be completed, at minimum, once each shift or once each clinic visit, even if the clinic visit is for a specific problem. The nurse may assist with an ear examination by properly restraining the child in a position that will enable safe and quick assessment by the health care provider (Figure 22-5). Obtaining vital signs is a priority. Often the first sign of shock or body stress in infants or

children is tachycardia (a rapid heartbeat). However, a fall in blood pressure may be a *late* sign of shock in children because of a compensatory mechanism that is activated early. Therefore hypotension in an infant or child is considered an acute emergency. Extreme irritability or pupils that are unequal in response to light should be reported immediately. The anterior fontanel, which is usually open until age 18 months, should be palpated. A *sunken* fontanel may indicate dehydration, whereas a *bulging* fontanel indicates increased intracranial pressure (ICP). A fontanel that feels *flat* to the contour of the head is normal. Increased ICP in the older child and adult is manifested by a rise in systolic blood pressure and a widening pulse pressure, irregular respirations, and bradycardia. In the infant, however, the open fontanels allow brain swelling to occur without these classic signs, and a decreased level of consciousness may be the only manifestation of increased ICP.

Bradycardia (a slow heartbeat) is always treated as a medical emergency in infants and young children. Unlike adults, infants and children cannot increase the stroke volume of their heart for a more effective cardiac output when the heart slows and must rely on increased rate alone to increase output. Therefore fatigue and heart failure may result. Mottling of the skin of the ex-

| box 22-1 | *Principles of Using Restraints for Children* |

Restraints may be used for infants and children to facilitate examinations or treatments and to maintain safety. The reason for the restraint must be explained to the parents and the child. *Restraints are used only when necessary. They are not a substitute for close observation, and should involve the fewest joints possible* in order to enable free movement, which is necessary for growth and development. Excessive restraints can result in the infant or child fighting the restraint, thereby wasting energy and increasing oxygen consumption needs. Parents should be taught the importance of fastening safety straps on infants who are in high chairs, shopping carts, and infant seats.

THE MUMMY RESTRAINT

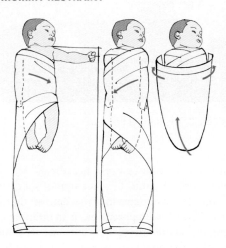

Place a small, light blanket flat on the bed with the top at the infant's shoulders.

Fold the blanket over the body and under the arm at the opposite side, tucking in the excess under the infant.

Place the other arm at the side and fold the blanket over the body, tucking the excess under the infant. The weight of the infant holds the restraint in place.

Separate the bottom of the blanket and fold upward toward the shoulder, tucking the sides under the infant's body.

The arms should be in anatomical position. This restraint provides a feeling of snug security for the infant. It may be used for jugular venipunctures, nasogastric tube insertion, and other procedures.

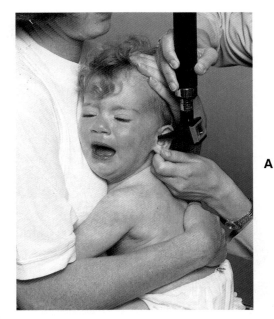

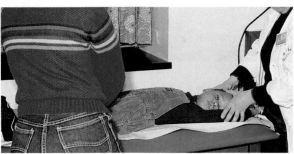

FIGURE **22-5** Positioning the child for an ear examination. **A,** The parent or nurse can hold the infant close with one hand immobilizing the head. **B,** The nurse holds the arms above the child's head and prevents movement of the head with the thumbs. The parent or assistant can hold the hips or thighs.

tremities may be normal in infants because of their immature temperature control mechanisms. Maintaining warmth during observation is essential for infants. Because of their large body surface area and high metabolic rate, they are prone to fluid loss and hypothermia as well as cold stress.

An accurate weight should be recorded because the dosage of medications for infants and children is based on milligrams per kilogram of body weight (see Figure 12-11). The temperature of infants may be taken via the axilla or in the ear (see Figure 22-8). The lungs should be clear to auscultation, and the chest should move symmetrically. Bowel sounds should be active in all four quadrants, and the abdomen should not be distended or tender to palpation. The skin should be observed for rashes or lesions.

table 22-1	*Average Pulse Rates at Rest*			
AGE	**AVERAGE (PER MINUTE, AWAKE)**		**UPPER LIMITS OF NORMAL (PER MINUTE)**	
Newborn	125		190	
1-11 months	120		160	
2 years	110		130	
4 years	100		120	
6 years	100		115	
8 years	90		110	
10 years	90		110	
	GIRLS	**BOYS**	**GIRLS**	**BOYS**
12 years	90	85	110	105
14 years	85	80	105	100
16 years	80	75	100	95
18 years	75	70	95	90

Modified from Behrman, R.E., Kliegman, R., & Jenson, H.B., (2000). *Nelson's textbook of pediatrics* (16th ed.). Philadelphia: W.B. Saunders.

Pulse and Respirations

The nurse counting a pulse feels the wave of blood as it is forced through the artery. The pulse rate varies considerably in different children of the same age and size. The pulse rate and respiratory rate of the newborn are high (Tables 22-1 and 22-2). Both pulse and respiratory rates gradually slow down with age until adult values are reached.

The pulse of the older child is taken just like that of an adult. Apical pulses are advised for children under 5 years of age (see Figure 12-10). The apical pulse is heard through a stethoscope at the apex of the heart. The nurse counts the rate for 1 full minute. Another common site is the radial pulse (at the thumb side of the wrist just above the radial artery). Actually, the pulse may be assessed in any area where a large artery lies close to the skin, especially if the artery runs across a bone and has little soft tissue around it. The following are the most common sites: radial, temporal (just in front of the ear), mandibular (on the lower jawbone), femoral (in the groin), and carotid (on each side of the front of the neck). The carotid pulse may not be appropriate in infants with chubby necks.

The child's respirations are counted in the same way as for an adult. The nurse notes the number of times the chest or abdomen rises and falls for 1 minute. The rate and character of respirations are important in determining the patient's general condition. The relationship of the pulse rate to the temperature and respiratory rate should be assessed; the pulse will rise as the temperature rises because of the increased cardiac output and increased oxygen consumption needs that occur with an elevated temperature.

table 22-2	*Normal Respiratory Ranges for Children*
AGE	**RATE PER MINUTE**
Birth to 1 month	30-40
1 month to 1 year	26-40
1 to 2 years	20-30
2 to 6 years	20-30
6 to 10 years	18-24
Adolescent	16-24

Blood Pressure

Blood pressure is defined as the pressure of the blood on the walls of the arteries. It is an index of elasticity of arterial walls, peripheral vascular resistance, efficiency of the heart as a pump, and blood volume. Common sites for measuring blood pressure in children are the brachial artery, popliteal artery, and posterior tibial artery (Figure 22-6).

Auscultation. Auscultation of blood pressure is done the same way as for an adult but with a pediatric stethoscope and blood pressure cuff. The cuff should be long enough to encircle the extremity. The width of the cuff should cover two thirds of the upper arm. The following sizes are suggested: birth to 1 year, 1½ inches; 2 to 8 years, 3 inches; and 8 to 12 years, 4½ inches. Pressure is normally slightly higher in the lower extremities. The American Heart Association designates the muffled tone as the most accurate index of diastolic pressure but recommends recording both that and the final distinct sound as the complete record; thus 120/80/78. Nurses

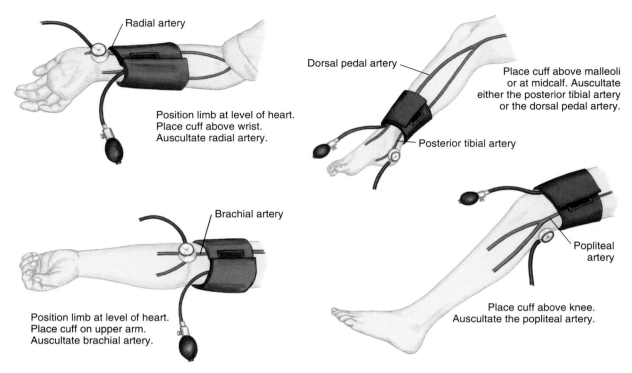

Radial artery

Position limb at level of heart.
Place cuff above wrist.
Auscultate radial artery.

Dorsal pedal artery

Place cuff above malleoli
or at midcalf. Auscultate
either the posterior tibial artery
or the dorsal pedal artery.

Posterior tibial artery

Brachial artery

Position limb at level of heart.
Place cuff on upper arm.
Auscultate brachial artery.

Popliteal artery

Place cuff above knee.
Auscultate the popliteal artery.

FIGURE **22-6** Common sites for measuring blood pressure in children: brachial artery, popliteal artery, posterior tibial artery. Blood pressure may be taken with a manometer and stethoscope or by an electronic machine using a cuff with a sensor that provides a digital readout of the blood pressure. A stethoscope is not necessary when this method is used.

should clarify this with the physician or institution to ensure uniformity. To determine *pulse pressure,* the diastolic reading is subtracted from the systolic. This usually varies from 20 to 50 mm Hg. Widening pulse pressure may be a sign of increased ICP. The American Medical Association has recommended that mercury manometers not be used when taking the blood pressure of patients. Digital manometers are environmentally safer.

Palpation. Palpation is one of the oldest methods of measuring blood pressure. The cuff is applied and inflated above the expected pressure. The fingers are placed over the brachial or radial artery. The systolic pressure is recorded at the point when the pulse reappears. Diastolic pressure is unobtainable. This method is useful in newborns.

Electronic or ultrasonographic measurement. This is a noninvasive type of blood pressure monitoring that ultrasonically detects motion of the arterial wall. A transducer with an attached cuff is secured over an artery, usually the brachial, femoral, or popliteal. The cuff is inflated above systolic pressure and is then gradually reduced. The transducer transmits vascular sounds, and the measurement appears on a digital readout. Both sys-

tolic and diastolic pressures are recorded. Electronic blood pressure machines do not require auscultation with a stethoscope. A cuff is applied, the machine is turned on, and a digital reading is obtained, usually in less than 1 minute.

Some hospitals require blood pressure measurements for all children, whereas others require them only for older children. The nurse explains what is about to happen, for example, "This will hug your arm and feel tight for a few seconds." The child is allowed to examine the sphygmomanometer and cuff.

Blood pressure is lower in children than in adults. If a patient needs blood pressure measurements throughout hospitalization, the nurse observes the previous readings before charting the current one. Many factors account for variations in blood pressure, including time of day, gender, age, exercise, pain, and emotion. A blood pressure taken when a child is frightened or crying is not accurate. If a significant change is observed, the blood pressure should be rechecked. Abnormal readings are charted and reported to the nurse in charge. Tables 22-3 and 22-4 show normal blood pressure readings for boys and girls (age 1 to 18 years).

table 22-3 | *Normal Blood Pressure Readings for Boys*

	SYSTOLIC BLOOD PRESSURE PERCENTILE						DIASTOLIC BLOOD PRESSURE* PERCENTILE				
AGE	5TH	10TH	50TH	90TH	95TH	AGE	5TH	10TH	50TH	90TH	95TH
1 day	54	58	73	87	92	1 day	38	42	55	68	72
3 days	55	59	74	89	93	3 days	38	42	55	68	71
7 days	57	62	76	91	95	7 days	37	41	54	67	71
1 mo	67	71	86	101	105	1 mo	35	39	52	64	68
2 mo	72	76	91	106	110	2 mo	33	37	50	63	66
3 mo	72	76	91	106	110	3 mo	33	37	50	63	66
4 mo	72	76	91	106	110	4 mo	34	37	50	63	67
5 mo	72	76	91	105	110	5 mo	35	39	52	65	68
6 mo	72	76	90	105	109	6 mo	36	40	53	66	70
7 mo	71	76	90	105	109	7 mo	37	41	54	67	71
8 mo	71	75	90	105	109	8 mo	38	42	55	68	72
9 mo	71	75	90	105	109	9 mo	39	43	55	68	72
10 mo	71	75	90	105	109	10 mo	39	43	56	69	73
11 mo	71	76	90	105	109	11 mo	39	43	56	69	73
1 yr	71	76	90	105	109	1 yr	39	43	56	69	73
2 yr	72	76	91	106	110	2 yr	39	43	56	68	72
3 yr	73	77	92	107	111	3 yr	39	42	55	68	72
4 yr	74	79	93	108	112	4 yr	39	43	56	69	72
5 yr	76	80	95	109	113	5 yr	40	43	56	69	73
6 yr	77	81	96	111	115	6 yr	41	44	57	70	74
7 yr	78	83	97	112	116	7 yr	42	45	58	71	75
8 yr	80	84	99	114	118	8 yr	43	47	60	73	76
9 yr	82	86	101	115	120	9 yr	44	48	61	74	78
10 yr	84	88	102	117	121	10 yr	45	49	62	75	79
11 yr	86	90	105	119	123	11 yr	47	50	63	76	80
12 yr	88	92	107	121	126	12 yr	48	51	64	77	81
13 yr	90	94	109	124	128	13 yr	45	49	63	77	81
14 yr	93	97	112	126	131	14 yr	46	50	64	78	82
15 yr	95	99	114	129	133	15 yr	47	51	65	79	83
16 yr	98	102	117	131	136	16 yr	49	53	67	81	85
17 yr	100	104	119	134	138	17 yr	51	55	69	83	87
18 yr	102	106	121	136	140	18 yr	52	56	70	84	88

From the Second Task Force on Blood Pressure Control in Children, National Heart, Lung and Blood Institute, Bethesda, MD.
*K4 was used for ages less than 13; K5 was used for ages 13 and over.

Temperature

Body temperature is regulated by the hypothalamus and aided by mechanisms such as sweating, vasoconstriction or vasodilation, and muscle activity (sweating). Fevers are most commonly caused by infection, response to vaccines, or environmental factors. Fever is an adaptive response during which germ reproduction decreases and inflammatory responses increase; therefore it may aid in the recovery process. However, there is an increase in oxygen consumption and cardiac output in response to fever.

Fever is most often defined as a body temperature over 38° C (100.4° F). The management of fever in a neonate is usually more aggressive than the management of fever in the older infant or child. The main

complication of fever in infants and young children is the development of febrile seizures. A fever of 39° C (102.2° F) requires medical intervention in infants and children with cardiac, lung, central nervous system, or metabolic problems. The main reasons for treating fevers below 39° C (102.2° F) are to prevent febrile seizures and promote comfort.

When evaluating the degree of illness in a febrile child, the response of the child to cuddling, alertness, hydration, sociability, and quality of cry should be assessed and recorded. A quiet, lethargic child who does not respond readily to the environment may be acutely ill. Because dehydration is a common problem in infants and children, skin turgor should be assessed (see

table 22-4 | *Normal Blood Pressure Readings for Girls*

AGE	SYSTOLIC BLOOD PRESSURE PERCENTILE					AGE	DIASTOLIC BLOOD PRESSURE* PERCENTILE				
	5TH	10TH	50TH	90TH	95TH		5TH	10TH	50TH	90TH	95TH
1 day	46	50	65	80	84	1 day	38	42	55	68	72
3 days	53	57	72	86	90	3 days	38	42	55	68	71
7 days	60	64	78	93	97	7 days	38	41	54	67	71
1 mo	65	69	84	98	102	1 mo	35	39	52	65	69
2 mo	68	72	87	101	106	2 mo	34	38	51	64	68
3 mo	70	74	89	104	108	3 mo	35	38	51	64	68
4 mo	71	75	90	105	109	4 mo	35	39	52	65	68
5 mo	72	76	91	106	110	5 mo	36	39	52	65	69
6 mo	72	76	91	106	110	6 mo	36	40	53	66	69
7 mo	72	76	91	106	110	7 mo	36	40	53	66	70
8 mo	72	76	91	106	110	8 mo	37	40	53	66	70
9 mo	72	76	91	106	110	9 mo	37	41	54	67	70
10 mo	72	76	91	106	110	10 mo	37	41	54	67	71
11 mo	72	76	91	105	110	11 mo	38	41	54	67	71
1 yr	72	76	91	105	110	1 yr	38	41	54	67	71
2 yr	71	76	90	105	109	2 yr	40	43	56	69	73
3 yr	72	76	91	106	110	3 yr	40	43	56	69	73
4 yr	73	78	92	107	111	4 yr	40	43	56	69	73
5 yr	75	79	94	109	113	5 yr	40	43	56	69	73
6 yr	77	81	96	111	115	6 yr	40	44	57	70	74
7 yr	78	83	97	112	116	7 yr	41	45	58	71	75
8 yr	80	84	99	114	118	8 yr	43	46	59	72	76
9 yr	81	86	100	115	119	9 yr	44	48	61	74	77
10 yr	83	87	102	117	121	10 yr	46	49	62	75	79
11 yr	86	90	105	119	123	11 yr	47	51	64	77	81
12 yr	88	92	107	122	126	12 yr	49	53	66	78	82
13 yr	90	94	109	124	128	13 yr	46	50	64	78	82
14 yr	92	96	110	125	129	14 yr	49	53	67	81	85
15 yr	93	97	111	126	130	15 yr	49	53	67	82	86
16 yr	93	97	112	127	131	16 yr	49	53	67	81	85
17 yr	93	98	112	127	131	17 yr	48	52	66	80	84
18 yr	94	98	112	127	131	18 yr	48	52	66	80	84

From the Second Task Force on Blood Pressure Control in Children, National Heart, Lung and Blood Institute, Bethesda, MD.
*K4 was used for ages less than 13; K5 was used for ages 13 and over.

Figure 12-13). Measures to reduce fever may promote comfort for the child. Acetaminophen and ibuprofen are the medications used. Parents should be carefully instructed regarding the correct dosage.

Body temperature measurement can be oral, axillary, or tympanic. There are several types of thermometers. The American Medical Association has recommended that thermometers containing mercury not be used. The electronic thermometer, the plastic strip thermometer, and the tympanic membrane sensor are commonly used in the pediatric unit. The electronic thermometer works quickly and is ideal because the plastic sheath is replaceable. The plastic strip changes color according to sensed temperature changes (Figure 22-7). Tympanic

thermometers (Figure 22-8) have a blunt tip that is covered with a disposable cover and can be inserted into the ear. They record temperature from the tympanic membrane (eardrum) by an infrared emission. This site is of importance because the hypothalamus (temperature-regulating center) and the eardrum are perfused by the same circulation. Table 22-5 shows normal temperature ranges.

Oral temperature. The procedure is the same as for adults and may be appropriate for older children.

Axillary temperature. Axillary temperatures are usually taken for newborns and/or according to unit policy. The thermometer is held in the axilla with the infant's arm pressed against the side. Traditionally, an axillary

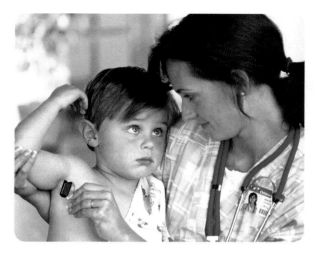

FIGURE **22-7** Skin sensor thermometer. This sensor adheres to the armpit on intact skin for up to 48 hours. Raising the arm will facilitate reading the temperature level. The last dot to turn black indicates the correct temperature. The sensor is intended for single use and is disposable. The temperature range of this continuous-reading thermometer is 35.0° to 40.0° C (95.0° to 104.0° F).

table 22-5	*Normal Temperature Ranges for Children*
METHOD	**RANGE**
Oral	36.4°-37.4° C (97.6°-99.3° F)
Rectal	37.0°-37.7° C (98.6°-100.0° F)
Axillary	35.8°-36.6° C (96.6°-98.0° F)
Ear	36.9°-37.5° C (98.4°-99.5° F)

brane. (Core body temperature is the estimated temperature of the internal body organs.) The tympanic temperature is generally 0.2° to 1.2° F lower than the rectal temperature. The tympanic technique is accurate for all ages. However, some brands of tympanic thermometers have ear probes that do not fit well into the auditory canal of infants under age 3 months. These thermometers should be used only for infants over 3 months of age.

Gently pulling the pinna (earlobe) *down and back* in infants under 3 years of age and *slightly up and back* in children over 3 years of age straightens the auditory canal and provides a more accurate temperature reading. The probe of the thermometer should be aimed at the opposite eyebrow. The accuracy of the tympanic temperature is not affected by illness such as otitis media. A table of Celsius and Fahrenheit temperature equivalents appears in Appendix E. Nursing Care Plan 22-1 reviews the care of a child with a fever.

Weight

Weight must be accurately recorded on admission (Figure 12-11). The weight of a patient provides a means of determining progress and is necessary to determine the dosage of certain medications. The way in which the nurse weighs the child depends on the age.

The infant is weighed completely naked in a warm room. A fresh absorbent pad or scale paper is placed on the scale. This prevents cross-contamination (the spread of germs from one infant to another). The scale is balanced to compensate for the weight of the pad. The infant is placed gently on the scale. The nurse's hand is held slightly above the infant to prevent falling. Once the exact weight appears on the digital readout, the infant is removed from the scale, wrapped in a blanket, and soothed. The weight is immediately recorded. The scale paper is disposed of in the proper receptacle.

The older child is weighed in the same manner as an adult. A paper towel is placed on the scale for the patient to stand on. The patient is generally weighed in a hospital gown. The shoes are removed. If the child is unable to stand on the scales, it may be necessary for the nurse to hold the child and read the combined weights. The nurse is then weighed and subtracts that number from the combined weight to obtain the patient's weight.

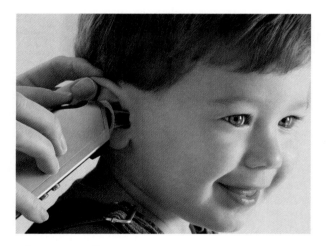

FIGURE **22-8** The tympanic thermometer. Note that the nurse is pulling the pinna of the ear up and back before inserting the ear thermometer in a child over age 3 years to straighten the auditory canal so that the infrared ray reaches the tympanic membrane. If the auditory canal is not straightened, the infrared ray will reach the walls of the ear canal, providing an inaccurate body temperature.

temperature is considered 1° F lower than an oral temperature. The nurse always records the route used.

Measuring body temperature. The tympanic thermometer measures core body temperature by detecting the infrared energy emitted from the tympanic mem-

The Child with a Fever

PATIENT DATA: A 6-year-old child is admitted with a diagnosis of dehydration and a fever of 39.6° C (103.3° F) and is unable to retain food because of nausea and vomiting.

SELECTED NURSING DIAGNOSIS *Deficient fluid volume: potential for dehydration due to increased metabolic rate*

Outcomes	Nursing Interventions	Rationales
The child will not become dehydrated as evidenced by good skin turgor, moist mucous membranes, no weight loss.	1. Increase fluid intake; offer juice, water, popsicles, yogurt, as age appropriate.	1. Body's metabolic rate increases with fever. Children have a higher proportion of body water; therefore more water can be lost rapidly. Body systems such as the kidneys are immature at some ages.
Child's temperature will be between 36.1° and 37.4° C (97.0° and 99.3° F).	1. Administer tepid sponge bath for fever of 40.0° C (104.0° F).	1. Tepid baths help to reduce fever and may make the child more comfortable.
	2. Determine vital signs before sponge bath.	2. Provides baseline data.
	3. Retake vital signs 30 minutes after procedure.	3. Retaking of vital signs will determine if fever is decreasing.
	4. Expose skin to air after procedure; prevent shivering.	4. Promotes evaporation and cooling of skin.
	5. Administer antipyretic medications according to physician's instructions.	5. Frequently, child with a fever also has a headache and painful joints; antipyretic medications will relieve these discomforts and reduce fever.
Injury during treatments will be prevented.	1. Keep side rails raised.	1. Side rails provide safety from falls.
	2. Observe child frequently.	2. Frequent observation will detect subtle changes and possibly reduce complications.
	3. Remain with child if tub bath is given.	3. Threat of drowning is always present with small children and water.
Parent will understand and verbalizes nature and treatment of fever. Parent will verbalize understanding of how to read a thermometer. Parent will verbalize understanding of potential for convulsion. Parent will understand how to give appropriate care during a convulsion.	1. Explain nature of fever (not always bad); too-vigorous control may mask signs of illness.	1. Potential benefits of fever have been cited; it is thought to enhance the body's defense mechanisms and to increase antibody activity.
	2. Emphasize removal of clothes when child has fever.	2. Removal of clothing cools child.
	3. Call physician if child looks sick or acts in a way different from normal.	3. Degree of fever does not always reflect the severity of disease.
	4. Demonstrate how to read a thermometer.	4. This gives parents a sense of control; accuracy of fever will be ensured on discharge.
	5. Discuss with parent potential for convulsion.	5. Only a small number of children convulse with fever; however, discussion is advisable.
	6. Review management of a convulsion.	6. Knowledge allays anxiety.
	7. Discourage use of alcohol sponge baths, which may cause toxicity and skin irritation.	7. Alcohol sponge bath may still be suggested by older relatives.
	8. Discourage use of cold water.	8. Cold water may cause shivering and raise body temperature.

?CRITICAL THINKING QUESTION

A mother states her child has developed a fever after receiving an immunization and requests antibiotic treatment. What data collection and parent teaching is indicated?

Occasionally a child is weighed while wearing a cast. The nurse records this as, for example, "weight 34 pounds with cast on right arm." It is often desirable to record the weight in pounds as well as kilograms. Some parents find pounds a more familiar term. Kilograms is used to calculate safe dosages of medications.

Height

The child's height is measured along with weight. The infant's height must be measured while the infant is lying on a flat surface alongside a metal tape measure or yardstick. The knees should be pressed flat on the table. The measurement is taken from the top of the head to the heels and recorded (see Figure 15-2).

Head Circumference

Head circumference increases rapidly during infancy as a result of brain growth. It is generally measured on infants and toddlers and on all children with neurological defects. The tape measure is placed around the head slightly above the eyebrows and ears and around the occipital prominence of the skull (see Figure 12-5). The measurement is recorded.

COLLECTING SPECIMENS

URINE SPECIMENS

A urine specimen is usually obtained from the newly admitted patient. Certain general principles of collecting specimens are observed, as follows:

- Explain the procedure to the child (as age appropriate).
- Use a clean container or urine collection device.
- Check frequently for results.
- Label all specimens clearly and attach the proper laboratory slip.
- Record in nurses' notes and on intake and output sheet.

Figure 22-9 shows how to apply newborn and pediatric urine collectors and how to recover a specimen.

In small infants a cotton ball may be placed at the opening of the collector. When the infant voids into the cotton ball, the small volume of urine can be retrieved by aspirating the cotton ball with a syringe. Urine collected directly from ultra-absorbent disposable diapers may yield inaccurate protein pH and specific gravity measurements because of the chemicals in the diaper.

Obtaining a Clean-Catch Specimen

Special sterile containers are available for clean-catch specimens; the manufacturer's directions should be fol-lowed. All require cleansing of the perineum with an antiseptic. Rinsing and drying the perineum is important to prevent contamination of urine from the antiseptic. Wiping is done from front to back. After the urine stream has started, the midstream specimen is caught in the sterile container. The nurse's participation is either direct or supervisory depending on the child's age or the availability of a parent. Adolescents, who may be embarrassed by carrying a urine specimen through the halls, may be given a bag or other suitable camouflage. The specimen should be sent to the laboratory promptly.

Obtaining a 24-Hour Specimen

At times a 24-hour urine specimen may be requested to determine the rate of urine production and measure the excretion of specific chemicals from the body. The nurses on each shift must closely supervise this test to maintain its accuracy, because lost specimens necessitate restarting the test. Problems can arise if the collection device does not adhere to the skin properly; therefore the nurse must be alert for this occurrence. Diversions suitable to the child's age are used. A sign is attached to the infant's crib to alert personnel of a 24-hour urine collection. The average daily amount of urine excreted, by age, is given in Table 22-6.

Testing for Albumin

The nurse working in a physician's office or clinic may also be requested to test urine for albumin (protein). Normally, little or no albumin is found in the urine of a healthy child. Reagent strips especially intended for this purpose are available. The nurse dips the end of the strip into urine and compares the strip with a special color chart. Specific instructions accompany test materials.

STOOL SPECIMENS

Stool specimens are obtained from older children as from adults. This is embarrassing for most children, who are "turned off" by the suggestion. The ambulatory child can use a bedpan placed beneath a toilet seat. It is difficult for a child to tell the nurse that the sample has been collected. The nurse can acknowledge these feelings by giving the child permission to express them without being critical, for example, "I know this must be embarrassing for you. It is for grown-ups too, but we need this because. . . ." and so on. An infant's stool specimen can be obtained from the infant by scraping the specimen from the diaper with a tongue depressor and placing it in the specimen container. Some specimen containers contain a level of liquid. The label indicates a "fill line." The amount of infant stool needed for

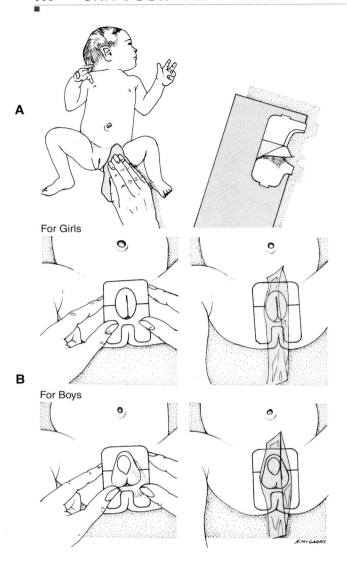

A

For Girls

B

For Boys

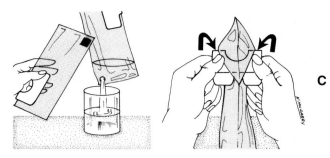

C

FIGURE **22-9** Applying newborn and pediatric urine collectors. Key points are as follows: **A,** The skin must be clean and perfectly dry. Avoid oils, baby powders and lotion soaps, which may leave a residue on the skin and interfere with the ability of the adhesive to stick. **B,** Application must begin on the tiny area of skin between the anus and the genitalia. The narrow "bridge" on the adhesive patch keeps feces from contaminating the specimen and helps to position the collector correctly. **C,** Recovering the specimen. The nurse can drain the urine bag collector into a clean beaker or specimen bottle by removing the tab in the lower corner, or the specimen can be sealed inside the collector itself by folding the sticky adhesive sides together. Then the collector with specimen is placed into a paper or plastic cup.

table 22-6	*Average Daily Excretion of Urine*	
AGE	**FLUID OUNCES**	**MILLILITERS**
First and second days	1-2	30-60
Third to tenth days	3-10	100-300
Tenth day to 2 months	9-15	250-450
2 months to 1 year	14-17	400-500
1 to 3 years	17-20	500-600
3 to 5 years	20-24	600-700
5 to 8 years	22-34	650-1000
8 to 14 years	27-47	800-1400

a specimen is the amount which, when placed into the container, results in the fluid level rising to the "fill line."

Some specimens must be sent to the laboratory while they are warm. The specimen container is labeled properly, placed in a plastic bag, and the laboratory slip attached. The nurse charts the time, color, amount, and consistency of the stool; the purpose for which it was collected (e.g., blood, ova, parasites, or bacteria); and any related information.

BLOOD SPECIMENS
Positioning the Child

Positioning the child for blood drawings is extremely important. The nurse is often asked to assist in these procedures. Figure 22-10 depicts how to position the patient for a femoral venipuncture. Both the jugular and the femoral veins are large; therefore the patient is frequently checked to ensure that there is no bleeding. These sites are used mainly when other areas have been exhausted. The infant is soothed accordingly, because crying and thrashing may precipitate oozing. The nurse charts the site used, the name of blood test, and any untoward developments.

LUMBAR PUNCTURE

The nurse sometimes assists the physician with a lumbar puncture, which is also referred to as a *spinal tap*. It

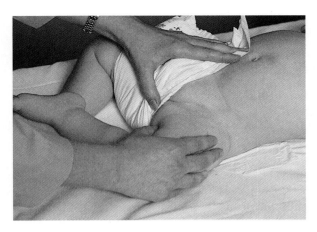

FIGURE **22-10** An infant positioned for femoral venipuncture. This position exposes the groin area.

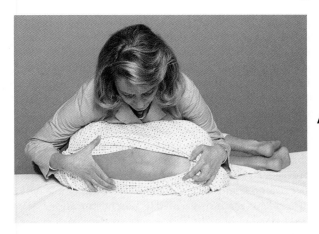

A

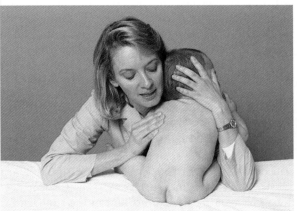

B

is done to obtain spinal fluid for examination or to reduce pressure within the brain in conditions such as hydrocephalus or meningitis. Disposable lumbar puncture sets are used.

Normal spinal fluid is clear like water. The pressure ranges from 60 to 180 mm Hg. It is somewhat lower in infants. The procedure for children is essentially the same as for adults. The main difference lies in the patient's ability to cooperate with positioning. The nurse explains that the child must lie quietly and will be helped to do this. Sensations during a lumbar puncture include a cool feeling when the skin is cleansed and a feeling of pressure when the needle is inserted. The way in which the child is held can directly affect the success of the procedure.

The child lies on the side with the back parallel to the side of the treatment table. The knees are flexed, and the head is brought down close to the flexed knees. The nurse can keep the child in this position by placing the child's head in the crook of one arm and the knees in the crook of the other arm. The nurse's hands are then clasped together at the front of the child. The nurse leans forward, gently placing the chest against the patient (Figure 22-11).

Once the child is positioned, the physician prepares the lower back using sterile technique. A vial of local anesthetic may be necessary unless this is provided in the sterile setup. The top of the vial is cleansed with an alcohol sponge. Once the area has been locally anesthetized, the physician inserts a special hollow needle into the patient's lower back and collects the spinal fluid in two or three test tubes. When the procedure is completed, a sterile bandage is placed over the injection site, and the child is comforted. Specimens are labeled and taken to the laboratory with the appropriate requisition form.

FIGURE **22-11** A child positioned for a lumbar puncture. **A,** An older child may be placed in a side-lying fetal position and held firmly by the nurse. **B,** Placing an infant in a sitting position allows for flexion of the lumbar spine. The nurse hugs the child for support and security.

The adolescent may avoid postlumbar puncture headache by lying flat for some time. The nurse charts the date and time of the lumbar puncture and the name of the attending physician. Also charted are the amount of fluid obtained, its character (e.g., cloudy or bloody), whether or not specimens were sent to the laboratory, and the patient's reaction to the procedure.

PHYSIOLOGICAL RESPONSES TO MEDICATIONS IN INFANTS AND CHILDREN

Medication administration is a primary responsibility of the nurse. It is important for the nurse to understand that the responses of infants differ from those of children and that the responses of infants and children differ from those of adults. These concepts must also be communicated to the parents, who often administer over-the-counter medications to their growing child. The most common over-the-counter medication administered by parents to infants and children is acetaminophen (Tylenol). A physician or health care provider may advise the parents to "give a teaspoon of acetaminophen to their young child." However, the parents who purchase the medication may choose Tylenol drops instead of Tylenol elixir. The 1-teaspoon dose of Tylenol *elixir* is the dose ordered. However, 1 teaspoon of Tylenol *drops* is a massive overdose and can harm the young child. These types of accidents can be prevented by parent education.

Understanding the differences in drug absorption, distribution, metabolism, and excretion between children and adults is essential to provide safe pediatric medication administration. Age is the most important variable in predicting response to any drug therapy. The functions of various organs in the body mature as the child grows and develops.

ABSORPTION OF MEDICATIONS IN INFANTS AND CHILDREN
Gastric Influences

In the neonate there is an absence of free hydrochloric acid in the stomach. The acid content of the stomach reaches adult levels by age 2 years. Therefore medications that require an acid medium in the stomach for absorption may not be completely absorbed if the child is under 2 years of age. The administration of such medications near the time of formula feedings will further decrease the acid content of the stomach. After 2 years of age, the ingestion of orange juice increases gastric acidity, causing more effective absorption of medication that requires an acid medium to absorb.

Intestinal Influences

Children under 5 years of age have a more rapid intestinal transit time than adults. Medication may have moved out of the small intestines before it is completely absorbed. Therefore delayed or timed-release oral medication may not be fully absorbed by children younger than 5 years of age. The presence of pancreatic enzymes may be low under 1 year of age. Some medications depend on pancreatic enzymes to help to absorb the drug.

Topical Medications (Ointments)

Pediatric patients have a thin stratum corneum that allows topical medications to be absorbed. The larger skin surface area also increases the amount of absorption of topical medication as compared to adults. The use of a plastic diaper can also cause increased absorption of a topically applied medication in the diaper area of the skin. Hydrocortisone and hexachlorophene may produce adverse systemic responses when applied to the buttocks and covered with a plastic diaper.

Parenteral Medications

Poor peripheral perfusion in the young infant will slow intramuscular (IM) drug absorption. IM drugs administered to infants and children under 4 years of age should be water soluble to prevent precipitation. In neonates, medication may pass through the blood-brain barrier more easily than in older children and adults. Therefore medications that depress respiration may have a more powerful effect on neonates than in adults.

METABOLISM OF MEDICATIONS IN INFANTS AND CHILDREN

Most medications are metabolized in the liver. Because the liver and enzymes do not function at a mature level until 2 to 4 years of age, drugs generally metabolize more slowly in the infant and young child compared to the adult. Medications given at frequent intervals to infants and children may result in toxic levels and responses.

EXCRETION OF MEDICATIONS IN INFANTS AND CHILDREN

Many medications such as penicillin and digoxin depend on the kidney for excretion. The immature kidney function prevents effective excretion of drugs from the body in infants under 1 year of age.

The combination of slow stomach emptying (delays medication from being absorbed), rapid intestinal transit time (may prevent the full amount of medication from being absorbed), unpredictable liver function (may impair metabolism of the drug), and inability to effectively excrete medications via the kidney can result in altered responses to medication and a high risk for toxicity.

NURSING RESPONSIBILITIES IN ADMINISTERING MEDICATIONS TO INFANTS AND CHILDREN

It becomes a legal and ethical responsibility of the nurse to understand that growing children differ in their ability to respond to medications. Nurses must observe for toxic symptoms whenever medications are administered and *document positive and negative responses.* Close attention must be paid to pediatric dose calculations. Every medication administered should have the safety of the dose prescribed calculated before administration. The official sources for safe dosage levels for

box 22-2 *Selected Age-Appropriate Techniques of Giving Medications to Children*

INFANT

Apply bib.

Support and elevate head and shoulders.

Plastic disposable syringe is accurate and safe for oral medications.

Depress chin with thumb to open mouth.

Slowly insert medication along the side of the infant's mouth; this helps to prevent gagging.

Allow time for swallowing.

The recommended site for IM injections is the vastus lateralis muscle.

Avoid using the buttocks, because the gluteal muscles are undeveloped in infants and there is danger of injury to sciatic nerve.

As a rule of thumb, give no more than 1 ml of solution in a single site; if in doubt, confer with another nurse or physician.

Soothe infant after procedure is completed.

TODDLER

May require help of another person.

May require some type of restraint if no assistance is available.

Let child explore an empty medicine cup.

Explain reasons for the medication.

Crush tablets if they are not chewable.

If child is cooperative, he or she may hold the medicine cup.

Allow the child to drink at his or her own pace.

When giving IM medications, carry out the injection quickly and gently.

Be prepared to find that resistive behavior is at its peak, particularly kicking, crying, and thrashing about.

Be prepared to be surprised, because some toddlers are very cooperative.

PRESCHOOL

Chewable tablets and liquids are preferred.

Regression in pill taking may be seen.

Watch for loose teeth that may be swallowed.

Avoid prolonged reasoning.

Involve parents if appropriate.

Provide puppet play to help child express frustrations concerning injections.

Praise child after procedure.

SCHOOL AGE

Child can take pills and capsules; instruct child to place pill near the back of the tongue and immediately swallow water.

Emphasize swallowing of fluid to distract the child from swallowing the pill.

Some children continue to have a difficult time swallowing pills, and other forms of the medication should be explored (many come in suspensions); never ridicule the child.

Child can be unpredictable from day to day in cooperation; allow more time for giving pediatric medication.

Always ascertain that the child is fully awake (particularly after nap time and during the night shift).

Always inform the child of what you are about to do.

Remain with the fearful child after the procedure until he or she regains composure.

When this is not possible or appears prolonged, enlist the help of auxiliary personnel.

ADOLESCENT

Prepare the adolescent with explanations suitable to his or her level of understanding.

Always ensure privacy.

Teach the adolescent what side effects to report.

Identify adolescents on contraceptives to avoid drug interactions (may have been too embarrassed to provide information during history or may be attempting to keep secret from significant others).

Remain with patient until medication is consumed (particularly if patient has a behavior disorder).

Anticipate mood swings in compliance.

Consider possibility of adolescent addiction (drugs, alcohol) even though this may not be a presenting problem; many medications are altered by such conditions.

various age-groups is provided by the manufacturer's pocket insert, the *Physician's Desk Reference (PDR)*, or other current drug reference book. One method of determining safe dosage for infants and children is described in Box 22-3 on p. 511. Parent teaching is essential to ensure compliance when the child is sent home. Instructions should include the following:

- The importance of administering the medicine.
- The importance of completing the prescribed

course of treatment.

- Techniques of measuring the amount of medication to give in each dose. The use of the teaspoon in the home is not advisable when administering medication to infants and children. Inexpensive and accurate measuring devices are available in pharmacies.
- Techniques of administering medications to their infant or child, as follows:

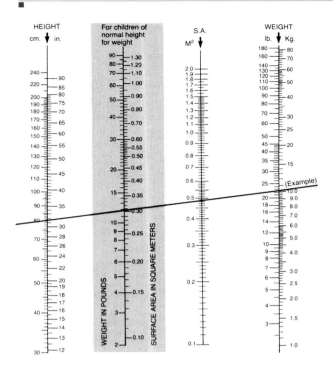

FIGURE **22-12** Nomogram for estimating surface area. The body surface area of the child is at the point where the height and weight levels intersects the surface area column. If the patient is of average size, the surface area can be deduced on the basis of weight alone (see shaded box).

CALCULATING PEDIATRIC DRUG DOSAGES
Body Surface Area

Most pediatric medications are prescribed in milligrams per kilogram of body weight per 24 hours. A hospital drug reference is usually available on the unit to enable the nurse to determine the safety of a particular dose. If there is any question, one should consult the charge nurse, the physician who wrote the order, or the hospital pharmacist. The nurse should not be interrupted when preparing medications.

The physician calculates a particular dosage of a medication for each child. One method, calculation by body surface area (BSA), is considered to be the most accurate. In this method, a nomogram is used (Figure 22-12).

On the nomogram, the child's height is located on the left scale and the weight on the right scale. A line is drawn between the two points. The point at which the line transects the surface area (SA) gives the BSA of the individual child. If the patient's size is roughly average, the SA can also be estimated from the weight alone by using the enclosed area of Figure 22-12. The results are inserted into a formula. The average adult BSA is approximately 1.7 M^2, as follows:

$$\frac{BSA \text{ (child)}}{BSA \text{ (adult)}} \times \text{Average adult dose} = \text{Child's dose}$$

CALCULATING THE SAFE DRUG DOSE
Milligrams per Kilogram (mg/kg)

For adults, most medications have an "average dose." There is no average dose in pediatrics because the weight of the child can vary between 2 pounds to 150 pounds, and at different ages the ability to metabolize and excrete drugs may be limited. Therefore it is necessary for the nurse to calculate if the ordered dose is safe. The mg/kg protocol can be used by the nurse when calculating safe doses for an infant or child. For example, the physician orders 25 mg of a medication to be administered. The nurse checks the *PDR* or other current drug reference book and finds that the safe dose for that medication is 2 to 4 mg/kg. This child weighs 7 kg. Using the highest safe dose, the nurse inserts the actual weight of the child in kilograms (kg) into the formula so that the formula now reads as follows: the safe dose of *this* medication for *this* child is 4 mg × 7 kg, or 28 mg. The physician's order does not exceed 28 mg, and therefore the dose that he or she ordered is safe to give. If the physician's order had exceeded the computed safe dose, the nurse would call his or her supervisor or the physician.

Using a dropper or syringe or measured cup
Not mixing medication with formula, food, or water
Shaking medication before administering
Refrigerating unused portions of medication if indicated
- Techniques of encouraging child compliance include the following:
  Allowing toddlers and young children autonomy of assisting with taking their own medication by squirting the contents into their own mouth or drinking it from the cup
  Providing praise for cooperation and perhaps a chart of stars or stickers for compliance
  Providing a good-tasting liquid or an ice-pop following administration of a medication that has a bad taste
- The importance of writing a schedule and documenting the administration to avoid forgetting or double-dosing.

Selected tips in giving medication to children at various ages are offered in Box 22-2.

box 22-3 *Formula for Dimensional Analysis*

$$\frac{\text{Unit}}{\text{Dosage on hand}} \times \frac{\text{Dosage wanted}}{\text{Unit to give}}$$

Dimensional Analysis

Dimensional analysis is one method of calculating dosages using basic arithmetic and algebra (Box 22-3). Some examples are given in this section.

EXAMPLE: A physician orders 0.025 g of a drug. Each tablet is 12.5 mg. How many tablets will you give? You know that 1000 mg = 1 g. Therefore:

$$\frac{\text{Unit}}{\text{Dosage on hand}} \times \frac{\text{Dosage wanted}}{\text{Unit to give}}$$

$$\frac{1000 \text{ mg}}{1 \text{ g}} \times \frac{0.025 \text{ mg}}{? \text{ mg}} = 1000 \times 0.025 = 25 \text{ mg}$$

You will give 25 mg. Remember that each tablet is 12.5 mg:

$$\begin{array}{cc} \text{What you have} & \text{What you want to give} \\ \dfrac{1 \text{ (tab)}}{12.5 \text{ mg}} \times & \dfrac{25 \text{ mg}}{? \text{ tab}} = 2 \text{ tablets} \end{array}$$

You would give two tablets.

EXAMPLE: A physician orders 5 mg of a drug. The label reads 10 mg/2 ml. How many ml are you going to give?

$$\frac{\text{Unit}}{\text{Dose}} = \frac{2 \text{ ml}}{10 \text{ mg}} = \frac{5 \text{ mg}}{? \text{ ml}} = \frac{10}{10} = 1 \text{ ml}$$

You will give 1 ml.

Determining Whether a Dose is Safe for an Infant

A physician orders 200 mg q6h. The *PDR* states that a 40-mg/kg dose is a safe dose for infants. This infant weighs 12 pounds.

$$\begin{array}{cccc} \text{Dose} & \text{Convert pounds} & \text{Weight of} & \text{What child is} \\ \text{ordered} & \text{to key} & \text{child} & \text{receiving} \\ \dfrac{200 \text{ mg}}{\text{Dose}} \times & \dfrac{2.2 \text{ lb}}{1 \text{ kg}} \times & \dfrac{1 \text{ infant}}{12 \text{ lb}} = & 36.6\text{-mg/kg dose} \end{array}$$

Because the 36.6 mg does not exceed the stated safe dose of 40 mg/kg, the dose ordered is safe for this child.

Besides knowing the correct amount and route of a drug, the nurse must also be aware of the toxic side effects that might occur. The absorption, distribution,

table 22-7 *Drug-Environment Interactions*

DRUGS	INTERACTS WITH	INTERACTION
Imipramine (Tofranil), phenothiazines, griseofulvin, tetracyclines, chlorothiazide (Diuril)	Sun	Skin rash when child is exposed to the sun
Vitamin C	Air	Decomposes when exposed to air

metabolism, and excretion of drugs differ substantially in children, who also react more quickly and violently to medication. Drug reactions are therefore not as predictable as they are in adult patients. The drug's impact on normal growth and development must be considered. Drug inserts must be read carefully to determine the suitability of a particular drug for children. *Drugs should be given only by the route indicated.*

Double-checking with another nurse may be required in some hospitals when administering drugs such as digoxin (Lanoxin), insulin, or heparin. *The child should be correctly identified by using the hospital ID band. The nurse must always know what medications the patient is receiving, whether or not the nurse personally administers them.* See Box 22-2 for further age-appropriate techniques of administering pediatric medications.

AVOIDING DRUG INTERACTIONS
Selected Drug-Environment Interactions

Some medications can cause skin reactions when the child is exposed to the sun (phototoxicity). Parents should be advised to keep their child protected from the sun while he or she is taking these medications. Drugs that decompose when exposed to the air or light are dispensed in darkened bottles. These drugs should not be purchased in the large economy size because deterioration might occur to tablets before all are used up. Table 22-7 lists some examples of drug-environment interactions.

Selected Drug-Drug Interactions

The nurse should be alert to possible interactions between drugs prescribed and between prescription drugs and drugs that parents may purchase without a prescription. Table 22-8 is a partial list of some common drug-drug interactions.

table 22-8 | *Selected Drug-Drug Interactions*

DRUG	INTERACTS WITH	INTERACTION
Antacids	Steroids	Decreased absorption
	Digoxin	Decreased absorption
	NSAIDs	Decreased absorption
	Tetracycline	Decreased absorption
	Theophylline	Increased toxicity
Barbiturates	Oral contraceptives	Decreased protection
	Steroids	Decreased steroid effectiveness
	Influenza vaccine	Barbiturate toxicity
	Theophylline	Decreased theophylline effect
Bleomycin	Oxygen	Increased lung toxicity
Erythromycin	Phenytoin	Decreased phenytoin effect
	Theophylline	Increased theophylline toxicity
Isoniazid	Antacid	Decreased absorption
	Phenytoin	Increased phenytoin toxicity
	Valproate	Hepatic and central nervous system toxicity
Phenytoin	Alcohol	Acute toxicity
	Antacid	Decreased phenytoin effect
	Antidepressants (tricyclic)	Increased phenytoin toxicity
	Contraceptives	Decreased protection
	Steroids	Decreased steroid effect
	Digoxin	Decreased digoxin effect
	Folic acid	Decreased phenytoin effect
	Isoniazid	Increased phenytoin toxicity
	Theophylline	Decreased effect of both medications
	Valproate	Increased phenytoin toxicity

table 22-9 | *Selected Drug-Food Interactions*

DRUG	INTERACTS WITH	INTERACTION
Aminoglycosides Gentamycin Penicillin Tetracycline	Any food	Decreased absorption rate
Theophylline	High-protein foods Low carbohydrate diet	Decreased time of drug activity in body
Monoamine (MAO) inhibitors (phenelzine [Nardil], tranyl-cypromine [Parnate], isocarbox-azid [Marplan])	Tyramine-containing foods such as yogurt, processed meats, beer	Possible hypertensive crises
Iron supplements	Starch, egg yolks	Decreased iron absorption
Antihypertensives	Licorice or natural licorice extract	Can counteract effect of antihypertensive drugs
Vitamin C	Foods high in vitamin B_{12}	Decreased absorption of vitamin B_{12} if both vitamins are taken together

Selected Drug-Food Interactions

The nurse should be aware that food and nutrients can influence the absorption, metabolism, and excretion of certain drugs. Foods that influence gastrointestinal motility or the pH of gastric secretions can affect absorption, thus lessening the drug's therapeutic value. Table 22-9 lists some drug-food interactions.

ADMINISTERING ORAL MEDICATIONS

The administration of medication by mouth is preferred in children but is not always possible because of vomiting, malabsorption, or refusal. Children younger than 5 years of age find it difficult to swallow tablets or capsules. Most pediatric medications are available in liquid, suspension, or chewable tablets. Only scored tablets should be divided. Suspensions must be fully shaken before use.

Medications may need to be disguised in a pleasant-tasting medium when the medication is bitter or otherwise unpalatable. Cherry syrup or jelly may be used. The use of important sources of nutrients, foods, or liquids (e.g., orange juice) for this purpose is discouraged because the child may develop a distaste for these foods. The medication is never referred to as "candy." Medication is administered slowly, especially if the child is crying. *The child's head and shoulders are elevated to prevent aspiration.* Toddlers may attempt to push away the medicine cup. In anticipation of this response, the nurse holds the child, with hands restrained, in the nurse's lap in a semi-sitting position (Figure 22-13). "Chasers" of water, fruit juice, frozen ice pops, or carbonated beverage are appreciated. The patient's age and diet are considered when choosing a chaser.

If a nasogastric tube is in place, the nurse tests for proper placement of the tube *before* pouring medication into the funnel. A small amount of water is administered afterward to cleanse the tube. The procedure is recorded on the intake and output (I&O) sheet.

For infants, an oral syringe is an excellent device for measuring small quantities. It is easily transported, and medication can be given directly from the syringe. The syringe is placed midway back at the side of the mouth. A bib is placed on an infant before performing the procedure. Medication should not be placed in a bottle of juice or water; if some of the contents are refused, there is no way to determine how much of the drug was consumed. A Medibottle, a device that consists of a syringe attached to a nipple, can be used for infants who will suck the medication from the nipple as the plunger of the syringe is slowly depressed (Figure 22-14).

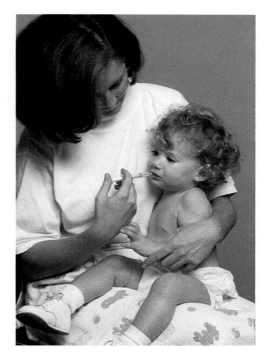

FIGURE **22-13** The syringe or cup method of administering oral medications to infants or children. The nurse may hold the child on the lap and restrain the child's hands as shown to prevent the medication from spilling. The child's legs can be restrained by placing them between the knees of the nurse.

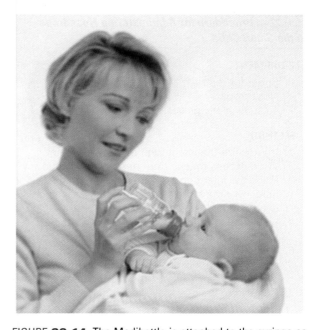

FIGURE **22-14** The Medibottle is attached to the syringe so the infant can suck on the nipple to consume the medication. The nurse controls the flow with gentle pressure on the syringe barrel.

A plastic medicine dropper is useful, and the drug manufacturer may provide one with the medication. It is used only for the medication specified; it is not intended for measuring other liquids. A drug ordered in teaspoons should be measured in milliliters to ensure accuracy (5 ml = 1 teaspoon). The nurse administering medications on the pediatric unit must keep the medicine tray or cart in sight at all times. This prevents other patients from upsetting or ingesting the contents.

ADMINISTERING PARENTERAL MEDICATIONS
Nosedrops, Eardrops, and Eyedrops

Except for a few differences, the principles for administering nosedrops, eardrops, and eyedrops to children are essentially the same as for adults. Infants and small children need to be restrained in a mummy restraint (see Box 22-1).

Nosedrops. The procedure for administering nosedrops to a small child is listed in Box 22-4.

Eardrops. The health care provider may prescribe a drug to be instilled into the ear to relieve pain. If the drops were refrigerated, they are allowed to warm to room temperature. In *children under 3 years of age,* the pinna of the infected ear is drawn *down and back* to

---

box 22-4 *Procedure for Administering Nosedrops to the Small Child*

EQUIPMENT
- Sheet for restraint
- Nosedrops
- Tissues, clean gloves

METHOD
1. Immobilize the infant with mummy restraint.
2. Wipe excess mucus from nose with a tissue.
3. Place the infant on his or her back, with the head over the side of the mattress or the neck extended over a pillow.
4. Encircle the infant's cheeks and chin with left arm and hand to steady.
5. Instill drops with the right hand.
6. Keep infant in this position for 1/2 to 1 minute to allow the drops to reach the proper area.
7. Remove restraints. Make the infant comfortable.
8. Chart the following: time, name of nosedrops, strength, number of drops instilled, how the patient tolerated the procedure, and untoward reactions.

---

straighten the canal, and the correct number of drops are instilled. In *older children,* the ear lobe is pulled *upward and backward* to obtain the same result. Gentle massage of the area in front of the ear may facilitate entry of the drops. The patient remains supine for a few minutes to permit the fluid to be absorbed. The nurse charts the following: time, name of drug, number of drops administered, area (right or left ear), untoward reactions, and whether or not the patient obtained relief.

Eyedrops/creams. Ophthalmic medication is administered to a child in the same manner as for the adult. The child is informed of the need for the medication. The patient is identified, and the orders and the label on the bottle are checked for correct medication and concentration. The nurse ascertains which eye requires treatment, that is the right eye (O.D.), left eye (O.S.), or both eyes (O.U.). The hands are washed before and after the procedure, and clean gloves are worn. With the thumb and index finger, gentle pressure is applied in opposite directions to open the eye. The older child is instructed to "look up." Supporting the hand on the patient's forehead, the medication is instilled into the center of the lower lid (conjunctival sac). (See Figure 6-25.) The child is instructed to close the eye but not to squeeze it, because this could expel some of the solution.

Ointment is applied in the same conjunctival sac as eyedrops. The mummy restraint is applied when only one nurse is available and the patient is an infant. Occasionally children refuse to open their eyes. The nurse must use ingenuity to coax reluctant children. It may help to involve the parents.

Rectal Medications

Some drugs, such as sedatives and antiemetics, come in the form of suppositories. Children's suppositories are long and thin in comparison with the cone-shaped types administered to adults. Wearing a rubber glove or finger cot, the nurse inserts the lubricated suppository well beyond the anal sphincter about half as far as the forefinger will reach. The nurse applies pressure to the anus by gently holding the buttocks together until the child's desire to expel the suppository subsides.

Subcutaneous and Intramuscular Injections

Most medications given to infants and children are given by the oral or intravenous (IV) route. However, some medications must be given by the subcutaneous route (SC or SQ), such as insulin for diabetic children. Some medications must be given via the intramuscular route (IM), such as immunizations or vitamin K to newborn infants. The site and technique of injection can affect the absorption rate and the effect of the drug on the child.

The subcutaneous route. In subcutaneous (SC) injections, absorption occurs by slow diffusion into the capillaries. If a medication such as epinephrine is given IM instead of SC, a life-threatening cardiac arrhythmia could occur. If the extremity in which the SC medication was given is exercised immediately before or after an SC injection, the absorption rate is increased. (If insulin is the drug injected, hypoglycemia could occur because of the rapid absorption.) Sites should be rotated. Irritating solutions should not be injected SC.

The intramuscular route. An intramuscular (IM) injection places medication into the skeletal muscle below the subcutaneous tissue. The medication spreads among the muscle's elastic fibers and absorbs rapidly. Aspirating the plunger after insertion and observing for a flashback of blood will confirm placement of the needle. A flashback of blood should not occur if the needle is correctly placed into the muscle. Accidental injection into a vein can cause a toxic response. Accidental injection into the subcutaneous tissue can cause tissue necrosis.

Intramuscular sites. IM injections are given into the vastus lateralis muscle of the thigh in all infants (Figure 22-15). The site is free of major nerves and blood vessels, but small nerve endings can cause the injection to be painful. The ventrogluteal site places the medication into the gluteus medius and minimus muscles, which are free of major nerve and blood vessels. This site can be used in children after they have been walking for 1 year.

The dorsogluteal site involves a high risk for sciatic nerve injury or piercing of a major blood vessel. This site is small and poorly developed in infants and is not used for IM injections. The *deltoid* site in the upper arm has a small muscle mass that limits the amount of medication that can be injected at one time. There are major blood vessels in this area, and the radial nerve can be injured. The deltoid muscle is not a preferred site for children under age 6 years. However, absorption of medication is more rapid in the deltoid than in the buttock or the thigh.

Reducing the pain of injections. Nurses can take the time to reduce the discomfort associated with injections. *Positioning* the patient properly can minimize muscle tenseness and ease the procedure. The child can lie face down or on the side with the upper leg placed in front of the lower one to relax the muscles. For a vastus lateralis injection, the child's toes should be turned so that the hip rotates internally. The child can flex the elbow and support the arm for a deltoid injection. A *topical anesthetic* such as EMLA (see Chapter 21) can be used when the time of injection can be planned in advance. Storing alcohol sponges in the refrigerator or rubbing the site with an ice cube before injection will numb the site. The current design of many syringes minimizes accidental needle punctures to the caregiver that can spread infections and increase risk of blood-borne pathogen exposure. The needle should be inserted rapidly while the child is distracted. The medication is injected slowly to minimize the increasing pressure within the muscle. Rapid removal of the needle and mild massage or exercise of the extremity will increase absorption and comfort.

The size of the syringe and of the needle vary with the size of the child, volume of medication prescribed,

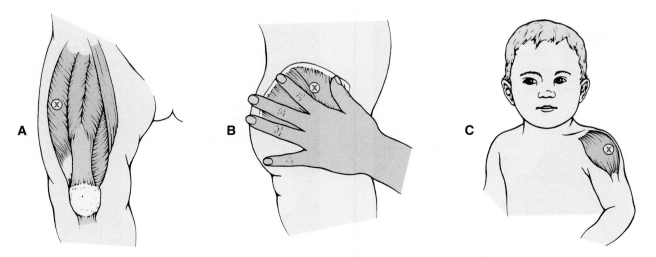

FIGURE **22-15** Appropriate sites for IM injection in children. **A,** The thigh. **B,** Ventrogluteal. **C,** Deltoid. The vastus lateralis **(A)** is preferred in children under 3 years of age.

amount and general condition of the muscle tissue, frequency of injections, and viscosity (thickness) of the drug. A small needle gauge, such as 25 to 27, and a length of 0.5 to 1 inch is commonly used. As a general rule, 1 ml is the maximum volume to be given in one site to infants and small children. Small or premature infants may tolerate even less. For volumes less than 1 ml, a tuberculin syringe or low-dose syringe is preferred. Some syringes are designed to automatically retract the needle into the syringe after injections, and some have a plastic sleeve (Figure 22-16) to pull over the needle after use. This eliminates the practice of re-capping the needles and reduces the risk of accidental needle sticks.

The nurse should anticipate some protest from children about injections. Whenever possible, a second person should assist by distracting and restraining the child. The child's first injection is particularly important because it establishes the pattern for future reactions (Figure 22-17). The school-age child may assist in selecting the site, if possible. This helps to increase feelings of mastery and control. Injections are more of a threat to toddlers and preschool children, who are too young to understand their necessity. The nurse should be careful not to shame the uncooperative child. Fortunately, the necessity for administering IM injections to children is decreasing because most medications can now be given orally, rectally, or intravenously.

Intravenous Medications

An IV injection places the drug directly into the bloodstream in a faster, more predictable time frame.

Medications given by the IV route are being administered routinely in pediatric patients. In some cases this prevents repeated IM injections. Other drugs are effective only if given by this method. The medication is also absorbed more rapidly, which is of value. Each hospital has its own policies about who may start IV lines or add medications to an established line. The nurse monitors the IV site carefully for infiltration, inflammation, and patency.

IV medications can cause phlebitis, and the nurse must observe the child's IV site hourly for reddened areas or signs of inflammation. Infiltration is a risk for children who are active, and the site should be observed hourly because children cannot communicate the burning or pain that may accompany infiltration. Leakage at the IV site, a tense tissue turgor, and cool, blanched skin around the IV site may indicate infiltration; the nurse manager should be notified. Because the medication reaches the heart and brain within seconds, adverse reactions can occur quickly. The nurse must be aware of the side effects associated with the drug administered. A rapid rate of flow of IV solution can cause fluid overload (manifested by increased pulse or blood pressure, distended neck veins, and puffy eyes), or a slow rate of infusion can result in clot formation that obstructs the patency of the IV line. The nurse should monitor the rate of the IV flow, refill the burettes hourly (Figure

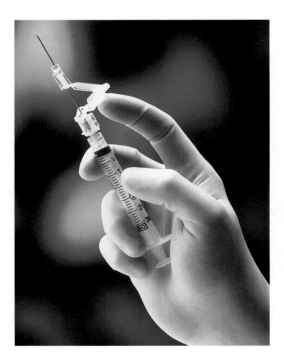

FIGURE **22-16** This syringe has a plastic sleeve that covers the needle after medication is administered. This helps to protect the nurse from an accidental needle stick.

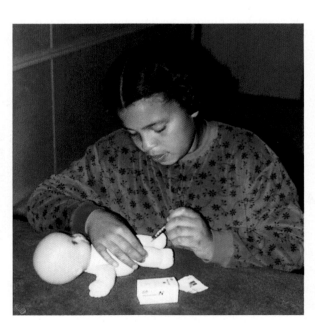

FIGURE **22-17** By giving injections to dolls or puppets, children can be prepared for this procedure and may be less frightened by it. (Photo courtesy of Pat Spier, RN-C.)

22-18), observe the condition of the IV site, and identify the responses of the child.

Sites for IV infusion in children are illustrated in Figure 22-19. A pediatric armboard is used (Figure 22-20) to restrain the extremity used for IV access, and the insertion site is secured and covered to prevent tampering by the child or parents. The child with an IV in the extremity or the scalp will benefit from being held and rocked and need not have his or her whole body immobilized. Infusion pumps are used in pediatrics to control the administration of small volumes of fluid and to prevent changes in rate resulting from changes in position or activity of the infant or child. A pacifier should be provided for infants who are given nothing by mouth (NPO status) to fulfill their developmental need for sucking.

Long-term peripheral venous access devices (VADs)

Heparin or saline lock. A heparin lock or saline lock is a device that keeps a vein open for long-term intermittent medicine administration. It allows children to be more ambulatory because they are free of IV tubing. Repeated "sticks" can be avoided when a patient has a heparin or saline lock in place. The apparatus consists of an IV needle attached to a 3¼-inch plastic tube plugged by a resealable rubber insert. This rubber top allows the insertion of a needle so that blood can be drawn or medications administered. The original needle remains in place and is periodically flushed with heparin or saline solution to prevent clotting.

Central venous access devices. A peripherally inserted central catheter (PICC) is inserted for moderate-length therapy. The median, cephalic, or basilic vein is used in the antecubital area and threaded into the superior vena cava. Specially trained RNs may insert the PICC line. Dressings are changed per established protocol, the insertion site is assessed, and care is taken to prevent dislodgement during this procedure.

Long-term central venous access devices

Hickman, Groshong, and Broviac catheters. Hickman, Groshong, and Broviac catheters are tiny, flexible tubes that can be inserted into a vein in the chest to establish a long-term IV site. Medications, chemotherapy, IV fluids, and blood products can be given through the catheter. They can also be used for hyperalimentation, or total parenteral nutrition. The pediatric Broviac catheter is used for children. The line is inserted while the patient is under local or general anesthesia. It remains in the patient from 1 month to 1 year or even longer.

The child or parents are taught how to care for the catheter during hospitalization so they may continue the procedure at home under the supervision of home

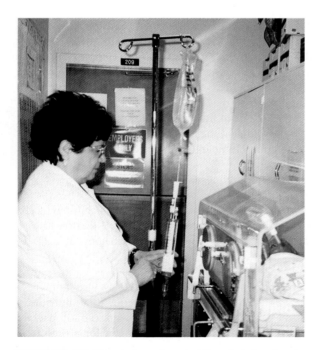

FIGURE **22-18** The graduated control (burette) chamber delivers micro drops, making it easier to calculate the rate and amount of fluids absorbed by infants and children. The burette is filled with the amount of solution to be administered in 1 hour. The IV pump will sound an alarm when the level in the burette is low, reminding the nurse to assess the IV site. The burette is then refilled and the site reevaluated every hour.

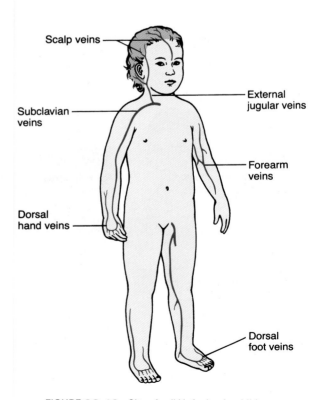

FIGURE **22-19**   Sites for IV infusion in children.

care nurses. Some catheters are flushed daily or weekly with heparin or saline solution. Activities of daily living are not curtailed; however, the physician should be contacted about any unusual change in activity. The exit site should be kept dry. The patient and family must participate in the home care, and the presence of the catheter may impact the child's self-image. A light shirt with a pocket, worn inside out, provides a place for any excess tubing and covers the area to protect it from the fingers of a curious child. If a catheter leak occurs, the tubing should be taped, a clamp applied, and medical intervention obtained.

Implanted ports. Infusion ports that can be implanted under the skin are also available (Port-A-Cath, MediPort, Infuse-A-Port, Groshong venous port). These small plastic devices are generally implanted under the skin beneath the clavicle. A small catheter is threaded from the port into a large central vein. The procedure is performed using a local or general anesthetic. Blood samples can be obtained, and medicines are injected by a puncture through the skin into the port. Special needles are provided by the manufacturer. The use of a local or topical anesthetic makes the skin puncture painless. The advantage is that nothing protrudes from the body that can be dislodged, and it is less apparent. This is es-

pecially important for the self-conscious young adolescent. Activities such as swimming need not be curtailed because the skin is intact. Vigorous contact sports are curtailed, and the child should be cautioned not to play with the bulge created by the device. Removal requires minor surgery.

Nursing Care of a Child Receiving Parenteral Fluids

Parenteral (*para,* "beside or apart from" and *enteron,* "intestine") fluids are those given by some route other than the digestive tract. They are necessary when sickness is accompanied by vomiting or loss of consciousness or when the gastrointestinal system requires rest. The extremity in which the IV is inserted is restrained on an armboard, and the insertion site is secured and covered. If the infant is on NPO status, a pacifier should be offered. Diversional therapy will prevent the child from focusing on the IV tubing and using it as a toy. The infant should be picked up, rocked, and played with.

IV pumps prevent a change in IV infusion rate when positions or activity change. The IV pump allows the administration of microdrops of IV solution so that a slow rate of infusion can be maintained. Adult IV sets administer 15 drops per 1 ml. Pediatric IV sets administer 60 drops per 1 ml. A burette is attached between the IV tubing and the pump and enables the nurse to fill the burette with the amount of solution to be administered in 1 hour (see Figure 22-18). The infusion pump sounds an alarm to alert the staff that the burette must be refilled; this allows the nurse to monitor the IV site hourly. The nurse observes the child hourly for the following:

- The rate of flow of the solution
- Swelling at the needle site
- Low volume in the bag or the need to refill the burette
- Pain or redness at the site of insertion
- Moisture at or around the site

An accurate I&O record is kept for all children receiving IV fluids. Nursing guidelines for IV therapy at various stages of development are described in Table 22-10.

Total Parenteral Nutrition

Total parenteral nutrition (TPN) is also known as *hyperalimentation* and provides the total nutritional needs for infants and children who cannot use the gastrointestinal tract for nourishment for a prolonged period (Figure 22-21). It allows highly concentrated solutions of proteins, glucose, and other nutrients to infuse directly into a large vessel such as the superior vena cava. In general, these concentrated solutions are not given through peripheral veins. The nursing responsibilities are similar to those for other IV infusions. The

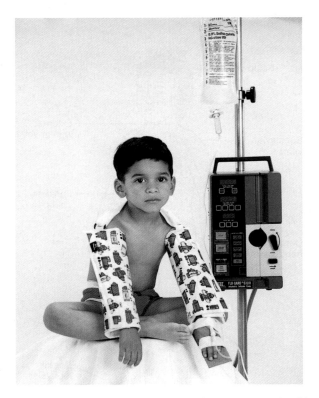

FIGURE **22-20** The armboard immobilizes the arm during IV therapy and permits movement.

solution is prepared by the pharmacist and is sterile. Monitoring vital signs, I&O, and laboratory reports are essential nursing responsibilities.

Hypoglycemia, hyperglycemia, and electrolyte imbalances can occur. Before discontinuing TPN therapy, the rate is *gradually* decreased, and the child monitored for adverse responses. Parents may need extensive teaching and return demonstrations if they are expected to care for their child receiving TPN treatment at home. Community agencies should be contacted to aid and support the family.

ADAPTATION OF SELECTED PROCEDURES TO CHILDREN

NUTRITION, DIGESTION, AND ELIMINATION

A gavage feeding may be ordered when an infant cannot take food or fluids by mouth but the gastrointestinal tract is functioning. A *gavage* feeding places nutrients directly into the stomach so that natural digestion can occur. This can be accomplished by placing a nasogastric tube into the stomach via the nose and securing it in place with tape or using the oral route, reinserting a new tube with each feeding. When long-term feeding is required, a gastrostomy may be performed and a tube inserted directly into the stomach (Figure 22-22).

Gastrostomy

A **gastrostomy** (*gastro*, "stomach" and *stoma*, "opening") is designed to introduce food directly into the stomach through the abdominal wall by means of a surgically placed tube or button (Box 22-5). It is used in infants or children who cannot have food by mouth because of anomalies or strictures of the esophagus or who are severely debilitated or in a coma. Cleansing of the skin around the tube prevents irritation from formula or gastric secretions. The nurse observes and reports vomiting or abdominal distention. Brown or green drainage may indicate that the tube has slipped through the pylorus into the duodenum. This could cause an obstruction and is reported immediately.

✴NURSING **TIP**

One way of determining fluid loss in infants is to weigh the dry diaper, mark the weight on the outside of the diaper, and then weigh the wet diaper. Subtract the weight of the dry diaper from the weight of the wet diaper, and record results on the I&O record. Include both urine and liquid stools (1 g = 1 ml of output).

Enema

Administering an enema to a child is essentially the same as for adults; however, the type, amount, and distance for inserting the tube require modifications. In addition, a child's bowel is more easily perforated under pressure. An isotonic solution (saline) is used in children. Tap water enemas are contraindicated. Plain water is hypotonic to the blood and could cause rapid fluid shift and overload if absorbed through the intestinal wall. The type of solution intended is always ascertained. Commercial enemas specific for the child may be used; however, some are not recommended for infants and children. The amount of fluid varies somewhat in procedure recommendations. The smaller the child, the less solution is used.

The exact amount for infants should be prescribed by the health care provider's order. Guidelines range from a low of 50 ml for infants to a high of 500 to 750 ml for the adolescent. The nurse consults the procedure manual for the institution's guidelines. The tube is inserted from 1 to 4 inches (0.4 to 1.6 cm) according to the size and age of the child. Infants and small children may be unable to retain the solution; therefore it may be necessary to hold the buttocks together for a short time.

RESPIRATION
Tracheostomy Care

A **tracheostomy** is a surgical procedure in which an opening is made in the trachea to enable the patient to breathe. This artificial airway may be necessary in emergency situations, may be an elective procedure, or may be combined with mechanical ventilation. Some of the childhood conditions that may require tracheostomy are acute epiglottitis, head injury, and burns. Nursing care is indispensable to the survival of the child, because blockage of the tube by mucus or other secretions can lead to suffocation. In many hospitals the child is placed in the intensive care unit immediately after surgery because this is a critical period that requires frequent suctioning and close observation. The child is placed on heart and respiratory monitors. When the child's condition stabilizes, the child is transferred to a general unit.

The child is placed in an area of high visibility. This is important because small children communicate their needs by crying and the tracheostomy prohibits vocalization. Whenever possible, one person is assigned to the child and to work with the parents. The nurse reinforces preoperative teaching and explains what happened; for example, "You were having a lot of trouble breathing. This operation is called a tracheostomy and helps you to breathe more easily. A small opening has been made in your neck. A hollow tube was inserted to

| table 22-10 | *Nursing Guidelines for Pediatric IVs at Various Stages of Development* | | |

DEVELOPMENTAL CHARACTERISTICS*	IV PLACEMENT (IDEAL SITES)	PREPARATION OF CHILD	FAMILY INVOLVEMENT
INFANT (FIRST YEAR)			
Infant is dependent on others for all needs. Needs to feel physically safe through close relationship with one care-giving person (usually the mother). Trust develops through needs being met consistently. Mistrust and anxiety develop when needs are met inconsistently. Stranger anxiety begins at approximately 6 to 8 months.	Scalp vein (best site); foot, hand, forearm	It is best not to feed infant immediately before IV insertion (vomiting and aspiration possible).	Prepare family about need for IV therapy, insertion procedure, appearance of infant with IV, and fluid needs. Encourage family to continue providing infant with tactile and verbal stimulation and tender, loving care. Demonstrate safe ways to hold an infant with an IV. Encourage questions and clarify misconceptions.
TODDLER (AGE 1 TO 3 YEARS)			
Discovers and explores self and surrounding world. Enjoys new mobility skills. Develops egocentric thinking and need for parallel play. Tolerates short separations from mother. Transitional objects (security blanket, special toy) provide some comfort. Oppositional syndrome ("no" stage). Separation anxiety is an important problem in hospitalized toddlers separated from mother (ages 8 to 24 months).	Hand, arm, foot. Important: From this age-group on, the less dominant extremity should be used for the IV whenever possible. Determine handedness before IV insertion.	Prepare child immediately before procedure (child has limited attention span and is likely to become more anxious if prepared sooner). Give very simple explanation in concrete terms. Show equipment to be used. Do not offer choice. See preparation for preschool age (below) and assess ability of each child to understand.	Prepare family about need for IV therapy, insertion procedure, and appearance of child with IV. Whether parents remain with the child during the procedure varies. If they stay with the child, their role is to comfort rather than to assist with restraining. Demonstrate to parents how to safely handle child with IV.
PRESCHOOL (AGE 4 TO 6 YEARS)			
Magical thinking, based on what the child would like to believe. Cannot always distinguish fantasy from reality. Fears intrusive procedures. Castration fears common. Develops conscience (guilt), while asserting independence and mastering new skills. Learning to share.	Hand, forearm (less dominant)	Prepare child just before procedure. Using small bottle, tubing, and doll or stuffed animal, explain in literal terms the need for IV and insertion procedure. Allow child to see and touch equipment. Explain how child can help with procedure by cleaning site, opening packages, taping, and so on. Allow some control in the situation. Say you will help child to hold still and that it is OK to cry.	As with toddlers, parents may or may not stay with the child during the procedure. If they stay, they should provide comfort and support, but they should not be asked to restrain the child for IV insertion. Reinforce the child's need for honest, simple explanations. Reassure parents that the child can still play and be active, even with the IV.

Modified from Guhlow, L.J., & Kolb, J. (1979). Pediatric IVs: Special measures you should take. *RN, 42,* 40. Published in RN, the full-service nursing journal. Copyright 1979 Medical Economics Company Inc, Oradell, NJ. Reprinted by permission.

IV, Intravenous line.

*Each stage builds on the earlier ones, and during hospitalization many children regress to behaviors appropriate to earlier levels of development.

†No child should be restricted to bed simply because of having an IV!

RELATED NURSING ACTIONS	PROTECTION OF IV SITE	MOBILITY CONSIDERATIONS†	SAFETY NEEDS
Restrain the infant during insertion. Comfort and cuddle during and after insertion. Observe carefully during insertion for problems of vomiting, aspiration, and so on. Firmly restrain the extremity with IV (see next column). Use of pacifier diminishes stress, especially for infants who are on NPO status.	IV may be secured with tape and is wrapped. Extremity may be restrained by using a small armboard or a sandbag.	Keep restraints as loose as possible to allow for motion. Release any restrained extremities hourly for range of motion (ROM). Mitten hands with cotton and Stockinette to prohibit infant from grasping the IV. Restraining all extremities is rarely necessary. Remember infant's need for sensory stimulation.	Maintain strict intake and output (I&O). Secure IV tubing out of range of kicking legs and flailing arms. Check restraints frequently for effectiveness and presence of adequate circulation.
Restraining the toddler for an IV usually requires more than one person. Reassure the child through verbal and tactile stimulation during procedure. Provide toys such as pegs to hammer for therapeutic expression of anger after procedure and throughout hospitalization.	See Infant (above). A securely anchored IV is essential for the normally active toddler. Even the best site protection will not remain effective unless it is coupled with close nursing supervision and distracting activities for the child.	Toddlers cope with the world and learn about it through action. Therefore minimum restraints should be used, and tying the child in bed is to be avoided. Parental presence during waking hours permits the child to be constantly supervised and makes restraints unnecessary in many cases. However, be careful to avoid setting up a situation in which the child associates parent's departure with punishment by restraint.	Child is unaware of danger at this age and will not know that movement of IV causes pain. Constant supervision is needed when the child is out of bed. Frequently remind the child not to touch the IV, but do not expect compliance. Distracting activities accomplish much more than does a scolding for handling the IV. Tape connections on tubing if the child continues to handle tubing. Keep tubing clamps out of reach.
Tell child IV is not being given as punishment. *Never* bribe or threaten with IVs (e.g., "Drink, or you'll get another IV.") Praise for cooperation or any efforts in that direction. Maintain patient privacy. Do not start an IV in view of other patients, visitors, or staff. Child needs support to cope with intrusiveness of this procedure. Show understanding.	See Infant (above). As with toddlers, securely anchored IVs are essential but inadequate unless coupled with close supervision and age-appropriate activities.	Preschoolers need maximum mobility to master surroundings. Provide a range of out-of-bed activities whenever possible.	Child will be curious about IV. Child is capable of understanding instructions to not touch it but needs frequent reminders. IV clamps should be out of reach or taped over. Constant supervision is needed when the child is out of bed. Child is liable to take off down the hall, heedless of pole, bottle, and so on. Short attention span limits duration of cooperation with instructions.

Continued

table 22-10 | *Nursing Guidelines for Pediatric IVs at Various Stages of Development—cont'd*

DEVELOPMENTAL CHARACTERISTICS*	IV PLACEMENT (IDEAL SITES)	PREPARATION OF CHILD	FAMILY INVOLVEMENT
SCHOOL AGE (AGE 7 TO 11 YEARS)			
Struggles between mastery of new skills and failure. Enjoys school, learning skills, games with rules. Needs to succeed. Fears body mutilation. May feel need to be brave. Can understand hospital rules. World now expanding beyond family. Peer group becomes important. Competitiveness.	Hand, forearm (less dominant)	Prepare child ahead of time but on same day of insertion. Carefully explain and demonstrate equipment and reasons for IV therapy, letting patient watch or help set up equipment. Ask child for questions about need for IV and procedure. Give child choices and let child help in procedure whenever possible. Tell child crying is OK because needles hurt, and you will help in holding still.	Whenever possible, family and child should be prepared together so that family can reinforce what the child has been told. Stress to the family the child's need for some independence in activities of daily living, even with an IV. Parental presence or participation in IV insertion may be appropriate, but child's preference should be considered primary.
ADOLESCENT (AGE 12 TO 18 YEARS)			
Vacillates between needs for independence and dependence. Adult cognitive abilities, deductive reasoning. Coping mechanisms: rationalization, intellectualization. Peer acceptance is very important. Egocentric, rebellious at times, especially against parents and authority figures. Very concerned with body image, body changes, sexuality, and role. Searching for "who I am."	Hand, forearm (less dominant)	Prepare patient several hours to a day before procedure, if possible. Needs time between preparation and insertion to absorb explanations and ask questions. For most adolescents, approach discussions on an adult level. Explain need for IV therapy and expected duration, and show equipment. May need much support for acceptance of therapy.	Explain therapy needs and duration as with patient. Decision regarding parental presence during procedure should be patient's, not parents'. Stress to family participation in decisions affecting child's care.

Modified from Guhlow, L.J., & Kolb, J. (1979). Pediatric IVs: Special measures you should take. *RN, 42,* 40. Published in RN, the full-service nursing journal. Copyright 1979 Medical Economics Company Inc, Oradell, NJ. Reprinted by permission.
IV, Intravenous line.
*Each stage builds on the earlier ones, and during hospitalization many children regress to behaviors appropriate to earlier levels of development.
†No child should be restricted to bed simply because of having an IV!

keep the area open. It is frightening not to be able to speak. When you are better, the hole will close by itself and your voice will return." An explanation of suction might be, "We have to keep the area in your neck open. This tube goes into the throat and clears it." The use of suction can be shown in a glass of water. The child is prepared for the unfamiliar sound. "You might feel like gagging, but afterward you will feel better. I know this is difficult for you and I'm sorry."

The nursing care of the child with a tracheostomy is a significant responsibility. The anatomical differences between children and adults and the small child's inability to communicate through writing increase the need for close observation. In addition, toddlers often have short, stubby necks that become easily irritated. It may be helpful to place a reminder on the intercom at the clerk's desk or in other suitable areas indicating that this patient cannot cry or speak. The nurse's touch and quiet voice and the presence of significant others help to make the child feel secure. Routines are incorporated by repeating familiar stories. A favorite article, such as a blanket or toy, is kept nearby. A supply of teaching aids and of dramatic play material is made available. Puppets are particularly valuable.

RELATED NURSING ACTIONS	PROTECTION OF IV SITE	MOBILITY CONSIDERATIONS†	SAFETY NEEDS
Approach child expecting cooperation (this age-group likes to please adults), but expect that child will need help holding still. Allow the child to clean the site with alcohol swab and to cut tape before insertion. Praise cooperative efforts. Give child step-by-step explanation of procedure as it progresses. Child may like to take some responsibility in keeping I&O.	Child will need less protection than younger children owing to interest in making IV work correctly. May naturally protect extremity with IV. Some children appreciate a warning sign—"Hands Off," on a piece of tape over the IV as a reminder. Use the child's natural curiosity and interest in learning. Tell child the rules of safe IV handling.	Show patient and family how to safely manipulate IV for out-of-bed activities (walking in hall with pole, keeping tubing out of wheelchair wheels, and so on).	Remind patient periodically about necessary caution with IV. Show patient the clamps and caution against handling them. Teach patient signs of IV problems. Enlist child's help in the interest of good compliance, but do not entirely depend on it. Tape tubing connections. Child may forget about IV. Emphasize need for caution in some activities, especially if play includes other children.
Be aware of IV adding to patient's dependency status and need for some control. Encourage child to keep own I&O, help in counting drip rate, and so on.	See School Age (above). If patient is very active, will need well-protected, well-anchored IV, because movements may be more forceful and strength may be greater than those of younger patients.	See School Age (above). Encourage mobility as much as possible as a means of independence for the adolescent.	Be aware of possibility of adolescent rebellion showing itself in lack of cooperation with therapy. These patients may rebel if feeling threatened and may be very manipulative in testing behaviors. Consistent limits, clearly communicated to patient, parents, and staff, are needed. Instruct patient about signs of infiltration, phlebitis, and so on.

Tracheostomy tube. Maintaining patency of the tracheostomy tube is of utmost importance. Plastic or Silastic tubes are generally used because they are flexible and reduce crust formation. They are lightweight and disposable, and most do not have inner cannulas. Cuffed tubes are not usually necessary in infants and small children, because their air passages are smaller and the tracheostomy tube provides a sufficient seal. The surgeon chooses a tracheostomy tube that is appropriate for the patient's neck size and condition. Administering oxygen by manual resuscitator (bagging) before or after the procedure helps to prevent hypoxia.

Suctioning. Selection of a suction catheter is important. The nurse chooses one that does not block the tube during suctioning. The diameter should be about half the size of the tracheostomy tube. Hands are washed before proceeding. The nurse uses sterile gloves for the procedure, and all equipment used in the care of a tracheostomy should be sterile. Suction is applied as the catheter is *withdrawn.* The tube is rotated to allow the removal of secretions on all sides. With Y-tube technique, suction is achieved by closing the port with the thumb. A drop of saline solution may be inserted before suctioning to aid in loosening secretions. Because variations in this procedure exist and modifications are often required, the nurse must understand what is intended for the particular patient and must ask for clarification of specific procedures of the institution.

Suctioning is done periodically and when necessary. Indications for suctioning include noisy breathing,

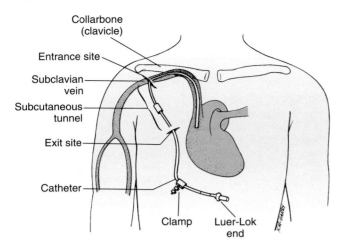

FIGURE **22-21** Catheter placement for total parenteral nutrition (TPN).

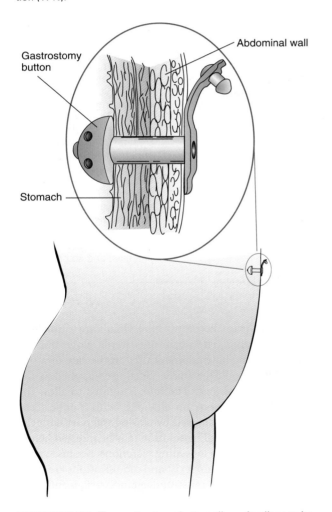

FIGURE **22-22** The gastrostomy button allows feedings to be administered directly into the stomach through the abdominal wall.

box 22-5   *Procedure for Gastrostomy Tube Feeding*

EQUIPMENT
- Tray, gloves
- Warmed formula
- Funnel or syringe barrel
- Syringe for aspiration
- 15 to 30 ml of water to flush tube as ordered

NOTE: Equipment should be sterile for preterm and newborn infants.

METHOD
1. Position child comfortably either flat or with head slightly elevated if not contraindicated. Provide pacifier to relax infant.
2. Check residual stomach contents by attaching syringe to gastrostomy tube and aspirating. If amount of residual is large (10 to 25 ml for newborns, over 50 ml for older children), replace residual and decrease present formula by equal amount or delay feeding for a short time. (This may vary according to the pediatrician's protocol.) Overloading the stomach can cause reflux and increases the danger of aspiration. If residual continues or increases, report this to the physician. If no residual is obtained, inject 2 to 5 ml of air into the tubing while listening via the stethoscope placed on the abdomen for a "whoosh" sound indicating that air has entered the stomach.
3. Attach the syringe barrel (if not already present for continuous infusion) to the gastrostomy tube. If the tube has more than one lumen, be sure to use the port labeled for *food or formula*. Fill with formula. Remove clamp. This prevents air from entering the stomach and causing distention.
4. Elevate the receptacle. Allow the formula to flow slowly by gravity—*force should not be used*.
5. Continue to add formula to the syringe before it empties completely (to prevent excess air from entering the tubing).
6. Clamp the tube as the final formula or water is passing through the lower part of the syringe. (NOTE: In infants, some physicians may prefer that the gastrostomy tube remain open at all times to produce a safety valve in the event that the infant vomits. In such cases, the tube is elevated above the patient's body.)
7. Whenever possible, hold the patient quietly after feeding. Reposition in Fowler's position or on right side to promote gastric emptying.
8. Record the type (gastrostomy feeding), the amount given, the amount and characteristics of residual, and how the child tolerated the procedure. Record input and output on the chart.

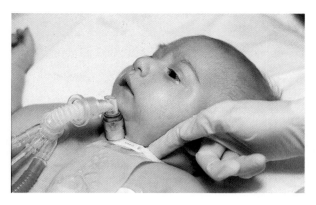

FIGURE **22-23** Tracheostomy. The tracheostomy ties should be snug but should allow one finger to be inserted to ensure that it is not too tight.

bubbling of mucus, and moist cough or respirations. Patients can rapidly become hypoxic during suctioning, and therefore it is limited to no more than 15 seconds. Two or three breaths for reoxygenation are allowed between suctioning. The depth of suctioning is important. In general, suctioning is limited to the length of the tracheostomy tube or slightly beyond to stimulate coughing. The catheter is cleared with sterile water between insertions. Unnecessary suctioning is avoided. The suction catheter is discarded after use. Disposing of water after suctioning prevents the growth of opportunistic organisms.

Tracheal stoma. The tracheal stoma is treated as a surgical wound. The area is kept free of secretions and exudate to minimize the risk of infection. Cotton-tipped applicators dipped in half-strength hydrogen peroxide and saline solution can be used to remove crusted mucus. Tapes around the child's neck should be loose enough to allow one finger to be easily inserted. The knot is placed to the side of the neck (Figure 22-23). The condition of the skin beneath the tape is assessed. The tape is changed as necessary. Two people are used for this procedure, one to hold the outer cannula and the other to change the tape. When feeding the infant, the nurse covers the tracheostomy with a bib or moist piece of gauze to prevent aspiration of food particles.

Observing for complications. The nurse observes the patient for symptoms such as restlessness, rising pulse rate, fatigue, apathy, dyspnea, sternal retractions, pallor, cyanosis, and inflammation or drainage around the incision. Possible complications include tracheoesophageal fistula, stenosis, tracheal ischemia, infection, atelectasis, cannula occlusion, and accidental extubation. Baseline monitoring of the patient is done on each shift and before suctioning. The patient's mental status, respirations, pulse rate and rhythm, and chest sounds are of particular importance. Accurate recording of observations is essential to evaluation. The time and frequency of suctioning, the character of secretions, the relief afforded the patient, the behavior, the appearance of the wound, and other pertinent data are recorded.

A sterile hemostat is kept at the bedside for emergency use. Accidental *extubation,* or expulsion of the tube, is uncommon but can occur from severe coughing if the tapes are too loose. Patency of the airway is maintained by spreading the edges of the wound with the sterile clamp until a duplicate sterile tube is inserted. An extra tracheostomy tube and the equipment needed for its replacement are always kept in a visible, easily reached area at the bedside for use in such emergencies. As the child's condition improves, he or she is weaned from the tube. The opening gradually closes by granulation. Children whose tubes must remain in place for a longer time may require periodic tube changes.

Additional nursing measures. Additional nursing measures include frequent changes of position, use of elbow restraints, oral feedings unless contraindicated, and careful bathing to prevent water from entering the tube. Range-of-motion exercises are a must for long-term patients, and in acute cases arm restraints are removed one at a time to allow for passive exercises. The diet is ordered by the health care provider. Although patients may initially have nothing by mouth, they progress to a soft or normal diet as the condition improves. The Fowler's position is preferred during feedings. The older child can cooperate by holding the head flexed with the chin down. This decreases swallowing difficulties, because the esophagus opens and the airway narrows.

Discharge. Certain patients are discharged with a tracheostomy. This is anticipated, and instruction and demonstration for the parents begin early. Parents who are comfortable with the procedure during hospitalization will feel more secure when the child returns home. Information about parent groups and visiting nurse and other referrals are made before discharge.

Oxygen Therapy

Box 22-6 reviews selected considerations for the child receiving oxygen. See Chapter 13 for care of a child in an incubator.

Safety considerations. All equipment used for oxygen therapy must be inspected periodically. Combustible materials and potential sources of fire are kept away from oxygen equipment. These materials are essentially the same as for adults; for the child, however, friction toys are also to be avoided because the sparks

box 22-6 *Selected Considerations for the Child Receiving Oxygen*

GENERAL CONSIDERATIONS

Signs of respiratory distress include an increase in pulse and respiration, restlessness, flaring nares, intercostal and substernal retractions, and cyanosis. In addition, children with dyspnea often vomit, which increases the danger of aspiration. Maintain a clear airway by suctioning if needed. Organize nursing care so that interruptions are kept at a minimum. Observe children carefully because vision may be obstructed by mist and young children are unable to verbalize their needs.

NEWBORN

Oxygen may be provided via hood, which may be used in the warming unit.

Oxygen may be provided via Isolette; keep sleeves closed to decrease oxygen loss.

Oxygen must be warmed to prevent neonatal stress from cold.

Analyze oxygen concentration carefully to avoid retrolental fibroplasia or pulmonary disease.

Parents are the primary focus of preparations; help to develop good parenting skills and self-confidence in their ability to care for the infant who is ill.

INFANT

Nose may need to be suctioned by bulb syringe to remove mucus.

Infant may benefit from use of infant seat; secure seat to bed frame, watch for slumping in seat.

Make sure crib sides are up; a canopy often gives the illusion of safety.

Avoid the use of baby oil, A and D ointment, petroleum jelly (Vaseline) or other oil- or alcohol-based substances.

Anticipate stranger anxiety at around 6 to 8 months of age; infant clings to parents and turns away from nurse.

An extremely irritable infant may benefit from comforting in parent's lap followed by sleeping in tent; clarify at report time.

Infants can often be removed from oxygen for bathing and eating; determine before proceeding.

TODDLER

Anticipate that a toddler will be distressed by a tent.

Anticipate regression.

When toddlers are restless and fussy, they may pull tent and covers apart.

Toddler cannot tell nurse if tent is too hot or too cold.

Change clothing and bed linen when damp.

Toddler may be comforted by a transitional object such as a blanket.

Parents may have suggestions as to how to keep toddler happy in the tent.

PRESCHOOL

Tent plastic distorts view.

Because thought processes are immature in preschool children, reality and fantasy are inseparable.

Prepare child for all procedures to decrease fear.

Anticipate that child will feel lonely and isolated.

Child will enjoy stories, puppets, and dramatic play.

If extremely restless and anxious, child may benefit from holding parent's hand through small opening in zippers.

It is helpful if the child can be out of the tent for meals.

SCHOOL AGE

School children usually are less frightened by the tent; fears center around body mutilation and loss of control.

Preparation information continues to focus on what the child will see, hear, feel, and be expected to do.

Child may benefit from writing a story about the experience; nurse reviews story with child and clarifies misconceptions; posting story on unit affirms child's self-esteem and mastery (always ask permission to post).

Allow child to make realistic choices before, during, and after procedures.

Draw "what it feels like to be in a tent" and discuss.

ADOLESCENT

Adolescent needs more time to process information and needs to know the results of blood studies and other tests.

Nurse remains available to the patient to answer questions as they arise.

Trust is extremely important as the adolescent attempts to move beyond the nuclear family.

Anticipate problems of being restricted by apparatus.

May feel weird when visited by peers; waivers between feeling self-confident and feeling ineffective.

Reiterate no smoking and other safety precautions with patient and peers.

Include patient in therapy; he or she may be able to manage own oxygen needs.

Review safe use of oxygen in the home if required for comfort and survival.

they can create could ignite. Nylon or wool blankets are not to be used. One should know where the nearest fire extinguisher is located. Parents are alerted to the precautions and to the presence of "no smoking" signs.

Infection control is extremely important. It is imperative that cross-infection via unclean equipment be prevented. Humidifiers and nebulizers, which are warm and moist, serve as an excellent medium for the growth of disease-producing organisms. Although most masks, tents, and cannulas that come into direct contact with the child are disposable, other pieces of mechanical equipment cannot be discarded. They require periodic cleansing if therapy is extended and terminal cleansing according to product direction. The respiratory therapy department should be contacted as necessary.

Prolonged exposure to high oxygen concentrations can be toxic to some body tissues (e.g., the retina in preterm infants and the lungs in the general population) but particularly in children with pulmonary diseases such as asthma or cystic fibrosis. It is therefore necessary to measure oxygen concentrations at regular intervals with an oxygen analyzer. This is usually done by the respiratory therapist; however, the nurse must ensure that the procedure is carried out on assigned patients. Readings are obtained close to the child's head. The amount of oxygen administered depends on the child's arterial oxygen concentration. Blood gas determinations (PO_2 and PCO_2) ensure safe and accurate therapy. Noninvasive pulse oximeters that measure blood oxygen tension via the skin are available (see Figure 13-6).

Oxygen is a dry gas and requires the addition of moisture to prevent irritation of the respiratory tract. High-humidity concentrations may be achieved by the use of jet humidifiers on several oxygen units. Compressed air rather than oxygen may also be used for this purpose. *Oxygen therapy is terminated gradually.* This allows the patient to adjust to *ambient* (environmental) oxygen. The nurse slowly reduces liter flow, opens air vents in Isolettes, or opens zippers in croup tents. The child's response is closely monitored. An increase in restlessness and in pulse and respirations indicates that the child is not tolerating withdrawal from the oxygen-enriched environment.

Methods of administration. Oxygen is administered to children as age appropriate via Isolette, nasal cannula, mask, hood, or tent. Regardless of the method used, the child is observed frequently to determine the effectiveness of the oxygen therapy. The desired goals include decreased restlessness and improved breathing, vital signs, and color. High concentrations of oxygen can be delivered by way of a plastic hood (see Figure 13-5). Warmed, humidified oxygen is delivered directly over the child's head. It may be used in a warming unit.

Mist tent. A mist tent (Figure 22-24) provides an atmosphere of fine particles of water suspended in a cool air or oxygen environment. The zippered openings in the clear plastic canopy facilitate easy access and observation of the child. A nebulizer can be attached to provide medicated inhalation therapy. The child should be dressed warmly when inside the tent to prevent hypothermia. The oxygen concentration should be checked periodically, and a pulse oximeter assessment of oxygen saturation should be monitored.

A physician's order often reads "keep O_2 saturation at 93%." This means that if the O_2 saturation on the pulse oximeter reads above 93%, the oxygen liter flow can be lowered and the child carefully monitored. If the O_2 saturation level reads below 93%, the liter flow can be gradually increased and the child closely monitored until the reading reaches 93% (see Chapter 13 for pulse oximeter). A parent at the bedside stroking the infant through the zippered opening in the canopy can have a calming effect. Keeping a child dry in a high-humidity tent can be a challenge. Frequent linen and clothing changes are essential.

Low-flow oxygen. Low-flow oxygen is a method of oxygen delivery used for children with chronic lung disease (e.g., cystic fibrosis) who are oxygen dependent for prolonged periods. These children react poorly to high oxygen concentrations. Approximately 1 or 2 liters per minute of oxygen are administered via nasal cannula or a "blow-by" catheter that is placed on the upper lip just below the nostrils (Figure 22-25). Because this type of oxygen delivery is used for prolonged periods, parent teaching concerning home management is a nursing responsibility.

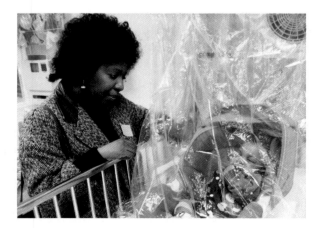

FIGURE **22-24** This infant is in an infant seat to maintain Fowler's position while in a mist tent. This method of oxygen administration allows the parent and child to see each other.

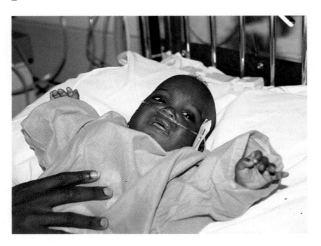

FIGURE **22-25** Child receiving blow-by oxygen therapy via nasal catheter. The prongs may be placed below (blow-by) or in the nares, and the loop is slipped over the ears to stabilize the position. The cannula can be taped to the side of the child's face to prevent slipping.

Management of Airway Obstruction

An emergency treatment known as the *Heimlich maneuver* is recommended to dislodge food or foreign bodies from the airway. This technique works on the principle that forcing the diaphragm up causes residual air in the lung to be forcefully expelled, resulting in popping the obstruction out of the airway.

Older child standing or sitting. The nurse stands behind the standing or sitting victim and wraps the arms around the victim's waist, with one hand made into a fist (Figure 22-26). The thumb side rests against the victim's abdomen, slightly above the navel and well below the tip of the sternum (xiphoid process). The fist is grasped with the other hand and pressed into the victim's abdomen with a quick upward thrust. From 6 to 10 thrusts may be necessary to dislodge the object. Each thrust should be a separate and distinct movement. The child may be placed in a side-lying position for the recovery phase.

Older child lying down (conscious or unconscious). The child is positioned on his back. The nurse kneels at the child's feet if the child is on the floor or stands at the child's feet if the child is on a table. The heel of one hand is placed on the child's abdomen in the midline, slightly above the navel and well below the rib cage. The fist is grasped with the other hand and pressed into the victim's abdomen with a quick upward thrust. The 6 to 10 thrusts are repeated as needed. Thrusts are directed upward into the midline and not to either side of the abdomen. The smaller the child, the gentler the procedure.

Infant. The nurse should determine airway obstruction. If the object is visualized, it is removed, trying not to push the object deeper into the throat. If this approach is unsuccessful, the infant is positioned prone with the head lower than the trunk. Support the head and neck with one hand and straddle the infant face down over the forearm, which is supported on the nurse's thigh (see Figure 22-26). Resting the infant on the thigh, the nurse performs five forceful back blows between the shoulder blades with the heel of one hand. After delivering the back blows, the free hand is placed on the infant's back so that he or she is sandwiched between the two hands; the infant is then turned on his or her back, with the head still lower than the trunk. Five thrusts are delivered in the midsternal region in the same manner as for external chest compressions, but at a slower rate (3 to 5 seconds). This is repeated until the foreign body is expelled. The nurse should not perform abdominal thrusts because this may cause injury to the infant's abdominal organs. Conventional cardiopulmonary resuscitation (CPR) can be initiated when the airway is cleared. Because all student nurses are required to have basic CPR certification, the technique is not reviewed at this time.

PREOPERATIVE AND POSTOPERATIVE CARE

Children are particularly fearful of surgery and require both physical and psychological preparation at the child's level of understanding. Listening to the child is especially valuable to clarify misunderstandings. The child is asked to point to the operative site on a body outline. "Show me what they are going to fix." Anesthesia is explained and the child allowed to play with a mask (Figure 22-27). Children and adults need reassurance.

Nursing interventions after surgery are aimed at assisting the child to master a threatening situation and minimizing physical and psychological complications. Tables 22-11 and 22-12 summarize preparation for surgery and postoperative care. Parents are included in all aspects of preoperative and postoperative care.

When adults are prepared for surgery, they are usually kept on NPO status from the midnight before the scheduled surgery date. The surgery may be done in the morning or afternoon. Infants should not be maintained on NPO status for longer than 4 to 6 hours because of the high risk for dehydration. It is a nursing responsibility to check that the test procedure or surgery is scheduled as early as possible in the morning to avoid a prolonged wait. Pacifiers should be provided to infants who are on NPO status to meet their developmental need for sucking.

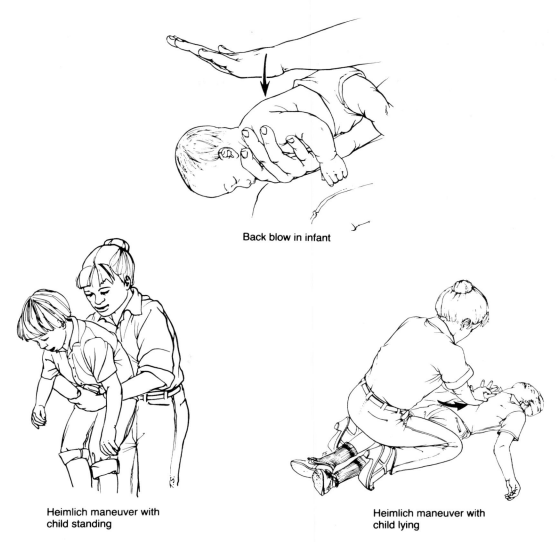

Back blow in infant

Heimlich maneuver with
child standing

Heimlich maneuver with
child lying

FIGURE **22-26** Procedures for clearing an airway obstruction.

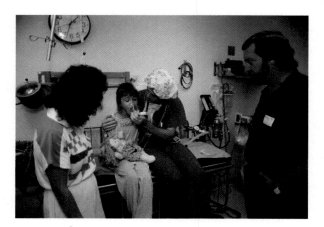

FIGURE **22-27** Preparing the child for the sights and sounds
of surgery. The parents may be present during early induction
of anesthesia to relieve anxiety during the preoperative period.

| table 22-11 | *Comparative Summary of Preparation of the Adult and Child for Surgery* | | |

PROCEDURE	ADULT	CHILD	MODIFICATION
Consent	Yes	Yes	Parent or legal guardian
Blood work	Yes	Yes	Age-appropriate restraint
Urinalysis	Yes	Yes	Age-appropriate collection (U-bag) Assist school child Age-appropriate instructions
Evaluate for respiratory infection, nutritional status	Yes	Yes	Use more objective observations in infants and toddlers because of child's limited verbal skills
Allergies	Yes	Yes	Indicate clearly on chart
Nothing by mouth (NPO)	Yes	Yes	Increase fluids before NPO Length of time may vary with age and type of surgery (4 to 12 hours) If surgery is late, place appropriate notice on child: "Do not feed me" Remove "goodies" from bedside stand No gum or hard candy Supervise hungry ambulatory patients carefully
Vital signs	Yes	Yes	Approach child carefully, explain, demonstrate Allow more time
Void before surgery	Yes	Preferred	Not always possible in infants and toddlers
Bath	Yes	Yes	Hospital gown, may wear underwear or pajama bottoms depending on age, type of surgery
Identification	Yes	Yes	ID bracelet
Teeth	Yes	Yes	Check for loose teeth, orthodontic appliance
Skin preparation	Yes	Possible	May be done in operating room
Nails	Yes	Yes	Trim, remove nail polish
Glasses or contact lenses	Yes	Yes	Have children and adolescents remove glasses or contact lenses
Enemas	Possible	Possible	Not routine
Transportation	Yes	Yes	Crib or stretcher Parents may accompany to operating room door
Emotional preparation	Yes	Yes	Preoperative tour Group and individual puppet play Body drawings of parts involved Play selected by child as mode of expression Support parents during surgery
Sedation	Yes	Yes	Usually 20 minutes before surgery
Record all pertinent data	Yes	Yes	Essentially the same with pediatric modifications as indicated by the above

table 22-12 | *Comparative Summary of Postoperative Care of the Adult and Child*

PROCEDURE	ADULT	CHILD	MODIFICATION
Return from recovery room	Yes	Yes	Notify parents Smaller patients generally in crib Age-appropriate safety precautions
Note general condition, alertness	Yes	Yes	Infant and toddler cannot verbalize fear or pain
Vital signs	Yes	Yes	Every 15 to 30 minutes until stable Blood pressure is sometimes omitted for infant
Evaluate for shock	Yes	Yes	Essentially the same
Assess operative site for bleeding, dressing intactness	Yes	Yes	Essentially the same Elevate casted extremities Circle drainage
Restraints	Possible	Probable	May be necessary to protect IV Remove periodically for range of motion
Connect dependent drainage (urinary catheter, nasogastric tubes, oxygen)	Yes	Yes	Prepare child for sight and noises of equipment, draw pictures to clarify purpose
Position patient	Yes	Yes	Prop on side unless contraindicated, no pillow
Intravenous (IV)	Yes	Yes	Should have pediatric adapting device and infusion pump Monitor rate meticulously, because infants and small children respond quickly to fluid shifts Measure and record intake and output
Assess elimination	Yes	Yes	Bowel and bladder
Relief of pain	Yes	Yes	Hold, comfort small children unless contraindicated Be sensitive to behavioral changes such as increase in irritability, crying, regression, nail biting, passivity, withdrawal Administer pain relievers Involve parents in care Provide transitional object such as blanket, favorite toy, pacifier Be aware of transcultural considerations that provide familiarity and comfort
Nothing by mouth (NPO)	Yes	Yes	Until fully awake Infants are started on clear fluids by bottle unless contraindicated Avoid brown or red liquids, which may be confused with old or fresh blood Monitor bowel sounds
Consider diet	Yes	Yes	Advance from clear to full liquids to soft to regular diet
Observe for complications	Yes	Yes	Turn, cough, deep-breathe; dangle feet; ambulate early; less of a problem in children Splint operative site with hands when child coughs

key points

- The nurse must be especially conscious of safety measures on the children's unit, particularly the following: keeping crib sides up when the child is unattended, careful application of restraints, safe transport, and proper identification of the child.
- The parents are included in both planning and implementing care. Children are prepared for and encouraged to express their feelings about treatments.
- Weights must be accurate because medication is often calculated according to the child's weight.
- The correct-size blood pressure cuff must be used for children to obtain an accurate reading. It should cover two-thirds of the upper arm.
- Special urine collection devices are used for newborns and infants.
- Proper positioning of the child for jugular and femoral puncture is important. Because these are large veins, the infant is frequently checked for bleeding after these procedures.
- Medications for children must be adapted to size, age, and body surface. The absorption, distribution, metabolism, and excretion of drugs differ substantially in children. Their reactions to drugs are less predictable.

- The recommended IM injection site for children under age 3 years is the vastus lateralis.
- Careful observation of the child receiving IV fluids is necessary because overload of fluids in an infant can lead to cardiac failure. IV pumps such as the IVAC pump are used to monitor infusions. Intake and output sheets must be accurate.
- When administering eardrops to children under 3 years of age, the pinna of the ear is pulled down and back to straighten the ear canal. In the older child, the pinna of the ear is pulled up and back.
- The nurse must monitor the rate of the IV flow, refill the burettes, observe the condition of the IV site, and assess the response of the child hourly.
- A pacifier should be offered to infants whose status is NPO (nothing by mouth).
- Weighing a wet diaper and subtracting the dry weight of a similar diaper is one method of recording the output of infants.

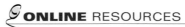

ONLINE RESOURCES

Electronic Medical Library: http://www.statref.com
Pediatric Information: http://www.drgreene.com
Trauma Information: http://www.trauma.org

REVIEW QUESTIONS   *Choose the most appropriate answer.*

1. Which of the following approaches is best when administering an oral medication to a young child?
   1. "Would you please take your medicine now, David?"
   2. "Look how good Johnny took his medication. Can you do that too, David?"
   3. "You must take your medicine now if you want to get better."
   4. "It's time for your medication, David. Would you like water or juice after it?"

2. The preferred site for an intramuscular injection in infants is:
   1. Dorsogluteal
   2. Ventrogluteal
   3. Vastus lateralis
   4. Deltoid

3. The physician orders 10 mg of Demerol for an infant after surgery. The label reads, 50 mg/1 ml. You would administer:
   1. 2.0 ml
   2. 0.8 ml
   3. 0.5 ml
   4. 0.2 ml

4. When preparing an enema for a young child, the nurse would select which of the following solutions?
   1. Tap water
   2. Saline
   3. Oil retention
   4. Fleet's solution

5. The best method to reduce the pain of a scheduled injection for a pediatric patient is to:
   1. Administer oral analgesics before the scheduled time of injection
   2. Use distraction techniques such as music
   3. Apply topical medication, such as EMLA, before the scheduled time of injection
   4. Reassure the child that it won't hurt for very long

23 The Child with a Sensory or Neurological Condition

objectives

1. Define each key term listed.
2. Discuss the prevention and treatment of ear infections.
3. Outline the nursing approach to serving the hearing-impaired child.
4. Discuss the cause and treatment of amblyopia.
5. Compare the treatment of paralytic and nonparalytic strabismus.
6. Review the prevention of eyestrain in children.
7. Discuss the functions of the 12 cranial nerves and nursing interventions for dysfunction.
8. Describe the symptoms of meningitis in a child.
9. Discuss the various types of epilepsy and the nursing responsibilities during a seizure.
10. Describe four types of cerebral palsy and the nursing goals involved in care.
11. Outline the prevention, treatment, and nursing care for the child with a Reye's syndrome.
12. Formulate a nursing care plan for the child with a decreased level of consciousness.
13. Prepare a plan for success in the care of a mentally retarded child.
14. Describe three types of posturing that may indicate brain damage.
15. Describe signs of increased intracranial pressure in a child.
16. Describe the components of a "neurological check."
17. State a method of determining level of consciousness in an infant.
18. Identify the priority goals in the care of a child who experienced near-drowning.

key terms

amblyopia (ăm-blē-Ō-pē-ă, p. 540)
athetosis (ăth-ē-TŌ-sĭs, p. 554)
aura (ĀW-ră, p. 549)
clonic movement (p. 549)

concussion (p. 559)
dyslexia (p. 540)
encephalopathy (ĕn-sĕf-ă-LŎP-ă-thē, p. 542)
enucleation (ē-nū-klē-Ā-shŭn, p. 542)
epicanthal folds (p. 539)
extensor posturing (p. 560)
flexor posturing (p. 560)
generalized seizures (p. 549)
grand mal (p. 549)
hyperopia (hī-pĕr-Ō-pē-ă, p. 540)
idiopathic (ĭd-ē-ō-PĂTH-ĭk, p. 549)
intracranial pressure (ICP) (p. 542)
ketogenic diet (p. 553)
mental retardation (p. 557)
myringotomy (mĭr-ĭng-GŎT-ō-mē, p. 536)
neurological check (p. 542)
nystagmus (nĭs-TĂG-măs, p. 548)
opisthotonos (ō-pĭs-THŎT-ō-nŏs, p. 546)
otoscope (p. 534)
papilledema (păp-ĭl-ă-DĒ-mă, p. 548)
paroxysmal (păr-ŏk-SĬZ-măl, p. 549)
partial seizures (p. 552)
petit mal (p. 549)
postictal (pōst-ĬK-tăl, p. 549)
posturing (p. 560)
sepsis (SĔP-sĭs, p. 545)
shaken baby syndrome (p. 560)
sign language (p. 538)
status epilepticus (p. 553)
strabismus (stră-BĬZ-mĕs, p. 540)
tonic movement (p. 549)

THE EARS

The ear, which can be considered a part of the nervous system, contains the receptors of the eighth cranial (acoustic) nerve. The ear performs two main functions: hearing and balance. Figure 23-1 summarizes ear, eye, and neurological differences between children and adults. The three divisions of the ear are the external ear, the middle ear, and the inner ear (Figure 23-2). In the newborn the tympanic membrane is almost horizontal

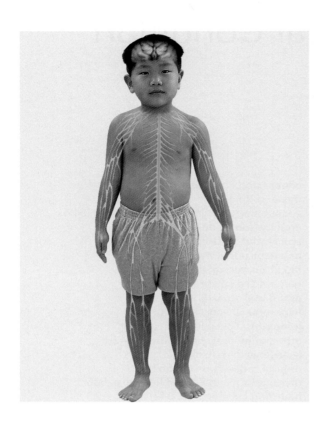

EARS

- The eustachian tube in infants is shorter, wider, and straighter than in older children and adults, and this may contribute to infections.
- In newborns and young infants, the walls of the ear canal are pliable because of underdeveloped cartilage and bony structures.

EYES

- Infants' eyes may occasionally cross until about 6 weeks of life.
- Tears are scant or absent for the first 2 to 4 weeks of life.

NERVOUS SYSTEM

- Brain and nerve cell growth and specialization are most rapid from birth until about 4 years of age.
- The suture lines and fontanels of the infant allow for molding during birth and also help compensate for increases in intracranial pressure.
- By the end of the first year, the brain has increased in weight about $2^1/_2$ times. Brain growth is almost complete by 2 years of age. Measuring head circumference in infants helps determine neurologic growth.
- Myelinization of nerve tracts in the central nervous system accelerates after birth and follows the cephalocaudal and proximodistal sequence. This allows for progressively more complex neurological and motor functions.

FIGURE **23-1** Summary of ear, eye, and neurological differences between the child and the adult.

and is more vascular than in the adult. It has a dull and opaque appearance and an inconsistent light reflex. The eustachian tube is shorter and straighter in the infant than in the adult. Three functions of the eustachian tube are *ventilation* of the middle ear, *protection* from nasopharyngeal secretions and sound pressure, and *drainage*. Middle-ear infections are common during early childhood.

When nurses examine the ear, they observe both the exterior and the interior. Ear alignment is observed. The top of the ear should cross an imaginary line drawn from the outer canthus of the eye to the occiput (see Figure 12-6). Low-set ears may be associated with kidney disorders and mental retardation. The outer ear and the area around it are inspected for cleanliness and

drainage. The inner ear is examined with an otoscope. One method of restraint used when assisting with the examination of the inner ear is to lay the child on a table with the arms held alongside the head, which is turned to the side. Another method of positioning a child for an ear examination is placing the child in the lap of the adult (see Figure 22-5).

NURSING **TIP**

Before instilling ear drops in *infants,* gently pull the pinna of the ear *down and back.* In *children,* gently pull the pinna of the ear *up and back* to straighten the external auditory canal.

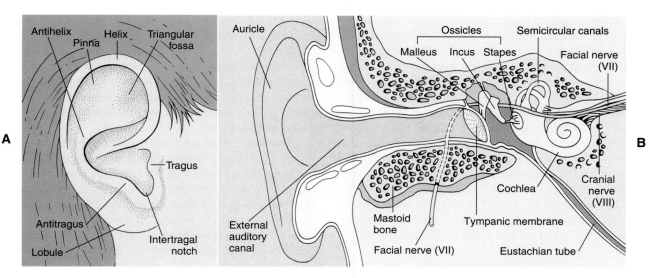

FIGURE **23-2** Anatomy of the ear. **A,** The normal external ear—the auricle (pinna) and tragus—is shown with common landmarks labeled. **B,** There are three divisions of the ear: the outer ear, the middle ear, and the inner ear. In the newborn the mastoid process and bony part of the external canal are not fully developed, leaving the *tympanic membrane* vulnerable to injury. Newborns can hear as soon as amniotic fluid is drained by the first sneeze. In infants the *eustachian tube* is shorter, wider, and straighter than in adults. Pooling of fluids such as milk in the throat of an infant who falls asleep with a bottle of milk can contribute to ear infections. The eustachian tube connects the middle ear and the pharynx and serves to vent the middle ear. The external auditory canal is more angulated (curved) in infants, and therefore pulling the pinna (auricle) is required to straighten the canal for an accurate tympanic temperature.

OTITIS EXTERNA

An acute infection of the external ear canal is called *otitis externa* and is often referred to as *swimmer's ear* because prolonged exposure to moisture is often the precipitating factor. Pain and tenderness on manipulating the pinna or tragus of the ear are specific signs of this type of infection (see Figure 23-2). The ear canal may be erythematous, but the tympanic membrane is normal. A foreign body, cellulitis, diabetes mellitus, or herpes zoster should be ruled out. Irrigation and topical antibiotics or antivirals are the treatment of choice. The health care provider may insert a loose cotton gauze (wick) into the outer third of the ear canal. The wick is kept moist with frequent drops of the appropriate medicated solution.

ACUTE OTITIS MEDIA (AOM)

Pathophysiology. Otitis media (*ot,* "ear," *itis,* "inflammation of," and *media,* "middle") is an inflammation of the middle ear. The middle ear is a tiny cavity in the temporal bone. Its entrance is guarded by the sensitive tympanic membrane, or eardrum, which transmits sound waves through the "oval window" to the inner ear, which contains the organs of hearing and balance. The middle ear opens into air spaces, or sinuses, in the mastoid process of the temporal bone. It is also connected to the throat by a channel called the eustachian tube. These structures—the mastoid sinuses, the middle ear, and the eustachian tube—are lined by mucous membranes. As a result, an infection of the throat can easily spread to the middle ear and mastoid. The eustachian tube also protects the middle ear from nasopharyngeal secretions, provides drainage of middle ear secretions into the nasopharynx, and equalizes air pressure between the middle ear and the outside atmosphere. These protective functions are diminished when the tubes are blocked. Unequalized air pressure within the ear creates a negative pressure that allows organisms to be swept up into the eustachian tube.

Otitis media occurs most often after an upper respiratory tract infection and usually affects children between 6 and 24 months of age and in early childhood. It is caused by various organisms, of which *Streptococcus pneumoniae* and *Hemophilus influenzae* are the most common.

Infants are more prone to middle-ear infections than are older children and adults because their eustachian tubes are shorter, wider, and straighter. When infants lie flat for long periods, microorganisms have easy access from the eustachian tube to the middle ear. Feeding methods may have a bearing on middle ear infection when the pooling of fluids, such as milk in the throat of an infant who falls asleep with a bottle of milk, provides a source for growth of organisms. The infant's *humoral* (*humor,* "body fluid") defense mechanisms are immature. Children in passive smoking environments have more respiratory infections because of the effect of secondary smoke on the protective cilia that line the nose. Day care attendance can contribute to the risk of upper respiratory infections and otitis media because of increased exposure to ill children.

> ⚡**NURSING TIP**
> Signs and symptoms of ear infection can include the following:
> - Rubbing or pulling at the ear
> - Rolling the head from side to side
> - Hearing loss
> - Loud speech
> - Inattentive behavior
> - Articulation problems
> - Speech development problems

Manifestations. The symptoms of otitis media are pain in the ear, which is often very severe; irritability; and diminished hearing. Fever, which may be as high as 40° C (104° F), headache, vomiting, diarrhea, and febrile convulsions may also occur. Earaches in infants may be manifested by general irritability, frequent rubbing or pulling at the ear, and rolling of the head from side to side. The older child can point to the place that is tender. Visualization of the tympanic membrane via otoscope reveals a reddened and bulging membrane.

If an abscess forms, a rupture of the eardrum may result, and drainage from the ear may be evident. When this happens, the pressure is relieved and the child is more comfortable. Some amount of hearing loss may result from the rupture. Otitis media is considered chronic if the condition persists for more than 3 months. Recurrent attacks can lead to serious complications. Chronic otitis media can lead to *cholesteatoma* (*chole,* "bile," *steato,* "fat," and *oma,* "tumor"), a cystlike sac filled with keratin debris. This may occlude the middle ear and erode adjacent ossicle bones, causing hearing loss. This

condition is best treated by an otolaryngologist. Complications of repeated attacks of acute otitis media can include the development of chronic otitis media with effusion (fluid accumulation). Hearing loss can result. Treatment may be indicated because hearing loss may impair cognitive and language development that can hamper the education and communication abilities in developing children.

Treatment. When an infection is evident, treatment is directed toward finding the causative organism and relieving the symptoms. A throat culture may be taken to determine the specific organism. Broad-spectrum antibiotics may be given orally and should be continued until the prescribed amount of medication has been taken. Analgesics are given to relieve pain. Antihistamines and decongestants are not effective in treating acute otitis media.

> ⚡**NURSING TIP**
> Instruct caregivers that the child's condition may improve dramatically after antibiotics are taken for few days. To prevent recurrence, caregivers must continue to administer the medication until the prescribed amount has been completed.

Surgical treatment. Surgical intervention may be necessary when medical treatment is unsuccessful. The physician may incise the tympanic membrane to relieve pressure and to prevent a tear by spontaneous rupture. This is called a myringotomy (*myringa,* "eardrum" and *otomy,* "incision of"). A *tympanic (TM)* button or tympanostomy ventilating tube (PE, pressure equalizer) may be inserted. This may fall out spontaneously within 6 to 12 months. In some children, the tubes may need to be reinserted to continue ventilation. Care is taken to avoid getting water in the ears while bathing or showering. All children should be followed up to make sure that the condition is resolved and to evaluate any hearing loss that may have occurred.

Comfort measures. Antipyretics may be given to reduce fever and a warm compress may be applied locally as comfort measures. If the eardrum has ruptured, the child is placed on the affected side. Cold may also be beneficial. An ice pack may be prescribed to reduce edema and pressure. The skin around the ears must be kept clean and protected from any drainage to prevent tissue breakdown. Parents are instructed not to insert cotton swabs into the ears.

HEARING IMPAIRMENT

Pathophysiology. Approximately 1 in 1000 newborns is born with some type of hearing impairment. This number may increase to 2 in 1000 for hearing loss occurring during childhood. Hearing-impaired children present special challenges to the health care team. Hearing loss can affect speech, language, social and emotional development, and behavior and academic achievement. The nurse should have a basic understanding of how to approach and work with a hearing-impaired child.

The inner ear is fully formed during the early months of prenatal life. If an expectant mother contracts German measles or other viral infection during this period, the child may be born with a hearing loss; this is termed *congenital deafness.* Deafness can also be *acquired.* Infectious diseases such as measles, mumps, chickenpox, or meningitis, can result in various degrees of hearing loss. The common cold, some medications, exposure to loud noise levels, certain allergies, and ear infections may also be responsible. Hearing problems can also be temporary if they are caused by cerumen (wax) accumulation. Some rattles and squeaky toys can emit sounds as loud as 110 decibels. (Above 80 decibels can cause damage.) These types of toys should not be held close to the infant's ear.

Early diagnosis and treatment of hearing-impaired children are important to prevent adverse physical and mental complications from developing. Members of the health care team concerned with the child who is hearing impaired include the physician, otologist (ear specialist), audiologist, speech therapist, specially trained teacher, social worker, psychologist, school nurse, and members of the child's family.

The various degrees of hearing loss range from a complete *bilateral* loss (which affects both ears) to a loss so mild that the problem is never recognized. Hearing loss can result from defects in the transmission of sound to the middle ear, from damage to the auditory nerve or ear structures, or from a mixed hearing loss that involves both a defect in nerve pathways and interference with sound transmission. If hearing loss is complete, the child misses all the pleasures of sound and has difficulty in communication (children learn to talk by imitating what they hear). Behavior problems may arise because these children do not understand directions. They may become aggressive with other children in their attempt to communicate. If they are ridiculed by playmates, personality development will be affected. Unless these children are helped early in life, they may become socially isolated.

Partial bilateral deafness may be responsible for behavior problems and poor progress in school. It is most commonly caused by chronic ear infections, such as otitis media, or by blockage of the eustachian tube. Children who have hearing losses in one ear are less affected if hearing in the other ear is normal.

NURSING **TIP**

When addressing a hearing-impaired child, the nurse should do the following:
- Be at eye level with the child.
- Be face-to-face with the child.
- Establish eye contact.
- Talk in short sentences.
- Avoid using exaggerated lip or face movement.

Diagnosis and treatment. The American Academy of Pediatrics recommends a goal of universal detection of hearing impairment in infants before 3 months of age, with interventions started no later than 6 months of age to minimize problems with growth and development. The *evoked otoacoustic emissions (OAE)* test is a preferred method for neonatal testing. The *brainstem auditory evoked response (BAER)* test records brain wave responses generated by the auditory system. These tests are easily administered to the newborn infant, and many hospitals routinely screen newborns for hearing ability before discharge. Lack of response by the infant to sounds, music, or the *startle reflex* in infants under 4 months of age are the first signs that may alert the parents or nurse to the possibility of hearing impairment. Early diagnosis and prompt treatment are primary requisites, regardless of the child's age. Complete bilateral deafness is usually discovered during infancy. Partial deafness may be unrecognized until the child begins school. Many hearing problems are detected by the school nurse administering standard hearing tests.

Tympanometry measures ear pressure but is difficult to perform adequately on an active infant or small child. A tuning fork is used to evaluate for air conduction (Rinne test) or bone conduction (Weber test). This type of test requires the child to be cooperative and able to communicate what is heard or felt. Diagnosis of hearing loss can be confirmed by a Visual Reinforcement Audiometry (VRA), which identifies sensitivity to sounds in young infants.

Many hearing defects are amenable to medical or surgical treatment. Hearing aids can amplify sound waves. Surgically placed *cochlear implants* are used for some children with nerve damage. Children who suffer a severe loss of hearing need more extensive help from personnel at an auditory training center. These children must begin treatment as soon as the hearing loss is discovered.

Nursing care. Various methods are used to bring the child into the world of sound. Lip reading, sign language, writing, visual aids, and amplified sound are but a few examples. The parents are instructed in means of communication that coincide with those used by the teachers.

The nurse must be aware of the symptoms of deafness in the child. Newborns are observed for their response to auditory stimuli. The Brazelton Neonatal Behavioral Assessment Scale evaluates the infant's orientation response to the sound of a voice (see p. 287). The persistence of the Moro reflex beyond 4 months of age may also be an indication of deafness. The infant who makes no verbal attempts by 18 months of age should undergo a complete physical examination. Indifference to sound, behavior problems, or poor school performance may also be signs of deafness. The nurse inquires into the facilities that are available in the community for such a child.

The hearing-impaired child in the hospital needs the same opportunities to communicate as the child who does not have this disability. The nurse smiles when approaching the child. Body language communicates a lot, especially if there is a severe communication problem. The nurse faces the child when speaking and is positioned at eye level with the child. The nurse must ensure that the child sees him or her before touching to avoid startling the child. Sign language is the use of hand signals that correspond to words and assist in communication with a deaf child. Previously developed speech patterns may regress during hospitalization. Visual aids, writing, or drawing can be used to enhance communication.

If a hearing aid is indicated, the child is equipped with one and taught how to use it. Regular checkups ensure that the hearing aid is working properly. A hearing aid is expensive and invaluable to the child. It is put in a safe place when not in use. When the child goes to surgery, it is given to the parents or placed in the hospital safe. The pockets of hospital gowns are checked before the gowns are placed in the laundry.

The National Hearing Aid Center provides information about hearing aids. Hearing aids are designed to fit in the ear, behind the ear, on eyeglass frames, or on the body with wires to the ear. The nurse should check ear hygiene and be sure hairs are not caught on the end of the hearing aid to ensure a proper fit and to minimize noise and whistling problems. Teaching safe battery handling and storage and promoting self-care are important nursing responsibilities.

Home care of the hearing-impaired child should include speech therapy. Flashing lights should be installed in the home to alert the child to doorbells and other sound-based devices. Telecommunication devices for the deaf (TDD) are available to enable telephone communication. Closed captioning devices for television are available to the child who can read.

The school nurse can help the family nurture socialization skills. Some hearing-impaired children attend special schools for the deaf, and some are mainstreamed into the general school population. Each hearing-impaired child and each family unit should be followed by the multidisciplinary health care team.

> ### NURSING TIP
> Emphasize to parents the need to supervise the care and storage of hearing aid batteries to prevent accidental ingestion. When inserting the ear piece of a hearing aid, be sure that the ear canal is free of hair.

BAROTRAUMA

Today many children travel with their family via airplanes and may react to a change in altitude and barometric pressure. During airplane descent, children should be encouraged to yawn or chew on gum to promote swallowing. Infants should be bottle-fed juice or water to promote swallowing, which produces autoinflation and relief of symptoms. Systemic decongestants can be taken before air travel and timed so that their peak effectiveness occurs during airplane descent.

Adolescents may participate in recreational underwater diving that can cause barometric pressure stress to the ear and result in severe earaches and other serious problems. Underwater diving should be slow during the descent phase to minimize negative pressure buildup. Sensory hearing loss and vertigo with nausea and vomiting may be early signs of decompression sickness when it occurs during the ascent phase of diving. The diver should be referred for medical care. Upper respiratory infections or tympanic membrane perforation are contraindications to diving because vertigo, nausea, vomiting, and disorientation can occur with dangerous results.

THE EYES

The eye is the organ of vision. The anatomy of the eyeball is depicted in Figure 23-3. The eyes begin to develop as an outgrowth of the forebrain in the 4-week-old embryo. At birth the eye is 65% of adult size. The new-

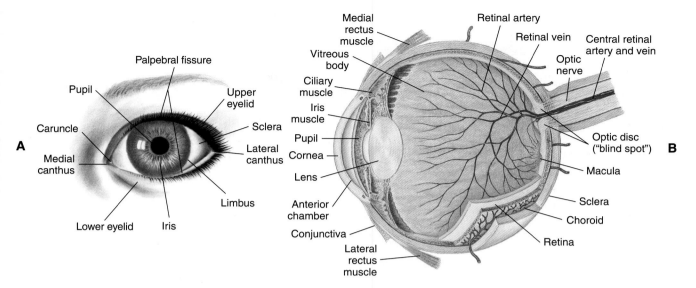

FIGURE **23-3** The normal eye. **A,** External view. **B,** Internal view showing relationship of the optic nerve, eye muscles, and chambers of the eye.

born's sight is not mature, but the newborn can see. Visual acuity is estimated to be in the range of 20/400. This improves rapidly and may reach 20/30 to 20/20 by 2 or 3 years of age (Behrman, Kliegman, & Jenson, 2000). The shape of the newborn's eye is less spherical than the adult's eye. The eyes may appear crossed in the early weeks of life, but alignment and coordination are usually achieved by 3 to 6 months of age. Tears are not present until 1 to 3 months of age. *Depth perception does not begin to develop until about 9 months of age.* The American Academy of Pediatrics (AAP) recommends that all children undergo preschool visual screening during well-child visits between 2 and 3 years of age.

On physical examination the nurse observes the eyes to see if they are symmetrical and are an equal distance from the nose. Epicanthal folds (*epi,* "upon" and *canthus,* "angle") are folds of skin that extend on either side of the bridge of the nose and cover the inner eye canthus. Some folds are broad and cover a large portion of the inner eye, causing the eye to appear crossed. Large epicanthal folds occur as part of some chromosomal anomalies. Pupils are observed for size, shape, and movement. Their reaction to light is observed by shining a penlight into the eye and quickly removing it. The healthy pupil constricts (gets smaller) as the light approaches and dilates (gets larger) as it disappears (see Figure 23-14). Older children are given explanations concerning the examination. They are allowed to hold the ophthalmoscope and to turn it off and on.

> **NURSING TIP**
> At birth the quiet, alert infant will respond to visual stimuli by cessation of movement. Visual responsiveness to the mother during feeding is noted. The infant's ability to focus and follow objects in the first months of life should be documented. Coordination of eye movements should be achieved by 3 to 6 months of age.

VISUAL ACUITY TESTS

The ability of an infant to fixate and focus on an object can be demonstrated by 6 weeks of age. The object should not emit a sound to be sure the infant is turning toward a sight stimulus rather than a sound stimulus. Visual acuity can be tested by 2½ to 3 years of age.

There are a variety of visual acuity charts (Figure 23-4). The Snellen alphabet chart and the Snellen E version for preschoolers who have not learned the alphabet are commonly used to assess the ability to see near and far objects. Picture cards are also useful for children who do not know letters.

The Titmus machine is often used for school-age children and adolescents. Directions for testing are standardized and must be carefully adhered to for proper results. Computerized tests, such as the random-dot stereogram, are also useful in the visual screening of children. Visual acuity is important in the learning process. Retinopathy of prematurity (ROP) is discussed in Chapter 13.

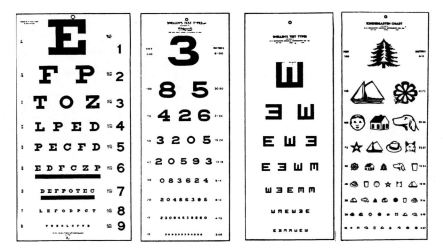

FIGURE **23-4** Various types of visual acuity charts. The "E" chart is often used for young children who can "show which way the fingers of the E are pointing."

DYSLEXIA

Dyslexia (*dys* "difficult" and *lexis,* "diction") is a reading disability that involves a defect in the cortex of the brain that processes graphic symbols. Although an eye evaluation is recommended when a child has mirror vision or word reversal, the problem does not involve any local eye defect. Correcting vision problems will aid in optimal visual function, but treatment for dyslexia involves remedial instruction.

AMBLYOPIA

Pathophysiology. Amblyopia (lazy eye) is a reduction in or loss of vision that usually occurs in children who strongly favor one eye. If both retinas do not receive a clearly defined image, bilateral amblyopia may result. However, it is more common for one eye to be affected. When abnormal binocular interaction occurs (such as crossed eyes or strabismus), the prognosis depends on how long the eye has been affected and on the age of the child when treatment begins. The earlier the treatment is given, the better the results. One commonly accepted diagnostic sign is that vision in the normal eye is at least two Snellen lines (E charts) better than that in the affected eye. There are various types of amblyopia. Strabismus is the most common; however, dissimilar refractory errors can also result in this condition. Because amblyopia occurs as a result of sensory deprivation of the affected eye, children are at risk for developing the problem until visual stability occurs, usually by 9 years of age.

Treatment and nursing care. Early detection and prompt treatment are essential. The goal of treatment is to obtain normal and equal vision in each eye. Treatment consists of eyeglasses for significant refractive errors (hyperopia, myopia) and patching (occlusion) of the *good eye.* The good eye is patched to force the use of the affected eye. Daytime patching may be instituted. Part-time occlusion is sufficient in some cases. Occlusion therapy is often difficult to maintain. The nurse can be of help by explaining the importance of the procedure and by offering support, but the child is often subjected to teasing by peers. Providing a safe place to express feelings is important to promoting a healthy self-image. In most cases an opaque contact lens or a contact lens of sufficiently high power to blur the vision in the better eye is used (Behrman et al., 2000).

STRABISMUS

Pathophysiology. Strabismus (cross-eye), also known as *squint,* is a condition in which the child is not able to direct both eyes toward the same object. There is a lack of coordination between the eye muscles that direct movement of the eye. When the eyes cannot coordinate sight together, the brain will disable one eye to provide a clear image. The disabled eye can develop permanent visual impairment because of sensory deprivation (amblyopia). Normal binocular vision is the goal that must be accomplished by early intervention *before the eye matures.*

There are several types of strabismus. *Nonparalytic strabismus* (concomitant) involves a constant deviation in the gaze related to faulty insertion of the eye muscle. One eye always looks crossed. The extraocular muscles are normal. *Paralytic strabismus* (nonconcomitant) involves a paralysis or weakness in the extraocular muscle. Double vision is experienced. Deviation of the gaze occurs with movement, when the eye attempts to focus. To avoid double vision *(diplopia)* the child will tilt his or her head or squint when focusing on an object. Strabismus may be present at birth or may be acquired after a disease or injury. This type of strabismus can occur after head trauma or a neurological disease. It is important to note that epicanthal folds can give a false impression of strabismus.

Treatment. In nonparalytic strabismus the refractory error is usually corrected with eyeglasses. When paralytic strabismus is seen during early infancy, the physician may recommend that the unaffected eye be covered by a patch until the infant is old enough to wear glasses. The affected eye may improve through use and often becomes normal. Eye exercises and glasses are effective ways of treating the condition medically. If they do not help, surgery should be considered. It is generally performed when the child is 3 or 4 years of age. Early correction is necessary to prevent amblyopia. If strabismus is left untreated, blindness may result in the affected eye because the brain tends to obliterate the confusing double image.

Nursing care. The child undergoing surgery for strabismus may be hospitalized for only a brief period. The surgery involves structures outside the eyeball; therefore the child is allowed to be up and about postoperatively. Eye dressings are kept at a minimum, and elbow restraints may be sufficient to keep the child from touching the dressings.

Prevention of eyestrain. Children who are beginning to read need books with large type in which the letters are spaced far apart. The lighting must be adequate and without glare. Chairs and desks must be of the proper height.

Symptoms that may indicate eyestrain include inflammation, aching or burning of the eyes, squinting, a short attention span, frequent headaches, difficulties with schoolwork, or an inability to see the blackboard. It is important for the nurse to *observe* the child for eyestrain, to *teach* proper eye care, to *prevent* complications of eyestrain or strabismus, to *refer* as needed for follow-up care, and to assist in *rehabilitation.*

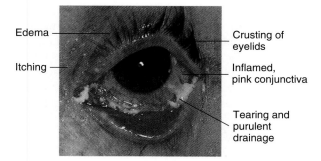

FIGURE **23-5** Acute bacterial conjunctivitis. Signs of conjunctivitis are evident in this highly contagious infection.

CONJUNCTIVITIS

Conjunctivitis (conjungere, "to join together" and *itis,* "inflammation") is an inflammation of the conjunctiva or the mucous membrane that lines the eyelids. It is caused by a wide range of bacterial and viral agents, allergens, irritants, toxins, and systemic diseases (Figure 23-5). Conjunctivitis that occurs with viral exanthems such as measles are usually self-limiting. It is common in childhood and may be infectious or noninfectious. The acute infectious form is commonly referred to as *pinkeye.* Conjunctivitis can also result from an obstruction of the lacrimal duct. In general, the common forms of conjunctivitis respond to warm compresses and topical antibiotic eye drops or eye ointments. Ointments blur vision and are not generally used during daytime hours in the ambulatory child.

The nurse instructs parents to administer the eye medication for the prescribed time to prevent recurrence. Parents and older children are taught to wipe secretions from the *inner canthus downward and away from the opposite eye.* Because conjunctivitis spreads easily, affected children should use separate towels and be instructed to wash their hands frequently. *Ophthalmia neonatorum,* an acute conjunctivitis in the newborn, is discussed in Chapter 6. Allergic conjunctivitis is often associated with allergic rhinitis *(rhin,* "nose" and *itis,* "inflammation") in children with hay fever. Symptoms include itching, tearing of one or both eyes, and edema of the eyelids and periorbital tissues. The child may appear distracted and irritable.

HYPHEMA

Hyphema, the presence of blood in the anterior chamber of the eye, is one of the most common ocular injuries. It can occur from either a blunt or a perforating injury. Blows from flying objects (e.g., baseball, snowball) or forceful coughing or sneezing can cause this condition. These accidents are common among active school-age children. Hyphema appears as a bright red or dark red spot in front of the lower portion of the iris.

Treatment includes bed rest and topical medication. The head of the bed is elevated 30 to 45 degrees to decrease intraocular pressure and decrease intracranial pressure if there is an associated head injury. The condition generally resolves itself without residual problems.

RETINOBLASTOMA

Pathophysiology. Retinoblastoma is a malignant tumor of the retina of the eye. There are hereditary and spontaneous forms. The average ages at diagnosis are 12 months for bilateral tumors and 21 months for unilateral tumors (Behrman et al., 2000). Gene-mapping techniques have shown chromosome 13 to be affected in hereditary forms. Chromosome 13 is also known to cause other congenital defects.

Manifestations. A yellowish white reflex is seen in the pupil because of a tumor behind the lens. This is called the *cat's eye reflex* or *leukokoria* (*leuk,* "white" and *kore,* "pupil"). This may be accompanied by loss of vision, strabismus, hyphema and, in advanced tumors, pain. Metastasis to the unaffected eye is common in unilateral tumors. When retinoblastoma is suspected in children, an examination is performed using an anesthetic so the pediatric ophthalmologist may carefully examine the fundus of the eye.

Treatment and nursing care. The standard treatment for unilateral disease is enucleation (removal) of the eye if there is no possibility of saving the vision. Small tumors are treated with laser photocoagulation to destroy the blood vessels supplying the tumor. Larger tumors can be treated with chemotherapy or external beam irradiation.

On return from surgery for enucleation, the child has a large pressure dressing on the eye. Elbow restraints may be necessary to prevent removal of the dressing. The bandage is observed for bleeding, and the vital signs are assessed. In a few days the surgeon removes the dressing and applies an eye patch. Other structures of the eye, such as the lids, lashes, and tear glands, are not affected. An eye prosthesis is fitted when the socket has healed. Instructions for care of the prosthesis are provided at the time of final fitting. Providing education and emotional support of the child and family and referral to the multidisciplinary health care team is essential.

THE NERVOUS SYSTEM

The nervous system is the body's communication center; it receives and transmits messages to all parts of the body. It also records experiences (memorization) and integrates certain stimuli (learning). The anatomy of the nervous system is depicted in Figure 23-6. Neural tube development occurs during the third to fourth week of fetal life. This eventually becomes the central nervous system (CNS). The fusing process of the neural tube is critical. Its failure to fuse may lead to congenital conditions such as spina bifida or anencephaly (Chapter 14). Most neurological disabilities in childhood result from congenital malformation (birth defects), brain injury, or infection. The 12 cranial nerves and their functions are shown in Figure 23-7.

CNS dysfunction may be detected by a neurological check (see Box 23-9 and Table 23-6), skull x-ray films, electroencephalogram (EEG), computed tomography (CT), magnetic resonance imaging (MRI), electromyography, and other methods. The reflexes of the newborn are good indicators of neurological health. A decreased level of consciousness in the ill child may be an indication of a neurological problem. Box 23-1 describes the causes of altered level of consciousness. In the finger-nose test (used to determine coordination), the child is asked to extend the arm and then to touch his or her nose with his or her index finger. This is done with the eyes opened and closed. The inability to balance on one foot in a school-age child requires further follow-up. The 12 cranial nerves, selected dysfunction, and nursing interventions are described in Table 23-1.

REYE'S SYNDROME

Pathophysiology. Reye's syndrome is an acute noninflammatory encephalopathy (pathology of the brain) and *hepatopathy* (pathology of the liver) that follows a viral infection in children. There may be a relationship between the use of aspirin (acetylsalicylic acid) during a viral flu or illness such as chickenpox (varicella) and the development of Reye's syndrome. For this reason, aspirin is generally contraindicated for the pediatric population. Some studies show that a genetic metabolic defect triggers Reye's syndrome when the stress of a viral illness produces vomiting and hypoglycemia.

> NURSING **TIP**
> Discourage the use of aspirin and other medications that contain salicylates in children with flulike symptoms. Advise parents to read medication labels carefully to determine their ingredients.

Manifestations. Liver cell pathology causes an accumulation of ammonia in the blood. Toxic levels of ammonia cause cerebral manifestations (e.g., cerebral edema, increased intracranial pressure [ICP]), which results in neurological changes such as altered behavior, altered level of consciousness, seizures, and coma.

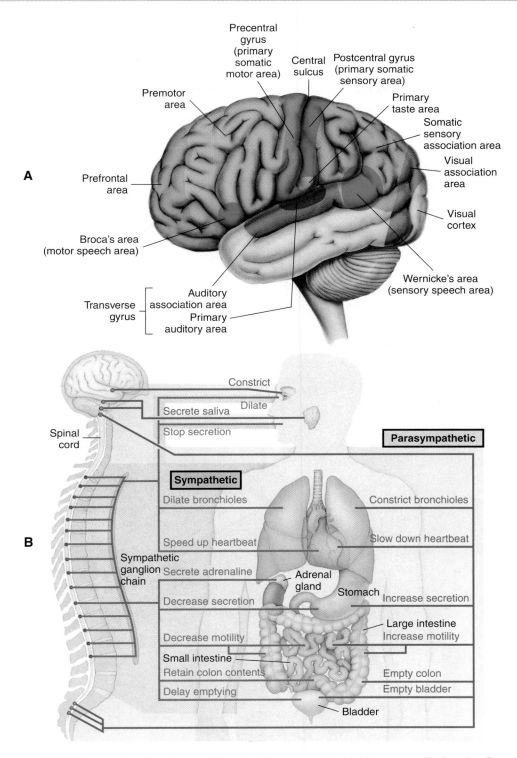

FIGURE **23-6** **A,** Functional areas of the brain. Each area of the brain has a specific function. Damage to the local area can cause loss of that function. **B,** The nervous system. The innervation of target organs by the autonomic nervous system. The sympathetic pathways are shown in orange and the parasympathetic pathways are shown in green.

In children, the sudden onset of effortless vomiting and altered behavior (e.g., lethargy, combativeness) or altered level of consciousness after a viral illness is characteristic of Reye's syndrome. The results of blood tests assessing liver function will be abnormal. In infants, diarrhea, hypoglycemia, tachypnea with apneic episodes, and seizures may occur approximately 1 week after a respiratory illness. See Box 23-2 for the characteristic signs and symptoms of Reye's syndrome.

Prevention. The education of the public concerning the dangers of using salicylate-containing medications during viral illnesses such as varicella in children may have contributed to the decline in the occurrence of Reye's syndrome. The availability of the varicella vaccine may also have an impact on the reduced incidence of Reye's syndrome.

Treatment. Early treatment can result in complete recovery. However, progression to the acute stage is often

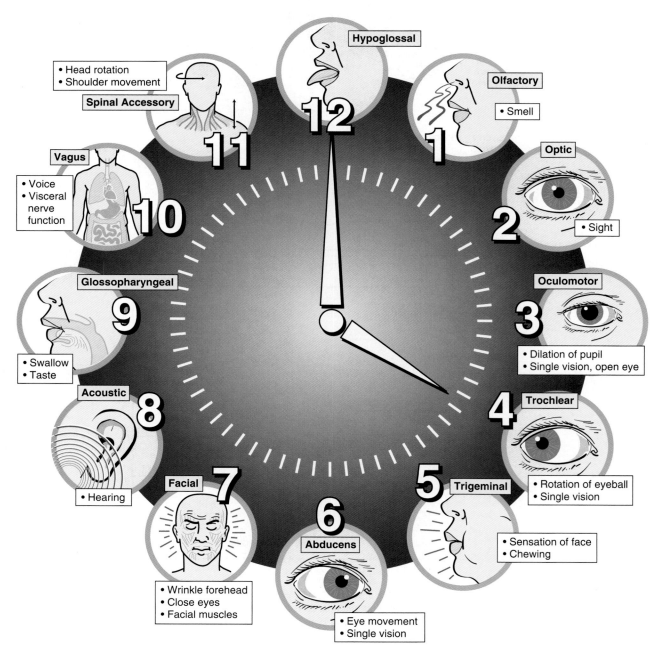

FIGURE **23-7** The 12 cranial nerves and their functions.

rapid and unpredictable. The goals of treatment include reducing ICP and maintaining a patent airway, cerebral oxygenation, and fluid and electrolyte balance.

Frequent assessment of vital signs and a careful assessment of neurological status are essential. Observation for signs of bleeding is important because liver dysfunction causes blood-clotting abnormalities. Parental education and support are necessary. Encouraging parents to participate in their child's care helps to reduce the parents' and child's level of anxiety.

---

box 23-1 | *Causes of Altered Level of Consciousness (LOC)*

- A fall to 60 mm Hg or below of PaO_2
- A rise above 45 mm of $PaCO_2$
- Low blood pressure causing cerebral hypoxia
- Fever (1-degree rise in fever increases oxygen need by 10%)
- Drugs (sedatives, antiepileptics)
- Seizures (postictal state)
- Increased ICP

SEPSIS

Sepsis *(bacteremia)* is bacteria in the bloodstream that cause severe systemic response (Box 23-3). Sepsis may follow an infection such as meningitis, or it may result from a primary infection. Children who are immunocompromised, have neutropenia, or are in intensive care to receive invasive therapy are at risk for developing sepsis. Sepsis causes a systemic inflammatory response syndrome (SIRS) as a reaction to the endotoxin of the bacteria that results in tissue damage. Complications of SIRS include shock and multiorgan system failure, leading to death.

Manifestations. Manifestations of sepsis include fever, tachypnea, tachycardia, hypotension, and neurological signs such as lethargy. Laboratory tests may include positive blood cultures, reduced fibrinogen and thrombocyte levels, and anemia. The presence of immature white blood cells and neutropenia are ominous signs. The nursing responsibilities include monitoring neurological status and vital signs and observing for shock. Intravenous antibiotics are prescribed. To prevent sepsis, immunization against *H. influenzae* type B(Hib)

---

table 23-1 | *The 12 Cranial Nerves: Selected Dysfunctions and Nursing Interventions*

CRANIAL NERVE	DYSFUNCTION	NURSING INTERVENTIONS
I Olfactory	Inability to smell	Appetite may be suppressed; present food attractively.
II Optic	Inability to control pupil reflex	Protect eyes from glaring lights.
III Oculomotor	Double vision	Cover eyes.
IV Trochlear	Inability to move eyes	When communicating, remain in child's view.
V Trigeminal	Difficulty in chewing	Provide soft foods.
VI Abducens	Inability to control corneal reflex	Have eye ointment or eye patch on hand to protect cornea.
VII Facial	Inability to close eye	Protect eyes with moist dressing.
VIII Acoustic	Inability to hear	Maintain body language for communication.
IX Glossopharyngeal	Inability to taste or to control gag and cough reflexes	Provide visually attractive food. Keep tracheotomy tray and suction at bedside.
X Vagus	Difficulty in talking or swallowing; visceral malfunction	Provide means of communication. Assess for aspiration. Assess body system functions and vital signs.
XI Spinal accessory	Controls head, turn, and shrug shoulders	Provide position change and support.
XII Hypoglossal	Controls tongue movement, thick speech	Have suction ready; observe ability to chew and swallow. Provide method of communication.

| box 23-2 | *Characteristic Manifestations of Reye's Syndrome in Children* |

A viral illness 1 week before presentation of symptoms such as the following:

- Persistent, effortless vomiting
- Diarrhea, hypoglycemia, lethargy, or combative behavior
- Tachypnea with apneic episodes in infants
- Absence of fever or jaundice

LABORATORY TEST RESULTS

- Elevated AST and ALT levels
- Elevated serum ammonia level
- Elevated blood urea nitrogen (BUN) and creatinine (related to dehydration from vomiting) levels
- Normal bilirubin levels
- Hypoglycemia
- A percutaneous liver biopsy is diagnostic but may be difficult to do if the child is gravely ill

ALT, Alanine aminotransferase; *AST*, aspartate aminotransferase.

| box 23-3 | *Sepsis* |

This chart shows the progression of primary bacteremia or local infection to sepsis and septic shock with complications. Early treatment of suspected sepsis can prevent these complications.

Bacteria

Local Infection   Bacteremia

Sepsis

Systemic inflammatory response syndrome (SIRS)

Septic shock

Multiorgan system failure

Death

Modified from Behrman, R., Kliegman, R., & Jenson, H.B. (2000). *Nelson's textbook of pediatrics* (16th ed.). Philadelphia: W.B. Saunders.

is recommended for all children between 2 months and 4 years of age.

MENINGITIS

Pathophysiology. Meningitis is an inflammation of the meninges (the covering of the brain and spinal cord). Various organisms can cause bacterial meningitis. Organisms may invade the meninges *indirectly* by way of the bloodstream (sepsis) from centers of infection such as the teeth, sinuses, tonsils, and lungs, or *directly* through the ear (otitis media) or from a fracture of the skull.

Bacterial meningitis is often referred to as *purulent,* that is, pus-forming, because a thick exudate surrounds the meninges and adjacent structures. This can lead to certain sequelae such as subdural effusion and, less frequently, hydrocephalus. The peak incidence for bacterial meningitis is between 6 and 12 months of age. Meningococcal meningitis is readily transmitted to others. Meningitis is less common in children older than 4 years of age. *H. influenzae* is the most common causative agent. *H. influenzae* type B vaccines are available for infants. The approaches to nursing care for all types of meningitis are similar.

Manifestations. The symptoms of purulent meningitis result mainly from intracranial irritation. They may be preceded by an upper respiratory infection and several days of gastrointestinal symptoms such as poor feeding. Severe headache, drowsiness, delirium, irritability, restlessness, fever, vomiting, and stiffness of the neck (nuchal rigidity) are other significant symptoms. A characteristic high-pitched cry is noted in infants. Convulsions are common. Coma may occur fairly early in the older child. In severe cases, involuntary arching of the back caused by muscle contractions is seen (Figure 23-8). This condition is called *opisthotonos* (*opistho,* "backward" and *tonos,* "tension"). The presence of *petechiae* (small hemorrhages beneath the skin) suggests meningococcal infection. Diagnosis is confirmed by examination of the cerebrospinal fluid (CSF).

NURSING **TIP**

A rash with petechiae that develops in a child who is acutely ill and lethargic must be referred for immediate follow-up care.

Treatment. At the first indication of meningitis, the physician performs a spinal tap (lumbar puncture, see Chapter 22) to obtain a specimen of CSF for laboratory testing. The spinal fluid may be clear in the early stages of the illness, but it rapidly becomes cloudy. The CSF pressure is increased, and further laboratory analysis indicates a high white cell count, an increase in protein, and a decrease in glucose.

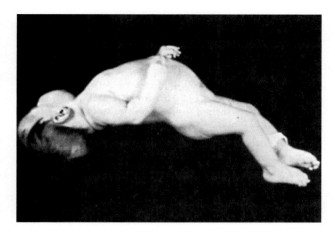

FIGURE **23-8** The opisthotonos position. An involuntary arching of the back and extension of the neck are seen in children with brain injury or meningeal irritation. Note that the back is arched so that the head is on an even level with the heels.

The child is placed in isolation until 24 hours after antibiotic therapy has been administered. An intravenous (IV) line is established for the administration of antibiotics and to restore fluid and electrolyte balance. Antibiotics are selected on the basis of culture and sensitivity laboratory results. Antibiotics are usually administered for a minimum of 10 to 14 days. A sedative may be given to make the child less restless. An anticonvulsant such as phenytoin (Dilantin) may also be required to decrease the risk of seizure activity.

Nursing care. The single room is prepared in accordance with hospital protocol (see Appendix A). Nursing responsibility includes performing a neurological check and maintaining an accurate recording of the child's vital signs and intake and output. The nurse should also organize care so that the child is disturbed as little as possible.

The child with meningitis may be overly sensitive to stimuli; therefore the room should be dimly lit and the noise kept to a minimum. The nurse carefully raises and lowers the sides of the crib to avoid jarring the bed. The nurse avoids startling the child by using a soft voice and gentle touch. These precautions are also explained to the parents.

Frequent monitoring of the child's vital signs is necessary. A slowed pulse rate, irregular respirations, and increased blood pressure are reported immediately because they could indicate increased ICP. Fever may be controlled by antipyretics, sponge baths, or a hypothermia (cooling) mattress. The nurse observes the child for additional or subtle signs of increased ICP, especially a change in alertness or muscle twitchings. The joints are

also observed for swelling, pain, and immobility. Oxygen is given as ordered.

The child's intake and output are carefully observed and recorded. Careful attention is given to maintaining the IV line. Good oral hygiene is essential during this stage, when the child is receiving nothing by mouth. As the child's condition improves, the diet progresses from clear fluids to an age-appropriate diet. A special formula may be given when nasogastric feedings are necessary. During the convalescent period, oral fluids are encouraged unless contraindicated. The nurse promptly reports a decrease in output of urine (oliguria), which could signal urinary retention. Bowel movements are recorded each day to detect constipation and avoid fecal impaction (an accumulation of feces in the rectum). The nurse continues to monitor neurological status and to record and report findings such as weakness of the limbs, speech difficulties, mental confusion, and behavior problems. The child should be assessed for developmental deficiencies. When recovery is uneventful, the child may be discharged home. The parents are taught the principles of intermittent IV therapy that can be accomplished in the home setting with visits from a home health agency nurse.

>NURSING **TIP**_____
When a spinal tap is planned, the infant can be sedated and EMLA cream can be applied to the area to reduce discomfort during needle insertion.

ENCEPHALITIS

Pathophysiology. Encephalitis (*encephalo,* "brain" and *itis,* "inflammation") is an inflammation of the brain. The condition is known as encephalomyelitis (*myelo,* "spinal cord") when the spinal cord is also infected. This disorder can be caused by "togaviruses" (RNA viruses) and herpesvirus types 1 and 2; it can be the aftermath of disorders such as upper respiratory tract infections, German measles (rubella), or measles (rubeola) or, rarely, an untoward reaction to vaccinations such as diphtheria, pertussis, and tetanus (DPT); it may also result from lead poisoning. Other etiological agents include bacteria, spirochetes, and fungi.

>NURSING **TIP**_____
Encephalitis may occur as a complication of childhood diseases such as measles, mumps, or chickenpox. It is crucial that children receive the immunizations available for the diseases that are preventable.

Manifestations. The symptoms of encephalitis result from the CNS response to irritation. Characteristically, the history is that of a headache followed by drowsiness that may proceed to coma. Because coma is sometimes prolonged, encephalitis is sometimes referred to as "sleeping sickness." Convulsions are seen, particularly in infants. Fever, cramps, abdominal pain, vomiting, stiff neck (nuchal rigidity), delirium, muscle twitching, and abnormal eye movements are other manifestations of the disease.

Treatment and nursing care. The treatment is supportive and is aimed at providing relief from specific symptoms. Sedatives and antipyretics may be prescribed. Seizure precautions are taken. Adequate nutrition and hydration are maintained. The nurse provides a quiet environment, good oral hygiene, skin care, and frequent changes of position. Oxygen is given as ordered, and the mouth and nose are kept free of mucus by gentle aspiration. Bowel movements are recorded daily because the child may be constipated from the lack of activity. Preventing the secondary effects of immobilization is paramount.

The nurse closely observes the child for neurological changes. Fatality rates and residual effects are higher among infants than among older children. Speech, mental processes, and motor abilities may be slowed, and permanent brain damage and mental retardation can result. Growth and development and hearing evaluations should be monitored. Parents are encouraged to help with the care of the child as soon as the condition is stable. They are instructed about the nursing procedures for home care and any required follow-up care.

BRAIN TUMORS

Pathophysiology. Brain tumors are the second most common type of neoplasm in children (the first is leukemia). The majority of childhood tumors occur in the lower part of the brain (cerebellum or brainstem). The etiology of these tumors is unknown. They occur most commonly in school-age children.

Manifestations. The signs and symptoms are directly related to the location and size of the tumor. Most tumors create increased ICP with the hallmark symptoms of headache, vomiting, drowsiness, and seizures (Figure 23-9). Nystagmus (constant jerky movements of the eyeball), strabismus, and decreased vision may be evidenced. Papilledema (edema of the optic nerve) may occur. Other symptoms include ataxia, head tilt, behavioral changes, and cerebral enlargement, particularly in infants. Deviations in vital signs are noticeable when the tumor presses on the brainstem.

Treatment and nursing care. Diagnosis is determined by clinical manifestations, laboratory tests, CT, MRI, and EEG. Angiography is used to assist in the surgical approach by identifying the tumor's blood supply. Radiotherapy, chemotherapy, or surgery may be indicated. Preoperative emphasis is placed on carefully explaining various procedures and on familiarizing the child and family with the recovery room, intensive care unit (ICU), and hospital personnel. The nurse explains that the child will have part or all of his or her head shaved. The size of the postoperative dressing is carefully explained. Applying a similar dressing to a doll may be helpful to the child.

Postoperative care is usually provided in the ICU. Adjuncts to care may include using a hypothermia (cooling) blanket or a mechanical respirator. Parents must be prepared for the appearance of the child after surgery. Empathetic family support and appropriate referral are offered.

Radiation treatment may be prescribed. The radiologist outlines the areas to be treated on the child's head.

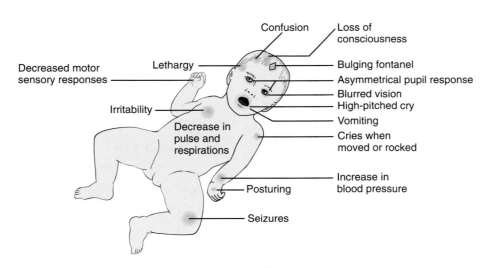

FIGURE **23-9** Signs of increased ICP in infants and children.

These marks are not to be washed off. Small doses of radiation are given over a period of weeks. Chemotherapy regimens may follow irradiation.

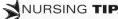

NURSING **TIP**

The timing of information is important when preparing the child for various procedures.

SEIZURE DISORDERS

Seizures are the most commonly observed neurological dysfunction in children. The etiology varies (Box 23-4). Seizures are sudden, intermittent episodes of altered consciousness that last seconds to minutes and may include involuntary tonic and clonic movements. A tonic movement is a stiffening (contraction) of muscles. A clonic movement is an alternating contraction and relaxation of muscles.

Febrile Seizures

Febrile seizures are a transient condition common in children between 6 months and 5 years of age. There may be a genetic predisposition explaining why children in the same family have this problem. The seizure occurs in response to a rapid rise in temperature—often above a level of 38.8° C (102° F). Because the seizure lasts a short time and is no longer present when the child reaches a hospital, causes other than fever may need to be ruled out. Simple febrile convulsions are treated by

---

box 23-4 | *Causes of Seizures in Children*

Etiology of seizures can be any of the following:

Intracranial
- Epilepsy
- Congenital anomaly
- Birth injury
- Infection
- Trauma
- Degenerative diseases
- Tumor
- Vascular disorder

Extracranial
- Fever
- Heart disease
- Metabolic disorders
- Hypocalcemia
- Hypoglycemia
- Dehydration and malnutrition

Toxic
- Anesthetics
- Drugs
- Poisons

---

teaching the parent to control the fever by appropriate use of antipyretics (e.g., acetaminophen) and cooling measures (e.g., removing heavy blankets and clothing). Parents should be reassured that the condition is self-limiting. The use of phenobarbital is not effective and may decrease cognitive function. Valproic acid (Depakene) produces side effects. These drugs are not recommended for first-time treatment. Rectal or oral diazepam (Valium) for the duration of a febrile illness may be prescribed if febrile convulsions recur. Side effects such as lethargy, irritability, or ataxia (lack of muscular coordination) should be reported. Febrile seizures rarely develop into epilepsy and have an excellent prognosis without residual problems.

Epilepsy

Pathophysiology. The term *epilepsy* (chronic recurrent convulsions) comes from the Greek *epilepsia,* which means "seizure." In the past, words such as *fit, spell,* and *blackout* were used to describe this entity. These terms are nonspecific and tend to create confusion.

Epilepsy is a disorder manifested by a variety of symptom complexes. It is characterized by recurrent paroxysmal (sudden, periodic) attacks of unconsciousness *or* impaired consciousness that may be followed by alternate (tonic) contraction and (clonic) relaxation of the muscles *or* abnormal behavior. It is a disorder of the CNS in which the neurons or nerve cells discharge in an abnormal way. These discharges may be focal or diffuse. The site of general discharge can sometimes be ascertained by observing the child's symptoms during the attack. When the cause is unknown, the term idiopathic epilepsy is used.

The nurse observes and records the following: the child's activity immediately before the seizure; body movements; changes in color, respiration, or muscle tone; incontinence; and the parts of the body involved. When possible, the seizure is timed. The child's appearance, behavior, and level of consciousness after the seizure are also documented. Table 23-2 describes the first aid response and nursing responsibilities during a seizure.

Types of epilepsy. Childhood epilepsy is classified into partial seizures and generalized seizures.

Generalized seizures. Generalized seizures involve a loss of consciousness. The most common generalized seizure is the *tonic-clonic* or grand mal. A grand mal epilepsy has three distinct phases: (1) An aura (subjective sensation), (2) a tonic/clonic seizure, followed by (3) postictal lethargy, a short period of sleep. Petit mal, or *absence,* seizures often are recognized when an intelligent child is referred for medical evaluation because of unexplained failure to achieve in school. The reason for

table 23-2 *Seizure Recognition and First Aid Response*

SEIZURE TYPE	WHAT IT LOOKS LIKE	OFTEN MISTAKEN FOR	WHAT TO DO	WHAT NOT TO DO
1. General: Generalized tonic-clinic (also called *grand mal*)	Sudden cry (or aura), fall, rigidity, followed by muscle jerking; shallow, irregular breathing; possible loss of bladder or bowel control; usually lasts seconds to minutes, followed by some confusion, a period of sleep (postictal lethargy), and then return to full consciousness	Heart attack, stroke	Look for medical identification. Protect from nearby hazards. Observe and record stages and manifestations. Following seizure, maintain patent airway, turn on side, loosen clothing, reassure person. If multiple seizures, or if one seizure lasts longer than 5 minutes, call ambulance (911). If person is pregnant, injured, or diabetic, call for aid at once.	Do not put any hard implement in the mouth. Do not try to hold tongue; it cannot be swallowed. Do not try to give liquids during or just after seizure. Do not restrain person.
2. Absence (also called *petit mal*)	A blank stare, beginning and ending abruptly, lasting only a few seconds; most common in children; may be accompanied by rapid blinking, some chewing movements of the mouth; person is unaware of what is going on during the seizure but quickly returns to full awareness once it has stopped; may result in learning difficulties if not recognized and treated	Daydreaming, lack of attention, deliberate ignoring of adult instructions	No first aid necessary, but if this is first observation of seizure(s), medical evaluation should be recommended.	
A. Partial: Simple partial (also called *Jacksonian*)	Jerking may begin in one area of body such as the arm, leg, or face; cannot be stopped, but person stays awake and aware;	Acting out, bizarre behavior, hysteria, mental illness, psychosomatic illness, parapsychological or mystical experience, tics	No first aid necessary unless seizure becomes generalized, then first aid as indicated.	

	jerking may proceed from one area of the body to another and sometimes spreads to become a generalized seizure		No immediate action needed other than reassurance and emotional support. Medical evaluation should be recommended.	Do not grab hold unless sudden danger (such as a cliff edge or an approaching car) threatens. Do not try to restrain person. Do not shout. Do not expect verbal instructions to be obeyed.
B. Complex partial (also called *psychomotor* or *temporal lobe*)	Usually starts with blank stare, followed by chewing, followed by random activity; person appears unaware of surroundings, may seem dazed and may mumble; is unresponsive; actions are clumsy, not directed; may pick at clothing, pick up objects, try to take off clothes; may run, appear afraid; may struggle or flail at restraint; once pattern established, same set of actions usually occurs with each seizure; can last 1 to 2 minutes; no memory of actions or behavior	Disorderly conduct	Speak calmly and reassuringly to person and others. Guide person gently away from obvious hazards. Stay with person until completely aware of environment. Offer to help getting home.	
3. Atonic seizures (also called *drop attacks*)	More frequent occurrence in the morning with jerking motions on awakening; suddenly collapses; after 10 seconds to 1 minute, person recovers and can stand and walk again	Clumsiness, normal childhood stage; lack of good walking skills; drunkenness	No first aid needed (unless hurt during fall), but the person should be given a thorough medical evaluation.	

school failure is found to be absence seizures, which cause a temporary loss of awareness that results in a lack of continuity in the learning environment.

Other types of general seizures include *myoclonic spasms,* where repetitive muscle contractions occur, and *infantile spasms,* which occur in infants under 1 year of age and are manifested by a jackknife posture for frequent but brief periods.

Partial seizures. Partial seizures account for 40% of childhood convulsions. Consciousness may be intact or slightly impaired. Simple partial seizures (jacksonian) are often mistaken for alterations in behavior or "tics," which usually involve only the face or shoulders. Complex partial seizures can be manifested by motor activities, sensory signs, or psychomotor (behavioral) activity.

Treatment. Initially, treatment is aimed at determining the type, site, or cause of the disorder. Diagnostic measures include a complete history and physical and neurological examinations. Skull radiography and CT or MRI scans are used to establish the presence or absence of tumors, skull abnormalities, hematomas, and intracranial calcifications. The electroencephalogram (EEG) is also a valuable tool in diagnosing seizures. It is especially helpful in differentiating between an absence seizure and a complex partial seizure. Prolonged EEG monitoring (24 hours) is another diagnostic technique.

Laboratory studies such as complete blood count (CBC), determinations of serum calcium and blood urea nitrogen (BUN), and tests to rule out lead poisoning or other metabolic disorders are done. Anticonvulsant medications are prescribed when epilepsy is the diagnosis (see Table 23-3). The drug of choice depends on the type of seizure, and the goal is the use of only one drug that will control the seizures with the fewest side effects.

The duration of therapy is based on the individual child. Initially, the physician prescribes the lowest dose of anticonvulsant medication likely to control the seizures. Drowsiness, a common side effect of many anticonvulsants, may interfere with the child's activities. Careful recording of seizure activity and compliance with the drug regimen are of particular importance in determining a suitable program. The medication is given at the *same time each day,* generally with meals or at bedtime.

If it is necessary for the child to take medication during school hours, the parents sign a consent form so that the school nurse can monitor the administration. The responses of the nurse and teacher, particularly during

| table 23-3 | *Properties of Selected Anticonvulsant Drugs* |

DRUG	SIDE EFFECTS	COMMENTS
Carbamazepine (Tegretol)	Blurred vision, diplopia, drowsiness, vertigo	Few side effects, fewer sedative properties
Phenobarbital (Luminal)	Drowsiness, irritability, hyperactivity	Altered sleep patterns, often combined with other drugs
Phenytoin (Dilantin)	Ataxia, insomnia, nystagmus, gum overgrowth, hirsutism (hairiness), rash, nausea, vitamin D and folic acid deficiencies	Generally effective and safe; may cause cognitive impairment; regular massaging of gums decreases hyperplasia; used in combination with phenobarbital or primidone
Valproic acid (Depakene)	Gastrointestinal disturbance, liver toxicity, amenorrhea, weight gain	Take with food or use enteric-coated preparations; potentiates action of phenobarbital and other drugs
Primidone (Mysoline)	Aggressive behavior, personality changes, anorexia, fatigue, dermatitis	May be used alone or in combination; side effects minimized by starting with small amounts
Ethosuximide (Zarontin)	Anorexia, gastrointestinal upset	
Clonazepam (Rivotril)	Drowsiness, excess salivation	
Topiramate (Topamax)	Cognitive depression, fatigue	
Gabapentin (Neurontin)	Weight gain and somnolence	
Lamotrigine (Lamictal)	Ataxia, rash, photosensitivity, and drowsiness	Given with valproic acid

NOTE: The physician determines the child's medication by the type of seizure and other factors. The goal is to achieve the best control with the minimum dosage and the least number of side effects. An important aspect of nursing intervention includes reinforcing the need for drug supervision and compliance.

and after a seizure, will have a significant effect on the attitude of classmates toward the child.

Abrupt withdrawal of anticonvulsant medications is the most common cause of status epilepticus (prolonged seizures). In the hospital the nurse clarifies with the physician whether anticonvulsants are to be withheld if the child is to be given nothing by mouth (NPO). When children are old enough, they can assume responsibility for their own medications. They should wear a medical identification bracelet. During puberty and adolescence, the dosages may need to be adjusted to meet growth needs. Anticonvulsant drugs should not be taken during pregnancy because birth defects can occur. Premenstrual fluid retention in girls can sometimes trigger seizures. Surgery is being performed on children who are unresponsive to anticonvulsants and who have a well-defined focus of seizure activity in the brain.

The ketogenic diet is sometimes prescribed for children who do not respond well to anticonvulsant therapy. It is high in fats and low in carbohydrates and produces ketoacidosis in the body, which appears to reduce convulsive episodes. A reduction of fluid intake tends to increase the ketogenic effect. The use of this diet is limited because it is boring and requires strict adherence to intake, and compliance tends to be a problem.

Rebellion against medical routine is not uncommon during adolescence. Some states do not allow controlled epileptics to obtain a driver's license, which is disheartening to the child. Other states have stipulations regarding the amount of seizure-free time required before licensing. Excess intake of fluids, particularly alcoholic beverages, can trigger a seizure. Parents can obtain valuable information and support from the Epilepsy Foundation of America. Other major resources include the Department of Vocational Rehabilitation, the Department of Public Health, the Department of Social Services, and other community agencies. The greatest untapped resource for persons with epilepsy is often within themselves. In a comprehensive multidisciplinary treatment approach, team members help the child to mobilize his or her inner resources to deal with the lifelong treatment and to lead a fully productive normal life.

A fundamental principle of comprehensive epilepsy management is that the child become an active member of the health care team. The child with epilepsy can lead a normal life with a few safety guidelines. Restriction of physical activity is not necessary, but adult supervision during swimming or bathing is advisable. A family assessment is helpful in establishing rapport and setting realistic short-term and long-term goals. Too much attention to seizures by well-meaning adults can make control difficult. The child may learn to use the threat of a seizure to manipulate caregivers. Teaching should include first-aid treatment for seizures (see Table 23-2), the importance of compliance with long-term medication regimens, and general reassurance that the child can lead a normal life. Medications used in the treatment of epilepsy are outlined in Table 23-3. The gum hypertrophy (Figure 23-10) that occurs as a side effect of phenytoin (Dilantin) will require meticulous oral hygiene and special care, especially if orthodontic treatment is necessary. Death or serious injury rarely occurs from a seizure, and it does not cause mental deterioration. The Individuals with Disabilities Education Act (IDEA) guarantees children with disabilities the right to publicly financed educational programs in the least restrictive environment.

> ### NURSING **TIP**
> The nurse is responsible for maintaining seizure precautions for a child diagnosed with a seizure disorder:
> - Keep side rails up.
> - Pad all sharp or hard objects around the bed.
> - Make sure child wears a medical ID bracelet.
> - Provide supervision during potentially hazardous play, such as swimming.
> - Avoid triggering factors.
> - Teach the importance of compliance with the medication regimen.

Status epilepticus. A prolonged seizure that can result in brain hypoxia and does not respond to treatment for 30 minutes or more is called status epilepticus. A common cause is sudden stopping of epilepsy medication or generalized infection. Treatment includes managing airway, providing oxygen, observing and documenting details of the seizure, and providing IV therapy.

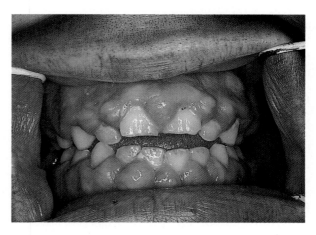

FIGURE **23-10** Phenytoin-induced gum hyperplasia.

Diazepam and phenytoin or a pentobarbital drug may be given intravenously. The child may need to be supported on a ventilator until seizures are controlled.

> **NURSING TIP**
>
> The following are common triggering factors for seizures:
> - Flashing of dark/light patterns
> - Startling movements
> - Overhydration
> - Photosensitivity

OTHER CONDITIONS CAUSING DECREASED LEVEL OF CONSCIOUSNESS

Several conditions are mistaken for epilepsy because they involve paroxysmal altered levels of consciousness. These conditions do not respond to antiepileptic drugs.

Benign Paroxysmal Vertigo

This condition occurs in children under 3 years of age, who often develop ataxia and fall. Nausea, vomiting, and complaints of motion sickness and migraine headache follow. The condition responds to dimenhydrinate (Dramamine) medication.

Night Terrors

Night terrors occur in children between 5 and 7 years of age. The child may sleepwalk, thrash, scream, and be unaware of his or her surroundings. A period of sleep follows. Brief treatment with diazepam (Valium) or imipramine (Tofranil) may be helpful, but family dysfunction should be investigated.

Breath-Holding Spells

Breath holding can result in cyanosis or extreme pallor. Episodes of breath holding are most common between 2 and 5 years of age. The child loses consciousness, and the parents are frightened. Counseling parents to avoid reinforcing the behavior by refusing to play with or hold the child after the episode is helpful.

Cough Syncope

Cough syncopes are paroxysmal coughing spells, usually at night, that result in a diminished cardiac output, cerebral hypoxia, and loss of consciousness. The condition usually occurs in asthmatic children. Prevention involves avoidance of bronchoconstriction.

Prolonged QT Syndrome

A sudden loss of consciousness associated with vigorous exercise is caused by a heart problem and can result in loss of consciousness and death. It usually occurs during adolescence and arises from a defect in chromosome 11. Beta-blockers may be lifesaving. Knowledge of cardiopulmonary resuscitation (CPR) and exercise restriction are essential.

Rage Attacks, or Episodic Dyscontrol Syndrome

Rage attacks are sudden recurrent attacks of violent physical behavior. These attacks appear out of control and are followed by fatigue, remorse, and amnesia. The EEG is usually normal. This condition is often mistaken for complex partial seizure epilepsy.

CEREBRAL PALSY

Pathophysiology. Cerebral palsy (CP) refers to a group of nonprogressive disorders that affect the motor centers of the brain. It is not fatal in itself, but currently there is no cure. It is one of the most common disabling conditions seen in children and occurs in as many as 4 per 1000 live births (Behrman et al, 2000). This disease is precipitated by many factors, some of which are birth injuries, neonatal anoxia, subdural hemorrhage, and prenatal infections. Studies indicate that more than one third of children with CP weighed less than 2500 g at birth. Lead poisoning, head injuries, and febrile illness are sometimes responsible during the toddler period In some children, no single cause can be found, yet recent studies indicate that a congenital problem may exist.

Manifestations. The symptoms of CP vary with each child and may range from mild to severe. Mental retardation sometimes accompanies this disorder; however, many children with CP have normal intelligence. The disease is suspected during infancy if there are feeding problems, convulsions not associated with high fever, and developmental delays. Developmental milestones are not achieved at the expected age level. Diagnostic tests may include a spinal tap, EEG, pneumoencephalography, CT, and screening for metabolic disorders. Brain tumors must also be ruled out. Early recognition is important for appropriate referrals.

There are four types of CP (Table 23-4). Two of the more common are those marked by spasticity and athetosis (Figure 23-11). These conditions occur in about 75% of the cases. *Spasticity* is characterized by tension in certain muscle groups. The stretch reflex is present in the involved muscles. When the child tries to move the voluntary muscles, jerky motions result. Eating, walking, and other coordinated movements are difficult to accomplish. The lower extremities are usually involved. The legs cross and the toes point inward. The arms and trunk may also be affected. In athetosis the child has involuntary, purposeless movements that in-

table 23-4 | *Types of Cerebral Palsy*

TYPE	CHARACTERISTICS
Spastic	Involves damage to the cortex of the brain Spasms occur with movement Related to cerebral asphyxia
Athetoid	Involves damage to the basal nuclei ganglion Continuous writhing involuntary movements Often associated with hyper-bilirubinemia
Ataxic	Uncoordinated movements and ataxia from a lesion in the cerebellum
Mixed	Usually a combination of spastic and athetoid

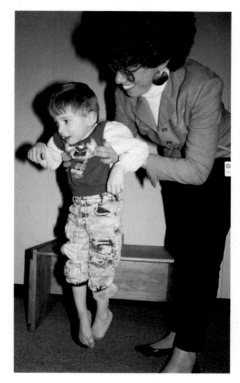

FIGURE **23-11** A child with spastic cerebral palsy. Note the legs crossing in a scissors-like pattern when the child is supported in vertical suspension.

terfere with normal motion. Speech, sight, and hearing defects or convulsions may be complications. The success in preventing kernicterus in the newborn by effective treatment of hyperbilirubinemia has reduced the incidence of the athetoid type of CP.

Treatment and nursing care. The goal of treatment of children with CP is to assist them in making the most of their assets and to guide them in becoming well-adjusted adults, performing at their maximum ability. Both short-term and long-term goals must be realistic. Parents need help in accepting the child and should not be deceived into expecting miraculous cures from treatment. Early diagnosis can result in fewer physical and emotional problems. Botulinum toxin has been used successfully to manage spasticity problems, and levodopa has helped control some athetoid symptoms.

Parents must be informed of community resources available to them. The family's religious affiliation should not be overlooked because it can be a source of support and help during times of stress. The long course of this disability can place a financial burden on the family. Caregivers need respite care from time to time in order to enhance their coping skills.

The specific treatment is highly individualized and depends on the severity of the disability. It is not uncommon for the parents of children with CP to become the experts in caring for their child. Therefore the parent should be an integral part of the health care team.

Good skin care is essential for the child with CP. The nurse observes the skin for redness and other evidence of pressure sores. All precautions are taken to prevent the formation of *contractures* (degeneration or shortening of the muscles because of lack of use), which could

result in permanent loss of function of the part involved (e.g., leg, arm, or finger). The nurse encourages these children to do as much as they can for themselves. When they bathe, they are encouraged to put their muscles and joints through the normal range of motion. The nurse must use judgment in assessing their capabilities and assist only in those areas where they are lacking.

Other measures necessary to prevent deformities include frequent changes of position, the use of splints, and the carrying out of passive, range-of-motion, and stretching exercises. The nurse must also ensure that the child maintains good posture while in bed. This is done through the use of footboards and the proper positioning of pillows and other comfort devices.

Braces are often used to treat this disability. A brace is a mechanical aid that supports weakened muscles or limbs. All braces are routinely checked for correct alignment, loose or missing parts, and the condition of straps and buckles. The child needs assistance to adjust to this unfamiliar device. Wheelchairs and crutches are designed to fit the child.

Orthopedic surgery may be indicated and may be followed by an extensive period of rehabilitation. The nurse must remember that the child is in a continuous state of psychological and physical growth during this period. Interest, or a lack of it, may have a decided effect on the personality of the child in later years.

Feeding problems can lead to nutritional deficiencies. Vitamin, mineral, or protein supplements may be indicated for some children. Swallowing and sucking may be difficult. Vomiting is common because the gag reflex is overactive. The entire body may become tense. The nurse must be especially careful to feed the child slowly to prevent aspiration. It is difficult for these infants to adjust to solid foods, and it takes a great deal of patience on the part of parents and nurses to help the child to adapt to this new experience (Box 23-5 and Figure 23-12). As the children grow, they can be taught to manage special feeding equipment so they are able to eat independently. They are also taught such activities as dressing and combing their hair. Dental care is discussed in Chapter 15.

The physically challenged child needs opportunities to play alone and with other children. Games suited to ability, such as finger painting, are fun and allow freedom of expression. Activities that require fine muscular movements of the hand cause frustration in the child whose arms and hands are affected by the disease. The nurse can learn a great deal from the parents about the types of play the child enjoys. Children with CP tire easily but find it difficult to relax. They use a great deal of energy to accomplish the simplest of tasks, and they do not respond well to being hurried or overly stimulated.

Educational opportunities geared to the child's abilities are essential. Public Law 94-142 mandates that public schools provide education for disabled children. The

---

box 23-5 *General Modifications/Precautions in Pediatric Feeding Techniques for Children with Cerebral Palsy*

1. Proper positioning and support of the head and back are essential before feeding solid foods.
2. Place small amounts of food on a spoon to avoid choking.
3. Avoid tilting the head back during feeding of solid foods because this will place the swallowing mechanisms out of alignment.
4. Do not touch the tip of the child's tongue with the spoon, because this can activate the tongue extrusion reflex.
5. Use rubber-coated spoons for children with hyperactive bite reflex to protect the teeth from injury.
6. Gently stroke the angle of the jaw below the ears to relax the bite of a child who has clamped down on a spoon.
7. Gently stroke, in a circular motion, the area under the chin to stimulate chewing when food is held in the mouth.
8. Gently press upward under the chin to stimulate swallowing when fluid is held in the mouth.
9. To help a disabled child drink from a cup, cut the top portion of the paper or plastic cup away to provide space for the nose. This will enable the cup to be tilted without the child's head being tilted back.
10. Avoid excessive pressure on the back of the head when positioning a disabled child for feeding to avoid reflex responses in the body/torso position.

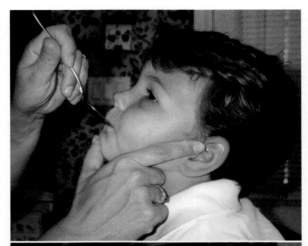
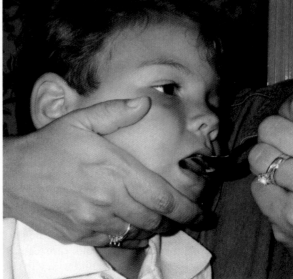

FIGURE **23-12** Feeding the disabled child. **A,** Manual jaw control is supplied anteriorly. **B,** Manual jaw control is provided from the side.

child's mental capacity is determined not just in the light of the intelligence quotient (IQ) itself but also by the demonstrated potential of the individual.

Preschools and summer camps for exceptional children are available. These programs vary in quality and extent of services. Parents are also referred to the United Cerebral Palsy Association, a national organization that provides education and support services. The expanding role of nurses in the home and schools may further assist in mainstreaming these children into educational and social situations (Box 23-6).

Successful experiences help to improve a child's self-concept; repeated failures are demoralizing and may lower self-esteem. The health care team works to bring satisfaction to these children by making it possible for them to succeed. The amount of confidence and self-respect that a disabled child has depends a great deal on a supportive environment.

Mental health needs of the physically challenged child. The requirements for good mental health in the physically challenged child do not differ from those of other children. They need to have their basic human needs satisfied and people who are genuinely interested in them. The disabled child must participate to the fullest extent in family, school, and community activities. Friendships with other disabled and nondisabled peers are encouraged. Extended family and the community are important resources. Educational programs are integrating the disabled more fully into the community. Barrier-free buildings and modifications that improve accessibility contribute positively to these efforts.

COGNITIVE IMPAIRMENT
Mental Retardation

Mental retardation has been defined as below-average mental functioning (IQ below 75) and a deficit in adaptive behavior manifested during the developmental period (before 18 years of age) (Box 23-7).

Definition. In 1992 the American Association of Mental Retardation refocused the definition of mental retardation away from only the IQ to the relationship of the cognitively impaired person functioning within an environment. The classification involves four levels of support systems needed for activities of daily living (ADLs): the need for intermittent support, limited support, extensive support, or pervasive (total) support. Mental retardation has many descriptive labels. The specific terminology most often used in the medical field is *mental retardation,* or *cognitive impairment.* The education system most often uses *mentally handicapped, mentally deficient, mentally disabled, mentally impaired,* or *mentally challenged.* The educational system uses criteria for classroom placement and eligibility for available resources. U.S. federal law provides for services from birth to 21 years of age. Public law requires providing the least restrictive environment for learning and mainstreaming with nonimpaired students whenever possible.

When a child is diagnosed as mentally retarded, it is important to correlate growth and development with mental functioning. For example, abstract thinking does not begin to appear before 12 years of age. *A child classified as mentally retarded is not necessarily retarded in all areas of mental functioning* (Box 23-8). There are numerous tests to measure intelligence. One test that is often given to children and adolescents is the Stanford-Binet.

Intelligence in children is difficult to evaluate and is best tested on an individual basis. Personality tests such as picture story tests, ink blot tests, drawing tests, and sentence completion tests may also be administered. All such tests have their limitations, and of course their accuracy is subject to the abilities of the person interpreting them. Nonetheless, the tests are of value when used in conjunction with a thorough study of the child's physical, mental, emotional, and social development.

---

box 23-6 | *Treatment Protocol for Cerebral Palsy*

1. Establish communication.
2. Establish locomotion.
3. Use and optimize existing motor functions.
4. Provide intellectual stimulation.
5. Promote socialization.
6. Provide technology to encourage self-care and promote growth and development.
7. Provide multidisciplinary approach to care.

---

box 23-7 | *American Association on Mental Retardation (AAMR) Definition of Mental Retardation*

Two levels: mild or severe
Intellectual functioning below IQ of 75

Limitations in at least two of the following 10 areas of adaptive behaviors:

1. Communication
2. Self-care
3. Home living
4. Social skills
5. Community use
6. Self-direction
7. Health and safety
8. Functional academics
9. Leisure
10. Work

There are many causes of mental retardation. Some conditions that can develop during the neonatal period are phenylketonuria, hypothyroidism, fetal alcohol syndrome, Down syndrome, malformations of the brain (e.g., microcephaly, hydrocephalus, craniosynostosis), and maternal infections such as cytomegalovirus (CMV). Birth injuries or anoxia during or shortly after delivery may also cause mental retardation. Conditions such as meningitis, lead poisoning, neoplasms, and encephalitis can cause mental retardation in a child or adult of any age. Heredity is a factor in mental retardation. It is also possible that living in a physically and emotionally deprived environment causes the child to be mentally retarded.

A diagnosis of mental retardation is determined after a thorough study is made. The American Psychiatric Association provides a DSM-IV listing that defines diagnostic criteria for mental retardation. Conditions such as epilepsy, CP, severe malnutrition, emotional disturbances, blindness, deafness, and speech disorders must be ruled out. In certain cases, early recognition and intervention can lessen or prevent mental retardation.

Other symptoms of mental retardation are associated with milestones of the growth process. Children who do not achieve milestones at the expected age may be cognitively impaired. Unusual clumsiness and failure to respond to stimuli are also early indications. Sometimes this disorder is not discovered until the child enters school. Each case must be frequently reevaluated according to the child's individual progress. The goal of care is to normalize the child and family as much as possible.

The importance of success in the approach to the mentally retarded child. We cannot all run at the same speed, sing with the same ability, dance as gracefully, or draw as skillfully as some of our peers. Yet most of us get by. However, problems can develop if one is not good in something such as reading, writing, and spelling (which, in our culture, is very important). The problems usually relate to the consequences of chronic failure.

The pediatric nurse must assist the parents to understand that providing experiences that the child can be successful in and concentrating on his or her strengths rather than weaknesses are the keys to dealing with a child who is developmentally different. A child who experiences consistent failure becomes angry. The anger causes behavior difficulties that can cloud the problem and the therapy.

NURSING TIP

The mentally retarded child needs to develop a sense of accomplishment. Do not "take over" projects because of your own need to assist or speed up the process.

Management and nursing goals. An individualized plan of care with goals and objectives is vital to managing mentally retarded children and helping their families. The initial step is to present the findings to the family and to provide the emotional support necessary to cope with a disabled child. The child's competence and adaptive behaviors should be discussed along with the deficiencies. Introduction to the multidisciplinary team for long-term management is important. Play therapy should be prescribed to nurture growth and development. The Special Olympics introduce healthy competition to the cognitively and physically impaired child. Receptive and expressive communication skills are developed with professional help.

Nurses must be familiar with the resources of the community so that they can direct the family to them. The local chapter of the National Association for Retarded Citizens may provide information and support. Summer camps, such as those run by the Easter Seal Society, provide stimulation and opportunities for socialization to children with mental and physical disabilities. The child guidance clinic or the psychological services of a nearby college or hospital may be used. Arrangements for proper dental care must be made because some children may be unable to cooperate with the necessary procedures.

The nurse caring for the mentally retarded child in the hospital must know the child's stage of maturation and ability. A detailed history, including a habit and care sheet, is completed. Self-help activities are documented. Home routines are to be followed as closely as possible to avoid the reversal of gains already made. Good communication between the parents and the nurse can help

---

box 23-8 | *Elements Involved in Mental Functioning*

LEVEL OF CONSCIOUSNESS
Attention
Short-term and long-term memory
Perceptions

THOUGHT PROCESSES
Insight
Judgments
Affect
Mood

EXPRESSIVE LANGUAGE
Vocabulary
Abstract thinking
Intelligence

to make the transition from home to hospital as smooth as possible for the child. A positive approach is recommended when obtaining information about the child from the parents. A request such as, "Tell me about Carla's eating habits" is preferable to "Does she feed herself?" and is likely to yield more helpful information.

NURSING TIP

Nursing responsibilities to disabled children are as follows:
- Emphasize the *strengths* present.
- Maintain communication with the family.
- Avoid labels; use simple terms.
- Contact the school nurse; plan for school needs.
- Provide daily experiences in which the child can succeed.
- Refer to local, state, and national support groups.

NURSING TIP

Many mentally retarded children have a normal facial appearance. Many children with unusual faces are not mentally retarded.

Prevention. The outlook is good for continued success in the prevention of mental retardation. Nurses can contribute to this by promoting genetic counseling, immunizations, newborn screening, and good prenatal care (Table 23-5). Comprehensive programs for early assessment and treatment of mentally retarded persons must also be promoted. The nurse can serve as an advocate for the child and/or adolescent to help ensure that his or her rights are upheld.

NURSING TIP

Cognitively impaired children have the same psychosocial needs as all other children but cannot express or respond as other children do.

HEAD INJURIES

Head injuries are the major cause of death in children older than 1 year of age. More physical force is needed to produce brain trauma when the head is in a fixed position than when it is freely moving—a fact that supports the use of infant car seats. The incidence of head injury among children is high. A concussion is a temporary disturbance of the brain that is usually followed by a period of unconsciousness. It jars the brainstem and is often

| table 23-5 | *Interventions Currently Available to Prevent Mental Retardation* |

FACTOR	INTERVENTION
NEARLY TOTAL ELIMINATION	
Congenital rubella	Early immunization, antibody screening
Phenylketonuria, galactosemia, congenital hypothyroidism	Newborn screening, dietary management, replacement therapy
Kernicterus	Reduction of sensitization
MAJOR REDUCTION	
Tay-Sachs disease	Carrier screening, prenatal diagnosis in high-risk persons
Morbidity from prematurity	Newborn intensive care nurseries
Measles encephalitis	Early vaccination
SIGNIFICANT REDUCTION	
Neural tube defects	Prenatal folic acid supplements
Lead intoxication	Screening for lead levels, improvement in environment, chelation when necessary
Fetal alcohol syndrome	Public education
Morbidity from head injury	Automobile child restraints, safety helmets and equipment
Child neglect and abuse	Parenting classes and family life education through the schools
SPECIAL ASSISTANCE AND RELIEF	
Multiple disabilities, hearing, speech, Down syndrome	Early identification, support for families, genetic counseling of special risks

Modified from Levine, M.D., Carey, W.B., & Crocker, A.C. (1999). *Developmental-behavioral pediatrics.* Philadelphia: W.B. Saunders.

accompanied by a loss of memory for events that occurred immediately before (retrograde amnesia), during, and after the accident. A *skull fracture* indicates that the skull bone is broken or depressed. Bleeding may occur, resulting in pressure being exerted on the brain.

The response of the child to a head injury may differ from that of the adult. The location and type of skull fracture may not correlate with clinical findings. Careful clinical assessment is essential to determine the extent of brain injury. The surface area of a child's scalp is large and very vascular. Significant blood loss can result from scalp lacerations.

> ✶NURSING **TIP**
> A concussion with resulting amnesia and confusion can be more serious than the presence of a fractured skull with no clinical symptoms.

Pathophysiology. A skull fracture, brain concussion, contusion, or intracranial hemorrhage may occur at the time of injury. Hypoxia, increased ICP, cerebral edema, and infection can occur within a few days. Hypoxia causes the brain to need increased energy, which results in increased cerebral blood flow. This increased blood flow (hyperemia) increases cerebral edema. If the ICP rises too high, cerebral perfusion diminishes and brain damage or death results. If the fontanels are open, the tolerance for increased ICP is higher in infants. Older children and adults do not have this advantage.

A child who sustains a mild bump to the head, retains consciousness, and does not vomit may have a covered ice pack applied to the site. During the first night after a bump on the head, parents are advised to be sure that they can arouse the child at least once, because intracranial bleeding occasionally occurs from a minor injury. They should be advised to contact a physician if the child appears confused, has trouble seeing or speaking, or walks unsteadily. Confusion and amnesia after any head injury may indicate a concussion even if consciousness is not lost.

Infants who are roughly shaken (shaken baby syndrome) can sustain retinal, subarachnoid, and subdural hemorrhages in the brain and high-level cervical spine injuries, resulting in permanent disability or death. A child who has suffered a blow to the head is often brought to the hospital for overnight observation to rule out or confirm the extent of injury. The child may experience all or some of the following symptoms: headache (manifested by fussiness in the toddler), drowsiness, blurred vision, vomiting, and dyspnea. In severe cases, the child may be completely unconscious. Decerebrate (extensor) posturing or decorticate (flexor) posturing may be evident (Figure 23-13). In decerebrate (extensor) rigidity,

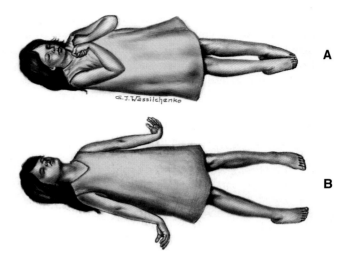

FIGURE **23-13** Posturing. Pathological posturing that may occur in the children with severe brain damage. **A,** Decorticate (flexor) posturing. **B,** Decerebrate (extensor) posturing.

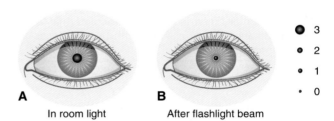

A In room light   B After flashlight beam

FIGURE **23-14** The response of the pupil of the eye to a flashlight beam. **A,** The pupil of the eye is a "3" in room light. **B,** The pupil of the eye is a "1" after a flashlight beam is directed at the eye. The letters "B," "S," and "N" may be used to denote *b*risk movement, *s*low movement, or *n*onmovement of the pupil response. This illustration would be recorded 3/1 B. The other eye should respond symmetrically. Sluggish movement, nonmovement, or asymmetrical response should be reported immediately.

all four limbs are extended and the hands are pronated. This may indicate brainstem injury. In decorticate (flexor) rigidity, the arms, wrists, and fingers are flexed. Plantar flexion occurs in the feet. This may indicate damage to the cortex of the brain. These pathological postures (posturing) are seen with severe brain injury.

A careful history is obtained to determine any preexisting conditions and to ascertain the exact circumstances of the accident. Of particular importance is the child's state of consciousness immediately after the accident.

The nurse observes the child for signs of increasing ICP. Four components of a cranial or neurological check are as follows: (1) level of consciousness, (2) pupil and eye movement (Figure 23-14), (3) vital signs, and (4) motor activity (Box 23-9).

box 23-9 *Neurological Monitoring of Infants and Children*

Many subtle clues to a change in neurological status in infants and children can be missed unless the nurse aggressively assesses them. The lack of the child's ability to communicate and cooperate poses a challenge in the neurological assessment of infants, but a knowledge of normal growth and development aids the nurse in evaluating the status of his or her little patient. For example, we know that an infant should turn his or her head toward the spoken word by age 6 months. However, assessing after a full feeding may cause a delayed response that may not be pathological.

PAIN STIMULI

There are two types of pain stimuli: *central,* a response of the brain, and *peripheral,* a response of the spinal cord. The pain stimulus should continue for 30 seconds to determine the optimal function response.

Central pain stimulus
1. *Trapezius muscle.* Firmly pinch large muscle mass at the angle where the neck and shoulder meet.
2. *Suborbital pressure.* Exert firm pressure on the "notch" that can be located under the center of the eyebrow.

LEVEL OF CONSCIOUSNESS

In children and adolescents we can determine the difference between arousal, awareness, orientation, and memory. In infants, the Glasgow Coma Scale is used (see Table 23-6).

AROUSAL AWARENESS

Child responds to his or her name, which is indicative of basic cerebral function.

Child can interact with environment, indicating cerebral cortex functioning.
1. *Orientation.* Determine awareness of person, place, or time. Use open-ended or multiple-choice questions rather than questions that can be answered by "yes" or "no."
2. *Attention span.* Although attention span can differ with the age of child, the child would not normally fall off to sleep in the middle of a response requiring rearousal stimuli. This should be recorded if it occurs.
3. *Language.* Understanding the level of language development is essential in determining if the language pattern is normal or abnormal. Speaking clearly and recognizing familiar objects is a skill that is age related in the pediatric setting.
4. *Irritability, lethargy, and vomiting.* These are clinical symptoms of increased intracranial pressure (ICP) in infants, in addition to signs such as a bulging fontanel.
5. *Memory.* A child's ability to recognize family members or repeat what he or she had for breakfast is a valid observation for memory.

CRANIAL NERVE RESPONSES

Cranial nerve responses are valuable in determining priority of need related to survival and safety.
1. *Olfactory (I).* A strong-smelling substance under the nose of an alert infant will elicit a grimace or startle response.
2. *Optic (II).* Infant is able to fix on object and follow a short distance. Pupils react equally to light.
3. *Oculomotor (III).* Pupils respond to light. In "doll's-eye test," eyes move away from direction head is rotated; infant is able to open eyes.
4. *Trochlear (IV).* Infant is able to move eyes and follow object.
5. *Trigeminal (V).* Infant turns head in response to stroking cheek.
6. *Abducens (VI).* Corneal reflex is present; eyes follow past midline.
7. *Facial (VII).* Wrinkles brow; symmetrical facial movements; closes eyes when crying.
8. *Auditory (VIII).* Tested via auditory screening machine; infant turns head toward sound source.
9. *Glossopharyngeal (IX).* Elicits a positive gag reflex, moves tongue in mouth.
10. *Vagus (X).* Infant has ability to swallow and a lusty cry and cough.
11. *Accessory (XI).* Turn infant's head to one side and infant will return head to midline.
12. *Hypoglossal (XII).* Infant able to suck and swallow; tongue protrusion is present.

MOTOR RESPONSE

Symmetrical spontaneous body movements are an important observation to record. Asking the child to follow a simple motor request is more accurate than a hand grasp, because in some age-groups a hand grasp is a *reflex* rather than a *voluntary response*. A purposeful voluntary motor response is a more valuable observation than a reflex response to remove irritants such as an attempt to pull out a nasogastric tube.

POSTURING

In children and adolescents, posturing can indicate a change in neurological status that requires immediate notification of the physician.

Decorticate (flexor). Flexion of the arms to center to body and flexing of wrists indicate partial brain

Continued

box 23-9 *Neurological Monitoring of Infants and Children—cont'd*

function (indicates injury to the cerebral cortex of the brain) (Figure 23-13).

Decerebrate (extensor). Arms are extended along the side of the body and the hands are pronated. This indicates brainstem function only (Figure 23-13).

Opisthotonos position. Hyperextension of the neck and arching of the spine is a position assumed by infants with cerebral pathology (Figure 23-8).

EYES (see Figure 23-14)

The pupils of the eyes should be observed for size, equality, and response to light. It may be best to evaluate the eye in a slightly darkened room so the pupils may be somewhat dilated and the response to sudden light from a flashlight can be readily assessed.

Pupils that remain *pinpoint* can indicate damage to the pons or part of the brainstem or can indicate drug toxicity.

Bilateral dilated pupils can be indicative of hypoxia or intoxication with atropine-like drugs.

Pupils that are *unequal* in size can signal brain herniation; *immediate action is required.*

Pupillary response to light can be brisk, sluggish, or absent. Recording should indicate the size of the pupil in normal light (e.g., 3), size of pupil after flashlight intervention (e.g., 1), and how fast the change occurred (B, brisk; S, sluggish/slow; A, absent). A normal recording for pupillary response would be as follows: R 3/1 B; L 3/1 B.

Keep in mind that infants and children who are blind will not have a meaningful light response test.

When the pupil constricts in response to light, be sure that constriction is maintained and that the eye does not dilate again before light is removed.

FONTANEL

A bulging anterior fontanel is indicative of increased ICP.

SCALP VEIN DISTENTION

Scalp veins distend because of the obstruction of flow from the bridging veins of the scalp to the sagittal sinus.

ATAXIA; SPASTICITY OF LOWER EXTREMITIES

Occur with damage to the corticospinal pathways.

MORO/TONIC NECK WITH WITHDRAWAL REFLEXES

In infants, an absence of these reflexes can occur with increased ICP.

Children are handled gently and are inspected for injuries to other areas. They are placed in a crib or bed in accordance with their age. Side rails are raised, because seizures are not uncommon. The head of the bed is slightly elevated to decrease cerebral edema.

NURSING **TIP**

The presence of asymmetrical pupils after a head injury is a medical emergency.

Level of consciousness. Changes in level of consciousness are particularly meaningful and require immediate medical attention. The child's alertness on admission is recorded for use as baseline data. The response should be correlated with the child's developmental age. Parents can be helpful in providing information about the child's usual capabilities. In general, children should be oriented to person, time, and place (according to developmental capabilities). The nurse asks, "What is your name?" and "Where are you?" Older children may know the day of the week. The child should recognize parents. The nurse points to the mother and asks, "Who is this?" The child should be able to follow simple commands, such as "Turn over."

When the child does not respond to verbal stimuli, the upper arm is gently pinched and the response is observed. The presence or absence of crying or speech is noted. It is not unusual for children to fall asleep, but they should be easily aroused. The nurse records changes in sleeping posture, movements of extremities, and any signs of tremors or restlessness. The bladder is observed for distention, which can contribute to irritability. Incontinence in the child who is toilet-trained is significant. The child's behavior is described in the nurse's notes. The Glasgow Coma Scale is valuable in determining various levels of consciousness. Table 23-6 shows a scale modified for infants.

Vital signs. An increase in blood pressure and a decrease in pulse and respiration are evidence of increased ICP. Temperature elevations may result from inflammation, systemic infection, or damage to the hypothalamus, which regulates body temperature. Mild elevations caused by trauma are not uncommon during the first 2 days after a head injury.

Motor activity. Because nerves energize the muscle tissue, any damage to the nervous system affects body movement. The quality and strength of muscle tone are observed in all four extremities. The child should be able to move the legs and push against the nurse's hands with both feet. The face should be symmetrical. The child can smile and frown. Drooping of the eyes *(ptosis)*, inability to close the eyes tightly, and drooping of the corner of the mouth are considered pathological. The child should be able to raise the arms and extend the palms upward and downward. Abnormal posturing is described and recorded.

Nursing care. Nursing care includes examination of wound swelling if a laceration of the head is present. The type and amount of drainage from the ears and nose are recorded. The nurse checks for *nuchal* (neck) rigidity, which might indicate infection such as meningitis. Occipital-frontal circumference of the head is monitored in infants, as are tension of the fontanels and the presence of a high-pitched cry. Fluids are carefully monitored to control *cerebral edema*. Feeding difficulties should be noted as the child's diet is increased. The child is observed for signs of shock, which can also occur. Children whose condition has remained stable are discharged. Parents are instructed about any additional observations and follow-up care.

> ### NURSING TIP
> A positive glucose (Dextrostix) test can determine if watery nasal discharge is CSF or a concurrent cold (rhinorrhea).

NEAR-DROWNING

Accidental drowning or near-drowning is the fourth leading cause of death for U.S. children under 19 years of age. Near-drowning is defined as survival beyond 24 hours after submersion. Proper supervision and environmental safety precautions are the best measures to prevent drowning. In adolescents the use of illicit drugs and alcohol during recreational swimming contributes to drowning incidents. The priorities include the immediate treatment of *hypoxia, aspiration,* and *hypothermia.*

Cardiorespiratory survival has increased with advances in emergency medical treatment by paramedics on site and the technology available in intensive care units in the hospital. However, CNS injury remains the major cause of death or long-term disability.

Submersion of more than 10 minutes with failure to regain consciousness at the scene or within 24 hours is an ominous sign and indicates severe neurological deficits if the child survives. Respiratory and cardiovascular support, controlled rewarming, and maintenance of adequate cerebral oxygenation are priorities of care (see Nursing Care Plan 23-1). The parents need to be offered support, explanations of the therapy, and referral to social services, religious, or community agencies for follow-up.

table 23-6	*The Glasgow Coma Scale Modified for Infants*

AGE IN MONTHS	RESPONSE
1	1. None 2. Crying to stimuli 3. Crying spontaneously 4. Blinks when eyelashes are touched 5. Throaty noises
2	1. None 2. Crying to stimuli 3. Shuts eyes to light 4. Smiles when caressed 5. Babbles—single vowel sounds
3	1. None 2. Crying to stimuli (moans) 3. Stares to response and looks at environment 4. Smiles to sound stimulation 5. Coos, chuckles, *vowels* in a prolonged way
4	1. None 2. Crying to stimuli (moans) 3. Turns head to sound 4. Smiles spontaneously or when stimulated, laughs when socially stimulated 5. Modulating voice and perfect vocalization of vowels
5 and 6	1. None 2. Crying to stimuli (moans) 3. Localizes general direction of sound 4. Discriminates family members 5. Babbles to people, toys
7 and 8	1. None 2. Crying to stimuli (moans) 3. Recognizes familiar voices and family 4. Babbles 5. "Ba," "Ma," "Da"
9 and 10	1. None 2. Crying to stimuli (moans) 3. Recognizes (smiles or laughs) 4. Babbles 5. "Mama," "Dada"
11 and 12	1. None 2. Crying to stimuli (moans) 3. Recognizes—smiles 4. Babbles 5. Words (specifically "Mama" and "Dada")

In the older child, the best verbal, motor, and eye-opening responses are scored and recorded.

Modified from Zimmerman, S.S., & Gildea, J.H. (1985). *Critical care pediatrics.* Philadelphia: W.B. Saunders; and Behrman, R.E., Kliegman, R.M., & Jensen, H.B. (2000) *Nelson's essentials of pediatrics* (3rd ed.). Philadelphia: W.B. Saunders.

NURSING CARE PLAN 23-1

The Child with Altered Level of Consciousness

PATIENT DATA: A 4-year-old child fell into a pool while playing, hitting his head on the pool deck. Cardiopulmonary resuscitation re-established a heartbeat and spontaneous respirations. The child is admitted with signs of increased intracranial pressure, including a decreased level of consciousness and an absence of the gag reflex.

SELECTED NURSING DIAGNOSIS *Ineffective airway clearance/ineffective breathing pattern related to decreased level of consciousness*

Outcomes	Nursing Interventions	Rationales
Child will demonstrate effective airway clearance and breathing pattern as evidenced by patent airway, age-appropriate respiratory rate (RR), lungs clear to auscultation, ability to breathe on his or her own without mechanical assistance.	1. Observe airway for patency.	1. Diminished oxygenation can lead to cerebral anoxia and/or death.
	2. Observe for presence/absence of gag/swallow reflex, RR, rhythm, and effort; note any irregularities.	2. Inability to protect the airway can lead to aspiration pneumonia. A marked increase or decrease in respiratory pattern can be a sign of impending respiratory failure.
	3. Auscultate breath sounds, noting and reporting any adventitious breath sounds.	3. Adventitious breath sounds are indicative of accumulated respiratory secretions, thereby increasing the risk for pneumonia or atelectasis.
	4. Provide meticulous pulmonary toilet to prevent respiratory compromise.	4. Good oral hygiene, suctioning of oral secretions, cleaning of buccal cavity, and turning child every 2 hours will help to prevent respiratory problems.

SELECTED NURSING DIAGNOSIS *Risk for impaired skin integrity related to physical immobility*

Outcomes	Nursing Interventions	Rationales
Child will maintain intact skin without signs or symptoms of tissue breakdown or decubitus formation.	1. Inspect all skin surfaces, noting areas of erythema, blanching, or edema. Pay particular attention to all bony prominences and areas in direct contact with the bed.	1. Lying in one position for extended periods increases the risk of tissue breakdown and decubitus formation.
	2. Reposition every 2 hours. Place child in prone position periodically (unless contraindicated by medical condition).	2. Repositioning helps to improve circulation and relieves pressure areas.
	3. Bathe child daily and keep bedding free of wrinkles and crumbs.	3. Bathing increases circulation because of the massaging of the skin with the washcloth. Having a bed free of wrinkles and crumbs prevents additional areas of potential skin breakdown and decubitus formation.

NURSING CARE PLAN 23-1—cont'd

SELECTED NURSING DIAGNOSIS *Compromised family coping related to loss of well-being of child*

Outcomes	Nursing Interventions	Rationales
Parent/family will demonstrate effective coping skills as evidenced by expressing a realistic understanding of child's illness and active participation in child's care.	1. Assess level of anxiety or concern of parent(s) and/or family members. 2. Provide opportunities for instruction on how to care for the ill child. 3. Reinforce and/or clarify medical explanation of child's condition and prognosis. 4. Identify community agencies and support services within the community available to the family.	1. Provides data to determine type of assistance or support that is needed. 2. Enhances feelings of control/involvement in the health care of the child. 3. Ensures parent/family has a clear understanding of information received. 4. Provides family with sources of emotional and spiritual support in time of crises.

?CRITICAL THINKING QUESTION

After resuscitation in the emergency department, the child has regained consciousness, is interacting with the mother, and has stable vital signs. The mother states, "Now that my child is OK I want to take him home." What is the best response of the nurse?

⟩NURSING TIP

All children who experience near-drowning should be admitted for a 24-hour observation period of close monitoring.

key points

- Infants are more prone to ear infections than are older children because their eustachian tubes are shorter, wider, and straighter.
- When instilling ear drops in infants, gently pull the pinna *down* and back. In children, the pinna is gently pulled *up* and back.
- In paralytic strabismus the *unaffected* eye is patched.
- Level of consciousness is the most important indicator of neurological health.
- Nursing care of the unconscious child includes assessing the child for increased intracranial pressure (ICP), maintaining an open airway, providing adequate nutrition and fluids, positioning, maintaining flexibility of joints, and preventing injury.
- Do not give aspirin or other salicylates to children with symptoms of influenza or chickenpox because the drug is linked to Reye's syndrome, a serious and life-threatening illness.
- Meningitis is an inflammation of the meninges that cover the brain and spinal cord.
- A high-pitched cry may be indicative of increased ICP.
- A seizure is a symptom of an underlying pathologic condition.

- Grand mal seizures have an aura, tonic and clonic phases, and postictal lethargy.
- Decerebrate, decorticate, or opisthotonos posturing indicates brain damage.
- The response of the pupils to light and level of consciousness are essential assessments to determine brain injury.
- The Glasgow Coma Scale is used to determine level of consciousness in infants and children.
- "Shaken baby syndrome" can result in subdural hematoma and death.
- Confusion and amnesia after a head injury may indicate concussion even if consciousness is not lost.
- The four types of cerebral palsy are spastic, athetoid, ataxic, and mixed.
- Mental retardation involves three components: intelligence, adaptive behavior, and onset before 18 years of age.
- The priority of care for a child who has experienced near-drowning is to prevent hypoxia, aspiration, and hypothermia.

⟩ONLINE RESOURCES

Pediatric Head Injuries:
http://www.pediatric-emergency.com/headtrauma.htm
Sight and Hearing Association:
http://www. sightandhearing.org
National Hydrocephalus Foundation:
http://www.nhfonline.org/index.html

REVIEW QUESTIONS   *Choose the most appropriate answer.*

1. Symptoms of an earache in an infant include:
   1. External drainage, pain, and decrease in temperature
   2. Tugging at the ear and rolling head from side to side
   3. Crying and pointing to affected ear
   4. Redness of the cheeks and cyanosis of ear

2. The medical term for crossed eyes is:
   1. Strabismus
   2. Amblyopia
   3. Myopia
   4. PERRLA

3. Reye's syndrome affects the:
   1. Stomach and intestine
   2. Islet of Langerhans
   3. Liver and brain
   4. Heart and blood vessels

4. Mental retardation can be prevented by:
   1. Administering the Stanford-Binet test
   2. A blood test at birth
   3. Careful preschool developmental screening
   4. A urine test at age 6 months

5. The seizure in which the child cries out, falls to the floor, becomes rigid, and then has a convulsion is termed:
   1. Petit mal
   2. Myoclonic
   3. Grand mal
   4. Atonic

objectives

1. Define each key term listed.
2. Demonstrate an understanding of age-specific changes that occur in the musculoskeletal system during growth and development.
3. Discuss the types of fractures commonly seen in children and their effect on growth and development.
4. List two symptoms of Duchenne's muscular dystrophy.
5. Describe three types of child abuse.
6. Identify symptoms of abuse and neglect in children.
7. Differentiate between Buck extension and Russell traction.
8. Describe two topics of discussion applicable at discharge for the child with juvenile rheumatoid arthritis.
9. Describe the symptoms, treatment, and nursing care for the child with Legg-Calvé-Perthes disease.
10. Compile a nursing care plan for the child who is immobilized by traction.
11. Describe a neurovascular check.
12. Describe the management of soft tissue injuries.
13. State two cultural or medical practices that may be misinterpreted as child abuse.
14. Describe three nursing care measures required to maintain skin integrity in an adolescent child in a cast for scoliosis.

key terms

arthroscopy (p. 569)
Bryant's traction (p. 570)
Buck extension (p. 570)
compartment syndrome (p. 573)
compound fracture (p. 570)
contusion (kŏn-TŪ-zhŭn, p. 569)
epiphysis (ă-PĬF-ă-sĭs, p. 570)
gait (p. 568)
genu valgum (JĒ-nū VĂL-găm, p. 568)
genu varum (JĒ-nū VĂR-ăm, p. 568)
greenstick fracture (p. 570)

hematoma (hē-mă-TŌ-mă, p. 569)
Milwaukee brace (p. 582)
neurovascular checks (p. 573)
Russell traction (p. 570)
shin splint (p. 585)
spiral fracture (p. 570)
sprain (p. 569)
strain (p. 570)

OVERVIEW

The musculoskeletal system supports the body and provides for movement. The muscular and skeletal systems work together to enable a person to sit, stand, walk, and remain upright. In addition, muscles move air into and out of the lungs, blood through vessels, and food through the digestive tract. They also produce heat, which aids in numerous body chemical reactions. Bones act as levers and provide support. Red blood cells are produced in the bone marrow, and minerals such as calcium and phosphorus are also stored there. Figure 24-1 describes some differences between the child's and adult's skeletal and muscular systems.

The musculoskeletal system arises from the mesoderm in the embryo. A great portion of skeletal growth occurs between the fourth and eighth weeks of fetal life. As the limbs elongate before birth, muscle masses form in the extremities. The Ballard scoring system (see Figure 13-2) is one measure of assessing neuromuscular maturity at birth. Testing various reflexes is another.

Locomotion develops gradually and in an orderly manner in the growing child. A marked slowing down of growth is always a signal for investigation.

OBSERVATION OF THE MUSCULOSKELETAL SYSTEM IN THE GROWING CHILD

To assess the musculoskeletal system of the growing child and to identify deviations, the nurse must have a basic understanding of the effect of growth, neurologi-

567

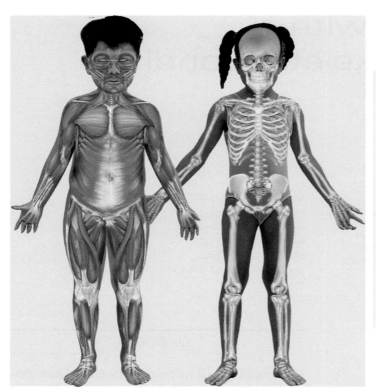

FIGURE **24-1** Some musculoskeletal system differences between the child and the adult. The muscular system consists of the large skeletal muscles that enable movement as well as the cardiac muscle of the heart and the smooth muscle of the internal organs. The skeletal system consists of bones and cartilage. This system helps to support and protect the body.

MUSCULOSKELETAL SYSTEM

- Skeletal growth is most rapid during infancy and adolescence. Assessing growth and development is an integral part of the physical examination for children.
- The bones of children are more resilient, tend to bend, and may deform before breaking.
- The blood supply to bone in children is rich; therefore healing occurs more quickly. Their periostium is thick, and osteogenic activity is high.
- Epiphyseal plate fractures in children can disrupt the growth of bones.
- Musculoskeletal problems may be growth related.
- Rapid growth of the skeletal frame of children can cause deformities to become more severe.

cal development, and motor milestones at various ages. The newborn hip has limited internal rotation range of motion (ROM). The legs are maintained in a flexed position, and the lower leg has an internal rotation (internal tibial torsion) caused by the effects of uterine positioning; this can last 4 to 6 months. The general curvature of the newborn spine is a C shape from the thoracic to the pelvic level and changes with the mastery of motor skills to a double S curve in childhood (see Figure 17-1). The newborn's feet normally turn inward *(varus)* or outward *(valgus),* but the turning-in self-corrects when the sole of the foot is stroked. The toddler's feet appear flat because of the presence of a fat pad at the arch. Any delay in neurological development can cause a delay in the mastery of motor skills, which can result in altered skeletal growth.

Assessment of the musculoskeletal system includes observation, palpation, ROM, and gait assessment in children who can walk. Children who do not walk independently by 18 months of age have a serious delay and should be referred to a health care provider for follow-up.

OBSERVATION OF GAIT

The toddler who begins to walk has a wide, unstable gait. The arms do not swing with the walking motion. By 18 months of age the wide base narrows and the walk is more stable. By 4 years of age the child can hop on one foot, and arm swings occur with walking. By 6 years of age the gait resembles the adult walk with equal stride lengths and associated arm swing. The trunk is centered over the legs and movement is symmetrical. When a child favors one side, pain may be present. Toe walking after 3 years of age can indicate a muscle problem.

In most cases, excessive in-toeing or pointing of the toe inward will clear by 4 years of age. These children trip and fall easily. Teaching proper sitting and body mechanics is the treatment of choice. Participation in ballet classes and roller-blading will enhance hip flexibility. If the problem does not resolve, a brace may be prescribed. Failure to treat can result in hip, knee, or back problems in adulthood.

Young children appear bowlegged (genu varum) or knock-kneed (genu valgum), with the knees turned inward until 5 years of age. Bowing is seldom pathological. The ligaments that support the arch are not mature before 6 years of age, and therefore the child may appear to have flat feet. If the condition interferes with walking, an orthotic appliance can be prescribed for the child to wear inside the shoes. When the flat foot is painful, a referral for follow-up examination should be initiated. The role of the nurse is to reassure parents that unless there is associated pain or a problem with motor or nerve functions, many minor abnormal-appearing alignments will spontaneously resolve with activity.

OBSERVATION OF MUSCLE TONE

The nurse should assess symmetry of movement and the strength and contour of the body and extremities. The strength of the extremities can be tested by having the child push away the examiner's hand with his or her foot or hand.

Neurological examination. A neurological assessment is a vital part of a comprehensive musculoskeletal examination. An assessment of reflexes, a sensory assessment, and the presence or absence of spasms should be noted.

DIAGNOSTIC TESTS AND TREATMENTS
X-ray Studies

Radiographs are taken to confirm a suspected pathologic condition, and the affected area is compared with the unaffected area.

Bone scans. Bone scans are helpful in identifying pathological conditions that may not clearly be seen on a routine x-ray, such as septic arthritis or tumors.

Computed tomography. Computed tomography (CT) provides a cross-sectional picture of the bone and its relationship to other structures within the area of examination.

Magnetic resonance imaging. Magnetic resonance imaging (MRIs) do not involve harmful radiation. They produce detailed pictures of the brain, spinal cord, and soft tissue lesions, including a slipped femoral epiphysis.

Ultrasound. Ultrasound does not involve harmful radiation or aftereffects. It is used to rule out foreign bodies in soft tissues, joint effusions, and developmental dysplasia of the hip.

Laboratory Tests and Treatments

A complete blood count (CBC) and erythrocyte sedimentation rate (ESR) may rule out septic arthritis or osteomyelitis. Human leukocyte antigen (HLA) B-27 may help diagnose rheumatological disorders.

A thorough history is necessary to determine the basis for musculoskeletal problems, which are often insidious. The nurse determines the history of injury; location of pain; when symptoms started; any weakness,

numbness, or loss of function in an extremity; and whether the problem is affecting the daily activities of the child. An arthroscopy is commonly performed on adolescents with sports injuries. The physician is able to look inside the joint (usually the knee) to determine the extent of injury. The area is inspected, foreign particles are removed, or repairs are made to the torn menisci. A bone biopsy may reveal a malignancy. Muscle biopsy may detect muscular dystrophy.

Traction, casting, and splints are used in accordance with the patient's needs. Three types of skin traction are often used for the lower extremities of children: *Bryant's traction, Buck extension,* and *Russell traction.* Children with musculoskeletal disorders may require lengthy hospitalization. Immobility causes a slowing down of body metabolism. Nursing interventions focus on maintaining body functions. ROM exercises and the use of a trapeze prevent muscle atrophy. Foods high in roughage stimulate the digestive tract and prevent constipation. Respiratory exercises prevent pneumonia. These and other measures can prevent complications that can lengthen hospitalization for the child. (Clubfoot and congenital hip dysplasia are discussed in Chapter 14. Rickets is discussed in Chapter 27.)

MUSCULOSKELETAL SYSTEM DIFFERENCES BETWEEN THE CHILD AND ADULT

The pediatric skeletal system differs from the adult in that bone is not completely ossified, epiphyses are present, and the periosteum is thicker and produces callus more rapidly than in the adult. The lower mineral content of the child's bone and greater porosity increase the bone's strength. However, rotational or angular forces can stress ligaments that insert at the epiphyseal area of the bone, and injury to the epiphysis can affect bone growth. Because of the presence of the epiphysis and hyperemia caused by the trauma, bone overgrowth is common in healing fractures of children under 10 years of age.

PEDIATRIC TRAUMA

Soft tissue injuries usually accompany traumatic fractures in the child at play or the adolescent involved in sports activities and include the following:

- **Contusions.** A tearing of subcutaneous tissue that results in hemorrhage, edema, and pain. The escape of blood into the soft tissue is referred to as a hematoma, or "black and blue mark."
- **Sprain.** When the ligament is torn or stretched away from the bone at the point of trauma, there may be resulting damage to the blood vessels, muscles, and nerves. Swelling, disability, and pain are major signs of a sprain.

- **Strain.** A microscopic tear to the muscle or tendon occurs over time and results in edema and pain.

Prevention of Pediatric Trauma

Accidents are common in childhood, but much can be done to prevent morbidity and mortality. Parents are responsible for maintaining a safe environment for their children. Nurses are responsible for educating parents and schoolteachers on how to prevent accidental injury and maintain a safe environment.

The proper use of pedestrian safety, car seat restraints, bicycle helmets and other athletic protective gear, pool fences, window bars, deadbolt locks, and locks on cabinets can prevent unnecessary injury to children. Pediatric trauma can cause permanent disability or premature death. Nursing assessment and interventions can assist the injured child toward recovery. The nurse also has a community responsibility to support legislation that would maintain safe environments for children.

Treatment of Soft Tissue Injuries

Soft tissue injuries should be treated immediately to limit damage from edema and bleeding. A cold pack and elastic wrap will reduce edema and bleeding, relieve pain, and should be applied at *alternating 30-minute intervals.* (After a 30-minute period, ischemia can occur and impede the tissue perfusion.) Elevating the extremity above heart level reduces edema. When an elastic bandage is used for compression, a priority nursing responsibility is to perform frequent neurovascular checks to ensure adequate tissue perfusion.

> ⭐NURSING **TIP**
> Principles of managing soft tissue injuries include the following:
> - **R**est
> - **I**ce
> - **C**ompression
> - **E**levation

TRAUMATIC FRACTURES AND TRACTION

Pathophysiology. A fracture is a break in a bone and is mainly caused by accidents. It is characterized by pain, tenderness on movement, and swelling. Discoloration, limited movement, and numbness may also occur. In a *simple fracture* the bone is broken, but the skin over the area is not. In a compound fracture a wound in the skin accompanies the broken bone, and there is an added danger of infection. A greenstick fracture is an incomplete fracture in which one side of the bone is

broken and the other is bent. This type of fracture is common in children because their bones are soft, flexible, and more likely to splinter. In a complete fracture the bone is entirely broken across its width. Figure 24-2 illustrates various types of fractures. When an x-ray film reveals multiple fractures in various stages of healing, child abuse should be suspected.

A fracture heals more rapidly in a child than it does in an adult. The child's periosteum is stronger and thicker, and there is less stiffness on mobilization. Injury to the cartilaginous epiphysis, which is found at the ends of the long bones, is serious if it happens during childhood because it may interfere with longitudinal growth. Care of a child in a cast is discussed in Chapter 14. Casts may be made of plaster or fiberglass.

Fractures of the femur in early childhood. The femur (the thigh bone) is the largest and strongest bone of the body. It is one of the most prevalent serious breaks that occur during early childhood. A spiral fracture of the femur is caused by a forceful twisting motion. When the history of an injury does not correlate with x-ray findings, child abuse should be suspected because spiral fractures can be the result of manual twisting of the extremity. The child complains of pain and tenderness when the leg is moved and cannot bear weight on it. Clothes are gently removed, starting at the uninjured side and proceeding to the injured side. It may be necessary to cut the clothes. X-ray films confirm the diagnosis. Skin traction is used to reduce the fracture and keep the bones in proper alignment.

Bryant's traction is used for treating fractures of the femur in children under 2 years of age or under 20 to 30 pounds. Weights and pulleys extend the limb as in the Buck extension; however, the legs are suspended vertically (Figure 24-3). The weight of the child supplies the countertraction.

Fractures and traction in the older child. Traction is used when the cast cannot maintain alignment of the two bone fragments. Skeletal muscles act as a splint for the fracture. Traction aligns the injured bone by the use of weights and countertraction. Immobilization is maintained until the bones fuse.

Buck skin traction (Buck extension) is a type of skin traction used in fractures of the femur and in hip and knee contractures. It pulls the hip and leg into extension. Countertraction is supplied by the child's body; therefore it is *essential* that the child not slip down in bed and that the bed not be placed in high Fowler's position. Buck extension is sometimes used preoperatively, either unilaterally or bilaterally, to reduce pain and muscle spasm associated with a slipped capital femoral epiphysis. Russell traction is similar to Buck extension. In Russell traction, however, a sling is positioned under the knee, which suspends the distal thigh above the bed

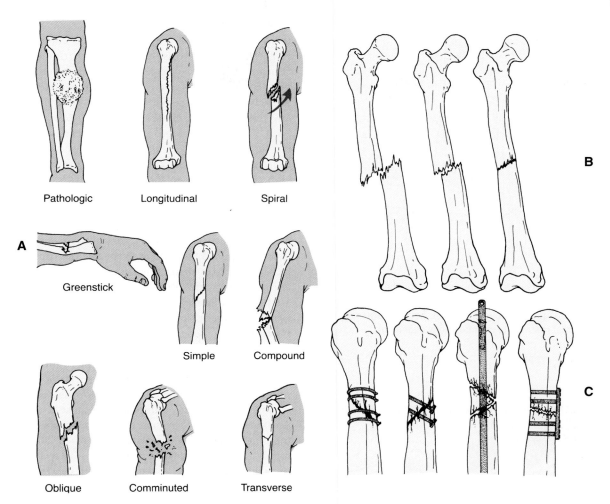

FIGURE **24-2 A,** Types of fractures. **B,** Reduction of a fractured bone. A gradual pull is exerted on the distal (lower) fragment of the bone until it is in alignment with the proximal fragment. **C,** Various methods of internal fixations, using plates, pins, nails, and screws to hold fragments of bone in place.

(Figure 24-4). Skin traction is applied to the lower extremity. Pull is in two directions, vertically from the knee sling and longitudinally from the foot plate (Figure 24-5). This prevents posterior subluxation of the tibia on the femur, which can occur in children in traction. *Split Russell traction* uses two sets of weights, one suspending the thigh and the other exerting a pull on the leg, with weights at the head and foot of the bed. Balanced suspension using the *Thomas splint* and *Pearson attachments* is used to treat diseases of the hip as well as fractures in older children and adolescents. It may be used both before and after surgery.

In *skeletal traction* a Steinmann pin or Kirschner wire is inserted into the bone, and traction is applied to the pin. Daily care of the pin site is essential. "Ninety-ninety" traction with a boot cast or sling on the lower leg may be used (Figure 24-6). *Crutchfield,* or *Barton, tongs* may be used in the skull to provide cervical traction

(Figure 24-7). Skeletal traction carries the added risk of infection from skin bacteria that may cause osteomyelitis. The child in traction experiences certain effects as a result of immobilization (Figure 24-8). Visitors are important to the child in traction and a school tutor should be contacted so that the child will be able to return to class after healing occurs.

NURSING **TIP**

The checklist for traction apparatus includes the following:
- Weights are hanging freely.
- Weights are out of reach of the child.
- Ropes are on the pulleys.
- Knots are not resting against pulleys.
- Bed linens are not on traction ropes.
- Countertraction is in place.
- Apparatus does not touch foot of bed.

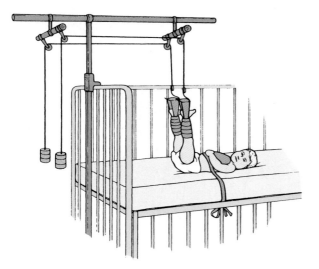

FIGURE **24-3** Bryant's traction is used for the young child who has a fractured femur. Note that the buttocks are slightly off the bed to facilitate countertraction. Active infants may require a jacket restraint to maintain body alignment.

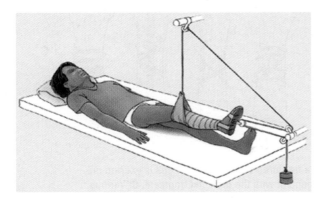

FIGURE **24-4** Russell skin traction. A skin traction system applied to the lower extremity using a foot plate and a knee sling. When the foot plate and knee sling each have their own separate weight attached to it, it is known as a *split Russell traction.*

Nursing responsibilities with Bryant's traction. The nurse observes the traction ropes to be sure they are intact and in the wheel grooves of the pulleys and that the child's body is in good position. The legs should be at right angles to the body, with the buttocks raised sufficiently to clear the bed. Elastic bandages should be neither too loose nor too tight. A jacket restraint may be used to keep the child from turning from side to side. The weights are not removed once applied. *Continuous traction is necessary.* The weights must hang free, and the pull of the weights must not be obstructed by room furnishings, such as a chair. The weights are *not* lifted or supported when the bed is moved.

The nurse performs a neurovascular check to the toes to see that they are warm and that their color is good (Figure 24-9). Cyanosis, numbness, or irritation from attachments, tight bandages, severe pain, or absence of pulse in the extremities are reported immediately to the nurse in charge. A specific and serious complication of any traction is *Volkmann's ischemia* (*ischein,* "to hold back" and *haima,* "blood"), which occurs when the circulation is obstructed. Because the legs are elevated overhead, there is gravitational vascular drainage. Arterial occlusion can cause anoxia of the muscles and reflex vasospasm, which when unnoticed could result in contractures and paralysis.

The child is bathed, and back and buttock care is given. A sheepskin padding may also be used. The sheets are pulled taut and are kept free of crumbs. The jacket restraint is changed when it is soiled. The child is encouraged to drink lots of fluids and to eat foods that are high in roughage to prevent constipation caused by a lack of exercise. Stool softeners may be necessary. A fracture pan is used for bowel movements, and a careful record is kept of eliminations. Deep-breathing exercises are encouraged to prevent the collection of fluids in the lungs caused by the child's immobility. These exercises may be done by blowing bubbles or blowing a pinwheel.

Diversional therapy is important because hospitalization may be lengthy. Toys may be securely suspended over the child's head so they are within easy reach. The child's crib is taken to the playroom when possible so he or she can experience the excitement of the activities there.

Tapes, compact discs (CDs), stories, and other forms of entertainment are important aspects of a total nursing care plan. Pain control is essential. Parents are encouraged to visit the child as often as possible. With proper treatment the prognosis for the child with this condition is good.

> ## NURSING **TIP**
> The checklist for the patient in traction includes the following:
> - Body in alignment
> - Head of bed no higher than 20 degrees (for countertraction)
> - Heels of feet elevated from bed
> - ROM of unaffected parts checked at regular intervals
> - Antiembolism stockings or foot pumps in place as ordered
> - Neurovascular checks performed regularly
> - Skin integrity monitored regularly
> - Pain relieved by medication reported
> - Measures to prevent constipation
> - Use of trapeze for change of position encouraged

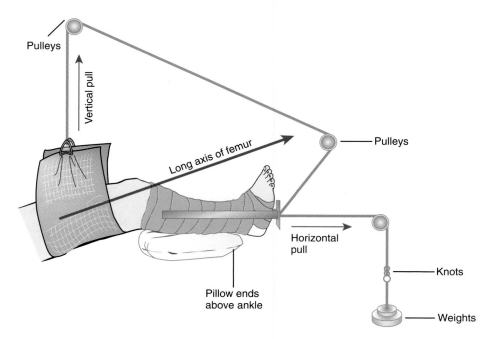

FIGURE **24-5** Forces involved in traction. The placement of pulleys and angle of the joints determine the line of pull. In this case the combined vertical and horizontal pull results in a pull on the long axis of the femur to reduce fracture displacement.

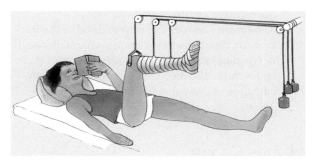

FIGURE **24-6** 90 degree—90 degree skeletal traction. A wire pin is inserted into the distal segment of the femur. The lower leg may be placed in a boot cast or is supported by a sling.

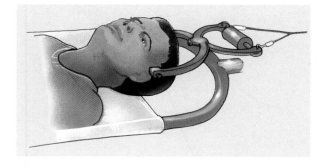

FIGURE **24-7** Cervical traction. A special bed may be used to turn a patient who is in cervical traction.

Neurovascular checks. A priority nursing responsibility in the care of a child with a fracture who in is traction or has a cast or Ace bandage in place is to perform neurovascular assessments or **neurovascular checks** at regular intervals. Aspects to check include the following:

- *Pain.* The location and quality of pain should be assessed and recorded. Pain control strategies and medication should be initiated as soon as possible. Pain at the trauma site that does not respond to medication may indicate a serious complication called **compartment syndrome.**

Compartment syndrome is a term used to describe *ischemia* to an extremity caused by pressure on the tissues as a result of excessive edema. Surgery (fasciotomy) may be needed to reduce the pressure and increase tissue perfusion.

- *Pulse.* The quality of the pulse on the affected extremity should be compared to that on the unaffected extremity. A strong pulse indicates good blood flow necessary for healing.
- *Sensation.* Reduced sensation to touch (numbness or tingling) at a site distal to the fracture may indicate poor tissue perfusion and should be reported.

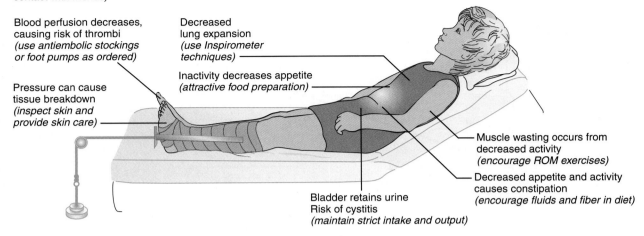

Prolonged treatment requires absence from school
*(request home tutor, maintain written or E-mail
contact with friends)*

Blood perfusion decreases,
causing risk of thrombi
*(use antiembolic stockings
or foot pumps as ordered)*

Decreased
lung expansion
*(use Inspirometer
techniques)*

Pressure can cause
tissue breakdown
*(inspect skin and
provide skin care)*

Inactivity decreases appetite
(attractive food preparation)

Muscle wasting occurs from
decreased activity
(encourage ROM exercises)

Decreased appetite and activity
causes constipation
(encourage fluids and fiber in diet)

Bladder retains urine
Risk of cystitis
(maintain strict intake and output)

FIGURE **24-8** Overcoming the effects of traction on a child.

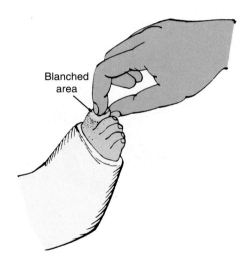

Blanched
area

FIGURE **24-9** Checking circulation to the toes or fingers. To
check circulation (capillary refill), squeeze or press a toe or finger to blanch the skin. If the circulation is adequate, the color
should return in less than 3 seconds when the pressure is released. 1. If the toes do not blanch, congestion may be present
and should be reported to the physician. 2. If the blanching persists after pressure is released, the circulation is impaired. The
physician must be notified. 3. Report to the physician if extreme
pain results from touching or moving the toes.

- *Color.* Pallor at the site distal to the fracture can
  indicate arterial insufficiency, whereas cyanosis of
  the site distal to the fracture can indicate venous
  stasis. Adequate blood supply and vascular
  drainage are essential for optimum healing.

- *Capillary refill.* A compressed nail bed should
  return to its original color in less than 3 seconds.
  The findings should be compared with the unaffected extremity and the results recorded frequently (see Figure 24-9).
- *Movement.* The toes and fingers distal to the fracture site should be tested for movement. Because
  nerve injury can occur as a complication of skeletal fractures, the movement associated with specific nerve supply should also be tested (Figure
  24-10).

> **NURSING TIP**
>
> The "neurovascular check" for tissue perfusion is
> performed on the toes or fingers distal to an injury or
> cast and includes the following:
> - Peripheral pulse
> - Color
> - Capillary refill time
> - Warmth
> - Movement and sensation

Nursing Care Plan 24-1 describes interventions for
the child in traction.

Compartment syndrome. *Compartment syndrome* is
a progressive loss of tissue perfusion because of an
increase in pressure caused by edema or swelling that
presses on the vessels and tissues. Circulation is compromised, and the neurovascular check is abnormal.

COMMON FRACTURES: HOW TO TEST FOR NERVE DAMAGE

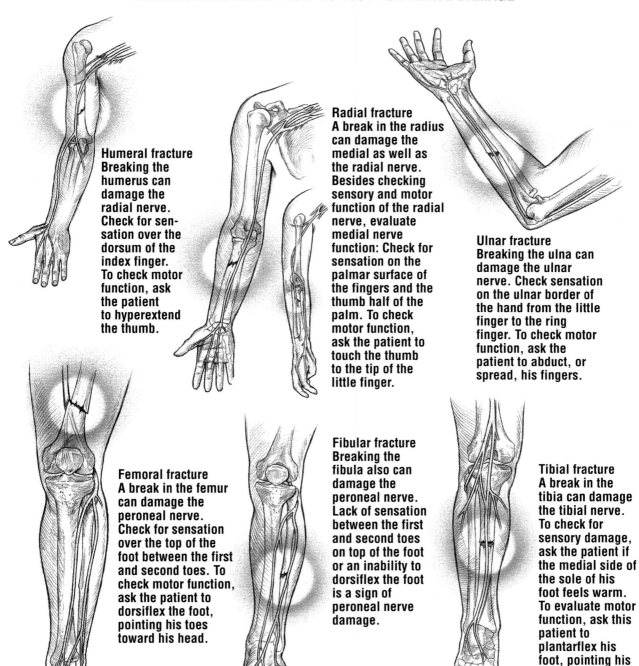

Humeral fracture
Breaking the humerus can damage the radial nerve. Check for sensation over the dorsum of the index finger. To check motor function, ask the patient to hyperextend the thumb.

Radial fracture
A break in the radius can damage the medial as well as the radial nerve. Besides checking sensory and motor function of the radial nerve, evaluate medial nerve function: Check for sensation on the palmar surface of the fingers and the thumb half of the palm. To check motor function, ask the patient to touch the thumb to the tip of the little finger.

Ulnar fracture
Breaking the ulna can damage the ulnar nerve. Check sensation on the ulnar border of the hand from the little finger to the ring finger. To check motor function, ask the patient to abduct, or spread, his fingers.

Femoral fracture
A break in the femur can damage the peroneal nerve. Check for sensation over the top of the foot between the first and second toes. To check motor function, ask the patient to dorsiflex the foot, pointing his toes toward his head.

Fibular fracture
Breaking the fibula also can damage the peroneal nerve. Lack of sensation between the first and second toes on top of the foot or an inability to dorsiflex the foot is a sign of peroneal nerve damage.

Tibial fracture
A break in the tibia can damage the tibial nerve. To check for sensory damage, ask the patient if the medial side of the sole of his foot feels warm. To evaluate motor function, ask this patient to plantarflex his foot, pointing his toes down.

FIGURE **24-10** Checking for nerve damage. Nerve damage can result from trauma, and the motor sensory status of the extremity should be assessed and recorded frequently.

NURSING CARE PLAN 24-1

The Child in Traction

PATIENT DATA: A 6-year-old child is admitted with a fractured femur after falling from a tree while playing. His leg is placed in Steinmann pin traction.

SELECTED NURSING DIAGNOSIS   *Impaired physical mobility related to fixation devices*

Outcomes	Nursing Interventions	Rationales
Child will demonstrate how to obtain help via call bell. Child will not develop complications of immobility as evidenced by intact skin, absence of respiratory and urinary infections. Child will have a bowel movement on a regular basis.	1. Draw picture of fracture for child and explain traction apparatus. 2. Place call bell within easy reach of child. 3. Change position as traction allows every 2 hours. 4. Encourage exercise through play by doing pull-ups on trapeze apparatus. 5. Institute range-of-motion (ROM) exercises on unaffected extremities. 6. Encourage self-care. 7. Encourage deep breathing with incentive spirometer or a toy. 8. Observe for urinary tract infection. 9. Provide high-fiber diet and stool softeners. 10. Provide adequate fluids; monitor intake and output.	1. An understanding of condition and of the type of traction used reduces anxiety and promotes compliance with treatment protocol. 2. It is frightening to be immobilized; a call bell provides reassurance that help is at hand. 3. Position changes every 2 hours help to prevent skin breakdown. 4. Exercise will help to prevent atrophy, joint contractures, and muscle weakness. 5. Unaffected limbs need exercise to prevent stiffness, muscle atrophy, and deformities. 6. Promote self-directed wellness. 7. Deep-breathing exercises help to prevent pneumonia and atelectasis. 8. Kidney filtration slows down with immobilization; immobility causes minerals (e.g., calcium) to leave bones and pool in renal pelvis; stasis of urine is likely to occur, causing renal calculi. 9. Bulk improves stool consistency and prevents constipation. Stool softeners prevent straining during defecation. 10. Increased fluids are necessary to hydrate body, and they decrease the risk of urine stasis and constipation.

SELECTED NURSING DIAGNOSIS   *Acute pain related to issue trauma*

Outcomes	Nursing Interventions	Rationales
Child will be comfortable as evidenced by a decrease in irritability, crying, body posturing, and anorexia. Older child verbalizes relief of pain.	1. Administer pain medication before activity and before pain escalates. 2. Allow choice in method of pain relief, if possible. 3. Encourage child to hold favorite possession; provide pacifier for toddler.	1. Child may be unable to verbalize pain. Premedication for pain allows for muscle relaxation and participation in activities. 2. Allowing some choice, if there is one, promotes self-control. 3. Favorite possessions and a pacifier are comforting, particularly to a small child.

NURSING CARE PLAN 24-1—cont'd

Outcomes	Nursing Interventions	Rationales
	4. Distract child with music box or tapes as age appropriate.	4. Distraction from a problem reduces stress and tension.
	5. Listen and communicate with child.	5. Listening to child gives nurse clues about amount of pain; nonverbal cues are important in infants and toddlers.
	6. Use touch as a comfort measure.	6. Touch is particularly important in infants and toddlers but is comforting for all ages; proceed with caution if there is reason to suspect abuse.
	7. Involve family in supporting child's ability to cope with pain.	7. Child trusts family; family members may be able to suggest favorite types of comfort for child.
	8. Consider cultural background in relation to pain expression.	8. In some cultures, showing pain is considered cowardly.
	9. Monitor vital signs.	9. A change in vital signs can indicate pain, infection, or poor tissue perfusion.
	10. Provide support and education to family members.	10. Family members who understand and participate in care can help the child to develop effective coping skills.

SELECTED NURSING DIAGNOSIS   *Risk for impaired skin integrity related to immobility, traction, poor circulation*

Outcomes	Nursing Interventions	Rationales
Skin will remain intact with no evidence of breakdown.	1. Inspect skin regularly.	1. Provides for early assessment of developing skin problems.
Circulation of affected extremity will be adequate as evidenced by normal capillary refill, equal and strong peripheral pulses, and sensation and motion in extremity.	2. Check capillary refill of nail beds in affected extremity.	2. Impaired tissue perfusion will result in an increased capillary refill time.
	3. Have child wiggle toes or fingers of affected extremity to determine sensation and motion.	3. Wiggling toes and fingers determines mobility and sensation.
	4. Inspect restraining devices and elastic bandages for wrinkles or looseness.	4. Excessive tightness or wrinkles in bandages can cause swelling and irritation of underlying tissue.
	5. Use sheepskin underneath hips and back.	5. Sheepskin may protect susceptible areas, such as bony prominences about sacrum.
	6. Monitor traction device, including ropes, pulleys, and weights.	6. To maintain effective traction, weights must be hanging freely, ropes must be securely on pulleys, and the traction device must be free of friction.
	7. Maintain body alignment.	7. Proper body alignment maintains a pull on the long axis of the bone.
	8. Inspect pin sites for redness, swelling, or discharge; provide pin care according to protocol.	8. Early intervention can prevent infection; pin care removes debris that can lead to infection or osteomyelitis.

Continued

NURSING CARE PLAN 24-1—cont'd

SELECTED NURSING DIAGNOSIS *Delayed growth and development related to separation from family and friends*

Outcomes	Nursing Interventions	Rationales
Child's developmental level will be maintained.	1. Allow child to choose age-appropriate games. 2. Encourage peer contact. 3. Involve child-life specialist or schoolteacher to provide appropriate learning activities.	1. Allowing child to choose activities increases active participation. 2. Children, particularly those of school age and adolescents, must remain in contact with their peers to prevent feeling isolated. 3. Maintaining age-appropriate studies will allow the child to rejoin peers in school.

?CRITICAL THINKING QUESTION

The nurse enters the room of a child who is in skeletal traction for a fractured femur. He is sitting in a high Fowler's position watching television and eating snacks. What nursing observations relating to the traction would the nurse make, and what interventions are necessary?

OSTEOMYELITIS

Pathophysiology. Osteomyelitis is an infection of the bone that generally occurs in children younger than 1 year of age and in those between 5 and 14 years of age. Long bones contain few phagocytic cells (white blood cells [WBCs]) to fight bacteria that may come to the bone from another part of the body. The inflammation produces an exudate that collects under the marrow and cortex of the bone.

Staphylococcus aureus is the organism responsible in 75% to 80% of cases in children over 5 years of age, and *Hemophilus influenzae* is the most common cause in young children. This incidence may be reduced by the widening practice of routine infant immunization against this organism. Other organisms include group A streptococci and pneumococci. *Salmonella* and *Pseudomonas* are organisms often involved in adolescents who are intravenous (IV) drug users. Osteomyelitis may be preceded by a local injury to the bone, such as an open fracture, burn, or contamination during surgery. It may also follow a furuncle, impetigo, and abscessed teeth. In neonates a heel puncture or scalp vein monitor can be the predisposing site of infection. Infective emboli may travel to the small arteries of the bone, setting up local destruction and abscess. For this reason, a careful search for infection in other bones and soft tissues is necessary.

The vessels in the affected area are compressed, and thrombosis occurs, producing ischemia and pain. The collection of pus under the periosteum of the bone can elevate the periosteum, which can result in necrosis of that part of the bone. If the pus reaches the epiphysis of the bone in infants, infection can travel to the joint space, causing septic arthritis of that joint.

Local inflammation and increased pressure from the distended periosteum can cause pain. Older children can localize the pain and may limp. Younger children and infants will show decreased voluntary movement of that extremity. Associated muscle spasms can cause limited active ROM. The child may refuse to stand or walk. Signs of local inflammation may be present. A detailed history may reveal possible sources of primary infection. Blood cultures to identify the organism may be valuable if the child has not been given antibiotics for the primary infection. A urine test for the presence of bacterial antigens and a tissue biopsy may be helpful to establish the diagnosis.

Manifestations. There is an elevation in WBC count and sedimentation rate. X-ray films may initially fail to reveal infection. A bone scan may be diagnostic.

Treatment and nursing care. Prompt and vigorous treatment is essential to ensure a favorable prognosis. Intravenous antibiotics are prescribed for a 4- to 6-week period. The high doses required indicate a nursing responsibility to monitor the infant or child for toxic responses and to ensure long-term compliance. The joint may be drained of pus arthroscopically or surgically to reduce pressure and avoid bone necrosis. The joint is immobilized in a functional position. A complication should be suspected if fever lasts beyond 5 days. Early passive ROM exercises after the splint is removed may be advisable to reduce the occurrence of contracture. The use of appropriate pain-relieving medications and gentle handling to minimize pain is essential. The child should be positioned comfortably with the limb supported by pillows or blanket rolls.

Routine cast or splint care, including frequent neurovascular checks is a nursing responsibility. Bed rest is followed by wheelchair access, but weight bearing should be avoided. Diversional therapy, physical therapy, and tutorial assistance for school-age children should be provided so they can return to their class and classmates after discharge. Close interaction with home care providers is indicated.

DUCHENNE'S OR BECKER (PSEUDOHYPERTROPHIC) MUSCULAR DYSTROPHY

Pathophysiology. The muscular dystrophies are a group of disorders in which progressive muscle degeneration occurs. The childhood form (Duchenne's muscular dystrophy) is the most common type. It has an incidence of about 0.14 in 3600 liveborn male infants of all races and ethnic groups. It is a sex-linked inherited disorder that occurs only in boys.

Manifestations. The onset is generally between 2 and 6 years of age; however, a history of delayed motor development during infancy may be evidenced. The calf muscles in particular become hypertrophied. The term *pseudohypertrophic* (*pseudo,* "false" and *hypertrophy,* "enlargement") refers to this characteristic. Other signs include progressive weakness as evidenced by frequent falling, clumsiness, contractures of the ankles and hips, and Gower's maneuver (a characteristic way of rising from the floor). Intellectual impairment is common.

Laboratory findings show marked increases in blood creatine phosphokinase levels. Muscle biopsy reveals a degeneration of muscle fibers and their replacement by fat and connective tissue. A *myelogram* (a graphic record of muscle contraction as a result of electrical stimulation) shows decreases in the amplitude and duration of motor unit potentials. Electrocardiographic (ECG) abnormalities are also common. The disease becomes progressively worse, and wheelchair confinement may occur. Death usually results from cardiac failure or respiratory infection. Mental retardation is not uncommon.

Treatment and nursing care. Treatment at this time is mainly supportive to prevent complications and maintain the quality of life. A multidisciplinary team should provide psychological support, nutritional support, physiotherapy, social/financial assistance, and, when necessary, respite and hospice care.

Compared with other children with disabilities, some children with muscular dystrophy may appear passive and withdrawn. Early on, depression may be seen because the child cannot compete with peers. Social and emotional pressures on the child and family are great.

LEGG-CALVÉ-PERTHES DISEASE (COXA PLANA)

Pathophysiology. Legg-Calvé-Perthes disease is one of a group of disorders called the *osteochondroses* (*osteo,* "bone," *chondros,* "cartilage," and *osis,* "disease") in which the blood supply to the epiphysis, or end of the bone, is disrupted. The tissue death that results from the inadequate blood supply is termed *avascular necrosis* (*a,* "without," *vasculum,* "vessels," and *nekros,* "death"). Legg-Calvé-Perthes disease affects the development of the head of the femur. Its cause and incidence are unknown. The disease is seen most commonly in boys between 5 and 12 years of age. It is more common in Caucasians. This disease is unilateral in about 85% of cases. Healing occurs spontaneously over 2 to 4 years; however, marked distortion of the head of the femur may lead to an imperfect joint or degenerative arthritis of the hip in later life. Symptoms include a painless limp and limitation of motion. X-ray films and bone scans confirm the diagnosis.

Treatment. Legg-Calvé-Perthes disease is a self-limiting disorder that heals spontaneously. The treatment involves keeping the femoral head deep in the hip socket while it heals and avoiding weight bearing. This is accomplished through the use of ambulation-abduction casts or braces that prevent subluxation (*sub,* "beneath" and *luxatio,* "dislocation") and enable the acetabulum to mold the healing head in such a way that it does not become deformed. This treatment may be preceded by bed rest and traction. The prognosis in Legg-Calvé-Perthes disease is fair. Some affected people may require hip joint replacement procedures as adults.

Nursing care. Nursing considerations depend on the age of the patient and the type of treatment. The general principles of traction, cast, and brace care are used when immobilization of the child is necessary. Teaching and counseling are directed toward a holistic understanding of and interest in the individual child and family. Total immobility or partial mobility is particularly trying for children. The natural inclination to compete physically is thwarted. In some cases surgical immobilization is required. Preoperative and postoperative care and care of a patient in a cast are discussed in Chapters 14 and 22.

OSTEOSARCOMA

Pathophysiology. Osteosarcoma (*osteo,* "bone," *sarx,* "flesh," and *oma,* "tumor") is a primary malignant tumor of the long bones. The two most common types of bone tumors in children are osteosarcoma and Ewing's tumor. The mean age of onset of osteosarcoma is between 10 and 15 years of age. Children who have had radiation therapy for other types of cancer and children with retinoblastoma have a higher incidence of this disease. Metastasis occurs quickly because of the high vascularity of bone tissue. The lungs are the primary site of metastasis; brain and other bone tissue are also sites of metastasis.

Manifestations. The patient experiences pain and swelling at the site. In adolescents this is often attributed to injury or "growing pains." The pain may be lessened by flexing the extremity. Later a pathological fracture may occur. Diagnosis is confirmed by biopsy. A complete physical examination, including CT and a bone scan, is done. Radiological studies help to confirm the diagnosis.

Treatment and nursing care. Treatment of the patient with osteosarcoma consists of radical resection or amputation surgery. Internal prostheses are available for most sites. Long-term survival is possible with early diagnosis and treatment.

The nursing care is similar to that for other types of cancer. Problems of body image are particularly important to the self-conscious adolescent. If amputation is necessary, the family and patient will need much support. The nurse anticipates anger, fear, and grief. Immediately after surgery the stump dressing is observed frequently for signs of bleeding. Vital signs are monitored. The child is positioned as ordered by the surgeon.

Phantom limb pain is likely to be experienced. This is the continued sensation of pain in the limb even though the limb is no longer there. It occurs because nerve tracts continue to report pain. This pain is very real, and an analgesic may be necessary. Rehabilitation measures follow surgical recovery.

EWING'S SARCOMA

Pathophysiology. Ewing's sarcoma was first described in 1921 by Dr. James Ewing. It is a malignant growth that occurs in the marrow of the long bones. It occurs mainly in older school-age children and early adolescents. When metastasis is present on diagnosis, the prognosis is poor. Without metastasis there is a 60% survival rate. The primary sites for metastasis are the lungs and bones.

Treatment and nursing care. Amputation is not generally recommended for Ewing's sarcoma because the tumor is sensitive to radiation therapy and chemotherapy. This is a relief to the child and family. The child is warned against vigorous weight bearing on the involved bone during therapy to avoid pathological fractures. Patients must be prepared for the effects of radiation therapy and chemotherapy. The nurse supports the family members in their efforts to gain equilibrium after such a crisis.

JUVENILE RHEUMATOID ARTHRITIS

Pathophysiology. Juvenile rheumatoid arthritis (JRA) is the most common arthritic condition of childhood. It is a systemic inflammatory disease that involves the joints, connective tissues, and viscera, and it differs somewhat from adult rheumatoid arthritis. It is not a rare disease. In 1998 approximately 70,000 children in the United States were diagnosed with JRA (Jackson & Vessey, 2000). The exact cause is unknown, but infection and an autoimmune response have been implicated.

Manifestations and types. JRA has three distinct methods of onset: systemic (or acute febrile), polyarticular, and pauciarticular. The *systemic* form is manifested by intermittent spiking fever above 39.5° C (103° F) persisting for over 10 days, a nonpruritic macular rash, abdominal pain, an elevated erythrocyte sedimentation rate (ESR), C-reactive protein in laboratory tests, and possibly an enlarged liver and spleen. It occurs most often in children ages 1 to 3 years and 8 to 10 years. Joint symptoms may be absent at onset but will develop in most patients.

The *polyarticular* form can involve five or more joints, often small joints of the hands and feet, which become swollen, warm, and tender. This form occurs throughout childhood and adolescence and predominantly affects girls. Approximately 40% of patients with JRA have the polyarticular type.

The *pauciarticular* form is limited to four or fewer joints, generally the larger ones such as the hips, knees, ankles, and elbows. It occurs in children under 3 years of age (mostly in girls) and in children over 13 years of age (mostly in boys). Approximately 35% of patients with JRA have the pauciarticular form.

Children with pauciarticular disease may be at risk for iridocyclitis (*irido,* "iris," *cycl,* "circle," and *itis,* "inflammation"), an inflammation of the iris and ciliary body of the eye also known as *uveitis.* Symptoms include redness, pain, photophobia, decreased visual acuity, and nonreactive pupils. All children with pauciarticular arthritis need periodic slit-lamp eye examinations. There are no specific tests or cures for JRA. The duration of the symptoms is important, particularly when they have lasted longer than 6 weeks.

Diagnosis is determined by clinical manifestations, x-ray studies, laboratory results, and exclusion of other disorders. Aspirated joint fluid is yellow to green, appears cloudy, and has a low viscosity.

Treatment. The goals of therapy are as follows:

- Reduce joint pain and swelling
- Promote mobility and preserve joint function
- Promote growth and development
- Promote independent functioning
- Help the child and family to adjust to living with a chronic disease

Treatment is supportive and is started as early as possible to limit permanent disability. Medications include nonsteroidal antiinflammatory drugs (NSAIDs), immune suppressant drugs, methotrexate, and IV immunoglobulins to reduce the effects of high dose steroids on growth. Oral and injectible gold and slow-acting antirheumatic drugs such as sulfasalazine (Azulfidine) or auranofin (Ridaura) are toxic drugs that require close monitoring. Cytotoxic agents such as chlorambucil or cyclosporin can have long-term side effects and are used only for resistant cases. Long-term care includes physical and occupational therapy and psychological support. Research concerning a soluble form of tumor necrosis factor (TNF) receptor, etanercept (Enbrel), shows promise for the future treatment of JRA.

Nursing care. The nurse functions as a member of a multidisciplinary health care team that includes the pediatrician, rheumatologist, social worker, physical therapist, occupational therapist, psychologist, ophthalmologist, and school and community nurses. The child may be hospitalized during an acute episode or for an unrelated illness. Treatment consists of administering medications and providing warm tub baths, joint exercises, and rest. The physical therapist oversees the type and amount of exercise performed. Daily ROM exercises and play activities that incorporate specific routines help to preserve function, maintain muscle strength, and prevent deformities. One must be careful to avoid traumatizing an inflamed joint. Morning tub baths and the application of moist hot packs help to lessen stiffness. Resting splints may be ordered to prevent flexion contractures and preserve functional alignment. Proper body alignment with regular changes to the prone position (unless contraindicated) facilitates comfort. Either no pillow or a small flat pillow is advised for under the head. Measures to alleviate boredom are instituted.

Home care. The patient is discharged with written instructions for home care. These are reviewed with family members to determine their level of understanding. A firm mattress or bed board is necessary to support the joints. Age-appropriate tricycles and pedal cars promote mobility and exercise. Modifications in daily living, such as elevation of toilet seats, installation of handrails, Velcro fasteners, and so on, may be necessary. The importance of regular eye examinations is empha-

sized. Parents should be assisted in planning nutritional meals. Weight gain is to be avoided because it places further stress on the joints. Unnecessary physical restrictions should be avoided because these can lead to rebellion. Swimming is an excellent form of exercise.

School attendance is encouraged. Excessive absence from school, particularly for nonspecific complaints, may suggest that the child is depressed or overly preoccupied with the illness. In such cases the meaning of the illness to the child and family and its effect on daily life must be explored. Parents need assistance in establishing limits. Consistently negative behavior of the child in social situations can present more problems than the actual disability. Overindulgence and preferential treatment often compromise the child's potential for happiness and independence. Siblings of chronically ill children may resent the special attention given to the patient. They may be torn by loyalty to the brother or sister and their own need to be with others. Parents need ongoing counseling and the services of various community resources.

This long-term disease is characterized by periods of remission and exacerbations. Nurses can serve as advocates for the child, that is, they can help alleviate stress by recognizing the impact of the disease and by openly communicating with the child, family, and other members of the health care team. Nurses support the child and family members and instill hope.

TORTICOLLIS (WRY NECK)

Pathophysiology. Torticollis (*tortus,* "twisted" and *collium,* "neck") is a condition in which neck motion is limited because of shortening of the sternocleidomastoid muscle. It can be either congenital or acquired and can also be either acute or chronic. The most common type is a congenital anomaly in which the sternocleidomastoid muscle is injured during birth. It is associated with breech and forceps delivery and may be seen in conjunction with other birth defects, such as congenital hip.

Manifestations. In congenital torticollis the symptoms are present at birth. The infant holds the head to the side of the muscle involved. The chin is tilted in the opposite direction. There is a hard palpable mass of dense fibrotic tissue (fibroma). This is not fixed to the skin and resolves by 2 to 6 months of age. Passive stretching and ROM exercises and physical therapy may be indicated. Feeding and playing with the infant can encourage turning to the desired side for correction. Operative correction is indicated if the condition persists beyond age 2 years.

Acquired torticollis is seen in older children. It may be associated with injury, inflammation, neurological disorders, and other causes. Nursing intervention is primarily that of detection. Infants who have limited head movements require further investigation.

SCOLIOSIS

Pathophysiology. The most prevalent of the three skeletal abnormalities shown in Figure 24-11 is *scoliosis*. Scoliosis refers to an S-shaped curvature of the spine. During adolescence, scoliosis is more common in girls. Many curvatures are not progressive and may require only periodic evaluation. Untreated progressive scoliosis may lead to back pain, fatigue, disability, and heart and lung complications. Skeletal deterioration does not stop with maturity and may be aggravated by pregnancy.

Causes. There are two types of scoliosis: functional and structural. *Functional* scoliosis is usually caused by poor posture, not by spinal disease. The curve is flexible and easily correctable. Structural or fixed scoliosis is caused by changes in the shape of the vertebrae or thorax. It is usually accompanied by rotation of the spine. The hips and shoulders may appear uneven. The patient cannot correct the condition by standing in a straighter posture.

There are many causes of *structural* scoliosis. Some are congenital and develop in utero. These are noticeable at birth or during periods of rapid growth. *Neuromuscu-*lar scoliosis is the result of muscle weakness or imbalance. It is seen in children with cerebral palsy, muscular dystrophy, and other conditions. The cause of *idiopathic* scoliosis is unknown; there may be a hereditary link.

Treatment. Treatment is aimed at correcting the curvature and preventing more severe scoliosis. Curves up to 20 degrees do not require treatment but are carefully followed. Curves between 20 and 40 degrees require the use of a Milwaukee brace (Figure 24-12). This apparatus exerts pressure on the chin, pelvis, and convex (arched) side of the spine. It is worn approximately 23 hours a day and is worn *over* a T-shirt to protect the skin. An underarm modification of the brace (the Boston brace) is proving effective for patients with low curvatures. It is less cumbersome and is more acceptable to the self-conscious young person. Transcutaneous electrical muscle stimulation (TENS) and exercise have not proven to be effective in the treatment of scoliosis (Behrman, Kliegman, & Jenson, 2000).

Hospitalization is required for curves of more than 40 degrees and for patients in whom conservative measures are not successful. A spinal fusion is performed. This is sometimes done in stages. A Harrington rod, Dwyer instrument, or Luque wires may be inserted for immobilization during the time required for the fusion to become solid. Halo traction may be used when there is associated weakness or paralysis of the neck and trunk muscles (Figure 24-13); it is also used in treating cervical fractures and fusions.

> **NURSING TIP**
> Insertion of a Harrington rod or other metal device may delay a patient at an airport security scanner because the metal could activate the alarm.

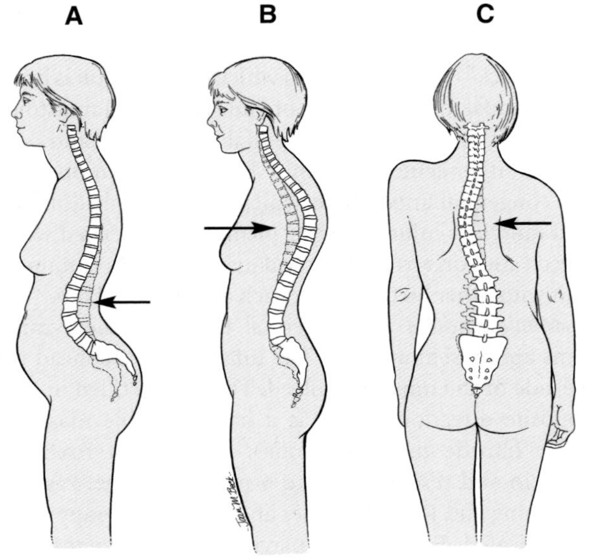

FIGURE **24-11** Abnormal spinal curvatures. **A,** Lordosis, known as "sway back," is commonly seen during pregnancy. **B,** Kyphosis, known as "hunchback," is an increased roundness in the thoracic curve commonly found in the elderly. **C,** Scoliosis, an abnormal side-to-side curvature of the spine, is commonly found in adolescents.

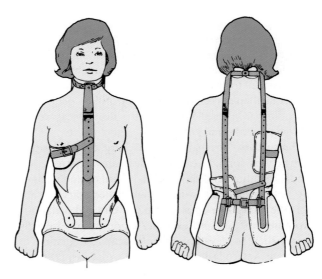

FIGURE **24-12** The Milwaukee brace.

Nursing care

Community nursing. The management of scoliosis begins with screening. This is done before middle school. It should be a part of every yearly physical examination given to prepubescent youngsters. Camp nurses also need to be aware of symptoms. Early recognition is of utmost importance in detecting mild cases amenable to nonsurgical treatment.

The adolescent is prepared by explaining the purpose of the procedure and by being reassured that it merely entails observing the back while standing and bending forward. Adolescents must know that it is simple, quick, and painless and that privacy will be afforded. They are instructed to wear clothing that is easy to remove, such as a pullover top. Boys disrobe to the waist, girls generally to the bra. No slip or undershirt should be worn.

The procedure consists of the nurse examining the spine from the front, side, and back while the adolescent stands erect and then observing the back as the adolescent bends forward. One looks initially for general body alignment and *asymmetry* (lack of proportion). In scoliosis, one shoulder may be higher than the other, a scapula may be prominent, the arm-to-body spaces may be unequal, or a hip may protrude; one arm may appear longer than the other when the person bends forward. Referrals are made as indicated to those who must obtain further treatment.

The adolescent may be admitted for extensive correction by spinal fusion. The nurse's knowledge of preadolescent and adolescent developmental tasks is imperative, because therapy often conflicts with these tasks.

Routine preoperative nursing care of the adolescent is necessary for spinal fusion. This includes instructing the adolescent and family about the purpose and extent of the cast or brace that may be prescribed. It is important that the nurse evaluate and document the adolescent's neuromuscular status at this time so that it may be used as a basis for comparison after the procedure is completed.

Much postoperative nursing care is directly related to combating the physical results of immobilization (see Figure 24-8). The body systems become sluggish because of inactivity. This is evidenced in the gastrointestinal tract by anorexia, irregularity, and constipation. Allowing the adolescent to select foods with the aid of the dietitian is helpful in improving appetite. Increasing fluid intake reduces constipation. Cranberry juice helps to neutralize the alkaline content of urine and decreases the possibility of bladder infection.

The adolescent and parents are introduced to the multidisciplinary health care team. Postoperative exercise, physical therapy, and promotion of adolescent school and developmental tasks are essential aspects of nursing care.

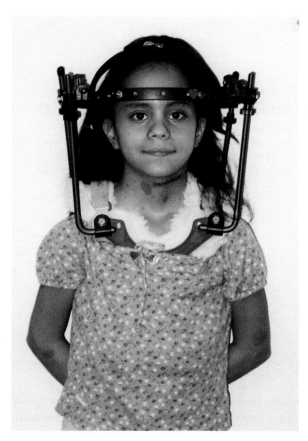

FIGURE **24-13** Halo traction. This halo jacket and apparatus is used for cervical fractures and spinal disorders. (Photo courtesy of Pat Spier, RN-C.)

SPORTS INJURIES

A high percentage of adolescent males and females participate in athletic activities. The American Academy of Pediatrics recommends that a complete physical examination be given at least every other year during adolescence and that sports-specific examinations be given for those involved in strenuous activity on entry into junior or senior high school. Such examinations should be updated by an annual questionnaire. The family history and an orthopedic screening are important in identifying risk factors.

Prevention. Several factors help to prevent sports injuries. Some of these are adequate warm-up and cool-down periods; year-round conditioning; careful selection of activity according to physical maturity, size, and skill necessary; proper supervision by adults; safe, well-

table 24-1	*Common Sports Injuries*

TYPE	DESCRIPTION
Concussion	Any blow to the head followed by alterations in mental functioning should be treated as a possible concussion; observe carefully for sequelae
"Stingers" or "burners"	A common neck injury when a player hits another in the head in such sports as football or soccer; caused by brachial plexus trauma; feels like an electrical jolt; usually mild and disappears suddenly; restrict sports activity until symptoms disappear; reassess protective gear
Injured knee	Usually a result of stress on the knee ligaments; potentially serious; should be evaluated by an experienced trainer or physician; may require arthroscopy
Sprain or strained ankle	May injure growth plate; x-ray films important in adolescent
Muscle cramps	Caused by injury, alterations in blood flow, or electrolyte deficiencies; important to warm up before activity; ensure fluid intake is adequate
Shin splints	Pain and discomfort in lower leg caused by repeated running on a hard surface such as concrete; avoid such activity; use well-fitting shoes; decrease inflammation by rest

fitting equipment; and avoidance of participation when in pain or injured. Proper diet and fluids are also necessary. A few of the more common injuries are listed in Table 24-1. The nurse has a major role in educating and directing parents to sources of accurate information to ensure that the physical, emotional, and maturational levels of the adolescent are appropriate for the activity (Table 24-2). Parents are encouraged to inquire about the capabilities of personnel and the availability of emergency services before the beginning of the competition.

FAMILY VIOLENCE

Violence has become a problem that affects children of all social classes across the nation. Family violence includes spousal abuse and child abuse, neglect, and maltreatment. Community violence is seen in neighborhoods where even non–gang-related adolescents arm themselves with guns and knives for protection. Preschoolers who are repeatedly allowed to watch violent programs on television or play aggressive computer games may be learning antisocial coping skills they will use as they grow and mature. The time spent watching television and the content of the programs should be controlled by parents so that television exposure results in the acquisition of knowledge, skills, and information that will motivate learning. In homes where spousal and/or child abuse occurs, children learn the behaviors they will practice when they become adults, and the abuse cycle continues. Parents who are abusive are not

box 24-1	*Factors that May Contribute to or Trigger Child Abuse*

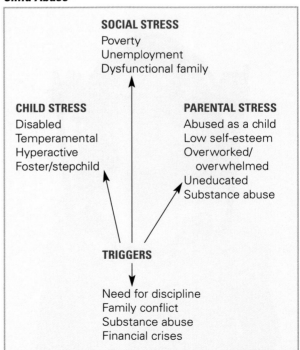

Abusive parents may love their child but respond to stress and triggers that provoke abusive behavior.

usually psychotic or criminal. They may have a knowledge deficit about child care needs and child growth and development. Abusive parents are often without a support system and are perhaps alone, angry, in crisis, or have unrealistic expectations (Box 24-1).

table 24-2 *Selected Sports Activities and Their Risks*

SPORT	RISK
Gymnastics	Common problems associated with children engaging in gymnastics are delayed menstruation and eating disorders. Trauma and overuse injuries of the large joints and spine are common. Prevention includes muscle strengthening exercises, flexibility exercises, and wrist braces. Nutritional needs and education are essential.
Ballet	Common problems associated with ballet include delayed menarche and eating disorders. There is a high risk for stress fractures, strains, shin splints, and spinal deviations. Prevention includes nutrition planning and education and skilled coaching.
Wrestling	Placement in a wrestling match is based on weight. A bingeing and purging behavior is commonly found in athletes participating in wrestling. Concussions, neck strains, and spinal injuries are common. Skin dermatitis and infection occurs from contact with floor mats. Skilled coaching, nutrition education, and planning are important.
Football	Improvement in techniques, protective equipment, and game exercises have decreased serious injuries in children participating on football teams.
Hockey	A contact sport involving physical collisions and often puck and stick injuries. Proper protective equipment and sporting rules decrease the seriousness of injuries.
Basketball, volleyball	Jumping sports that involve injury risk to ankles, knees, and fingers. Ankle sprain, tendonitis, stress fractures, and blisters are common complications of these sports.
Running	Involves repeated poorly absorbed foot impact. Muscle fatigue, environmental temperature, and running surface contribute to injuries. Engaging in proper exercises before running, using good impact-absorbing shoes, cross-training, and adequate rest are essential. Shin splints involve pain over the anterior tibia and result from tearing the collagenous fibers that connect muscle to bone. Shoe orthotics, running on a soft surface, cross-training, and rest are the priorities of management.
Skiing	Injuries are usually related to falls. Better equipment, controlled slope conditions, and separation of skill levels contribute to a decreased rate of injury.

CHILD ABUSE

The term *battered child syndrome* was coined by Kempe in his landmark paper published in 1962 by the *Journal of the American Medical Association.* It refers to "a clinical condition in young children who have received serious physical abuse, generally from a parent or foster parent." The impact of Kempe's research was considerable and focused the attention of physicians on unexplained fractures and signs of physical abuse. Today, most authorities consider Kempe's definition narrow and have broadened it to include neglect and maltreatment.

According to the National Center on Child Abuse and Neglect, the incidence of the following aspects of child abuse has been increasing:

- *Emotional abuse:* intentional verbal acts that result in a destruction of self-esteem in the child; can include rejection or threatening the child
- *Emotional neglect:* an intentional omission of verbal or behavioral actions that are necessary for

development of a healthy self-esteem; can include social or emotional isolation of a child
- *Sexual abuse:* involves an act that is performed on a child for the sexual gratification of the adult
- *Physical neglect:* the failure to provide for the basic physical needs of the child, including food, clothing, shelter, and basic cleanliness
- *Physical abuse:* the deliberate infliction of injury on a child; suspected when an injury is not consistent with the history or developmental level of the child

The temperament of the child and the parent can be a causal factor in child abuse. Children who are different from others in any way are at particular risk. This includes preterm infants, sick or disabled children, and merely unattractive children. Unwanted or illegitimate infants and stepchildren are especially vulnerable. It has been noted that people are often reluctant to report occurrences in middle- and upper-income families or when the incident involves friends or relatives.

FEDERAL LAWS AND AGENCIES

By 1963 the United States Children's Bureau drafted a model mandatory state reporting law that has been adopted in some form in all states. This law aids in establishing statistics and is based on the need to provide therapeutic help to both child and family. Immunity from liability is provided for persons reporting suspected cases. Most states have penalties for failure to report suspected child abuse. Referrals usually are made to the local child protective services, and a case worker is assigned.

NURSING TIP

Reporting Suspected Abuse or Neglect

A citizen can report suspected child abuse or neglect by contacting the child protective services in the yellow pages of the telephone directory under "Social Service Organizations." This can be done anonymously. After obtaining the facts, the agency informs the parents that a report is being filed and checks the condition of the child. A visit must be initiated within 72 hours. In most cases, this is accomplished within 48 hours or earlier if the situation is life threatening. All persons who report suspected abuse or neglect are given immunity from criminal prosecution and civil liability if the report is made in good faith. Many professionals, such as physicians, nurses, and social workers, *must report child abuse.*

NURSING CARE AND INTERVENTION

Nursing interventions for high-risk children is of utmost importance (Box 24-2). One approach currently taken is to identify high-risk infants and parents during the prenatal and perinatal periods. Predictive questionnaires are being used as screening tools in some clinics. Many hospitals also provide closer follow-up of mothers and newborns. Maternal-infant bonding and its significance to later parent-child relationships have been explored.

Nurses in obstetrical clinics have the opportunity to observe parents and their abilities to cope. The history of the parent(s), desirability of the pregnancy, number of children already in the family, financial and personal stability of the family, types of support systems, and other factors may have a bearing on how the parents accept the new offspring. Pertinent observations include a description of parent-newborn interaction. Both verbal and nonverbal communications are important, as is the level of body and eye contact. Lack of interest, indifference, or negative comments about the sex, looks, or temperament of the infant could be significant.

In other areas a cooperative team approach is necessary. This may include services such as family planning, protective services, day care centers, homemakers, parenting classes, self-help groups, family counseling, child advocates, and a continued effort to reduce the incidence of preterm birth. Other related areas include financial assistance, employment services, transportation, emotional support and encouragement, and long-term follow-up care.

Individual nurses can help to detect child abuse by maintaining a vigilant approach in their work settings. Record keeping should be *factual* and *objective*. The pediatric nurse should make a point of reviewing old records of their patients, which may reveal repeated hospitalizations, x-ray films of multiple fractures, persistent feeding problems, a history of failure to thrive, and a history of chronic absenteeism in school. Neglect or delay in seeking medical attention for a child or failure to obtain immunization and well-child care can be significant findings. Children who seem overly upset about being discharged must be brought to the attention of the health care provider. Runaway teenagers are often victims of abuse.

The abused child is approached quietly, and preparation for any treatment is carefully explained in advance. The number of caretakers should be kept to a minimum. The child may be able to express some hostility and fear through play or drawing. It is not unusual for these children to be unresponsive or openly hostile or to show affection indiscriminately. Direct questioning is kept to a minimum. Praise is used when appropriate. Activities that promote physical and sensory development are encouraged. The nurse avoids speaking to the child about the parents in a negative manner. Other professionals are consulted about setting limits for poor behavior.

The nurse must acknowledge that there are always two victims in cases of child abuse: the child *and* the abuser. Because of personal problems, the abuser often leads an isolated life. Some have been battered or neglected children themselves. Many have unrealistic expectations about the child's intelligence and capabilities. There may be a role reversal in which the child becomes the comforter. Although removing the child from the home is one answer, many authorities believe this can be more detrimental in the long run.

Being open to parents during this type of crisis is difficult but essential if the nurse wishes to be part of the solution rather than part of the problem. When place-

box 24-2 *Nursing Interventions for Abused and Neglected Children and Adolescents*

TEACH CHILD ANXIETY-REDUCING TECHNIQUES

Gradual relaxation
Relaxation to music
Visual imagery
Exercise
Talking with safe, appropriate people about feelings
Choosing, building, and maintaining positive support
  systems
Ensuring personal safety
Setting boundaries
Establishing a safe, supportive relationship
Clarifying expectations and rules
Self-soothing techniques

ASSIST CHILD IN MANAGING HIS OR HER FEELINGS

Teach child to identify feelings.
Teach child to express feelings appropriately.
Teach child to modulate and control feelings.
Teach child to identify events that elicit strong positive
  and negative feelings.
Teach child to express feelings verbally instead of
  physically.
Teach child to normalize feelings resulting from abuse.
Teach child to share feelings appropriately with peer
  group.
Teach child to find commonality and support within
  group for feelings resulting from abuse.

TEACH CHILD ASSERTIVENESS SKILLS

Teach child to identify differences between
  assertiveness, passivity, and aggression.
Teach child to practice assertiveness skills.
Teach child to identify boundaries.
Teach child to understand when someone violates
  boundaries.
Teach child to practice responses when someone
  violates boundaries.

ASSIST CHILD IN DEVELOPING PROBLEM-SOLVING SKILLS

Provide simple problem-solving model.
Increase awareness of child's control and decision
  making.
Teach child to generate a list of possible solutions to
  problem situations.
Help child look at consequences of each solution.
Help child make best choice.
Help child give self positive and gentle negative
  feedback.
Coach problem solving with actual situations as much
  as possible.
Teach good touch/bad touch.
Teach refusal skills.
Teach age-appropriate sexual expression.
Teach the effects of substance abuse.

ASSIST CHILD IN VALUE BUILDING AND CLARIFICATION

Define values.
Identify role of values.
Assist child in identifying and verbalizing values.
Help link child's values to child's actions.
Assist child in development of values.
Help child practice value-based decision making.

ASSIST CHILD IN ENHANCING HIS OR HER COPING MECHANISMS

Teach child to practice positive self-talk.
Help child set realistic expectations for self.
Assist child in learning to nurture self.
Teach child to practice relaxation.
Teach child to practice assertiveness and appropriate
  expression of feelings.
Assist child in learning to accept defeat and failure.
Help child identify and build skills and hobbies.
Encourage child to identify and focus on strengths.
Help child set and accomplish goals.
Assist child in developing organizational skills.

Data from Bowden, V.R., Dickey, S.B., Greenberg, C.S. (1998). *Children and their families: The continuum of care.* Philadelphia: W.B. Saunders.

ment in a foster home is necessary, parents experience grief, loss, and remorse. The child also mourns the loss of the family, even though there has been abuse. The nurse should be aware of the child's needs and facilitate the expression of feelings of loss. The nurse who recognizes the potential for violence within us all is better able to respond to this complex problem.

NURSING **TIP**

Bruises heal in various stages that are indicated according to color (1 to 2 days, *swollen,* tender; 0 to 5 days, *red/purple;* 5 to 7 days, *green;* 7 to 10 days, *yellow;* 10 to 14 days, *brown;* 14 to 28 days, *clear*). It is important to ask yourself, "Does the bruise match the caregiver's explanation of what happened?"

CULTURAL AND MEDICAL ISSUES

Multiple factors should be considered when evaluating the child. A culturally sensitive history is essential. The nurse should be aware that what appears to be a cigarette burn could be a single lesion of impetigo. Mongolian spots can be mistaken for bruises. A severe diaper rash caused by a fungal infection can look like a scald burn. In some cases, loving parents can injure infants when shaking them to wake or feed them. They are not aware of the danger of "shaken baby syndrome."

Some cultural practices can be interpreted as physical abuse if the nurse is not culturally aware of folk healing and ethnic practices. For example, "coining" of the body by the Vietnamese to allay disease can cause welts on the body (Chapter 33). Burning small areas of the skin to treat enuresis is practiced by some Asian cultures. Forced kneeling is a common Caribbean discipline technique. Yemenite Jews treat infections by placing garlic preparations on the wrists, which can result in blisters. The Telugu people of Southern India touch the penis of a child to show respect.

The nurse should document all signs of abuse and interaction as well as verbal comments between the child and parents (Figure 24-14). Child protective services should oversee any investigation that is warranted. Providing support to parents and child, an opportunity to talk in privacy, and planning for follow-up care are basic nursing responsibilities. Parent education concerning growth and development is valuable.

key points

- The age, neurological development, and motor milestones achieved will influence the nursing assessment of the musculoskeletal system in a growing child.
- The normal gait of a toddler is wide and unstable. By 6 years of age the gait resembles an adult walk.
- Immobility causes a slowing down of body metabolism.
- Injury to the epiphyseal plate at the ends of long bones is serious during childhood because it may interfere with longitudinal growth.
- In a compound fracture a wound in the skin accompanies the broken bone, and there is added danger of infection.
- Any delay in neurological development can cause a delay in mastery of motor skills, which can result in altered skeletal growth.
- Children who do not walk by 18 months of age should be referred for follow-up care.
- Rest, ice, compression, and elevation are the principles of managing soft tissue injuries.
- Pain over a muscle area that does not respond to medication may indicate a complication known as *compartment syndrome*.
- A *neurovascular check* includes color, warmth, capillary refill time, movement, pulse, sensation, and pain.
- Tutorial assistance should be provided to school-age children who are hospitalized or immobilized for long periods of time.

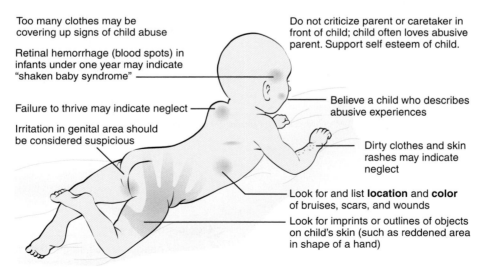

Too many clothes may be covering up signs of child abuse

Retinal hemorrhage (blood spots) in infants under one year may indicate "shaken baby syndrome"

Failure to thrive may indicate neglect

Irritation in genital area should be considered suspicious

Do not criticize parent or caretaker in front of child; child often loves abusive parent. Support self esteem of child.

Believe a child who describes abusive experiences

Dirty clothes and skin rashes may indicate neglect

Look for and list **location** and **color** of bruises, scars, and wounds

Look for imprints or outlines of objects on child's skin (such as reddened area in shape of a hand)

Divide the body into four planes Front, Back, Right side, and Left side.
Injuries occurring in more than one plane should be considered suspicious.

FIGURE **24-14** Assessing for child abuse. The nurse should be alert for inconsistent statements about injuries; bruises at various stages of healing; delay in seeking care; and a history that is not compatible with injury or development.

- A complication of any traction is an arterial occlusion termed Volkmann's ischemia.
- Legg-Calvé-Perthes disease affects the blood supply to the head of the femur.
- Juvenile rheumatoid arthritis is the most common arthritic condition of childhood.
- Medical treatment of scoliosis includes bracing, exercise, and the use of transcutaneous electrical nerve stimulation (TENS).
- Adolescents who participate in sports are subject to injuries such as concussions and ligament injuries. Activities must be selected carefully according to physical maturity, size, and skill required.

- A spiral fracture of the femur or humerus may be a sign of child abuse.
- Child abuse may be physical, emotional, or sexual or may involve neglect.

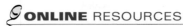ONLINE RESOURCES

Pavlik Harness: http://www.ccmckids.org/departments/orthopaedics/orthoed7.htm

Limp and Joint Pain: http://www.vh.org/Providers/ClinRef/FPHandbook/Chapter12/19-12.html

Scoliosis: http://www.kidshealth.org/kid/health_problems/bone/scolio.html

---

REVIEW QUESTIONS   *Choose the most appropriate answer.*

1. A disorder in which the blood supply to the epiphyses of the bone is disrupted is called:
   1. Muscular dystrophy
   2. Cerebral palsy
   3. Congenital hip dysplasia
   4. Legg-Calvé-Perthes disease

2. The term used when the circulation to a part of the body is obstructed is:
   1. Ischemia
   2. Ischesis
   3. Anemia
   4. Infarction

3. Buck extension is an example of:
   1. Skin traction
   2. Skeletal traction
   3. Balanced traction
   4. Bryant's traction

4. An S-shaped curvature of the spine seen in school-age children is:
   1. Sclerosis
   2. Sciatica
   3. Scabies
   4. Scoliosis

5. A yellow bruise is approximately:
   1. 2 days old
   2. 5 to 7 days old
   3. 7 to 10 days old
   4. 10 to 14 days old

25 The Child with a Respiratory or Cardiovascular Disorder

objectives

1. Define each key term listed.
2. Distinguish the differences between the respiratory tract of the infant and that of the adult.
3. Describe the normal process of respiration.
4. Identify three methods of preventing the spread of infection.
5. Review the signs and symptoms of respiratory distress in infants and children.
6. Discuss the nursing care of a child with pneumonia.
7. Compare bed rest for a toddler with bed rest for an adult.
8. Discuss the nursing care of a child with croup.
9. Describe the treatment and nursing care of an infant with respiratory syncytial virus (RSV).
10. Recall the characteristic manifestations of allergic rhinitis.
11. Discuss how sinusitis in children is different from that in adults.
12. Recognize the precautions involved in the care of a child diagnosed with epiglottitis.
13. Assess the control of environmental exposure to allergens in the home of a child with asthma.
14. Express five goals of asthma therapy.
15. Interpret the role of sports and physical exercise for the asthmatic child.
16. Examine the prevention of sudden infant death syndrome (SIDS).
17. Recall four nursing goals in the care of a child with cystic fibrosis.
18. Review the prevention of bronchopulmonary dysplasia (BPD).
19. Discuss the postoperative care of a 5-year-old who has had a tonsillectomy.
20. Devise a nursing care plan for the child with cystic fibrosis, including family interventions.
21. List the general signs and symptoms of congenital heart disease.
22. Differentiate between patent ductus arteriosus, coarctation of the aorta, atrial septal defect, ventricular septal defect, and tetralogy of Fallot.
23. Discuss six nursing goals relevant to the child with heart disease.
24. Discuss hypertension in childhood.
25. Differentiate between primary and secondary hypertension.
26. List the symptoms of rheumatic fever.
27. Discuss the prevention of rheumatic fever.
28. Describe a heart-healthy diet for a child over 2 years of age.
29. Identify factors that can prevent hypertension.

key terms

alveoli (ăl-VĒ-ō-lī, p. 598)
atelectasis (ă-tĕ-LĔK-tă-sĭs, p. 608)
carbon dioxide narcosis (p. 591)
carditis (kăhr-DĪ-tĭs, p. 625)
chorea (kă-RĒ-ă, p. 625)
clubbing of fingers (p. 609)
coryza (kō-RĪ-ză, p. 591)
Croupette (kroo-pĕt, p. 595)
dysphagia (dĭs-FĀ-jē-ă, p. 594)
hemodynamics (hē-mō-dī-NĂM-ĭks, p. 617)
hypothermia (hī-pō-THĔR-mē-ă, p. 617)
Jones criteria (p. 626)
laryngeal spasm (p. 595)
meconium ileus (mē-kō-nē-ĕm ĬL-ē-ăs, p. 609)
orthopnea (ŏr-thŏp-NĒ-ă, p. 595)
Pediatric Advanced Life Support (PALS) (p. 624)
polyarthritis (p. 625)
polycythemia (pŏl-ē-sī-THĒ-mē-ă, p. 621)
pulse pressure (p. 620)
pursed-lip breathing (p. 614)
reactive airway disease (RAD) (p. 598)
shunt (p. 617)
stenosis (p. 620)
stridor (STRĪ-dŏr, p. 594)
stroke volume (p. 623)
surfactant (sŭr-FĂK-tănt, p. 591)
tachycardia (tăk-ē-KĂR-dē-ă, p. 597)
tachypnea (tăk-ĭp-NĒ-ă, p. 597)
"tet" spells (p. 621)
thoracotomy (thō-ră-KŎT-ō-mē, p. 616)
ventilation (p. 591)

RESPIRATORY SYSTEM

DEVELOPMENT OF THE RESPIRATORY TRACT

Pulmonary structures differentiate in an orderly fashion during fetal life. This makes it possible to determine at what point a particular defect may have occurred. The laryngotracheal groove appears at 2 to 4 weeks' gestation. The trachea and the esophagus originate as one hollow tube; gradually, by 4 weeks' gestation, a septum forms to completely separate them. If the septum fails to form completely, a tracheoesophageal fistula occurs (see Chapter 27). By the seventh week of fetal life the diaphragm forms and separates the chest from the abdominal cavity. If the diaphragm fails to close completely, a *diaphragmatic hernia* allows the abdominal contents (intestines, spleen, stomach) to enter the chest cavity and prevents the lungs from expanding fully. Alveoli and capillaries, which are necessary for gas exchange in the human body, are formed between 24 and 28 weeks' gestation.

At the twenty-fourth week the formed alveolar cells begin to produce surfactant. Surfactant is composed of *lecithin* and *sphingomyelin* and prevents the alveoli from collapsing during respirations after birth. A premature birth is accompanied by problems with respiratory gas exchange. During fetal life the lungs are filled with a fluid that has a low surface tension and viscosity; this is rapidly absorbed after birth. Spontaneous respiratory movements occur in the fetus, although gas exchange occurs via placental circulation. When surfactant is present in the lungs, the respiratory movements force some of the surfactant into the amniotic fluid. At about 35 weeks' gestation, the lecithin component is twice that of the sphingomyelin component. The analysis of the lecithin/sphingomyelin ratio (L/S ratio) by amniocentesis (see Table 5-1) is one method of determining fetal maturity and the ability of the fetus to survive outside the uterus.

NORMAL RESPIRATION

The process of normal respiration is described in Figure 25-1.

VENTILATION

Ventilation, the process of breathing air into and out of the lungs, is affected by the following elements that interact:

- *Intercostal muscles, diaphragm, ribs.* These allow chest expansion and contraction. Expansion of the chest lowers pressure in the chest cavity, and air flows from the higher pressure of the atmosphere into the lower pressure of the chest cavity. The opposite occurs during expiration.
- *Brain.* The vagus nerve and the respiratory centers in the medulla of the brain regulate rhythmic respiratory movements. Signals sent to the respiratory center will increase or decrease respiratory rates.
- *Chemoreceptors.* These sensors respond to changes in the oxygen saturation of the blood by sending a signal to the pons in the brainstem, which is stimulated to increase respirations when the oxygen (O_2) saturation is low.

NOTE: A high carbon dioxide (CO_2) level in the blood and a low O_2 saturation stimulate the brain to increase the respiratory rate. In chronic lung disease, however, the receptors become tolerant to the high CO_2 and low O_2 concentration in the blood. Administration of supplemental oxygen increases the O_2 saturation level and may result in a decreased respiratory effort (carbon dioxide narcosis), leading to respiratory failure. The differences between the respiratory tract of the growing child and that of the adult are shown in Table 25-1.

Procedures that may be performed on the child with a respiratory condition include throat and nasopharyngeal cultures, bronchoscopy, lung biopsy, arterial blood gas (PO_2, PCO_2) and pH analysis, pulse oximetry, and various pulmonary function tests (PFTs). Chest x-ray films, computed tomography, radioisotope scan, bronchogram, and angiography may prove useful depending on symptoms. The inspection, percussion, and auscultation procedures performed by the nurse are of utmost value in data collection.

NASOPHARYNGITIS

Pathophysiology. A cold, also known as acute coryza, is the most common infection of the respiratory tract. It is caused by one or a number of viruses, principally the rhinoviruses, which are spread from one child to another by sneezing, coughing, or direct contact. The age, state of nutrition, and general health of the child contribute to the susceptibility level.

The rhinovirus is spread by contact with contaminated fingers touching the conjunctiva of the eyes or mucous membranes of the mouth. Routine handwashing practices, especially before rubbing the nose or sucking the fingers, can prevent the spread of the common cold.

The common cold differs from allergic rhinitis in that a child who has allergic rhinitis has no fever, no purulent nasal discharge, and no reddened mucous membranes. Sneezing, watery eyes, and itching are the primary manifestations of *allergic rhinitis*. In the older child or adolescent, persistent nasopharyngitis may be related to inhaled cocaine or other drug abuse.

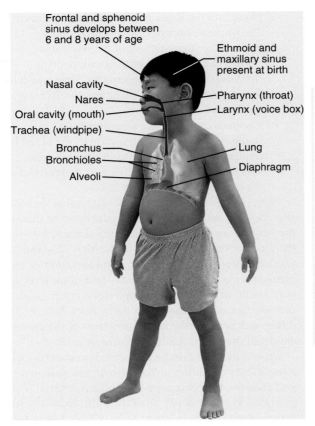

Frontal and sphenoid sinus develops between 6 and 8 years of age

Ethmoid and maxillary sinus present at birth

Nasal cavity
Nares
Oral cavity (mouth)
Trachea (windpipe)
Bronchus
Bronchioles
Alveoli

Pharynx (throat)
Larynx (voice box)
Lung
Diaphragm

FIGURE **25-1** Summary of respiratory tract in children. The ribs and the diaphragm allow for inspiration of air. Air enters the body through the *nares,* or nostrils. The mucous membranes and cilia that line the respiratory tract warm, moisten, and filter the air as it passes to the *pharynx.* The pharynx contains the tonsils, which assist in infection control. The *larynx* at the upper end of the trachea contains the epiglottis, glottis, and vocal cords, which prevent food and fluids from entering the trachea and allow voice sounds. The *trachea* is encircled by smooth muscle and cartilage to maintain patency and carries the air to the bronchi and then to the smaller bronchioles. The bronchioles continue to divide and lead to small, thin air sacs (alveoli) that are kept open on inspiration by the air contained in them. During expiration when the air sacs collapse, *surfactant* prevents the walls from sticking together, allowing for reinflation. Gas exchange occurs in the alveoli by diffusion to the bloodstream. The volume of air inhaled with each breath is related to body size.

RESPIRATORY SYSTEM

- Respiratory rates are higher in children. Diaphragmatic abdominal breathing is common in infants.
- Oxygen consumption is high in children in proportion to body size; metabolic rate is higher than in adults.
- Airway diameter is smaller in children, which increases the potential for obstruction.
- Mucous membranes of airways are highly vascular and are susceptible to trauma, edema, and spasm.
- Surfactant is lacking in preterm infants, which contributes to respiratory distress syndrome.
- Accessory muscles of respiration are not as strong in children, particularly in infants.
- Chest wall retractions are common in infants with respiratory problems because the chest wall is supple.

Manifestations. The symptoms of a cold in an infant or small child are different from those in an adult. Children's air passages are smaller and more easily obstructed. The virus causes inflammation and edema of the membranes of the upper respiratory tract, which damages cilia and prevents the drainage of mucus. Fever as high as 40° C (104° F) is not uncommon in children under 3 years of age. Nasal discharge, irritability, sore throat, cough, and general discomfort are present, and there may be vomiting and diarrhea. The diagnosis is complicated by the fact that many infectious diseases resemble the common cold during their onset. Complications of a cold include bronchitis, pneumonitis, and ear infections.

Treatment and nursing care. There is no cure for the common cold. Treatment should begin early, when a cold is suspected. The following treatment is designed to relieve symptoms:

- *Rest.* Fatigue should be avoided. Confinement to bed for a child does not always result in physical rest. In pediatrics, "bed rest" means providing play therapy that promotes minimal activity. The nurse should consider the age and developmental level of the child and the activity level involved in the play when designing appropriate activities and guiding parents in the home care of their child.
- *Clear airways.* Congested nasal passages cause discomfort and prevent sucking of formula.

table 25-1 *Differences in the Respiratory Tract of the Growing Child and the Adult*

HOW INFANT DIFFERS FROM ADULT	SIGNIFICANCE
The infant relies primarily on the abdominal muscles and the diaphragm for breathing. The intercostal muscles only stabilize the chest wall.	Assessment of respiration is best accomplished by monitoring the rise and fall of the abdomen until 3 years of age, when thoracic breathing begins. Adult-type breathing patterns are typically developed by 7 years of age. Substernal retraction is a sign of respiratory distress in infants.
In infants, the diaphragm is attached higher than in the adult and is stretched longer, limiting its ability to contract forcefully.	Abdominal distention from formula or gas can interfere with movement of the diaphragm.
The infant depends on the accessory muscles for respiratory efforts.	Muscle fatigue can result in respiratory arrest.
Infants are nose breathers and do not breathe through the mouth unless crying.	Swelling of the nasal mucosa will interfere with sucking and cause irritability.
In infants, the tissue below the vocal cords is not firm, and portions of the larynx are very narrow.	Any edema or swelling can cause respiratory obstruction.
In infants, the cartilage that maintains the patency of the airway is soft, not firm.	Vagal nerve stimulation or muscle constriction can cause collapse of the airway and respiratory obstruction.
The larynx and trachea are higher in the chest in infancy and descend slowly as the child grows.	Positioning the infant or child for airway clearance and resuscitation is different than for adults. Excess flexion or extension of neck can cause respiratory obstruction.
Alveoli in the lung divide and thin as the child grows and develops, resulting in increased surface area for gas exchange. The number of alveoli present at puberty is nine times that found in the infant.	Less surface area in the alveoli is available for gas exchange, which predisposes infants and young children to respiratory distress.
Lung growth is inhibited by phenobarbital and excess insulin.	Drugs and disease can inhibit lung development.
Infants and young children have a small airway diameter.	Edema or muscle spasm can rapidly cause respiratory obstruction.
Newborns and infants produce less respiratory mucus (which serves as a cleansing agent).	Infants and children are more susceptible to respiratory infections.
Infants have less developed smooth muscle lining the airway than do older children and adults.	Bronchospasm may not occur in infants, and therefore wheezing may not be a presenting sign of a narrowed airway.
In infants, the respiratory rate is higher and the breathing pattern is irregular.	Meaningful assessment of respiration must be related to the age of the child. Irregular respirations with short periods of apnea is normal for a young infant but abnormal in an adult.

Because fluid consumption is essential to prevent fever and dehydration, the airways must be cleared before feeding and before bedtime to provide a restful sleep. The nurse can teach the parents that instilling a few drops of saline solution into the nose and then suctioning with a bulb syringe (Chapter 12, Figure 12-8) is the best way to clear the nostrils. Medicated nosedrops can be irritating to the mucosa of a young child's nasal passages. Nosedrops with an oily base should be avoided because they are readily aspirated and can cause respiratory problems. Rebound congestion can be avoided by limiting the use of nosedrops to no more than 3 days.

- *Adequate fluid intake.* Anorexia is common in children with nasopharyngitis. Fluids should be encouraged to prevent dehydration. Cool, bland liquids are usually tolerated well in a child who has a sore throat.
- *Prevention of fever.* Ibuprofen (Motrin) or acetaminophen (Tylenol) can be administered when a high fever accompanies a cold. Parents should be cautioned to check the label of the medication for appropriate dosages. The safe dosage for Tylenol *elixir* differs from that of Tylenol *drops.*
- *Skin care.* A petroleum-based ointment can be applied to the nares and upper lip to prevent skin irritation from a nasal discharge.

Moist air soothes the inflamed nose and throat. An electric cold air humidifier is safe and convenient. It must be cleaned and disinfected daily. If a great deal of moisture is indicated (as in croup), the infant may be taken to a small room, such as the bathroom, and the hot water faucets or shower can be turned on to produce sufficient steam.

The older child is taught the proper way to remove nasal secretions from the nose. The mouth is opened slightly, and secretions are gently blown through both nostrils at the same time. This method prevents the infection from being forced into the eustachian tubes. Children must be taught to cover the mouth and nose when sneezing and to wash their hands afterward. Tissues must be properly discarded. Antibiotics are not effective against the common cold because it is viral in origin.

ACUTE PHARYNGITIS

Pathophysiology. Acute pharyngitis is an inflammation of the structures in the throat. This infection is common among children between 5 and 15 years of age. In 80% of cases the causative organism is a virus. Group A beta-hemolytic streptococcus (strep throat) occurs in 20% of the cases. The bacterium *Hemophilus influenzae* is common in children under 3 years of age.

Manifestations, treatment, and nursing care. Symptoms include fever, malaise, dysphagia (*dys,* "difficult" and *phagia,* "swallowing"), and anorexia. It is difficult to distinguish viral from bacterial types by symptoms only. Conjunctivitis, rhinitis, cough, and hoarseness with a gradual onset and persisting no longer than 5 days are characteristic of viral pharyngitis. In a child over 2 years of age, streptococcal pharyngitis characteristically includes high fever (40° C [104° F]) and difficulty in swallowing, and it may last longer than 1 week. A strep throat is determined by throat culture. When the culture is positive, antimicrobial therapy such as penicillin is administered. It is prescribed orally for 10 days. Compliance may be a problem; therefore the nurse carefully

explains to parents the need for the child to finish all of the medication. Erythromycin may be prescribed if the child is allergic to penicillin. Acetaminophen may be taken to relieve soreness of the throat. If the child is old enough to gargle, a solution of warm water and salt may be used.

Prompt treatment of strep throat is important to avoid serious complications such as rheumatic fever, glomerulonephritis, peritonsillar abscess, otitis media, mastoiditis, meningitis, osteomyelitis, or pneumonia. The persistence of a positive streptococcal culture after careful follow-up and therapy may indicate that the child is a group A beta-hemolytic streptococcus carrier. However, it may also mean that the child did not complete the 10-day course of medication or that a drug-resistant organism has evolved. The child with strep throat is no longer infectious to others once drug therapy has begun and fever has decreased.

SINUSITIS IN CHILDREN

The frontal sinuses are present at 8 years of age but may not be fully developed until age 18. Some ethmoid sinus cells are present at birth. The sphenoid sinus is present by 3 years of age and is fully developed by age 12. The maxillary sinuses are present at birth and develop as long as teeth are erupting. The proximity of this sinus to the tooth roots often results in tooth pain when the sinus is infected. The maxillary and ethmoid sinuses are most often involved in childhood sinusitis. Signs and symptoms of sinusitis in children are different from those in the adult. An acute sinusitis is suspected when an upper respiratory infection lasts longer than 10 days, with a daytime cough. Halitosis is often present. Untreated sinusitis can lead to periorbital cellulitis because the infection spreads from the ethmoid sinus to the subperiosteal space around the eye. Treatment involves a 10- to 14-day course of antibiotic therapy.

CROUP SYNDROMES

Pathophysiology. *Croup* is a general term applied to a number of conditions whose chief symptom is a "barking" (croupy) cough and varying degrees of inspiratory stridor (a harsh, high-pitched sound). When the larynx is involved, the clinical picture becomes more intense because of possible alterations in respiratory status, such as airway obstruction, acute respiratory failure, and hypoxia (Figure 25-2). Acute spasmodic laryngitis is the milder form of the syndrome. Acute laryngotracheobronchitis is the most common. It is also referred to as subglottic croup because edema occurs *below* the vocal cords. Croup can be benign or acute. Benign croup is frightening but rarely life threatening. Acute croup can develop into a respiratory emergency.

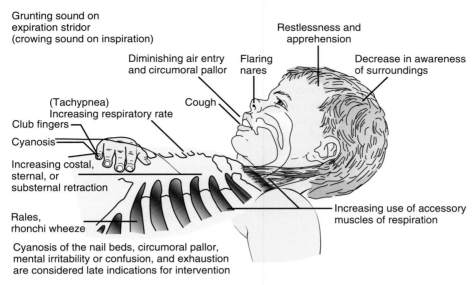

Grunting sound on
expiration stridor
(crowing sound on inspiration)

Restlessness and
apprehension

Diminishing air entry
and circumoral pallor

Flaring
nares

Decrease in awareness
of surroundings

(Tachypnea)
Increasing respiratory rate

Cough

Club fingers

Cyanosis

Increasing costal,
sternal, or
substernal retraction

Increasing use of accessory
muscles of respiration

Rales,
rhonchi wheeze

Cyanosis of the nail beds, circumoral pallor,
mental irritability or confusion, and exhaustion
are considered late indications for intervention

FIGURE 25-2 Signs of respiratory distress in infants and children.

Benign Crouplike Conditions

Congenital laryngeal stridor (laryngomalacia). Some infants are born with a weakness of the airway walls and a floppy epiglottis that causes a stridor (crowlike noise) on inspiration. There may be inspiratory retractions. The symptoms lessen when the infant is placed prone or propped in the side-lying position. Respiratory infection and crying may cause the symptoms to become frightening to the parents. The condition usually spontaneously clears as the child grows and the muscles strengthen. The nurse should provide reassurance and suggest slow, small feedings and a prone or side-lying position for the infant.

Spasmodic laryngitis (spasmodic croup). Spasmodic croup usually occurs in children between 1 to 3 years of age and can be caused by a virus, allergy, or psychological trigger. Very often, gastroesophageal reflux (GER) will trigger an attack. Spasmodic croup has a sudden onset, usually at night, and is characterized by a barking, brassy cough and respiratory distress. The child appears anxious, and the parents become frightened. The attack lasts a few hours, and by morning the child appears normal and is in no distress. Increasing humidity and providing fluids are helpful treatment measures.

Acute Croup

Laryngotracheobronchitis. The viral condition laryngotracheobronchitis is manifested by edema, destruction of respiratory cilia, and exudate, resulting in respiratory obstruction. A mild upper respiratory infection usually precedes the development of a characteristic barking or brassy cough. Stridor develops, and classic symptoms of respiratory distress follow (see Figure 25-2). The infant prefers to be held upright or sit up in bed (orthopnea). Crying and agitation worsen the symptoms. Hypoxia can develop and be accompanied by tachycardia and diminished breath sounds.

Treatment and nursing care. When the child is treated at home, parents are often instructed to increase humidity levels around the child. This can be accomplished by using an electric cold water humidifier. The humidifier must be emptied, washed, and disinfected each day to prevent the growth of microorganisms that occur in stagnant tap water. The child can also be taken into the bathroom, where the hot water in the shower is turned on to increase humidity. The child inhales the moist air, which usually relieves the respiratory distress and laryngeal spasm (constriction of laryngeal muscles).

When continuing symptoms of respiratory distress require hospitalization, the child may be placed in a mist tent, or Croupette (see p. 527). The cool air, well saturated in microdroplets that can enter the small airway of a child, causes mucosal cooling and vasoconstriction and relieves the respiratory obstruction and distress. Recent studies, however, have shown that the value of mist tent therapy in the acutely ill child is unproven (Bjornson & Johnson, 2001). Intravenous (IV) fluids are prescribed to prevent dehydration and to decrease the risk of vomiting and aspiration that can occur after a coughing episode. Organization of care is essential to enable the child to have long periods of rest. The child is placed on a cardiorespiratory monitor (CRM), and the vital signs are observed closely. Oxygen is given to reduce hypoxia (see Chapter 22). Oxygen saturation is monitored, and saturation levels are maintained above 90% (see Chapter 13 for sensor application).

Opiates are contraindicated because they depress respiration. Sedatives are contraindicated because increased restlessness is a primary sign of increased respiratory obstruction, and sedatives can mask signs of restlessness. Nebulized epinephrine may be used to relieve the symptoms of respiratory obstruction (Figure 25-3). The American Academy of Pediatrics (AAP) recommends that corticosteroids be prescribed to reduce the edema caused by inflammation and to prevent further destruction of ciliated epithelium in children hospitalized with croup, providing there is no history of recent exposure to varicella (chickenpox).

> ✳ NURSING **TIP**_____
> Respiratory illness is always potentially more serious in children than in adults.

Epiglottitis

Pathophysiology. Epiglottitis is a swelling of the tissues *above* the vocal cords, that is, supraglottic swelling. This results in narrowing of the *airway inlet,* with the possibility of total obstruction. It is caused by *H. influenzae* type B and most often occurs in children 3 to 6 years of age. It can occur in any season. The course is rapid and progressive. *Epiglottitis is a life-threatening medical emergency.* Blood gases fluctuate, and there is leukocytosis.

Manifestations. The onset of epiglottitis is abrupt, and the child presents with classic symptoms. The child insists on sitting up, leans forward with the mouth open, and drools saliva because of the difficulty in swallowing. The child appears wide-eyed, anxious, and restless, and he or she may emit a froglike croaking sound on inspiration. Cough is absent. Inspection of the throat shows an enlarged, reddened edematous epiglottis much like a "beefy-red thumb." However, the examining tongue blade may trigger a laryngospasm and result in sudden respiratory arrest. *Therefore it is a primary nursing responsibility to be sure there is a tracheotomy set at the bedside before any examination of the throat is attempted.*

Treatment. The treatment of choice is immediate tracheotomy or endotracheal intubation and oxygen to prevent hypoxia, brain damage, and sudden death caused by respiratory arrest. Parenteral antibiotic therapy usually results in a dramatic improvement within a few days.

Prevention. The AAP recommends that *H. influenzae* type B conjugate vaccines be administered beginning at 2 months of age as part of a regular immunization program for all children. This type of program results in a decreased incidence of acute epiglottitis in children.

Bronchitis

Pathophysiology. A study of the respiratory system reveals that the air tubes leading to the lungs resemble an upside-down tree. The trachea is the main trunk, with the bronchi, bronchioles, and alveoli as branches. These passages proceed from large to small and are lined with a continuous membrane. If there is an infection of the bronchial tree, it is seldom confined to one area but more often involves other structures.

Acute bronchitis is an infection of the bronchi. It seldom occurs as a primary infection but is usually secondary to a cold or communicable disease. It is caused by a variety of organisms. Poor nutrition, allergy, and chronic infection of the respiratory tract may precipitate this condition. Most patients are under 4 years of age.

Manifestations. The gradual onset of an unproductive "hacking" cough is preceded by an upper respiratory infection, or cold. The cough may become productive with purulent sputum. Children under 7 years of age cannot voluntarily cough and usually swallow their sputum.

Treatment. The use of cough suppressants before bedtime may be helpful in promoting restful sleep. Antihistamines, cough expectorants, and antibiotics are usually not helpful. Most children recover uneventfully with symptomatic care at home.

Bronchiolitis

Pathophysiology. Acute bronchiolitis is a viral infection of the small airways (bronchioles) in the lower res-

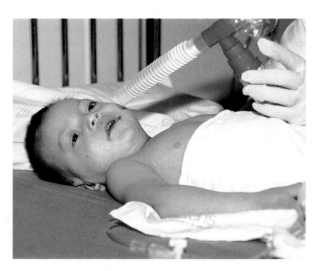

FIGURE **25-3** A child receiving aerosol therapy (medicated nebulizer treatments).

piratory tract. It occurs in infants and children 6 months to 2 years of age, with a peak at 6 months of age. The small diameter of the bronchioles in the infant are susceptible to obstruction when inflammation results in edema and excess mucus. The obstruction often leads to atelectasis. The gas exchange in the lungs becomes impaired, and hypoxia can occur.

Manifestations. An upper respiratory infection, or cold, with a mild fever and serous (clear) nasal discharge is followed by the development of a wheezing cough and signs of respiratory distress (see Figure 25-2). The increase in respiratory rate interferes with successful feeding, and the infant becomes irritable and dehydrated. The respiratory syncytial virus (RSV) is the causative organism in 50% of cases in infants. An apneic episode is usually the cause of hospitalization. Infants who have bronchiolitis may develop a hyperreactive airway or asthma later in life (see Figure 25-5).

Treatment and nursing care. The treatment of an infant with bronchiolitis is symptomatic and similar to that of the child with croup (see p. 595). A semi-Fowler's position with a slightly hyperextended neck facilitates respirations. Oral feedings are often supplemented by IV fluids. Intake and output are recorded. Bronchodilating aerosol therapy (see Figure 25-3) and high-humidity tents are prescribed. Frequent assessment of vital signs and monitoring of oxygen saturation levels are essential.

RESPIRATORY SYNCYTIAL VIRUS

Respiratory Syncytial Virus (RSV) is responsible for 50% of cases of bronchiolitis in infants and young children and is the most common cause of viral pneumonia. RSV is the single most important respiratory pathogen in infancy. RSV occurs worldwide and causes annual epidemics during the winter months. Most children are infected with RSV before their fourth birthday, and reinfection is common, especially in children attending day care centers. Infants between 2 and 7 months of age can become seriously ill with this condition because their airways are so small and prone to obstruction by the thick mucus produced. Older children and adults are not as seriously ill and continue to go to work or school, becoming carriers and spreading the infection.

Transmission. RSV is spread by direct contact with respiratory secretions, usually by contaminated hands to the mucous membranes (eyes, mouth, nose). RSV survives for more than 6 hours on countertops, tissues, and soap bars. RSV is not spread via the airborne route. The incubation period is approximately 4 days.

Hospital cross infection is a major problem, because caregivers may be carrying the organism. For this reason, an infant diagnosed with RSV infection is placed on standard contact (isolation) precaution to prevent the spread of RSV to other sick children.

RSV immunoglobulin may be used for preterm newborns with bronchopulmonary dysplasia who are at risk for infection.

Diagnosis. An examination of nasopharyngeal washings for RSV antigens can be done while the child waits in the admitting unit so that the diagnosis is established before the infant is admitted to the pediatric unit.

Treatment and nursing care. The care of infants with RSV infection should be assigned to personnel who are not caring for patients at high risk for adverse response to RSV. Infection control techniques (see Appendix A) are used to prevent the spread of infection to others on the unit. Contact isolation precautions are used to prevent fomite spread. Frequent handwashing is essential. Liquid soap dispensers should be available at the sink because the organism survives for a long time on a dry bar of soap.

Support of the infant and family. Effective communication skills are necessary to provide support for parents of the infant who is seriously ill. The parent can be familiarized with the mist tent and encouraged to participate in the care and feeding of the infant.

Symptomatic care. An ineffective breathing pattern is the priority nursing diagnosis for an infant hospitalized with RSV infection. Reporting tachypnea (increased respiration) and tachycardia (increased heart rate) is essential because these vital sign changes may be indicative of hypoxemia. It is also important to auscultate breath sounds and report wheezing, rales, or rhonchi. A child who has been wheezing and suddenly has a "quiet chest" on auscultation may be at risk for respiratory arrest. The higher pitched the wheeze, the more constricted is the airway. Signs of respiratory distress (see Figure 25-2) should be assessed and reported. Oxygen saturation levels are monitored and oxygen is administered at levels needed to maintain a minimum of 90% to 95% saturation. Suctioning of mucus may be required to maintain a patent airway. Monitoring IV fluids and recording intake and output are essential to prevent dehydration. Urine output should be a minimum of 1 to 2 ml/kg/hr for infants and children. Pedialyte or Ricelyte are examples of clear liquid electrolyte formulas prescribed for infants at risk of dehydration. The child should be weighed daily to detect early signs of dehydration. Inhaled bronchodilators or steroids are not helpful with RSV infections.

Antiviral medication. Antiviral medication such as ribavirin (Virazole) may be prescribed for use with severely ill infants or infants who have heart or lung problems that place them at high risk for serious complications. The medication has been found to be effective in the treatment of RSV infection but is rarely used pro-phylactically because of its serious side effects. The medication is administered by fine-droplet aerosol mist while the infant is in a mist tent. It is administered 18 to 24 hours a day for a minimum of 3 days. If the infant is on a ventilator, the nurse must monitor the ventilator tubes, which may be warped by ribavirin. Caregivers and visitors who are of childbearing age, pregnant, or breastfeeding should not care for infants receiving riba-virin, because teratogenic effects have been reported. The ribavirin mist can cause precipitation on the sur-face of plastics, and therefore caregivers with contact lenses may develop conjunctivitis because of the lens changes. When providing care to an infant receiving ri-bavirin therapy, the nurse should turn off the nebulizer and allow the mist to settle before opening the mist tent and providing care. Linen removed from the bed should be slowly rolled and carefully folded to avoid releasing droplets of ribavirin into the air.

An IV immune globulin (RespiGam) may be pre-scribed for high-risk infants to prevent complications from RSV disease. (American Academy of Pediatrics, 2000). RespiGam is administered intravenously and re-quires close observation for fluid volume overload. Routine immunizations may need to be postponed for 9 months if antiviral medication for RSV is prescribed. Intramuscular palivizumab (Synagis) can also be given to high-risk infants and does not interfere with mumps-measles-rubella (MMR) or varicella vaccines.

> ★NURSING **TIP**_____
> Caregivers who are pregnant or wear contact lenses should not give direct care to infants who are receiving ribavirin aerosol therapy.

Complications. Infants who have a small airway size and are severely ill and hospitalized with RSV infection may be at risk for wheezing and reactive airway disease (RAD) later in life. Some studies (Behrman, Kliegman, & Jenson, 2000) have shown that the inflammation caused by RSV injures the respiratory epithelial cells, re-sulting in exposed sensory nerve fibers that respond eas-ily to environmental irritants.

PNEUMONIA

Pathophysiology. Pneumonia or pneumonitis is an inflammation of the lungs in which the alveoli (air sacs) become filled with exudate and surfactant may be re-duced. The affected portion of the lung does not receive enough air. Breathing is shallow. As a result, the blood-stream is denied sufficient oxygen.

Pneumonia may occur as the initial or *primary* dis-ease, or it may complicate another illness, in which case it is termed *secondary* pneumonia. There are many types of pneumonia. Classification may be by causative organ-ism (i.e., bacterial or viral) or by the part of the respira-tory system involved (i.e., lobar or bronchial). Group B streptococci are the most common cause of pneumonia in newborns, whereas *Chlamydia* are the most common cause of pneumonia in infants 3 weeks to 3 months of age. The incidence of *H. influenzae* type B infection has been decreasing with current immunization programs. RSV, rhinovirus, adenovirus, and pneumococcus are other organisms that are responsible for pneumonia in infants and children. Immunocompromised children may develop pneumonia caused by a gram-negative or-ganism such as *Pneumocystis carinii* or fungi.

Toddlers often aspirate small objects such as peanuts or popcorn and develop pneumonia as a result; there-fore such foods are to be discouraged for this age-group. *Lipoid pneumonia* occurs when the infant inhales an oil-based substance into the airways. It is less common to-day because children are seldom given cod liver oil or castor oil routinely, as they were in the past. Nosedrops with an oil base must not be used for children because the oil can be aspirated and cause lipoid pneumonia. A toddler who drinks kerosene may also develop a type of pneumonia. *Hypostatic pneumonia* may occur in pa-tients who have poor circulation in their lungs and re-main in one position too long. The child recovering from anesthesia must be turned frequently to stimulate circulation through the lungs. Early ambulation also ac-complishes this.

Manifestations. The symptoms of pneumonia vary with the patient's age and the causative organism. They may develop suddenly or may be preceded by an upper respiratory tract infection. The cough is dry at first, but it gradually becomes productive. Fever rises as high as 39.5° to 40° C (103° to 104° F) and may fluctuate widely during a 24-hour period. The respiratory rate may in-crease (tachypnea) to 40 to 80 breaths/min in infants and 30 to 50 breaths/min in older children. Respirations are shallow in an attempt to reduce the amount of chest pain. The chest pain may be caused by a pleural irritation or a musculoskeletal irritation from frequent coughing. *Sternal retractions* may be seen when the assisting mus-cles of respiration are used. The nostrils may flare. The child is listless, has a poor appetite, and tends to lie on the affected side. X-ray films confirm the diagnosis and de-termine whether there are complications such as atelec-tasis. A differential white blood cell count is routinely performed. Blood specimens show a marked increase in the number of white blood cells (16,000 to 40,000/mm^3). Cultures may be taken from the nose and throat.

Treatment. Treatment depends on the causative or-ganism. Antipyretics are given to reduce fever. Oxygen is administered for dyspnea or cyanosis. When this treatment is begun early, the child is less restless and does not require as many sedatives or drugs to relieve pain. Because drug therapy has become so effective, many uncomplicated cases can be treated at home. Fluid intake should be increased, particularly clear fluids and "flattened" soft drinks. Erythromycin sulfisoxazole (Pediazole) may be prescribed for infants younger than 6 months of age, but amoxicillin is the drug of choice for children up to 5 years of age.

Rest, fluids, and a cough suppressant before bedtime are the basics of home care. Parent education concerning the need to complete all medication prescribed is essential. Tobacco use in the environment should be avoided, and the need for *H. influenzae B* (Hib) immunizations is stressed. The use and disposal of tissues, covering the mouth during a cough, and modeling of proper handwashing techniques are preventive measures the nurse should teach the family.

Nursing care. Nursing care in all types of pneumonia is basically the same. The age of the patient determines the nurse's approach and the type of equipment used. (The newborn receives oxygen in the Isolette, whereas the older child requires a Croupette or a larger tent.) Rest is an important part of the treatment. The nurse must be organized so that the child is not disturbed unnecessarily. Planned, quiet activities for the child are recommended (Pictorial Pathway 25-1).

The nurse checks the vital signs at regular intervals. When a child is flushed with fever, heavy clothing and blankets should be removed. The nurse encourages the child to take fluids, flavored ice pops, or small sips of water frequently. If vomiting persists, parenteral fluids are given.

TONSILLITIS AND ADENOIDITIS

Pathophysiology. The tonsils and adenoids, located in the pharynx (throat), are made of lymph tissue and are part of the body's defense mechanism against infection. The symptoms of tonsillitis includes difficulty in swallowing and breathing. Enlarged adenoids block the nasal passage, resulting in mouth breathing. Other symptoms are similar to those of nasopharyngitis. Nursing care involves providing a cool mist vaporizer to keep the mucous membranes moist; salt water gargles; throat lozenges (if age appropriate); a cool, liquid diet; and acetaminophen to promote comfort. Antibiotics are not usually prescribed unless a throat culture is positive for the streptococcal organism.

Treatment. The removal of the tonsils and adenoids, referred to as a "T&A," is usually not recommended for children under 3 years of age. It is thought that the condition may correct itself if surgery is postponed, because the tissues become smaller as the child grows. A *tonsillectomy* (removal of the palatine tonsils) is indicated only if persistent airway obstruction or difficulty in breathing occurs. The surgery is not performed during an acute infectious episode because inflamed tissue responds poorly to surgery.

Children are prepared for the surgery with age-appropriate explanations. Wording should be carefully selected, because young children may associate being "put to sleep" for the operation with their sick pet being "put to sleep" and never heard from again. Same-day surgery is the usual setting for a tonsillectomy, with the child returning home after a few hours. The presence of loose teeth should be reported to the anesthesiologist because there may be a danger of aspiration during the surgical procedure. Identification bands are applied, and routine preoperative care is initiated and documented.

Postoperative care. To facilitate drainage immediately after surgery, the child is placed partly on the side and partly on the abdomen, with the knee of the uppermost leg flexed to hold the position. The child is watched carefully for evidence of bleeding, such as an increase in pulse and respirations, restlessness, frequent swallowing (which may be from blood trickling down the back of the child's throat), or vomiting of bright red blood. An ice collar may be applied for comfort. The child's face and hands are wiped with a warm washcloth, and the hospital gown and linen are changed whenever necessary. Small amounts of clear liquids are given as tolerated. Red- or brown-colored juices are avoided because they make it difficult to evaluate the content of emesis and the presence of blood. A Popsicle may appeal to the child. If these are well tolerated, progression to a soft diet is begun. The child is kept quiet for the remainder of the day. A small child may nestle on a parent's lap. Coughing, clearing the throat, and blowing the nose are avoided to decrease the risk of precipitating bleeding at the operative site. Appropriate pain relief is important and will minimize crying, which may further irritate the throat. Hemorrhage is the most common postoperative complication. The nurse should not assume that because the surgery is minor it does not involve certain risks.

Written instructions are given to the parents when the child is discharged. The child should be kept quiet for a few days and should receive nourishing fluids and soft foods. After this, the child may continue to take a nap or to have a rest period so that he or she has sufficient convalescent time. Acetaminophen may be given to reduce throat discomfort. The child must be protected from exposure to infections. Gargling and highly seasoned food should be avoided during the first postoperative week.

PICTORIAL PATHWAY 25-1 | *Care of a Child with Pneumonia*

Nursing Diagnosis: Ineffective breathing pattern as evidenced by rapid respiration rate; retractions; nasal flaring
Deficient knowledge related to home care as evidenced by unfamiliarity with suction, MDI, medication
NIC: Airway management
NOC: Ventilation

	1	2	3	4	5
Medications	IV antibiotics	Heplok (Saline-lok)	Oral antibiotics	Oral antibiotics	Discharge to home
Monitors	O$_2$ saturation (Continuous apnea monitor)	O$_2$ saturation	O$_2$ saturation checks		
Nutrition	NPO	As tolerated	As tolerated	Full diet for age	
Respiratory Treatment	O$_2$ and nebulized treatment	O$_2$ and nebulized treatment	Intermittent nebulizer treatments	Metered-dose inhaler	

NURSING **TIP**

After a tonsillectomy, milk and milk products may coat the throat and cause the child to "clear" the throat, further irritating the operative site.

NURSING **TIP**

Frequent swallowing while the child is sleeping is an early sign of bleeding after a tonsillectomy.

ALLERGIC RHINITIS

Allergic rhinitis is an inflammation of the nasal mucosa caused by an allergic response. It often occurs during specific seasons and is referred to as *hay fever*. Allergic rhinitis is not a life-threatening condition and does not require hospitalization, but it occurs in 10% of children and accounts for many school absences.

Pathophysiology. The mast cells in the nasal mucosa respond to an antigen by releasing mediators such as histamine, which cause edema and increased mucous secretion. A generalized parasympathetic response can

PICTORIAL PATHWAY 25-1 | *Care of a Child with Pneumonia—cont'd*

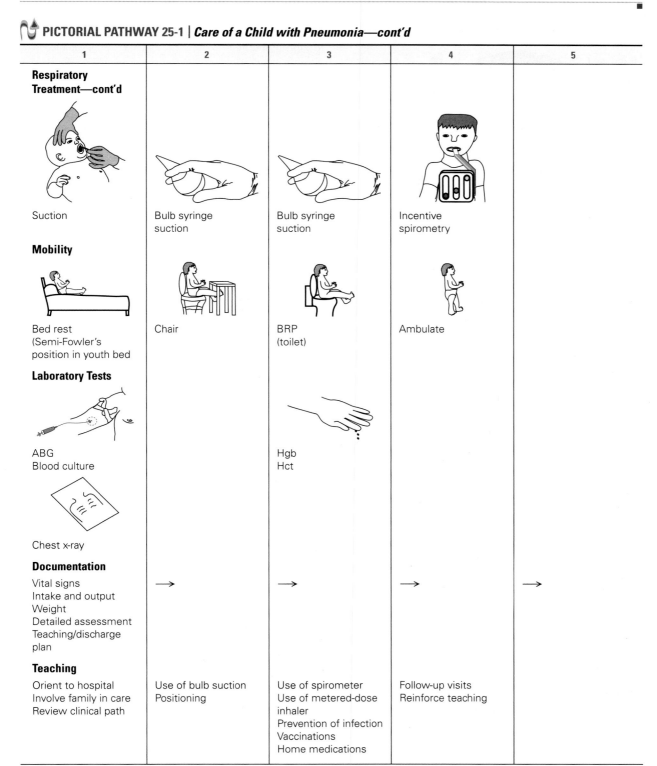

	1	2	3	4	5
Respiratory Treatment—cont'd	Suction	Bulb syringe suction	Bulb syringe suction	Incentive spirometry	
Mobility	Bed rest (Semi-Fowler's position in youth bed	Chair	BRP (toilet)	Ambulate	
Laboratory Tests	ABG Blood culture Chest x-ray		Hgb Hct		
Documentation	Vital signs Intake and output Weight Detailed assessment Teaching/discharge plan	→	→	→	→
Teaching	Orient to hospital Involve family in care Review clinical path	Use of bulb suction Positioning	Use of spirometer Use of metered-dose inhaler Prevention of infection Vaccinations Home medications	Follow-up visits Reinforce teaching	

follow. The child may have a genetic predisposition to develop the allergy, and exposure to the allergen triggers the response.

Manifestations. The characteristic signs of allergic rhinitis include nasal congestion, a clear, watery nasal discharge, sneezing, and itching of the eyes (Figure 25-4).

Diagnosis. Laboratory tests of the mucous membranes of the nose reveal the presence of eosinophils, and skin testing may be positive for specific allergens (skin sensitization testing). The history shows seasonal

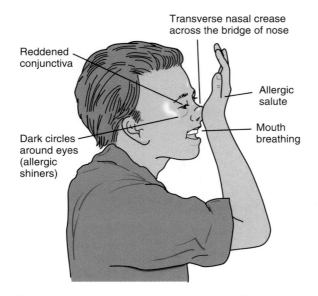

Reddened conjunctiva

Transverse nasal crease across the bridge of nose

Allergic salute

Mouth breathing

Dark circles around eyes (allergic shiners)

FIGURE **25-4** The allergic salute. Signs of allergic rhinitis include a typical rubbing of the nose in response to nasal discharge *(allergic salute),* darkened circles under the eyes *(allergic shiners)* caused by an obstruction of lymphatic and vein flow, and a *transverse crease* across the bridge of the nose resulting from the allergic salutes.

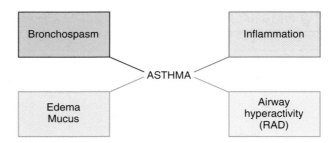

Bronchospasm

Inflammation

ASTHMA

Edema Mucus

Airway hyperactivity (RAD)

FIGURE **25-5** There are four main components of asthma, and the medication prescribed by the physician is specifically designed to deal with the component manifested by the individual child. Inhaled corticosteroids may be prescribed for children with reactive airway disease (RAD), whereas inhaled bronchodilator is the treatment of choice for bronchospasm. A child with asthma can manifest one or more of the components of the asthma syndrome.

occurrence, family history of allergy or asthma, typical appearance, and absence of fever or purulent drainage.

Treatment. Symptomatic treatment revolves around the use of antihistamine (nonsedating) medications and decongestants to reduce edema of the nasal mucous membranes without creating sedation, which can interfere with learning. Topical medications should not be used because of a "rebound effect" that occurs with long-term use. Prophylactic therapy with cromolyn inhalants or glucocorticoid nasal sprays may be prescribed if antihistamines are not effective, but this type of medication requires daily dosing and parent and child compliance. Immunotherapy for identified allergens may be prescribed.

The main goals of the nurse are to help the parent identify the difference between the allergy and a cold and to provide a referral for medical care and support during the long-term allergy testing and immunotherapy process. Teaching the family about controlling the environmental exposure to allergens is very important. Dust control, prevention of contact with animal dander, the use of air-conditioners and high-efficiency particulate air (HEPA) filters in the home, and the planning of vacation locales that do not present pollen challenges are some of the vital issues to discuss with the family. Leukotriene antagonist drugs have also been effective in the treatment of allergic rhinitis (Behrman et al., 2000).

ASTHMA

Pathophysiology. Asthma is a syndrome caused by increased responsiveness of the tracheobronchial tree to various stimuli that results in reversible, *paroxysmal* (intermittent) constriction of the airways (Figure 25-5). The term *asthma* is a Greek word for panting or breathlessness. Asthma is the principal cause of chronic illness in children. It is the leading cause of school absenteeism, emergency department visits, and hospitalization. Although it may occur at any age, about 80% of asthma sufferers have their first symptoms before 5 years of age. Before puberty, about twice as many boys as girls are affected; thereafter the sex incidence is equal.

Asthma is a recurrent and reversible obstruction of the airways in which bronchospasm, mucosal edema, and secretion and plugging by mucus contribute to significant narrowing of the airways and subsequent impaired gas exchange (Figure 25-6). Both large and small airways may be involved. The onset of asthma may be triggered by house dust, animal dander, wool, feathers, pollen, mold, passive smoking, strong odors (as from wet paint, wood stoves, or fireplaces), and certain foods. Vigorous physical activity (especially in cold weather) and rapid changes in temperature and humidity may precipitate an attack. Viral infections are also responsible. Emotional upsets, which affect smooth muscle and vasomotor tone (*vas,* "vessel" and *motor,* "mover"), are closely intertwined with the condition. Whatever the precipitating cause, the response of the airways is similar. As the attack worsens, arterial blood gases change. Pco_2 rises and the blood pH falls, increasing respiratory acidosis and producing a strain on the heart. Children who are prone to allergies often develop asthma. Some children who suffer from infantile eczema (see Chapter 29) develop asthma as they grow older. A family history of allergies is often seen.

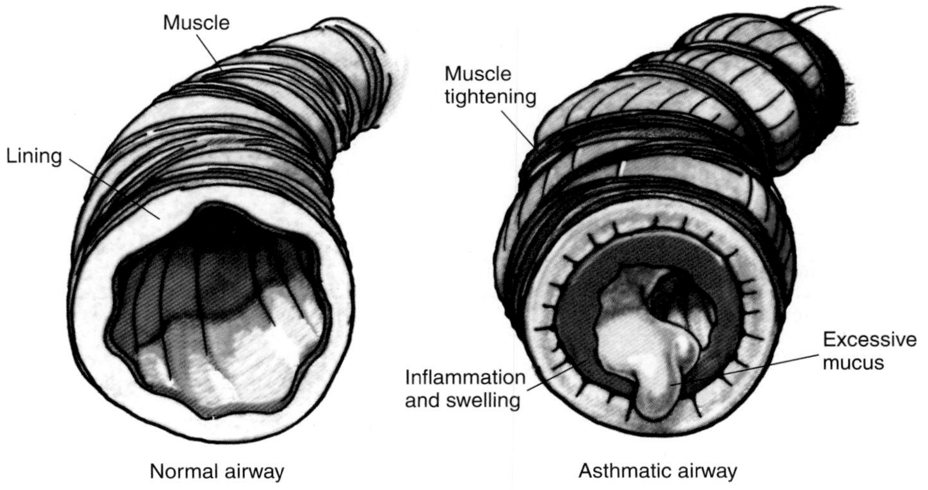

FIGURE **25-6** An asthmatic airway compared to a normal airway.

Diagnosis. A history, physical examination, and response to bronchodilator therapy are the first diagnostic tools. An elevated eosinophil blood level is typical. Eosinophils in the sputum are also diagnostic. Allergy skin testing and a radioallergosorbent test (RAST) are measures that can identify a sensitivity to allergens. Exercise testing and pulmonary function tests help to diagnose asthma and to assess the progress of the syndrome.

Asthma is rarely diagnosed in infancy; the increased susceptibility of infants to respiratory obstruction and dyspnea in response to many different illnesses results from the following:

- Decreased smooth muscle of an infant's airway
- Presence of increased mucous glands in the bronchi
- Normally narrow lumen of the normal airway
- Lack of muscle elasticity in the airway
- Fatigue-prone and overworked diaphragmatic muscle on which infant respiration depends

The symptom of wheezing in infancy can be caused by gastroesophageal reflux (GER), cystic fibrosis, or chronic aspiration often seen in developmentally delayed infants, or it may be a manifestation of a milk or food allergy.

Manifestations. The symptoms of asthma may begin slowly or abruptly. They may be mild, moderate, or severe. Obstruction is most severe during expiration because the airways become smaller during this phase of respiration. The trapped air in the lung causes hyperinflation and results in increased effort for breathing. This increased work of breathing can eventually put a strain on the heart. The hypoxia and resulting acidosis can then cause general pulmonary vasoconstriction that damages alveoli, decreases surfactant, and causes a chronic respiratory problem.

In acute episodes the patient coughs, wheezes, and has difficulty breathing, particularly during expiration. The child may complain that his or her chin, neck, or chest itches. Signs of air hunger, such as flaring of the nostrils, and the use of the accessory muscles of respiration (chest and abdominal muscles) may be evident. Orthopnea appears. The child is restless, perspires, and sometimes complains of abdominal pain; participation in activities decreases. Pulse and respirations are increased, and rales (abnormal respiratory sounds) may be heard in the chest. Inflammation of the nose and sinuses may accompany asthma.

Asthma attacks often happen during the night and are frightening for both the child and the parents. Repeated attacks over a long period of time may lead to emphysema. Chronic asthma is manifested by discoloration beneath the eyes (allergic shiners), slight eyelid eczema, and mouth breathing (see Figure 25-5).

Laboratory studies may reveal eosinophilia (increased blood eosinophils). Pulmonary function tests assess the degree of respiratory obstruction. Exercise testing may reveal bronchoconstriction with prolonged physical exercise.

Treatment and long-term management (Box 25-1). The main goals of asthma therapy are as follows:

- Maintain a near-normal pulmonary function.
- Maintain a near-normal activity level.
- Prevent chronic signs and symptoms.
- Prevent exacerbations that require hospital treatment.
- Prevent adverse responses to medication.
- Promote self-care and monitoring consistent with developmental level.

Medications. Bronchodilators or antiinflammatory agents may be prescribed.

box 25-1 *Management of Asthma*

Appropriate drug therapy		Measurement of lung function
Follow-up care	Patient education	Environmental control of
Routine immunizations		allergens and irritants
Influenza vaccine		

table 25-2 *Asthma Drug Interactions*

ASTHMA DRUG	INTERACTING SUBSTANCE	EFFECT
Ephedrine	Antihypertensive drugs	Decrease antihypertensive effects
	Antidepressants—monoamine oxidase inhibitors (MAOIs) such as isocarboxazid (Marplan), phenelzine (Nardil), tranylcypromine (Parnate)	Can cause a rise in blood pressure
	Antacids	Increase serum level of ephedrine
	Ammonium chloride expectorants	Reduce effectiveness of ephedrine
	Steroids	Lessen steroid effectiveness
Epinephrine	Antidepressants—tricyclics (e.g., imipramine [Tofranil], amitriptyline [Elavil]) and MAOIs	Can cause tachycardia, high blood pressure, and cardiac arrhythmia
	Beta-adrenergic blockers such as propranolol (Inderal)	Can cause high blood pressure
	Digitalis	Can cause cardiac arrhythmia
Theophylline	Allopurinol (Zyloprim)	Can cause tachycardia and Zyloprim toxicity
	Antibiotics (erythromycin)	Can cause theophylline toxicity
	Antibacterials (ciprofloxacin [Cipro])	
	Rifampin	Decreases effectiveness of theophylline
	Cimetidine (Tagamet)	Can cause theophylline toxicity
	Phenytoin (Dilantin)	Can decrease effect of both drugs
	Phenobarbital	Decreases effect of theophylline
	Ephedrine	Can cause arrhythmia and nervousness
	Beta-blockers, such as propranolol (Inderal)	Decreases effect of theophylline
	Oral contraceptives	Can increase theophylline blood levels
	High-fat foods	Increase absorption of theophylline

Bronchodilators. Albuterol (Ventolin, Proventil), metaproterenol (Alupent), and terbutaline (Brethaire) are examples of bronchodilators used for the long-term management of asthma in children. The drug is inhaled with the aid of a metered dose inhaler (MDI). If a child has difficulty coordinating or inhaling the dose, a spacer device can be added. The nurse should teach the family how to use the devices and the precautions concerning frequency of doses. Theophylline is given orally, usually at night, in a liquid, tablet, or powder form that is sprinkled on a teaspoon of applesauce. The nurse should observe for signs of theophylline toxicity, which include restlessness, tremor, headache, tachycardia, abdominal pain, hypotension, and diuresis; the nurse should also instruct the patient and family about drug-drug interactions (Table 25-2). Periodic serum levels must be taken to ensure safety. Toxicity can lead to convulsions and death. The family must be taught to tell the health care provider when the last dose of theophylline was given when seeking medical care for asthma problems.

Antiinflammatory drugs. *Cromolyn sodium* (Intal) is a nonsteroidal antiinflammatory medication that is inhaled using a spinhaler, a device that delivers the drug. Its use is as a *prophylactic,* or preventive medication. It cannot be used as a therapeutic drug for the emergency care of respiratory distress. Cromolyn sodium is prescribed before exercise if a child has exercise-induced asthma to enable the child to participate in the activity. Daily doses are prescribed to ensure an adequate blood level. *Nedocromil* (Tilade), another antiinflammatory, may be prescribed. *Corticosteroids* are steroid antiinflammatory medications that decrease inflammation. Inhaled preparations have fewer side effects than oral preparations and are used when bronchodilators are not effective. An increased appetite and euphoria are side effects of most steroids.

Slow inhalation of an inhaled drug enables the drug to reach the lower airway. Rapid inhalation loses some of the dose, which is deposited on the sides of the pharynx. Nebulized inhalation therapy (often referred to as med-nebs) is administered by the respiratory therapist in the hospital. Home care units are available (see Figure 25-3).

Other drugs approved for use with asthmatic children include zafirlukast (Accolate) or zileuton (Zyflo) for children age 12 years and montelukast (Singulair) for children as young as 6 years of age.

Nursing care. The general control of the environment is explained to the child and family. Avoiding pet dander, mold, smoking, and dust is essential. Stuffed toys are not desirable. Humidity in living areas of the house should be controlled between 25% and 50%, because excess humidity (above 50%) promotes mold growth. Dust collectors such as carpets, upholstery, or drapes should not be in the bedroom of an asthmatic child. Mattress covers, foam rubber pillows, and cotton blankets are preferred. Wool, down, and feather-stuffed items should be avoided. Upholstery, drapes, and carpets can be sprayed every 3 months with benzyl benzoate (Acarosan) to kill dust mites, followed by cleaning and vacuuming. The use of HEPA filters in the bedroom and in the vacuum is advisable. Children can be taught to monitor their own lung function with the use of a peak flowmeter at home (Figure 25-7). Involvement in self-care aids in compliance and results in better control of asthmatic symptoms.

Very often the parents and teachers exclude the child from physical activity in school because of the fear of triggering an asthmatic attack. School personnel must be taught by the school nurse the types of activities that are best tolerated by the asthmatic child. Swimming is best tolerated probably because of the high humidity in the air inhaled, and the exhaling of air underwater is similar to "pursed-lip" exhaling. Sports such as baseball, short sprints, and gymnastics are well tolerated because the activity is intense but short. Prolonged intense activity, such as jogging, lap running, race running, or basketball, is less tolerated by individuals with asthma. Pre-exercise puffs of a prescribed inhaler and a warm-up before vigorous exercise can enable the child to participate more fully in age-appropriate school physical exercise. Many Olympic athletes have successfully managed their asthma symptoms. The promotion of normal growth and development is a basic goal in asthma care, and participation with peers is important.

The child is hospitalized for more severe asthma attacks. The nurse limits conversation with the child during the emergency period to questions that can be answered "yes" or "no." Oxygen reduces hypoxia and improves the patient's color. It is administered by nasal prongs, hood, or facial mask.

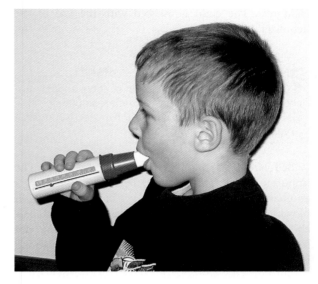

FIGURE **25-7** Using the peak flowmeter. Assessments should be done daily at home. The reading in the morning should be within 20% of the evening reading.

If the child is in respiratory distress on admission, oxygen is administered per the physician's protocol, and the child is positioned comfortably. One method is to place a pillow on the overbed table and have the child extend the arms over it, elbows bent. This is comfortable and allows maximum use of the accessory muscles of breathing. Lung sounds are assessed for rhonchi, wheezing, or rales. Arterial blood gases and vital signs are monitored. The child is evaluated for clinical improvement (quieter, slower respirations, relaxed facial expressions, cessation of retractions). Oral fluids are encouraged because they help to liquefy secretions and are needed to compensate for fluid loss from dyspnea and diaphoresis. Carbonated beverages, such as ginger ale and colas, are avoided when the child is wheezing. Beverages are served at room temperature because cold liquids can trigger reflex bronchospasm. Milk products are avoided because they tend to increase the production of mucus. Intake and output should be recorded. The patient is observed for cracked lips, the absence of tears, poor skin turgor, and a decrease in urine output, all of which signal dehydration.

A well-balanced diet and adequate fluids are necessary for general health. Ample time is allowed for meals because respiratory distress may interfere with eating. The nurse organizes tasks so that the child obtains sufficient rest. The child is assisted with the use of the nebulizer.

✶NURSING **TIP**
Oxygen is a drug, and administration should be correlated with monitoring of oxygen saturation levels. Too little oxygen can result in hypoxia; too much oxygen can result in lung damage.

Self-care. The child is gradually taught self-care. The importance of exercise to strengthen vulnerable lungs is emphasized. *Pursed-lip breathing* (blowing out as if blowing a kiss) and biofeedback are also helpful. The child is taught to observe "personal triggers" that are forewarnings of an attack. He or she is taught how to use the peak expiratory flowmeter. Other aspects of care include how to administer MDIs and understanding medications and their possible side effects. Specific information about how often and when to use inhalers is paramount. The child is encouraged to discuss daily school routines. The health care provider is seen regularly to evaluate progress and readjust the medications as needed. *The nurse reviews the signs of respiratory infection with the child and where, when, and whom to call for help.* Early attention to symptoms may prevent escalation of the disease.

Metered dose inhalers. Routine monitoring of airway obstruction should be part of comprehensive asthma management. A child of age 6 years can self-test with adult supervision. A diary of peak flow readings (PFR) should be brought to the physician at each follow-up visit (Figure 25-8). The nurse should be alert to the fact that compliance may be a problem with older children and adolescents who may cause false results by manipulating the unit.

An MDI consists of a pump that is a mouthpiece and an actuator (or holder) into which a medicine canister is inserted. Pushing down on the actuator releases a dose of medication (puff), which is inhaled through the mouthpiece. This delivers the medicine directly to the lungs without systemic side effects. The use of a spacer slows the movement of the medicine, allowing more time to inhale the medicine. Some spacers reduce the need for hand-press-breath inhalation coordination. Aerochambers with masks are available for infants. Dry powder inhalers are becoming popular as more medications are coming in powder form. The child should be taught to rinse the mouth after steroid inhalation to prevent the development of candidiasis. Activators should be cleaned regularly.

Most near-empty inhaler canisters will float in a bowl of water. Measuring the canister content level enables the child to request a refill and avoid missing medication

---

| box 25-2 | *Teaching the Use of a Metered Dose Inhaler* |

1. Insert the metered dose inhaler (MDI) canister into the holder.
2. Shake the MDI vigorously.
3. Exhale a normal breath.
4. Close mouth around the mouthpiece (or hold 2 to 4 cm from mouth).
5. Push down on the canister for one puff.
6. Inhale deeply and slowly for 3 to 5 seconds.
7. Hold the breath for 10 seconds.
8. Remove MDI from mouth.
9. Exhale slowly from the nose.

---

doses. Inhalers are designed to be used with an open-mouth technique or a closed-mouth technique (Box 25-2). A nebulizer machine can be used in the home when inhalers are not appropriate for the individual child.

The nurse should help the child see connections between triggers, medicines, and signs of respiratory distress. For example, did the peak flow drop after contact with a cat or rabbit? Does the peak flow always change with a cold? Any time there is a change in peak flow, the child should know to look for what triggered it.

During every clinic visit, the nurse should have the child demonstrate the use of the inhaler or spacer and reinforce the principles involved. Inhaler therapy with specific "leukotriene modifiers" may be replacing corticosteroid inhalers for preventive therapy in asthma.

Status Asthmaticus

Status asthmaticus is continued severe respiratory distress that is not responsive to drugs, including epinephrine and aminophylline. *This is a medical emergency.* The child requires immediate admission to the intensive care unit (ICU). Oxygen is administered via nasal cannula because mist in a mist tent can cause coughing or wheezing. Vital signs and the flow of IV medications are carefully monitored. Complying with the prescribed medical regimen, promptly seeking medical care when indicated, minimizing exposure to known allergens, wearing medical identification bracelets, and having a written crisis plan of management can minimize the life-threatening occurrence of status asthmaticus.

✶NURSING **TIP**
The principles of asthma treatment are as follows:
- Daily monitoring
- Symptom diary
- Treatment plan with active participation of the child
- Identification and avoidance of triggers

SAMPLE DIARY:

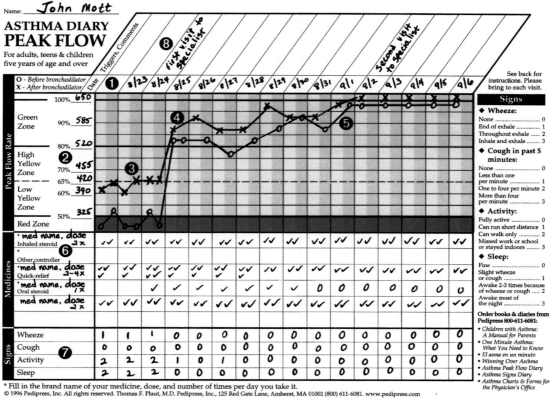

This asthma diary can help you learn about asthma and asthma medicines. With this information, you and your doctor can work out a written plan that will help you care for your (child's) asthma at home.

❶ **DATE:** Fill in date above the grid.

❷ **ASTHMA CARE ZONES:**

• *Green Zone:* Your current treatment plan is effective.

• *High Yellow Zone:* Avoid triggers and change your medication routine.

• *Low Yellow Zone:* Intensify treatment if your peak flow score does not increase into the high yellow zone within 10 minutes after inhaling a quick-relief medicine, or if it falls back into the low yellow zone within four hours.

• *Red Zone:* Take emergency medicine and see your doctor or go to the Emergency Room if your peak flow score does not increase into the low yellow zone within 10 minutes after inhaling a quick-relief medicine, or if it falls back into the red zone within four hours.

Put your (child's) personal best peak flow score here: _____. This is the top of the *Green Zone.* Find your (child's) personal best score on the table below. List it and the numbers below it on the front of this sheet.

If your (child's) personal best peak flow score has not yet been determined, use the average peak flow score for your (child's) height from a standard chart, e.g., *Children with Asthma,* page 100.

If your (child's) personal best peak flow score reaches a higher level on two separate days, start a new section by drawing a thick

vertical line to indicate the change. Enter the new numbers from the chart below.

❸ **DAY/NIGHT COLUMNS:** Use the clear column for daytime scores (7 AM-7 PM) and the shaded column for nighttime scores (7 PM-7 AM).

❹ **PLOT PEAK FLOW SCORE:** Use an *"O"* to plot scores blown before taking an inhaled bronchodilator and an *"X"* to plot scores blown after taking an inhaled bronchodilator. Estimate placement of mark between zone lines.

❺ **PEAK FLOW TREND:** Connect the O's with a line to illustrate a trend. Do the same thing for the X's.

❻ **MEDICINES:** Enter the name, dose, and number of doses per day for each medicine. Put one check mark (✔) in the box for each dose given.

❼ **SIGNS:** Sign scores are listed on the right side of diary. Enter each score by time of day. Cough is assessed during a five minute period.

❽ **COMMENTS:** Enter comments above the date such as *"Exposed to cigarette smoke," "Had cold," "Rabbit in school"* and *"Painting bedroom."*

◆ **RELATIONSHIPS:** Try to see connections between triggers, medicines and signs. For example, did peak flow drop after contact with a cat or a rabbit? Does peak flow always change with a cold? If not, why not? Any time there is a change in peak flow, you should look for a trigger.

◆ **ILLNESS:** If you (or your child) are sick, and you want to record peak flow more often, use several sections to record each day.

FIGURE **25-8** The asthma diary. The clear column is for daytime peak flow reading (PFR) score, and the shaded column is for nighttime peak flow scores. An X indicates PFR following inhaler therapy. An O indicates PFR without inhaler therapy. A check mark indicates medication taken. Asthma triggers/comments are recorded. The diary is brought to each follow-up clinic visit.

CYSTIC FIBROSIS

Pathophysiology. Cystic fibrosis (CF) is a major worldwide cause of serious chronic lung disease in children. It occurs in approximately one in 3000 live births of Caucasian infants and one in 17,000 births of African-American infants in the United States. It is most prevalent in persons of Northern and Central European descent. It is an inherited recessive trait, with both parents carrying a gene for the disease. There is a defect in chromosome number 7 that is thought to have developed many years ago as a protective response of the human body against cholera. As the body mutated chromosomes to develop a resistance to cholera, the change in the gene resulted in a defect that caused CF.

The basic defect in CF is an endocrine gland dysfunction that includes (1) increased viscosity (thickness) of mucous gland secretions, and (2) a loss of electrolytes in sweat because of an abnormal chloride movement. CF is considered a *multisystem* disease because the thick, viscid secretions affect the following:

- *The respiratory system.* Small and large airways are obstructed by the thick secretions, resulting in difficulty breathing. The accumulation and stasis of the thick secretions create a medium for growth of organisms that cause repeated respiratory infections. The thick secretions in the lungs and response of tissues to infections cause hypoxia

that can result in heart failure. Emphysema, wheezes, and respiratory distress are common.

- *The digestive system.* The thickened secretions prevent the digestive enzymes from flowing to the gastrointestinal tract, resulting in poor absorption of food and general growth failure. Bulky, foul-smelling stools that are frothy because of the undigested fat content are characteristic. Thick, impacted feces can cause rectal prolapse. Pancreatic, liver, and biliary obstruction occur.
- *Skin.* Loss of electrolytes (sodium and chloride) in the sweat causes a "salty" skin surface. Loss of electrolytes via the skin predisposes the child to electrolyte imbalances during hot weather.
- *Reproductive system.* Thick secretions can decrease sperm motility. Thick cervical mucus can inhibit sperm from reaching the fallopian tubes.

Manifestations. The manifestations of CF are illustrated in Figure 25-9.

Lung involvement. The air passages of the lungs become clogged with mucus. There is widespread obstruction of the bronchioles. It is difficult for the child to breathe; expiration is especially difficult. More and more air becomes trapped in the lungs *(obstructive emphysema),* and small areas of collapse (atelectasis) may occur. Eventually the chest assumes a barrel shape, with increased diameter across the front and back. The right

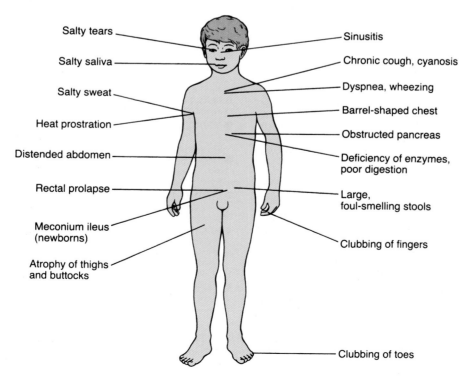

Salty tears — Sinusitis

Salty saliva — Chronic cough, cyanosis

Salty sweat — Dyspnea, wheezing

Heat prostration — Barrel-shaped chest

Distended abdomen — Obstructed pancreas

— Deficiency of enzymes, poor digestion

Rectal prolapse — Large, foul-smelling stools

Meconium ileus (newborns) — Clubbing of fingers

Atrophy of thighs and buttocks

Clubbing of toes

FIGURE **25-9** Manifestations of cystic fibrosis.

ventricle of the heart, which supplies the lungs, may become strained and enlarged. Clubbing of the fingers and toes (Figure 25-10), a compensatory response indicating a chronic lack of oxygen, may be present. *Staphylococcus* and *Pseudomonas* infections can easily occur in the lungs and provide a suitable medium for the organisms' growth. This causes more thickening of the abnormal secretions, irritates and damages lung tissues, and further increases lung obstruction.

Dyspnea, wheezing, and cyanosis may occur. The child is irritable and tires easily. Gradually, there is a change in physical appearance. Evidence of obstructive emphysema, atelectasis, and fibrosis of lung tissue may also be present. The prognosis for survival depends on the extent of lung damage. However, this is only part of the picture, because CF also affects the pancreas and sweat glands.

Pancreatic involvement. The pancreas lies behind the stomach. Some of its cells secrete pancreatic enzymes that drain from the pancreatic duct into the duodenum at the same area in which bile enters. Changes occurring in the pancreas result from obstruction by thickened secretions that block the flow of pancreatic digestive enzymes. As a result, foodstuffs, particularly fats and proteins, are not properly digested and used by the body.

In infants the stools may be loose. Because of impaired digestion and food absorption, the feces of the child become large, fatty, and foul-smelling. They are usually light in color. The child does not gain weight despite a good appetite and may look undernourished. The abdomen becomes distended, and the buttocks and thighs *atrophy* (waste away) as fat disappears from the main deposit sites.

A condition known as meconium ileus exists when the intestine of the newborn becomes obstructed with abnormally thick meconium while in utero. This condition is caused by the absence of pancreatic enzymes that normally digest proteins in the meconium. The abnormal, puttylike stool sticks to the walls of the intestine, causing blockage. The presenting symptoms develop within hours after birth. The absence of stools and the presence of vomiting and of abdominal distention lead one to suspect intestinal obstruction. X-ray films confirm the diagnosis.

Sweat glands. The sweat, tears, and saliva of the patient with CF become abnormally salty because of an increase in sodium chloride levels. Up to about 20 years of age, more than 60 mEq/liter of sodium chloride in sweat is diagnostic of CF when one or more criteria are present. Levels of 40 to 60 mEq/L are highly suggestive. The analysis of sweat is a major aid in diagnosing the condition. The *sweat test* is the best diagnostic study. Because these children lose large amounts of salt through perspiration, they must be watched for heat prostration. Liberal amounts of salt should be given with food, and extra fluids and salt should be provided during the hot weather.

Complications. CF is often responsible for rectal prolapse in infants and children partly because of poor muscle tone in the rectal area and because of the excessive leanness of the buttocks of the patient.

As the disease progresses, the liver may become hard, nodular, and enlarged. Cor pulmonale (*cor,* "heart" and *pulmon,* "lung"), heart strain caused by improper lung function, is often a cause of death. There is a deficiency of vitamin A because the child is unable to absorb fats from which this vitamin is obtained. Sexual development may be delayed in these patients. Males are generally sterile, but sexual function is unimpaired. Adolescent girls may experience secondary amenorrhea during exacerbations.

Treatment and nursing care

Respiratory relief. (Oxygen therapy is discussed in Chapter 22.) Antibiotics may be given as a preventive measure against respiratory infection; however, this treatment is controversial. Nursing Care Plan 25-1 summarizes interventions for the CF patient. Intermittent aerosol therapy is administered to provide medication to the lower respiratory tract and to promote the evacuation of secretions. An inhaler that acts as a mucus clearance device can be used in the home care of these children. Expectorants, especially the iodides, are also used to thin secretions. Bronchodilators are used to increase the width of the bronchi, allowing free passage of air into the lungs. Human recombinant dornase alfa (Pulmozyme) in a single daily aerosol dose is effective in improving pulmonary function.

Postural drainage and chest-clapping therapy are also of value (Figure 25-11). These are performed by the physical or respiratory therapist during hospitalization. When postural drainage and chest clapping are done

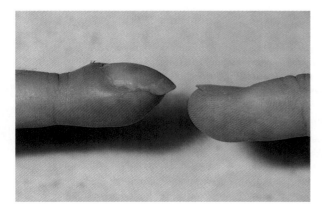

FIGURE **25-10** Clubbing of the fingers, a sign of chronic hypoxia.

The Pediatric Patient with Cystic Fibrosis

PATIENT DATA: A 5-year-old child diagnosed with cystic fibrosis is admitted to the unit. The child has loose, foul-smelling stools, a persistent cough with some nasal flaring, and chest retractions.

SELECTED NURSING DIAGNOSIS   *Risk for ineffective airway clearance related to inability to clear mucus from respiratory tract secondary to cystic fibrosis as evidenced by thick mucus production, unproductive/minimal cough, and adventitious breath sounds (wheezes, crackles, dyspnea, tachypnea, cyanosis)*

Outcomes	Nursing Interventions	Rationales
Child will have an effective airway as demonstrated by effective cough, thin respiratory secretions, age-appropriate respiratory rate and effort, and O_2 saturation $\geq 92\%$ on room air.	1. Observe respiratory status (rate, depth, effort, breath sounds, oxygen saturation, and skin color) *at least* every 4 hours.	1. Allows for early detection and intervention of changes in child's respiratory status.
	2. Administer humidified O_2 as ordered by physician; monitor O_2 saturation frequently.	2. Humidification helps to thin and loosen secretions. In chronic obstructive respiratory diseases, the respiratory center in the brain becomes tolerant of low O_2 saturation in the blood. Administering high concentrations of O_2 to a child with chronic lung disease can lead to carbon dioxide narcosis.
	3. Administer bronchodilators and expectorants as ordered by physician.	3. These medications help the thinning, loosening, and expectoration of respiratory mucus.
	4. Encourage age-appropriate oral intake of fluids.	4. Helps to decrease the viscosity (thickness) of secretions.
	5. Perform chest physiotherapy treatments (CPT) and postural drainage (PD) every 4 hours or as needed. Perform CPT/PD 1 hour before or 2 hours after meals.	5. CPT/PD helps to mobilize secretions and to increase oxygenation. Performing 1 hour before or 2 hours after meals lessens the risk of vomiting and/or aspiration.
	6. Teach the child how to do coughing and deep-breathing exercises. Use play therapy whenever possible. For example, using an inspirometer, "blow up" the fingers of a clean glove.	6. Children under age 7 years cannot voluntarily produce an effective cough. Coughing and deep-breathing exercises help expand the lungs and mobilize secretions.
	7. Teach parents/caregivers *not* to give over-the-counter (OTC) medications, especially cough suppressants, to the child with cystic fibrosis.	7. Cough suppressant medication inhibits the cough reflex, leading to retained secretions and the possibility of respiratory infection.

SELECTED NURSING DIAGNOSIS   *Imbalanced nutrition: less than body requirements related to decrease in the availability of pancreatic enzymes; poor intestinal absorption of nutritional intake; anorexia secondary to cystic fibrosis as evidenced by decreased oral intake, weight loss/failure to thrive, diarrhea, steatorrhea, or constipation*

Outcomes	Nursing Interventions	Rationales
Child will be able to ingest age-appropriate nutrition and maintain weight or gain height and weight according to the normal growth and development charts. Stools will be of	1. Determine child's normal feeding patterns, dietary likes and dislikes, and activity level.	1. Knowing the child's preferences and activity level will aid in the plan of care with regard to feeding the child.
	2. Administer pancreatic replacement enzymes and fat-soluble vitamin supplements as directed by the	2. Digestive and nutritional therapy consists of replacement of pancreatic enzymes and dietary adjustments.

Outcomes	Nursing Interventions	Rationales
normal color, consistency, and amount for age.	physician before meals and snacks.	Administering supplemental fat-soluble vitamins is necessary because of the inability of the body to absorb fats.
	3. Teach the child (and parents) *not* to chew the capsules or "beads"; to swallow the medication whole; if powder form, sprinkle over a nonfat, nonprotein food, such as applesauce. Do not mix enzymes with hot (heated) foods, high-starch, or high-acid–containing foods. Wipe any powder from oral mucosa or lips.	3. Pancreatic enzymes are inactivated by heat, and acids are known to degrade the enzymes. Wipe the excess powder off mucosa to prevent excoriation or breakdown of mucosal membranes.
	4. Note the color, consistency, amount, and frequency of stools. Notify the physician of any changes (i.e., diarrhea, constipation, or steatorrhea).	4. Pancreatic enzymes are known to cause constipation if taken in high doses or steatorrhea from malabsorption of fats and proteins because of low intake of the enzymes.

SELECTED NURSING DIAGNOSIS *Interrupted family processes related to chronicity of disease, need for outside support, and the risk of life-threatening complications as evidenced by frequent physician office visits or hospitalizations, a diminished focus on other siblings in home, and the need for therapeutic interventions and compliance and home care routines*

Outcomes	Nursing Interventions	Rationales
Family members will verbalize their feelings about the impact cystic fibrosis has on them; will be able to comply with the therapeutic treatment plan; and will use available resources within their community to assist in the care and treatment of their child.	1. Determine the educational level and amount of knowledge each family member has on cystic fibrosis *before* planning any family interventions or teaching sessions.	1. Educational level will help to determine the type of teaching methods to be used (i.e., written, visual, hands-on, auditory). Having this information in advance helps the nurse to map out the plan of care and teaching. It also prevents the repetition of the same information or guides the nurse as to the amount of teaching/information required or needed by the family.
	2. Determine the level of impact that the disease has had on the family.	2. Guides the nurse in selecting appropriate referrals to community or support agencies needed by the family.
	3. Teach and/or review with family the skills required in the daily care of the child with cystic fibrosis. For example, assessing respiratory rate and status, CPT/PD methods, monitoring stools, skin care, medication administration.	3. Return demonstration enables the nurse to evaluate the ability of the family to provide effective home care.

?CRITICAL THINKING QUESTION

The father of a child diagnosed with cystic fibrosis visits his child in the hospital. He states that he thinks the hospital food does not agree with his child because he notices the child has a loose stool with a very bad odor. None of his other children have that type of stool. He brought some loperamide (Imodium) pills from the drugstore to give to the child. What is the best response of the nurse?

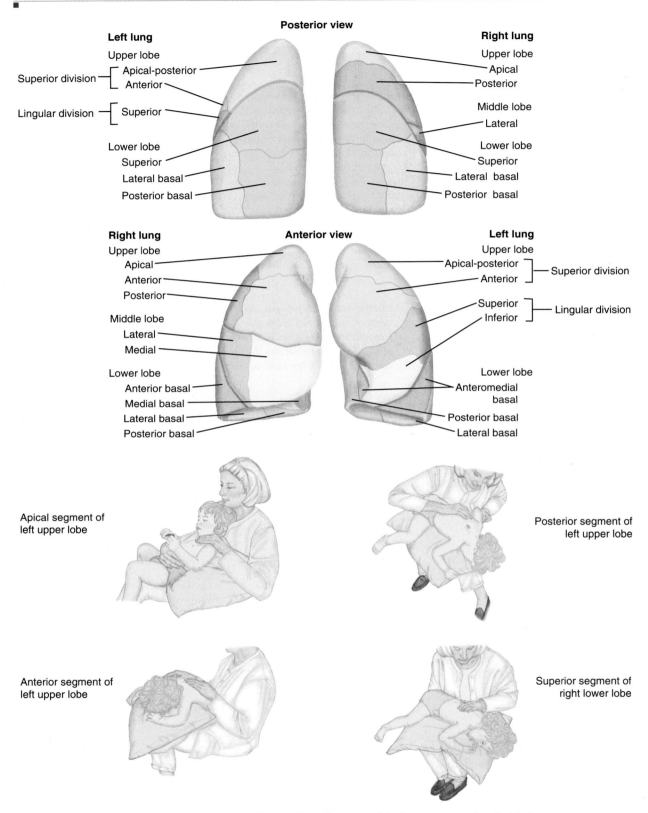

FIGURE **25-11** Postural drainage. The positions for postural drainage are correlated with the segment being drained.

Correct hand position for percussion

Infant percussion device

Cup the hand to trap a pocket of air that will transmit vibrations through the chest wall to the secretions that need to be dislodged.

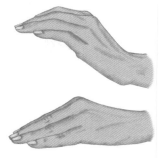

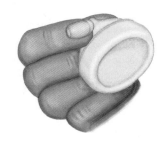

Clap the cupped hand in rapid sequence over a lung segment. Elbow should be flexed and the wrist relaxed while creating a rapid, popping action.

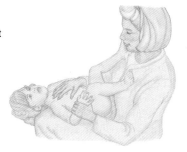

Posterior basal segment of right lower lobe

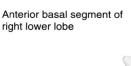
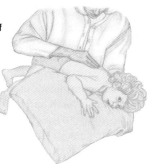

Lateral basal segment of right lower lobe

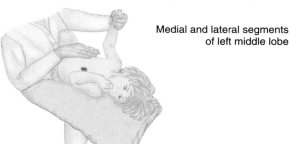

Anterior basal segment of right lower lobe

Medial and lateral segments of left middle lobe

Lingular segments (superior and inferior) of left upper lobe

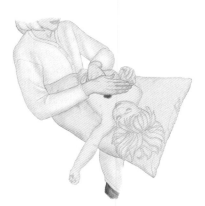

FIGURE **25-11,** cont'd.   For legend see opposite page.

properly, the secretions in the chest are moved up and out. This should be explained to the parents so they will continue this valuable procedure when the child comes home. Instructions may need to be repeated frequently to encourage full cooperation of the parents and child. These procedures are done after nebulization and at least 2 hours after eating. General exercise is good for the patient because it stimulates coughing. Play activities such as somersaults and headstands within the child's endurance limits are therapeutic.

Breathing exercises may also be recommended for the older child. Pursed-lip breathing is one technique that is simple and effective. The patient is instructed to inhale through the nose, then to exhale through the mouth with the lips pursed as if whistling. Exhalation should be at least twice as long as inhalation. (If it takes 3 seconds to breathe in, 6 seconds are taken to allow all the air to escape.) The child is taught not to force the air out but to let it escape naturally.

Prevention of respiratory infections is essential. The child is isolated from patients and personnel who may harbor infections. The period of hospitalization is kept brief, if possible, to avoid cross-infection. This child must be given the necessary immunizations against childhood diseases (see Chapter 31).

An oral pancreatic preparation, such as pancrelipase (Pancrease), is given to the child with each meal and snack to replace the pancreatic enzymes the child's body cannot produce. This medication is considered specific for the disease because it helps the child to digest and absorb food, thus improving the condition of the stools. If the child is ill and not eating, the medication is withheld. When meals are erratic, such as during vacations, medication is given when the largest amount of food will be consumed. High doses have been associated with the development of gastrointestinal strictures and the child should be monitored. Vitamins A, D, E, and K, iron, and zinc supplements are also prescribed.

> ⭐NURSING **TIP**
> Chest physiotherapy should be done *between* meals.

Diet. The maintenance of adequate nutrition is essential. The diet is high in protein and calories. Supplemental enzymes are given with the food to aid in digestion, and fat-soluble vitamins are prescribed. The child should be weighed daily. Intake and output are recorded. Children should have free access to salt, although a regimented salt supplementation is no longer recommended. Infants can breastfeed with added enzyme intake. Formula-fed infants do best with a higher calorie-per-ounce formula, such as Pregestimil or Alimentum. Parenteral alimentation (TPN) may be indicated in some cases.

> ⭐NURSING **TIP**
> Pancreatic enzyme powder should be given with applesauce or other nonstarch, nonfat nonprotein food.

General hygiene. The nurse must pay special attention to the skin of the child with CF. The diaper area is cleansed after each bowel movement. An ointment to protect the skin is advisable because the character of the stool subjects the diaper area to irritation. The buttocks are exposed to air when a rash occurs. Because the child has little fat and muscle, the position must be changed frequently, especially if the child is weak and cannot get out of bed. Frequent changes of position also prevent the development of pneumonia.

The child wears light clothing to avoid becoming overheated; it should be loose to allow freedom of movement. Good oral hygiene is necessary, because the teeth may be in poor condition because of dietary deficiencies. Mouth care is given after postural drainage because foul mucus may be raised, leaving an unpleasant taste in the patient's mouth.

Long-term care. The goals of care include minimizing pulmonary complications, ensuring adequate nutrition, promoting growth and development, and assisting the family to adjust to the chronic care required at home. This is extremely taxing financially, physically, and emotionally. The parents must distribute their time and energy within the family yet give careful attention to their sick child or, sometimes, children. How do they keep from spoiling the child? Do they limit the normal activities of the remaining children to spare the sick one? What about birthday parties, camping, scouts, pets, and epidemics at school? What does a trip to the shore or mountains entail? When do the parents find time for themselves? Coping techniques must be developed and used.

Parents need explicit instructions regarding diet, medication, postural drainage, prevention of infection, rest, and continued medical supervision. Many families require the assistance of a social worker to secure funds for equipment and drugs. Genetic counseling is also advised.

Emotional support. The child who is chronically ill finds it hard to accept restricted activity. The amount and types of diversion required vary in CF because the disease affects children of all ages and varies in severity.

It is thought that children benefit from simple, straightforward answers to questions about their illness.

An uncomplicated diagram might be helpful. They should know why they must take medications with each meal, use the nebulizer, and have postural drainage. They should see and handle the unfamiliar equipment necessary for care.

The young child finds it more difficult to be separated from parents during hospitalization. Even when the prognosis is grave, a child's courage is sustained if parents are there. Rooming-in is encouraged whenever possible. Close contact by mail, telephone, or E-mail with school, church, and clubs is important for the school-age child. It is helpful for patients to develop an activity that they enjoy, such as piano or art. This increases feelings of worth and provides outlets for feelings. Consideration must be given to ways of fostering love, acceptance, trust, fair play, security, freedom of choice, creativity, and maintenance of self-identity.

BRONCHOPULMONARY DYSPLASIA

Pathophysiology. Bronchopulmonary dysplasia (BPD) is a fibrosis, or thickening, of the alveolar walls and the bronchiolar epithelium caused by oxygen concentrations above 40% or by the mechanical pressure ventilation given to newborns for a prolonged time. Swelling of the tissues causes edema, and the respiratory cilia are paralyzed by the high oxygen concentrations and lose their ability to clear mucus from the airways. Respiratory obstruction, mucus plugs, and atelectasis follow.

Prevention. Respiratory distress in the newborn is the major reason why oxygen and ventilators are used for prolonged periods. The main cause of respiratory distress in the newborn is prematurity. Therefore the prevention of preterm births is the best way to prevent BPD. The goal of treatment for respiratory distress in the newborn should be to administer only the amount of oxygen required to prevent hypoxia at the minimum ventilator pressures needed to prevent tissue trauma.

Symptoms. Symptoms of chronic respiratory distress (see Figure 25-2) include the following:

- Wheezing
- Retractions
- Cyanosis on exertion
- Use of accessory respiratory muscles
- Clubbing of the fingers
- Failure to thrive
- Irritability caused by hypoxia

Treatment. Once BPD has developed, the goal of therapy is to reduce inflammation of the airway and to wean the infant from the mechanical ventilator. The infant may become oxygen dependent and develop reactive airway bronchoconstriction. Right-sided heart failure may also develop. Fluid restriction, bronchodilators, and diuretics may be prescribed. A tracheostomy may be also needed. Infants with BPD often develop respiratory stridor and retractions with even minor respiratory infections that result in repeated hospitalizations. Ongoing home care is required, and respiratory problems persist through adulthood. Maintaining optimum growth and development is a challenge. Education and support of the family for a technology-dependent child at home are essential, and a multidisciplinary health care team approach is essential.

> ## NURSING **TIP**
> When oxygen is used in the home, the family should be taught safety precautions to prevent fire and injury.

SUDDEN INFANT DEATH SYNDROME

Sudden infant death syndrome (SIDS) is clinically defined as the sudden, unexpected death of an apparently healthy infant between 2 weeks and 1 year of age, for which a routine autopsy fails to identify the cause. It is also referred to as "crib death." The peak incidence is between 2 and 4 months of age. The clinical features of the disease remain constant: (1) death occurs during sleep, and (2) the infant does not cry or make other sounds of distress. It has occurred even when the parents were sleeping in the same room. The occurrence of SIDS has decreased by 38% between 1992 and 1996 when the "back to sleep" program was implemented. Approximately 2500 infants died of SIDS in the United States in 1998 (Behrman et al., 2000).

SIDS is thought to be caused by a brainstem abnormality of cardiorespiratory control. Overheating, irregular respiratory patterns, and decreased arousal responses are contributing factors. Increased risk factors for SIDS may include maternal smoking or cocaine use that causes hypoxia of the fetus, preterm birth, and poor postneonatal care. A face-down sleeping position may cause rebreathing of expired air or airway occlusion. Wrapping the infant who is placed face down may increase the risk for SIDS by preventing the infant from lifting and turning the face to the side. Medications, such as caffeine and theophylline, have been used in selected groups of high-risk infants with apnea problems, and research is ongoing (Behrman et al., 2000).

Prevention. For high-risk infants, home apnea monitors have been used to warn parents of an impending problem and enable them to try to resuscitate the infant manually. All parents should have cardiopulmonary resuscitation education. However, frustration with frequent alarm malfunctions and noncompliance have made this intervention less effective. In 1996 the AAP recommended that all healthy infants be placed in the supine (back-lying) position on firm mattresses to prevent SIDS. The use of soft pillows or fluffy blankets for the infant to lie on is discouraged because it can prevent the infant from raising and turning his or her head. A national educational media campaign for this recommended positioning of infants has decreased the occurrence of SIDS.

> ### NURSING TIP
> The AAP recommends that all healthy infants be placed on their backs for sleep to help prevent the occurrence of SIDS.

Nursing care. In talking with grieving parents after the death of their infant, the nurse must convey some important facts: that the infant died of a disease entity called sudden infant death syndrome, that currently the disease cannot be predicted or prevented, and that they are *not* responsible for the child's death. Grieving parents need time to say good-bye to their child. They are encouraged to hold and rock the infant, shed tears, and assist in burial preparations. This process is conducive to the resolution of grief.

Parents experience much guilt and are catapulted into a totally unexpected bereavement that requires numerous explanations to relatives and friends. Often needless blame has been placed on one parent by the other or by relatives. The family baby-sitter and physician may also be targets of attack. Emergency department personnel must be especially sensitive and supportive during this crisis. There have been crib deaths for which parents have been mistakenly charged with child abuse.

CARDIOVASCULAR SYSTEM

The cardiovascular system consists of the heart, the blood, and the blood vessels. See Figure 3-6 for changes that occur in cardiovascular circulation at birth. As the heart beats, blood, oxygen, and nutrients are transported to all tissues of the body, and waste products are removed. Because of anatomical and physiological immaturity, the cardiovascular system of the child differs from that of the adult. Figure 25-12 summarizes some of these differences.

The cardiovascular system develops between the third and the eighth week of gestation. It is the first system to function in intrauterine life. When cardiovascular development is incomplete, heart defects occur. Fetal circulation is designed to serve the metabolic needs during intrauterine life and also to permit safe transition to life outside the womb.

SIGNS RELATED TO SUSPECTED CARDIAC PATHOLOGY

Although signs and symptoms of specific congenital heart defects relate to the specific pathology involved, several signs and symptoms are common to most infants with congenital cardiac problems. When the nurse assesses the child, the following observations should be reported:

- Failure to thrive and/or poor weight gain
- Cyanosis, pallor
- Visually observed pulsations in the neck veins
- Tachypnea, dyspnea
- Irregular pulse rate
- Clubbing of fingers
- Fatigue during feeding or activity
- Excessive perspiration, especially over forehead

CONGENITAL HEART DISEASE

Congenital heart defects may be caused by genetic or maternal factors (e.g., drug intake or rubella illness) or environmental factors. Fetal echocardiography can detect cardiac malformations in high-risk cases. Acquired heart disease occurs *after* birth, as a result of a defect or illness.

Pathophysiology. Congenital heart defects are not a problem for the fetus because the fetal-maternal circulation compensates for all fetal oxygen needs. However, at birth, the infant's circulatory system must provide for the child's own oxygen needs. Any heart defect or patent (open) fetal pathways in the cardiovascular system after birth produce signs and symptoms that indicate an anatomical heart defect. Congenital heart disease occurs in approximately 8 out of 1000 births, and 50% of these infants evidence signs and symptoms before the first year of life. Some defects, such as mitral valve prolapse, may not be manifested until later in life.

Of the congenital anomalies, heart defects are the principal cause of death during the first year of life. Therefore nurses must stress the need for good prenatal care and impress on parents the value of regular checkups at well-baby clinics. Many organic heart murmurs have been detected early in infancy at periodic checkups.

Diagnosis and treatment. The appearance of clinical symptoms and results of diagnostic tests aid in the diagnosis of congenital heart disease (Table 25-3). The treatment of most cardiac defects is surgical. A thoracotomy (chest incision) is performed, and the use of a cardiopulmonary bypass machine and hypothermia during

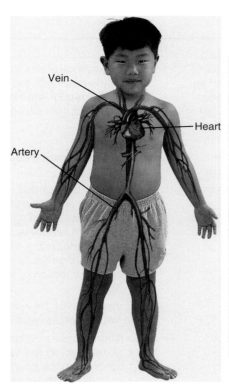

CARDIOVASCULAR SYSTEM

- Pulse, respiration, blood pressure, and hematologic values vary with the age of the child.
- Chest walls are thin in infants and young children because of the relative lack of subcutaneous and muscle tissue compared with older children. "Innocent" murmurs can be heard in structurally normal hearts.
- The newborn's circulation differs from fetal circulation; if adaptations do not take place, congenital heart problems may arise.
- Capillary function is immature in newborns. It takes several weeks for the small capillaries to expand and contract in response to external temperatures.
- The heart rate is higher in newborns and infants than in adults.
- Children have limited ability to increase stroke volume in response to decreased cardiac output.
- Most heart conditions in children result from defects in embryonic structure.

FIGURE 25-12 Summary of some cardiovascular system differences between the child and the adult. The cardiovascular system consists of the heart, blood, and blood vessels. As the heart beats, blood, oxygen, and nutrients are transported to all the tissues of the body, and waste products are removed.

the procedure minimize blood loss and enhance patient response. Hypothermia (*hypo,* "under" and *thermal,* "heat") reduces the temperature of body tissues, resulting in a decreased need for oxygen. The cardiopulmonary bypass machine provides oxygenation of the body tissues while the surgeon stops the heart to perform surgery. Heart transplants may be the treatment of choice in cases such as a three-chambered heart.

Classification. Congenital heart defects can be divided into two categories: cyanotic and acyanotic. A more accurate classification is based on the effect of the defect on blood circulation. The study of blood circulation is termed hemodynamics (*hemo,* "blood" and *dynamics,* "power"). Blood always flows from an area of high pressure to an area of low pressure and takes the path of least resistance. Physiologically, defects can be organized into (1) lesions that increase pulmonary blood flow, (2) lesions that obstruct blood flow, and (3) lesions that decrease pulmonary blood flow. There are also mixed lesions. A shunt refers to the flow of blood through an abnormal opening between two vessels of the heart. Figure 25-13 compares the normal heart and the heart with various congenital defects.

Defects That Increase Pulmonary Blood Flow

Congenital heart defects that cause the blood to *return to the right ventricle and recirculate through the lungs* before exiting the left ventricle through the aorta are known as defects that *increase pulmonary blood flow.* For example, the defect in the atrial septum in the fetus allows blood to flow from the right atrium through the defect into the left atrium, providing a bypass of the lungs. After birth, the pressure is higher in the left atrium; if the atrial opening persists, the blood flows *back* into the right atrium *(left-to-right shunt)* and then *recirculates* to the lungs, causing increased pulmonary flow. Some defects that increase pulmonary flow are atrial septal defect, ventricular septal defect, and patent ductus arteriosus (see Figure 25-13). In heart defects that result in increased pulmonary flow because of a left to right shunt, the oxygenated blood recirculates to the lungs, and cyanosis is rare.

NURSING **TIP**

In congenital heart disease, cyanosis is *not always* a clinical sign.

| table 25-3 | *Diagnostic Tests Used in Congenital Heart Defects* |

TEST	DEFINITION	VALUE
Angiocardiography (selective)	Serial x-ray films of the heart and great vessels after injection of an opaque substance; a radiopaque catheter is moved into the heart chambers, and contrast medium is injected in specific areas	Abnormal communications in the heart can be observed; the course of the blood through the heart and great vessels can be traced
Aortography	X-ray films of the aorta after the injection of an opaque material	Useful in revealing patent ductus arteriosus
Radionuclide angiocardiography	Noninvasive nuclear procedure that permits visualization of the course of blood through the heart	May be used as a precardiac catheterization screening study; provides assessment of congenital and acquired cardiovascular lesions and monitors the effects of therapy; an IV device is necessary to permit injection of the radionuclide
Barium swallow	Barium given by mouth	Shows indentation of the esophagus by the aorta or other vessels
Cardiac catheterization	A radiopaque catheter is passed through the femoral artery directly into the heart and large vessels	Reveals blood pressure within the heart; physicians can examine the heart closely with the tip of the catheter to detect abnormalities; blood samples can be obtained to determine oxygen content
Chest x-ray film	A radiographic image of a body structure	Provides a permanent record; shows abnormalities in the shape and position of heart
Cineangiocardiography	Motion pictures of images recorded by fluoroscopy	Useful recording and monitoring device
Echocardiography	The use of ultrasound to produce an image of sound waves of the heart; transducer placed directly on chest; sounds are analyzed	Noninvasive procedure; localizes murmurs; determines if heart is structurally normal
Electrocardiogram	Tracing of heart action by electrocardiography	Detects variations in heart action and shows the condition of the heart muscle; may also be used as a monitoring device during cardiac catheterization
Magnetic resonance imaging (3-dimensional imaging)	Noninvasive imaging technique that uses low-energy radio waves in combination with a magnetic field to generate signals that produce tomographic images	Very useful in diagnosing coarctation of the aorta

Atrial septal defect. Atrial septal defect (ASD) involves an abnormal opening between the right and left atria. Blood that already contains oxygen is forced from the left atrium back to the right atrium. Most patients do not have symptoms. The defect may be recognized when a murmur is heard during a routine health examination. Cardiac catheterization, electrocardiogram, and echocardiography may be performed to help to confirm the diagnosis. The surgical repair involves a median *sternotomy* (*sternum*, and *otomy*, "cutting"). Closure is sim-

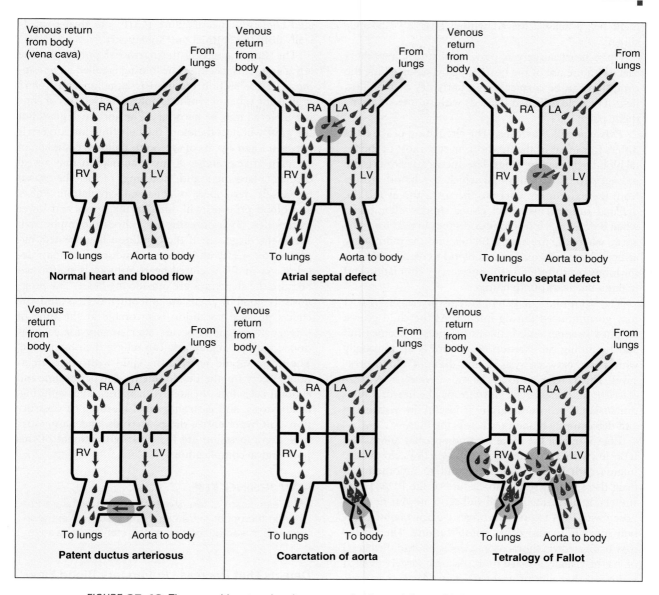

FIGURE **25-13** The normal heart and various congenital heart defects. *RA,* Right atrium; *RV,* right ventricle; *LA,* left atrium; *LV,* left ventricle.

ilar to that for ventricular septal defect (see the following discussion). Continued cardiology follow-up is necessary. Prognosis is excellent.

Ventricular septal defect. Ventricular septal defect (VSD) is the most common heart anomaly. As the name suggests, there is an opening between the right and left ventricles of the heart. Increased pressure within the left ventricle forces blood back into the right ventricle (left-to-right shunt). A loud, harsh murmur combined with a systolic thrill is characteristic of this defect. The condition may be mild or severe. It is often associated with other defects. Many children with small

defects may experience spontaneous closure during the first year of life as a result of growth.

Treatment includes close observation of the growing child. Antibiotic prophylaxis is necessary for dental care and minor surgical procedures to prevent bacterial endocarditis. The child is encouraged to live a normal life and undergoes frequent electrocardiographic and physical examinations to detect hypertrophy of the heart. If the septal defect is large, symptoms of pulmonary disease or heart failure may occur. Early surgical intervention has a low risk for most infants and the prognosis is excellent. Normal growth and development are usually achieved within 1 or 2 years after surgery.

Open heart surgery is performed under hypothermia. With the use of the heart-lung bypass machine the condition can be corrected in a fairly dry or bloodless field. The hole is ligated (closed) with sutures or a synthetic patch.

Patent ductus arteriosus. The circulation of the fetus differs from that of the newborn in that most of the fetal blood bypasses the lungs. The ductus arteriosus is the passageway (shunt) through which the blood crosses from the pulmonary artery to the aorta and avoids the deflated lungs. This vessel closes shortly after birth; when it does not close, blood continues to pass from the aorta, where the pressure is higher, into the pulmonary artery. This causes oxygenated blood to recycle through the lungs, overburdening the pulmonary circulation and making the heart pump harder.

The symptoms of patent ductus arteriosus (PDA) may go unnoticed during infancy. As the child grows, dyspnea is experienced, the radial pulse becomes full and bounding on exertion, and there is an unusually wide range between systolic and diastolic blood pressures. This is referred to as the pulse pressure. A *characteristic machinery-type murmur* may be heard. A two-dimensional echocardiogram is useful in visualizing and determining blood flow across the PDA.

PDA is one of the more common cardiac anomalies. It occurs twice as frequently in girls as in boys. Premature infants with hypoxia often respond to indomethacin drug therapy that results in closure of the PDA. Heart surgery is performed on all full-term newborns diagnosed with PDA to prevent congestive heart failure, emboli formation, and other complications. The ductus may be ligated via thoracotomy (incision into the chest) or via the visually assisted thoracoscopic surgery (VATS) technique that eliminates the need for a large chest incision. The prognosis is excellent.

Obstructive Defect

Some congenital cardiac defects can obstruct blood flow from the ventricles because of a stenosis (narrowing) of a vessel.

Coarctation of the aorta. The word *coarctation* means "a tightening." In coarctation of the aorta, there is a constriction or narrowing of the aortic arch or of the descending aorta (the blood meets an obstruction) (see Figure 25-13). Hemodynamics consists of increased pressure proximal to the defect and decreased pressure distally. The characteristic symptoms are a *marked difference in the blood pressure and pulses of the upper and lower extremities.* The patient may not develop symptoms until late childhood. Treatment depends on the type and severity of the defect. Infants who have associated congestive heart failure (CHF) are treated medically until the optimal time for surgery.

The surgeon resects the narrowed portion of the aorta and joins its ends. The joining is called an *anastomosis.* If the section removed is large, an end-to-end graft using tubes of synthetic polyester (Dacron) or similar material may be necessary. The aorta will grow but the graft will not; therefore the best time for surgery is between 2 and 4 years of age. Some children complain of leg pain after exercise. X-ray examination may reveal cardiac enlargement and "notching" of the ribs caused by vessels developed as collateral circulation. Pulses and blood pressure will differ in the upper and lower extremities. Two-dimensional echocardiography can aid in the diagnosis. If the condition is untreated, hypertension, CHF, and infective endocarditis may develop. As in PDA, closed-heart surgery is performed because the structures are outside the heart. The prognosis is good if there are no other defects and the child's physical condition is favorable at the time of surgery. If restenosis occurs after surgery for coarctation, a balloon angioplasty can relieve the obstruction. The nurse should observe the child with postcoarctation surgery for the development of hypertension and abdominal pain associated with nausea and vomiting, leukocytosis, and gastrointestinal bleeding or obstruction. Antihypertensive drugs, steroids, and nasogastric tube decompression are the priority treatment of this postsurgical complication.

⚡NURSING **TIP**

A significant difference in the blood pressure between the upper extremities and the lower extremities is a characteristic sign of coarctation of the aorta.

Defects That Decrease Pulmonary Blood Flow

A *decrease* in pulmonary blood flow occurs when a congenital heart anomaly allows blood that has not passed through the lungs (unoxygenated blood) to enter the aorta and general circulation. Cyanosis caused by the presence of unoxygenated blood in the circulation is a characteristic feature of this type of congenital heart anomaly.

Tetralogy of Fallot. Tetra means "four." In *tetralogy of Fallot* there are four defects: (1) stenosis or narrowing of the pulmonary artery, which decreases the blood flow to the lungs; (2) hypertrophy of the right ventricle, which enlarges because it must work harder to pump blood through the narrow pulmonary artery; (3) dextroposition (*dextro,* "right" and *position*) of the aorta, in which the aorta is displaced to the right and blood from both ventricles enters it; and (4) VSD (see Figure 25-13).

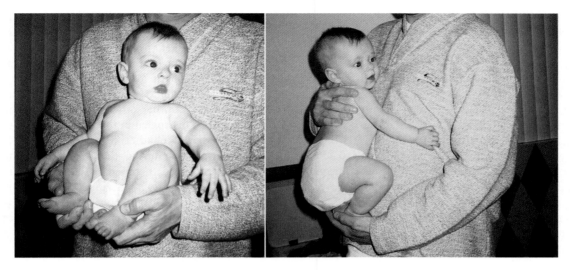

FIGURE **25-14** Tet position. Infants and children with tetralogy of Fallot can have paroxysmal hyper-cyanosis or "tet" spells. Placing the child in the tet position (a knee-chest position) will relieve these symptoms. Older children will spontaneously squat when a tet spell occurs.

When venous blood enters the aorta, the infant displays symptoms of cardiac problems. Cyanosis increases with age, and *clubbing of the fingers and toes* is seen. The child rests in a "squatting" position to breathe more easily. This position increases systemic venous return. Feeding problems, growth retardation, frequent respiratory infections, and severe dyspnea on exertion are prevalent. The red blood cells (RBCs) of the body increase, causing polycythemia (*poly,* "many," *cyt,* "cells," and *hema,* "blood") to compensate for the lack of oxygen.

Narrowing of the pulmonary artery causes CHF as a result of the increased muscular force necessary to propel blood through the narrowed orifice. When unoxygenated blood enters the general circulation, *hypoxia* occurs and may be manifested by cyanosis.

In response to chronic hypoxia, *clubbing of the fingers* results (see Figure 25-10). As a response to chronic hypoxia, the body produces more RBCs, causing polycythemia. *Failure to thrive* results from decreasing energy and ability to eat and increased oxygen consumption. Multiple hospitalizations, cyanotic skin, and limited energy can impede growth and development both physically and socially.

Paroxysmal hypercyanotic episodes, or "tet" spells, occur during the first 2 years of life. Spontaneous cyanosis, respiratory distress, weakness, and syncope occur. They can last a few minutes to a few hours and are followed by lethargy and sleep. Parents and day care personnel must be instructed to place the child in a knee-chest position when a tet spell occurs (Figure 25-14). Often the child will pause and voluntarily squat in posi-

tion until the attack abates. Recovery from the tet spell is usually rapid.

Diagnosis of tetralogy of Fallot is confirmed by chest x-ray that shows a typical *boot-shaped heart.* An electrocardiogram, three-dimensional echocardiography, and cardiac catheterization aid in confirming the diagnosis.

Complications such as cerebral thrombosis caused by polycythemia (thickened blood as a result of increased RBCs) is a problem, especially if dehydration occurs. Iron deficiency anemia develops because of decreased appetite and increased energy required to suck or eat. Bacterial endocarditis can occur and is prevented with prophylactic antibiotic therapy.

Treatment is designed to increase pulmonary blood flow to relieve hypoxia. A Blalock-Taussig surgical procedure can be performed successfully on newborns or premature infants. Open heart surgery with total correction of all defects is usually done on the older, stable child with excellent results. In some cases, IV prostaglandin E therapy can open a constricted ductus arteriosus and allow for oxygenation of the body until surgery is performed.

NURSING **TIP**

The four defects in tetralogy of Fallot are as follows:
- Pulmonary artery stenosis
- Hypertrophy of the right ventricle
- Dextroposition of aorta
- VSD

Defects That Cause Mixed Pathology

Hypoplastic left heart syndrome. In hypoplastic left heart syndrome there is an underdevelopment of the left side of the heart, usually resulting in an absent or nonfunctional left ventricle and hypoplasia of the ascending aorta. This condition can be diagnosed before birth and placed on a transplant list early so that surgery can be performed soon after birth. The initial survival of the infant depends on a patent foramen ovale and ductus arteriosus to provide a pathway for oxygenated blood to the general body system. Other serious congenital anomalies may be present and the infant should be carefully assessed.

Symptoms include a grayish blue color of the skin and mucous membranes and signs of CHF, including dyspnea, weak pulses, and a cardiac murmur. Survival beyond the first month of life without intervention is rare. With the advent of successful heart transplants, however, the prognosis of these infants is much brighter and emphasis is placed on maintaining life and hope until an appropriate heart is available for transplant. After a transplant, immunosuppressive therapy to prevent organ rejection is required.

General Treatment and Nursing Care of Children with Congenital Heart Defects

Recent technological advances have enabled therapeutic catheterization procedures for valvuloplasty, angioplasty, and other corrections of pediatric heart pathologies as an alternative to open heart surgery. After the procedure the nursing care involves monitoring vital signs, observing for thrombosis formation, and performing neurovascular checks of the limb, including pedal pulses. Emotional support of the family and education concerning what to do and expect during and after therapy is a nursing responsibility. In most cases, hospitalization after cardiac catheterization is limited to 2 or 3 days. Parents must be guided to understand that the child should not be overprotected and restricted from normal activities related to optimum growth and development. Fear and anxiety can be transferred from the parents to the child. Education concerning general health, hygiene, dental care, balanced diet, and routine immunizations should be emphasized. Immunizations after cardiac transplantation must be placed on hold. Immunizations are not recommended before cardiac surgery because immunosuppressants are used to prevent rejection of the transplanted heart, and the child's ability to manufacture antibodies in response to routine immunizations will be impaired. Dental health care in children with heart disease is important to prevent bacteremia, which can cause bacterial endocarditis. Antibiotics are usually required before dental care. Competitive sports are avoided in children with congenital heart disease because the pressure for a team win can influence the child's need to stop activity if specific symptoms arise. Some children benefit from being transported to school so that energy can be consumed *during* school activities rather than by walking to school.

Nutritional guidance is aimed at preventing anemia and promoting optimal growth and development. Parents should be instructed in the techniques of preventing dehydration in children with polycythemia. Family trips or vacations during the hot summer months require attention to the child's fluid needs to replace fluid loss from sweating. Vacations to high altitudes or very cold environments may cause adverse responses in a child who is already hypoxic or has cardiac problems.

Cardiac surgery—if needed to repair a defect that causes heart failure—is generally performed at a regional medical center where the necessary costly equipment is available. Chest tubes may be used postoperatively to remove secretions and air from the pleural cavity and to allow reexpansion of the lungs. These are attached to underwater-seal drainage systems or a commercially manufactured disposable system such as Pleur-Evac. Units for infants and older children are available. This system must be *airtight* to prevent collapse of the lung. Drainage bottles *are always kept below the level of the chest* to prevent the backflow of secretions. This is especially important during transportation. *Two rubber-shod Kelly clamps must be available at all times* for emergency clamping of tubes. These are applied to the tubes as close as possible to the child's chest if a break in the system occurs.

Postoperative cardiac care usually takes place in an ICU, where high-technology monitoring minimizes complications. The licensed vocational nurse will have contact with the child who is returning for postoperative checkups or is on a home care program after discharge. Providing routine supportive care, encouraging appropriate medical follow-up, and designing activities that promote optimal growth and development are primary goals of care.

ACQUIRED HEART DISEASE

Acquired heart disease is a cardiac problem that occurs *after* birth. It may be a complication of a congenital heart disease or a response to respiratory infection, sepsis, hypertension, or severe anemia. *Heart failure* is defined as a decrease in cardiac output necessary to meet the metabolic needs of the body.

Congestive Heart Failure

Manifestations. Manifestations of CHF depend on the side of the heart affected (Figure 25-15). Signs differ somewhat and are more subtle in infants. Some of these

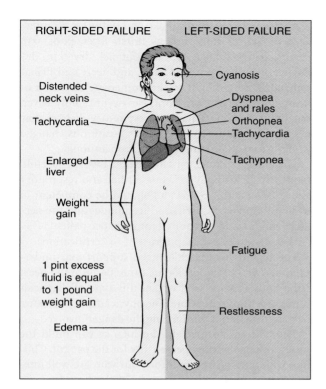

RIGHT-SIDED FAILURE   LEFT-SIDED FAILURE

Cyanosis

Distended
neck veins

Dyspnea
and rales

Tachycardia

Orthopnea
Tachycardia

Tachypnea

Enlarged
liver

Weight
gain

Fatigue

1 pint excess
fluid is equal
to 1 pound
weight gain

Restlessness

Edema

FIGURE **25-15** Congestive heart failure. The *right side* of the heart moves unoxygenated blood to pulmonary circulation. A failure results in the backup of blood in the systemic venous system. The *left side* of the heart moves oxygenated blood from the pulmonary circulation to the systemic circulation. A failure results in backup into the lung. When the body tries to compensate for the problems, peripheral vasoconstriction occurs and results in cold/blue hands and feet, tachycardia, and tachypnea. Although heart failure may start as a right-sided or left-sided failure, eventually *both* sides become involved.

signs are cyanosis, pallor, rapid respiration, rapid pulse, feeding difficulties, fatigu a weak cry, excessive perspiration (especially to the forehead), failure to gain weight, edema, and frequent respiratory infections.

⚡NURSING **TIP**

Early signs of CHF in infants that should be reported are as follows:
- Tachycardia at rest
- Fatigue during feedings
- Sweating around scalp and forehead
- Dyspnea
- Sudden weight gain

Cyanosis. When observing color, the nurse notes whether the cyanosis is general or localized. If it is localized, the exact location is recorded in the nurse's notes, for example, hands, feet, lips, or around the mouth. Is the cyanosis deep or light? Is it constant or transient? Sometimes color improves during crying, and sometimes it gets worse; this is significant. If overt cyanosis is not apparent in the African-American infant, the palms of the hands and bottoms of the feet are observed. Clubbing of the fingers and toes (see Figure 25-10) as a result of blood pooling in the capillaries of the extremities in children with chronic hypoxia may be evident. The skin may be very pale or may be mottled. Sweating, particularly of the head, may be seen.

Rapid respiration. Rapid respiration is called *tachypnea*. A rate of over 60 breaths/min in a newborn at rest indicates distress. The amount of dyspnea does vary. In more acute cases, dyspnea is accompanied by flaring of the nostrils, mouth breathing, grunting, and sternal retractions (see Figure 25-2). The infant has more trouble breathing when flat in bed than when held upright. Air hunger is evidenced if the child is irritable and restless. The cry is weak and hoarse.

Rapid pulse. A rapid pulse is termed *tachycardia*. An increase in pulse rate is one of the first signs of CHF. The heart is pumping harder in an effort to increase its output and provide increased oxygen to all the tissues of the body. Cardiac output can be increased by one of two mechanisms: tachycardia or increased stroke volume. Stroke volume is the amount of blood ejected during one contraction. Because infants and small children have a limited ability to increase stroke volume, their heart rate increases. The heart is pumping harder to get sufficient oxygen to all parts of the body.

Feeding difficulties. When the nurse feeds these infants, they tire easily and may stop after sucking a few ounces. When placed in the crib, they cry and appear hungry. They may choke and gag during feedings; the pleasure of sucking is spoiled by their inability to breathe.

Poor weight gain. The child fails to gain weight. A sudden increase in weight may indicate edema and the beginning of heart failure.

Edema. Blood flow to the kidneys is decreased, and the glomerular filtration rate slows. This causes both fluid and sodium to be retained. The nurse watches for puffiness about the eyes and, occasionally, in the legs, feet, and abdomen. Urine output may decrease.

Frequent respiratory tract infections. Resistance is very low. Slight infections can be highly dangerous because the heart and lungs are already compromised. Immunizations are reviewed and updated as needed. The nurse prevents exposure to other children who have upper respiratory tract infections and other illnesses.

Treatment and nursing care. The nursing goals significant to the care of children with heart failure are to (1) reduce the work of the heart, (2) improve respiration, (3) maintain proper nutrition, (4) prevent infection, (5) reduce the anxiety of the patient, and (6) support and instruct the parents.

The nurse must organize care so that the infant is not unnecessarily disturbed. A complete bath and linen change for an infant with a serious heart defect may not be a priority. The infant is fed early if crying and late if asleep. The physician orders the position in which the infant is placed. In some cases the knee-chest position facilitates breathing; in other cases, a position with the head elevated (Fowler's position) may be helpful. Older infants may be placed in infant seats.

Feedings are small and frequent. A soft nipple with holes large enough to prevent the infant from tiring is provided. In some cases, nasogastric tube feedings are advantageous because they are less tiring for the child. Oxygen is administered to relieve dyspnea. As breathing becomes easier, the infant begins to relax. A soft voice and gentle care is soothing. Whenever possible, the infant is held and comforted during feedings.

Digitoxin and digoxin (Lanoxin) are common oral digitalis preparations. In pediatric patients, Lanoxin is preferred because of its rapid action and shorter half-life. These agents slow and strengthen the heartbeat. The nurse counts the patient's pulse for 1 full minute before administering them. A resting apical pulse is most accurate. As a rule, *if the pulse rate of a newborn is below 100 beats/min the medication is withheld* and the physician is notified. In older children the pulse rate should be above 70 beats/min. Because the pulse rate varies with the age of the child, it is ideal for the physician to specify in the written drug order at what heart rate the nurse should withhold the drug. When this is not done, the nurse obtains clarification. The physician is notified when the drug is withheld.

The physician is contacted if the patient vomits. Digitalis administration is not repeated until the physician confirms it is safe to do so. Tachycardia and irregularities in the rhythm of the pulse are significant and should be reported. Symptoms of toxicity include nausea, vomiting, anorexia, irregularity in rate and rhythm of the pulse, and a sudden change in pulse. If the infant is discharged while still receiving medication, the parents are taught how to take the pulse and what signs to be alert for when administering the drug.

Diuretics such as furosemide (Lasix) or chlorothiazide (Diuril) are useful in reducing edema. Careful monitoring of serum electrolyte levels prevents electrolyte imbalance, particularly potassium depletion. Parents of older patients are taught to recognize foods high in potassium, such as bananas, oranges, milk, potatoes, and prune juice. Diapers are weighed to determine urine output. Daily weighing of the infant also helps the physician determine the effectiveness of the diuresis.

An accurate record of intake and output is essential. Signs of dehydration such as thirst, fever, poor skin turgor, apathy, sunken eyes or fontanel, dry skin, dry tongue, dry mucous membranes, and decreased urination should be brought to the immediate attention of the nurse in charge. Pneumonia can occur rapidly. Fever, irritability, and an increase in respiratory distress may indicate this condition. The child's position is changed regularly to help prevent hypostatic pneumonia.

The nurse working in a cardiac unit assesses the child frequently for complications of cardiac and respiratory failure (see Figure 25-15) and should be competent in cardiopulmonary resuscitation techniques and the necessary modifications required for pediatric patients (Pediatric Advanced Life Support [PALS] certification).

The parents of the child need support and understanding over a long period of time. Because the heart is the body's major vital organ, this type of diagnosis causes much apprehension . The physician must reassure the parents without minimizing the danger involved.

The patterns formed during infancy can build the framework of a healthy personality for the patient. Children who have heart conditions but who are well integrated into family life have a decided advantage over children who are made to think they are invalids. Routine naps and early bedtime provide adequate rest for most children.

As children grow, they usually set their own limits on the amount of activity they can handle. Prompt treatment of infections is important. A suitable diet with adequate fluids is necessary. Eating iron-rich foods is encouraged. Dental care should be regular. All-day attendance in school may be too tiring for the child; therefore special provisions may be necessary. The child needs careful evaluation before any type of minor surgery is performed.

Detailed discharge planning and coordination of community services are of value to the family.

RHEUMATIC FEVER

Pathophysiology. Rheumatic fever (RF) is a systemic disease involving the joints, heart, central nervous system (CNS), skin, and subcutaneous tissues. It belongs to a group of disorders known as *collagen diseases.* Their common feature is the destruction of connective tissue. RF is particularly detrimental to the heart, causing scarring of the mitral valves. Its peak incidence is between 5 and 15 years of age. RF is common worldwide in lower income groups and where overcrowded conditions exist. It is more prevalent during the winter and spring, and carrier rates among school-age children are believed to be higher during these seasons. Genetic factors have implicated an abnormal immune response.

RF is an autoimmune disease that occurs as a reaction to a group A beta-hemolytic *Streptococcus* infection of the throat. The disease almost disappeared during the 1960s and 1970s; since the late 1980s, however, a resurgence has occurred in the United States. This has emphasized the need for more aggressive diagnosis and treatment of streptococcal pharyngitis.

Manifestations. Symptoms of RF range from mild to severe and may not occur for 1 to 3 weeks after a strep throat infection (Figure 25-16). The classic symptoms are *migratory polyarthritis* (wandering joint pains), *skin eruptions, chorea* (a nervous disorder), and *inflammation of the heart.* Subcutaneous nodules may appear beneath the skin but are less common in children. Abdominal pain, often mistaken for appendicitis, sometimes occurs. Fever varies from slight to very high. Pallor, fatigue, anorexia, and unexplained nosebleeds may be seen. RF tends to *recur,* and each attack carries the threat of further damage to the heart. The recurrences are most frequent during the first 5 years after the initial attack, and they decline rapidly thereafter.

Migratory polyarthritis. The polyarthritis (*poly,* "many," *arthr,* "joint," and *itis,* "inflammation of ") seen in RF is distinctive in that it does not result in permanent deformity to the joint. It involves mainly the larger joints: knees, elbows, ankles, wrists, and shoulders. The joints become painful and tender and are difficult to move. The symptoms last for a few days, disappear without treatment, and frequently return in another joint. This pattern may continue for a few weeks. The symptoms tend to be more severe in older children. The joint may be visibly swollen and inflamed. On diagnosis, salicylates are administered to relieve the pain.

Skin eruptions. *Erythema marginatum,* the rash seen in RF, consists of small red circles with red-colored margins, a pale center, and wavy lines appearing on the trunk and abdomen. They appear and disappear rapidly and are significant in diagnosing the disease.

Sydenham's chorea. Chorea is a disorder of the CNS characterized by involuntary, purposeless movements of the muscles. It may occur as an acute rheumatic involvement of the brain. Sydenham's chorea is primarily seen in prepubertal girls.

Attacks of chorea, which begin slowly, may be preceded by increased tension and behavioral problems. The child becomes "clumsy," may stumble and spill things, and may have difficulty buttoning clothes and writing. When the facial muscles are involved, grimaces occur. The child may laugh and cry inappropriately. In severe cases the patient may become completely incapacitated, and deterioration in speech may be noticeable. Treatment of Sydenham's chorea is directed toward the relief of symptoms. The condition usually disappears spontaneously within weeks to months. Medication may also be required. The presence of Sydenham's chorea alone can support the diagnosis of RF.

Rheumatic carditis. Carditis, an inflammation of the heart, is a manifestation of RF that can be fatal. It occurs more often in the young child. The tissues that cover the heart and the heart valves are affected. The heart muscle (myocardium) may be involved, as may the pericardium and endocardium. The *mitral valve,* which is located between the left atrium and left ventricle, is often involved. Vegetations form that interfere with the proper closing of the valve and disturb its normal function. When this valve becomes narrowed, the condition is called *mitral stenosis.* Myocardial lesions called *Aschoff's bodies* are also characteristic of the disease. The burden on the heart is great because it must pump harder to circulate the blood. As a result, it may become enlarged. Symptoms of poor circulation and heart failure may appear.

The child has an irregular low-grade fever, is pale and listless, and has a poor appetite. Moderate anemia and weight loss are apparent. The child may experience dyspnea on exertion. The pulse and respiration rates are out of proportion to the body temperature. The physician may detect a soft murmur over the apex of the heart.

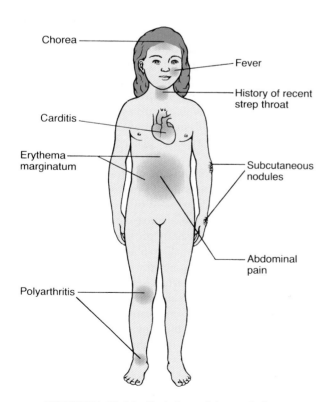

Chorea

Carditis

Erythema marginatum

Polyarthritis

Fever

History of recent strep throat

Subcutaneous nodules

Abdominal pain

FIGURE **25-16** Manifestations of rheumatic fever.

Diagnosis. The diagnosis of RF is difficult to make, and for this reason the Jones criteria have been developed and modified over the years (Box 25-3). The presence of two major criteria or one major and two minor criteria, supported by evidence of recent streptococcal infection, indicates a high probability of rheumatic fever. A careful physical examination is done, and a complete history of the patient is obtained. Certain blood tests are helpful. The erythrocyte sedimentation rate is elevated. Abnormal proteins, such as C-reactive protein, may also be evident in the blood serum. Leukocytosis may occur but is not regularly present. Antibodies against the streptococci (measured by ASO titer) may also be detected. Additional studies may include chest x-rays, throat culture, and pulmonary function tests. The electrocardiogram, a graphic record of the electrical changes caused by the beating of the heart, is very useful. Changes in conductivity, particularly a prolonged P-R interval (first-degree heart block), may indicate carditis. These tests are repeated throughout the course of the disease so that the physician may determine when the active stage has subsided.

Treatment and nursing care. Treatment is aimed at preventing permanent damage to the heart. This is accomplished by antibacterial therapy, physical and mental rest, relief of pain and fever, and management of cardiac failure should it occur. Initial antibacterial therapy is directed toward eliminating the streptococcal infection. Penicillin is the drug of choice (given for a 10-day period) unless the patient is sensitive to it, in which case erythromycin is substituted.

---

box 25-3 | **Modified Jones Criteria**

MAJOR CRITERIA
Carditis
Polyarthritis
Erythema marginatum
Chorea
Subcutaneous nodules

MINOR CRITERIA
Fever
Arthralgia
Previous history of rheumatic heart disease
Elevated erythrocyte sedimentation rate
Leukocytosis
Altered P-R interval on electrocardiogram
Positive C-reactive protein

A positive diagnosis of rheumatic fever cannot be made without the presence of two major criteria, or one major and two minor criteria, plus a history of streptococcal infection.

Elimination of infection through medication is followed by long-term *chemoprophylaxis* (prevention of disease by drugs); intramuscular benzathine penicillin G is given monthly to children with a history of RF or evidence of rheumatic heart disease for a minimum of a 5-year period or until 18 years of age. Oral administration is considered for patients with minimal involvement whose reliability about taking medications can be determined. Erythromycin is recommended for long-term therapy for children who cannot tolerate penicillin. Financial assistance may be available to patients and their families. Local heart associations, rehabilitation services, and state and municipal health departments are sources of such aid.

Antiinflammatory drugs are used to decrease fever and pain. Aspirin is the drug of choice for joint disease without evidence of carditis. The use of steroids is reserved for severe cardiac symptoms or when aspirin does not relieve cardiac pain. Concerns during therapy include aspirin toxicity and the effects of aspirin on blood clotting. Mild signs of Cushing's disease, such as moon face, acne, and hirsutism (increased hairiness), should be anticipated with the use of steroids. More severe reactions such as gastric ulcer, hypertension, overwhelming infection, and toxic psychosis may occur. Phenobarbital is effective in reducing chorea. Padded side rails are used to protect the patient who experiences spasms. If CHF occurs, symptomatic treatment is given.

Bed rest during the initial attack is recommended until the erythrocyte sedimentation rate (ESR) returns to normal levels. The amount of work the heart must do must be limited by resting the entire body. In this way the circulation of the heart is slower, and the heart does not need to work as fast or as hard as when a child is active. The nurse should teach parents and children the need for rest and the types of play activity appropriate during home care.

Nursing activities should be organized to ensure as few interruptions as possible to prevent tiring the patient. A bed cradle can be used to prevent pressure on painful extremities. Care includes special attention to the skin, especially over bony prominences; back care; good oral hygiene; and small, frequent feedings of nourishing foods. Maintaining healthy teeth and preventing cavities are of special importance. The patient with RF is particularly susceptible to *subacute bacterial endocarditis,* which can occur as a complication of dental or other procedures likely to cause bleeding or infection. Prophylactic antibiotic treatment is required before any dental procedure. Nutrition consists of small servings from the basic food groups. These are increased as the child's appetite improves. A record of fluid intake and output is kept, because overhydration may tax the heart. All efforts are made to provide emotional support for the child and family. Provisions should be made for the child to continue school studies.

Prevention. Prevention of infection and prompt treatment of group A beta-hemolytic streptococcal infections can prevent the occurrence of RF. All throat infections should be cultured. Once a diagnosis of strep throat is established, the nurse stresses the need to complete antibiotic therapy even if symptoms disappear and the child "feels better." Close medical supervision and follow-up care are essential. The prognosis is favorable.

SYSTEMIC HYPERTENSION

Pathophysiology. Hypertension, or high blood pressure, is being seen more often during childhood and adolescence. Blood pressure is a product of peripheral vascular resistance and cardiac output. An increase in cardiac output or peripheral resistance results in an increase in blood pressure. Systemic blood pressure increases with age and is correlated with height and weight throughout childhood and adolescence. (See Chapter 22 for normal blood pressure measurements in infants and children.) *Significant hypertension* is considered when measurements are persistently at or above the 95th percentile for the patient's age and sex. The hypertension is referred to as *secondary* when the cause of the increased pressure can be explained by a disease process. Renal, congenital, vascular, and endocrine disorders represent the majority of illnesses that account for secondary hypertension. *Primary,* or *essential, hypertension* implies that no known underlying disease is present. Nevertheless, heredity, obesity, stress, and a poor diet and exercise pattern can contribute to any type of hypertension.

There is increasing evidence that essential hypertension, although not generally seen until adolescence or adulthood, may have its roots in childhood. The prevention of this is significant in reducing stroke or myocardial infarction as a person ages. The assessment of blood pressure levels should be part of every physical examination during childhood. Hypertension is more prevalent in children whose parents have high blood pressure. High blood pressure in children is usually discovered during a routine physical examination. Measuring blood pressure in young children requires careful attention to cuff size (see Chapter 22).

NURSING **TIP**

The blood pressure cuff should encircle two thirds of the length of the upper arm for an accurate blood pressure assessment.

Treatment and nursing care. Treatment and nursing care involve nutritional counseling, weight reduction, and an age-appropriate program of aerobic exercise. Adolescents should be counseled concerning the adverse effects of drugs, alcohol, and tobacco on blood pressure. Drug therapy to reduce high blood pressure may not be effective in adolescents, who often are noncompliant with long-term regimens.

The focus of treatment for secondary hypertension is the underlying disease causing the high blood pressure.

Prevention. The main focus of a hypertensive prevention program is patient education. The nurse can work with school personnel to promote awareness of the problem at parent-teacher association (PTA) meetings. Community health fairs should offer blood pressure screening opportunities. Blood pressure measurement must be part of every routine physical examination. Risk factors such as obesity, elevated serum cholesterol levels, sedentary lifestyle, and drug, alcohol, or tobacco use should be discussed.

HYPERLIPIDEMIA

Hyperlipidemia refers to excessive lipids (fat and fatlike substances) in the blood. Because there is evidence that the factors responsible for degenerative vascular disease may begin in childhood and may be somewhat controllable, considerable interest has developed in screening children for risk factors and in attempting to change these risks (Table 25-4).

Children with a parental history of cholesterol levels exceeding 240 mg/dl or a family history of early cardiac death (under age 55 years) should have their cholesterol levels tested. However, screening only those children who are identified as high risk may not reach all children who need follow-up care. Therefore an active preventive program for all children and adolescents is essential. Lifelong healthy eating habits should be nurtured early and practiced by the entire family. A step-one dietary program involves no more than 300 mg of cholesterol per day and no more than 30% of total dietary calories from fat. Children under 2 years of age should not have a fat-restricted diet because calories and fat are necessary for CNS growth and development. The AAP recommendations for heart-healthy guidelines are presented in Box 25-4.

table 25-4 | *Average Plasma Cholesterol and Triglyceride Levels in Childhood*

	CHOLESTEROL	TRIGLYCERIDES
Newborn	68	35
1 to 9 years	155-165	55-65
10 to 14 years	160	62-72
15 to 19 years	150-160	73-78

box 25-4 *Heart-Healthy Guidelines for Children*

INFANTS

Provide breast milk or formula for 1 year.

Provide rice or other single-grain cereal from 4 to 6 months.

Provide a balanced mixture of cereal, vegetables, fruits, and meats for the second 6 months of life.

Baby foods are labeled regarding calories and nutrient composition; avoid foods with added sugar or salt; most baby foods, with the exception of combined foods and desserts, do not have these additives.

Infants do not need desserts to grow; infant fruits are more nutritious.

Fats do not need to be restricted in healthy infants.

TODDLERS AND PRESCHOOLERS

Avoid excessive fats, salt, and refined sugars.

Avoid salty snacks and sweet desserts.

Offer heart-healthy snacks of vegetables, fruits, and finger foods.

Offer a variety of foods from the basic food groups.

Discourage the consumption of large amounts of milk, which can lead to nutritional imbalances.

SCHOOL-AGE CHILDREN

Provide heart-healthy school lunches.

Role-model good daily exercise.

Screen children with family history of congenital heart disease (cholesterol, triglycerides, blood pressure).*

Avoid obesity.

Discourage smoking.

ADOLESCENTS

Emphasize the importance of heart-healthy foods to improve endurance and good body image.

Avoid a sedentary lifestyle.

Discourage the excessive intake of dietary saturated fat, sodium, sugar, and excess calories.

Be a nonsmoking parent as a model for the adolescent.

Assess stress management capabilities; counsel accordingly.

Screen periodically for serum cholesterol elevations and blood pressure measurements.

Provide serial monitoring of adolescents deemed to be at high risk (sustained high blood pressure readings on at least three separate occasions).

*Children over 2 years of age with a family history of hyperlipidemia or early atherosclerotic heart disease should undergo routine screening for hyperlipidemia.

NURSING **TIP**

Hospitalization provides an excellent opportunity for the nurse to review heart-healthy information. Reviews of family history, lifestyle, and eating patterns are suitable interventions, even in the absence of high risks.

KAWASAKI DISEASE

Kawasaki disease (KD) (mucocutaneous lymph node syndrome) occurs worldwide and is the leading cause of acquired cardiovascular disease in the United States. It usually affects children under age 5 years. Studies have shown that KD may be a reaction to toxins produced by a previous infection with an organism such as the staphylococci. KD is not spread from person to person. The diagnosis is made by clinical signs and symptoms, because specific laboratory findings are not diagnostic. KD causes inflammation of the vessels in the cardiovascular system. The inflammation weakens the walls of the vessels and often results in an *aneurysm* (an abnormal dilation of the wall of a blood vessel). Aneurysms can cause thrombi (blood clots) to form, resulting in serious complications. Approximately 40% of untreated children develop aneurysms of the coronary vessels, which can be life threatening.

Manifestations. The onset is abrupt with a sustained fever, sometimes above 40° C (104° F), that does not respond to antipyretics or antibiotics. The fever lasts for more than 5 days. Conjunctivitis without discharge, fissured lips, a "strawberry tongue" (enlarged reddened papilla on the tongue), inflamed mouth and pharyngeal membranes, and enlarged nontender lymph nodes are seen. An erythematous skin rash develops, with swollen hands and desquamation (peeling) of the palms and soles (Figure 25-17). The child is very irritable and may develop signs of cardiac problems.

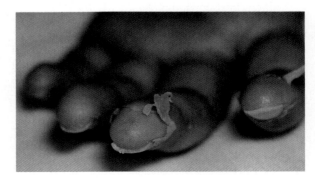

FIGURE **25-17** Peeling of the fingertips. The typical appearance of fingertip or toe-tip peeling in the subacute phase of Kawasaki syndrome.

Treatment and nursing care. IV gamma globulin given early in the illness can prevent the development of coronary artery pathology. Salicylate therapy (aspirin) is prescribed for its antithrombus properties. Warfarin (Coumadin) therapy may be prescribed if aneurysms are detected to prevent clot formation.

Nursing care is symptomatic and supportive. Parent teaching should be reinforced concerning the need to postpone active routine immunizations for several months after the administration of immune globulin, which is an immunosuppressant.

Long-term, low-dose aspirin therapy may be prescribed to prevent clot formation. Compliance may be a problem for any long-term regimen in which medication must be taken when the child feels "well." The nurse should reinforce parent teaching concerning the recognition of cardiac problems and updating their CPR skills.

key points

- Routine handwashing practices can prevent the spread of the common cold.
- Quiet play may be more restful than confinement to bed for toddlers and young children.
- Nosedrops with an oil base should be avoided.
- Laryngomalacia and acute spasmodic laryngitis are benign forms of croup.
- Laryngotracheobronchitis and epiglottitis are acute types of croup.
- A Croupette, or mist tent, provides moist air supersaturated with microdroplets that can enter the small airway of a child and relieve respiratory distress.
- A tongue blade examination of the throat can cause sudden respiratory arrest in a child with epiglottitis.
- Frequent swallowing while the child is sleeping is an early sign of bleeding immediately after a tonsillectomy.
- Coughing, clearing the throat, and blowing the nose should be avoided in the immediate postoperative period after a tonsillectomy.
- Swimming and sports activities that involve intermittent activity are well tolerated by asthmatic children.
- Cystic fibrosis is a multisystem disease characterized by an increased viscosity of mucous gland secretions.
- Bulky, frothy, foul-smelling stools are characteristic of cystic fibrosis.

- The maxillary and ethmoid sinuses are most often involved in childhood sinusitis.
- Periorbital cellulitis is a complication of childhood sinusitis.
- Signs and symptoms of congenital heart abnormalities in infants include dyspnea, difficulty with feedings, choking spells, recurrent respiratory infections, cyanosis, poor weight gain, clubbing of the fingers and toes, and heart murmurs.
- The nursing goals significant to the care of children with heart failure are to (1) reduce the work of the heart, (2) improve respiration, (3) maintain proper nutrition, (4) prevent infection, (5) reduce the anxiety of the parent, and (6) support growth and development.
- *Congenital heart defects* may be caused by genetic factors, maternal factors such as drug use or illness, or environmental factors. *Acquired heart disease* occurs *after* birth as a response to a defect or illness.
- Congenital heart defects that result in a recirculation of blood to the lungs do not usually produce cyanosis as a clinical sign.
- A congenital heart defect can cause an increase in pulmonary blood flow, a decrease in pulmonary blood flow, or an obstruction of blood flow.
- A difference in the blood pressure between the arms and the legs is characteristic of coarctation of the aorta.
- The defects in tetralogy of Fallot include pulmonary artery stenosis, hypertrophy of the right ventricle, dextroposition of the aorta, and a ventricular septal defect.
- Hypercyanotic "tet" spells are relieved by placing the child in a knee-chest position.
- Signs of congestive heart failure in infants include tachycardia, at-rest fatigue during feedings, and perspiration around the forehead.
- The major Jones criteria diagnostic of rheumatic fever include polyarthritis, erythema marginatum, Sydenham's chorea, and rheumatic carditis.
- Chest tube drainage systems must always be kept below the level of the chest.
- A child under age 2 years should *not* have a fat-restricted diet.

ONLINE RESOURCES

Micromedex: http://www.micromedex.com

Asthma Statistics: http://rover.nhlbi.nih.gov/health/prof/lung/asthma/asthstat.htm

Guidelines for the Diagnosis and Management of Asthma: http://www.nhlbi.nih.gov/guidelines/asthma/asthgdln.pdf

REVIEW QUESTIONS *Choose the most appropriate answer.*

1. Which of the following is a priority nursing diagnosis in a child admitted with acute asthma?
   1. Risk for infection
   2. Imbalanced nutrition
   3. Ineffective breathing pattern
   4. Disturbed body image

2. Which of the following signs or symptoms observed in a sleeping 2-year-old child immediately after a tonsillectomy requires reporting and follow-up care?
   1. A pulse of 110 beats/min
   2. A blood pressure of 96/64 mm Hg
   3. Nausea
   4. Frequent swallowing

3. The nurse is reinforcing teaching concerning the use of a cromolyn sodium inhaler for a 10-year-old with asthma. An accurate concept to emphasize would be:
   1. You should use the inhaler whenever you feel some difficulty in breathing.
   2. You should use the inhaler between meals.
   3. You should use the inhaler regularly every day even if you are symptom free.
   4. You can discontinue using the inhaler when you are feeling stronger.

4. When administering digoxin (Lanoxin) to an infant, the medication should be withheld and the physician notified if:
   1. The pulse rate is below 60 beats/min
   2. The infant is dyspneic
   3. The pulse rate is below 100 beats/min
   4. The respiratory rate is above 40 breaths/min

5. An infant with tetralogy of Fallot is experiencing a tet attack involving cyanosis and dyspnea. Which position should the infant be placed in?
   1. Fowler's
   2. Knee-chest
   3. Trendelenburg's
   4. Prone

26 The Child with a Condition of the Blood, Blood-Forming Organs, or Lymphatic System

objectives

1. Define each key term listed.
2. Summarize the components of the blood.
3. Recall normal blood values of infants and children.
4. List two laboratory procedures commonly performed on children with blood disorders.
5. Compare and contrast four manifestations of bleeding into the skin.
6. List the symptoms, prevention, and treatment of iron-deficiency anemia.
7. Recommend four food sources of iron for a child with iron-deficiency anemia.
8. Recognize the effects on the bone marrow of increased red blood cell production caused by thalassemia.
9. Review the effects of severe anemia on the heart.
10. Devise a nursing care plan for a child with sickle cell disease.
11. Examine the pathology and signs and symptoms of sickle cell disease.
12. Describe four types of sickle cell crises.
13. Discuss the nursing care of a child receiving a blood transfusion.
14. Recall the pathology and signs and symptoms of hemophilia A and B.
15. Identify the nursing interventions necessary to prevent hemarthrosis in a child with hemophilia.
16. Discuss the effects of chronic illness on the growth and development of children.
17. Plan the nursing care of a child with leukemia.
18. Review the nursing care of a child receiving a transfusion.
19. Recall the stages of dying.
20. Contrast age-appropriate responses to a sibling's death and the nursing interventions required.
21. Formulate techniques the nurse can use to facilitate the grieving process.
22. Discuss the nurse's role in helping families to deal with the death of a child.

key terms

alopecia (ăl-ō-PĒ-shē-ă, p. 643)
Christmas disease (p. 640)
ecchymosis (ĕk-ĭ-MŌ-sĭs, p. 641)
erythropoietin (ĕ-rĭth-rō-POI-ă-tĭn, p. 631)
hemarthrosis (hē-măr-THRŌ-sĭs, p. 640)
hematoma (hē-mă-TŌ-mă, p. 641)
hematopoiesis (hē-mă-tō-poi-Ē-sĭs, p. 631)
hemosiderosis (hē-mō-sĭd-ĕr-Ō-sĭs, p. 637)
lymphadenopathy (lĭm-făd-ĕ-NŎP-ă-thē, p. 632)
oncologist (p. 641)
petechiae (pē-TĒ-kē-ē, p. 632)
purpura (PŬR-pū-ră, p. 632)
respite care (RĔS-pīt kăr, p. 650)
sickle cell crises (p. 636)
Sickledex (p. 636)
splenomegaly (splē-nō-MĔG-ă-lē, p. 632)

The blood and blood-forming organs make up the hematological system. *Blood dyscrasias* or disorders occur when blood components fail to form correctly or when blood values exceed or fail to meet normal standards. Blood is vital to all body functions. Plasma and blood cells are formed at about the second week of gestation, primarily in the yolk sac. Later it forms in the spleen, liver, thymus, lymph system, and bone marrow. In the fetus, blood is formed primarily in the liver until the last trimester of pregnancy.

During childhood the red blood cells (RBCs) are formed in the marrow of the long bones (such as the tibia and femur); by adolescence, hematopoiesis (blood formation) takes place in the marrow of the ribs, sternum, vertebrae, pelvis, skull, clavicle, and scapula. The rate of RBC production is regulated by erythropoietin. This substance is produced by the liver of the fetus, but at birth the kidney takes over erythropoietin production.

The lymphatic system includes lymphocytes, lymphatic vessels, lymph nodes, spleen, tonsils, adenoids, and the thymus gland. The lymphatic system drains regions of the body to lymph nodes, where infectious organisms are destroyed and antibody production is stimulated. Lymph nodes are not palpable in the newborn, but the cervical, axillary, and inguinal nodes may be palpable by childhood. Lymphadenopathy is an enlargement of lymph nodes that is indicative of infection or disease. Figure 26-1 summarizes some of the differences between the child's and the adult's lymphatic system.

Figure 26-2 depicts the main types of blood cells in the circulating blood. Circulating blood consists of two portions: plasma and formed elements. The formed elements are erythrocytes, leukocytes (white blood cells [WBCs]), and thrombocytes (platelets). Erythrocytes primarily transport oxygen and carbon dioxide to and from the lungs and tissues. Leukocytes act as the body's defense against infections. Thrombocytes, along with portions of blood plasma, are involved with blood coagulation. In the young child, every available space in the bone marrow is involved with blood formation.

Lymphocytes, unlike other WBCs, are produced in the lymphoid tissues of the body. They travel in the circulation but are more commonly found in the lymph tissue. They are released into the body to fight infection and provide immunity. Their numbers greatly increase in chronic inflammatory conditions. The spleen is the largest organ of the lymphatic system. One of the main functions of the spleen is to bring blood into contact with lymphocytes. Aside from trauma and rupture, the most commonly seen pathological condition of the spleen is enlargement. This is termed splenomegaly. The spleen enlarges during infections, congenital and acquired hemolytic anemias, and liver malfunction.

Bone marrow aspiration is a procedure helpful in determining disorders of the blood. Numerous blood counts are used as well. Many are specific to a particular disease. The skin is sometimes an indicator of certain conditions of the blood. Petechiae (pinpoint hemorrhagic spots) and purpura (large petechiae) are often seen and should alert the nurse to the possibility of blood dyscrasia. The physician examines the liver and spleen by palpation and percussion to determine if they are enlarged.

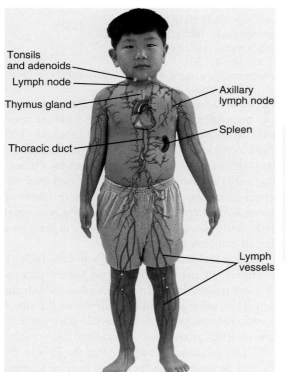

Tonsils and adenoids
Lymph node
Thymus gland
Thoracic duct
Axillary lymph node
Spleen
Lymph vessels

LYMPHATIC SYSTEM

- The increased size of tonsils and adenoids is normal in preschool and school-age children and is one of the body's defense mechanisms.
- The thymus gland is important in the development of the immune response in newborns.
- Preterm and term infants are at greater risk for viral and bacterial infections because of immature T-cell activity.

FIGURE **26-1** Summary of lymphatic system differences between the child and the adult. The lymphatic system is a subsystem of the circulatory system. It returns excess tissue fluid to the blood and defends the body against disease.

ANEMIAS

Anemia can result from many different underlying causes. A reduction in the amount of circulating hemoglobin reduces the oxygen-carrying ability of the blood. A hemoglobin level below 8 g/dl results in an increased

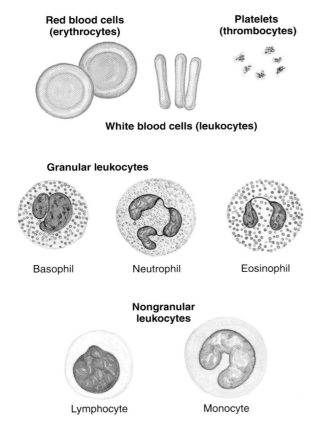

Red blood cells (erythrocytes)

Platelets (thrombocytes)

White blood cells (leukocytes)

Granular leukocytes

Basophil   Neutrophil   Eosinophil

Nongranular leukocytes

Lymphocyte   Monocyte

FIGURE **26-2** The formed elements of the blood. RBCs (erythrocytes), WBCs (leukocytes), and platelets (thrombocytes) constitute the formed elements of the blood.

cardiac output and a shunting of blood from the periphery of the body to the vital organs. Pallor, weakness, tachypnea, shortness of breath, and congestive heart failure can result. Table 26-1 reviews normal blood values in infants and children.

IRON-DEFICIENCY ANEMIA

Pathophysiology. The most common nutritional deficiency of children in the United States today is anemia caused by insufficient amounts of iron in the body. The incidence is highest during infancy and adolescence—two rapid growth periods. Anemia (*an,* "without" and *emia,* "blood") is a condition in which there is a reduction in the amount and size of the RBCs or in the amount of hemoglobin, or both. Iron-deficiency anemia may be caused by severe hemorrhage, the child's inability to absorb the iron received, excessive growth requirements, or an inadequate diet. Researchers have also found that feeding whole cow's milk to infants can precipitate gastrointestinal bleeding, resulting in anemia.

Prevention of iron-deficiency anemia begins with good prenatal care to ensure that the mother has a suitable intake of iron during pregnancy. During the first few months after birth the newborn relies on iron that was stored in the system during fetal life. Preterm infants may be deprived of a sufficient supply, because iron is obtained late in the prenatal period. In addition, the iron stores of low-birth-weight infants and infants from multiple births are relatively small.

The highest incidence of iron-deficiency anemia occurs from the ninth to the twenty-fourth month. During this rapid growth period, the infant outgrows the limited iron reserve that was in the body; in addition, iron-fortified formula and infant cereals may have been eliminated from the diet. Poorly planned meals or feeding problems also contribute to this deficiency. The mother

| table 26-1 | *Normal Blood Values During Infancy and Childhood* |

AGE	RBCs (g/dl)	HEMATOCRIT (%)	LEUKOCYTES (WBC/mm^3)	NEUTROPHILS (%)	LYMPHOCYTES (%)	EOSINOPHILS (%)	MONOCYTES (%)
Neonate	16.5	50	12,000	40	63	3	9
3 months	12	36	12,000	30	48	2	5
6 months to 6 years	12	37	10,000	45	48	2	5
7 to 12 years	13	38	8,000 to 10,000	55	38	2	5
Adult	14 to 16	42 to 47	8,000 to 10,000	55	35	3	7

may sometimes rely too heavily on bottle feedings to avoid conflict at meals. Unfortunately, milk contains very little iron. Instead, the amounts of solid food should be increased and the amount of milk decreased. Boiled egg yolk, liver, leafy green vegetables, Cream of Wheat, dried fruits (apricots, peaches, prunes, raisins), dry beans, crushed nuts, and whole-grain bread are good sources of iron. Iron-fortified cereals eaten out of the box provide a nutritious snack. Unfortunately, not all the iron found in a food source is absorbed by the body. The bioavailability of iron in vegetables is less than in meat.

Manifestations. The symptoms of iron-deficiency anemia are pallor, irritability, anorexia, and a decrease in activity. Many infants are overweight because of excessive consumption of milk (so-called "milk babies"). Blood tests for anemia may include RBC count, hemoglobin, hematocrit, morphological cell changes, and iron concentration. The stool may be tested for occult blood. A dietary history is also obtained. Sometimes a slight heart murmur is heard. The spleen may be enlarged.

Untreated iron-deficiency anemias progress slowly, and in severe cases the heart muscle becomes too weak to function. If this happens, heart failure follows. Children with long-standing anemia may also show growth retardation and cognitive changes. Screening procedures are suggested at 9 and 24 months for full-term infants and earlier for low-birth-weight infants.

Treatment. Iron-deficiency anemia responds well to treatment. Iron, usually ferrous sulfate, is given orally two or three times a day *between meals*. Vitamin C aids in the absorption of iron; therefore giving juice when administering iron is suggested. Liquid preparations are taken through a straw to prevent temporary discoloration of the teeth. (Some available iron preparations do not have this disadvantage.) The toddler needs solid foods that are rich sources of iron. An iron-dextran mixture (Imferon) given intramuscularly is also highly effective. It must be injected deep in a large muscle using the Z-track technique to minimize staining and tissue irritation.

Parent education. Parents need explicit instructions on proper foods for the infant. The nurse stresses the importance of breastfeeding for the first 6 months and the use of iron-fortified formula throughout the first year of life (the absorption of iron from human milk is much better than from cow's milk). The amount of milk consumed during the day and night is determined. Solid food intake is reviewed, and specific iron-enriched nutrients are suggested. The nurse considers financial, ethnic, and family preferences in teaching plans. Behavior concerns at mealtime may also need to be addressed.

The stools of infants who are taking oral iron supplements are tarry green. An absence of this finding may indicate poor parental compliance with therapy. Oral iron preparations are not to be given with milk, which interferes with absorption. To increase absorption, these preparations should be given between meals, when digestive acid concentration is highest. It is important to emphasize that both dietary changes and supplemental iron therapy are necessary to eradicate iron-deficiency anemia. Good dietary practices must be lifelong to maintain good health. Parents are encouraged to return for periodic evaluation of the child's blood status. Nursing Care Plan 26-1 specifies interventions for the child with iron-deficiency anemia.

> ⧩NURSING **TIP**_____
> Avoid iron poisoning in children by keeping preparations well out of reach. Educate parents about this hazard.

SICKLE CELL DISEASE

Pathophysiology. Sickle cell disease is an inherited defect in the formation of hemoglobin. It occurs mainly in African-American populations, but it is also carried by some people of Arabian, Greek, Maltese, Sicilian, and other Mediterranean races. Many researchers believe that the gene for sickle cell disease developed in these populations as protection against malaria. Sickling (clumping) caused by decreased blood oxygen may be triggered by dehydration, infection, physical or emotional stress, or exposure to cold. Laboratory examination of the affected child's blood shows that the RBC has changed its shape to resemble that of a sickle blade, from which the name of the disorder is derived (Figure 26-3).

Sickle cells contain an abnormal form of hemoglobin termed *hemoglobin S* (the sickling type). The membranes of these cells are fragile and easily destroyed. Their crescent shape makes it difficult for them to pass through the capillaries, causing a pile-up of cells in the small vessels. This clumping may lead to a *thrombosis* (clot) and cause an obstruction. *Infarcts,* or areas of dead tissue, may result when the tissue is denied proper blood supply. These generally develop in the spleen but may also be seen in other areas of the body, such as the brain, heart, lungs, gastrointestinal tract, kidneys, and bones. The patient feels acute pain in the affected area.

There are two types of sickle cell disease: an asymptomatic (*a,* "without" and *symptoma,* "symptom") version *(sickle cell trait),* and much more severe forms that require intermittent hospitalization *(sickle cell anemia).*

NURSING CARE PLAN 26-1

The Child with Iron-Deficiency Anemia

PATIENT DATA: A parent brings a 10-month-old boy to the clinic. The child is pale and listless. Laboratory results show iron deficiency anemia. The parent states that the child loves to drink milk.

SELECTED NURSING DIAGNOSIS   *Deficient knowledge (parents) related to cause and treatment of anemia*

Outcomes	Nursing Interventions	Rationales
Parents will verbalize an understanding of the importance of dietary factors and iron supplements in the prevention and treatment of this condition. Infant will ingest iron-rich formula plus two servings of iron-fortified cereal and iron supplement, if prescribed.	1. Encourage breastfeeding.	1. Absorption of iron from human milk is much better than that from cow's milk.
	2. Encourage iron-rich formula for full first year.	2. Cow's milk contains little iron.
	3. Dispel the myth that milk is a perfect food.	3. Parents often rely too heavily on milk because it is easier than preparing solid foods, which the infant may initially dislike; ingestion of large amounts of milk may interfere with absorption of iron supplements.
	4. Give iron supplement between meals with juice.	4. Vitamin C aids in the absorption of iron.

SELECTED NURSING DIAGNOSIS   *Imbalanced nutrition: less than body requirements related to iron-poor diet*

Outcomes	Nursing Interventions	Rationales
Patient's hemoglobin level will improve with therapy; there will be no recurrence of anemia.	1. Review 24-hour dietary history.	1. Nurse can determine what foods are missing and quantities of food ingested; this information can be used as a baseline for teaching.
	2. Review height and weight chart.	2. Determines child's status in relation to norms; compares patient's present measurements with former rate of growth and progress.
	3. Review solid food intake and suggest iron-rich foods as age appropriate.	3. Solid foods high in iron must be increased as age appropriate (egg yolk, liver, leafy green vegetables, Cream of Wheat, dried fruits, whole-grain bread, iron-fortified cereal).
	4. Educate parents as to how to administer the iron supplement.	4. Usually given orally two or three times a day between meals. Supplements are easily forgotten because evidence of improvement is slow and signs of disease may not be noticeable. Poisoning can result from overdose.
	5. Stress the importance of compliance with the dietary regimen to prevent recurrence.	5. Dietary changes must be lifelong to maintain good health.

?CRITICAL THINKING QUESTION

The mother of a child diagnosed with anemia comes to the clinic and states she is worried about the pallor and lack of energy her child continues to show. She states she works outside the home but has her child in "good day care" that provides good meals. What further questions would be appropriate for the nurse to ask in this interview?

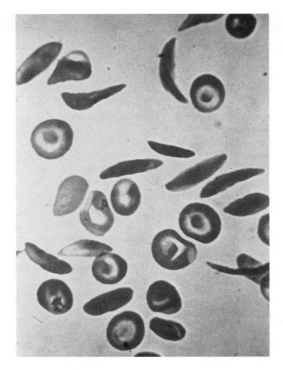

FIGURE **26-3** Scanning electron micrograph of erythrocytes. Note that the normal RBC is round. The sickle-shaped cell can clump as it flows through the circulation, causing a vaso-occlusive sickle cell crisis.

Sickle cell trait. This form of the disease occurs in about 10% of the African-American population in the United States. The blood of the patient contains a mixture of normal (hemoglobin A) and sickle (hemoglobin S) hemoglobins. The proportions of hemoglobin S are low because the disease is inherited from only one parent. The physician can distinguish sickle cell trait from the more severe disease by electrophoresis study of the patient's RBCs and hemoglobin. Sickling is more rapid and extreme with sickle cell disease. In sickle cell trait the hemoglobin and RBC counts are normal.

Sickle cell trait does not develop into sickle cell disease. Although there is no need to treat the patient with sickle cell trait, the patient *is* a carrier, and genetic counseling is important.

Sickle cell anemia. This severe form of sickle cell disease results when the abnormality is inherited from both parents (Figure 26-4). *Each offspring* has a one-in-four chance of inheriting the disease (not one of four children). In general, the clinical symptoms do not appear until the last part of the first year of life. There may be an unusual swelling of the fingers and toes. The symptoms of sickle cell disease are caused by enlarging bone marrow sites that impair circulation to the bone

and the abnormal sickle cell shape that causes clumping, obstruction in the vessel, and ischemia to the organ that vessel supplies.

There is chronic anemia. The hemoglobin level ranges from 6 to 9 g/dl or lower. The child is pale, tires easily, and has little appetite. These manifestations of anemia are complicated by characteristic episodes of sickle cell crises, which are painful and can be fatal. Specific types of crises have been defined. They differ in pathology and may require somewhat different treatments (Table 26-2). Unfortunately, in some cases the sickle cell crisis is the first obvious manifestation of the condition. The patient appears acutely ill. There is severe abdominal pain. Muscle spasms, leg pains, or painful swollen joints may be seen. Fever, vomiting, hematuria, convulsions, stiff neck, coma, or paralysis can result, depending on the organs involved. Children with sickle cell disease have a risk for stroke as a complication of a vaso-occlusive sickle cell crisis.

The sickle cell crises recur periodically throughout childhood; however, they tend to decrease with age. Patients should be kept in good health between episodes. Immunizations of these children are particularly important, including the *Hemophilus influenzae*, hepatitis A and B, and pneumococcal vaccine. Patients should refrain from becoming overly tired. They also should avoid situations such as flying in an unpressurized airplane or exercising at a high altitude, because oxygen concentrations are already reduced in their blood. Extra stress and exposure to cold may lower resistance, causing additional problems. Overheating, which can lead to dehydration, is also to be avoided. Oral intake of iron is of no value.

NURSING **TIP**

During sickle cell crises, anticipate the child's need for tissue oxygenation, hydration, rest, protection from infection, pain control, blood transfusion, and emotional support for this life-threatening illness.

Diagnosis. Sickle cell disease can be detected before birth by chorionic villi sampling. Early diagnosis by mandatory screening of all newborns in the United States allows early detection before symptoms occur. The sickling test (Sickledex) is commonly used for screening. Hemoglobin electrophoresis ("fingerprinting") is used when the result is positive. This procedure separates and records the various peptide patterns of the blood. It distinguishes between patients with the trait and those with the disease.

Treatment and nursing care. When the infant or child is hospitalized during a crisis, the treatment is support-

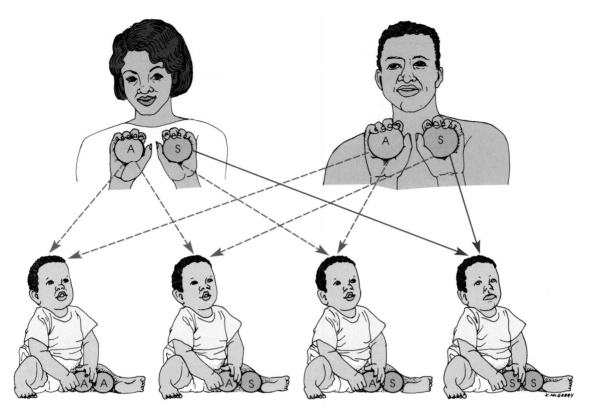

FIGURE **26-4** Transmission of sickle cell disease from parents to children. Parents who are carriers of the sickle cell trait do not show symptoms of the disease because hemoglobin A (the normal form of hemoglobin) in their RBCs protects them from hemoglobin S (the sickling form). When two carriers become parents, however, the possibilities are as follows: One child in four will inherit all normal hemoglobin (AA) and thus be free of the disease; two children in four will inherit both hemoglobin A and hemoglobin S and thus become carriers (AS) of the trait (like their parents); and one child in four will inherit all sickling hemoglobin (SS) and thus be affected by sickle cell disease.

ive and symptomatic. The patient is confined to bed. Analgesics are given to relieve pain. Children in severe pain may need a continuous intravenous (IV) infusion containing a narcotic. Meperidine (Demerol) is not recommended for children with sickle cell disease because of the risk of normeperidine-induced seizures (American Pain Society, 1999). A patient-controlled analgesia (PCA) pump enables children over 7 years of age to maintain control and participate in care. Every effort is made to combat dehydration and acidosis. Small blood transfusions may be administered to increase the hemoglobin count, but the results are only temporary. Packed RBCs are often given for this purpose. An accurate record of intake and output is kept. The patient's body position is changed frequently but gently.

Sickle cell disease may take a wide variety of courses. As always, the individual patient's progress is followed.

Sometimes it is difficult to distinguish between a sickle cell crisis causing ischemia in the abdominal area from abdominal pain caused by appendicitis. The nurse must remember that pain experienced by a child with sickle cell disease may also be caused by an unrelated condition.

Prevention of infection and dehydration are important goals in the care of a child with sickle cell disease. Multiple transfusions of packed cells may be required to maintain adequate hemoglobin levels. The nurse should observe the child for reactions to the blood transfusion. Hemosiderosis (the deposit of iron into organs and tissues in the body) is a complication of this type of hemolytic disease.

The main goals of therapy are to prevent sickling, dehydration, hypoxia, and infection, which can cause a sickle cell crisis. Erythropoietin and some chemotherapy regimens can increase the production of fetal hemo-

table 26-2 *Types of Sickle Cell Crises*

TYPE	COMMENT
Vasoocclusive (painful crises)	Most common type; there is an obstruction of blood flow by cells, infarctions, some degree of vasospasm. Dactylitis, painful joints and extremities, abdominal pain (infarction or bleeding within liver, spleen, abdominal lymph node), central nervous system strokes, pulmonary disease, priapism are present.
Splenic sequestration	Large amounts of blood pool in liver and spleen. Spleen becomes massive. Circulatory collapse and shock are present. Children between 8 months and 5 years of age are particularly susceptible. Death may occur within hours of appearance of symptoms. Minor episodes may resolve spontaneously. Splenectomy may be indicated for children who have one or more severe crises.
Aplastic crises	Bone marrow stops producing red blood cells (RBCs); a number of infections may precipitate this (usually viral). Child may be transfused with fresh packed RBCs if severe anemia occurs.
Hyperhemolytic	Rapid rate of hemolysis is superimposed on an already severe process; rare. Functional hyposplenism and overwhelming infection occur. Progressive fibrosis of spleen reduces its function; patient becomes more susceptible to infection.

Data from Dickerman, J., & Lucey, J. (1985). *Smith's The critically ill child* (3rd ed.). Philadelphia: W.B. Saunders; and Jackson, P., & Vessey, J. (2000) *Primary care of the child with a chronic condition* (3rd ed.). Philadelphia: W.B. Saunders.

globin and reduce complications. Bone marrow transplantation and gene replacement therapy may hold a promising cure (Jackson & Vessey, 2000).

Surgery. The approach to splenectomy in children with sickle cell disease has been conservative. A recurrence of acute splenic sequestration becomes less likely after age 5 years. Routine splenectomy is not recommended because the spleen generally atrophies on its own because of fibrotic changes that take place in patients with sickle cell disease.

THALASSEMIA

Pathophysiology. The thalassemias are a group of hereditary blood disorders in which the patient's body cannot produce sufficient adult hemoglobin. The RBCs are abnormal in size and shape and are rapidly destroyed. This abnormality results in a chronic anemia. The body attempts to compensate by producing large amounts of fetal hemoglobin. These disorders are caused by a deficiency in the normal synthesis of hemoglobin polypeptide chains. They are categorized according to the polypeptide chain affected as alpha-, beta-, gamma-, or delta-thalassemia.

The most common variety of thalassemia involves impaired production of beta chains and is known as *beta-thalassemia*. This variety consists of two forms: thalassemia minor and thalassemia major. Thalassemia major is also called Cooley's anemia. Thalassemia occurs mainly in persons of Mediterranean origin, such as Greeks, Syrians, Italians, and their descendants elsewhere. The term is derived from the Greek *thalassa*, which means "sea." Thalassemia can also occur from spontaneous mutations.

Thalassemia minor. Thalassemia minor, also termed *beta-thalassemia trait*, occurs when the child inherits a thalassemia gene from only one parent (heterozygous inheritance). It is associated with mild anemia. Hemoglobin concentration averages 2 to 3 g/dl, lower than age-related values. These patients are often misdiagnosed as having an iron-deficiency anemia. Symptoms are minimal. The patient is pale, and the spleen may be enlarged. The patient may lead a normal life, with the illness going undetected. This condition is of genetic importance, particularly if both parents are carriers of the trait. Prenatal blood samples can detect thalassemia major in such cases.

Thalassemia major (Cooley's anemia). When two thalassemia genes are inherited (homozygous inheritance), the child is born with a more serious form of the disease. A progressive, severe anemia becomes evident within the second 6 months of life.

The child is pale and hypoxic, has a poor appetite, and may have a fever. Jaundice, which at first is mild, progresses to a muddy bronze color resulting from *hemosiderosis*, a deposit of iron (released by blood cell destruction) into the tissues. The liver enlarges, and the spleen grows enormously. Abdominal distention is great, which causes pressure on the organs of the chest. Cardiac failure caused by the profound anemia is a constant threat. Bone marrow space enlarges to compensate for an increased production of blood cells. Hematopoietic (*hema,* "blood" and *poiesis,* "to make") defects and a massive expansion of the bone marrow in the face and skull result in changes in the facial contour that give the child a characteristic appearance (Figure 26-5). The teeth protrude because of an overgrowth of the upper jawbone; the bone becomes thin and is subject to pathological fracture.

Diagnosis is aided by a family history of thalassemia, radiographic bone growth studies, and blood tests. Hemoglobin electrophoresis is helpful in diagnosing the type and severity of the various thalassemias. Prenatal screening and diagnosis are available, and genetic counseling is advised.

Treatment and nursing care. The goals of care for children with thalassemia are to (1) maintain hemoglobin levels to prevent overgrowth of bone marrow and resultant deformities, and (2) provide for growth and development and normal physical activity. Prevention or early treatment of infection is important. Some patients require splenectomy. Bone marrow transplantation holds promise for the future treatment of this condition (Jackson & Vessey, 2000).

The mainstay of treatment for thalassemia major is frequent blood transfusions to maintain the hemoglobin level above 10 g/dl. As a result of repeated blood transfusions, excessive deposits of iron may be stored in the tissues. This is termed *hemosiderosis* and is seen especially in the spleen, liver, heart, pancreas, and lymph glands. Deferoxamine mesylate (Desferal), an iron-chelating agent, is given to counteract hemosiderosis. Severe splenomegaly may occur in some children. Splenectomy may make the patient more comfortable, increase the ability to move about, and allow for more normal growth. After surgery, these children are given prophylactic antibiotics to prevent infection.

Nursing measures adhere to the principles of long-term care. The observation of the patient during a blood transfusion is discussed on pp. 644 and 645. Monitoring of vital signs is necessary to detect irregularities of the

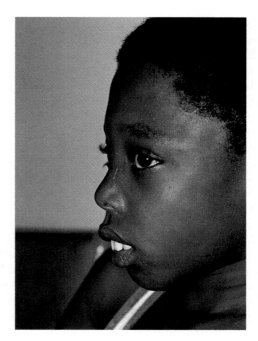

FIGURE **26-5** Appearance of child with thalassemia major (Cooley's anemia). Note the overgrowth of the upper jaw bone (maxillary hyperplasia).

heart. Whenever possible, the same nurse cares for the patient during transfusions, blood tests, and other unpleasant procedures to provide security. Children are taught to regulate their activities according to their own tolerance.

The emotional health of the child and parents needs special consideration by the nurse. Every attempt to ease the strain of this prolonged illness must be made. Home care arrangements can be provided through community agencies. The family can be referred to the Cooley's Anemia Foundation for support and education. Older children need special support to accept changes in their body image caused by the disease. Suggestions applicable to the care of the chronically ill child are discussed throughout the text. Care of the dying child is discussed on pp. 650 to 654.

BLEEDING DISORDERS

HEMOPHILIA

Pathophysiology. Hemophilia is one of the oldest hereditary diseases known to humanity. In this disorder the blood does not clot normally, and even the slightest injury can cause severe bleeding. It has been called the disease of kings because it has occurred in the children of several royal families in Russia and Europe. This congenital disorder is confined almost exclusively to males but is transmitted by symptom-free females.

Hemophilia is inherited as a sex-linked recessive trait. It is termed *sex-linked* because the defective gene is located on the X, or female, chromosome. Different combinations of genes account for the fact that some children inherit the disease, some become carriers, and others neither inherit nor carry the trait. New mutations do occur, and the reason for this is unclear. The sex of the fetus can be determined by amniocentesis. Fetal blood sampling detects hemophilia. Some carrier women can also be identified.

There are several types of hemophilia. More than 10 identified factors in the blood are involved in the clotting mechanism. A deficiency in any one of the factors will interfere with normal blood clotting. The two most common types of hemophilia are *hemophilia B* or Christmas disease, (a factor IX deficiency) and *hemophilia A* (a deficiency in factor VIII). This discussion is limited to classic hemophilia, or hemophilia A, which accounts for approximately 84% of cases.

Hemophilia A is caused by a deficiency of coagulation factor VIII, or antihemophilic globulin (AHG). The severity of the disease depends on the level of factor VIII in the plasma of the patient's blood. Some patients' lives are endangered by minor injury, whereas a child with a mild case of hemophilia might just bruise a little more easily than the normal person. The degree of severity tends to remain constant within a given family. The aim of therapy is to increase the level of factor VIII to ensure clotting. It is possible to determine the level of factor VIII in the blood by means of a test called the *partial thromboplastin time (PTT)*, which can help to diagnose and assess the child's condition. Prenatal diagnosis by amniocentesis is possible.

> ✸ NURSING **TIP**
> A classic symptom of hemophilia is bleeding into the joints (hemarthrosis).

Manifestations. Hemophilia can be diagnosed at birth because maternal factor VIII cannot cross the placenta and be transferred to the fetus. It is usually not apparent in the newborn unless abnormal bleeding occurs at the umbilical cord or after circumcision. As the child grows older and becomes more subject to injury, the slightest bruise or cut can induce extensive bleeding. Normal blood clots in about 3 to 6 minutes. In a patient with severe hemophilia, however, the time required for clotting may be 1 hour or longer.

Anemia, leukocytosis, and a moderate increase in platelets may be seen in the hemorrhaging child. There may also be signs of *shock.* Spontaneous hematuria is seen. Death can result from excessive bleeding anywhere in the body, but particularly when hemorrhage into the brain or neck occurs. Severe headache, vomiting, and disorientation may reflect cranial bleeding. Bleeding into the neck can cause airway obstruction. Bleeding into the ears and eyes can affect hearing and vision. Bleeding into the spinal column can lead to paralysis.

The circumstances leading to diagnosis may be the inability of a parent to stop a child's bleeding from a cut around the mouth or gums. A deciduous tooth loss may precipitate problems in a child who has a bleeding disorder. *Hematomas* may develop after immunization. An injured knee, elbow, or ankle presents particular problems. Hemorrhage into the joint cavity, or hemarthrosis (*hema*, "blood," *arthron*, "joint," and *osis*, "condition of"), is considered a classic symptom of hemophilia. The effusion (*ex*, "out" and *fundere*, "to pour") into the joint is very painful because of the pressure buildup. Repeated hemorrhages may cause permanent deformities that could incapacitate the child. This deformity is sometimes referred to as an ankylosis (*ankyle*, "stiff joint" and *osis*, "condition of").

Treatment and nursing care. In a newborn with a family history of hemophilia, circumcision, heel sticks, and intramuscular injections are delayed to prevent bleeding and tissue injury. The principal therapy for hemophilia is to prevent bleeding by replacing the missing factor. The development of recombinant antihemophilic factor, a synthetic product, has eliminated the need for repeated blood transfusions and its accompanying dangers (such as human immunodeficiency virus [HIV] and hepatitis infection). The missing factor is replaced by reconstituting the product with sterile water and administering it through an implanted IV port. Once the parents and child are taught how to administer the medication, treatment is carried out in the home. Diagnosed infants may receive prophylactic factor replacements at regular intervals to prevent hemarthrosis. Desmopressin acetate (DDAVP) is a nasal spray that can stop bleeding. It may be the treatment of choice for mild cases of hemophilia. Aminocaproic acid (Amicar) is an antifibrinolytic agent that can control bleeding that may occur because of dental care or other oral bleeding.

Prophylactic factor replacement combined with specific treatment before planned invasive procedures such as dental extraction or minor surgery, as well as education concerning the prevention of injuries that can cause bleeding, enable the hemophiliac child to live a normal life. Because young children often fall while playing, the joints of the knees, hips, and elbows can be protected by padding their play outfits. Appropriate sports activities should be selected to avoid undue injury and the risk of bleeding episodes. When bleeding does occur, the traditional approach to care includes *rest*, *ice*, *compression*, and *elevation* (RICE). A medical alert identification band should be worn at all times.

Home care programs are the treatment of choice. These greatly reduce the cost of treatment and decrease the risk of psychological trauma. A multidisciplinary approach to care assists families to develop healthy coping strategies to deal with a child who has a chronic illness. The multidisciplinary approach to care is facilitated by Hemophilic Treatment Centers (HTC), which are funded by the government to meet the comprehensive needs of these children.

It is difficult for parents not to be overly protective. Children may resent being unable to participate in athletic activities with peers or may attempt to conceal their problem from others. Schooling should not be interrupted so that friendships are maintained with peers. The struggle to protect these children and still foster independence and a sense of autonomy may seem monumental to parents who work away from home. Allowing children to participate in decision making about their care and focusing on their strengths are helpful.

Parent groups and professional counseling may provide support to enable children and parents to develop a healthy attitude toward the child's medical condition.

⚡NURSING **TIP**

Drugs that contain salicylates are contraindicated for children with hemophilia.

PLATELET DISORDERS

The reduction or destruction of platelets in the body interferes with the clotting mechanism. Skin lesions that are common to these disorders include petechiae, a bluish, nonblanching, pinpoint-sized lesion; purpura, groups of adjoining petechiae; ecchymosis, an isolated bluish lesion larger than a petechiae; and hematoma, a raised ecchymosis.

IDIOPATHIC (IMMUNOLOGICAL) THROMBOCYTOPENIC PURPURA

Pathophysiology. Idiopathic (immunological) thrombocytopenic purpura (ITP) is an acquired platelet disorder that occurs in childhood. It is the most common of the purpuras, a group of disorders affecting the numbers of platelets or their function. The cause is unknown, but it is thought to be an autoimmune system reaction to a virus. Platelets become coated with antiplatelet antibody, are "perceived" as foreign material,

and are eventually destroyed by the spleen. ITP occurs in all age-groups, with the main incidence seen between 2 and 4 years of age.

Manifestations. The classic symptoms of ITP include being easily bruised, which results in petechiae (pinpoint hemorrhagic spots beneath the skin) and purpura (hemorrhage into the skin). Approximately 30% of the patients also have nosebleeds. There may have been a recent history of rubella, rubeola, or viral respiratory infection. The interval between exposure and onset is about 2 weeks. The platelet count is below 20,000/mm^3 (normal range is between 150,000 and 400,000/mm^3). Diagnosis is confirmed by bone marrow aspiration to rule out leukemia. The bruises of ITP must be distinguished from those of child abuse.

Treatment and nursing care. When platelet counts are low, the greatest danger is spontaneous intracranial bleeding. Neurological assessments are therefore a priority of care. Treatment is not indicated in most cases of ITP. Spontaneous remission occurs in about 6 weeks to 4 months. A few children progress to chronic ITP. Drugs that interfere with platelet function should be avoided to prevent bleeding. These include aspirin, phenylbutazone (Butazolidin), and phenacetin (an ingredient of acetylsalicylic acid), and caffeine (APC). Activity is limited during the acute stage to avoid bruises from falls and trauma. Nursing considerations for the more acutely ill child focus on observing the patient for signs of bleeding. The child should use soft toothbrushes for oral hygiene to minimize tissue trauma. Packed RBCs may be administered when there has been a large amount of blood loss. Platelets are usually not given because they are destroyed by the disease process. Steroids such as prednisone may be prescribed. IV gamma globulin may be used to elevate platelet counts. In some patients, infusion with anti-D antibody may be an effective treatment when there is no active bleeding present. A splenectomy may be indicated for cases of chronic ITP. Complications of ITP include bleeding from the gastrointestinal tract, hemarthrosis, and intracranial hemorrhage. Mortality in childhood ITP is less than 1%. All children must be immunized against the viral diseases of childhood, which help to prevent this complication.

DISORDERS OF WHITE BLOOD CELLS

LEUKEMIA

Pediatric oncologists (physicians who specialize in the treatment of tumors) are challenged with the treatment of cancer in children because irradiation, surgery, and chemotherapy often have adverse effects on growth and development. Most children with cancer are treated in large medical centers to maximize the availability of high technology and newer treatment methods.

Risk for development of cancer. The incidence of leukemia increased after the atomic bombs were dropped in Japan. It is obvious that both genetic and environmental factors play a role in the development of childhood cancer. Exposure of the fetus to diagnostic x-rays, therapeutic irradiation for brain tumors, the use of fluoroscopy, ultraviolet (sun) exposure, and some drugs have been associated with the increase in cancer rates. RNA and DNA virus infections have also shown a relationship to the development of leukemia and other cancers.

Pathophysiology. Leukemia (*leuko,* "white" and *emia,* "blood") is a malignant disease of the blood-forming organs of the body that results in an uncontrolled growth of immature WBCs. The immature cells are termed *blasts,* or stem cells. This term comes from the Greek *blastos,* meaning "germ" or "formative cell." The nurse may see the terms *lymphoblasts* or *myeloblasts* referred to in descriptive histories. Leukemia is the most common form of childhood cancer. It was considered fatal in the past, but the prognosis has improved greatly with modern treatments and medication. Approximately 2000 new cases of childhood leukemia are diagnosed in the United States every year. About 40 children per million under 15 years of age are affected. Chromosomal abnormalities can be identified in 80% of cases of acute lymphocytic leukemia.

The leukemias involve a disruption of bone marrow function caused by the overproduction of immature WBCs in the marrow. Although the WBC count can be as high as 50,000 to 100,000, the cells are immature and do not function as healthy WBCs do to fight infection. Increased susceptibility to infection results. The WBCs take over the centers that are designed to form RBCs, and *anemia* results. When the WBCs infiltrate and take over the marrow centers that form platelets, the reduced platelet counts cause *bleeding tendencies.* The invasion of the bone marrow causes weakening of the bone, and pathological *fractures* can occur.

Leukemia cells can infiltrate the spleen, liver, and lymph glands, resulting in fibrosis and diminishing their function. The cancerous cells invade the central nervous system and other organs, draining these organs of their nutrients and finally causing metabolic starvation of the body. Leukemias are classified according to the type of WBC affected: (1) acute lymphocytic (ALL); (2) acute nonlymphocytic (ANLL); or (3) acute myelocytic (AML). This discussion focuses on the most common childhood leukemia, ALL.

Manifestations. The most common symptoms during the initial phase of leukemia are low-grade fever, pallor, bruising tendency, leg and joint pain, listlessness,

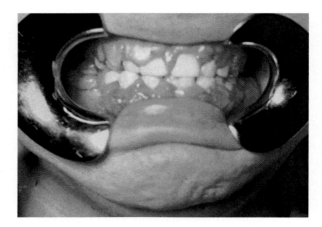

FIGURE **26-6** The mouth lesions of leukemia.

abdominal pain, and enlargement of lymph nodes. These symptoms may develop gradually or may be sudden in onset. As the disease progresses, the liver and spleen become enlarged. The skin may have an unusual lemon yellow color. *Petechiae* and *purpura* may be early objective symptoms. Anorexia, vomiting, weight loss, and dyspnea are also common. The kidneys and testicles may enlarge, and the patient may develop hematuria.

Because the WBCs are not functioning normally, bacteria easily invade the body. Ulcerations develop around the mucous membranes of the mouth and anal regions and have a tendency to bleed (Figure 26-6). Anemia becomes severe despite transfusions. The child may die as a direct result of the disease or from secondary infection. The symptoms are the same regardless of the type of WBC affected, and they vary widely with each patient depending on the parts of the body involved.

Diagnosis. The diagnosis of leukemia is based on the history and symptoms of the patient and the results of extensive blood tests that demonstrate the presence of leukemic blast cells in the blood, bone marrow, or other tissues. Because many WBCs and RBCs are formed in the bone marrow, a bone marrow aspiration is commonly performed. A piece of bone marrow is aspirated from the sternum or, more often in children, from the iliac crest. A special needle is used to obtain the sample, and the marrow is studied in the laboratory (Figure 26-7). X-ray films of the long bones show changes. After the diagnosis has been confirmed, a spinal tap determines central nervous system involvement. Kidney and liver function studies are also performed because normal functioning of these organs is absolutely necessary for chemotherapy to be safely used in treating the disease.

Treatment and nursing care. Long-term care is given on an outpatient basis whenever possible. The treat-

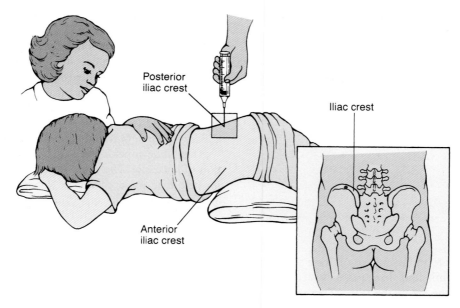

FIGURE **26-7** Bone marrow aspiration. Because many WBCs and RBCs are formed in the bone marrow, a bone marrow aspiration can determine the type and quantity of cells present and help to rule out or to confirm a serious disease.

ment of a child with cancer involves the multidisciplinary health care team (pediatrician, pathologist, oncologist, nurse, radiotherapist, nutritionist, psychologist, and school personnel). As with any diagnosis of cancer, the child with leukemia is usually referred to a specialized center where facilities for required care are available. Chemotherapy is carried out in specialized units with specially trained and certified personnel.

Although chemotherapy may be effective in reducing leukemic cells, the side effects as well as the long-term effects of treatments must be addressed. In chemotherapy, bone marrow suppression requires that the family be taught about infection prevention. Adequate hydration should be emphasized to minimize kidney damage. Active routine immunizations must be delayed while the child is receiving immunosuppressive drugs, because the body will not be able to manufacture antigens as expected. Parents should report any exposure to infections such as chickenpox so that immunoglobulin can be administered. Chickenpox can be life-threatening to a child who is immunosuppressed. Nausea and vomiting are common complications of chemotherapy and result in decreased appetite, weight loss, and generalized weakness. Presenting the child's favorite foods in an attractive manner may help stimulate the appetite. Total parenteral nutrition (TPN) may be indicated to support nutritional needs. An intake and output record is maintained, and meticulous oral hygiene is given.

The nurse should refer parents to available support groups. The Ronald McDonald house and hospice programs help parents and families cope with this illness. Because hair loss (alopecia) is a side effect of chemotherapy, the child can be offered a hat or a wig to help preserve a positive body image. School tutoring and counseling should be continuous in the hospital setting and in the home during home care to provide optimum growth and development.

The development of specific chemotherapeutic agents for acute leukemia has significantly changed the survival time. The overall cure rate for childhood ALL is 80% (Behrman, Kliegman, & Jenson, 2000). Components of chemotherapy include (1) an induction period, (2) central nervous system prophylaxis for high-risk patients, (3) maintenance, (4) reinduction therapy (if relapse occurs), and (5) extramedullary disease therapy.

The list of medications for treatment of this disease is growing (Box 26-1). A combination of drugs used to induce remissions includes prednisone, vincristine sulfate, and daunorubicin or L-asparaginase. They work within 4 to 6 weeks in about 95% of children with ALL. The therapeutic effects of these drugs are of short duration, and therefore it is necessary to use additional drugs that help to maintain the remissions. The steroid prednisone has the side effects of masking the symptoms of infection, increasing fluid retention, inducing personality changes, and causing the child's face to appear moon

box 26-1 *Drugs Used to Treat Acute Lymphocytic Leukemia*

L-Asparaginase
Cyclophosphamide (Cytoxan)
Cytarabine (Ara-C)
Daunorubicin (Cerubidine)
Doxorubicin (Adriamycin)
Etoposide (VePesid)
6-Mercaptopurine (Purinethol)
Methotrexate
Pegaspargase
Prednisone
Vincristine (Oncovin)

shaped. Methotrexate and 6-mercaptopurine are useful in maintaining remissions because they act against chemicals vital to the life of the WBC. These powerful medications produce side effects of varying degrees, such as nausea, diarrhea, rash, hair loss *(alopecia)*, fever, anuria, anemia, and bone marrow depression. Peripheral neuropathy may be signaled by severe constipation caused by decreased nerve sensations to the bowel. The nurse should consult a pharmacology text for information about the particular drugs used for the patient to anticipate potential problems.

A bone marrow transplant may be useful. An autologous transplant uses the child's own bone marrow that has been purged of malignant cells. An allogeneic bone marrow transplant is taken from a donor who matches the child. Transplanted marrow rejection is a risk. When the child is hospitalized, "reverse isolation" precautions may prevent nosocomial infections.

Children's anxiety often centers on their symptoms. They fear that the treatments necessary to correct their problems may be painful, as indeed some are, such as venipunctures, bone marrow aspirations, and blood transfusions. Their trust in others is in a precarious balance. Nurses must inform children of what they are about to do and why it is necessary. The explanation is given in terms the child will understand.

The child may ask the nurse the inevitable question, "Am I going to die?" One suggestion is to reply with a question, such as "Why do you ask that? Do you feel sick today?" This may encourage the child to verbalize feelings. The pediatric nurse who gives patients permission to discuss their concerns will find opportunities to clear up misconceptions and to decrease children's feelings of isolation.

The patient is frequently observed for signs of infection. Particular attention is given to potential sites of infection, such as the patient's mucous membranes and puncture breaks in the skin from laboratory or therapeutic procedures. Pierced ears or other body parts are observed for inflammation. Vital signs are observed for subtle variances, because steroid therapy may mask these indicators. The patient is turned often and is observed for skin breakdown, particularly in the perianal area. Nutritious meals and supplemental feedings that are high in protein and calories are offered. Parents and children are taught what to look for and report.

Thrombocytopenic bleeding is a common complication of leukemia. The nurse observes the patient's skin for petechiae and ecchymosis. Nosebleeds are common and are treated by the application of cold and pressure.

The mouth is inspected daily for ulcerations and bleeding from the gums. It may be rinsed with a prescribed solution of one part hydrogen peroxide to four parts saline solution. Commercial mouthwashes are used with caution because they may alter normal flora and may cause fungal overgrowth. A Water-Pik is helpful in massaging and toughening the gums. If the child is comatose, mouth care supplies are kept at the bedside. A soft toothsponge is helpful. The nurse may also clean food particles from the patient's teeth with a piece of gauze wrapped around the finger. Lip balm is applied to dry, cracked lips.

NURSING TIP

Bleeding from the nose or mouth may be evidenced by a soiled pillowcase or sheet.

Care of a child receiving a transfusion. Platelets and packed RBCs may be given to the child. Hemolytic reactions caused by mismatched blood are rare. Nevertheless, the registered nurse should positively identify donor and recipient blood types and groups on labels and the patient's chart with another licensed professional. Blood is infused through a blood filter to avoid impurities. Medications are *never* added to blood. Blood is administered *slowly*. The IV site is frequently checked for infiltration. The patient is observed for *signs of transfusion reaction*, which include chills, itching, rash, fever, headache, and pain in the back. If such a reaction occurs, the tubing should be clamped off immediately, the line kept open with normal saline solution, and the nurse in charge notified.

Transfusions with piggyback setups are common. Blood, normal saline, or other suitable IV solutions are connected by a stopcock. When blood must be stopped, tube patency can be maintained by opening the saline line. Necessary emergency medications can thus be administered and the site preserved for future infusions. An *autosyringe* may be used to administer small amounts of blood. The line is flushed with normal saline solution before and after instillation.

Circulatory overload is always a danger with children. *An infusion pump is routinely used to regulate blood flow.* Dyspnea, precordial pain, rales, cyanosis, dry cough, and distended neck veins are indicative of circulatory overload. Apprehension can also be a warning signal of air emboli or electrolyte disturbance. The nurse must maintain a high level of alertness for such signs, particularly in children whose conditions warrant repeated transfusions. If a reaction occurs, the blood bag and tubing are saved and returned to the blood bank. Most transfusion reactions occur within the first 10 minutes of administration; nevertheless, the patient is carefully monitored throughout this treatment. Diphenhydramine (Benadryl) may be ordered for allergic reactions. Aminophylline may be ordered for wheezing. Oxygen may be necessary to relieve dyspnea and cyanosis. Blood transfusions administered through central lines must be warmed by a blood warmer to prevent cardiac arrhythmias. Baseline data (temperature, pulse, respiration, and blood pressure) are established before transfusion, and the nurse monitors for changes. It is helpful if the parents remain with the child during this time. Suitable diversions minimize boredom.

NURSING **TIP**

If a blood transfusion reaction occurs, stop the infusion, keep the vein open with normal saline solution, and notify the charge nurse. Take the patient's vital signs and observe closely.

HODGKIN'S DISEASE

Pathophysiology. Hodgkin's disease is a malignancy of the lymph system that primarily involves the lymph nodes. It may metastasize to the spleen, liver, bone marrow, lungs, or other parts of the body. The presence of giant multinucleated cells called *Reed-Sternberg cells* is diagnostic of the disease. Hodgkin's disease is rarely seen before 5 years of age, with the incidence increasing during adolescence and early adulthood. It is twice as common in boys as in girls.

Manifestations. The presenting symptom of Hodgkin's disease is generally a painless lump along the neck. Characteristically, there are few other manifestations. In general the swelling is first noted by the patient or parents. In more advanced cases, there may be unexplained low-grade fever, anorexia, unexplained weight loss, night sweats, general malaise, rash, and itching. Diagnosis is confirmed by x-ray films, body scan, lymphangiogram, and a biopsy of the node. The stages of Hodgkin's disease are defined in Table 26-3.

table 26-3 *Criteria for Staging of Hodgkin's Disease*

STAGE	CRITERIA
I	Disease restricted to single site or localized in a group of lymph nodes; asymptomatic
II	Two or more lymph nodes in the area or on the same side of the diaphragm
III	Involves lymph node regions on both sides of the diaphragm, involves adjacent organ or spleen
IV	Diffuse disease, least favorable prognosis

Treatment. Well-established treatment regimens are now being used to combat this illness. Both radiation therapy and chemotherapy are used in accordance with the clinical stage of the disease. The combination of nitrogen mustard, vincristine sulfate (Oncovin), procarbazine hydrochloride, and prednisone is a common protocol. It is referred to as the MOPP regimen. Another drug combination currently being used is doxorubicin hydrochloride (Adriamycin), bleomycin, vinblastine sulfate, and dacarbazine (ABVD). Cure is primarily related to the stage of disease at diagnosis. Long-term prognosis is excellent.

Nursing care. Nursing care is mainly directed toward the symptomatic relief of the side effects of radiation therapy and chemotherapy. Education of the patient and family is paramount because most patients are cared for in the home. The nurse should explain the myriad of diagnostic tests to be performed and prepare the child for the typical procedures and aftereffects. After a lymphangiogram, for example, the skin and urine may take on a bluish color.

Children and parents should be prepared to deal with the impact on self-image. The school nurse should be contacted to implement a schedule that will promote growth and development while preventing overfatigue. A common side effect of irradiation is malaise. The adolescent tires easily and may be irritable and anorectic. The skin in the treated area may be sensitive and must be protected against exposure to sunlight and irritation. After treatment, a sun-blocking agent containing para-aminobenzoic acid (PABA) should be used to prevent burning. The attending physician may prescribe an ointment to relieve itching. Nothing should be applied to the treatment area without the recommendation of the physician. There may be diarrhea after abdominal irradiation. The patient *does not* become radioactive during or after therapy.

After splenectomy, the patient faces the long-term risk of serious infection. This risk is explained to the

table 26-4 *The Effects of Chronic Illness on Growth and Development**

AGE	FEATURE	EFFECT
Infancy	Trust	A visible defect can delay bonding. Prolonged illness may separate the child from the family. Irritability promotes parental negativity.
Toddler	Autonomy	Physical restrictions impede the development of motor and language skills. Toilet training may be delayed. Actual fear may erode self-confidence. Separation anxiety occurs.
Preschooler	Initiative	Impaired ability to experience the world outside of the family impedes social skills. Overprotective parents delay learning self-discipline. Child may develop to a negative body image. Child develops a sense of guilt at his or her inability master tasks.
School age	Industry	Loss of grade level in school because of illness and inability to participate or compete can lead to a sense of inferiority. Sense of independence and accomplishment can be lost. Being different from peers may impede the child's sense of belonging.
Adolescent	Identity	Adolescent feels a loss of control and an inability to conform with peers. The developing self-concept may become negative. The adolescent may grieve for a lost ability. Enforced dependence may impair plans for future goals. Rebellion results in decreased compliance.

*Chronic illness can impede growth and development. The nurse should reinforce teaching concerning the developmental needs of chronically ill children at different age levels to promote self-acceptance and a positive self-esteem.

parents and adolescent. Temperature elevations of must be monitored carefully. There may also be infection with little or no fever as a result of masking by certain medications. In such cases, cultures of blood, urine, sputum, or stool may need to be taken. Parents or the adolescent are instructed to feel free to call the clinic, particularly if there is a change in the condition or if there is apprehension or confusion about symptoms. Medication readjustments should not be attempted unless specifically advised by the physician.

Emotional support of the adolescent is age appropriate. Nurses must particularly be prepared for periods of anger, which may be directed at them. Suitable outlets, such as the use of a punching bag, allow for the safe direction of anger. Routine use helps to prevent a buildup of tension. Activity is generally regulated by the patient. The physician advises the patient if special precautions are necessary.

The appearance of secondary sexual characteristics and menstruation may be delayed in pubescent patients. Sterility is often a side effect of the treatment. This can be a source of anxiety. Adolescents may be interested in sperm banking before immunosuppressive therapy is initiated. The nurse respects the patient concerns and can be most effective by listening empathetically (Nursing Care Plan 26-2).

NURSING CARE OF THE CHRONICALLY ILL CHILD

CHRONIC ILLNESS

Chronic illness during childhood often impacts growth and development (Table 26-4). Specific programs that foster feelings of security and independence within the limits of the situation are essential. Behavior problems are lessened when patients can verbalize specific concerns with persons sensitive to their problems. To be in school and to be considered one of the group is very important to children. If they feel rejected by and different from their peers, they may be prone to depression. Hospital school programs provide familiarity and enable patients to keep pace with their classmates. The recreational therapist may also be helpful in combating boredom and providing outlets for tension.

Nurses must help patients to accept their body with all its strengths and imperfections. They must develop an awareness of the adolescent's particular fears of forced dependence, bodily invasion, mutilation, rejection, and loss of face, especially within peer groups. The nurse anticipates a certain amount of reluctance to adhere to hospital regulations, which reflects the adolescent's need for self-determination. Recognizing this as an asset rather than a liability enables the nurse to respond creatively.

NURSING CARE PLAN 26-2

The Adolescent Receiving Cancer Chemotherapy

PATIENT DATA: An adolescent is admitted for initiation of chemotherapy. She appears thin, anxious, and fearful. She asks if she is going to die.

SELECTED NURSING DIAGNOSIS   *Deficient knowledge concerning prevention of infection due to myelosuppression*

Outcomes	Nursing Interventions	Rationales
Patient will remain free of infection as evidenced by temperature of 37.1° to 37.6° C (98.7° to 99.6° F); skin and mucous membranes will show no signs of irritation or inflammation. Patient's hemoglobin level will improve with therapy; there will be no recurrence of anemia.	1. Instruct patient about the body's immune system and immunotherapy as age appropriate; use visual aids.	1. A malignant process depresses the immune system at the onset of disease; chemotherapy further suppresses it and causes some physical changes that increase chances of infection.
	2. Monitor WBC count and interpret blood values at patient's level of understanding.	2. Leukopenia (decreased WBCs), which predisposes patient to infection, and thrombocytopenia (decreased platelets), which predisposes patient to bruising and bleeding, are the most serious side effects. Anemia caused by decreased erythrocyte count is also a side effect but is more easily treated.
	3. Place the patient in a private room, avoid crowds, and practice proper handwashing and good personal hygiene; monitor temperature.	3. Bone marrow suppression as a side effect of chemotherapy or radiation predisposes the child to anemia, infection, and bleeding. In addition to treatment effects, patients with leukemia are particularly vulnerable because their bone marrow is depressed as a result of disease; neutropenia may result. Infection can be life threatening.
	4. Observe the mouth and perianal area for infection and bleeding.	4. Ulcerations of mouth and anus are common; meticulous rectal care will prevent natural microbial flora (*Escherichia coli*) from being introduced by a break in the mucosa. Enemas and rectal temperatures are avoided because of this. Stomatitis is a common side effect of chemotherapy.
	5. Use a soft toothbrush, Water-Pik, and soothing mouthwashes.	5. Protecting membranes decreases the likelihood of capillary damage and of mucous membrane breakdown.
	6. Limit exposure to direct sunlight.	6. Photosensitivity is a side effect of some chemotherapeutic drugs.

Continued

NURSING CARE PLAN 26-2—cont'd

SELECTED NURSING DIAGNOSIS *Risk for impaired tissue integrity due to platelet deficit from bone marrow suppression*

Outcomes	Nursing Interventions	Rationales
Patient shows no signs of bleeding, as evidenced by stable vital signs and absence of hematuria, petechiae, and ecchymosis.	1. Observe for hematuria, hematemesis melena, epistaxis, petechiae, and ecchymosis.	1. Bleeding from these sites can occur because of myelosuppression.
	2. Increase fluid intake.	2. Patient may be febrile; a liberal fluid intake also prevents hemorrhagic cystitis. Vomiting from chemotherapy may deplete fluid volume, and the patient may become dehydrated.
	3. Use local measures if necessary to control bleeding.	3. Direct pressure reduces small hemorrhages. Avoid puncture wounds whenever possible; bandages and old blood are promptly removed because they provide media for infection.
	4. Monitor platelet counts and assist the patient in types of safe activity when the count is low.	4. Children with low platelet counts are advised to temporarily avoid activities that might cause bleeding or injury (e.g., skateboarding, contact sports); aspirin is avoided because it destroys platelets.

SELECTED NURSING DIAGNOSIS *Imbalanced nutrition due to stomatitis, nausea, and vomiting*

Outcomes	Nursing Interventions	Rationales
Patient is able to eat frequent small meals; caloric intake is adequate for age.	1. Inspect mouth daily for ulcerations.	1. Mouth lesions may lead to anorexia; early treatment is necessary.
Nausea and vomiting will decrease; patient's weight will stabilize.	2. Serve bland, moist, soft diet.	2. Prevents trauma to mouth and lesions of the esophagus.
	3. Apply local anesthetics to ulcerated areas before meals.	3. Protects lesions and makes eating easier.
	4. Monitor weight.	4. Malnutrition may be present; weight loss is common owing to nature of treatments and side effects of medication, such as nausea and vomiting.
	5. Alert patient to expected reactions to treatment protocol.	5. Preparing patient in advance reduces anxiety.
	6. Give antiemetic before onset of nausea and vomiting.	6. Regularly scheduled antiemetics reduce discomfort of nausea and vomiting.
	7. Suggest appropriate relaxation techniques.	7. Symptoms can be controlled or lessened by relaxation techniques.

SELECTED NURSING DIAGNOSIS *Disturbed body image due to moon face, hair loss*

Outcomes	Nursing Interventions	Rationales
Patient will verbalize some satisfaction with appearance.	1. Allow the adolescent to ventilate feelings about his or her body.	1. Accept all feelings.

NURSING CARE PLAN 26-2—cont'd

Outcomes	Nursing Interventions	Rationales
Patient will participate in self-care. Patient will remain in contact with peers.	2. Provide continuity of care.	2. Teenagers need persons they can trust; continuity of care provides this.
	3. Use wigs, scarfs, eyebrow pencil, false eyelashes. Stress that hair loss is temporary. Suggest clothing that minimizes body changes and enhances appearance.	3. Looking and feeling attractive are morale boosters.
	4. Have the patient draw "How it feels to be sick," "How it feels to be well"; discuss.	4. Indirect communication is helpful for the self-conscious adolescent; drawing provides an outlet for the expression of feelings.
	5. Involve the patient in decision making.	5. Control is important to a teen.
	6. Provide an opportunity for groups.	6. Group identity is a task of adolescence.

SELECTED NURSING DIAGNOSIS   *Fear of death due to treatment or nature of disease*

Outcomes	Nursing Interventions	Rationales
Patient will express two concerns regarding life expectancy. Patient will express hope, although this may be changed from "hope" of cure to prolonged life.	1. Convey empathic understanding of patient's and family's worries, fears, and doubts.	1. Fear of death is like an elephant in a living room that everyone pretends does not exist; by refusing to discuss it, the family can pretend that it will not happen. Because no feelings are shared, each member suffers in isolation; sharing a threat lessens the burden and brings members closer; nevertheless, sharing cannot be forced on persons who are not ready for it.
	2. Determine the patient's perception of diagnosis, for example, "What are your concerns?" and "How can I help?"	2. Misconceptions abound in life-threatening illness because the patient is in crisis.
	3. Support "hope" by clarifying and by educating patient about the disease and side effects.	3. Hope is important to the patient and family members; it may be hope of celebrating a birthday or seeing a special friend; it may be hope that suffering will end.
	4. Avoid discounting the patient by making statements such as "I know exactly how you feel" or "You shouldn't feel that way" or by changing the subject.	4. Expression of feelings is the basis for identifying effective coping methods.
	5. Have patient draw and discuss "the strongest feeling I've had today."	5. The patient can distance himself or herself from feelings through drawings. This makes the feelings less threatening.

?CRITICAL THINKING QUESTION

An adolescent receiving cancer chemotherapy has withdrawn from contact with her peers and states she is not interested in attending school. What is the best response of the nurse?

DEVELOPMENTAL DISABILITIES

Children who have a developmental disability that affects their intellect or ability to cope face some unique difficulties. They may often be overprotected, unable to break away from supervision, and deprived of necessary peer relationships. The pubertal process with its emerging sexuality concerns parents and may precipitate a family crisis.

HOME CARE

Most children with acute and chronic conditions are cared for in the home. Home health care and other community agencies work together to provide holistic care. Respite care provides trained workers who come into the home for brief periods to relieve parents of the responsibility of caring for the child. This enables the parents to shop, do business transactions, or simply take a much-needed vacation. The school systems also share in the responsibility of care, which is crucial if a family is to be successful in home care. One mother, whose 13-year-old daughter has a severe developmental disability (cerebral palsy, blindness, scoliosis, mental retardation), offered the following suggestions for the health care worker assisting in the home:

- Observe how the parents interact with the child.
- Do not wait for the child to cry out for attention, because the youngster may be unable to communicate in this way.
- Watch for facial expressions and body language.
- Post signs above the bed denoting special considerations, such as "Never position on left side" and "Do not feed with plastic spoon."
- Listen to the parents and observe how they attend to the physical needs of the youngster.
- Do not be afraid to ask questions or discuss apprehensions you may feel about your ability to care for the child.
- Be attuned to the needs of other children in the home.
- Be creative in exploring avenues for socialization, because these adolescents are seldom invited to birthday or slumber parties.
- Explore community facilities or support groups that might benefit the family.

CARE OF THE CHRONICALLY ILL CHILD

The chronically ill child must be a contributing member to the family unit. The child and parent will often discard the health care practice when health care activities inhibit development and prevent peer socialization opportunities. The child must be treated normally, avoiding overprotection and overrestriction. Focusing on what the child can do and providing successful experiences is more effective than focusing on the disability.

Involvement of the entire family with the care of the chronically ill child aids in normal family interaction. Respite care opportunities are needed to provide parents with a normal spousal relationship. The child should be integrated into rather than isolated from the community and society. Nurses can assist the child and the family to develop strategies to cope with chronic illness and to promote optimum growth and development. The wellness of the child should be the center of the child's life, rather than the disability.

NURSING CARE OF THE DYING CHILD

FACING DEATH

Facing death is often a difficult personal issue for the nurse. The nurse must understand the grieving process; personal and cultural views concerning that process; the views of a parent losing a child; and the perceptions of the child facing death. Integrating these understandings and helping all involved to cope successfully involves a multidisciplinary approach. The response to a child's death is influenced by whether there was a long period of uncertainty before the death or whether it was a sudden unexpected event. The nurse must show compassion but function in a clinically competent, professional manner. Demonstrating a nonjudgmental approach when the personal or cultural practices of the family conflict with the nurse's own values presents a challenge. Sensitive, effective care can be provided only if the nurse is aware of these needs of the family. The nurse can facilitate the grief process by anticipating psychological and somatic responses and maintaining open communication. The family's efforts to cope, adapt, and grieve must be supported.

The response of the family to the death of the child may initially be manifested by somatic distress such as weakness, anguish, or shortness of breath. A family member may feel detached from the world and have a sense of unreality or disbelief. A sense of guilt and blame may follow ("I should have" or "I could have"). Hostility is a normal response and may drive away those who do not understand its normalcy in the acute grieving process. A restlessness and general irritability or inability to function may follow. Assistance in the care of other children or household responsibilities may be necessary. Nursing priorities include being a patient and family advocate, providing support, and facilitating the grieving process.

table 26-5 *A Child's Response to a Sibling's Death*

AGE	RESPONSE/UNDERSTANDING	PARENT GUIDANCE
Infant	Does not understand concept of death; reacts on emotional level to anxiety of parents	Maintain normal routine. Use a support network to assist in care.
Preschooler	Thinks death is temporary; may blame self for sibling's death	Use accurate terms and simple explanations. Reassure the child and *listen*.
School age	Realizes death is final; may be interested in details of death; may fear parents will die; may try to "take care of" parents	Respond to the child's need for reassurance and security. Refer to death using accurate terms. Allow the child to participate in the funeral and feel useful.
Adolescent	Can understand abstract concept of death but has feelings of own immortality; may express anger at death of sibling	Accept the adolescent's behavior. Encourage communication and discussion.

SELF-EXPLORATION

One important, if not the most important, task to prepare for working with the dying patient is self-exploration. Our own attitudes about life and death affect our nursing practice. Emotions buried deep within can form barriers to effective communication unless they are recognized and released. How nurses have or have not dealt with their own losses affects present lives and the ability to relate to patients. Nurses must recognize that *coping is an active and ongoing process.* At times nurses need compassionate detachment from patients and their families to become revitalized. We must find constructive outlets, such as exercise and music, to maintain equilibrium. An active support system consisting of nonjudgmental people who are not threatened by natural expressions of feelings is crucial. Proper channeling of these emotions can be a valuable part of the empathetic response to others. It is vital that nurses support one another in the work environment.

THE CHILD'S REACTION TO DEATH

Each child, like each adult, approaches death in an individual way, drawing on limited experience. Nurses must become well acquainted with patients and view them within the context of the family and social culture. Their anxiety often centers on symptoms. They fear that treatments may be painful. Nurses must be honest and inform patients about the upcoming procedures in terms the child will understand. Expressing feelings is encouraged: "You seem angry." Sufficient time should be given for a response. Children should be allowed to have as much control as possible regarding what happens to them. This is fostered by including them in decisions that concern their welfare. However, the child should not be offered a choice when there is none. Children often communicate symbolically. The nurse *listens* to what they say to adults, to their toys, and to other children. Crayons and paper are provided for self-expression.

Although age is a factor, the child's level of cognitive development, rather than chronological age, affects the response to death (Table 26-5). Children younger than 5 years of age are mainly concerned with separation from their parents and abandonment. (Even adults are threatened by thoughts of dying alone.) Preschool children respond to questions about death by relying on their experience and by turning to fantasy. They may believe death is reversible or that they are in some way responsible. Children do not develop a realistic concept of death as a permanent biological process until 9 or 10 years of age.

Dying adolescents face conflicts between their treatment regimens and their need to establish independence from their parents and conformity with their peers. This leads to anger and resentment, which are often displaced onto hospital staff members. An atmosphere of acceptance and nonjudgmental listening allows adolescents freedom to ventilate their hostility in a nonthreatening environment. Nursing Care Plan 26-3 specifies nursing interventions for the dying child.

NURSING **TIP**

Brothers and sisters often feel neglected and lonely. They are frustrated because they are unable to comfort their parents and loved ones. They need to be included in the plan of care.

NURSING CARE PLAN 26-3

The Dying Child

PATIENT DATA: The parents of a terminally ill school-age child sit stoic and silent at the bedside of their child. The child appears cranky and withdrawn and states he wants to go home and see his friends.

SELECTED NURSING DIAGNOSIS *Death anxiety (family members) due to potential death of child*

Outcomes	Nursing Interventions	Rationales
Parents will express two anxieties to the nurse. Communications among parents, other children, patient, and nurse remain open.	1. Remain available to family as child grows weaker.	1. Nurse's presence provides support.
	2. Give parents permission to talk and grieve about the upcoming death and to think about funeral arrangements if they choose.	2. Helps to prepare family for the inevitable; sorts out and identifies actual sources of feelings.
	3. Involve siblings in plans and progress of brother or sister.	3. Siblings will feel less isolated.
	4. Provide permission for laughter, play, friends (make every day count).	4. Laughter and play reduce tension.
	5. Suggest that overprotection and attention, even when provided out of love, can be detrimental to the dying child.	5. Child will feel more in control if not overprotected.
	6. Encourage family to maintain as normal a lifestyle as possible, and encourage each member to take time for his or her own needs (continue to go to hairdresser, a movie—whatever was previously enjoyed).	6. When all members are taking care of themselves, they will have more energy to cope with crises.
	7. Facilitate honesty about child's imminent death among family members and the patient.	7. Information helps to relieve anxiety.
	8. Explain that family members often cannot support one another, because each grieves in his or her own way.	8. Explaining this to the family helps to relieve the guilt stemming from irritability or anger.
	9. Recognize that grief is often expressed as anger.	9. Anger is a natural emotion; it is not fearsome in itself, although its expression may be. Family has a right to all feelings.
	10. Provide for ventilation of guilt ("If only I had taken her to the physician sooner" and the like).	10. Prevents accumulation or repression of guilt.
	11. Suggest meditation, progressive relaxation, guided imagery.	11. Helps to reduce stress.

SELECTED NURSING DIAGNOSIS *Anxiety (dying child) due to pain, isolation, lack of information*

Outcomes	Nursing Interventions	Rationales
Child will verbalize feelings of comfort; if nonverbal, child rests comfortably, with no crying. Child is not isolated.	1. Administer pain relievers as necessary.	1. Child may deny pain because of fear of treatment.

Continued

NURSING CARE PLAN 26-3—cont'd

Outcomes	Nursing Interventions	Rationales
Child will verbalized understanding of treatment, procedures, and outcome as age appropriate.	2. Encourage parents to hold, cuddle, and touch their child as condition permits.	2. Reduces anxiety, thereby reducing pain.
	3. Encourage visits from friends and siblings as age appropriate.	3. Provides emotional support and distraction from the disease.
	4. Decorate hospital room with cards, pictures, mementos; provide telephone as age appropriate.	4. Attractive environment promotes mental health.
	5. Investigate possibility of home or hospice care.	5. Familiar and stable environment may facilitate child's emotional healing.
	6. Explain all procedures.	6. Information relieves anxiety.
	7. Determine child's knowledge about impending death.	7. Nurse can determine level of understanding as age appropriate; this assists in communication.
	8. Answer all questions about death honestly; use open-ended questions to assist patient in the expression of feelings.	8. Conveys that all feelings are acceptable.
	9. Listen to what child says in play.	9. Children work through many fears in play.
	10. Assist child in drawing "a wish," "yesterday, today, tomorrow."	10. Drawings promote the release of feelings and a means of communication.
	11. Allow the child to grieve (behavior may be sulky, cranky, withdrawn).	11. Therapeutic grieving prevents depression.

SELECTED NURSING DIAGNOSIS   *Grieving related to death of child*

Outcomes	Nursing Interventions	Rationales
Family members will have an opportunity to say good-bye.	1. Provide time for family to be alone with the dead child as desired.	1. Family needs to say good-bye.
Family members will express feelings of grief, fear, anger, loss, and guilt.	2. Remain available; express your own loss and grief.	2. Parents derive comfort from knowing others loved their child.
	3. Assist parents in making decisions.	3. Even a simple decision such as when to telephone relatives becomes monumental at this stage.
	4. Offer a beverage.	4. Denotes concern.
	5. Determine spiritual need; refer to pastoral counseling if desired.	5. A belief in God provides strength for many persons; pastoral counselors are effective.
	6. Respect family's beliefs, worldview, and philosophy.	6. Many beliefs may be unconventional.
	7. Listen to expressions of grief.	7. Family needs to repeat story to work through grief.

?CRITICAL THINKING QUESTION

The parents of a child dying from a terminal illness stay in the corner of the child's room, hugging each other and crying. What would be the best nursing intervention?

THE CHILD'S AWARENESS OF HIS OR HER CONDITION

Surprising as it may seem, many investigators have shown that terminally ill children are generally aware of their condition, even when it is carefully concealed. This is reflected in their drawings and play and can be detected through psychological testing. Failure to be honest with children leaves them to suffer alone, unable to express their fears and sadness or even to say good-bye. The family should be referred as needed for support and social services.

PHYSICAL CHANGES OF IMPENDING DEATH

The physical changes that occur with impending death include cool, mottled, cyanotic skin and the slowing down of all body processes. There may be a loss of consciousness, but hearing is intact. Rales in the chest may be heard, which result from increased secretions pooling in the lungs. Movement and neurological signs lessen. If thrashing or groaning occurs, the patient is assessed for pain, and pain relief should be provided.

STAGES OF DYING

The stages of dying as detailed by Kubler-Ross (1975)—denial, anger, bargaining, depression, acceptance, and reaching out to help others—can be applied to parents and siblings as well as to the sick child. (Nurses may also respond with similar feelings.) It is important to accept and support each participant at whatever stage has been reached and not to try to direct progress. Nurses should be available and make their availability known (Box 26-2).

Parents are encouraged to assist in the care of their child. This is facilitated by hospice care and the movement toward supervised home care. It is therapeutic for children to be in their own surroundings whenever possible. Siblings involved in patient care feel less neglected, and the sacrifices they must make become more meaningful. Discussions before death allow them to make amends for their hostilities toward the sick child. The family's religious and spiritual philosophy can be a source of strength and support, as can caring neighbors and friends.

Statistics show a high correlation between the death of a child and divorce. Nurses must observe signs of tension between parents so that suitable intervention may be implemented. Each parent grieves in an individual time and way, often making it difficult for spouses to be supportive of each other. The suppression of strong feelings of guilt, helplessness, and outrage can be devastating. Feelings left unexpressed can cause depression and/or physical illness.

---

box 26-2 | *The Nurse's Role in Helping the Family Cope with the Dying Child*

Listen. Giving advice is a reflection of the nurse's need to "solve the problem."

Provide privacy. Family members need to express their emotions and comfort each other without being embarrassed.

Provide therapeutic intervention. Assess coping behaviors and work with clergy and social workers to meet immediate needs for patient comfort and family coping.

Provide information. Avoid the tenseness of waiting for test results. Be truthful to the child and family.

Use appropriate phrases and open-ended statements. When speaking with a sibling of a child who has died, avoid using terms such as "he isn't hurting anymore," "he is living with God or a deceased relative," or "he has passed away." These terms are confusing to children; explanations should be short, direct, and truthful.

Kubler-Ross (1969) reminds us that dying is the easy part. Helping patients to live until they die is the real challenge. She discusses this beautifully in *A Letter to a Child with Cancer,* which she wrote in response to a child's question, "What is life, what is death, and why do little children have to die?" A library may be consulted to locate this classic book and others published especially to help children and parents with dying and grief. There are several hospices in the United States that limit their services to children. St. Mary's Hospice in Bay Side, New York, is credited with being the first.

>NURSING **TIP**

Grandparents, teachers, and friends are also grieving. Be alert for the emotional responses of all significant others.

key points

- Circulating blood consists of two portions: plasma and formed elements.
- Bone marrow aspiration is one procedure that is helpful in determining disorders of the blood.
- The most common nutritional deficiency of children in the United States is iron-deficiency anemia.
- Sickle cell disease is an inherited defect in the formation of hemoglobin. The cells become crescent shaped and clump together.

- Massive expansion of the bone marrow in thalassemia causes changes in the contour of the child's skull and face.
- Hemophilia A results from a deficiency in coagulation factor VIII, and hemophilia B (Christmas disease) involves a deficiency of factor IX.
- Hemarthrosis (bleeding into the joints) is a characteristic sign of hemophilia A.
- Hemosiderosis (deposits of iron in the organs and tissues) is a complication of multiple transfusions in hemolytic blood disorders.
- Signs of transfusion reactions include chills, itching rash, fever, and headache.
- *Petechiae* are bluish pinpoint lesions on the skin. *Purpura* are groups of adjoining petechiae; *ecchymosis* is an isolated bluish lesion larger than petechiae, and a *hematoma* is a raised ecchymosis.
- Leukemia is the most common form of childhood cancer.
- Diagnostic procedures for patients with blood disorders are often invasive or painful. The nurse prepares and supports the patient and family during these procedures.
- Maintenance of schooling, adequate hydration and nutrition, prevention of infection, promotion of a positive self-image, and meticulous oral hygiene are essential components of nursing care of a leukemic child.
- Reed-Sternberg cells are diagnostic for Hodgkin's disease.
- Children who are chronically ill must be aided in mastering developmental tasks.
- The stages of dying according to Kubler-Ross include denial, anger, bargaining, depression, acceptance, and reaching out to help others.
- The nurse can help the family of a dying child by listening and assessing their needs; reinforcing information; providing privacy; and using appropriate phrases and open-ended statements.

ONLINE RESOURCES

Cooley's Anemia Foundation:
http://www.thalassemia.org

Hematology and Blood Disorders:
http://www.viahealth.org/disease/blood/itp.htm

Non-Hodgkin's Lymphoma:
http://www.oncologychannel.com/nonhodgkins

REVIEW QUESTIONS   *Choose the most appropriate answer.*

1. When the patient experiences apprehension and urticaria while receiving a blood transfusion, the nurse:
   1. Slows the transfusion and takes the patient's vital signs
   2. Observes the child for further transfusion reactions
   3. Stops the transfusion, lets normal saline solution run slowly, and notifies the charge nurse
   4. Stops what he or she is doing and obtains the patient's history

2. The role of platelets in the blood is to:
   1. Carry oxygen to the tissues
   2. Fight germs and overcome infection
   3. Help the body to stop bleeding
   4. Provide nutrition to the body

3. Which of the following principles should the nurse teach the parent concerning administering liquid iron preparations to her child with iron-deficiency anemia?
   1. Allow the preparation to mix with saliva and bathe the teeth before swallowing
   2. Warm the medication before administering
   3. Administer between meals
   4. Administer in the bottle of formula

4. Thalassemia major (Cooley's anemia) is treated primarily with:
   1. A diet high in iron
   2. Multiple blood transfusions
   3. Bed rest until the sedimentation rate is normal
   4. Oxygen therapy

5. Which of the following is a characteristic manifestation of Hodgkin's disease?
   1. Petechiae
   2. Erythematous rash
   3. Enlarged lymph nodes
   4. Pallor

objectives

1. Define each key term listed.
2. Discuss three common gastrointestinal anomalies in infants.
3. Interpret the nursing management of an infant with gastroesophageal reflux.
4. Discuss the postoperative nursing care of an infant with pyloric stenosis.
5. Explain why infants and young children become dehydrated more easily than do adults.
6. Differentiate between three types of dehydration.
7. Trace the route of the pinworm cycle and describe how reinfection takes place.
8. Review the prevention of the spread of thrush in infants and children.
9. Prepare a teaching plan for the prevention of poisoning in children.
10. List two measures to reduce acetaminophen poisoning in children.
11. Indicate the primary source of lead poisoning.

key terms

anasarca (ăn-ă-SĂR-kă, p. 672)
anthelmintics (ănt-hĕl-MĬN-tĭkz, p. 677)
colitis (p. 664)
colonoscopy (p. 657)
currant jelly stools (p. 662)
encopresis (ĕn-kō-PRĒ-sĭs, p. 666)
endoscopy (p. 656)
enterocolitis (ĕn-tĕr-ō-kō-LĪ-tĭs, p. 661)
guarding (p. 675)
herniorrhaphy (hĕr-nē-ŌR-ĕ-fē, p. 664)
homeostasis (hō-mē-ō-STĀ-sĭs, p. 670)
hypertonic (hī-pĕr-TŎN-ĭk, p. 671)
hypotonic (hī-pō-TŎN-ĭk, p. 671)
incarcerated (p. 663)
isotonic (ī-sō-TŎN-ĭk, p. 671)
McBurney's point (p. 675)
parenteral fluids (pĕ-RĔN-tĕr-ăl, p. 670)
peritoneal dialysis (pĕ-rĭ-tō-NĒ-ăl dī-ĂL-ĭ-sĭs, p. 680)
pica (PĪ-kă, p. 680)
plumbism (p. 680)
polyhydramnios (pŏl-ē-hī-DRĂM-nē-ōs, p. 658)
projectile vomiting (p. 658)
pruritus (proo-RĪ-tŭs, p. 657)
rebound tenderness (p. 675)
reflux (p. 665)
sigmoidoscopy (p. 657)
stenosis (p. 658)

OVERVIEW

The gastrointestinal (GI) tract transports and metabolizes nutrients necessary for the life of the cell. It extends from the mouth to the anus. Nutrients are broken down into absorbable products by enzymes from various digestive organs. The anatomy of the digestive tract, with some of the differences between the child and adult, is depicted in Figure 27-1. The primitive digestive tube is formed by the yolk sac and is divided into the foregut, midgut, and hindgut. The foregut evolves into the pharynx, lower respiratory tract, esophagus, stomach, duodenum, and beginning of the common bile duct. The midgut elongates in the fifth fetal week to form the primary intestinal loop. The remainder of the large colon is derived from the primitive hindgut. The liver, pancreas, and biliary tree evolve from the foregut. The anal membrane ruptures at 8 weeks' gestation, forming the anal canal and opening.

A number of procedures are available to determine GI disorders. Laboratory work, such as a complete blood count (CBC) with differential, will reveal anemia, infections, and chronic illness. An elevated erythrocyte sedimentation rate (ESR) is indicative of inflammation. A sequential multiple analysis (SMA 12) will reveal electrolyte and chemical imbalances. X-ray films include GI series, barium enema, and flat plates of the abdomen. Endoscopy allows direct visualization of the GI tract through a flexible lighted tube. Upper endoscopy permits visualization and biopsy of the esophagus, stomach, and duodenum. It is also valuable to remove foreign objects and cauterize bleeding vessels. Visualization

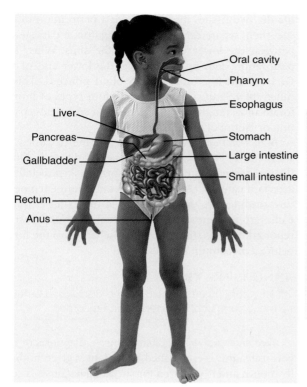

Oral cavity
Pharynx
Esophagus
Liver
Pancreas
Stomach
Gallbladder
Large intestine
Small intestine
Rectum
Anus

FIGURE **27-1** Some of the gastrointestinal system differences between the child and adult. The digestive system consists of the digestive tract and the glands that secrete digestive juices into the digestive tract. This system mechanically and chemically breaks down food and eliminates wastes.

GASTROINTESTINAL SYSTEM

- At birth the resistance of the newborn's intestinal tract to bacterial and viral infection is incompletely developed.
- As children grow, they have higher nutritional, metabolic, and energy needs.
- Children with nausea and vomiting dehydrate more quickly than adults with those symptoms.
- The infant's stomach is small and empties rapidly.
- Newborns produce little saliva until 3 months of age.
- Swallowing is reflex for the first 3 months.
- Hepatic efficiency in the newborn is immature, somtimes causing jaundice.
- The infant's fat absorption is poor because of a decreased pool of bile acid.

of the bile and pancreatic ducts is also possible through endoscopy. The lower colon is inspected by sigmoidoscopy. Colonoscopy provides visualization of the entire colon to the ileocecal valve. Stool cultures and rectal biopsy are also important diagnostic tools. Ultrasonography is a noninvasive procedure useful in visualizing intestinal organs and masses, particularly of the liver and pancreas. Some liver blood tests include alanine aminotransferase (ALT), aspartate aminotransferase (AST) prothrombin time (PT), and partial thromboplastin time (PTT). Liver biopsy may also be indicated. Overall malabsorption tests, such as the 72-hour fecal fat test and the Schilling test (which can determine the absorption capacity of the lower ileum) are also useful.

Symptoms of GI disorders may be manifested by systemic signs such as *failure to thrive* (FTT; failure to develop according to established growth parameters such as height, weight, and head circumference) or jaundice. Pruritus (itching) in the absence of allergy may indicate liver dysfunction. Local manifestations of a GI disorder include pain, vomiting, diarrhea, constipation, rectal bleeding, and hematemesis.

Nursing intervention focuses on providing adequate nutrition and freedom from infection, which can result from malnutrition or depressed immune function. Developmental delays in children should be investigated to determine whether they are related to the GI system. Skin problems in these patients may be related to pruritus from liver disease, irritation from frequent bowel movements, or other disorders. Pain and discomfort may occur during acute episodes; however, they may also result from medication side effects, or they may be referred pain. Cleft lip and cleft palate are discussed in Chapter 14. Anorexia is discussed in Chapter 32, and necrotizing enterocolitis is discussed in Chapter 13.

CONGENITAL DISORDERS

ESOPHAGEAL ATRESIA (TRACHEOESOPHAGEAL FISTULA, TEF)

Pathophysiology. Atresia of the esophagus is caused by a failure of the tissues of the GI tract to separate properly from the respiratory tract early in prenatal life.

The following are the four types of atresia (TEF):

- The upper esophagus and the lower esophagus (leading from the stomach) end in a blind pouch.
- The upper esophagus ends in a blind pouch; the lower esophagus (leading from the stomach) connects to the trachea.
- The upper esophagus is attached to the trachea; the lower esophagus (leading from the stomach) is also attached to the trachea.
- The upper esophagus connects to the trachea; the lower esophagus (leading from the stomach) ends in a blind pouch.

The diagnosis of this condition is based on clinical manifestations and confirmed by x-ray study.

Manifestations. The earliest sign of tracheoesophageal fistula (TEF) occurs prenatally when the mother develops polyhydramnios. When the upper esophagus ends in a blind pouch, the fetus cannot swallow the amniotic fluid, resulting in an accumulation of fluid in the amniotic sac (polyhydramnios). At birth the infant will *vomit* and *choke* when the first feeding is introduced. Because the upper end of the esophagus ends in a blind pouch, the newborn cannot swallow accumulated secretions and will appear to be drooling. Although drooling after age 3 months is related to teething, drooling in a newborn is pathological and is related to atresia. If the upper esophagus enters the trachea, the first feeding will enter the trachea and result in *coughing, choking, cyanosis,* and *apnea.* If the lower end of the esophagus (from the stomach) enters the trachea, air will enter the stomach each time the infant breathes, causing abdominal distention.

> **NURSING TIP**
> Drooling in the newborn is pathological because the salivary glands do not develop for several months.

Treatment and nursing care. The nursing goals involve preventing pneumonia, choking, and apnea in the newborn. Assessment of every newborn during the first feeding is essential. The first feeding usually consists of clear water or colostrum (if breastfed) to minimize the seriousness of aspiration should it occur. If symptoms are noted, the infant is placed on NPO status (nothing by mouth), suctioned to clear the airway, and positioned to drain mucus from the nose and throat. Surgical repair is essential for survival.

IMPERFORATE ANUS

Pathophysiology. Imperforate anus occurs in about 1 of every 5000 live births. The lower GI tract and the anus arise from two different tissues. Early in fetal life the two tissues meet and join; a perforation of tissue then separates them, allowing for a passageway between the lower GI tract and the anus. When this perforation does not take place, the lower end of the GI tract and the anus end in blind pouches. This is called *imperforate anus.* There are four types of imperforate anus, ranging from a stenosis to complete separation or failure of the anus to form.

Manifestations. A routine part of the newborn assessment is determining the patency of the anus. Often the first temperature of the newborn is taken rectally to ascertain patency. (All subsequent and routine temperature readings are usually taken via the axillary route.) Failure to pass meconium in the first 24 hours must be reported. Infants should not be discharged to the home before a meconium stool is passed.

> **NURSING TIP**
> Newborn infants should not be discharged before a meconium stool is observed and recorded.

Treatment and nursing care. Once a diagnosis of imperforate anus is established, the infant is given nothing by mouth and is prepared for surgery. Diagnosis is confirmed by x-ray study or magnetic resonance imaging (MRI). The initial surgical procedure may be a colostomy. Subsequent surgery can reestablish the patency of the anal canal.

PYLORIC STENOSIS

Pathophysiology. Pyloric stenosis (narrowing) is an obstruction at the lower end of the stomach (pylorus) caused by an overgrowth (hypertrophy) of the circular muscles of the pylorus or by spasms of the sphincter. This condition is commonly classified as a congenital anomaly; however, its symptoms do not appear until the infant is 2 or 3 weeks old. Pyloric stenosis is the most common surgical condition of the digestive tract in infancy (Figure 27-2). Its incidence is higher in boys than in girls, and it has a tendency to be inherited.

Manifestations. Vomiting is the outstanding symptom of this disorder. The force progresses until most of the food is ejected a considerable distance from the mouth. This is termed projectile vomiting, and it occurs immediately after feeding. The vomitus contains mucus and ingested milk. The infant is constantly hungry and will eat again immediately after vomiting. Dehydration as evidenced by sunken fontanel, inelastic skin, and decreased urination, as well as malnutrition can develop. An olive-shaped mass may be felt in the right upper quadrant of the abdomen. Ultrasonography or scintiscans are commonly used today for diagnostic purposes, because it is noninvasive and accurate. In

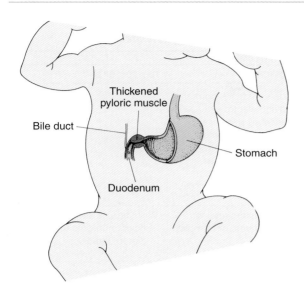

FIGURE **27-2** Pyloric stenosis. Hypertrophy or thickening of the pyloric sphincter blocks the stomach contents, causing the infant to regurgitate forcefully. Serious electrolyte imbalances ultimately occur, and surgery is necessary to correct the condition.

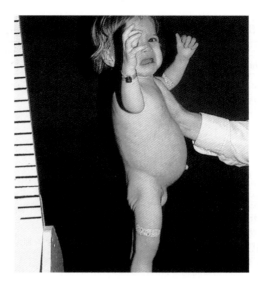

FIGURE **27-3** A child with celiac disease. Note that the classic profile of a child with a malabsorption syndrome is an enlarged abdomen with atrophy of the buttocks.

severe cases the outline of the distended stomach and peristaltic waves are visible during feeding.

Treatment. The surgery performed for pyloric stenosis is called a *pyloromyotomy* (*pylorus, myo,* "muscle," and *tomy,* "incision of"). The surgeon incises the pyloric muscle to enlarge the opening so that food may easily pass through it again. This is done as soon as possible if the infant is not dehydrated.

Nursing care. The dehydrated infant is given intravenous (IV) fluids preoperatively to restore fluid and electrolyte balance. If this is not done, shock may occur during surgery. Thickened feedings may be given until the time of operation in hopes that some nutrients will be retained. The physician prescribes the degree of thickness of the formula, which is given by teaspoon or through a nipple with a large hole. The infant is burped *before* as well as *during* feedings to remove any gas accumulated in the stomach. The feeding is done slowly, and the infant is handled gently and as little as possible. The infant is placed on the right side after feedings to facilitate drainage into the intestine. Fowler's position is preferred to aid gravity in passing milk through the stomach (see Fowler's sling, Figure 27-7). If vomiting occurs, the nurse may be instructed to *refeed* the infant. Charting of the feeding includes time, type, and amount offered; amount taken and retained; and type and amount of vomiting. The nurse also notes whether the infant appeared hungry after the feeding or if vomiting occurred again.

The nurse obtains and records a baseline weight and weighs the infant at about the same time each morning. Other factors to be charted include the type and number of stools and the color of urine and frequency of voiding (intake and output). Position is changed frequently because the infant is weak and vulnerable to pneumonia. All procedures designed to protect from infection must be strictly carried out.

The care of the infant after surgery includes a careful observation of vital signs and the administration of IV fluids. The wound site is inspected frequently (see Chapter 22 for postoperative care). The surgery involves cutting into the hypertrophied muscle but *not through the mucous membrane of the bowel;* therefore the infant will not need nasogastric decompression postoperatively and will be able to resume oral feedings shortly after recovering from anesthesia. The physician prescribes oral feedings of small amounts of glucose water that gradually increase until a regular formula can be taken and retained. Overfeeding is avoided, and the nurse reviews feeding techniques with parents. The diaper is placed low over the abdomen to prevent contamination of the wound site (Clinical Pathway 27-1).

CELIAC DISEASE

Pathophysiology. Celiac disease is also known as *gluten enteropathy* and *sprue* and is the leading malabsorption problem in children. The cause is thought to be an inherited disposition with environmental triggers (Figure 27-3).

CLINICAL PATHWAY 27-1 | *An Interdisciplinary Plan of Care for the Infant with Pyloric Stenosis*

PATIENT/FAMILY INTERMEDIATE OUTCOMES			
NURSING DIAGNOSIS	**DAY: ADMISSION**	**DAY: POSTOP 1**	**DAY: POSTOP 2**
Deficient fluid volume related to effects of persistent vomiting	Child shows improved fluid and electrolyte balance.	Child demonstrates normal fluid and electrolyte balance, as evidenced by normal urine output (1 mL/kg/hr), moist mucous membranes, good skin turgor, laboratory values within normal limits.	→
Imbalanced nutrition: less than body requirements related to persistent vomiting	Child stops vomiting.	Child ingests and retains small amounts of formula.	Child ingests and retains sufficient nutrients to meet dietary needs.
Acute pain related to incision, muscle cutting and manipulation during surgery		Child has signs of pain recognized and interventions are promptly implemented. Child experiences minimal levels of pain.	→
Deficient knowledge related to treatments, surgery, postoperative care	Parents verbalize understanding of treatments and surgery.	Parents verbalize understanding of postoperative pain management, feeding, and incision care.	Parents verbalize understanding of home care and follow-up needs.

CARE INTERVENTION CATEGORIES			
	DAY: ADMISSION	**DAY: POSTOP 1**	**DAY: POSTOP 2**
Consults	Surgical consult		
Labs	CBC, electrolytes Repeat electrolytes prn to monitor CL^- and CO_2 values		
Medications and IVs	IV fluids: maintenance and replacement Give acetaminophen with codeine or acetaminophen prn for pain	Saline or heparin lock IV when tolerating PO fluids.	Discontinue IV if tolerating PO fluids.

Modified from Bowden, V., Dickey, S., & Greenberg, C. (1998). *Children and their families: The continuum of care.* Philadelphia: W.B. Saunders.

Manifestations. Symptoms are not evident until 6 months to 2 years of age, when foods containing gluten are introduced to the infant. Gluten is found in wheat, barley, oats, and rye. Repeated exposure to gluten damages the villi in the mucous membranes of the intestine, resulting in malabsorption of food. The infant presents with failure to thrive. *Stools are large, bulky, and frothy* because of undigested contents. The infant is irritable. Diagnosis is confirmed by serum IgA test and small bowel biopsy. The characteristic profile of a child with a malabsorption syndrome is abdominal distention with atrophy of the buttocks.

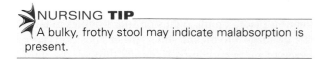

NURSING **TIP**

A bulky, frothy stool may indicate malabsorption is present.

Treatment and nursing care. The treatment involves a lifelong diet restricted in wheat, barley, oats, and rye. It is a nursing challenge to teach the family the importance of dietary compliance. A professional nutritionist or dietitian can aid in identifying foods that are gluten free. Long-term bowel pathology can occur if dietary compliance is not lifelong.

CLINICAL PATHWAY 27-1—cont'd

	CARE INTERVENTION CATEGORIES		
	DAY: ADMISSION	**DAY: POSTOP 1**	**DAY: POSTOP 2**
Nutrition	NPO	Give 10 ml oral electrolyte solution after recovered from anesthesia; start pyloric refeeding protocol (increasing feeding volumes from clear fluids to dilute to full-strength formula); repeat previous step if emesis × 1, notify surgeon if emesis × 2.	Give full-strength formula at normal feeding volumes.
Pain management	Give acetaminophen with codeine or plain (see Medications above) Flex knees; position to avoid stretching abdominal muscles Burp frequently to avoid abdominal distention	→	→
Procedures	Nasogastric (NG) tube to gravity drainage	Discontinue NG tube before starting feedings.	
Radiology	Sonogram of abdomen and barium study as needed to confirm diagnosis		
Teaching/discharge planning	Teach parents about pre-operative care routines Teach parents about surgical routines; review postoperative care	Teach parents methods of pain assessment and management; reintroduce feedings; provide incision care. Assess what supplies will be needed at home (medications, dressings) and ability of parents to obtain them.	Evaluate parent's ability to manage pain, feed, and care for incision; review techniques prn. Discharge child when full oral feedings are tolerated.
Vital signs/baseline parameters	Vital signs with blood pressure on admission and q 4 hr	→	→
	Daily weight	→	→
	Urine specific gravity each shift	→	→
	Intake and output	→	→

HIRSCHSPRUNG'S DISEASE (AGANGLIONIC MEGACOLON)

Pathophysiology. Hirschsprung's disease occurs when there is an absence of ganglionic innervation to the muscle of a segment of the bowel. This usually happens in the lower portion of the sigmoid colon. Because of the absence of nerve cells, there is a lack of normal peristalsis. This results in chronic constipation. Ribbonlike stools are seen as feces pass through the narrow segment. The portion of the bowel nearest to the obstruction dilates, causing abdominal distention (Figure 27-4). It is seen more often in boys than girls and has familial tendencies. The incidence is approximately 1 in 5000 live births.

There is a higher incidence in children with Down syndrome. The condition may be acute or chronic.

Manifestations. In the newborn, failure to pass meconium stools within 24 to 48 hours may be a symptom of Hirschsprung's disease. In the infant, constipation, ribbonlike stools, abdominal distention, anorexia, vomiting, and failure to thrive may be evident. Often the parent brings the young child to the clinic after trying several over-the-counter laxatives to treat the constipation without success. If the child is untreated, other signs of intestinal obstruction and shock may be seen. The development of enterocolitis (inflammation of the small bowel and colon) is a serious complication. It may

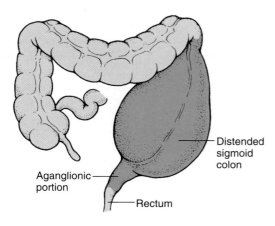

FIGURE **27-4** Hirschsprung's disease (megacolon). There is no ganglionic nerve innervation or peristalsis in the narrowed section. The adjacent bowel becomes enlarged, causing distention of the abdomen.

be signaled by fever, explosive stools, and depletion of strength. Diagnostic evaluation usually includes a barium enema and rectal biopsy, which shows a lack of innervation. Anorectal manometry tests the strength of the internal rectal sphincter. In this procedure a balloon catheter is placed into the rectum, and the pressure exerted against it is measured.

Treatment and nursing care. Megacolon is treated by surgery. The impaired part of the colon is removed, and an anastomosis of the intestine is performed. In newborns a temporary colostomy may be necessary, and more extensive repair may follow at about 12 to 18 months of age. Closure of the colostomy follows in a few months.

Nursing care is age dependent. In the newborn, detection is a high priority. As the child grows older, careful attention to a history of constipation and diarrhea is important. Signs of undernutrition, abdominal distention, and poor feedings are suspect.

Because the distended bowel in a child with megacolon provides a larger mucous membrane surface area that will come in contact with fluid inserted during an enema, an increased absorption of the fluid can be anticipated. For this reason, when a child is given an enema at home, normal saline solution, not tap water, is used. Tap water enemas in infants and small children can lead to water intoxication and death. Parents can obtain normal saline solution from the pharmacy without prescription, or they can make it at home by using one half of a teaspoon of noniodized salt to 1 cup of lukewarm tap water. The amount of fluid administered should be determined by the health care provider. The nurse stresses to parents the importance of adding salt to water. Postoperative care of children is discussed in Chapter 22.

INTUSSUSCEPTION

Pathophysiology. Intussusception (*intus,* "within" and *suscipere,* "to receive") is a slipping of one part of the intestine into another part just below it (Figure 27-5). It is often seen at the ileocecal valve, where the small intestine opens into the ascending colon. The *mesentery,* a double fan-shaped fold of peritoneum that covers most of the intestine and is filled with blood vessels and nerves, is also pulled along. Edema occurs. At first this telescoping of the bowel causes intestinal obstruction, but strangulation takes place as peristalsis forces the structures more tightly. This portion may burst, causing peritonitis.

Intussusception generally occurs in boys between 3 months and 6 years of age who are otherwise healthy. Its frequency decreases after age 36 months. Occasionally the condition corrects itself without treatment. This is termed a spontaneous reduction. However, because the patient's life is in danger, the physician does not waste time waiting for this to occur. The prognosis is good when the patient is treated within 24 hours.

Manifestations. In typical cases the onset is sudden. The infant feels severe pain in the abdomen, as evidenced by loud cries, straining efforts, and kicking and drawing of the legs toward the abdomen. At first there is comfort between pains, but the intervals shorten and the condition becomes worse. The child vomits. The stomach contents are green or greenish yellow (this results from bile stain), and the contents are described as bilious. Bowel movements diminish, and little flatus is passed. Movements of blood and mucus that contain no feces are common about 12 hours after the onset of the obstruction; these are termed currant jelly stools. The child's fever may run as high as 41.1° C (106° F), and signs of shock, such as sweating, weak pulse, and shallow, grunting respirations are evident. The abdomen is rigid.

Treatment and nursing care. Intussusception is an *emergency,* and because of the severity of symptoms, most parents contact a physician promptly. The diagnosis is determined by the history and physical findings. The physician may feel a sausage-shaped mass in the right upper portion of the abdomen during bimanual rectal and abdominal palpation. Abdominal films also may indicate the mass. A barium enema is the treatment of choice, with surgery scheduled if reduction is not achieved. The recurrence rate after barium enema reduction is approximately 10%.

During the operation a small incision is made into the abdomen, and the wayward intestine is "milked" back into position. The intestine is inspected for gangrene; if all is well, the abdomen is sutured. Barring complications, recovery is straightforward. If the intestine cannot be reduced or if gangrene has set in, a bowel resection is done and the affected area is removed.

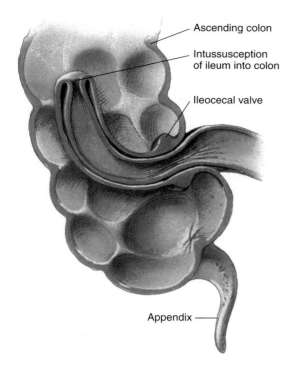

FIGURE **27-5** Intussusception. The most common type begins at or near the ileocecal valve, pushing into the cecum and on to the colon. At first the obstruction is partial, but complete obstruction occurs as the bowel becomes inflamed and edematous.

The cut end of the ileum is joined to the cut end of the colon; this is called an *anastomosis*. Routine preoperative and postoperative care is discussed in Chapter 22.

MECKEL'S DIVERTICULUM

Pathophysiology. During fetal life the intestine is attached to the yolk sac by the vitelline duct. A small blind pouch may form if this duct fails to disappear completely. This condition is termed Meckel's diverticulum. It usually occurs near the ileocecal valve, and it may be connected to the umbilicus by a cord. A fistula may also form. This sac is subject to inflammation, much like the appendix. This disorder is the most common congenital malformation of the GI tract. It is seen more often in boys.

Manifestations. Symptoms may occur at any age but appear most often before 2 years of age. Painless bleeding from the rectum is the most common sign. Bright red or dark red blood is more usual than tarry stools. Abdominal pain may or may not be present. In some persons it may exist without causing symptoms. Barium enema and radionuclide scintigraphy are useful in diagnosing Meckel's diverticulum. X-ray films are not helpful because the pouch is so small that it may not appear on the screen.

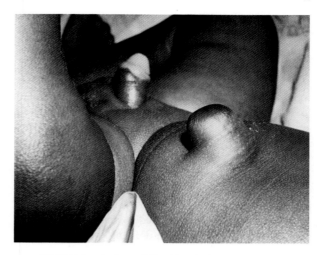

FIGURE **27-6** An umbilical hernia in an infant boy.

Treatment and nursing care. The diverticulum is removed by surgery. Nursing care is the same as for the patient undergoing exploration of the abdomen. Because this condition appears suddenly and bleeding causes parental anxiety, emotional support is of particular importance.

HERNIAS

Pathophysiology. An *inguinal* hernia is a protrusion of part of the abdominal contents through the inguinal canal in the groin. It is more common in boys than in girls. It is also commonly seen in preterm infants. An *umbilical* hernia is a protrusion of a portion of intestine through the umbilical ring (an opening in the muscular area of the abdomen through which the umbilical vessels pass, Figure 27-6). This type of hernia appears as a soft swelling covered by skin, which protrudes when the infant cries or strains. Hernias may be present at birth (congenital) or may be acquired, and they can vary in size. A hernia is called reducible if it can be put back into place by gentle pressure; if this cannot be done, it is called an irreducible or an incarcerated (constricted) hernia. Incarceration occurs more often in infants under 10 months of age. Hernias may be bilateral.

Manifestations. The infant with a hernia may be relatively free of symptoms. Irritability, fretfulness, and constipation are sometimes evident. The diagnosis is made when physical examination shows a mass in the area that reappears from time to time, particularly when the child cries or strains. A *strangulated* hernia occurs when the intestine becomes caught in the passage and the blood supply is diminished. This happens more often during the first 6 months of life. Vomiting and severe abdominal pain are present. Emergency surgery is necessary if strangulation occurs, and in some cases a bowel resection is performed.

Treatment and nursing care. Hernias are successfully repaired by the surgical operation called a herniorrhaphy. This is a relatively simple procedure and is well tolerated by the child. Most children are scheduled for same-day surgery units. The benefits of this method are both economic and psychological. Parents are instructed to bring the fasting child to the hospital about 1 hour before surgery. Parents remain with the child during the entire time except during the actual procedure. They are encouraged to assist in routine postoperative care.

Often no dressing is applied to the wound. Sometimes a waterproof collodion dressing, which looks like clear nail polish, is applied. Postoperative care is directed toward keeping the wound clean. Diapers are left open for this purpose. Wet diapers are changed frequently.

DISORDERS OF MOTILITY

GASTROENTERITIS

Pathophysiology. Gastroenteritis involves an inflammation of the stomach and the intestines; colitis involves an inflammation of the colon; *enterocolitis* involves an inflammation of the colon and the small intestine. The most common noninfectious causes of diarrhea involve food intolerance, overfeeding, improper formula preparation, or ingestion of high amounts of sorbitol (a substance found in sweetened "sugar-free" products). The priority problem in diarrhea is fluid and electrolyte imbalance and failure to thrive.

Treatment and nursing care. Treatment is focused on identifying and eradicating the cause. Nursing responsibilities include teaching parents and caregivers proper and age-appropriate diet and feeding techniques. The priority goal of care includes preventing fluid and electrolyte imbalance.

Oral rehydrating solutions such as Pedialyte, Lytren, Ricelyte, and Resol, are used for infants in small frequent feedings. Although formula feeding is withheld, breastfeeding can accompany oral rehydration therapy (ORT) because of its osmolarity, antimicrobial properties, and enzyme content.

The nursing care of gastroenteritis includes maintaining intake and output records and providing skin care and frequent diaper changes to prevent excoriation from the frequent stools. Parents should be taught good handwashing techniques, proper food handling, and principles of cleanliness and infection prevention. The infant should be weighed daily, observed for dehydration

or overhydration, and kept warm. Enteric precautions and standard precautions should be used to prevent the spread of infection (see Appendix A). Sometimes parents need help in interpreting food labels to avoid foods to which their child may be allergic. Box 27-1 lists some terms that often need clarification for the parents of a child who is food intolerant.

VOMITING

Pathophysiology. Vomiting, a common symptom during infancy and childhood, results from sudden contractions of the diaphragm and muscles of the stomach. It must be evaluated in relation to the child's overall health status. Persistent vomiting requires investigation because it results in dehydration and electrolyte imbalance. The continuous loss of hydrochloric acid and sodium chloride from the stomach can cause *alkalosis.* In this condition the acid-base balance of the body becomes disturbed because of a loss of chlorides and potassium. This can result in death if left untreated.

Manifestations. The child may vomit from various causes. Some stem from improper feeding techniques that should be assessed by the nurse. Sometimes the difficulty lies with formula intolerance. The introduction of foods of a different consistency may also precipitate this symptom.

Other causes of vomiting are systemic illness such as increased intracranial pressure or infection. Aspiration pneumonia is a serious complication of vomiting. In aspiration, vomitus is drawn into the air passages on inspiration, causing immediate death in extreme cases. Health professionals and laypersons should become familiar with lifesaving procedures such as cardiopulmonary resuscitation (CPR) for use in such emergencies.

Treatment and nursing care. To prevent vomiting the nurse must carefully feed and burp the infant. Treatments are avoided immediately after feedings. The infant is handled as little as possible after feedings. To prevent aspiration of vomitus the nurse places the infant on

---

box 27-1 *Clarifying Food Labels*

Ingredient	What It May Contain
Binder	Egg
Bulking agent	Soy
Casein	Cow's milk (often in canned tuna)
Coagulant	Egg
Emulsifier	Egg
Protein extender	Soy

the right side following feedings. When an older child begins to vomit, the head is turned to one side, and an emesis basin and tissues are provided.

Factors to be charted include time, amount, color (e.g., bloody, bile-stained), consistency, force, frequency, and whether or not vomiting was preceded by nausea or by feedings. IV fluids may be given. Oral fluids are withheld for a short time to allow the stomach to rest. Gradually, sips of water are given according to the infant's tolerance and condition. The infant's intake and output are carefully recorded so that the physician is able to compare the urine output with the total fluid intake.

Drugs such as trimethobenzamide (Tigan) or promethazine (Phenergan) may be prescribed when vomiting is persistent. They are available in rectal suppository form. The nurse lubricates the suppository and inserts it into the rectum, where it dissolves. Slight pressure is exerted over the anus for a short time to ensure that the suppository is not expelled. Charting includes the time administered and whether or not vomiting subsided.

GASTROESOPHAGEAL REFLUX

Pathophysiology. Gastroesophageal reflux (GER, or chalasia) results when the lower esophageal sphincter is relaxed or not competent, which allows stomach contents to be easily regurgitated into the esophagus.

The term *chalasia* is derived from the Greek word *chalasis,* which means "relaxation." Although many infants have this condition to a small degree, about 1 in 300 to 1 in 1000 have significant reflux and associated complications. The condition is associated with neuromuscular delay and is often seen in preterm infants and children with neuromuscular disorders, such as cerebral palsy and Down syndrome. In many infants the symptoms decrease around age 12 months, when the child stands upright and eats more solid foods.

Manifestations. Symptoms include vomiting, weight loss, and failure to thrive. The vomiting occurs within the first and second weeks of life. The infant is fussy and hungry. Respiratory problems can occur when vomiting stimulates the closure of the epiglottis and the infant presents with apnea. Aspiration of vomitus can also occur.

Treatment and nursing care. A careful history is taken. Of particular interest are when the vomiting started, type of formula, type of vomiting, feeding techniques, and the infant's eating in general. Tests used to determine the presence of GER include a barium swallow under fluoroscopy or esophagoscopy. Esophageal sphincter pressure may also be measured. Prolonged esophageal pH monitoring is one of the most definitive diagnostic tests and helps to determine the acuity of the disease and the course of treatment.

Therapy depends on the severity of symptoms. Some parents need only reassurance and education about feeding the infant. The routine includes careful burping, avoiding overfeeding (which distends the stomach), and proper positioning. Medication and surgical intervention may be required in infants with more complicated GER. Parents are instructed to burp the infant well. Feedings are thickened with cereal (1 teaspoon to 1 tablespoon of cereal per ounce of formula). After being fed, the infant is placed in an upright position or propped on the right side. The body is inclined about 30 to 40 degrees, and the infant is held in place by a Fowler's sling (Figure 27-7). Sitting upright in an infant seat is not recommended because it increases intra-abdominal pressure. The upright prone position has been recommended for the infant with GER. This is an exception to the supine (back) sleep position recommended for healthy infants. Medications that relax the pyloric sphincter and promote stomach emptying may be used, such as metoclopramide (Reglan). The medication is administered before meals. Side effects such as drowsiness or restlessness can occur. Cimetidine (Tagamet) or ranitidine (Zantac) may be prescribed to reduce stomach acid and prevent the development of esophagitis.

DIARRHEA

Pathophysiology. Diarrhea in the infant cannot be defined in the same way as diarrhea in the adult. The number of stools per day is not often significant in the infant. Diarrhea in infancy is a sudden increase in stools from the infant's normal pattern, with a *fluid*

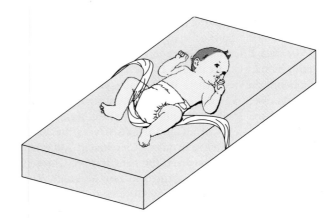

FIGURE **27-7** Fowler's sling. Fowler's sling is used to maintain Fowler's position and to prevent the infant from sliding down to the foot of the bed. The bed is in Fowler's position; the rolled blanket is tucked under the mattress on each side at armpit level; when the infant is in the side-lying position or prone, the legs *straddle* the sling to maintain positioning.

consistency and a *color* that is green or contains mucus or blood. *Acute sudden diarrhea* is most often caused by an inflammation, an infection, or a response to a medication, food, or poisoning. *Chronic diarrhea* lasts for more than 2 weeks and may be indicative of a malabsorption problem, long-term inflammatory disease, or allergic responses. *Infectious diarrhea* is caused by viral, bacterial, or parasitic infection and usually involves gastroenteritis.

> ⚡NURSING **TIP**_____
> Green, watery stools may indicate diarrhea in infants.

Manifestations. The symptoms of diarrhea may be mild or extremely severe. The stools are watery and are expelled with force (explosive stools). They may be yellowish green. The infant becomes listless, refuses to eat, and loses weight. The temperature may be elevated, and the infant may vomit. Dehydration is evidenced by sunken eyes and fontanel and by dry skin, tongue, and mucous membranes. Urination may become less frequent. In severe cases the excessive loss of bicarbonate from the GI tract results in acidosis.

Infectious diarrhea in infants is commonly caused by the rotavirus that often occurs in day care centers; by *Escherichia coli,* which is caused by lack of hygiene or poorly cooked foods; by *Salmonella* from contaminated food or pet (especially turtles) contact; by *Shigella;* and by other organisms. *Clostridium difficile* infection often follows prolonged antibiotic therapy. *Giardia lamblia* is an intestinal protozoan that causes diarrhea. It is spread by contaminated water, unsanitary conditions, and fecal contamination by animals. Prevention is important and centers around teaching the basics of hygienic practices, handwashing, and the use of disinfectants.

Treatment and nursing care. Mild diarrhea in older children may be treated at home under a physician's direction, provided there is a suitable caregiver. Treatment is essentially the same. The intestine is rested by reducing the intake of solid foods. Clear fluids, fruit juice, gelatin, and carbonated drinks have a low electrolyte content and are avoided. Caffeinated sodas act as a diuretic and can worsen the dehydration. Chicken broth is often high in sodium and not advisable. The BRAT diet (bananas, rice, applesauce, and toast) is not nutritionally sound enough to support growth and development. ORT solutions such as Pedialyte or Infalyte in liquid or frozen (ice pop) form are preferred, with the gradual introduction of a soft, bland diet. A regular intake is usually resumed within 2 to 3 days. Nursing Care Plan 27-1 provides nursing interventions for the care of a child with diarrhea.

CONSTIPATION

Pathophysiology. Constipation is difficult or infrequent defecation with the passage of hard, dry fecal material. There may be associated symptoms, such as abdominal discomfort or blood-streaked stools.

Manifestations. The frequency of bowel movements varies widely in children. There may be periods of diarrhea or encopresis (constipation with fecal soiling). Constipation may be a symptom of other disorders, particularly obstructive conditions. Diet, culture, and social, psychological, and familial patterns may also influence its occurrence. The use of laxatives and enemas should be discouraged. Most children use the bathroom every day, but they may be hurried and have an incomplete bowel movement. Some children are embarrassed or even afraid to use school or public bathrooms.

Treatment and nursing care. Evaluation begins with a thorough history of dietary and bowel habits. Some infants respond to formula with a high iron content by developing constipation. Changing to a low-iron formula may be helpful. The frequency, color, and consistency of the stool are noted. The nurse inquires about any medication the child may be taking. The parents are asked to define what they mean by constipation. Parent teaching concerning the prevention of constipation is essential.

Dietary modifications include adding more roughage in the diet. Foods high in fiber include whole-grain breads and cereals, raw vegetables and fruits, bran, and popcorn for older children. Increasing fluid intake is also important. A stool softener such as docusate sodium (Colace) may be prescribed. The child is encouraged to try to move the bowels at the same time each day to establish a routine. The child should not be hurried. Increased exercise may help sedentary children.

FLUID AND ELECTROLYTE IMBALANCE
Principles of Fluid Balance in Children

Infants and small children have different proportions of body water and body fat from those of adults (Figure 27-8), and the water needs and water losses of the infant (per unit of body weight) are greater. In children under 2 years of age, *surface area* is particularly important in fluid and electrolyte balance because more water is lost through the skin than through the kidneys. The surface area of the infant is from two to three times greater than that of the adult in proportion to body volume or body weight. *Metabolic rate* and *heat production* are also two to three times greater in infants per kilogram of body weight. This produces more waste products, which must be diluted to be excreted. It also stimulates respiration, which causes increased evaporation through the lungs.

The Child with Gastroenteritis (Diarrhea/Vomiting)

PATIENT DATA: An 11-month-old infant is admitted with a history of diarrhea for several days and vomiting related to food ingestion. A diaper rash is evident, and skin tissue turgor is poor.

SELECTED NURSING DIAGNOSIS — *Deficient fluid volume related to diarrhea and/or vomiting as evidenced by weight loss, output greater than intake, emesis, liquid stools, decreased urine output, abdominal distension/rebound tenderness, excoriation of perianal mucosa, hypotension, increased pulse rate, change in skin turgor, lethargy, irritability*

Outcomes	Nursing Interventions	Rationales
Infant/child's weight will be within 5% of normal baseline.	1. Weigh infant/child daily.	1. Daily *accurate* weights are necessary to ascertain the amount of fluids lost through liquid stools and/or vomiting.
Bowel movements will be reduced in number within 24 hours of nursing intervention.		
Urine output will be above 1 ml/kg/hr.	2. Monitor vital signs (e.g., temperature, pulse, respirations, blood pressure, and skin turgor).	2. Helps determine if the infant/child is responding appropriately to medical and nursing interventions.
Infant/child will be free from fluid/electrolyte imbalance.	3. Record intake and output accurately, including ice chips, IV fluids, gelatins, or other food products that become waterlike at room temperature.	3. Accurate recording of intake and output is necessary to determine the amount of fluid replacement required.
	4. Observe/monitor IV fluid administration.	4. Fluid depletion occurs very rapidly in infants and small children because they have different proportions of both body water and fat from an adult. IV fluids may be needed to prevent dehydration, electrolyte imbalance, shock, and death.
	5. Notify health care provider of decreased number of stools, ability to drink liquids without emesis; increased urine output, and improvement in vital signs and skin turgor.	5. Prevents overhydration of infant/child.
	6. Obtain fresh stool specimen, if ordered, and send to laboratory for analysis.	6. A fresh sample is required to determine if there are any ova (eggs) or parasites in the stool that could be the cause of the gastroenteritis.
	7. Resume oral liquids/foods gradually, starting with ordered rehydration fluids.	7. Rehydration fluids help to decrease the mobility of the colon, rests the intestinal tract, and decreases the risk of water toxicity.

SELECTED NURSING DIAGNOSIS — *Risk for impaired skin integrity related to frequency of stools as evidenced by excoriation of skin/tissue in perianal area, erythema, pain with each stooling; complaint of burning/pain in perianal area*

Outcomes	Nursing Interventions	Rationales
Infant/child will show improvement or resolution of erythema and exhibit tissue intact and free from secondary infection.	1. Change diapers/underwear as soon as a stooling occurs; cleanse perianal area with warm water using a soft cloth free of any alcohol.	1. Liquid stools generally contain high amounts of acids. The longer the stool is in contact with the infant/child's skin, the greater the risk of excoriated tissue. Alcohol can be very painful on impaired tissue.

Continued

NURSING CARE PLAN 27-1—cont'd

Outcomes	Nursing Interventions	Rationales
	2. Leave buttocks exposed to air whenever possible (usually *after* the diarrhea slows down or stops).	2. Air helps to keep the skin dry and free from any irritation such as diapers or underwear rubbing on the skin.
	3. Apply soothing balm or ointment to affected area (*after* thorough cleansing) sparingly.	3. The balm or ointment is a protective barrier on the infant/child's skin. If the ointment is placed on uncleansed skin, the infant/child is at increased risk of excoriation.
	4. If medicated powders are prescribed and/or used, teach the parent to put powder in the hand and then apply on the infant/child's buttocks and to keep powder container away from the infant/child.	4. If powder is "sprayed" onto the buttocks, the infant/child is at risk of inhaling the powder.

SELECTED NURSING DIAGNOSIS *Deficient knowledge (parents) related to diarrhea in infants/children as evidenced by lack of previous experience*

Outcomes	Nursing Interventions	Rationales
Parents will verbalize understanding of the dietary restrictions, potential complications, and method of treatment for gastroenteritis/diarrhea.	1. Instruct parents on proper methods of making, reconstituting, and storing formulas, oral fluid replacements, and foods.	1. Ensure that parents understand that improper handling or storing of food products can increase the risk of further gastroenteritis.
	2. Teach/reinforce proper handwashing techniques, especially after handling soiled diapers and clothing and before preparing and/or eating a meal.	2. Handwashing is the first in the line of defense in preventing the spread of infection.
	3. Explain that dehydration occurs rapidly in infants and small children. Because of this fact, the parents need to seek help from their health care provider early to prevent potential hospitalization and/or further complications.	3. Early detection and interventions prevent more severe complications from the dehydration that occurs with gastroenteritis.
	4. Teach parents that some over-the-counter remedies for vomiting and diarrhea can be harmful to infants and small children.	4. Absorbents such as kaolin and pectin may alter the consistency and appearance of stools, decreasing the frequency of evacuation; however, they may mask actual fluid loss.

CRITICAL THINKING QUESTION

An 11-month-old infant is brought to the clinic. The mother states he has watery diarrhea, and you notice that his eyes are sunken and that his skin turgor is only fair. The mother tells you she wants to give an antidiarrheal medicine that she has at home and asks how much to give. What is the best response of the nurse?

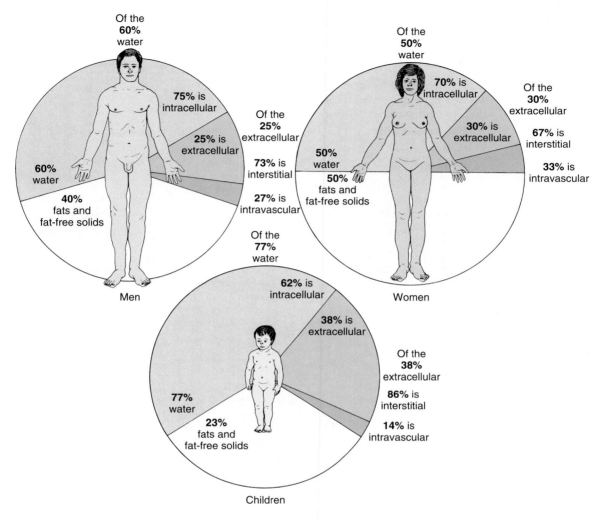

FIGURE **27-8** Relationship of body water and body solids to the body weight of the adult man and woman and the child.

Compared with adults, a greater percentage of body water in children under 2 years of age is contained in the extracellular compartment.

Fluid turnover is rapid, and dehydration occurs more quickly in infants than in adults (Table 27-1 and Box 27-2). The infant cannot survive as long as the adult in the presence of continued water depletion. A sick infant does not adapt as rapidly to shifts in intake and output because the kidneys lack maturity. They are less able to concentrate urine and require more water than an adult's kidneys to excrete a given amount of solute. Disturbances of the GI tract often lead to vomiting and diarrhea. Electrolyte balance depends on fluid balance and cardiovascular, renal, adrenal, pituitary, parathyroid, and pulmonary regulatory mechanisms. Many of these mechanisms are maturing in the developing child

and are unable to react to full capacity under the stress of illness, such as diarrhea and vomiting.

NURSING **TIP**

An accurate intake and output record must be kept for all children with vomiting or diarrhea.

Oral Fluids

ORT solutions such as Pedialyte or Infalyte are preferred to IV therapy. Nurses must use their ingenuity to coax sick children to take enough fluids because they may refuse food and water and do not understand their importance for recovery. Toddlers and infants are not capable of drinking by themselves. The busy nurse must find time to offer fluids and must be patient and gently

table 27-1 *Signs of Isotonic, Hypertonic, and Hypotonic Dehydration*

AREA OF ASSESSMENT	SIGNS OF DEHYDRATION		
	ISOTONIC	HYPERTONIC	HYPOTONIC
Weight loss	Mild dehydration: up to 5% weight loss Moderate dehydration: 5% to 10% weight loss Severe dehydration: over 10% weight loss		
Behavior	Irritable and lethargic	Irritable when disturbed; lethargic	Lethargic to delirious; coma
Skin turgor	Dead elasticity	Good turgor; "foam rubber" feel	Very poor turgor; clammy
Mucous membranes	Dry	Parched	Clammy
Eyeballs and fontanel	Sunken and soft	Sunken	Sunken and soft
Tearing and salivation	Absent or decreased	Absent or decreased	Absent or decreased
Thirst	Present	Marked	Present
Urine	Decreased output; serum globulin (SG) elevated	Normal to decreased output; SG elevated or decreased	Decreased output; SG elevated
Body temperature	Subnormal to elevated	Elevated	Subnormal
Respiration	Rapid	Rapid	Rapid
Blood pressure	Normal to low	Normal to low	Very low
Pulse	Rapid	Rapid	Rapid
Blood chemistry	BUN increased Na decreased K normal or increased Cl decreased pH usually decreased	BUN increased Na decreased K decreased Cl low during correction Ca decreased	BUN increased Na decreased K varies or increased Cl decreased

Data from Chinn, P. (1979). *Child health maintenance* (2nd ed.). St. Louis, Mosby. Data also from Barken, R., Rosen, P. (1999). *Emergency pediatrics.* St. Louis: Mosby. *BUN,* Blood urea nitrogen; *Na,* sodium; *K,* potassium; *Cl,* chloride, *Ca,* calcium.

persistent. Liquids are offered frequently and in small amounts. Brightly colored containers and drinking straws may help. ORT solutions are available in varied flavors and in frozen ice pop forms that are more acceptable to the young child. The nurse keeps an accurate record of the patient's intake and output. General hygiene and principles of preventing diarrhea are discussed with the parents.

Parenteral Fluids

Parenteral fluids (*para,* "beside or apart from" and *enteron,* "intestine") are those given by some route other than the digestive tract. They are necessary when sickness is accompanied by vomiting or loss of consciousness or when the GI system requires rest. Parenteral fluids are needed in severe cases of vomiting and diarrhea in which the loss of excessive water and electrolytes will lead to death if untreated. It also provides a means for the safe and effective administration of selective parenteral medications. Solutions given parenterally must

be sterile to prevent a general or local infection. The nurse must be aware of the importance of parenteral therapy and the assessments required.

The infant or child receiving parenteral fluids needs the nurse's warmth and affection. A pacifier should be used whenever infants are on NPO status. Parents should be encouraged to pick up and hold or rock their children who are receiving IV therapy. Arm boards prevent the child from pulling out the IV and protect the tubing. Parenteral therapy is discussed in Chapter 22.

DEHYDRATION

Pathophysiology. When a person is in good health, the intake and output of fluids are balanced and homeostasis (a uniform state) exists. This is accomplished by appropriate shifts of fluids and electrolytes across cellular membranes and by elimination of products of metabolism that are no longer needed or are in excess. The volume of blood plasma and interstitial and intracellular fluids remains relatively constant. Dehydration

box 27-2 | *Assessment of the Dehydrated Child*

HISTORY
Weight change
History of illness contacts
Stool and vomiting frequency

CLINICAL EXAMINATION
Daily weight
Skin turgor
Mucous membrane moisture
Fontanel fullness
Mental state

LABORATORY STUDIES
Complete blood count
Electrolytes
Blood urea nitrogen
Creatinine
Osmolarity
Glucose
Calcium

URINALYSIS
Specific gravity
pH
Glucose
Ketones
Amino acids
Other appropriate cultures

table 27-2 | *Average Daily Excretion of Urine*

AGE	FLUID OUNCES	MILLILITERS
First and second days	1-2	30-60
Third to tenth days	3-10	100-300
Tenth day to 2 months	9-15	250-450
2 months to 1 year	14-17	400-500
1 to 3 years	17-20	500-600
3 to 5 years	20-24	600-700
5 to 8 years	22-34	650-1000
8 to 14 years	27-47	800-1400

occurs whenever fluid output exceeds fluid intake, regardless of the cause.

Manifestations. Disorders of fluids and electrolytes—sodium (Na), potassium (K), calcium (Ca), and magnesium (Mg)—are more complex in growing children. A newborn's total weight is approximately 77% water, compared with 60% in adults (see Figure 27-8). This varies with the amount of fat. In addition, the daily turnover of water in infants is equal to almost 24% of total body water, compared with about 6% in adults. An infant's body surface in comparison with weight is three times that of the older child; therefore the infant is subject to greater evaporation of water from the skin. The younger the patient, the higher the metabolic rate and the more unstable the heat-regulating mechanisms. (Elevations in temperature also increase the rate of water loss.) Rapid respirations speed up this process; when diarrhea is present, additional fluid is lost in the stools. Immaturity of the kidneys impairs the infant's ability to conserve water. The average urine output in infants and children is seen in Table 27-2. Preterm and newborn infants are also more susceptible to dehydration from

variations in room temperature and humidity. When this is coupled with higher fluid losses, life-threatening deficits can ensue within a few hours.

Problems of fluid and electrolyte disturbance require evaluation of the type and severity of dehydration, clinical observation of the patient, and chemical analysis of the blood. The types of dehydration are classified according to the level of serum sodium, which depends on the relative losses of water and electrolytes. These types are usually termed isotonic (the patient has lost equal amounts of fluids and electrolytes), hypotonic (the child has lost more electrolytes than fluid), and hypertonic (more fluids are lost than electrolytes, Table 27-3). These classifications are important because each form of dehydration is associated with different relative losses from intracellular fluid (ICF) and extracellular fluid (ECF) compartments, and each requires certain modifications in treatment.

Treatment and nursing care. Maintenance fluid therapy replaces normal water and electrolyte losses, and deficit therapy restores preexisting body fluid and electrolyte deficiencies. The composition of IV fluids and the amount and rate of flow are important in preventing complications.

Shock (hypovolemia) is the greatest threat to life in isotonic dehydration. The electrolyte content of oral fluids is particularly significant in the care of infants and small children suffering from disorders of fluid balance and receiving infusions. Commercially prepared electrolyte solutions are available and are called oral rehydrating solutions. Children with hypotonic dehydration (excess water with sodium electrolyte depletion) are at risk for water intoxication. This can also occur if tap

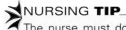

table 27-3 *Estimation of Dehydration*

| | DEGREE | | |
CLINICAL SIGN	MILD	MODERATE	SEVERE
Weight loss (%)	5	10	15
Behavior	Normal	Irritable	Hyperirritable to lethargic
Thirst	Slight	Moderate	Intense
Mucous membrane	May be normal	Dry	Parched
Tears	Present	+/−	Absent
Anterior fontanel	Flat	+/−	Sunken
Skin turgor	Normal	+/−	Decreased

From Graef, J., & Cone, T. (1988). *Manual of pediatric therapeutics* (4th ed.). Boston: Little, Brown; and Behrman, R.E., Kliegman, R.M., and Jenson, H.B. (2000). *Nelson textbook of pediatrics* (16th ed.). Philadelphia: W.B. Saunders.

water enemas are given to small children. Potassium is lost in almost all states of dehydration. Replacement potassium is administered only after normal urinary excretion is confirmed.

> ⋆NURSING **TIP**
> The nurse must document that at least one void has occurred before IV potassium is administered.

OVERHYDRATION

Pathophysiology. Overhydration results when the body receives more fluid than it can excrete. This can occur in patients with normal kidneys who receive IV fluids too rapidly. It also can occur in a patient receiving acceptable rates of fluid, especially when the patient's illness is related to disorders of fluid mechanism.

Manifestations. Edema is the presence of excess fluid in the interstitial (interstitium, "a thing standing between") spaces. Interstitial fluid is similar to plasma, but it contains little protein. In healthy persons, it responds well to shifts in fluid balance. Any factor causing sodium retention can cause edema. The flow of blood out of the interstitial compartments also depends on adequate circulation of blood and lymph. Low protein levels can also disturb osmotic cellular pressure, causing edema. This is seen in patients with nephrosis, in which large amounts of albumin are lost.

Trauma to or infections of the head can cause cerebral edema, which can be life threatening. Constrictive dressings may obstruct venous return, causing swelling, particularly in dependent areas. Anasarca (ana, "throughout" and sarx, "flesh") is a severe generalized edema.

Treatment and nursing care. Early detection and management of edema are essential. Taking accurate daily weights is indispensable, as is close attention to body weight changes. Vital signs, physical appearance, and

changes in urine character or output are noted. Edema in infants may first be seen about the eyes and in the presacral, occipital, or genital areas. In pitting edema, the nurse notices an impression in the skin that lasts for several seconds after exerting gentle pressure with the finger.

Infants receiving IV therapy have an IV and oral intake recorded. If the oral intake falls below prescribed rates, the IV rate is increased. If the oral intake exceeds prescribed levels, the IV rate is decreased or the IV is heparin/saline locked to maintain patency and avoid overhydration.

Electrolyte imbalance. The nurse must be able to assess the electrolyte needs of the child (Table 27-4). When fluid snacks or nourishment are ordered, the selection of fluid can influence the treatment given for dehydration. For example, if the child has a hypertonic type of dehydration (which means there is excess sodium) and the nurse offers the child tomato juice, the high sodium content of tomato juice will negatively impact the child's prescribed treatment. If the child has hypotonic dehydration (which means the child has deficient electrolytes) and the nurse offers plain water, this will also impact the child's care negatively. Therefore it is a nursing responsibility to correlate laboratory findings of the individual child with fluids and foods offered to the child.

NUTRITIONAL DEFICIENCIES

Because infancy is a period of rapid growth, poor nutrition is particularly dangerous at this time. Severe vitamin deficiencies are rare in prosperous countries; those that do occur are caused by poverty, ignorance, or neglect. Figure 27-9 shows a child, from the United States, with general, moderate malnutrition. Severe malnutrition is still rampant in many underdeveloped countries.

table 27-4 *Interpreting ABG Values*

	ACID	NORMAL	ALKALINE
pH	<7.35	7.35-7.45	>7.45
Respiratory parameter: $Paco_2$	>45	35-45	<35
Metabolic parameter: HCO_3	<22	22-26	>26

- Where the patient's pH falls indicates acidosis or alkalosis.
- If the pH falls in the same line as the HCO_3, the problem is *metabolic*.
- If the pH falls in the same box as $Paco_2$, the problem is *respiratory*.

INTERPRETING A SAMPLE PATIENT'S LABORATORY VALUES

	ACID	NORMAL	ALKALINE
pH	pH		
$Paco_2$		$Paco_2$	
HCO_3	HCO_3		

Interpretation
- The column the pH is in tells you *acidosis* is the problem.
- The HCO_3 (the metabolic parameter) is in the same line as the pH; therefore the problem is *metabolic acidosis*.

INTERPRETING A SAMPLE PATIENT'S LABORATORY VALUES

	ACID	NORMAL	ALKALINE
pH			pH
$Paco_2$			$Paco_2$
HCO_3		HCO_3	

Interpretation
Place the patient's laboratory values in the appropriate columns.
- The column the pH is in tells you *alkalosis* is the problem.
- The $Paco_2$ (the respiratory parameter) is in the same line as the pH; therefore the problem is *respiratory alkalosis*.

Modified from Mays, D. (1995). Turn ABGs into child's play. *RN, 58*(1), 37-38. Reprinted with permission. © 1995 Medical Economics.

Every person must be concerned with the plight of the starving child. Sometimes the infant's body is unable to use food even though the diet is adequate. An example of this is celiac disease, in which the intestines are unable to handle fats and starches. Severe malnutrition may also be seen in failure to thrive.

FAILURE TO THRIVE

Pathophysiology. Failure to thrive (FTT) describes infants and children who, without an obvious cause, fail to gain and often lose weight. This condition can be caused by physical (organic) pathology (OFTT), such as congenital heart disease or malabsorption syndromes. It may be caused by a lack of parent-infant interaction that can result from environmental factors, neglect, or lack of information concerning the nutritional needs of infants; this is nonorganic failure to thrive (NFTT).

Infants who fail to thrive are often admitted to the hospital for evaluation with presenting symptoms of weight loss or failure to gain, irritability, and disturbances of food intake such as anorexia or pica (abnor-mal consumption of nonfood materials). Vomiting, diarrhea, and general neuromuscular spasticity sometimes accompany the condition. The child has a complete work-up to identify organic reasons for FTT, and the cause is treated. FTT can be caused by environmental stresses. Children fall below the third percentile (some authorities suggest the fifth) in weight and height on standard growth charts. Their development is delayed. Children who fail to thrive seem apathetic. Some have a "ragdoll limpness" (hypotonia), and they often appear wary of their caregivers. Others appear stiff and unre-sponsive to cuddling. The personality of the infant may not foster maternal attachment. FTT with malabsorp-tion has been reported with frequency among autistic children and among institutionalized mentally retarded children.

Manifestations. With NFTT, there may be a distur-bance in the mother-child or caregiver-child relation-ship. The situation is complex and is often associated with marital discord, economic pressures, parental im-maturity, low stress tolerance, and single parenthood.

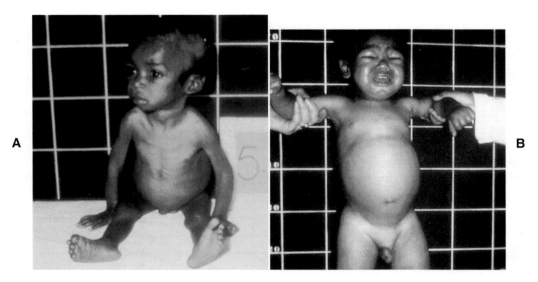

FIGURE **27-9 A,** Marasmus. A general nutritional-calorie deficiency. Note the profound wasting found in malnutrition. **B,** Kwashiorkor, caused by a protein deficiency. The infant has generalized edema with a white streak in the hair.

Alcohol and drug abuse can be present. Many mothers feel deprived and unloved and have conflicting needs. Infants suffer from the inability to establish a sense of trust in their caregivers. Their coping abilities are affected by a lack of nurturing. Outward neglect and physical abuse are not uncommon.

Prevention of environmental FTT consists chiefly of social measures such as parenting classes, family planning, and early recognition and support of families at risk. All children should receive routine health assessments. The pregnancy history may detect circumstances that may contribute to a lack of bonding, such as an unplanned pregnancy or desertion by the child's father. Planning interventions that will enhance parent-infant interaction is an important nursing responsibility.

Treatment and nursing care. Treatment involves a multidisciplinary approach in accordance with the circumstance; that is, the physician, nurse, social worker, family agency, and counselor may all participate. If no progress can be made, temporary or permanent placement of the child or children in a foster home may be required. During hospitalization, one nurse per shift is selected to increase nurturing and interaction with the infant and parent.

Treatment of the child who fails to thrive requires maturity on the part of the nurse. It is vital to support rather than reject the mother. Maternal attachment can be facilitated by listening and helping the mother to understand her feelings and frustrations and to explore her choices. The nurse encourages her to assist with the daily care of her child. The child's uniqueness and responses to the mother are stressed. The nurse points out

developmental patterns and provides anticipatory guidance in this area. Often the mother's lack of interest stems from her own insecurities. Parents Anonymous and parent aides are other resources.

The prognosis of this condition is uncertain. Emotional starvation, particularly in the early years, can be psychologically traumatic. Inadequacies in intelligence, language, and social behavior have been documented in children who fail to thrive.

KWASHIORKOR

Pathophysiology. Kwashiorkor is a protein deficiency. In many parts of the world, children still starve to death. There are no well-planned maternal and child health programs to elevate health standards in these localities. In some areas, superstition and ignorance prevent children from using nutritious foods found in their environment. In kwashiorkor, there is a severe deficiency of protein in the diet despite the fact that the number of calories consumed may be nearly adequate. It belongs to a class of disorders termed protein-energy malnutrition (see Figure 27-9).

Manifestations. Kwashiorkor occurs in children 1 to 4 years of age who have been weaned from the breast. Kwashiorkor means, in native dialect, "the disease of the deposed baby when the next one is born," indicating that the child no longer breastfeeds because a sibling is born and takes over the breast of the mother. Oral intake then is deficient in protein. The child fails to grow normally. The muscles become weak and wasted. There is edema of the abdomen that may become generalized. Diarrhea, skin infections, irritability, anorexia, and vomiting may be present. The hair becomes thin and dry. Because protein is the basis of melanin, a substance that provides color to hair, melanin becomes deficient. This is the reason the earliest sign of this protein malnutrition is a white streak in the hair of the child (depigmentation). The child looks apathetic and weak.

Treatment and nursing care. Treatment for kwashiorkor is mainly preventive. Although hunger may never be completely eradicated in the world, many private, public, and world health agencies sponsor programs to alleviate such suffering. Simple protein powder sprinkled on the culturally prepared meal will alleviate the problem. Early dietary treatment in established cases may prevent more serious growth retardation.

RICKETS

Pathophysiology. Rickets is a disease of infancy and childhood caused by deficient amounts of vitamin D. Vitamin D and exposure to sunshine are necessary for the proper absorption and metabolism of calcium and phosphorus, which are needed for the normal growth of bones.

Manifestations. The classic symptoms of rickets are bowlegs; knock-knees; beading of the ribs, called the *rachitic rosary;* and improper formation of the teeth.

Treatment and nursing care. The widespread use of vitamin supplements and the fortification of foods have largely eliminated the problem of rickets in North America. The nurse should guide parents concerning the need for an optimum, well-balanced diet, exercise, and exposure to outdoor sunlight.

SCURVY

Scurvy is a disease caused by insufficient fruits and vegetables that contain vitamin C in the diet. The symptoms of scurvy include joint pains, bleeding gums, loose teeth, and lack of energy. Good sources of vitamin C are citrus fruits and raw, leafy vegetables. Vitamin C is easily destroyed by heat and exposure to air. Small amounts of water should be used for cooking vegetables to prevent vitamin C from being destroyed, because it is also water soluble. It may be given to infants in the form of orange juice, which should not be boiled. Vitamin supplements prescribed for infants and children contain vitamin C. The vitamin is not stored in the body and requires a daily intake from food sources.

INFECTIONS

APPENDICITIS

The most common reason for emergency abdominal surgery in childhood is appendicitis, with over 80,000 cases each year in the United States. The average age of occurrence is 10 years of age. The challenge in diagnosing appendicitis is that rupture or perforation of the appendix can occur with serious complications within 36 hours after the onset of abdominal pain. A delay in diagnosis often occurs because the child is unable to localize or express the symptoms experienced.

Pathophysiology and manifestations. The appendix is a small appendage arising from the cecum; it is located on the right side of the abdomen. The lumen may become obstructed with fecal matter or with lymphoid tissue after a viral illness or with parasites. There is stasis, increased swelling, edema, and growth of organisms. The initial pain perceived is usually periumbilical and increases within a 4-hour period. When the inflammation spreads to the peritoneum, the pain localizes in the right lower quadrant (RLQ) of the abdomen. The appendix may become gangrenous or rupture, causing peritonitis and septicemia. Vomiting may occur after periumbilical pain starts. (In children with gastroenteritis, vomiting *precedes* abdominal pain.) Infrequent mucus diarrhea may occur because of intestinal irritation and perforated material. (Frequent watery stools are associated with gastroenteritis.) Fever is not a reliable sign of appendicitis in children. On examination, characteristic tenderness in the right lower quadrant known as **McBurney's point** will occur. Other diagnostic signs include the following:

- **Guarding:** There is a tightening of the abdominal muscles or rigidity of the abdomen on palpation.
- **Rebound tenderness:** Pressing the RLQ with rapid release of pressure causes severe pain.
- Pain on lifting the thigh while in the supine position is caused by muscle irritation.
- Pain in the RLQ when palpated and pain on rectal examination often occurs.

Laboratory tests may be done to confirm the diagnosis and rule out other possible diagnoses. A urinalysis will rule out a urinary tract infection. C-reactive protein levels will be increased after 12 hours if any infection is present. An abdominal x-ray study (KUB [kidney, ureter, bladder]) will show a right sided curvature of the spine, a dilated cecum with an air/fluid level, and a decrease in bowel gas in the RLQ (if ruptured). An ultrasound will show a thickened appendix and a soft tissue mass in the RLQ, and it is used to rule out an ovarian cyst in females who may exhibit similar clinical signs. A CT scan with rectal contrast (CTRC) is administered via the rectum to confirm the enlarged appendix. A culture of the stool may be done to rule out gastroenteritis. A laboratory evaluation of the white blood cell (WBC) count will show an increased WBC with neutrophils increased 75% but may not be helpful in diagnosing an unperforated appendix.

Treatment and nursing care. Observing the behavior of the child in relation to the developmental level and using pain perception scales can help assess the pain level. A warmed stethoscope should be used when auscultating the abdomen of a child; it is less frightening than the approaching fingers of the hand. The child and family are prepared for the diagnostic tests and possibility of surgery. An explanation of the reason for NPO status until the need for surgery is determined will help with compliance. The nurse should explain what to expect, discuss coping mechanisms, and provide referrals as necessary. Postoperative care is similar to that for any abdominal surgery. IV therapy is gradually replaced with fluids and food. A drain may be present at the wound site if perforation has occurred, and a frequent change of dressings may be necessary. Pain management, prevention of infection, and early ambulation are the primary goals.

THRUSH (ORAL CANDIDIASIS)

Pathophysiology. Thrush is an infection of the mucous membranes of the mouth caused by the fungus *Candida.* This organism is normally present in the mother's vagina and is nonpathogenic. However, the altered conditions in the vagina produced by pregnancy may lead to the development of monilial vaginitis. The mucous membranes of the infant's mouth may become infected by direct contact with this infection during delivery or by contact with the mother's or nurse's contaminated hands. Cross-infection of other newborns may result.

Manifestations. White patches that resemble milk curds appear on the tongue, inner lips, gums, and oral mucosa. They are painless but cannot be wiped away. Anorexia may be present. The systemic symptoms are mild if the infection remains in the mouth; however, it can pass along the mucous membranes into the GI tract, causing inflammation of the esophagus and stomach. Pneumonitis may also develop. *Epstein's pearls,* which are small, white, epithelial cysts that appear along both sides of the midline of the hard palate, are sometimes mistaken for thrush. These are harmless and gradually disappear.

Treatment and nursing care. A thrush infection responds well to the local application of an antibiotic suspension such as nystatin (Mycostatin). The mouth is swabbed three or four times a day between feedings with a sterile applicator moistened with the prescribed solution. With proper care, the condition disappears within a few days after its onset.

Newborns suspected of having thrush are cared for using isolation (standard) precautions. Individual feeding equipment is necessary, and the equipment should be sterile. Disposable bottles or prefilled formula bottles are used. Disposable nipples, pacifiers, and bottles are preferred.

Candida infection of the diaper area presents as a bright red, sharply demarcated diaper rash. Nystatin cream is often prescribed.

> ## NURSING **TIP**
>
> In the home, parents are taught to drop nystatin or other medication slowly into the *side of the infant's mouth.* Medication must remain in contact with "patches" as long as possible. Instruct parents to watch for dehydration (e.g., decrease in number of wet diapers) because of the infant's refusal to take fluids due to mouth discomfort.

WORMS

The main nursing responsibility is the education of the patient and family concerning the prevention of worm infestation through general hygiene, food handling, and environmental controls.

Enterobiasis (Pinworms)

Pathophysiology. Of the several varieties of worms that affect humans, the most common is the pinworm, *Enterobius vermicularis* (*enteron,* "intestine," *bios,* "life," and *vermis,* "wormlike"). It is seen more often in toddlers but can develop in older children and adults. The pinworm looks like a white thread about 1/3 inch. It lives in the lower intestine but comes out of the anus to lay its eggs, generally during the night. These eggs become infective a few hours after they have been deposited. This type of parasite spreads from one person to another particularly where large groups of children are in close contact with one another. The child becomes infected by ingesting the eggs. The route of entry is the mouth. Reinfection takes place by way of the rectum to the fingers to the mouth or by way of the rectum to the clothing to the fingers to the mouth.

Manifestations. The nurse or parent may notice that the child scratches the anal area and may complain of itching. There may be associated irritability and restlessness. Weight loss, poor appetite, and fretfulness during the night can develop. The rectal area may become irritated from scratching. A special pinworm diagnostic tape or paddle or a tongue blade covered with cellophane tape, sticky side out, may be placed against the anal region to obtain pinworm eggs (the Scotch tape test). This is done early in the morning, before the child has a bowel movement, bathes, or scratches the anal area with the fingers. The tape is put on a glass slide and examined under a microscope. The eggs are typical of pinworms.

Treatment and nursing care. Several effective anthelmintics (*anti,* "against" and *helminth,* "worms") are available. Mebendazole (Vermox) is a single-dose, chewable tablet and is the drug of choice for children over 2 years of age. Pyrantel pamoate (Antiminth) also controls the infestation. Pyrvinium pamoate (Povan) suspension, a one-dose treatment, is an alternative drug; nurses advise parents that Povan stains and turns the stools red.

The child must be taught to wash the hands well after bowel movements. The child's fingernails are kept short. A soothing ointment is applied to the rectal area. The patient should wear clean underwear that fits snugly to avoid scratching the anus with the fingers.

All symptomatic members of the family should be treated for this condition to prevent reinfection. Pregnant women should not take Vermox and should consult a physician before taking any alternative drug. The toilet seats in the home are scrubbed daily. Cloth diapers and bed linens are washed in hot water.

Ascariasis (Roundworms)

Ascaris lumbricoides is a roundworm, and infestation can be asymptomatic or cause abdominal pain. The infestation is estimated to affect 1 billion persons worldwide. Roundworms thrive in warm climates and among the impoverished. In the United States, it is seen more often in the Southern states and among immigrants and migratory workers living below poverty levels. It is caused by the unsanitary disposal of human feces and poor hygiene practices. An egg from an infected person can survive for weeks in the soil. The child ingests eggs from contaminated soil. The eggs develop into larvae in the intestine, penetrate the intestinal wall, and enter the liver, from which they circulate to the lungs and heart. The patient is generally without symptoms until the larvae reach the glottis, are coughed up, swallowed, and enter the small intestine. There they develop into adult male and female species. They survive on undigested food in the canal and produce eggs that are expelled in the child's feces. A chronic cough without fever is characteristic of this condition. Diagnosis is made by confirmation of the eggs in the patient's stool. The treatment of ascariasis is the same as that for enterobiasis (pinworms).

POISONING

Goals in the treatment of poisoning are as follows:
- Remove the poison.
- Prevent further absorption.
- Call the poison control center.
- Provide supportive care—seek medical help.

GENERAL CONCEPTS

Volume of a swallow. The volume of a swallow has been estimated to be 0.21 ml/kg. Thus a child age 2 to 3 years who takes one swallow may have ingested about 3 ml of poison.

Principles of care. Education of parents and children is the best way to prevent poisoning. The school and the clinic are the best resources to be used in an active accident prevention program.

Poison control centers. The telephone number of the poison control center is listed in the telephone directory and should be posted near the phone.

Ipecac syrup. Ipecac can be kept in the home out of the reach of children. Doses up to 15 ml may be given to children over 1 year of age with 200 ml of water to induce vomiting. Ipecac should *not* be used with corrosive, alkali, gasoline, and cleaning fluid ingestion or if child is not fully conscious. Table 27-5 indicates how to assess the type of toxic substance ingested according to the smell of the vomitus.

Activated charcoal. Activated charcoal will absorb poisons such as strychnine, atropine, malathion, and arsenic compounds. When activated charcoal is given together with ipecac, however, they neutralize each other and render both ineffective in the treatment of poisoning.

POISONOUS PLANTS

Many common plants used to landscape homes can be poisonous to the young child exploring in the backyard. Table 27-6 lists common poisonous plants and the symptoms they cause when ingested.

DRUGS

Drugs prescribed for family members and left within the reach of children are often the cause of accidental poisoning. Many over-the-counter medications are con-

table 27-5 *Detecting the Poison by Specific Odor of Vomitus*

ODOR OF VOMITUS	PROBABLE CONTENT
Sweet	Chloroform, acetone
Bitter almond	Cyanide
Pear	Chloral hydrate
Garlic	Phosphorus, arsenic
Shoe polish	Nitrobenzene
Violet	Turpentine

Note: The nurse should report and document the specific odor of vomitus, which can be helpful in determining the specific poison contained in the substance ingested.

table 27-6 *Common Household Plants That Are Poisonous*

PLANT	ACTION
Azalea Buttercup Marigold	Cause symtoms of aconitine poisoning
Lantana Jimsonweed	Cause symptoms of atropine poisoning
Sweet pea Black mountain laurel	Cause symptoms of curare poisoning
Apricot pits Peach pits Elderberry	Cause symptoms of cyanide poisoning
Camellia seeds Foxglove Oleander	Cause symptoms similar to digitalis poisoning
Goldenrod Nightshade Poinsettia	Cause sypmtoms of nitrate poisoning
Laurel Water hemlock	Cause symptoms of resin poisoning
Camellia Marigold Tulips Violets	Cause symptoms of salicylates poisoning

Note: These plants should not be used to landscape the backyard of homes with young children.

sidered harmless by parents but can be deadly to toddlers, even in small doses (Table 27-7).

Acetaminophen Poisoning

Acetaminophen overdose is listed along with other poisons commonly encountered in pediatrics in Box 27-3.

Pathophysiology. Acetaminophen (Tylenol) has now replaced aspirin as the most commonly ingested drug that causes toxicity. This is because it is so widely used and because aspirin associated with Reye's syndrome is no longer recommended for fever in children with flulike symptoms. Acetaminophen poisoning occurs most often from acute overdose rather than from the cumulative effects seen with aspirin. Because acetaminophen is metabolized in the liver, overdose results in hepatic destruction. With early treatment, most children recover without complications. Tylenol drops and Tylenol Elixir each have a different potency. When "1 teaspoon of Tylenol" is advised, the nurse must be sure the parent understands which preparation to purchase, or a massive overdose can occur.

Manifestations. Manifestations and treatment modalities that the nurse might anticipate in patients with acute poisoning are shown in Table 27-8.

Treatment and nursing care. The stomach is emptied by lavage or induced emesis from syrup of ipecac. Depending on the serum acetaminophen level, this may be followed by the *N*-acetylcysteine (Mucomyst) antidote. In small children, it may be administered directly into the nasogastric tube after lavage. Otherwise it is

table 27-7 *Over-the-Counter Drugs That Are Deadly to Toddlers*

GENERIC NAME	TRADE NAME	TOXICITY
Benzocaine	Orajel	Methemoglobinemia, seizures
Camphor	Vicks VapoRub Campho-Phenique	Central nervous system (CNS) depression Seizures
Diphenoxylate	Lomotil	CNS depression
Methyl salicylate	Oil of wintergreen Icy-Hot balm Arthritis ointments	Cardiovascular collapse
Phenylpropanolamine	Many decongestants (e.g., Afrin, Sudafed)	Hypertension Intracranial bleeding Cardiac arrhythmia
	Lindane	CNS depressant Seizures
Tetrahydrozoline hydrochloride	Visine Eye Drops	Tachycardia

Data from Osterhardt, K. (2000). The toxic toddler: Drugs that can kill in small doses. *Contemporary Pediatrics,* 17(3):73; Wong, D.L., Perry S.E., & Hockenberry-Eaton, M.J. (2002). *Maternal-child nursing* (2nd ed.). St. Louis: Mosby; and *Physician's Desk Reference* (2002). Medical Economics.

generally given orally every 4 hours for 72 hours. This medicine has a bad smell and taste, and the patient needs coaxing and support to assist with compliance. The medicine may be mixed with a soft drink or juice. Levels of liver enzymes (ALT and AST) are monitored. Prevention of overdose is of utmost importance. Even in uncomplicated cases the child is subjected to unpleasant, stressful procedures. Because parents are often informed that acetaminophen is "safer" than aspirin, they may be more careless in storing it.

Salicylate Poisoning

Pathophysiology. Aspirin (acetylsalicylic acid) poisoning is seen less often than in the past because of safety packaging and the increased use of acetaminophen. Nevertheless, aspirin is often used in many homes and may be stored carelessly on bedside stands or in a mother's purse. Oil of wintergreen (methyl salicylate) is also extremely hazardous when mistakenly administered as cough medicine or swallowed by the curious child. It is sometimes used as a home remedy

---

box 27-3 | *Poisons Commonly Encountered in Pediatrics*

ACIDS
Toilet bowl cleaners
Swimming pool pH adjustment solutions
Concentrated acids in hardware and paint stores

ALKALINES
Clinitest tablets
Drain-cleaning crystals
Dishwasher soaps
Industrial cleaners (brought home in unlabeled containers)

MEDICATIONS
Diet pills
Sleeping pills
Sedatives
Cold remedies
Birth control pills
Vitamin supplements, iron supplements
Diarrhea remedies (Lomotil)
Menstrual pain relievers
Antipyretics (aspirin, acetaminophen)
Oil of wintergreen

CYANIDE
Pesticides
Metal polishes
Photographic solutions
Fumigating products

ETHANOL
Alcoholic beverages
Cold remedies
Perfumes
Mouthwashes
Aftershave lotions

PETROLEUM DISTILLATES
Heavy greases, oils
Turpentine
Furniture polishes
Gasoline, kerosene

Lighter fluid
Insecticides
Home gardening products
Recently sprayed lawns

CARBON MONOXIDE
Accidental
Suicidal

LEAD
Paint
Air
Food
Ant poison
Unglazed pottery
Colored newsprint
Curtain weights
Fishing sinkers
Lead water pipes
Acid juices in leaded pottery

ARTHROPODS, INSECT STINGS
Spiders (brown recluse, black widow)
Certain scorpions
Insects (bees, wasps, hornets)

SNAKES
Rattlesnakes
Moccasins
Copperheads
Other snakes

POISONOUS PLANTS
Boston ivy
Split-leaf philodendron
Umbrella plant
Azalea
Daffodil
Foxglove
Mistletoe
Tulip
Others

table 27-8 *Anticipated Care for Poisoning*

SYMPTOMS	INTERVENTION
Absorption	Lavage, ipecac, activated charcoal
Central nervous system: restlessness, agitation, seizures, coma	Seizure precautions
Respiratory: airway obstruction, hypo-ventilation, hypoxia	Cardiopulmonary resuscitation, oxygen saturation monitoring, oxygen therapy, keep artificial airway handy
Cardiovascular: difficulties with electrolytes, blood urea nitrogen, creatinine, glucose	Monitor vital signs
Gastrointestinal: difficulty swallowing, abdominal pain	NPO status; possible gastrostomy
Kidney problems	Monitor intake and output; monitor IV lines
Need for increased elimination	Cathartic, forced diuresis, dialysis, hemoperfusion; monitor patient responses
Hypothermia or hyperthermia	Sponge baths, cooling blanket
Child: physical response or psychological trauma	Crisis intervention
Parents: guilt, anger, family dysfunction	Counseling, teaching, referral

for arthritic pain. Even a dose as small as 1 teaspoon can cause a child's death.

Manifestations. Salicylate acts rapidly but is excreted slowly. Ingestion of 150 mg/kg causes symptoms. Although most cases of aspirin poisoning are emergencies, a child may unknowingly be poisoned by the cumulative effect of aspirin. The use of several aspirin-containing products at once, such as over-the-counter cold remedies and aspirin, can be hazardous. Time-release aspirin is especially dangerous because the symptoms of poisoning are delayed and aspiration of the stomach is of little value. Therefore it is wise to read labels carefully and to administer aspirin sparingly. It is even better to use it only under a physician's direction.

Treatment and nursing care. Vitamin K is administered to control bleeding. Peritoneal dialysis (*peritoneum* and *dialysis,* "passing of a solute through a membrane") is a therapeutic measure used in acute renal failure. The therapy uses the principles of osmosis and diffusion through the semipermeable peritoneal membrane, with the purpose of removing toxic substances from the blood. Hemodialysis is another method used for essentially the same purpose.

The nurse must realize the danger of drug poisoning and must constantly practice and teach safety measures to prevent tragedies. Treatment, utility rooms, and drug baskets are scrutinized to ensure that nothing harmful is within the reach of ambulatory children.

LEAD POISONING (PLUMBISM)

Pathophysiology. Lead poisoning (plumbism) results when a child repeatedly ingests or absorbs substances containing lead. The primary source is paint from old, deteriorating buildings. The lead contents of food, water, and air have decreased substantially since 1990. Lead poisoning is most common in children between $1\frac{1}{2}$ and 3 years of age. The incidence is increased in tenement areas of large cities. Although the incidence is highest among the poor, lead poisoning is also found among suburban and middle-class children.

Children who chew on windowsills and stair rails ingest flakes of paint, putty, or crumbled plaster. Eating nonfood items is called pica. Food, particularly fruit juices consumed from improperly glazed earthenware, is another source. Lead poisoning among Mexican Americans may result from azarcon, a bright orange powder containing approximately 93.5% lead. Azarcon is used as a folk remedy to treat "empacho" and other digestive problems in infants. Lead poisoning among Hmong Laotian refugees may be caused by paylooah, a bright orange-red powder that may be used for fever or rash. Unwashed fresh fruit sprayed with insecticides and dust from enclosed shooting galleries are also culprits. Another source is dust in homes near lead-processing plants. "Spitballs" made from the colored section of newspaper comics is also a source of lead poisoning. Older synthetic venetian or vertical blinds used as window coverings, brightly colored metal vases, and lead crystal are also common sources for lead poisoning in the home when a toddler handles the item and then places the hands in the mouth.

Lead can have a lasting effect on the nervous system, especially the brain. The incidence is high among siblings of an affected child and recurrence is common. Mental retardation may occur in severe cases. In much of the United States, lead poisoning is a reportable disease. The Agency for Toxic Substances and Diseases Registry (ATSDR) provides information on this condition.

Manifestations. The symptoms occur gradually and range from mild to severe. Because the infant's or young child's central nervous system is extremely vulnerable, acute symptoms of encephalitis may follow a relatively short period of exposure. The lead settles in the soft tissues and bones and is excreted in the urine. In the beginning, weakness, weight loss, anorexia, pallor, irritability, vomiting, abdominal pain, and constipation may be seen. In later stages, signs of anemia and nervous system involvement, such as muscular incoordination, neuritis, convulsions, and encephalitis, are seen.

Treatment and nursing care. Blood and urine tests are performed to determine the amount of lead in the system. Lead is especially toxic to *the synthesis of heme* in the blood; heme is necessary for hemoglobin formation and for the functioning of renal tubules. Blood lead levels are the primary screening test. X-ray films of the bones show further deposits of lead. The child's history may reveal *pica,* a condition in which the child has a distorted appetite and eats a variety of things that most persons consider unpalatable, such as sand, grass, wool, glass, plaster, coal, animal droppings, and paint from furniture.

Treatment is aimed at reducing the concentration of lead in the tissues and blood. Chelating agents that render the lead nontoxic and increase its excretion in the urine are given in more severe cases. Calcium disodium edetate (calcium disodium versenate, CaEDTA) and dimercaprol are commonly used. CaEDTA may be given intravenously or as a deep intramuscular injection. Mild symptomatic lead poisoning may be treated with meso-2,3,-dimercaptosuccinic acid (DMSA). It can be given orally, has not been associated with serious side effects and, unlike CaEDTA, does not cause zinc depletion. British antilewisite (BAL) is also used but may not be given to children who have a peanut butter allergy or are taking supplemental iron. Complete deleading takes several months, and retreatment may be necessary when the child has an acute infection or other metabolic disturbance. The prognosis depends on the extent of poisoning. All children with elevated lead blood levels must be followed to evaluate developmental and intellectual milestone achievement. Providing an increased fluid intake and monitoring intake and output during therapy is an important nursing responsibility.

Prevention of this condition is foremost. Lead paint should not be used on children's toys or furniture. Instead, one should use paint marked for indoor use. Inexpensive lead detection kits are available at most home improvement stores. The kit contains a "crayon" that can be rubbed on the vertical blind or other items in the home; it turns a different color if significant lead is present. Lead level screening of children in high-risk areas is recommended.

FOREIGN BODIES

Approximately 80% of all foreign body ingestion occurs in children between 6 months and 3 years of age. About 80% of the foreign bodies ingested pass through the GI tract, but others require surgical removal. The high level of curiosity of the young child and the tendency to place objects in the mouth increase the susceptibility to accidental ingestion of a nonfood object. Unless the object is sharp or large, passage through the GI tract can take up to 4 to 6 days. The child is cared for at home, and the nurse should emphasize the importance of cutting and examining each stool until the object is passed successfully.

The nurse should caution parents not to use laxatives and to maintain a normal diet to avoid the intestinal spasms that may precipitate an obstruction. Parents should be instructed to notify the physician if abdominal pain or vomiting occurs. Follow-up care and teaching concerning safety in the environment and the prevention of ingested or inhaled foreign bodies are priority nursing responsibilities.

key points

- The newborn should be closely observed for signs of tracheoesophageal fistula, which includes coughing, choking, cyanosis, and apnea during feedings.
- Drooling in the newborn may be a sign of an obstructed esophagus (TEF).
- The first stool of the newborn should be documented to record the patency of the anus.
- Pyloric stenosis is caused by hypertrophy of the pyloric muscles and is manifested by projectile vomiting.
- Nursing care for the child with pyloric stenosis involves frequent assessment, careful feeding, positioning on the right side after feedings, and education and support of the parents.

- Large, bulky, frothy stools are characteristic of malabsorption syndromes.
- Celiac disease is caused by an intolerance to gluten in the diet.
- To prevent the development of water intoxication, tap water should not be used for enemas in children with megacolon.
- Intussusception is characterized by currant jelly stools.
- Hirschsprung's disease occurs when there is an absence of ganglionic innervation of the muscle of a bowel segment.
- The treatment of gastroesophageal reflux includes thickened feedings, burping, and maintaining Fowler's position.
- A diarrheal stool in an infant is manifested by a watery consistency and a greenish color with the possible presence of mucus or blood. Frequency of bowel movements, by itself, is not an indication of diarrhea in infants.
- Teaching parents basic hygienic practices, handwashing, and animal handling can prevent outbreaks of diarrhea.
- The functions of the gastrointestinal tract have a great influence on the fluid and electrolyte balance in infants and children.
- The higher daily exchange of water that occurs in infants leaves them less volume reserve when they are dehydrated.
- Oral rehydrating solutions are commercially prepared electrolyte solutions.
- Isotonic dehydration is the loss of equal amounts of water and electrolytes. Hypertonic dehydration is the loss of more water than electrolytes. Hypotonic dehydration is the loss of more electrolytes than water.
- Infants who are fed by the IV route should be picked up and held and allowed to suck on a pacifier.
- Kwashiorkor is a protein deficiency characterized by a depigmented (white) streak of hair.
- Disposable nipples, pacifiers, and bottles should be used for infants with thrush.
- Pinworm is diagnosed by a "Scotch tape test." Preventing the child from scratching the anal area is an essential part of breaking the cycle of worm reinfestation.
- A chronic productive cough without fever is part of the roundworm life cycle in children.
- The nurse should teach parents not to store poisonous substances in food containers.
- Prevention of accidental poisoning should be part of every parent teaching plan.
- Pica, the eating of nonfood items, is characteristic of children with lead poisoning.
- Lead poisoning (plumbism) can cause neurological damage.

ONLINE RESOURCES

Pyloric Stenosis:
http://cpmcnet.columbia.edu/dept/surgery/peds/pyl.html

Hirschsprung's Disease: http://www.pedisurg.com/PtEduc/Hirschsprung's_Disease.htm

Celiac Disease:
http://www.niddk.nih.gov/health/digest/pubs/celiac

REVIEW QUESTIONS   *Choose the most appropriate answer.*

1. The pathology of pyloric stenosis results from:
   1. Edema of the pyloric muscle
   2. Ischemia of the pyloric muscle
   3. Hypertrophy of the pyloric muscle
   4. Neoplastic obstruction

2. Which of the following menu selections is best for a child diagnosed with celiac disease?
   1. Pizza and chocolate cake
   2. Spaghetti and blueberry muffin
   3. Chicken sandwich on whole-wheat bread
   4. Corn tortilla and fresh fruit

3. After surgery for pyloric stenosis, the nurse could anticipate that the infant:
   1. Will have nasogastric suction for 24 hours
   2. Will be fed clear liquids within 6 hours
   3. Will remain NPO for 24 to 48 hours
   4. Will be fed formula within 4 hours

4. Pinworms are diagnosed by:
   1. Seeing the worm in the stool
   2. A blood antigen level
   3. A "Scotch tape test" in the early morning
   4. A stool laboratory examination obtained at the hour of sleep

5. Priority teaching for a parent of a child who ingested a foreign body includes:
   1. Encouraging the use of mild laxatives every night
   2. Slicing each stool passed to observe for the foreign body
   3. Encouraging a daily enema until the foreign body is passed
   4. Keeping the child NPO until the foreign body is passed

The Child with a Genitourinary Condition

objectives

1. Define each key term listed.
2. Differentiate between nephrosis and acute glomerulonephritis.
3. Name the functional unit of the kidney.
4. List four urological diagnostic procedures.
5. Discuss the skin care pertinent to the child with nephrosis.
6. Explain any alterations in diet applicable to the child with nephrosis.
7. Outline the nursing care for a child who is diagnosed as having Wilms' tumor.
8. Discuss the impact of genitourinary surgery on the growth and development of children at various ages.
9. Discuss the impact of undescended testes on fertility.

key terms

chordee (KŎR-dē, p. 687)
cryptorchidism (krĭp-TŎR-kĭ-dĭz-ĕm, p. 697)
cystometrogram (sĭs-tō-MĔT-rō-grăm, p. 686)
dysuria (dĭs-Ū-rē-ă, p. 686)
encopresis (ĕn-kō-PRĒ-sĭs, p. 684)
enuresis (ĕn-ū-RĒ-sĭs, p. 686)
epispadias (ĕp-ĭ-SPĀ-dē-ăs, p. 687)
frequency (p.686)
glomeruli (glō-MĔR-ū-lī, p. 690)
hydrocele (HĪ-drō-sēl, p. 694)
hydronephrosis (hī-drō-nĕ-FRŌ-sĭs, p. 688)
hyperkalemia (hī-pĕr-kă-LĒ-mē-ă, p. 693)
hypoalbuminemia (hī-pō-ăl-bū-mĭn-Ē-mē-ă, p. 690)
hypospadias (hī-pō-SPĀ-dē-ăs, p. 687)
micturition (mĭk-tū-RĬSH-ŭn, p. 686)
nephron (NĔF-rŏn, p. 683)
neutropenia (nū-trō-PĒ-nē-ă, p. 690)
nocturia (nŏk-TŪ-rē-ă, p. 686)
oliguria (ŏl-ĭ-GŪ-rē-ă, p. 686)
orchiopexy (ŏr-kē-ō-PĔK-sē, p. 697)
paraphimosis (păr-ă-fĭ-MŌ-sĭs, p. 687)
phimosis (fī-MŌ-sĭs, p. 686)

polyuria (pŏl-ē-Ū-rē-ă, p. 686)
pyelonephritis (pī-ă-lō-nĕ-FRĪ-tĭs, p. 688)
testicular torsion (tĕs-TĬK-ū-lăr TŌR-shŭn, p. 697)
ureteritis (ū-rē-tĕr-Ī-tĭs, p. 688)
urethritis (ū-rĕ-THRĪ-tĭs, p. 688)
urgency (p. 686)
vesicoureteral reflux (vĕs-ĭ-kō-ū-RĒ-tĕr-ăl RĒ-flŭks, p. 688)

DEVELOPMENT OF THE URINARY TRACT

The urinary system consists of two kidneys, two ureters, the urinary bladder, and the urethra. Figure 28-1 depicts these structures and how they differ in the developing child and in the adult. The function of the kidneys is to rid the body of waste products and to maintain body fluid homeostasis (Figure 28-2). The kidneys also produce substances that stimulate red blood cell formation in the bone marrow (e.g., erythropoietin-stimulating factor [ESF]), as well as renin, which regulates blood pressure. Microscopically, the functional unit of the kidneys is the nephron. Each kidney contains more than 1 million nephrons. Although the newborn's kidneys are immature, they function quite effectively. Nevertheless, the functional limitations must be considered carefully when the newborn is premature or ill. This applies especially to the administration of medications, formula, and parenteral fluids.

Soon after implantation, the embryonic mass differentiates into three distinct layers of cells: the *ectoderm*, *mesoderm*, and *endoderm*. The urinary and reproductive organs originate from the mesoderm. At approximately the third month of gestation the fetal kidney begins to secrete urine. The amount gradually increases as the fetus matures and is contained in a portion of the amniotic fluid volume. An absence or small amount of amniotic fluid may indicate genitourinary difficulties.

The kidney and urinary tract develop about the same time as the ears form during fetal life. There is an unexplained relationship between low-set ears in the

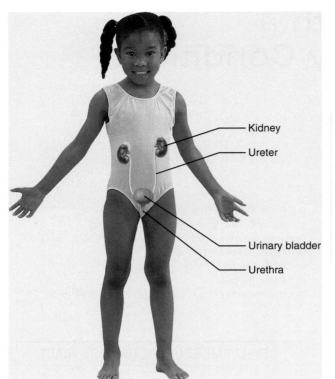

Kidney
Ureter

Urinary bladder
Urethra

URINARY SYSTEM

- Fluid is of greater importance to the body chemistry of infants and small children, because it constitutes a larger fraction of their total body weight.
- Glomerular filtration and absorption are relatively low until 1 to 2 years of age. Infants are more prone to fluid volume excess and dehydration.
- Kidneys are more susceptible to tramua in children, because they usually do not have as much fat padding.
- Kidney function is immature until after 2 years of age.

FIGURE **28-1** Summary of some urinary system differences between the child and the adult. The urinary system is the main excretory system. The kidneys remove wastes and excess materials from the blood and produce urine. This system helps to regulate blood chemistry.

newborn and urinary tract anomalies. When assessing the newborn, an imaginary line should be drawn between the outer canthus of the eye and the ear. The line should cross the tip of the earlobe. If the tip of the earlobe falls below this line, the assessment should be recorded and reported (see Figure 12-6).

DEVELOPMENT OF THE REPRODUCTIVE SYSTEMS

Figure 28-3 shows the female and male reproductive systems and lists some of the differences between children and adults. The reproductive system provides for perpetuation of the species. Each gender is equipped with gonads (which provide reproductive cells) and a set of accessory organs. The gonads (ovaries in the female and testes in the male) produce sex cells and hormones that affect the reproductive organs and other body systems.

Gender is genetically determined at the time of fertilization. The presence of a Y chromosome is essential for the development of the testes and their hormones. Sex differentiation occurs early in the embryo. The organs specific to the male or female child develop. Before this,

the embryo has neither male nor female characteristics. The development of the ovaries occurs later than that of the testes. By the twelfth week the external genitalia of the fetus are recognizably male or female.

Several tests are helpful in diagnosing conditions of the reproductive tract. These include a Papanicolaou (Pap) smear, serological blood tests, cultures, ultrasound procedures, pregnancy tests, and routine blood and urine tests. Sexual abuse in children may be manifested by behaviors such as urinary frequency, excessive masturbation, encopresis (fecal soiling beyond 4 years of age), severe nightmares, bedwetting, irritation or pain in the genital area, and a decrease in physical or emotional development. Suggestive posturing by young children or an explicit knowledge of sex acts shown by children under 8 years of age requires further investigation. Menstrual disorders and premenstrual syndrome are discussed in Chapter 11. Sexually transmitted diseases are discussed in Chapters 11 and 31.

NURSING **TIP**

Most newborns urinate within the first 24 hours of life. Recording and reporting the presence or absence of urination is very important.

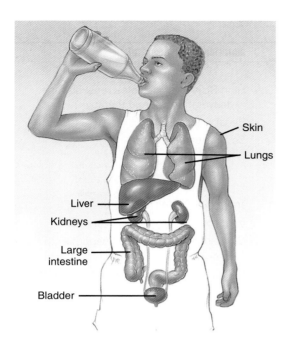

System	Organ	Excretion
Urinary	Kidney	Nitrogen compounds Toxins Water Electrolytes
Integumentary	Skin—sweat glands	Nitrogen compounds Water Electrolytes
Respiratory	Lung	Carbon dioxide Water
Digestive	Intestine	Digestive wastes Bile pigments Salts of heavy metals

FIGURE **28-2** The urinary system's chief function is to regulate the volume and composition of body fluids and excrete unwanted materials, but it is not the only system in the body that is able to excrete unneeded substances. The table in this figure compares the excretory functions of several systems. Although all of these systems contribute to the body's effort to remove wastes, only the urinary system can finely adjust the water and electrolyte balance to the degree required for normal homeostasis of body fluids.

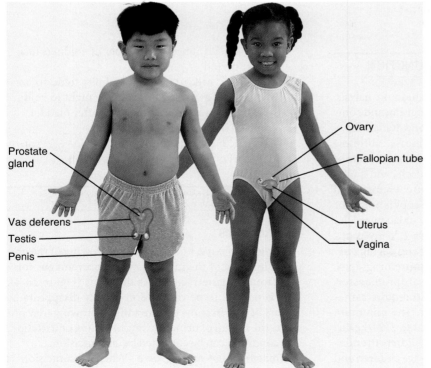

REPRODUCTIVE SYSTEM

- The gentials in preterm females may appear swollen. The labia minora may protrude beyond the labia majora.
- The testicles may appear large at birth in proportion to the size of the infant. They may fail to move into the scrotum, causing a condition termed "undescended testes."
- The foreskin may be tight at birth, causing phimosis.
- The sex organs do not mature until the onset of puberty.
- Secondary sex characteristics occur with the onset of puberty.

FIGURE **28-3** Summary of some reproductive system differences between the child and the adult male and female. Each reproductive system consists of gonads and associated structures. The reproductive system maintains sexual characteristics and perpetuates the species.

| table 28-1 | *Common Laboratory Tests for Urinary Tract Function* |

TEST	NORMAL LEVELS*	SIGNIFICANCE OR DEVIATION
BLOOD		
Blood urea nitrogen (BUN)	Newborn: 3-12 mg/dl Child: 5-18 mg/dl	High BUN level indicates renal disease, dehydration, steroid therapy
Uric acid	Child: 2-5 mg/dl	Renal disease
Creatinine	Infant: 0.2-0.4 mg/dl Child: 0.3-0.7 mg/dl Adolescent: 0.5-1.0 mg/dl	Severe renal disease
URINE		
Red blood cells	<2 million/mm^3	Trauma, infection, stones
Bacteria	Few	Infection
Casts	Occasional	Glomerular disease, pyelonephritis
White blood cells	<2	Infection
Ketones	0	Stress; diabetes mellitus
Glucose	0	Diabetes mellitus
Protein	0	Glomerular kidney disease
pH	Newborn: 5-7 Child: 4.8-7.8	Potassium deficiency, electrolyte imbalance
Specific gravity	Newborn: 1.001-1.020 Child: 1.001-1.030	Dehydration Overhydration, renal disease, pituitary malfunction

*Values for different age-groups are indicated only when relevant.

ASSESSMENT OF URINARY FUNCTION

Urological diagnostic procedures include urinalysis, ultrasonography, intravenous (IV) pyelogram, and computed tomography (CT) scan of the kidneys. Renal biopsy is used to diagnose the extent of kidney disease. A uroflow is an assessment procedure used to determine the rate of urine flow. The child voids into a receptacle, and a uroflowmeter graphs the volume and pressure. This is useful in diagnosing stricture or scarring. Cytoscopy is useful for investigating congenital abnormalities or acquired lesions in the bladder and lower urinary tract. X-ray examination of the bladder and urethra before and during micturition (voiding) is called voiding cystourethrography. The cystometrogram and urethral pressure profile assess bladder capacity and function. Both tests require catheterization and infusion of sterile water. The minimum urine output for infants and toddlers is 2 to 3 ml/kg/hr; for preschoolers and young school-age children, the minimum is 1 to 2 ml/kg/hr; and for school-age children and adolescents, the minimum is 0.5 to 1 ml/kg/hr. Common laboratory tests are reviewed in Table 28-1.

Terms commonly used to describe urinary dysfunction include the following:

- Dysuria: difficulty in urination
- Frequency: abnormal number of voidings in a short period
- Urgency: urge to void but inability to do so
- Nocturia: awakening during the night to void
- Enuresis: uncontrolled voiding after bladder control has been established
- Polyuria: increased urine output
- Oliguria: decreased urine output

ANOMALIES OF THE URINARY TRACT

PHIMOSIS

Pathophysiology. Phimosis is a narrowing of the preputial opening of the foreskin, which prevents the foreskin from being retracted over the penis (Figure 28-4). This is normal in newborns and usually disappears by 3 years of age. In some children this narrowing may obstruct the stream of urine, causing dribbling or irritation. The condition can be corrected by circumcision.

Treatment and nursing care. When circumcision is performed on an older boy, careful explanations and reassurance are provided. The nurse is sensitive to the child's embarrassment and fear. Postoperatively the penis is covered with a petroleum gauze. It is tender and may burn on urination.

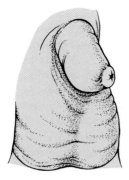

FIGURE **28-4** Phimosis. The foreskin is advanced and fixed; it cannot be retracted over the glans.

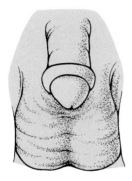

FIGURE **28-5** Paraphimosis. The foreskin is retracted and fixed; it cannot be returned to its original position. Constriction impedes circulation.

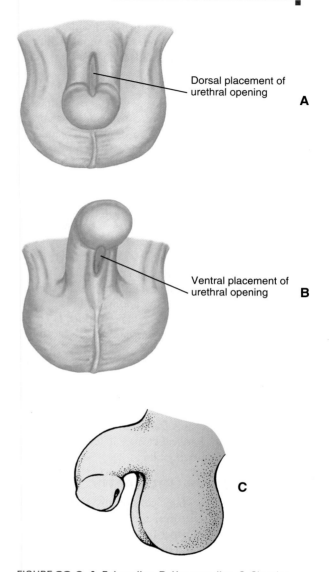

FIGURE **28-6** **A,** Epispadias. **B,** Hypospadias. **C,** Chordee.

Cleansing of the uncircumcised penis and retraction of the foreskin are discussed in Chapter 12. Forcible retraction of a tight foreskin is avoided because it can lead to paraphimosis (Figure 28-5). When this occurs, the foreskin cannot be returned to its normal position. There may be swelling and impaired circulation caused by the constriction. This condition requires immediate evaluation by a physician.

HYPOSPADIAS AND EPISPADIAS

Pathophysiology. Hypospadias is a congenital defect in which the urinary meatus is located not at the end of the penis but on the lower shaft. In mild cases it lies just below the tip of the penis, but it may be found at the midshaft or near the penile-scrotal junction. With epispadias, the opening of the urinary meatus is on the upper surface of the penis (Figure 28-6). Unlike epispadias, hypospadias is fairly common, occurring in 1 out of 250 to 500 newborn boys. Hypospadias may be accompanied by chordee, a downward curvature of the penis caused by a fibrotic band of tissue.

Treatment and nursing care. The alert nurse may discover hypospadias or epispadias in the nursery during neonatal assessment. In many mild cases surgery is not necessary for either condition unless the location and extent of the defect are such that the child will not be able to stand to void or the defect would cause psychological problems or difficulties in future sexual relations. Treatment consists of surgical repair and is usually performed before age 18 months. It is sometimes done in stages depending on the associated defects. Most techniques can be performed during same-day surgery. Routine circumcision is avoided in these children, because the foreskin may be useful in the repair. A urinary catheter may be required after surgery. Parents are instructed in the home care of the catheter. Medication for bladder spasms may be required.

This condition is corrected at a time in childhood when fears of separation and mutilation are great, and therefore attention is directed to psychological considerations. In the older child, questions about virility and reproduction may surface and need to be addressed.

EXSTROPHY OF THE BLADDER

Pathophysiology. In exstrophy of the bladder the lower portion of the abdominal wall and anterior wall of the bladder are missing. As a result, the bladder lies open and exposed on the abdomen. Exstrophy is caused by a failure of the midline to close during embryonic development. Other congenital anomalies may also be present. This anomaly occurs in 1 out of 40,000 live births and is more common in boys than in girls.

Manifestations. This disorder is noticeable by fetal sonogram. The defect may range from a small cutaneous fistula in the abdominal wall to complete exstrophy (the turning inside out of an organ). Urine leaks continually from the bladder. The skin around the bladder becomes excoriated. Other anomalies are common.

Treatment and nursing care. The bladder is covered with a plastic shield or appropriate dressing to protect its mucosa but allow for urinary drainage. This also protects the bladder from irritation by bedclothes or diapers. The skin is protected by a suitable ointment. Diapers are generally placed under rather than around the infant. The infant is positioned on his or her back or side so that urine drains freely. Antibiotics are given to prevent infection. Surgical closure is ideally performed during the first 48 hours of life.

OBSTRUCTIVE UROPATHY

Pathophysiology. Many conditions, such as calculi (stones), tumors, strictures, and scarring may cause an obstruction of the normal flow of urine. These conditions may be congenital or acquired, and blockage may be either partial or complete. One or both kidneys may be affected. The pathological changes depend on the nature and location of the problem. Hydronephrosis (*hydro,* "water" and *nephro,* "kidney") is the distention of the renal pelvis because of an obstruction. The pelvis of the kidney becomes enlarged and cysts form. This may eventually damage renal nephrons, resulting in deterioration of the kidneys. *Polycystic kidney* refers to a condition in which large, fluid-filled cysts form in place of healthy kidney tissue in the fetus. This is inherited as an autosomal recessive trait. Kidney damage can result in an inability of the kidney to concentrate urine, resulting in metabolic acidosis. Urine that is not excreted promptly can promote the growth of organisms that cause urinary tract infection.

Treatment and nursing care. Urinary diversion is necessary in certain conditions and may be accomplished by several procedures (Table 28-2). This type of surgery is a source of great apprehension for parents. The physical care of the child with a urinary stoma (artificially created opening or passage) presents hygiene problems, skin problems, and difficulties in leaving the infant in the care of others. Frequent trips to the health care provider add to the strain of everyday life.

Stress from the urinary diversion is age related. The toddler may be unable to attain independence in toilet training. The school-age child suffers from being different and may have a distorted body image. The adolescent may have lowered self-esteem and is concerned about sexuality. Parents with affected newborns grieve for the loss of a perfect child and experience concerns about the length and quality of the infant's life. The nurse anticipates the impact of this type of diagnosis and incorporates suitable psychological interventions into daily care. Providing emotional support and teaching parents how to prevent infection are priorities of care.

Assessing for a distended bladder. To assess for a distended bladder, the nurse gently palpates below the umbilicus, moving toward the symphysis pubis. The normal bladder is not palpable because it lies behind the symphysis pubis.

>NURSING **TIP**_____

The bladder capacity of a child can be approximated by the following formula:

Age in years +2 = Ounces of bladder volume or capacity

ACUTE URINARY TRACT INFECTION

Pathophysiology. Urinary tract infections (UTIs) are common in children. They are more common in girls than in boys (except during the neonatal period) and occur predominantly in children 7 to 11 years of age. Of all infections, 75% to 90% are caused by *Escherichia coli,* followed by *Klebsiella* and *Proteus* (Behrman, Kliegman, & Jenson, 2000). The nurse will see the following terms used to describe the location and problem of urinary tract disturbances:

- Urethritis: infection of the urethra
- *Cystitis:* inflammation of the bladder
- *Bacteriuria:* bacteria in the urine
- Pyelonephritis: infection of the kidney and renal pelvis
- Ureteritis: infection of the ureters
- Vesicoureteral reflux: backward flow of urine into the ureters

Several factors account for the preponderance of UTIs in girls. These include a shorter urethra, the location of the

table 28-2 | *Surgical Procedures Used in Urinary Diversion*

PROCEDURE	DEFINITION
Ureterostomy	Ureters are surgically implanted to the outside abdominal wall. This allows urine to drain into a collection device.
Ileal or colon conduit (artificial channel)	Conduit diverts urine at ureter, bypassing the bladder and urethra; ureters are removed from bladder and attached to the ileum or colon, which then acts as a bladder without voluntary control of voiding. Patient has a stoma, which is larger and not as prone to stenosis as a ureterostomy; child wears ileostomy appliance. NOTE: Urine from a conduit may appear cloudy from the secretions of the bowel conduit; this is not a sign of urinary tract infection.
Nephrostomy	Tube passes through the flank into the pelvis of kidney; this allows urine to be drained from the pelvis (bypassing ureter, bladder, and urethra; drains into ostomy bag).
Suprapubic tube placement	A suprapubic tube is placed above the symphysis pubis into the bladder to provide urinary drainage.
Vesicostomy (*vesico,* "bladder" and *stoma,* "passage")	A surgical opening is made into the bladder between umbilicus and pubis; the bladder wall is brought to the surface of the abdomen.

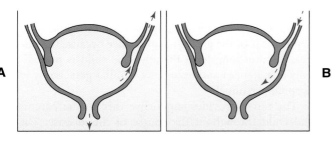

A   **B**

FIGURE **28-7** Vesicoureteral reflux. **A,** Congenital abnormalities of the junction between the bladder and the ureters can force urine to flow backward into the ureters during voiding. **B,** After voiding, residual urine from the ureter remains in the bladder.

urethra closer to the anus, the wearing of close-fitting nylon underwear, the use of bubble bath, the retention of urine, and vaginitis. Incest or other sexual abuse should be considered in young girls with repeated infections.

Certain chemical and physical factors are important. Normal urine is acidic. Alkaline urine favors pathogens. Urine that remains in the bladder for a prolonged time serves as an excellent medium for bacterial growth. In certain conditions such as *vesicoureteral reflux,* the urine is forced backward from the bladder and into the ureters during urination (Figure 28-7).

Manifestations. The signs and symptoms of UTI are age dependent. Infants often are brought for treatment with fever, frequent urination, foul-smelling urine, and persistent diaper rash. In the older child, urinary frequency, pain during micturition, onset of bedwetting in a previously "dry" child, and abdominal pain may be present.

The diagnosis depends on the culture of bacteria from the urine. The technique of collecting urine specimens is important to prevent false-positive results resulting from the growth of organisms that can occur in a warm environment or contaminated specimen bag. Specimens must be processed promptly or refrigerated (Roberts, 2000). A negative bacterial growth on a urine specimen rules out the diagnosis of UTI; a positive result, however, may result from a contaminated specimen bag and should be followed by a catheterized or suprapubic aspirated specimen (Roberts, 2000). Specimens should not be collected from the diaper because the chemicals and gels contained in the diaper fabric may alter the results of some tests. In toilet-trained children, a midstream urine specimen is obtained after cleansing the urethral meatus and rinsing with sterile water. Catheterization may be necessary to obtain a sterile specimen.

Treatment and nursing care. Infants under 1 year of age are usually hospitalized and given IV antibiotics until afebrile. Older children are treated at home with a 7- to 10-day regimen of oral antibiotics such as amoxicillin or ceftriaxone (Rocephin) and increased fluid intake. More than three UTIs in 1 year may require prophylactic antimicrobial treatment. Repeated UTIs can result in renal scarring, lead to decreased renal functioning, and contribute to the development of hypertension in adult-hood. Whenever there is lack of response to medication within 48 hours, an ultrasound examination may be indicated to rule out other causes. Acute cystitis is treated promptly to avoid developing pyelonephritis and kidney damage. Broad-spectrum antibiotics are usually initially prescribed.

Methods of preventing UTIs are taught to parents and to the patient, as age appropriate. The nurse stresses the need for proper amounts of fluid to maintain sterility and flushing of the bladder. Nursing Care Plan 28-1 presents the nursing considerations appropriate for these patients. The prognosis is excellent with prompt treatment. Monitoring vital signs, including blood pressure, and providing anticipatory guidance help decrease the stress levels of the children and parents.

NEPHROTIC SYNDROME (NEPHROSIS)

Pathophysiology. Nephrotic syndrome refers to a number of different types of kidney conditions that are distinguished by the presence of marked amounts of protein in the urine, edema, and hypoalbuminemia. Minimal change nephrotic syndrome (MCNS), found in approximately 85% of cases, is discussed in this section.

Nephrosis is more common in boys than in girls and is seen most often in children 2 to 7 years of age. The specific cause is unknown but may be related to a thymus T-cell dysfunction. The prognosis is good in steroid-responsive patients. Most children have periods of relapse until the disease resolves itself.

Manifestations. The characteristic symptom of nephrosis is *edema.* This occurs slowly; the child does not appear to be sick. It is first noticed around the eyes and ankles and later becomes generalized. The edema shifts with the position of the child during sleep. The child gains weight because of the accumulation of fluid. The abdomen may become distended *(ascites).* The child is pale, irritable, and listless and has a poor appetite. Blood pressure is usually normal.

Urine examination reveals massive albumin (protein) and a few red blood cells. The glomeruli, the working units of the kidneys that filter the blood, become damaged and allow albumin and blood cells to enter the urine. The level of protein in the blood falls; this is termed hypoalbuminemia (*hypo,* "below," *albumin,* and *emia,* "blood").

Treatment. The goals of treatment include minimizing edema, preventing infection, reducing the loss of protein in the urine, and preventing toxicity from the medication prescribed.

Control of edema. The child with nephrosis is given medications designed to reduce proteinuria and, consequently, edema. Steroid therapy is currently used for this purpose. Oral prednisone is initially given. The dosage is reduced for maintenance therapy, which continues for 1 to 2 months. Because steroids mask signs of infection, the patient must be watched closely for more subtle symptoms of illness. Children are prone to infection when absolute granulocyte counts fall below 1000 cells/mm^3. This is called neutropenia.

The child's skin is examined at sites of punctures, wounds, pierced ears, body piercings, and catheters. The nurse watches for temperature variations and changes in behavior. Suspicions are promptly reported because septicemia is life threatening. Prompt antimicrobial therapy is begun when an acute infection is recognized. Diuretics have not generally been effective in reducing nephrotic edema. Immunosuppressive therapy (i.e., cyclophosphamide [Cytoxan] and chlorambucil) is used for some steroid-resistant children.

Diet. A well-balanced diet attractively served is desirable because appetite is often poor. Parents are instructed to avoid adding salt to foods served whenever edema is present. Fluids are not usually restricted except when massive edema is present.

Nursing care. The nursing care of the child with nephrosis is of the greatest significance because the disease requires long-term therapy. The child is periodically hospitalized and becomes a familiar personality to hospital personnel.

The nurse provides supportive care to the parents and child throughout the course of this disease. The child is treated at home whenever possible and is brought to the hospital for special therapy only. Parents are instructed to keep a daily record of the child's weight, urinary proteins, and medications. Signs of infection, abnormal weight gain, and increased protein in the urine must be reported promptly. Good skin care is especially important during periods of marked edema. After the acute stage of the illness subsides, the child is allowed up and about to participate in normal childhood activities.

Positioning. The child is turned frequently to prevent respiratory infection. A pillow placed between the knees when the child is lying on the side prevents pressure on edematous organs. The child's head is elevated from time to time during the day to reduce edema of the eyelids and to make him or her more comfortable. Swelling impairs the circulation of the lacrimal secretions. It may therefore be necessary to bathe the eyes to prevent the accumulation of exudate.

Monitoring intake and output. The child's intake and output are strictly charted. This is the responsibility

NURSING CARE PLAN 28-1

The Child with a Urinary Tract Infection

PATIENT DATA: A school-aged female child is brought to the clinic complaining of burning on urination. Her mother states the child fears going to the bathroom because "it will hurt."

SELECTED NURSING DIAGNOSIS   *Impaired urinary elimination related to dysuria, incontinence*

Outcomes	Nursing Interventions	Rationales
Child will not complain of frequency, urgency, or pain on urination. Child will not strain or fret before voiding. Child will verbalize reasons for frequent bladder emptying.	1. Administer antibiotics as prescribed.	1. Antibiotics are chosen according to urine culture and sensitivity; phenazopyridine (Pyridium) may be given to decrease dysuria.
	2. Encourage complete bladder emptying; explain necessity for this, as age appropriate.	2. Retained urine in the bladder is very susceptible to the growth of organisms.
	3. Remind child to void frequently; anticipate incontinence.	3. Under normal conditions the bladder flushes away organisms by regularly ridding itself of urine; this prevents organisms from accumulating and invading nearby structures. The convalescent bladder is less resistant to invasion than is a healthy bladder.
	4. Encourage fluids.	4. Child may be febrile; increasing fluids decreases the concentration of solutes and alleviates urinary stasis.
	5. Keep accurate intake and output records.	5. This is essential to determine the progress of treatment, because the kidneys and bladder play an important part in fluid balance.
	6. Teach child how to collect urine specimens, if age appropriate.	6. Education ensures that the specimen will be correctly obtained without contamination.
	7. Provide privacy.	7. Children must be given the same courtesy as adults because they are sensitive and embarrassed by body exposure and bodily functions.

SELECTED NURSING DIAGNOSIS   *Deficient knowledge concerning hygiene measures useful in prevention of urinary tract infection*

Outcomes	Nursing Interventions	Rationales
Girl will demonstrate on doll how to wipe herself after voiding. Child will verbalize methods to accomplish this.	1. Instruct girl in importance of wiping self from front to back.	1. Good perineal hygiene avoids fecal contamination of urethra.
	2. Emphasize need to avoid bubble baths, water softeners.	2. The oils in these products are known to irritate urethra.
	3. Encourage the use of showers.	3. These hygienic measures are helpful in preventing infection.
	4. Explain the need for cotton underwear.	4. Cotton underwear is more absorbent.
	5. Suggest juices (e.g., apple, cranberry) to maintain acidity of urine.	5. Acidifying urine decreases the rate of bacterial multiplication; an acid-ash

Continued

NURSING CARE PLAN 28-1—cont'd

Outcomes	Nursing Interventions	Rationales
		diet of meats, cheese, prunes, cranberries, plums, and whole grains is also beneficial.
	6. Recommend frequent pad change for menstruating girls and proper genital cleansing during period.	6. Old pooled blood fosters the growth of organisms; proper cleansing helps to prevent irritation.

SELECTED NURSING DIAGNOSIS *Deficient knowledge (parents) concerning follow-up care*

Outcomes	Nursing Interventions	Rationales
Parents will verbalize necessity for continued supervision and medication.	1. Instruct parents to administer medication as prescribed and to continue for length of time recommended by the physician.	1. Typical course of antibiotic treatment is 7 to 10 days; emphasize the need to complete prescribed dosage.
	2. Suggest that patient avoid hot tubs or whirlpool baths.	2. May be potential sources of infection.
	3. Remind parents of necessity of adequate hydration for child.	3. Children dehydrate very quickly.
	4. Instruct parents that recurrence is most likely within 3 to 12 months after infection and is often asymptomatic.	4. Emphasize the need for routine office visits to test for asymptomatic infections.
	5. Explain necessity for periodic follow-up urine cultures.	5. Recurrence is common; a urine culture obtained approximately 1 week after medicine is discontinued will determine if medication has eradicated bacteria.

?CRITICAL THINKING QUESTION

A mother comes to the clinic with her 5-year-old child who has a urinary tract infection for the second time in 3 months. You notice that the child is wearing spandex sports shorts and carrying a doll. She is holding a bottled water container that is filled with fruit punch. What teaching interventions could the nurse initiate?

---

of the nurse, regardless of who feeds the patient. Parents are instructed to inform the nurse of how much fluid has been taken. The importance of keeping proper fluid balance sheets (i.e., intake and output records) for patients with diseases of the kidneys cannot be overemphasized.

As stated, the patient's urine must be carefully measured. Diapers may be weighed on a gram scale before application and after removal (1 g = 1 ml). The dry weights are marked on the diaper. A careful check of the number of voidings is of particular value. The character, odor, and color of the urine are also important. If a 24-hour urine collection is ordered, *every* voided specimen within that time must be saved or the test will not be valid. The specimens are collected in a large bottle or container that is correctly labeled. Some tests require that certain preservatives be added to the container; this matter is clarified before the procedure begins.

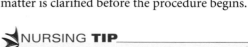
NURSING **TIP**

Remember to measure and record urine specimens sent to the laboratory.

Weight and protection from infection. The patient is weighed two or three times a week to determine changes in the degree of edema. The child is weighed on the same scale each time and at about the same time of day. Abdominal girth (circumference) should also be measured daily.

table **28-3** | *Comparison of Nephrosis with Acute Glomerulonephritis*

	NEPHROSIS	ACUTE GLOMERULONEPHRITIS
Cause	Unknown, may be a thymus T-cell dysfunction	Response to infection with group A beta-hemolytic streptococci
Edema	Massive edema Anasarca: whole-body edema Ascites: fluid in abdominal cavity	Periorbital edema (puffiness of eyes)
Blood pressure	Usually normal	Usually moderately elevated
Urine tests	Proteinuria Trace of blood	Trace of protein Hematuria (resolves within 1 month, but urinary symptoms may persist for 1 year)
Pallor	Degree of pallor is greater than expected in relation to the degree of anemia (appearance resulting from edematous tissue)	Pallor related to anemia

NOTE: The signs and symptoms of nephrosis and acute glomerulonephritis are similar. Careful analysis and comparisons reveal significant differences. Either condition can lead to renal failure and its consequences.

Nurses make every effort to protect the child from exposure to upper respiratory tract infections. Children who are up and about must not be allowed to wander into areas where they would be in danger of contracting an infection. *No vaccinations or immunizations should be administered while the disease is active and during immunosuppressive therapy.*

The vital signs of a patient with nephrosis are taken regularly. Ordinarily there is no temperature elevation unless an infection is present. Blood pressure remains normal. Parental guidance and support are given by all members of the nursing team. The child with nephrosis is kept under close medical supervision over an extended period. Prognosis is considered favorable.

ACUTE GLOMERULONEPHRITIS

Pathophysiology. Acute glomerulonephritis (AGN), formerly called *Bright's disease,* is an allergic reaction (antigen-antibody) to a group A beta-hemolytic streptococcal infection. It may appear after the patient has had scarlet fever or skin infections. The body's immune mechanisms appear to be important in its development. Antibodies produced to fight the invading organisms also react against the glomerular tissue. Glomerulonephritis is the most common form of nephritis in children, and it occurs most often in boys 3 to 7 years of age. Both kidneys are usually affected.

The nephron is the working unit of the kidneys. Nephrons number in the millions. Within the bulb of each nephron lies a cluster of capillaries called the glomerulus. It is these structures that are affected, as the name implies. They become inflamed and sometimes blocked, permitting red blood cells and protein (which are normally retained) to enter the urine. The kidneys become pale and slightly enlarged. Table 28-3 compares nephrosis with AGN.

The prognosis for AGN is excellent. Patients with mild cases of the disease may recover within 10 to 14 days. Patients with protracted cases may show urinary changes for as long as 1 year but have complete recovery. Observation for complications that involve hypertensive changes such as brain ischemia necessitate careful monitoring and care of each patient.

Manifestations. From 1 to 3 weeks after a streptococcal infection has occurred, the parent may notice that the child has periorbital edema upon awakening in the morning and that the child's urine is smoky brown or bloody. This is frightening to the parent and child, and most parents immediately seek medical advice. Urine output may be decreased. The urine specific gravity is high, and albumin, red and white blood cells, and casts may be found on examination. The blood urea nitrogen level is elevated, as are the serum creatinine and sedimentation rate. The serum complement level is usually reduced. Hyperkalemia (excessive potassium in the blood) may produce cardiac toxicity. Hypertension may occur.

Treatment and nursing care. Although children may feel well, activity is limited until gross hematuria subsides. The urine is regularly examined. Every effort is made to prevent children from becoming overly tired, chilled, or exposed to infection. As renal function is impaired, there is a danger of accumulating nitrogenous wastes and sodium in the body. Dietary sodium and fluid restrictions are based on the hypertension and edema present. Foods high in potassium, such as bananas, are restricted during periods of oliguria.

Nursing care is supportive. Prevention of infection, fatigue, maintenance of accurate intake and output records, and frequent monitoring of vital signs are essential.

Although glomerulonephritis is generally benign, it can be a source of anguish for the parents and child. If the patient is treated at home, the parents must plan activities to keep the child occupied with quiet activity. They must understand the importance of continued medical supervision, because follow-up urine and blood tests are necessary to assess progress toward recovery. All children with hypertension should be monitored for signs of increased intracranial pressure.

WILMS' TUMOR

Pathophysiology. Wilms' tumor, or *nephroblastoma* (*nephro,* "kidney," *blasto,* "bud," and *oma,* "tumor"), is one of the most common malignancies of early life. It is an embryonal adenosarcoma (*adeno,* "glandular," and *sarcoma,* "cancer of connective tissue") that is now known to be associated with certain congenital anomalies, particularly of the genitourinary tract. It is thought to have a genetic basis.

About two thirds of these growths are discovered before the child is 3 years of age. As with some other malignancies, there are few or no symptoms during the early stages of growth. A mass in the abdomen is generally discovered by a parent or by the physician during a routine checkup. X-ray examinations of the kidneys (most importantly, IV pyelograms) reveal a growth and verify the fact that the remaining kidney is normal. The tumor compresses kidney tissue and is usually encapsulated. Renal damage may cause hypertension. Chest x-ray films, ultrasound, bone surveys, liver scan, and CT may also be indicated. Wilms' tumor seldom affects both kidneys.

Treatment and nursing care. Treatment of Wilms' tumor patients consists of a combination of surgery, radiation therapy, and chemotherapy. The kidney and tumor are removed as soon as possible after the diagnosis has been confirmed. It is important to prepare the parents and the child for the extent of the incision, which is considerable.

General nursing measures for the comfort of the patient are carried out. One factor pertinent to this condition is *that all unnecessary handling of the abdomen is to be avoided* because it can cause the tumor to spread. The physician explains this to the parents, and in the hospital a sign is placed on the crib: "Do not palpate abdomen." Abdominal palpation, as part of the daily assessment, is omitted. Nursing Care Plan 28-2 outlines care for a child undergoing surgery of the renal system. Chemotherapy and radiation therapy after surgery are usually completed at a specialized cancer center.

HYDROCELE

Pathophysiology. A hydrocele (*hydro,* "water" and *cele,* "tumor") is an excessive amount of fluid in the sac that surrounds the testicle and causes the scrotum to swell (Figure 28-8). When the testes descend into the scrotum in utero, the *processus vaginalis* (a fold of tissue) precedes them. This tissue ordinarily fuses, separating the peritoneal cavity from the scrotum. When this

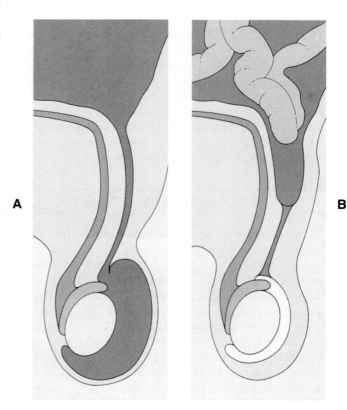

A   **B**

FIGURE **28-8** Hydrocele. **A,** Simple hydrocele. **B,** Hydrocele with herniation of the bowel into the scrotum.

NURSING CARE PLAN 28-2

The Child Undergoing Surgery of the Renal System

PATIENT DATA: A preadolescent boy is admitted for elective kidney surgery. The child asks his parents to stay and asks the nurse many questions about the planned surgery.

SELECTED NURSING DIAGNOSIS   *Anxiety related to surgical experience*

Outcomes	Nursing Interventions	Rationales
Parents will state two ways they are coping with the stress of this surgery. Child will verbalize an understanding of procedure, as age appropriate.	1. Provide surgical tour, include wake-up room.	1. Explanations and familiarity with physical surroundings may decrease apprehension.
	2. Encourage parents to remain with child, as appropriate.	2. Child is more secure when parents are close by.
	3. Explain mask and anesthesia equipment.	3. It is frightening to have something placed over the face; equipment is intimidating.
	4. Determine the small child's words for penis, urination.	4. This will promote understanding postoperatively.
	5. Provide support and reassurance.	5. Urinary surgery may raise anxiety about sexual function, which parents or patients are often unable to express.

SELECTED NURSING DIAGNOSIS   *High risk for ineffective airway clearance related to poor cough effort associated with postanesthesia, postoperative immobility, pain*

Outcomes	Nursing Interventions	Rationales
Child will maintain airway patency as evidenced by clear lung sounds, vital signs within normal range.	1. Assist child to turn, cough, deep breathe; reposition infants.	1. Prolonged postoperative immobility leads to decreased chest expansion, pooling of mucus in bronchi, and hypostatic pneumonia. In nephrectomy patients, the incision is close to the diaphragm, making breathing painful; allow infants to cry for a few seconds to ensure deep breathing; if secretions are present, coughing will generally follow. Ambulate as ordered.
	2. Monitor vital signs frequently.	2. Monitoring vital signs will assess cardiovascular function and tissue perfusion.
	3. Teach splinting of incision preoperatively.	3. Splinting incision lessens pain.
	4. Teach incentive spirometry preoperatively.	4. Spirometry promotes alveolar inflation, restores and maintains lung capacity, and strengthens respiratory muscles; it also provides immediate feedback about the effectiveness of deep breathing.
	5. Observe and medicate for bladder spasm and incisional pain.	5. Postoperative pain and discomfort may make patients reluctant to turn, cough, and deep breathe.

Continued

NURSING CARE PLAN 28-2—cont'd

SELECTED NURSING DIAGNOSIS *High risk for deficient fluid volume related to patient's age, surgery, catheters, refusal to drink*

Outcomes	Nursing Interventions	Rationales
Vital signs will remain within normal limits. Child's hydration and acid-base balance will remain stable as evidenced by laboratory reports.	1. Regulate IV fluids.	1. Child will probably take nothing by mouth for a brief period before and after surgery. IV fluids maintain hydration and replace lost electrolytes.
	2. Keep accurate intake and output records.	2. Careful monitoring of fluid intake and output will identify early renal complications.
	3. Weigh infants daily.	3. Daily weights in infants assist in monitoring underhydration or overhydration. Comparison with preoperative weight will assess infant's nutritional progress.
	4. Record separate output for each drainage tube.	4. An unexpected reduction in urine flow requires prompt intervention. Each catheter drains into its own collection bag, so that source of reduced flow will be immediately noticed.
	5. Observe tissue turgor and fontanels of infants.	5. Depressed fontanels, sunken eyeballs, lack of tears, dark circles around eyes, and poor skin turgor denote dehydration, which can occur quickly in infants and children.
	6. Begin clear oral fluids gradually.	6. Replacement of fluids and electrolytes by mouth is generally considered to be the safest method; clarify ambiguous orders, such as "force fluids," "restrict fluids," particularly in infants and small children with urological disorders, cardiac conditions, and so on.
Child's temperature will remain at or below 38° C (100.4° F); incision site will not be erythematous or foul-smelling.	1. Observe for signs of infection.	1. Fever, incisional tenderness, redness, drainage from incisions, and lethargy indicate infection.
	2. Observe and record patency, color, amount, and consistency of drainage.	2. Catheters can become plugged by mucus shreds, blood clots, and chemical sediment; plugging of conduits can lead to infection of urinary tract, urine stasis and, if obstruction persists, hydronephrosis.
	3. Obtain urine cultures as indicated.	3. Pathogens in urine are most specifically determined by culture; goal is to obtain urine that is uncontaminated by organisms outside the urinary tract.

NURSING CARE PLAN 28-2—cont'd

Outcomes	Nursing Interventions	Rationales
	4. Maintain aseptic closed drainage system.	4. Maintaining a closed drainage system aids in preventing infection; careful handwashing before and after handling of catheter or drainage system is also of importance.

?CRITICAL THINKING QUESTION

The parents of a postoperative patient who has had renal surgery appear anxious and upset. When questioned, they state that they both work, cannot afford to take the time off from work to stay with their child, and are also worried that he will fail in school and no longer be able to travel with his friends in a carpool. They don't know how they will manage. What is the best response of the nurse?

---

fusion does not take place, however, peritoneal fluid may enter the inguinal canal. Its appearance in the newborn is not uncommon, and in many cases the condition corrects itself by 1 year of age.

Treatment. A chronic hydrocele that persists beyond 1 year is corrected by surgery. Routine postoperative nursing care is given. This is outlined in Chapter 22. Same-day surgery may be arranged.

CRYPTORCHIDISM

Pathophysiology. The testes are the male sex glands. These two oval bodies begin their development in the abdominal cavity below the kidneys in the embryo. Their function is to produce spermatozoa (male sex cells) and male hormones, particularly testosterone. Toward the end of the seventh fetal month, the testes begin to descend along a pathway into the scrotum. If this descent does not take place normally, the testes may remain in the abdomen or inguinal canal. This condition is common in approximately 30% of low-birth-weight infants. When one or both testes fail to lower into the scrotum, the condition is termed cryptorchidism (*kryptos,* "hidden" and *orchi,* "testis"). The unilateral form is more common.

Because the testes are warmer in the abdomen than in the scrotum, the sperm cells begin to deteriorate. If both testes are affected, sterility results. *Inguinal hernia* often accompanies this condition. Secondary sex characteristics, such as voice change and growth of facial hair, are not affected because the testes continue to secrete hormones directly into the bloodstream. Acute scrotal pain may indicate a testicular torsion (twisting), which requires immediate surgery to preserve testicular function.

Treatment and nursing care. Occasionally, a testis or the testes spontaneously descend during the first year of life. Hormonal management before surgery consists of the administration of human chorionic gonadotropin (hCG). This hormone is useful as a diagnostic aid and may also precipitate the descent of the testes into the scrotal sac. If this does not occur, an operation called an orchiopexy (*orchio,* "testicle" and *pexy,* "fixation") is performed.

Although an orchiopexy improves the condition, the fertility rate among these patients may be reduced, even when only one testis is undescended. In addition, the incidence of testicular tumors is increased in these patients during adulthood. Parents are told to teach the growing child the importance of self-examination of the testes. When the child returns from surgery, care is taken to prevent contamination of the suture line, and scrotal support is maintained.

The psychological approach of the nurse to the patient and his family is important because of the embarrassment they may feel. People may ask the child why he is being operated on when there is no visible evidence of trauma. This problem is often compounded by the fact that the older child may have been told not to discuss his condition; in addition, his understanding of his problem and just what is going to happen in surgery may be vague. Therefore the nurse caring for the child should know what he has been told and how he feels about his operation to give emotional support. Terminology is clarified. The nurse assures the child that his penis will not be involved in the surgery.

The parents, too, may have anxieties that they cannot verbalize. It is difficult for many of them to communicate with their child about such matters. A thoughtful, sensitive nurse who tries to anticipate related feelings and fears promotes the child's adjustment.

IMPACT OF URINARY OR GENITAL SURGERY ON GROWTH AND DEVELOPMENT

Surgery of the urinary or genital tract impacts growth and development. Preschoolers may perceive the treatment as punishment. Separation anxiety during hospitalizations peak, and preventive strategies should be explained to the parents. The body image of the child must be assertively maintained whenever surgery is delayed beyond infancy. Between 3 and 6 years of age, the child becomes curious about sexual differences and may masturbate. Surgical interventions during this stage of development require guidance and preparation to minimize the negative impact on growth and development.

During home care, tub baths may be contraindicated, dressings to "private parts" of the body must be inspected daily, and restrictions on play activities that involve straddle toys (e.g., tricycles, rocking horses) are necessary. Adolescents may be concerned about the effects of surgery on their appearance and sexual abilities.

key points

- The functional unit of the kidney is the nephron.
- Children with hypospadias are born with the urethral opening on the undersurface of the penis.
- Bladder exstrophy is a serious congenital defect in which the bladder lies exposed on the lower portion of the abdominal wall. Surgical correction of this defect is lifesaving.
- Obstruction of the urinary tract may lead to hydronephrosis, a distention of the kidney pelvis. This is a serious condition because it could eventually lead to kidney failure if left untreated.
- To avoid fecal contamination of the urinary tract, girls are taught to wipe the perineal area from front to back after urination.
- Ascites is an abnormal collection of fluid in the peritoneal cavity. It is seen in advanced cases of nephrosis and in other conditions.

- The accurate charting of intake and output on patients with kidney problems is absolutely essential to their treatment and recovery. This includes ostomy and urinary drainage.
- Accurate blood pressure measurements will detect hypertension, a condition often associated with kidney problems.
- Normally urine flows from the ureters into the bladder, and almost no flow reenters the ureters.
- Repeated urinary tract infections or improper position of the ureters or sphincters in the bladder at birth may result in the reflux of urine into the ureters.
- Good health habits include assessing one's own body, including the genitalia.
- Early treatment of cryptorchidism is necessary to preserve testicular function.
- A hydrocele is an excessive amount of fluid in the sac that surrounds the testicle. It causes the scrotum to swell.
- Undescended testes *(cryptorchidism)* refers to a condition in which the testes do not lower into the scrotum during the fetal period but remain in the abdomen or inguinal canal after birth.
- The minimum urine output for infants and toddlers is 2 to 3 ml/kg/hr; for preschoolers, the minimum is 1 to 2 ml/kg/hr; and for school-age children and adolescents, the minimum is 0.5 to 1 ml/kg/hr.

ONLINE RESOURCES

Urinary Tract Infections: http://www.pediatrics.org/cgi/content/full/103/4/e54

Phimosis: http://www.healthsquare.com/ndfiles/nd0808.htm

Hypospadias: http://www.duj.com/hypospadias.html

Vesicoureteral Reflux: http://www.findarticles.com/cf_dls/g2601/0014/2601001452/p1/article.jhtml

REVIEW QUESTIONS   *Choose the most appropriate answer.*

1. The nurse understands that genitourinary surgery impacts growth and development. When caring for a 4-year-old child postoperatively, a priority nursing responsibility would include:
   1. Strategies to preserve child's body image
   2. Assurances that appearance and sexual function will not be affected
   3. Providing age-appropriate toys such as tricycles
   4. Preventing embarrassment by limiting family and friends visiting

2. The administration of prednisone to children with nephrosis creates the problem of:
   1. Intolerance of foods
   2. Increased risk of infection
   3. Increased periorbital edema
   4. Weight loss

3. Daily weights are obtained in children with nephrosis to monitor:
   1. Weight loss from low-protein diet
   2. Accuracy of fluid balance sheets
   3. Changes in the amount of edema
   4. Percentile on growth grid

4. A priority nursing responsibility in the care of a child with Wilms' tumor is to:
   1. Maintain accurate intake and output records
   2. Omit abdominal palpation during daily assessments
   3. Maintain strict bed rest
   4. Assess neurological function

5. Accurate fluid intake and output records are particularly important in patients with kidney disease because:
   1. They aid in assessing kidney damage
   2. They help to determine nutritional adequacy
   3. They are important in assessing hypertension
   4. They provide a reliable method of determining infection

objectives

1. Define each key term listed.
2. Recall the differences between the skin of the infant and that of the adult.
3. Describe two topical agents used to treat acne.
4. Summarize the nursing care for a child who has infantile eczema. State the rationale for each nursing measure.
5. Discuss the symptoms and treatment of pediculosis.
6. Differentiate among first-, second-, and third-degree burns in anatomical structures involved, appearance, level of sensation, and first aid required.
7. List five objectives of the nurse caring for the burned child.
8. Describe how the response of the child with burns differs from that of the adult.
9. Identify the principles of topical therapy.
10. Examine the emergency treatment of three types of burns.
11. Differentiate four types of topical medication.
12. Discuss the prevention and treatment of frostbite.

key terms

allergens (ĂL-ĕr-jĕnz, p. 707)
alopecia (ăl-ō-PĒ-shē-ă, p. 711)
autograft (AW-tō-grăft, p. 719)
chilblain (CHĬL-blān, p. 720)
comedo (KŌM-ĕ-dō, p. 705)
crust (p. 702)
Curling's ulcer (KŬR-lĭngz ŬL-sĕr, p. 717)
debridement (dă-BRĒD-măw, p. 717)
dermabrasion (dĕrm-ă-BRĀ-zhŭn, p. 706)
ecchymosis (ĕk-ĭ-MŌ-sĭs, p. 702)
emollient (ĕ-MŌL-ē-ŭnt, p. 707)
eschar (ĒS-kăhr, p. 717)
exanthem (ĕg-ZĂN-thăm, p. 702)
frostbite (p. 720)
heterografts (HĔT-ĕr-ō-grăftz, p. 719)
hives (p. 702)

homografts (HŌ-mō-grăftz, p. 718)
ileus (ĬL-ē-ŭs, p. 717)
isograft (ī-sō-grăft, p. 719)
macule (MĂK-ūl, p. 702)
Methicillin-resistant *Staphylococcus aureus* (MRSA) (mĕth-ĭ-SĬL-ĭn rē-zĭs-tĕnt stăf-ĭ-lō-kŏk-ŭs AW-rē-ŭs, p. 710)
papule (PĂP-ūl, p. 702)
pediculosis (pĕ-dĭk-ū-LŌ-sĭs, p. 712)
pruritus (proo-RĪ-tŭs, p. 707)
pustule (PŬS-tūl, p. 702)
sebum (p. 705)
stye (p. 703)
total body surface area (TBSA) (p. 713)
vesicle (VĔS-ĭ-k'l, p. 702)
wheal (wēl, p. 702)
xenograft (ZĒ-nō-grăft, p. 719)

SKIN DEVELOPMENT AND FUNCTIONS

The main function of the skin is protection. It acts as the body's first line of defense against disease. It prevents the passage of harmful physical and chemical agents and prevents the loss of water and electrolytes. It also has a great capacity to regenerate and repair itself. The skin and the structures derived from it, such as hair and fingernails, are known as the *integumentary system*. Figure 29-1 depicts these structures and how they differ in the developing child and in the adult.

Maintaining skin integrity is important to self-esteem and therefore has both a psychological and a physiological component. This is particularly evident in patients with facial disfiguration. Four basic skin sensations—pain, temperature, touch, and pressure—are felt by the skin in conjunction with the nervous system. The skin also secretes sebum, which helps to protect and maintain its texture. The outer surface of the skin is acidic, with a pH of 4.5 to 6.5 to protect the skin from pathological bacteria, which thrive in an alkaline environment.

The skin is composed of two layers: the epidermis (derived from the ectoderm) and the dermis (derived from the mesoderm). Vernix caseosa, a cheeselike sub-

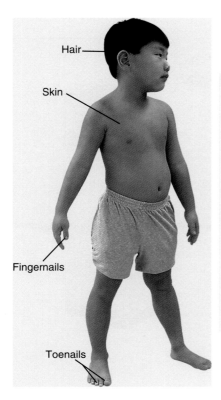

Hair

Skin

Fingernails

Toenails

INTEGUMENTARY SYSTEM

- The thin epidermis in infants blisters easily, absorption is dramatically greater, and infections occur more readily.
- Sebaceous glands do not begin producing sebum until about 8 to 10 years. Without lubrication, the skin is more dry and chaps more easily.
- Skin infections are more apt to produce systemic symptoms.
- Preterm and term newborns have less subcutaneous fat; therefore they are more sensitive to heat and cold.
- At birth, the skin is alkaline, increasing suseptibility to infection.
- The ability to perspire through the skin matures by 3 years of age, and axillary perspiration begins near puberty. Therefore thermoregulation may be a problem in children.

FIGURE **29-1** Summary of some integumentary system differences between the child and the adult. The integumentary system consists of the skin and the structures derived from it. This system protects the body, helps to regulate body temperature, and receives stimuli such as pressure, pain, and temperature.

stance, covers the fetus until birth. This protects the fetal skin from maceration as it floats in its watery home. The fetal skin is at first so transparent that blood vessels are clearly visible. Downy lanugo hair begins to develop at about 13 to 16 weeks, especially on the head. At 21 to 24 weeks the skin is reddish and wrinkled, with little subcutaneous fat. Adipose tissue forms during later weeks. At birth the subcutaneous glands are well developed, and the skin is pink and smooth and has a polished look. It is thinner than the skin of an adult.

SKIN DISORDERS AND VARIATIONS

Certain skin conditions in children may be associated with age, as in the case of milia in infants and acne in adolescents. A skin condition may be a manifestation of a systemic disease, such as chickenpox. Some lesions, such as strawberry nevi and mongolian spots, are congenital. Other skin lesions, such as those seen in rubella and fifth disease, are self-limited and do not require treatment.

There are great individual differences in skin texture, color, pH, and moisture. Skin color is an important diagnostic criterion in cases of liver disease, heart conditions, and child abuse and for overall assessment. Complete blood counts and serum electrolyte levels are helpful in diagnosing skin conditions. Skin tests are used in diagnosing allergies. The purified protein derivative (PPD) test is useful in screening for tuberculosis. Skin scrapings are used for microscopic examination. The Wood light is an instrument used to diagnose certain skin conditions. It reflects a particular color according to the organism present.

Hair condition is important to observe. Hair is inspected for color, texture, quality, distribution, and elasticity. Hair may become dry and brittle and may lack luster owing to inadequate nutrition. Hair may begin to fall out or even change color during illness or the ingestion of certain medications.

Skin conditions may be acute or chronic. The nurse should describe the lesions with regard to size, color, configuration (e.g., butterfly rash), presence of pain or itching, distribution (e.g., arms, legs, behind ears), and

box 29-1 *Terms Used to Describe Skin Conditions*

Macule: flat rash (freckles)

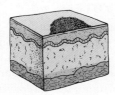

Papule: elevated area (pimple)

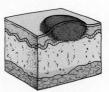

Vesicle: elevated, fluid-filled blister (cold sore, chickenpox)

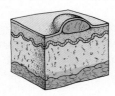

Pustules: elevated, pus filled (impetigo, acne)

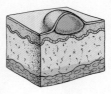

Crust: scab

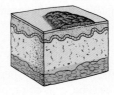

Ecchymosis: black and blue-purple mark (bruise)

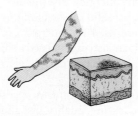

Wheal: raised red, irregular (mosquito bite, allergic reactions)

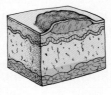

whether the rash is general or local. Hives, a general rash that appears abruptly, is often an allergic or medication reaction. The condition of the skin around the lesions is also significant, as is the skin turgor. Managing itching is a key component in preventing secondary infection from scratching. Dressings and ointments are applied as prescribed. Preventing infections is a consid-

eration in open wounds. Mongolian spots and physiological jaundice are covered in Chapters 12 and 14. The communicable diseases are discussed in Chapter 31.

Many childhood infectious diseases, such as measles, German measles, and chickenpox, involve the presence of an exanthem (a skin rash). Box 29-1 identifies terms used to describe some conditions of the skin that the

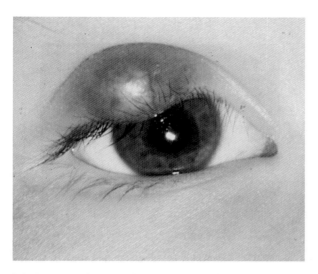

FIGURE **29-2** A stye or hordeolum is an inflammation of the sebaceous gland of the eyelid commonly seen in infants and children.

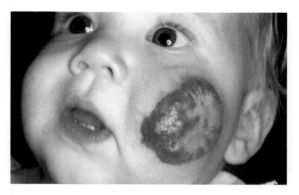

FIGURE **29-3** Strawberry nevus. This minor lesion can result in major psychological problems.

nurse may witness. Some rashes begin as one lesion and evolve into others. For example, the pattern of chickenpox rash is macule, papule, vesicle, and crust. A stye is an infection of the sebaceous gland of the eyelash (Figure 29-2).

CONGENITAL LESIONS

STRAWBERRY NEVUS

The strawberry nevus (Figure 29-3) is a common *hemangioma* (consists of dilated capillaries in the dermal space) that may not become apparent for a few weeks after birth. Although it is harmless and usually disappears without treatment, it is disturbing to parents, especially when it appears on the head or face. At first it is flat, but it gradually becomes raised. The lesion is bright red, elevated, and sharply demarcated. The lesions gradually blanch, with 60% disappearing spontaneously by 5 years of age and 90% disappearing by 9 years of age. Laser treatment or excision may be considered if the area becomes ulcerated. Parents are often quizzed about the growth by insensitive persons and may be advised of various unorthodox treatments. The nurse offers support and reassurance to parents and corrects misinformation.

PORT-WINE NEVUS

Port-wine nevi (Figure 29-4) are present at birth and are caused by dilated dermal capillaries. The lesions are flat, sharply demarcated, and purple to pink. The lesion darkens as the child gets older. If the area is small, cosmetics may disguise the lesion. If the area is large, laser surgery may be indicated.

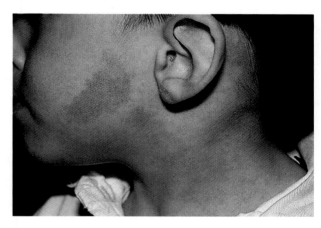

FIGURE **29-4** Port-wine stain.

INFECTIONS

MILIARIA

Pathophysiology. Miliaria (prickly heat) refers to a rash caused by excess body heat and moisture (Figure 29-5). There is a retention of sweat in the sweat glands, which have become blocked or inflamed. Rupture or leakage into the skin causes the inflamed response. It appears suddenly as tiny, pinhead-sized, reddened papules with occasional clear vesicles. It may be accompanied by *pruritus* (itching). It is seen in infants during hot weather or in newborns who sleep in overheated rooms. It often occurs in the diaper area or in the folds of the skin where moisture accumulates. Plastic enclosures on diapers hold in body warmth that results in a rash. This harmless condition may be reversed by removing extra clothing, bathing, skin care, and frequent diaper changes.

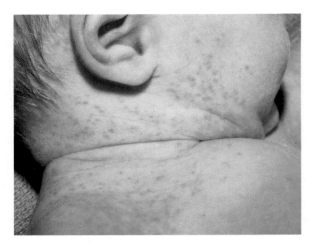

FIGURE **29-5** Miliaria. Note the many tiny pustular lesions in the folds of the neck.

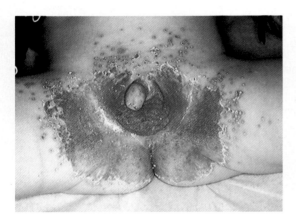

FIGURE **29-6** Intertrigo (candidiasis). Red, moist patches have sharply demarcated borders and some loose scales, usually in the genital area extending along the inguinal and gluteal folds. This lesion is aggravated by urine, feces, heat, and moisture.

INTERTRIGO

Pathophysiology. Intertrigo (*in,* "into" and *terere,* "to rub") is the medical term for chafing. It is a dermatitis that occurs in the folds of the skin (Figure 29-6). The patches are red and moist and are usually located along the neck and in the inguinal and gluteal folds. This condition is aggravated by urine, feces, heat, and moisture. Prevention consists of keeping the affected areas clean and *dry.* The child is allowed to be out of diapers to expose the area to air and light. Maceration of the skin can lead to secondary infections.

SEBORRHEIC DERMATITIS

Pathophysiology. Seborrheic dermatitis (cradle cap) is an inflammation of the skin that involves the seba-

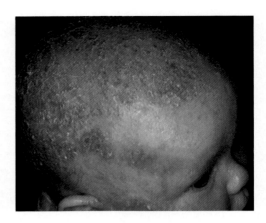

FIGURE **29-7** Seborrheic dermatitis (cradle cap). Thick, yellow, greasy adherent scales appear on the scalp and forehead. There is no itching (pruritus).

ceous glands (Figure 29-7). It is characterized by thick, yellow, oily, adherent, crustlike scales on the scalp and forehead. The skin beneath the patches may be red (erythematous). Less often it may involve the eyelids, external ear, and inguinal area. Secondary bacterial and yeast infections may occur. It is seen in newborns, in infants, and at puberty. In newborns it is commonly known as "cradle cap." It is seen in infants with sensitive skin, even when the head and hair are washed frequently. Seborrhea resembles eczema, but it usually does not itch and there is a negative family history. In adolescence it is more localized and is usually confined to the scalp. A condition resembling seborrheic dermatitis is common in children and adolescents infected with the human immunodeficiency virus (HIV).

Treatment. Treatment consists of shampooing the hair on a regular basis. Scales that are particularly stubborn in newborns may be softened by applying baby oil to the head the evening before and shampooing in the morning. The scalp is rinsed well. A soft brush is helpful in removing loose particles from the hair. The nurse teaches the parent how to shampoo an infant's head using the football hold (see Chapter 22, Figure 22-4). A dandruff-control shampoo is used for adolescents. Medications such as sulfur, salicylic acid, or hydrocortisone may be prescribed. Topical antifungal agents effective against *Pityrosporum* have also been suggested. The response to therapy is usually rapid.

DIAPER DERMATITIS

Pathophysiology. Diaper dermatitis (diaper rash) is a commonly seen condition that results when the skin becomes irritated by prolonged contact with urine, feces, retained laundry soaps, and friction (Figure 29-8).

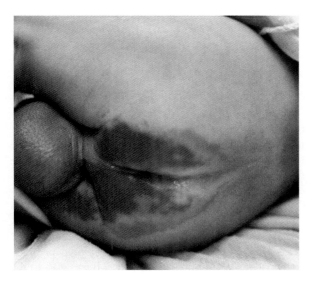

FIGURE **29-8** Diaper rash (diaper dermatitis). A red, moist maculopapular rash with poorly defined borders appears in the diaper area. The infant may have a history of infrequent diaper changes or the use of snug rubber/plastic pants. The inflammation results from ammonia, heat, and moisture.

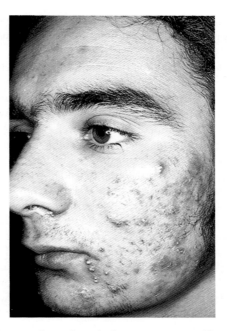

FIGURE **29-9** Acne. Acne is the most common skin problem of adolescence. An increase in sebaceous gland activity creates increased oiliness. Open comedones (blackheads) and closed comedones (whiteheads) are common. Severe acne includes papules and nodules. The lesions appear on the face, chest, back, and shoulders.

It may be seen in response to the addition of solid foods or with a change in breast or bottle feedings. Changes in detergent, water softeners, the use of wipes that contain fragrance or chemicals, or other household substances may precipitate the irritation. The rash may appear as a simple erythema (redness) or may be evidenced by scales, blisters, and ulcerations. Perianal involvement may be apparent if the infant has loose stools. A beefy red rash in the diaper area may be indicative of a *Candida* (thrush) infection and requires prompt treatment.

Treatment and nursing care. It is easier to prevent diaper rash than to cure it. This is accomplished by frequent diaper changes to limit the exposure to moisture. The diaper is periodically removed to expose the skin to light and air. With each diaper change, the perineal area is thoroughly cleansed (preferably with warm water) and gently dried. Plastic pants are avoided. After bowel movements, the area is cleansed with mild soap and water. The skin folds are thoroughly washed, rinsed, and dried. If a rash is persistent, the pediatrician may prescribe a light application of a mild hydrocortisone ointment. Superabsorbent disposable diapers reduce the occurrence of diaper rash, but frequent diaper changes and skin care remain essential. Petrolatum, A and D ointment, or zinc oxide ointment are protective ointments that can be applied between diaper changes and removed with mineral oil before reapplying after a diaper change.

ACNE VULGARIS

Pathophysiology. Acne is an inflammation of the sebaceous glands and hair follicles in the skin (Figure 29-9). Because of hormonal influence, the sebaceous follicles enlarge at puberty and secrete increased amounts of a fatty substance called sebum. Genetic factors and stress are also thought to play a part. The course of acne may be brief or prolonged (lasting 10 years or longer). Premenstrual acne in girls is not uncommon. The principal lesions include comedones, papules, and nodulocystic growths.

A comedo (plural, *comedones*) is a plug of keratin, sebum, or bacteria. Keratin is a protein substance and is the main constituent of epidermis and hair. There are two types of comedones: open and closed. In the open comedo, or *blackhead,* the surface is darkened by melanin. Closed comedones, or *whiteheads,* are responsible for the inflammatory process of acne. With continued buildup, the walls of the follicle rupture, releasing their irritating contents into the surrounding skin. A pustule may appear when this develops near the exterior. This process occurs no matter how carefully the teenager washes because surface bacteria are not involved in the pathogenesis. Acne is usually seen on the chin, cheeks, and forehead. It can also develop on the chest, upper back, and shoulders. It usually is more severe in winter.

Treatment. The basic treatment of acne has changed considerably over the past few years. It is no longer thought that certain foods trigger the condition; therefore the restriction of chocolate, peanuts, and cola drinks is unwarranted. A regular, well-balanced diet is encouraged. Patients who are not taking tetracycline or vitamin A benefit from sunshine. General hygienic measures of cleanliness, rest, and the avoidance of emotional stress may help to prevent exacerbations.

Routine skin cleansing is indicated, and greasy hair and cosmetic preparations should be avoided. Excessive cleansing of the skin can irritate and chap the tissues. Squeezing pimples ruptures intact lesions and causes local inflammation. The topical preparations recommended include benzoyl peroxide gels or lotions that dry and peel the skin and suppress fatty acid growth. Vitamin A acid (Retin-A) helps eliminate keratinous plugs. Vitamin A acid can increase sensitivity to the sun, so precautions should be taken when it is used. Tetracycline, erythromycin, doxycycline (Vibramycin), or minocycline (Minocin) may be given in conjunction with topical medications in more serious cases. Monilial vaginitis is a secondary complication sometimes seen when these drugs are used, and this should be explained to the unsuspecting adolescent girl.

Isotretinoin (Accutane) is given to patients with severe pustulocystic acne who have been unable to benefit from other types of treatment. It has many side effects; thus the patient must be carefully monitored with liver studies and lipid levels. *It is not prescribed during pregnancy or to those at risk for pregnancy because of the possibilities of fetal deformity.* Planing of the skin to minimize scarring (dermabrasion) is done selectively, because it is not always successful. Oral contraceptives (OC) such as Ortho Tri-Cyclen (norgestimate and ethinyl estradiol) may also be given because sebum production is controlled by androgens, and such OCs reduce androgen levels.

Acne is distressing to the adolescent, particularly when the face is extensively involved. Sometimes even a minimum problem is seen as disastrous when it happens before an important event. The self-conscious young person feels different and embarrassed. The nurse who is attuned to the feelings of individuals can provide understanding support. Although the adolescent is educated to assume responsibility for the regimen, including the parents helps to prevent conflict surrounding it. Drug-induced acne can occur in children taking long-term steroids, phenobarbital, phenytoin, lithium, vitamin B_{12}, or medications containing iodides or bromides.

> **NURSING TIP**
>
> Topical benzoyl peroxide and Retin-A neutralize each other when applied together.

HERPES SIMPLEX TYPE I

Pathophysiology. Herpes simplex type I, a viral infection, is commonly known as a *cold sore* or fever blister. It may begin by a feeling of tingling, itching, or burning on the lip. Vesicles and crusts form (Figure 29-10). Spontaneous healing occurs in about 8 to 10 days. Communicability is highest early in the formation and is spread by direct contact. Recurrence is common because the virus lies dormant in the body until it is activated by stress, sun exposure, menstruation, fever, and other causes. Patients must become familiar with their own personal triggers. Herpes can be serious in newborns and in the patients who are immunocompromised.

Treatment and nursing care. Topical acyclovir may reduce viral shedding and hasten healing. In the hospital, ointments are applied with gloved hands. Contact (standard) precautions should be followed (see Appendix A). Patients are instructed not to pick at lesions because this may produce spreading to other sites. They should not share lipstick and should avoid kissing while lesions are active. Sensitivity to the self-conscious adolescent who has a cold sore is important. Genital herpes caused by the herpes virus type II and spread by sexual intimacy is discussed in Chapter 11, Table 11-1. The distinction between the two types has become less clear because of an increase in the practice of oral-genital sex.

INFANTILE ECZEMA

Pathophysiology. Infantile eczema, or atopic dermatitis, is an inflammation of genetically hypersensitive

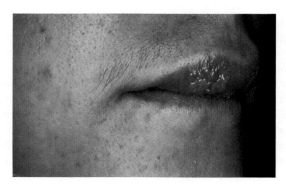

FIGURE **29-10** Herpes simplex (cold sores). These begin with skin tingling and sensitivity and erupt with tight vesicles, then pustules, and then a crust. Lesions commonly appear on the upper lip.

skin (Figure 29-11). The pathophysiology is characterized by local vasodilation in affected areas. This progresses to *spongiosis,* or the breakdown of dermal cells and the formation of intradermal vesicles. Chronic scratching produces weeping and results in lichenification, or coarsening, of the skin folds. The exact cause of this condition is difficult to pinpoint because it is believed to be caused mainly by allergy. Infantile eczema is rarely seen in breastfed infants until they begin to eat additional food. It seems to follow a definite familial history of allergies; emotional factors are often involved.

Eczema actually is a symptom rather than a disorder. It indicates that the infant is oversensitive to certain substances called allergens, which enter the body via the digestive tract (food), by inhalation (dust, pollen), by direct contact (wool, soap, strong sunlight), or by injections (insect bites, vaccines). Some children develop the triad of atopic dermatitis, asthma, and hay fever.

Manifestations. Although infantile eczema can occur at any age, it is more common during the first 2 years. The pruritic lesions form vesicles that weep and develop a dry crust. They are more severe on the face but may occur on the entire body, particularly in the skin folds. Eczema is worse in the winter than in the summer and has periods of temporary remission.

The infant scratches because the itching is constant, and he or she is irritable and unable to sleep. The lesions become easily infected by bacterial or viral agents. Infants and children with eczema should not be exposed to adults with cold sores because they may develop a systemic reaction with high fever and multiple vesicles on the eczematous skin. Eczema may flare up after immunization. Laboratory studies may show an increase in immunoglobulin E (IgE) and eosinophil levels.

Treatment and nursing care. Treatment of the child with infantile eczema is aimed at relieving pruritus (itching), hydrating the skin, relieving inflammation, and preventing infection. An emollient bath is sometimes ordered for its soothing effect on the skin. Oatmeal and a mixture of cornstarch and baking soda are examples of emollients prescribed. The infant's hair is washed with a soap substitute rather than a shampoo. Some dermatologists believe that bathing should be kept to a minimum. The physician may suggest that a bath oil such as Alpha Keri Therapeutic Bath Oil be used as the lesions begin to heal. This prevents the skin from becoming too dry. To be correctly used, bath oils should be added after the patient has soaked for a while and the skin is hydrated. In this way, moisture is sealed rather than excluded, as it is when oil is added before the patient gets into the tub.

Whenever possible, patients are treated at home because of the danger of infection in the hospital. When soap is used, a mild, nonperfumed soap such as Dove or Neutrogena is used. Glycerin-based lubricants are preferred over lanolin, which may be an irritant to an infant who is allergic to wool (Wong, Perry, & Hockenberry, 2002).

Corticosteroids may be administered systemically or locally. Antibiotics are needed if infection is present. Medication to help relieve itching is ordered for the patient. A child who is uncomfortable and unable to sleep may receive sedation.

The nurse plays a vital role in the treatment of patients with skin problems (Nursing Care Plan 29-1). The nurse should assess the family's ability to cope with the care of this child at home. Techniques of home bathing or application of soaks combined with quiet playtime enhances family coping. Control of itching is essential. Ointments are applied with a gloved hand to minimize contact with the skin. The fingernails of the child are kept short, and cotton gloves or socks can be used to prevent scratching. Appropriate dress is advised, as are using cotton fabric and avoiding wool and stuffed animals because of their allergy potential. Clothes should be laundered using mild soaps, avoiding products that contain fragrances or harsh chemicals. Parents should be taught the principles of general hygiene to avoid secondary infection of the open skin lesions. A hypoallergenic formula and a plan to identify possible food allergens are explained to parents. When a food allergen is the cause of eczema, stopping the food results in a clearing of the skin; however, restarting the food after a time may cause an anaphylactic reaction. The types of topical medications are listed in Table 29-1.

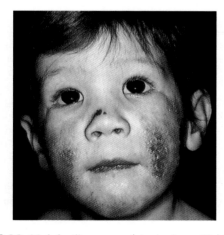

FIGURE **29-11** Infantile eczema (atopic dermatitis) is characterized by erythematous papules and vesicles with weeping, oozing, and crusts on the face and body. Severe itching is common. There is often a family history of allergy.

NURSING CARE PLAN 29-1

The Child with Eczema

PATIENT DATA: An 18-month-old child is brought to the clinic by his parents. The child has many open lesions on the skin and is diagnosed with eczema.

SELECTED NURSING DIAGNOSIS *Impaired skin integrity related to inflammation*

Outcomes	Nursing Interventions	Rationales
Child's skin will not show signs of irritation or infection.	1. Describe the types of lesions, configuration, and location.	1. Eczema has a typical pattern of distribution; vesicles, oozing, and crusting may denote infection.
	2. Provide supervision rather than restraints whenever possible.	2. Elbow restraints may assist in avoiding self-inflicted skin damage caused by scratching and picking; restriction of movement to infants has been related to learning difficulties and other problems; therefore judicious application of any restraint is necessary.
	3. Keep fingernails short.	3. Trimming fingernails and covering hands with "sock mittens" reduces excoriation from scratching.
	4. Administer medicated baths such as Aveeno.	4. Medicated baths soothe and rehydrate the skin.
	5. Apply wet dressings.	5. Wet dressings promote cooling of the skin, which decreases inflammation and itching (pruritus).
	6. Administer oral antibiotics and sedatives as prescribed.	6. Systemic antibiotics such as erythromycin may be prescribed if there is an infection; sedatives reduce itching.
	7. Apply steroid ointments as prescribed.	7. Steroid creams reduce inflammation.

SELECTED NURSING DIAGNOSIS *Risk for imbalanced nutrition: less than body requirements, related to irritability, sensitivity to certain foods*

Outcomes	Nursing Interventions	Rationales
Child will eat portions of each meal and maintain weight. Child will receive adequate nutrition as evidenced by growth charts and other parameters.	1. Serve hypoallergenic diet if prescribed.	1. This is a basic diet in which only one new food is added at a time to determine whether the infant is allergic to it.
	2. Determine specific food sensitivities from parents if child is not on a diet.	2. Parents have the most knowledge from experience with their child.
	3. Observe child for food sensitivities.	3. Any food can produce allergic symptoms, but some are thought to be highly allergenic. Certain antigens (foreign protein) may enter the bloodstream and activate antibody formation of the immune system. One reason this occurs during infancy is that an infant's gastrointestinal tract is immature. The allergy may be outgrown as body systems mature.

NURSING CARE PLAN 29-1—cont'd

Outcomes	Nursing Interventions	Rationales
	4. Administer vitamins and mineral supplements as prescribed.	4. Child may be deficient in nutrients owing to irritability and food restrictions. Adequate intake of vitamins and minerals is essential to the maintenance of healthy skin (particularly vitamins A, B, and C).
	5. Provide adequate fluids.	5. Adequate hydration prevents drying of the skin and pruritus, and it makes the skin less prone to breaks, which can become infected.

SELECTED NURSING DIAGNOSIS *Deficient knowledge (parents) related to nature of disorder*

Outcomes	Nursing Interventions	Rationales
Parents will verbalize understanding of potential allergens. Parents will state they have an understanding of the disease process.	1. Advise parents to remove articles that irritate skin (e.g., wool) and to provide loose cotton clothing.	1. Clothing with rough and tightly woven fibers will prevent natural evaporation from skin; wool may cause an allergic reaction. Sweating increases itching.
	2. Encourage parents to use mild detergents and to rinse clothes thoroughly.	2. Avoiding strong detergents and rinsing clothing thoroughly will prevent skin flare-ups.
	3. Expose child to sunlight, but monitor carefully.	3. Although sunlight is beneficial, overexposure to ultraviolet rays can seriously damage the skin. Infants and young children require special protection from the sun because their epidermis is thin; exposure time should be brief, even on hazy days.
	4. Help parents identify products in which wheat, milk, and eggs may not be readily apparent.	4. Food labels are read carefully to determine content.
	5. Advise parents to expect exacerbations and remissions.	5. Eczema is a chronic disease that takes time and energy to control.

❓CRITICAL THINKING QUESTION

The parents bring their child to the clinic. This child has a history of long-term asthma and eczema. The child is dressed in a wool jacket and is eating from a bag of peanuts. The mother states she has been using a lanolin lotion for dry skin that her friend gave her, but the child's skin lesions have only become worse. What teaching interventions by the nurse would be appropriate?

Parent teaching concerning topical therapy. Skin lesions can be pruritic (itchy), scaling, weeping, or crusted. Most skin lesions cause psychological stress, which should be addressed for both the parents and the child with the skin lesion. Prevention of secondary infection is essential, and the nurse should help the parent to understand the signs of inflammation or infection. When topical medication is applied, the lesions may change in form or color as they heal. Parents should be advised of changes to expect and when to seek follow-up advice. The nurse should teach parents the principles and techniques of applying topical medication, which includes the following:

- Absorption is best when an ointment is applied after a warm bath.
- Medication should be applied by stroking in the direction of hair growth. (Circular or rubbing motions can inflame hair follicles.)

table 29-1	*Types of Topical Medications*
TYPE	**DEFINITION**
Cream	A water-based emulsion of oil in water that is nongreasy for use on weeping lesions
Ointment	An oil-based emulsion of water in oil that is clear and greasy; used on dry skin; does not rub off easily
Lotion	A suspension of powder in water that should be shaken well before using; may be drying; often used on scalp lesions
Aerosol spray	Suspension of medication in an alcohol base; alcohol evaporates, leaving medication on the skin; effective for hairy areas
Gel	A clear, semisolid emulsion; liquefies when applied to skin
Bath oils	Bath oils are not used in pediatrics because they lubricate the sides of the tub, causing falls and injuries; the value of the treatment must be weighed against the risks involved; colloidal oatmeal baths may be soothing

- Teach how much ointment to apply (e.g., pea sized).
- The use of elbow restraints can prevent an infant from scratching while allowing freedom of movement.
- Do not use topical steroids when a viral infection is present.

Over-the-counter skin products. Parents should be guided in the use of over-the-counter products that affect skin health. Simple ointments such as petrolatum, A and D, and zinc oxide are helpful only if they are washed off completely between diaper changes. Frequent diaper changes are essential. High-absorbency disposable diapers decrease wetness of the skin and may help to prevent diaper dermatitis. Home-laundered diapers are not subject to high temperatures, and soaps often contain fragrances that may be irritating. Commercially prepared wipes sometimes contain perfumes and can leave the skin moist; warm water and a mild soap are less irritating. If paper towels are used, prints should be avoided because the color dyes can be irritating to the skin. Cortisone creams should be avoided because it may temporarily clear the rash but does not resolve the underlying cause that will prevent recurrence.

✴NURSING TIP_____

Parents should be taught that "kissing a wound to make it better" can introduce organisms that can cause infection.

STAPHYLOCOCCAL INFECTION

Pathophysiology. The genus of bacteria called *Staphylococcus* comprises common bacteria that are found in dust and on the skin. Under normal conditions, they do not present a problem to the healthy body's defenses. Skin infections may occur if the number of organisms increases in preterm infants and newborns, whose general resistance is low. An abscess may form, and infection may enter the bloodstream. This condition is called *septicemia*. Pneumonia, osteomyelitis, or meningitis may result. Primary infection of the newborn may develop in the umbilicus or circumcision wound. It may occur while the newborn is in the hospital or after discharge. This infection spreads readily from one infant to another. Small pustules on the newborn must be reported immediately.

Treatment and nursing care. Antibiotics effective against the appropriate strain of *Staphylococcus* are administered. Ointments may be locally applied. In past years the staphylococci that invaded the body developed resistance to the drugs in current use. Methicillin-resistant *Staphylococcus aureus* (MRSA) infections are resistant to certain antibiotics and are handled under strict isolation (standard) precautions. The use of disposable individual equipment for patients and aseptic techniques can decrease nosocomial spread.

Scalded skin syndrome is caused by *S. aureus*. The lesions begin with a mild erythema with sandpaper texture; vesicles appear and rupture and peeling occurs, exposing a bright red surface. The skin looks as though it has been scalded, and child abuse is often suspected. Intravenous (IV) antibiotics, strict isolation, and prevention of secondary infection are priorities. Maintaining warmth and fluid-electrolyte balance are also important in the plan of care. Healing usually takes place without scarring.

IMPETIGO

Pathophysiology. Impetigo is an infectious disease of the skin caused by staphylococci or by group A beta-hemolytic streptococci. It results when the organism

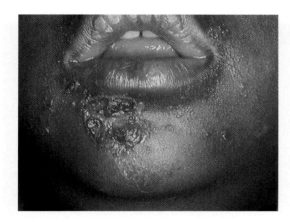

FIGURE **29-12** Impetigo. This consists of moist, thin-roofed vesicles with an erythematous base. The vesicles rupture to form a thick, honey-colored crust. It is a contagious bacterial infection of the skin that is most common in infants and children.

comes in contact with a break in the skin, such as an insect bite. The bullous form seen primarily in infants is usually staphylococcal, whereas nonbullous types are more commonly seen in children and young adults. Both organisms can usually be cultivated in the latter. The newborn is susceptible to this infection because resistance to skin bacteria is low. Impetigo tends to spread from one area of skin to another and is contagious.

Manifestations. The first symptoms of a bullous lesion are red papules (Figure 29-12). These eventually become small vesicles or pustules surrounded by a reddened area. When the blister breaks, the surface beneath is raw and weeping. The lesions may occur anywhere but are most often found around the nose and mouth and in moist areas of the body, such as the creases of the neck, axilla, and groin. A crust may form in older children, and scratching may cause further infection.

Treatment and nursing care. Systemic antibiotics are administered either orally or parenterally. Parents are instructed to wash the lesions three or four times daily to remove crusts. Ointments such as mupirocin (Bactroban) may be prescribed for topical application. Prevention of the disease by treating small cuts promptly is important.

The prognosis with proper treatment is good. Nursing care consists primarily of preventing this disease.

Education of parents includes reminding them of the necessity for prompt attention to minor cuts and bites. In diagnosed cases, compliance with the treatment regimen is needed to prevent the spread of infection to other children and family members. If the diagnosis is made in the newborn nursery, the infant is

isolated to prevent other newborns from becoming infected. Nephritis may occur as a complication of beta-hemolytic streptococcal infections.

FUNGAL INFECTIONS

Pathophysiology. Fungal infections are caused by closely related fungi that have a preference for invading the stratum corneum, hair, and nails. The word *tinea* comes from the Latin "worm." The common name for this infection is *ringworm.* Fungi are larger than bacteria. Some fungi may be transmitted from person to person and others from animal to person. The name denotes the part of the body involved.

Tinea capitis. Tinea capitis ("ringworm of the scalp") is seen in school-age children. It is characterized by patches of alopecia (hair loss). The hair loses pigment and may break off. The papules become pustules, which progress to red scales. There are areas of circular balding.

Diagnosis is made by history and appearance. Some strains of tinea capitis glow green under a *Wood's light.* This condition is treated with griseofulvin (Fulvicin, Grisactin), which is administered by mouth. It is given with or after meals to avoid gastrointestinal irritation and increase absorption. Suspensions should be well shaken. Parents are instructed to continue therapy as long as ordered and not to miss a dose. Exposure to the sun is avoided. Treatment may be necessary for 8 to 12 weeks. Children may go to school but are warned not to exchange hats, combs, or other personal items. Selenium sulfide shampoos are also used. This infection can be stubborn and may take several weeks to clear.

Tinea corporis. Tinea corporis ("ringworm of the skin") is evident as an oval scaly inflamed ring with a clear center. It is seen on the face, neck, arms, and hands (Figure 29-13). It can be transmitted by infected pets. Treatment consists of local application of an antifungal preparation such as haloprogin twice daily for 2 to 4 weeks. More severe cases may require treatment with oral griseofulvin.

Tinea pedis. Tinea pedis refers to *athlete's foot.* Lesions are located between the toes, on the instep, and on the soles. There is accompanying pruritus. It occurs more often in preadolescents and adolescents. It is diagnosed by direct microscopic scrapings of the lesions. Treatment consists of topical therapy with an antifungal preparation. Oral griseofulvin therapy may also be given. Adolescents are cautioned to avoid alcohol when taking this medicine because it may produce tachycardia and flushing.

Because this condition is aggravated by heat and moisture, the feet must be carefully dried, especially

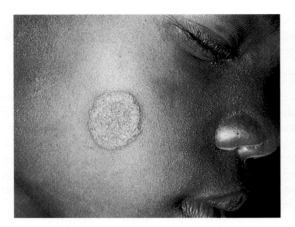

FIGURE **29-13** Tinea corporis (ringworm of the body). Scales, hyperpigmented in Caucasians and depigmented in dark-skinned children, appear on the face, chest, abdomen, or arms, forming multiple circular lesions with clear centers.

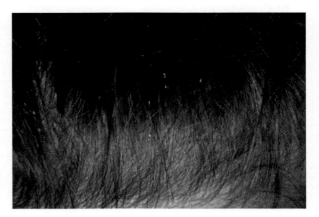

FIGURE **29-14** Pediculosis. White nits or eggs of the head lice are attached to the hair.

between the toes. Clean socks are worn. Shoes need to be well ventilated. Plastic shoes that retain heat are avoided. Recurrences are common.

Tinea cruris. Tinea cruris ("thigh") affects the groin area and is commonly referred to as "jock itch." It occurs on the inner aspects of the thighs and scrotum. The initial lesion is small, raised, and scaly. It spreads, and tiny vesicles occur at the margins of the rash. Local application of tolnaftate liquid (Tinactin, Aftate) or powder is effective. Stinging may occur when a spray solution is applied. General hygiene should be stressed.

PEDICULOSIS

The infestation of humans by lice is termed pediculosis. There are three types: pediculosis capitis (head lice), pediculosis corporis (body lice), and pediculosis pubis (crabs or pubic lice). The various types usually remain in the part of the body designated by their name. They are transmitted from person to person or by contact with contaminated articles. Their survival depends on the blood they extract from the infected person. Severe itching in the affected area is the main symptom. In all cases, treatment is aimed at ridding the patient of the parasite, treating the excoriated skin, and preventing the infestation of others. The most common form seen in children is head lice (Figure 29-14).

Pediculosis Capitis

Pathophysiology. Pediculosis capitis, commonly known as head lice, affects the scalp and hair. The louse lays eggs (nits) that attach to the hair and hatch within 3 or 4 days. Head lice are more common in girls than in boys because of hair length and the tendency to share combs and hair ornaments. The parasite may be acquired from hats, combs, or hairbrushes. It is easily transferred from one child to another and is seen most often in the school-age child and in preschool children who attend day care centers.

Manifestations. Children with pediculosis capitis suffer from severe itching of the scalp. They scratch their heads frequently and often cause further irritation. The hair becomes matted. Pustules and excoriations may be seen about the face. Nurses admitting patients to pediatric units should be on the alert for head lice. In particular, the nurse inspects the hairline at the back of the neck and about the ears. Crusts, pediculi, nits, and dirt may cause matting of the hair and a foul odor. When the condition is discovered, it is handled with discretion so as not to embarrass the child or parents.

Treatment and nursing care. Treatment is directed toward killing the lice, getting rid of the nits, and managing any infections of the face and scalp. Family members and playmates of the child should be examined and treated as necessary. Prescription shampoos such as RID or NIX are commonly used. Retreatment may be necessary in 1 week to 10 days. Lindane (Kwell) has also been used; however, it has more reported neurotoxic side effects (consult package insert).

If the eyebrows and eyelashes are involved, a thick coating of petroleum jelly (Vaseline) may be applied, followed by removal of the remaining nits. Nits on the head are removed by combing the hair with a fine-toothed comb dipped in a 1:1 solution of white vinegar and water. The hair is then washed. In some cases, recovery is hastened by cutting the hair. Contact (standard) precautions should be followed.

Children should be cautioned against swapping caps, head scarves, and combs. Parents are instructed to inspect the child's head regularly. Parents are encouraged to report infestations to the school nurse, because widespread outbreaks are periodically encountered.

SCABIES

Pathophysiology. Scabies is a parasitic infection caused by the itch mite, *Sarcoptes scabiei.* It is seen worldwide. It is caused by the adult female mite, who burrows under the skin and lays eggs. The mite has a round body and four pairs of legs and is visible by microscopic examination. A characteristic burrow is sometimes seen under the skin, particularly between the fingers. Burrows contain the eggs and feces of the mite. Itching is intense, especially at night. A vesiculopustular lesion can occur in children.

Scabies may occur anywhere on the body but is seldom seen on the face. It thrives in moist body folds, but in young children the lesions may appear on the head, palms, and soles of the feet. It is spread by close personal contact, including sexual relations. It is rarely transmitted by fomites because the isolated mite dies within 2 to 3 days.

Treatment and nursing care. Treatment consists of the application of permethrin (Elimite). It can be used for children older than 2 months of age. Parents are instructed to follow the directions carefully. All family members, baby-sitters, and close associates require treatment. Contact standard precautions are followed (Appendix A).

INJURIES

BURNS

Pathophysiology. Burns often occur during childhood. They are the leading cause of accidental death in the home for children between 1 and 4 years of age. Sometimes burns are a result of child abuse and neglect. The two times of day during which burns are most likely to occur are the early morning hours before parents awaken and after school.

Types of burns include the following:
- *Thermal:* due to fire or a scalding vapor or liquid
- *Chemical:* due to a corrosive powder or liquid
- *Electrical:* due to electrical current passing through the body
- *Radiation:* due to x-rays or radioactive substances

Burns can involve the skin or mucous membranes. When a child is burned by fire near the face, the flames may be *inhaled,* causing a burn of the mucous membrane lining the airway. Assessing for resulting edema and respiratory distress is a priority. When a formula or food is heated in the microwave oven, "hot spots" occur that can cause burns to the mucous membranes lining the mouth.

The differences in responses of children to a burn are as follows:
- The child's skin is thinner than that of the adult, lending to a more serious depth of burn with lower temperatures and shorter exposure than adults.
- The large body surface area of the child results in greater fluid, electrolyte, and heat loss.
- Immature response systems in young children can cause shock and heart failure.
- The increased basal metabolism rate (BMR) of a child results in increased protein and calorie needs.
- Smaller muscle and fat content in the body results in protein and caloric deficiencies when oral intake is limited.
- The skin is more elastic in children, causing pulling on the scarring areas and resulting in formation of a larger scar.
- The immature immune system predisposes the child to developing infections that complicate burn treatment.
- The prolonged immobilization and treatment required for burns adversely affects growth and development.

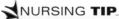
NURSING **TIP**

The small child is taught to stop, drop, and roll should the clothes become ignited.

Classification. The severity of a burn depends on the *area*, *extent*, and *depth* of involvement. The size of the burn is calculated as a percentage of total body surface area (TBSA). Age-related charts are used for children because their body proportions differ from those of adults and a standard (rule of nines) cannot be applied (Figure 29-15). The extent of destruction of the skin is described as partial thickness or full thickness. In partial-thickness burns, only part of the skin is damaged. Full-thickness burns are more extensive and may require skin grafting. The classification of and first aid treatment for burns are summarized in Table 29-2. One can survive a rather extensive superficial burn, whereas a deep burn involving a smaller surface area can threaten the patient's life. Table 29-3 discusses children's response to burn injuries.

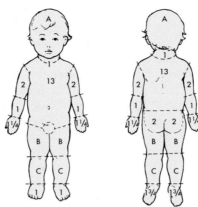

RELATIVE PERCENTAGES OF AREAS AFFECTED BY GROWTH

AREA	BIRTH	AGE 1 YR	AGE 5 YR
A = ¹/₂ of head	9¹/₂	8¹/₂	6¹/₂
B = ¹/₂ of one thigh	2³/₄	3¹/₄	4
C = ¹/₂ of one leg	2¹/₂	2¹/₂	2³/₄

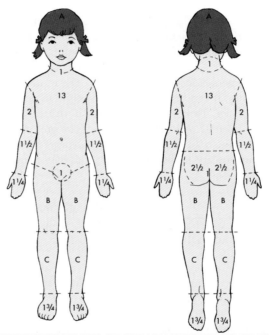

RELATIVE PERCENTAGES OF AREAS AFFECTED BY GROWTH

AREA	AGE 10 YR	AGE 15 YR	ADULT
A = ¹/₂ of head	5¹/₂	4¹/₂	3¹/₂
B = ¹/₂ of one thigh	4¹/₂	4¹/₂	4³/₄
C = ¹/₂ of one leg	3	3¹/₄	3¹/₂

FIGURE **29-15** Body surface area (BSA) charts. This chart is used to determine the developmentally related percentage of body surface area burned. The percent of BSA involved is the basis for determining the fluid and nutritional needs of the burned child. In children younger than 3 years of age, the "rule of nines" assigns the infant's head as 18% of total BSA (TBSA) and the lower extremities as 14% TBSA, with 9% assigned to each arm and 1¼% to the hands or palms.

table 29-2 *Classification and First-Aid Treatment of Burns*

DEGREE	ANATOMY AND DEPTH	APPEARANCE AND SENSATION	FIRST-AID TREATMENT
First (superficial)	Epidermis only	Skin red but blanches easily on pressure and refills quickly; painful, indicating tissue viability	Immerse in cold water to halt burning process; apply an antimicrobial ointment.
Second (partial thickness)	Epidermis and much of dermis; partial thickness	Blistered, moist, pink, or red; painful, indicating tissue viability	If area is small, treat as for first-degree burn and apply antimicrobial ointment; otherwise treat as for deep dermal burn.
Deep dermal (deep partial thickness)	Extends deep into dermis; partial thickness but can become full thickness with infection, trauma, or poor blood supply	Mottled; red, tan, or dull white; blisters; painful, indicating tissue viability	Immerse in cold water to halt burning process; cover with sterile dressing or clean cloth to prevent contamination and decrease pain from contact with air; avoid breaking blisters; seek medical attention immediately.
Third (full thickness)	Subdermal; involves entire skin and all its structures; full thickness	Tough, leathery, dry; does not blanch or refill; dull brown, tan, black, or pearly white; painless to touch, indicating death of tissue	Halt the burning process by immersing in cold water or rolling in blanket or rug; wrap in clean sheet or other sterile dressing; provide blanket for warmth; have victim lie down; *do not* apply ointment or any other substance to burned area; take patient to nearest emergency treatment center immediately.

Burns can also be complicated by fractures, soft tissue injury, or preexisting conditions such as diabetes, obesity, epilepsy, and heart or renal disease. Moderate burns are considered to be (1) partial-thickness burns involving 15% to 30% of body surface, or (2) full-thickness burns involving less than 10% of body surface. Major burns are (1) partial-thickness types involving 30% or more of body surface or (2) full-thickness burns involving 10% or more of body surface. Second- and third-degree burns must be regarded as open wounds that have the added danger of infection. The 6 "C's" of burn care include *c*lothing, *c*ooling, *c*leaning, *c*hemoprophylaxis, *c*overing, and *c*omforting or pain relief (Morgan & Luczon-Peterman, 2001). Burn treatment can be given in an outpatient clinic, in a general hospital, or at a specialized burn center.

Treatment

Care of electrical burns. When electricity is the cause of the injury, the child should be assessed for entry and exit lesions that may appear as a small erythematous area. The locations of the entry and exit wounds indicate the path of electricity through the body (Figure 29-16). Muscle damage can occur, and if the electrical current passed through the heart, cardiac muscle damage can result. Deep muscle damage can cause renal impairment from myoglobinuria. The child should be observed closely for responses with electrocardiographic (ECG) monitors, vital signs recorded, and cardiac enzymes assessed before discharge.

table 29-3 | *Response to Burn Injury in Children**

RESPONSE	EFFECT
Capillary permeability increases, and hypovolemia occurs.	There is a loss of plasma, proteins, and fluids; shock occurs.
Blood flow to vital organs increases, and blood flow to periphery of body and nonvital organs decreases.	Peristalsis ceases (ileus). Curling's ulcer can form in stomach.
Body metabolism increases to maintain heat.	Increased basal metabolic rate (BMR) can strain the heart by causing increased cardiac output.
Damage to red blood cells and hemolysis results in anemia.	Anemia causes increased cardiac output to maintain perfusion.
Open wounds of burn can predispose to infection. Dead tissue provides a medium for bacterial growth.	Immature immune system can be overwhelmed, and sepsis can result.
Waste products accumulate in the blood because of anemia and slow perfusion of nonvital organs.	Renal failure, cardiac failure, and pulmonary edema can complicate toxicity from burn injury.

*Thermal injuries produce both local and systemic effects.

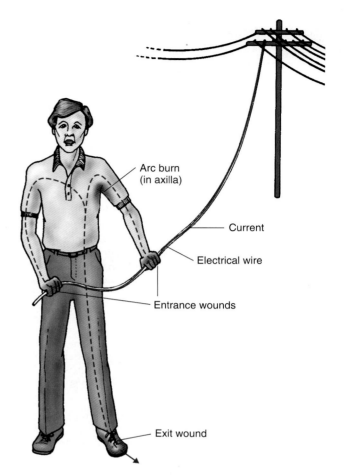

FIGURE **29-16** Mechanism of electrical injury. The electrical current enters the body and travels through the heart before exiting the body. All patients with electrical injuries should have their cardiac enzymes monitored to determine if heart damage has occurred.

> **NURSING TIP**
>
> Electrical burns of the mouth are common in small children, who put everything into their mouths. Biting into electrical cords is not unusual. Such wounds are usually deep and leave an entrance and exit burn. They are subject to bleeding for several weeks.

Emergency care. Community education programs emphasize the response to a child with a burn injury. The school nurse plays a major role in the education process, as follows:

- *Stop the burning process.* Stop, drop, and roll is the sequence of care. Rolling the child in a blanket smothers the flames. A caustic powder should be brushed off before water is used to wash the area; this prevents spreading contact with the caustic substance. Electricity should be turned off before touching a child who has been electrocuted.
- *Evaluate the injury.* Check the ABCs (*a*irway, *b*reathing, *c*irculation) of the victim. Cardiopulmonary resuscitation (CPR) is initiated as appropriate. Minor burns can be treated; major burns should be assessed by a physician.
- *Cover the burn.* The burned area should be covered with a clean cloth to minimize contact with air, reduce pain, minimize hypothermia, and prevent contamination of the wound. Burned clothing and jewelry should be removed because metal retains heat and continues the burn injury.
- *Transport to a hospital.* Do not give any fluids by mouth because peristalsis may have diminished

in response to the burn injury. If available, IV fluids and oxygen should be administered and the child comforted and reassured.

Care of minor thermal burns. Minor burns are treated at home and followed with clinic visits until healing is complete. The wound is cleansed and an antimicrobial ointment applied with a loose dressing. Blisters are not disturbed. Dressings are changed as prescribed, and the parent is advised to report any sign of infection. The status of tetanus immunization is reviewed and updated as needed. Pain relief is administered as needed. The wound of a minor burn is usually completely healed within 20 days. Evaluation of scarring and effect on range of motion (ROM) will determine future follow-up needs.

Care of major burns. The immediate treatment of shock in cases of severe burns is handled by the physician, nurse, and respiratory therapist and other specialists in the emergency department or, in some instances, the operating room. Priorities include establishing an airway in patients with facial burns or smoke inhalation, instituting IV lines, and assessing burn wounds and other, perhaps initially unrecognized, injuries. At times, some of these procedures are carried out simultaneously.

> ◥NURSING **TIP**_____
> A severe burn can cause a loss of function in two of the most important properties of the skin: the ability to protect against infection and the ability to prevent loss of body fluid.

Establishing an airway. Cyanosis, singed nasal hairs, charred lips, and stridor are indications that flames may have been inhaled. An endotracheal tube is inserted to maintain an adequate airway, although this is not required for all patients. This permits the delivery of humidified air with oxygen, easy removal of secretions from respiratory passages, and use of a pressure ventilator if needed. Sedation is administered with caution to avoid further respiratory embarrassment.

If eschar (*eschara,* "scab") from burns on the trunk inhibits respirations, an incision called an *escharotomy* is made to prevent the restriction of chest movement. Blood gas levels, including level of carbon monoxide, are ascertained. The child is placed on sterile sheets. Attendants wear face masks, a sterile gown, and gloves.

IV infusions are begun to prevent intravascular dehydration and electrolyte imbalance. Ringer's lactate solution is often used initially. Albumin or plasma may be used when capillary permeability is restored (within 24 to 48 hours).

Laboratory studies include hematocrit and sodium chloride, potassium, carbon dioxide, blood urea nitrogen, creatinine, and serum protein levels. Blood typing and cross-matching are performed. Fluid therapy requires close monitoring throughout hospitalization. To determine urine volume and characteristics, a urinary catheter is inserted and an intake and output record is maintained.

The loss of fluid causes renal vasoconstriction, leading to depressed glomerular filtration and oliguria. Acute renal failure can develop without adequate therapy. Urine output is observed hourly. It varies considerably, but on the average 20 to 30 ml/hr for patients older than age 2 years is considered adequate during the resuscitative stage. The patient's present weight is recorded and used as baseline data for determining adequacy of treatment.

A nasogastric tube is inserted and is attached to low wall suction. This empties the stomach and prevents complications such as gastric dilation, vomiting, and paralytic ileus (intestinal muscle paralysis). The patient has nothing by mouth for the first 24 hours. Sporadic bleeding as a result of Curling's ulcer (stress ulcer) is not uncommon in patients with severe burns; the administration of IV antacids such as cimetidine has helped to reduce its incidence.

Wound care. Cleaning a burn wound can be painful, and techniques of pain relief should be used. Chlorhexidine (Hibiclens) and povidone-iodine (Betadine) can inhibit the healing process and are not advised for use on open burn wounds. Mild soap and water with thorough rinsing is preferred. Residual crusts can be removed with mineral oil or daily applications of Polysporin (polymixin and bacitracin) topical cream. The black eschar of necrotic tissue can be debrided via whirlpool. Yellow eschar is not removed.

Immediate care of the wound itself includes cleansing and debridement (removal of dried crusts) of necrotic tissue. The loss of skin increases the threat of infection, and fluid loss caused by evaporation can be significant. The immune system is depressed. Strict asepsis is maintained, and the wound site is treated in accordance with the physician's instruction. A tetanus immunization history is obtained, and tetanus prophylaxis is administered as required. Low doses of antibiotics may be prescribed to prevent streptococcal infection.

A semi-open method of burn dressing may be used, although exposure methods may be useful on accessible areas such as the face. The wound is covered by a few layers of sterile gauze that has been saturated with antibacterial ointment or cream. The gauze is held in place by elastic netting (Figure 29-17). When the wound is being dressed, *no two burn surfaces should touch.* A sterile blanket may be used to prevent chilling. The wound is cleansed by tub baths or, in many cases, whirlpool baths

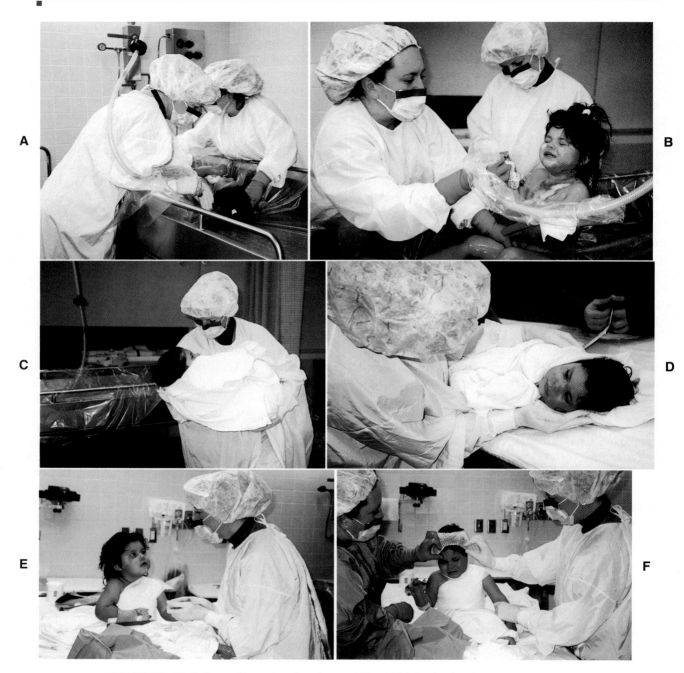

FIGURE **29-17** Collage of burn dressing change. This child is having her burn dressings changed and is undergoing whirlpool bath debridement. She is gently dried with sterile towels, and a pressure dressing is reapplied. (Photos courtesy of Pat Spier, RN-C.)

are used to soften necrotic areas and debride the wound. Surgical debridement is done when needed to cleanse the wound and prepare the new granulation tissue for grafting. The use of ointments such as Sulfamylon or Silvadene may be prescribed. A biologic dressing or a synthetic dressing may be used to prevent fluid loss and promote healing. The burn area is closed and resurfaced by grafting.

Skin grafts. Temporary grafts are used during the acute stage of recovery. They protect the wound from infection and reduce fluid loss but are eventually rejected by the body. Temporary grafts include homografts (usually tissue from disease-free cadavers) and hetero-grafts (tissues obtained from different species). Hetero-grafts are also referred to as xenografts (*xeno,* "foreign" and *graft,* "slice of skin").

Many grafts are derived from pigskin, which is available commercially either fresh or frozen; these biological dressings are often used in children and are called *porcine xenografts.* They are particularly useful in partial-thickness or deep dermal burns and have greatly improved burn management. Deep dermal wounds may be preceded by tangential (merely touching) excision, which is a surgical technique of removing burned eschar with a dermatome. Thin layers are shaved down to the live tissues, and temporary porcine grafts are applied.

There are two types of permanent grafts: *autografts* and *isografts.* An autograft (*auto,* "self") is healthy tissue obtained from another part of the patient's body. An isograft (*iso,* "equal") is obtained from the patient's identical twin or genotype. Permanent grafts are done during the rehabilitative stage of the patient's illness to improve appearance and function. The site from which the tissue has been removed is called the *donor area.*

Advances in grafting techniques have improved the overall prognosis in burn patients and have helped to minimize scarring. A split-thickness skin graft can be prepared with the use of a dermatome. For extensive burns, it is sometimes difficult to find enough intact skin for use. Special methods such as the Tanner mesh graft may be used. In this method a strip of split-thickness skin is run through a special cutting machine that makes multiple slits; this expands the skin to provide more coverage, in some cases as much as nine times the original area of the skin. The graft is sutured in place to maintain tension.

The "postage stamp" graft consists of small pieces of donor skin placed on the granulation tissue. Spaces between grafts allow for drainage and healing. Full-cover grafts are sheets of skin placed intact over the wound. These are cosmetically more effective than patch and mesh grafts but are not always available. The donor site is covered with xenograft or fine mesh gauze; it heals in about 2 weeks. Newly grafted areas are covered with sterile dressings. Every effort is made to prevent bleeding and infection. The areas surrounding the wound are observed for edema and impaired circulation.

Biological dressings. Biological dressings can be applied to a noninfected burn wound within 6 hours of the injury and will peel off as the wound heals. Dressing changes are not necessary. The dressings are made from neonatal foreskin fibroblast cells combined in a nylon mesh that is sterile and frozen for storage. Once thawed, they cannot be refrozen. The dressings, Briobane and TransCyte, and bismuth-impregnated petrolatum gauze contain human or pigskin products, and hypersensitivity should be considered before use. Elastic dressings may be used for a short time to hold it in contact with the wound or a splint to immobilize an involved joint. TransCyte is transparent so that outer dressings can be removed to assess the wound. The dressing should be covered with a plastic bag before daily baths or showers are taken. The dressing may change color as the wound heals.

Posthealing care. After basic healing has occurred, a nonperfumed moisturizer cream such as Eucerin, Nivea Moisturizing, or cocoa butter may be recommended to maintain skin moisture. Ointments containing lanolin are not advised. Sun block should be used to prevent hyperpigmentation of the newly healed skin. It may take 2 years for complete healing to occur. Systemic antihistamines such as diphenhydramine (Benadryl) or hydroxyzine (Atarax) may be prescribed to control itching. Bicarbonate of soda baths are soothing.

NURSING TIP
Disorientation, fever, and diminished bowel sounds may be early signs of sepsis.

Nursing care of the burned child. Children who have suffered extensive burns and survive the early dangers face a long period of hospitalization and require specialized care. The various aspects of nursing care differ with the age of the patient, the area of the burn, and the type of treatment used. Box 29-2 lists topical agents used in treating burn patients.

Protective isolation (standard precautions) is instituted. All instruments that come in contact with the wound must be sterile. Ointments are applied with a sterile gloved hand or sterile tongue depressor. Care must be taken to avoid injury to granulation tissue. If the wound is to be covered, a layer of fine mesh gauze is secured with sterile fluffs, followed by Kling bandages and a stockinette or elastic tubular netting.

The nurse reports signs of infection immediately. Signs of infections are elevations of temperature, pulse, and respiration; restlessness and confusion; pain; purulent drainage; and odor of wound dressing. A careful description of the wound in the nurse's notes facilitates daily comparison and determination of progress. All infection must be cleared before skin grafting can be performed.

The nurse remains alert for signs of fluid overload, in particular, behavioral changes and altered sensorium. Although initially restricted to prevent nausea and vomiting, oral fluids are necessary during the convalescent

box 29-2 *Topical Agents Used to Treat Burn Patients*

SILVER SULFADIAZINE CREAM 1% (SILVADENE)

Cream is effective against gram-negative and gram-positive bacteria and yeast (*Candida albicans*).

Do not use if patient is allergic to sulfa drugs.

Cream does not sting; it softens eschar.

Do not waste; cream is expensive.

Gently remove old cream before reapplying.

MAFENIDE ACETATE 10% (SULFAMYLON)

Agent is effective against gram-positive and gram-negative organisms.

Agent is painful because it draws water out of the tissues; pain may last 15 to 30 minutes or longer.

Remain with child after application for comfort and diversion.

Allergic rash is common.

Agent has a tendency to cake and is best used with hydrotherapy.

There is a potential for metabolic acidosis.

SILVER NITRATE 0.5% (AgNO$_3$)

Agent is effective against gram-negative organisms.

Dressing must be kept *wet* and changed frequently.

Agent stains unburned skin, linen, and most surfaces a dark brown or black.

Eschar becomes light brown.

BACITRACIN

Agent is a low-cost prophylactic antibiotic.

stages to prevent kidney damage and to maintain body fluid requirements. The nurse must use ingenuity to persuade the child to take sufficient amounts of fluids. An accurate record of intake and output of fluids is kept.

There is an increase in demands on the metabolism as it deals with this trauma, and more calories are spent as water evaporates from the wound site. Frequent feedings of foods high in calories, protein, and iron are therefore necessary. A high-protein diet, a normal diet with added amounts of meat, milk, eggs, fish, or poultry, is usually prescribed. Iron therapy may be initiated if anemia begins to develop. Eggnogs are nourishing between-meal drinks for burn patients with such needs. Small amounts are offered frequently. Vitamins A, B, and C and zinc sulfate are given to hasten healing and to stimulate the appetite. Gavage feedings may be necessary. Accurate daily records of foods consumed, calorie count, and patient's weight will help to determine the nutritional status.

The nurse bears in mind that other, unaffected parts of the body need exercise and proper positioning to prevent painful contractures. The child's position is changed every 2 to 4 hours unless contraindicated. A footboard is used to prevent foot drop. Support should be given by means of pillows, sandbags, and rolled towels as necessary.

The physical therapist attends to the child regularly for exercise and to keep the joints limber and healthy. The child begins to ambulate as soon as possible. Self-help activities and mobility are encouraged. Pressure splints or elasticized garments help to reduce scar tissue and are sometimes worn for months after discharge.

Emotional support. A burn injury is taxing to the child and parents. It requires long periods of hospitalization and frequent readmissions. The accident itself is terrifying for the child but is made even worse if caused by disobedience. Nurses encourage children to express their feelings. Analgesics are administered *before* painful procedures. The long-term patient requires diversions of various types. School tutors are requested and contact is maintained with peers through cards or e-mail.

Nurses give constant support to the parents, who usually feel guilty if the child was injured in an accident. Nurses indicate by their manner that they do not blame the parents for what has happened. Preparation for discharge begins early. The multidisciplinary health care team includes the physician, nurse, school nurse, schoolteacher, physiotherapist, and psychologist. Instructions are given regarding wound care, diet, exercise, and rest. Return appointments are made, and referral agencies are contacted. Methods to improve the physical appearance of the patient are discussed. The importance of burn prevention cannot be overemphasized. Figure 29-18 shows the difference in appearance of a scald burn wound from an accidental spill and a scald wound that was inflicted (child abuse).

NURSING TIP

In cases of car, house, or airplane fires, patients may face additional crises, such as the loss of relatives, pets, and possessions.

FROSTBITE

Frostbite is the result of freezing of a body part. Chilblain is a cold injury with erythema, vesicles, and ulcerative lesions that occur as a result of vasoconstriction. Education to prevent cold injury is essential for those living or visiting cold climates. School nurses play a vital role in educating parents and children. Adequate

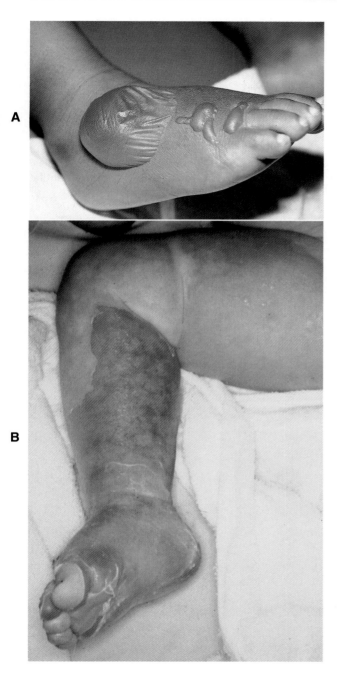

A

B

FIGURE **29-18** Scald burns. **A,** An accidental scald burn. Note the droplet pattern indicating a splash. **B,** Nonaccidental scald burn. An inflicted scald reveals severe extensive second-degree burns on the entire leg.

layered clothing, including hats and gloves (wool over cotton), is preferred.

In exposure to extreme cold, warmth is lost in the periphery of the body before the core temperature drops. Therefore, in extreme cases of exposure to freez-

ing temperatures, the head and torso should be warmed before the extremities to ensure survival with minimal consequences. Frostbitten extremities appear pale and hard and are without sensation. Dry clothing should be applied and muscle activity encouraged. Blankets or sleeping bags are initially used to start rewarming. Warm, moist oxygen; warming blankets; and warming baths are used. A deep purple flush appears with the return of sensation, which is accompanied by extreme pain. Pain relief and monitoring of vital signs are essential. Blistering and ulcers can occur and are treated with whirlpool soaks. Skin damage is similar to that incurred with burns. Frostbite can result in *necrosis* (death) of tissue and may require amputation of the extremity.

key points

- The skin is the body's first line of defense against disease.
- Certain skin conditions are symptoms of systemic disease.
- Common skin problems in infants are diaper dermatitis, seborrheic dermatitis, and atopic dermatitis (eczema).
- A strawberry nevus is an example of a hemangioma.
- Pediculosis is the term for lice. Lice may occur on the head, body, or pubic area.
- Tinea pedis, or athlete's foot, is prevented by drying the feet well, particularly between the toes, and wearing well-ventilated footwear.
- A severe burn can cause a loss of function in two of the most important properties of the skin: the ability to protect against infection and the ability to prevent the loss of body fluid.
- Electrical burns carry the risk of thrombosis and tissue damage in other parts of the body.
- The severity of a burn depends on the area, extent, and depth of involvement.
- Preventing infection is an important nursing intervention for patients with burns or any skin lesion.
- Frostbite can cause tissue damage similar to burns.
- Absorption of a topical hydrating medication is best when applied after a warm bath.
- Types of burns include thermal, electrical, chemical, and radiation.

ONLINE RESOURCES

Emergency Treatment of Burns:
http://www.shrinershq.org/prevention/burntips/
treatment.html
DermNet: http://www.dermnetnz.org/index.html
Eczema/Atopic Dermatitis:
http://www.aad.org/pamphlets/eczema.html

REVIEW QUESTIONS *Choose the most appropriate answer.*

1. Pain relief is important in the burn patient because:
   1. It prevents discomfort
   2. The child must be kept from crying
   3. Parents become upset
   4. Pain contributes to shock

2. Which of the following would be contraindicated in a patient with infantile eczema?
   1. Wrapping the infant in a wool blanket
   2. Covering hands with cotton mittens
   3. Using elbow restraints to prevent scratching
   4. Using open, wet dressings

3. A characteristic of third-degree burns not present in second-degree burns is:
   1. Lack of pain
   2. Blisters and warmth
   3. Redness
   4. Severe pain

4. Which of the following is contained in an emollient bath often prescribed for children with dermatitis?
   1. Bath oil
   2. Glycerine soap
   3. Oatmeal
   4. Salt or saline solution

5. The cause of infantile eczema may be the basis of a teaching plan for the child's parent. Infantile eczema is most likely caused by:
   1. An infection with *Staphylococcus aureus*
   2. A parasitic skin disease
   3. Poor hygiene
   4. An allergic response

The Child with a Metabolic Condition

objectives

1. Define each key term listed.
2. Relate why growth parameters are of importance to patients with a family history of endocrine disease.
3. Compare the signs and symptoms of hyperglycemia and hypoglycemia.
4. Differentiate between type I and type II diabetes.
5. List a predictable stress that the disease of diabetes has on children and families during the following periods of life: infancy, toddlerhood, preschool age, elementary school age, puberty, and adolescence.
6. Outline the educational needs of the diabetic child and parents in the following areas: nutrition and meal planning, exercise, blood tests, administration of insulin, and skin care.
7. List three precipitating events that might cause diabetic ketoacidosis.
8. List three possible causes of insulin shock.
9. Explain the Somogyi phenomenon.
10. Discuss the preparation and administration of insulin to a child, highlighting any differences between pediatric and adult administration.
11. List two benefits of exercise for the diabetic adolescent.
12. List the symptoms of hypothyroidism in infants.
13. Discuss the dietary adjustment required for a child with diabetes insipidus.

key terms

antidiuretic hormone (p. 725)
gestational diabetes (p. 728)
glucagon (p. 736)
glycosuria (glī-kō-SŪ-rē-ă, p. 728)
glycosylated hemoglobin test (HbA1c) (glī-kō-sī-lā-tĭd HĒ-mō-glō-bĭn tĕst, p. 728)
hormones (p. 723)
hyperglycemia (hī-pĕr-glī-SĒ-mē-ă, p. 728)
hypoglycemia (hī-pō-glī-SĒ-mē-ă, p. 735)
hypotonia (hī-pō-TŌ-nē-ă, p. 725)

ketoacidosis (kē-tō-ă-sĭ-DŌ-sĭs, p. 729)
lipoatrophy (lĭp-ō-ĂT-rō-fē, p. 734)
polydipsia (pŏl-ē-DĬP-sē-ă, p. 728)
polyphagia (pŏl-ē-FĀ-jē-ă, p. 728)
polyuria (pŏl-ē-Ū-rē-ă, p. 728)
Somogyi phenomenon (p. 736)
target organ (p. 723)
vasopressin (văz-ō-PRĔS-ĭn, p. 725)

OVERVIEW

The two major control systems that monitor the functions of the body are the nervous system and the endocrine system. These systems are interdependent. The endocrine, or ductless, glands regulate the body's metabolic processes. They are primarily responsible for growth, maturation, reproduction, and the response of the body to stress. Figure 30-1 depicts the organs of the endocrine system and outlines how this system in children differs from that in adults. Hormones are chemical substances produced by the glands. They pour their secretions directly into the blood that flows through them. An organ specifically influenced by a certain hormone is called a target organ. Too much or too little of a given hormone may result in a disease state. Most of the glands and structures of the endocrine system develop during the first trimester of fetal development.

Maternal endocrine dysfunction may affect the fetus; therefore an in-depth maternal history is a valuable tool in data collection. The absence or deficiency of an enzyme that has a role in metabolism causes a defect in the metabolism process; this can result in illness. Most inborn errors of metabolism can be detected by clinical signs or screening tests that can be performed in utero. Lethargy, poor feeding, failure to thrive, vomiting, and an enlarged liver may be early signs of an inborn error of metabolism in the newborn. When clinical signs are not manifested in the neonatal period, an infection or body stress can precipitate symptoms of a latent defect in the older child. Unexplained mental retardation, developmental delay, convulsions, an odor to body or

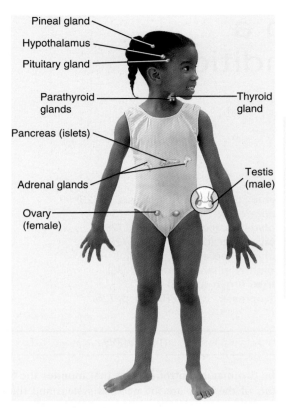

Pineal gland
Hypothalamus
Pituitary gland
Parathyroid glands
Pancreas (islets)
Adrenal glands
Ovary (female)
Thyroid gland
Testis (male)

FIGURE **30-1** Summary of some endocrine system differences between the child and the adult. The endocrine system consists of the ductless glands that release hormones. It works with the nervous system to regulate metabolic activities.

ENDOCRINE SYSTEM

- The endocrine system of the newborn is supplemented by maternal hormones that cross the placental barrier. In males and females, this may result in swelling of the breasts and genital changes.
- Hormone disturbances during childhood may cause disrupted growth patterns, resulting in short stature or gigantism.
- Congenital hypothyroidism may occur as a result of an absent, nonfunctioning thyroid gland.
- In childhood the pancreas may be deficient in insulin, causing type I (insulin-dependent) diabetes.

urine, or episodes of vomiting may be subtle signs of a metabolic dysfunction. Phenylketonuria (PKU), galactosemia, and maple syrup urine disease are discussed in Chapter 14. Cystic fibrosis is discussed in Chapter 25.

Radiographic studies to determine bone age are valuable diagnostic tools. Serum electrolytes and glucose, hormonal, and calcium level tests may be required. Phenylketonuria testing of newborns is an important screening device for identifying an enzyme deficiency. Chromosomal studies and tissue biopsy are other diagnostic tools. Sexual maturation and skin texture, pigment, and temperature may be indicators of specific disorders. Thyroid function tests may be required. Ultrasound is helpful in determining the size and character of the adrenal glands, ovaries, and other organs. A 24-hour urine specimen may reveal important data. The glucose tolerance test is commonly performed to detect or monitor diabetes. Genetic counseling can help prevent some disorders.

NURSING **TIP**

Growth hormone is administered at bedtime to simulate the natural timing of hormone release.

INBORN ERRORS OF METABOLISM

The term *inborn errors of metabolism* was coined at the turn of the century by Garrod. There are literally hundreds of these hereditary biochemical disorders that affect body metabolism. The pattern of inheritance is generally autosomal recessive. These conditions range from mild to severe.

TAY-SACHS DISEASE

Pathophysiology. Tay-Sachs disease involves a deficiency of *hexosaminidase,* an enzyme necessary for the metabolism of fats. Lipid deposits accumulate on nerve cells, causing both physical and mental deterioration. This is a disease found primarily in the Ashkenazic Jewish population. It is an autosomal recessive trait carried by 1 in 30 of the Ashkenazic Jewish population, resulting in an occurrence of 1 in 4000 live births.

Manifestations. The infant with Tay-Sachs disease is normal until about age 5 to 6 months, when physical development begins to slow. There may be head lag or an inability to sit. The disease progresses, and when deposits occur on the optic nerve, blindness may result.

Mental retardation eventually develops because the brain cells become damaged. Most children with Tay-Sachs disease die before 5 years of age from secondary infection or malnutrition.

Treatment and nursing care. There is no treatment for this devastating disease. The nursing care is mainly palliative. Most care is given in the home, with periodic hospitalization for complications such as pneumonia. Chapter 26 discusses the care of the dying child. Carriers can be identified by screening tests. Genetic and prenatal counseling have markedly decreased the occurrence of Tay-Sachs disease.

ENDOCRINE DISORDERS

HYPOTHYROIDISM

Pathophysiology. Hypothyroidism occurs when there is a deficiency in the secretions of the thyroid gland. It may be congenital or acquired. It is one of the more common disorders of the endocrine system in children. The thyroid gland controls the rate of metabolism in the body by producing thyroxine (T_4) and triiodothyronine (T_3). In congenital hypothyroidism the gland is absent or not functioning. The symptoms of hypothyroidism may not be apparent for several months.

Juvenile hypothyroidism is acquired by the older child. It may be caused by a number of conditions, the most common being lymphocytic thyroiditis. Often it appears during periods of rapid growth. Infectious disease, irradiation for cancer, certain medications containing iodine, and lack of dietary iodine (uncommon in the United States) may predispose the child. The symptoms, diagnosis, and treatment are similar to those mentioned for congenital hypothyroidism. Because brain growth is nearly complete by 2 to 3 years of age, mental retardation and neurological complications are not seen in the older child.

Manifestations. The infant with hypothyroidism is very sluggish and sleeps a lot. The tongue becomes enlarged, causing noisy respiration (Figure 30-2). The skin is dry, there is no perspiration, and the hands and feet are cold. The infant feels floppy when handled. This hypotonia also affects the intestinal tract, causing chronic constipation. The hair eventually becomes dry and brittle. If hypothyroidism is left untreated, irreversible mental retardation and physical disabilities result.

Treatment and nursing care. Early recognition and diagnosis are essential to prevent the developing sequelae. A screening test for hypothyroidism may be performed at birth. It consists of T_4 measurement and a thyroid-stimulating hormone (TSH) measurement when T_4 level is low. This is generally part of an overall screen for other metabolic defects. Treatment involves

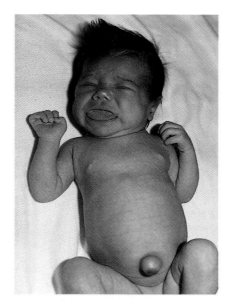

FIGURE **30-2** An infant with hypothyroidism. Note the large head and tongue, puffy face, broad nasal bridge, and relaxed abdominal muscles resulting in an umbilical hernia. The infant is not alert and feeds poorly.

the administration of the synthetic hormone sodium levothyroxine (Synthroid or Levothroid). Hormone levels are monitored regularly. Therapy reverses the symptoms and prevents further mental retardation but does not reverse existing retardation; therefore early detection of congenital hypothyroidism is very important.

The medication is taken at the same time each day, preferably in the morning. Parents are cautioned not to interchange brands. Children may experience reversible hair loss, insomnia, and aggressiveness, and their schoolwork may decline during the first few months of therapy. This is temporary. It may take 1 to 3 weeks to reach the full therapeutic effect. Medication is not to be discontinued because the replacement for hypothyroidism is lifelong. Parents are instructed about these measures and are advised to consult their physician before giving other medications.

COMMON METABOLIC DYSFUNCTIONS

Other common metabolic dysfunctions, their manifestations, and their treatment are discussed in Table 30-1.

DIABETES INSIPIDUS

Pathophysiology. Diabetes insipidus can be hereditary (autosomal dominant) or acquired as the result of a head injury or tumor. It is the result of posterior pituitary *hypofunction* that results in a decreased secretion of vasopressin, the antidiuretic hormone. A lack of antidiuretic hormone results in uncontrolled diuresis.

table 30-1 *Metabolic Dysfunctions*

GLAND	PROBLEM	INVOLVED HORMONE	MANIFESTATION	THERAPY
Pituitary— anterior	*Decreased* hypo-pituitarism	Growth hormone	Short stature, dwarfism	Synthetic growth hormone replacement
	Increased hyper-pituitarism	Growth hormone	Before epiphyseal closure, gigantism After epiphyseal closure, acromegaly Sexual precocity (puberty before 8 to 9 years of age)	Surgery, irradiation Radioactive implants Monthly hormone injection to control secretions until puberty
Pituitary— posterior	*Decreased* hypo-pituitarism	Decreased antidiuretic hormone	Diabetes insipidus (see p. 725)	Vasopressin by injection or nasal spray Provide adequate fluids
	Increased hyper-pituitarism (syndrome of inappropriate antidiuretic hormone secretion [SIADH])	Increased antidiuretic hormone	SIADH	Fluid restriction and hormone antagonists
Parathyroid	*Decreased* hypo-parathyroidism	Decreased parahormone	Decreased blood calcium and increased phosphorus, causing tetany and laryngospasm	Calcium gluconate, vitamin D supplements
	Increased hyperparathyroidism	Increased parathormone	Elevated blood calcium and lowered phosphorus levels, causing spontaneous fractures and CNS problems	Restore calcium balance, excise tumor
Adrenal	*Decreased* adrenal cortical insufficiency (Addison's disease)	Decreased steroids, sex steroids, epinephrine	Craving for salt, seizures, neurological and circulatory changes, decreased sexual development	Replace cortisol and body fluids, genetic sexual assessment
	Increased hyperadrenalism (Cushing's disease)	Increased cortisol	Cushing syndrome, hyperglycemia, electrolyte problems, pheochromocytoma	Depends on cause, tumor removal

The kidney does not concentrate the urine during dehydration episodes.

Manifestations. *Polydipsia* and *polyuria* are the initial signs. The infant cries and prefers water to milk formula. Loss of weight, growth failure, and dehydration occur rapidly. As the child grows older, enuresis may be a problem. Excessive thirst and the search for water overshadow the desire to play, explore, eat, learn, or sleep. Perspiration is deficient, and the skin is dry.

Treatment and nursing care. Treatment involves hormone replacement of vasopressin in the form of desmopressin by subcutaneous injection or DDAVP (desmopressin acetate) nasal spray. Parents should be taught to monitor for signs of overdosage, which include symptoms of water intoxication (edema, lethargy, nausea, central nervous system signs). Children with diabetes insipidus who are admitted to the hospital in an unconscious state and are unable to express thirst are at great

| table 30-2 | *Clinical Features of Type I and Type II Diabetes* | |

FEATURE	TYPE I (IDDM)	TYPE II (NIDDM)
Onset	Abrupt, can often state week of onset	Insidious, often found by screening tests
Body size	Normal or thin	Often obese
Blood glucose	Fluctuates widely with exercise and infection	Fluctuations are less marked
Ketoacidosis	Common	Infrequent
Sulfonylurea responsiveness	Rare	Greater than 50%
Insulin required	Almost all	Less than 25%
Insulin dosage	Increases until stable glucose control	May remain stable

IDDM, Insulin-dependent diabetes mellitus; *NIDDM*, non-insulin-dependent diabetes mellitus.

risk. A medical identification bracelet should be worn. School personnel should be advised of the child's needs. School protocol often limits children's access to bathrooms and water fountains, even during or after physical activity. Such restrictions could be life threatening to a child with diabetes insipidus. The nurse should contact the school nurse and physical education instructors and educate parents concerning the child's needs and the lifelong administration of the medication. Home care instructions should include recognizing the signs of water intoxication.

DIABETES MELLITUS

Pathophysiology. Diabetes mellitus (DM) is a chronic metabolic condition in which the body is unable to use carbohydrates properly because of a deficiency of insulin, an internal secretion of the beta cells of the pancreas. Insulin deficiency leads to an impairment of glucose transport (sugar cannot pass into the cells). The body is also unable to store and use fats properly. There is a decrease in protein synthesis. When the blood glucose level becomes dangerously high, glucose spills into the urine, and diuresis occurs. Incomplete fat metabolism produces ketone bodies that accumulate in the blood. This is termed *ketonemia.* Untreated diabetes can lead to coma and death.

Etiology. DM is considered to be an autoimmune disease that may involve a defect in chromosome number six. A trigger, or stressor (e.g., virus) causes a destruction of the beta cells in the islets of Langerhans of the pancreas, resulting in manifestation of the illness. It is the most common endocrine disorder of childhood and has a number of physical, emotional, and developmental consequences. Constant attention to dietary intake and daily administration of medication place a stress on the growing child. Long-term complications relating to kidney disease, blindness, circulatory prob-

lems, and neuropathy loom in the future for these children. Treatment is designed to optimize growth and development and to minimize complications.

Classification. Diabetes mellitus is not a single entity but rather a syndrome. To help eliminate confusion in terminology, the National Institutes of Health appointed an international committee, the National Diabetes Data Group, to classify the carbohydrate intolerance syndromes. Further refinements in classification will be necessary as more is learned about diabetes. The following categories are pertinent to this discussion of pediatric diabetes:

- *Type I, insulin-dependent diabetes mellitus (IDDM).* This was formerly termed juvenile-onset diabetes. It is characterized by insulin deficiency caused by an autoimmune destruction of the pancreatic beta cells. Childhood diabetes is usually of this type. Although there may be some insulin production during certain phases of the disease, patients eventually become insulin deficient. They are prone to ketosis.
- *Type II, non-insulin-dependent diabetes mellitus (NIDDM).* This is caused by insulin resistance or failure of the body to use the insulin. It was formerly called adult-onset diabetes. These persons are not usually dependent on insulin and rarely develop ketoacidosis. Although NIDDM may occur at any age, it generally develops after 40 years of age. Hypotension and obesity are common. Type II diabetes seen in young adults is sometimes called maturity-onset diabetes of youth. Table 30-2 lists the clinical features of types I and II.
- *Maturity-onset diabetes of youth (MODY).* MODY is transmitted as an autosomal dominant disorder that results in the production of an abnormal type of insulin that does not function properly. Onset occurs in early adulthood.

- **Gestational diabetes** is the appearance of symptoms for the first time during pregnancy (see Chapter 5).

Type I IDDM Diabetes

Incidence. Approximately 12 million Americans have diabetes. In the United States the annual incidence is about 10 to 12 new cases per 100,000 children (Behrman, Kliegman, & Jenson, 2000). The frequency is increasing. Contributing factors include (1) patients with diabetes are living into their reproductive years and having children, (2) cow's milk is being fed to children under 2 years of age, (3) obesity has increased, and (4) good prenatal care has decreased the mortality rates of mothers and infants. Specific viral infections can also trigger IDDM.

Symptoms of IDDM may occur at any time in childhood, but the rate of occurrence of new cases is highest among 5- and 7-year-old children and pubescent children 11 to 13 years of age. In the former group the stress of school and the increased exposure to infectious diseases may be responsible.

During puberty, increased growth, increased emotional stress, and insulin antagonism of sex hormones may be implicated. It occurs in both sexes with equal frequency. The disease is more difficult to manage in childhood because the patients are growing, expend a great deal of energy, have varying nutritional needs, and face a lifetime of diabetic management. Young children with IDDM often do not demonstrate the typical "textbook" picture of the disorder. The initial diagnosis may be determined when the child develops ketoacidosis. Therefore the nurse must be particularly astute in subjective and objective observations.

Manifestations. Children with diabetes present a classic triad of symptoms: polydipsia, polyuria, and polyphagia. The symptoms appear more rapidly in children. The patient complains of excessive thirst (polydipsia), excretes large amounts of urine frequently (polyuria), and is constantly hungry (polyphagia). An insidious onset with lethargy, weakness, and weight loss is also common. Anorexia may be seen. The child who is toilet trained may begin wetting the bed or have frequent "accidents" during play periods, may lose weight, and is irritable. The skin becomes dry. Vaginal yeast infections may be seen in the adolescent girl. There may be a history of recurrent infections. The symptoms may go unrecognized until an infection becomes apparent or coma results. Laboratory findings indicate glucose in the urine (glycosuria or glucosuria). Hyperglycemia (*hyper,* "above," *gly,* "sugar," and *emia,* "blood") is also apparent.

The honeymoon period. When IDDM is initially diagnosed and the child is stabilized on insulin dosage, the condition may appear to improve. Insulin requirements decrease, and the child feels well. This phenomenon supports the parent's phase of "denial" in accepting the long-term diagnosis of DM for their child. The "honeymoon period" lasts a short time (a few months), and parents must be encouraged to closely monitor blood sugar levels to avoid complications.

NURSING **TIP**

A period of remission, or the "honeymoon" phase of the disease, may occur within a few weeks of beginning insulin administration. There is a decline in insulin need and improved metabolic control. This phase, however, is temporary.

Diagnostic Blood Tests

Blood glucose. A random blood glucose level may be obtained at any time and requires no preparation of the patient. The results should be within the normal limits for both nondiabetics and diabetics in good control.

Fasting blood glucose. A fasting blood glucose level is a standard and reliable test for diabetes. The blood glucose level is measured in the fasting patient, usually first thing in the morning. The results of the test will not be accurate if the patient is receiving a dextrose intravenous solution. If the child is known to have diabetes, food and insulin are withheld until after the test. If a person's fasting blood glucose level is greater than 126 mg/dl on two separate occasions and the history is positive, the patient is considered to have diabetes and requires treatment.

Glucose tolerance test. Another test to determine the amount of sugar in the blood is the glucose tolerance test (GTT). The results are plotted on a graph (Figure 30-3). This procedure is time-consuming, and therefore parents and adolescents are advised to bring reading material, homework, headsets, and other activities to the physician's office or laboratory. A blood glucose concentration greater than 200 mg/dl is considered positive. Normal values may not return for more than 3 hours.

Glycosylated hemoglobin test. The glycosylated hemoglobin test (HbAlc) reflects glycemic levels over a period of months. Values are found to be elevated in virtually all children with newly diagnosed diabetes. This study also helps to confirm the results of blood and urine tests done either at home or by the physician. Glucose in the bloodstream constantly enters red blood cells and links with, or glycosylates, molecules of hemoglobin. The more glucose in the blood, the more hemoglobin becomes coated with glucose. The red blood cells carry this glucose until they are replaced by cells with fresh hemoglobin. This process takes about 3 to 4 months. Values vary according to the measurement used. Values of 6% to 9% represent very good metabolic control. Values above 12% indicate poor control.

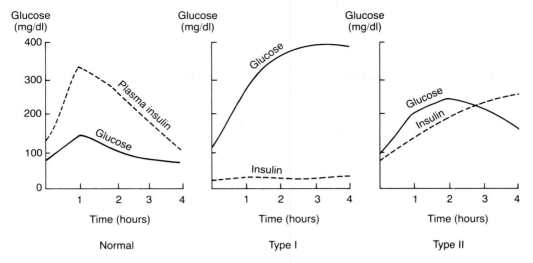

FIGURE **30-3** The glucose tolerance test: *Left,* Normal; *center,* type I diabetes; *right,* type II diabetes. The graphs show the relationship between the ingestion of glucose and the level of plasma insulin over 4 hours in a normal person and in persons with type I and type II diabetes.

Glycosylated hemoglobin (fructosamine) is a test used to measure blood glucose control over the preceding 7 to 10 days. C-peptide (connecting chains of insulin peptides) may also be measured to determine how much insulin the body is producing (endogenous). This is of particular value during the honeymoon period of the disease.

Diabetic Ketoacidosis

Diabetic ketoacidosis (DKA) is also referred to as *diabetic coma,* although a person may have DKA with or without being in a coma. It may result if a patient with diabetes contracts a secondary infection and does not follow proper self-care. It may also result if the disease proceeds unrecognized; this occurs fairly often in children with diabetes. Even minor infections, such as a cold, increase the body's metabolic rate and thereby change the body's demand for insulin and the severity of diabetes.

Symptoms of ketoacidosis are compared to those of hypoglycemia in Table 30-3. Diabetic teaching should include this information. The symptoms range from mild to severe and occur within hours to days.

Treatment and Nursing Care

The aims of treatment in type I diabetes are to (1) ensure normal growth and development through metabolic control; (2) enable the child to cope with a chronic illness, have a happy and active childhood, and be well integrated into the family; and (3) prevent complications. Complications can be minimized by maintaining the blood glucose at consistently normal levels. Teaching ideally begins when the diagnosis is confirmed. A

table 30-3 *Hyperglycemia and Hypoglycemia*

HYPERGLYCEMIA (KETOACIDOSIS)	HYPOGLYCEMIA
CAUSE	
Insulin underdose	Excess exercise
Food overdose	Too little food
	Insulin overdose
SIGNS AND SYMPTOMS	
Polyuria, polydipsia, polyphagia	Fatigue
	Hunger
Fruity odor to breath	Pale, clammy
Fatigue	Diaphoresis
Abdominal pain	Tremors
Red lips, flushed face	Lethargy
Dehydration	Headache
Disorientation	
Drowsiness progressing to coma	
Deep, rapid (Kussmaul) respirations	
TREATMENT	
Regular insulin	Administer glucagon, orange juice, or carbohydrates orally

planned educational program is necessary to provide a consistent body of information, which can then be individualized. The patient's age and financial, educational, cultural, and religious background must be considered. Many hospitals hold group clinics for diabetic patients and their relatives. These sessions are conducted by the multidisciplinary health care team and include the diabetes nurse educator, dietitian, and pharmacist. Patients who are living with the disease provide encouragement and help by sharing concerns. Health professionals become directly involved with the patient's progress and can offer necessary feedback and support. Continuous follow-up is essential.

Because children with diabetes are growing, additional dimensions of the disorder and its treatment become evident. Growth is not steady but occurs in spurts and plateaus that affect treatment. Infants and toddlers may have hydration problems, especially during illness. Preschool children have irregular activity and eating patterns. School-age children may grieve over the diagnosis and ask, "Why me?" They may use their illness to gain attention or to avoid responsibilities. The onset of puberty may require insulin adjustments as a result of growth and the antagonistic effect of the sex hormones on insulin. Adolescents often resent this condition, which deviates from their concept of the "body ideal." They have more difficulty in resolving their conflict between dependence and independence. This may lead to rebellion against parents and treatment regimens.

The impact of the disease on the rest of the family must also be considered. Parents may feel guilty for having passed on the disease. Siblings may feel jealous of the attention the patient receives. The sharing of responsibility by parents is ideal but not necessarily a reality. Some may have difficulty accepting the diagnosis and the more regimented lifestyle it imposes. Family members must cope with their individual reactions to the stress of the illness.

Children must assume responsibility for their own care gradually and with a minimum of pressure. Overprotection can be as detrimental as neglect. Parents who have received satisfaction from their child's dependence on them may need help "letting go." The diabetic camp experience is helpful in this respect. A medical identification bracelet should be worn.

The nursing management of childhood diabetes requires knowledge of growth and development, pathophysiology, blood glucose self-monitoring, nutritional management, insulin management, insulin shock, exercise, skin and foot care, infections, effects of emotional upsets, and long-term care. Nursing Care Plan 30-1 lists interventions for the child with diabetes.

Teaching Plan for Children with Diabetes Mellitus

The patient and family are instructed about the location of the pancreas and its normal function. The nurse explains the relationship of insulin to the pancreas, differentiating between type I and type II diabetes. All information is given gradually and at the level of understanding of the child and family. Audiovisual aids and pamphlets are incorporated into the session. If the patient is newly diagnosed, hospitalization offers opportunities for instruction.

Blood Glucose Self-Monitoring

Patients can test their own blood glucose level in the home. While still being supervised by and consulting with the physician, the patient can make rational changes in insulin dosage (sliding scale dosage) based on home blood glucose tests, nutritional requirements, and daily exercise. This is of great psychological value to the child, teenager, and parents because it reduces feelings of helplessness and complete dependence on medical personnel. Home glucose monitoring should be taught to all young patients and their caregivers. The patient must not only be skilled in the techniques but also understand the results and how to incorporate them into daily regimens. This means involving the entire health care team in ongoing supervision, demonstrations, and support. Although instructions come with the various products, patients need individual training.

Glucometer systems provide readouts and automatically store data by time and date. Some also keep track of diet and the amount of exercise for the day. This can be connected to a computer or computer printer for review. Records can be transmitted electronically to the physician.

Obtaining blood specimens has been simplified by the use of capillary blood-letting devices such as the Glucolet. This device automatically controls the depth of penetration of the lancet into the skin. Other brands include the Hamalet, Autoclix, Monoject, and Autolet. The sides of the fingertips are recommended testing sites because there are fewer nerve endings and more capillary beds in these areas. The best finger to use is the middle, ring, or little finger on either hand. The finger will bleed more easily if the child washes the hands in warm water for about 30 seconds. To perform the test, a drop of blood is put on a chemically treated reagent strip. The test strip with a drop of blood is inserted into the glucometer, and the blood glucose reading appears. Noninvasive devices to assess blood sugar levels have been developed (Figure 30-4).

Cost, convenience, and portability are factors to consider when selecting glucometers. Most products can be obtained at the local pharmacy. Newer and more precise instruments are being developed constantly. Frequency of use is determined by the amount of diabetes control required by the particular child.

NURSING CARE PLAN 30-1

The Child with Diabetes Mellitus

PATIENT DATA: A 10-year-old boy is admitted with new-onset diabetes mellitus. An insulin regimen is prescribed. The child states that he wishes to return to a normal life with his peers.

SELECTED NURSING DIAGNOSIS   *Risk for injury related to hypoglycemia or diabetic ketoacidosis(hyperglycemia)*

Outcomes	Nursing Interventions	Rationales
Child will be able to measure blood glucose level with glucometer, as age appropriate.	1. Teach child home glucose monitoring.	1. Self-care increases feelings of control.
Child will be adequately hydrated as evidenced by good tissue turgor and intake and output records.	2. Record vital signs regularly.	2. Vital signs detect infection and illness, which affect diabetes; in ketoacidosis, Kussmaul respirations may be seen until blood pH and serum bicarbonate normalize.
Child will be asymptomatic of hypoglycemia or hyperglycemia.	3. Monitor fluid intake and output.	3. Dehydration may occur as a result of vomiting, polyuria, and hyperglycemia.
	4. Serve meals and snacks on time.	4. Serving meals on time prevents hypoglycemia and minimizes hyperglycemia.
	5. Administer or have patient administer insulin as ordered.	5. Insulin is individualized to meet the response of patients. It cannot be taken by mouth because stomach juices would destroy it before it could be used.
	6. Determine level of consciousness.	6. Both hypoglycemia and hyperglycemia affect sensorium, depending on stage of reaction.
	7. Carefully observe patient for signs of hypoglycemia or hyperglycemia.	7. Many factors such as diet, increased exercise, or illness can contribute to the body's balance of insulin and glucose; changes in hormone levels that accompany menstruation can cause swings of high or low blood sugar levels.

SELECTED NURSING DIAGNOSIS   *Deficient knowledge regarding exercise*

Outcomes	Nursing Interventions	Rationales
Child will describe physical exercise program.	1. Determine child's activity level as age appropriate.	1. Exercise increases glucose utilization.
Child will be prepared for hypoglycemia should it occur.	2. Explain that exercise lowers the blood sugar level and in this respect acts like more insulin.	2. Patient may need to adjust insulin for days when involved in high-impact exercise.
	3. Instruct as to symptoms of hypoglycemia such as irritability, shakiness, hunger, headache, and altered levels of consciousness.	3. Early recognition and prompt treatment will prevent injury.

Continued

NURSING CARE PLAN 30-1—cont'd

Outcomes	Nursing Interventions	Rationales
	4. Teach child importance of carrying extra sugar when exercising or playing sports.	4. Taking sugar reverses symptoms of hypoglycemia.
	5. Teach child the dangers of swimming alone.	5. Child could drown if symptoms occur.

SELECTED NURSING DIAGNOSIS *Deficient knowledge regarding identification*

Outcomes	Nursing Interventions	Rationales
Child will state understanding of importance of wearing proper identification bracelet.	1. Child demonstrates proper identification.	1. Diabetes symptoms may be mistaken for other conditions, such as flu.
Family will acquire identification bracelet.	2. Encourage purchase of means of identification.	2. Child may be unconscious or too young to inform others of condition.

⚲CRITICAL THINKING QUESTION

A child comes to the clinic for follow-up after discharge from the hospital with a diagnosis of diabetic ketoacidosis. He states he is excited about returning to school and rejoining his cross-country team with his friends. His father states he wants his son to stay home and do more sedentary activities to avoid any more health problems. What is the best response of the nurse?

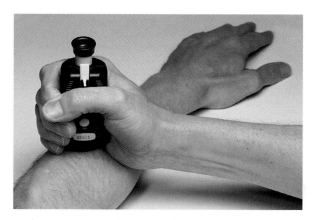

FIGURE **30-4** A noninvasive glucometer used to determine blood glucose values. A skin sensor is pressed firmly against the skin to obtain a transcutaneous noninvasive glucose level. Other glucometers have lancets that pierce the skin and obtain a blood sample that is placed on a sensor strip and analyzed within seconds.

Diet Therapy for Children with Diabetes Mellitus

Nutritional management. The triad of management of diabetes comprises a well-balanced diet, insulin, and regular exercise. The importance of glycemic control in decreasing the incidence of symptoms and complications of the disease has been established. The advent of blood glucose self-monitoring is affecting food intake in that diets can be fine-tuned and more flexible while the cornerstone of *consistency* (in amount of food and time of feeding) is maintained. Contrary to popular belief, there is no scientific evidence that persons with diabetes require special foods. In fact, if it is good for the diabetic, it is good for the entire family. The nutritional needs of diabetic children are essentially no different from those of nondiabetic children, with the exception of the elimination of concentrated carbohydrates (simple sugars). These cause a marked increase in blood glucose level and should generally be avoided.

The goals of nutritional management in children are to ensure normal growth and development, to distribute food intake so that it aids metabolic control, and to individualize the diet in accordance with the child's ethnic background, age, sex, weight, activity, family economics, and food preferences. Once a diet prescription is received from the physician, the dietitian assists the family in designing an individualized diet plan. The dietitian also explains the use of exchange lists.

Education of the patient is ongoing. Too much information given at one time may overwhelm the parents and discourage the child. Well-informed nurses can offer much reinforcement and support. They can clarify terms such as dietetic, sugar-free, juice-packed, water-packed, and unsweetened. Meal trays in the hospital provide an excellent opportunity for teaching. Children should bring their lunch to school. Respecting cultural patterns and personal preferences is important. The content of foods commonly found in fast-food chain restaurants is available through the American Diabetes Association.

The importance of fiber in diets is well documented. In the diabetic patient, soluble fiber has been shown to reduce blood sugar levels, lower serum cholesterol values, and sometimes reduce insulin requirements. Fiber appears to slow the rate of absorption of sugar by the digestive tract. Raw fruits and vegetables, bran cereals, wheat germ, beans, peas, and lentils are good sources of soluble fiber.

> **NURSING TIP**
> Instruct the patient and family to read food labels carefully. The word *dietetic* does not mean *diabetic*. Dietetic merely means something has been changed or replaced; for example, the food may contain less salt or less sugar.

Glycemic index, cholesterol, and artificial sweeteners. The glycemic index for selected foods has an impact on the manipulation of dietary needs. Because persons with diabetes have an increased risk for atherosclerosis, the reduction of serum cholesterol level is another concern. Most of the general public need to reduce their intake of animal fats. This is accomplished by consuming less beef and pork and more chicken, turkey, fish, low-fat milk (depending on the age of the patient), and vegetable proteins. The form of food is also significant. An apple, apple juice, and applesauce may precipitate different blood sugar responses. Portions, the type of processing, cooking, and combinations of foods have also been shown to have a bearing on these responses.

Aspartame (NutraSweet) was approved by the U.S. Food and Drug Administration (FDA) in 1981. It is used in items that do not require cooking. Aspartame is made of two amino acids, both of which contain insignificant amounts of carbohydrate. One granulation form is called Equal. Sorbitol, mannitol, and xylitol are sugars commonly found in foods called "sugar-free." These substances are absorbed more slowly into the bloodstream. Large amounts of sorbitol can cause diarrhea, and overuse should be avoided.

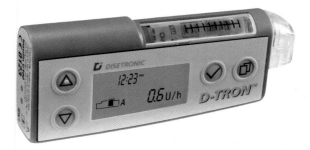

FIGURE **30-5** The insulin pump offers continuous subcutaneous insulin infusion without the need for frequent injections. A small, pager-size, battery-powered, programmable pump holds a syringe of insulin. A catheter attaches to a needle that is inserted into the subcutaneous tissue and secured with transparent tape.

> **NURSING TIP**
> Take snacks seriously—they are an important part of the day's food supply.

Insulin management. Insulin is used principally as a specific drug for the control of DM. When injected into the diabetic patient, it enables the body to burn and store sugar. Current data emphasize the importance of blood glucose control in the prevention of microvascular disease. Insulin turns excess glucose into fat (triglycerides), promotes fat storage, and causes the kidneys to store sodium and uric acid, which can lead to hypertension. More highly purified insulins are being developed to reduce complications. *Human insulin,* which is not made from humans but is produced biosynthetically in bacteria using recombinant DNA technology, is widely used. It is reported to be very similar to the body's natural insulin. One example is Humulin. Insulin pumps are used in certain patients (Figure 30-5).

The dose of insulin is measured in units, and special syringes are used in its administration. U-100 (100-unit) insulin is the standard form. All vials of U-100 insulin have color-coded caps, and all labels bear black printing on a white background. Bold letters indicate type: "R" for regular, "P" for protamine zinc insulin (PZI), "N" for neutral protamine Hagedorn (NPH) insulin, "L" for lente, "U" for ultralente, and "S" for semilente.

It is important to teach the parents and child about the administration of insulin. Insulin cannot be taken orally because it is a protein and would be broken down by the gastric juices. The usual method of administration is *subcutaneously* (Figure 30-6). When injected at a 90-degree angle, the short needle enters the subcutaneous space. This technique may be easier for the child to learn because it takes less coordination to administer than a

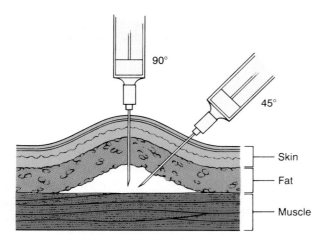

FIGURE **30-6** Subcutaneous injection of insulin.

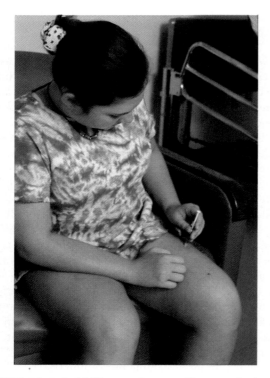

FIGURE **30-7** A child 7 years of age or older can take the responsibility for self-injection with proper supervision.

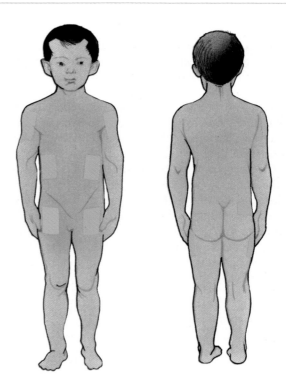

FIGURE **30-8** Sites of injection of insulin.

The site of the injection is rotated to prevent poor absorption and injury to tissues (Figure 30-8). Injection model forms made from construction paper and site rotation patterns are useful. One suggested site rotation pattern is to use one area for 1 week. A different site within that area is used for each injection. Injections should be about 1 inch apart. The young child can use a doll to practice self-injection.

Insulin should not be injected into an area that has a temporarily increased circulation. In such areas, a more rapid than expected absorption and effect can trigger hypoglycemia. For example, a more rapid circulation to the legs can be expected in a child who is riding a tricycle; therefore the thigh should not be selected as a site for injection. If a teen returns from playing tennis, the upper arm is avoided as an injection site.

Lipoatrophy (*lipo,* "fat" and *atrophy,* "loss of") and *lipohypertrophy* (*lipo,* and *hypertrophy,* "increase of") refer to changes that can occur in the subcutaneous tissue at the injection site. Proper rotation of sites and the availability of the newer purified insulins have helped to eliminate this condition. The child is taught to "feel for lumps" every week and to avoid using any sites that are suspicious.

The various types of insulin and their action are listed in Table 30-4. The main difference is in the

45-degree-angle technique. Automatic injection devices, the insulin pump, and needle-free injectors are fairly easy to use and promote independence in the child. In general, a child can be taught to perform self-injection after 7 years of age (Figure 30-7). The physician prescribes the type and amount of insulin and specifies the time of administration.

table 30-4 *Insulin*

| | | HYPOGLYCEMIC EFFECT | | |
	BRAND NAME(S)	ONSET (HR)	PEAK (HR)	DURATION (HR)
RAPID-ACTING	Lispro	15-30 min	30-90 min	2-4
Regular insulin	Humulin R	0.5-1	2-4	6-8
	Novolin R			
	Velosulin			
Semilente insulin	Semilente	1-1.5	5-10	12-16
INTERMEDIATE-ACTING				
Lente insulin	Humulin L	1-2.5	7-15	24
	Novolin L			
(NPH) insulin	Humulin N	1-1.5	4-12	24
	Insulatard			
	Novolin N			
LONG-ACTING				
Iletin 1		4-8	8-24	24-36
Ultralente insulin	Humulin U	4-8	10-30	>36
	Ultralente			
MIXTURES				
Novolin 70/30	Isophane insulin	Varied		
Humulin 50/50	supension			

Data from Skidmore-Roth, L.(2001). *Nursing drug reference*. St. Louis: Mosby; and Behrman, R., Kliegman, R., & Jenson, H. (2000). *Nelson's textbook of pediatrics* (16th ed.). Philadelphia: W.B. Saunders.

amount of time required for it to take effect and the length of protection time. The values listed in Table 30-4 are only *guidelines*. The response of each diabetic child to any given insulin dose is highly individual and depends on many factors, such as site of injection, local destruction of insulin by tissue enzymes, and insulin antibodies.

Regular insulin is less likely to cause allergic reactions. Both NPH, an intermediate type, and PZI, a long-lasting insulin, have had small amounts of chemicals added to prolong their action and to make them more stable. They offer protection over a period of hours, enabling the patient to do without repeated injections of unmodified insulin. They are cloudy and require mixing before being withdrawn from the vials. This mixing is done by gently rolling the bottle between the palms of the hands. Insulin is not used if it is discolored.

The physician often orders a combination of short-acting and intermediate-acting insulin; for example, "Give 10 units of NPH insulin and 5 units of regular insulin at 7:30 AM." This offers the patient immediate and longer-lasting protection. NPH or Lente insulin may be given in the same syringe as regular or crystalline insulin (Figure 30-9). Long-acting types of insulin are seldom given to children because of the danger of hypoglycemia during sleep. Stable, premixed insulins are available.

> ➤NURSING **TIP**
>
> When mixing insulin, always withdraw the regular insulin first and then add the long-acting insulin into the syringe.

Insulin shock. Insulin shock, also known as *hypoglycemia* (*hypo*, "below," *glyco*, "sugar," and *emia*, "blood"), occurs when the blood sugar level becomes abnormally low. This condition is caused by too much insulin. Factors that may account for this imbalance include poorly planned exercise, reduction of diet, and errors made because of improper knowledge of insulin and the insulin syringe.

Children are more prone to insulin reactions than adults because (1) the condition itself is more unstable in young people, (2) they are growing, and (3) their activities are more irregular. Poorly planned exercise is often the cause of insulin shock during childhood. Hospitalized patients who are being regulated must be observed frequently during naptime and at night. The nurse becomes suspicious of problems if unable to arouse the patient or if the child is perspiring heavily.

The symptoms of an insulin reaction, which range from mild to severe, are generally noticed and treated in the early stages. They appear suddenly in the otherwise

1. Wash your hands.
2. Gently rotate the intermediate insulin bottle.
3. Wipe off the tops of the insulin vials with an alcohol sponge.
4. Draw back an amount of air into the syringe equal to the total dose.
5. Inject air equal to the NPH dose into the NPH vial. Remove the syringe from the vial.

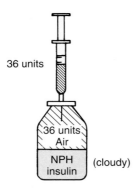

36 units

36 units Air

NPH insulin   (cloudy)

6. Inject air equal to the regular dose into the regular vial.

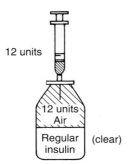

12 units

12 units Air

Regular insulin   (clear)

7. Invert the regular insulin bottle and withdraw the regular insulin dose.

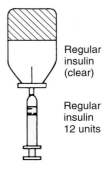

Regular insulin (clear)

Regular insulin 12 units

8. Without adding more air to the NPH vial, carefully withdraw the NPH dose.

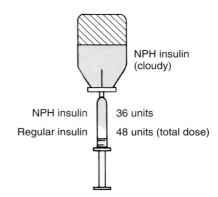

NPH insulin (cloudy)

NPH insulin   36 units

Regular insulin   48 units (total dose)

FIGURE 30-9 Mixing insulin. This step-order process avoids the problem of contaminating the regular insulin with the intermediate insulin. If contamination of the regular insulin does occur, the rapid-acting effect of this drug is dampened and is unreliable as a quick-acting insulin in an acute situation such as diabetic ketoacidosis.

well person. Examination of the blood would reveal a lowered blood sugar level. The child becomes irritable, may behave poorly, is pale, and may complain of feeling hungry and weak. Sweating occurs. Symptoms related to disorders of the nervous system arise because glucose is vital to the proper functioning of nerves. The child may become mentally confused and giddy, and muscular co-ordination is affected. If insulin shock is left untreated, coma and convulsions can occur.

The immediate treatment consists of administering sugar in some form, such as orange juice, hard candy, or a commercial product. The patient begins to feel better within a few minutes and at that time may eat a small amount of protein or starch (sandwich, milk, cheese) to prevent another reaction. Glucagon is recommended for the treatment of severe hypoglycemia. It quickly restores the child to consciousness in an emergency; the child can then consume some form of sugar or a planned meal.

The Somogyi phenomenon (rebound hypergly-cemia) occurs when blood glucose levels are lowered to a point at which the body's counterregulatory hormones (epinephrine, cortisol, glucagon) are released. Glucose is released from muscle and liver cells, which precipitates a rapid rise in blood glucose levels. It is generally the result of chronic insulin use, especially in patients who require fairly large doses of insulin to regulate their blood sugar levels. Hypoglycemia during the night and high glucose levels in the morning are suggestive of the phenomenon. The child may awaken at night or have frequent nightmares and experience early morning sweating and headaches. The child actually needs *less* insulin, not more, to rectify the problem.

The Somogyi phenomenon differs from the *dawn phenomenon,* in which early morning elevations of blood glucose occur *without* preceding hypoglycemia but may be a response to growth hormone secretion that occurs in the early morning hours. Together the Somogyi and dawn phenomena are the most common causes of instability in diabetic children. Testing blood glucose levels around 3 AM helps to differentiate the two conditions and assists in regulating insulin dosage.

Home Management of Children with Diabetes Mellitus

Exercise. Exercise is important for the patient with diabetes because it causes the body to use sugar and promotes good circulation. It lowers the blood glucose level, and in this respect it acts like more insulin. The diabetic patient who has planned vigorous exercise should carry extra sugar to avoid insulin reactions. The patient should also carry money for candy or a drink and, if possible, a cell phone. The blood glucose level is high directly after meals, and the child can participate in active sports at such times. Games enjoyed directly before meals should be less active. The diabetic child is able to participate in almost all active sports. Poorly planned exercise, however, can lead to difficulties.

Skin care. The patient is instructed to bathe daily and dry well, especially between the toes. Cleansing of the inguinal area, axillae, perineum, and inframammary areas is especially important because yeast and fungal infections tend to occur there. The skin is inspected for cuts, rashes, abrasions, bruises, cysts, or boils. These lesions are managed promptly. If skin is very dry, an oil such as Alpha Keri may be used in the bath water. Adolescents are taught to use electric razors. Exposing the skin to extremes in temperatures is avoided. Injection sites are inspected for lumps.

Foot care. Although circulatory problems of the feet are less common in children, proper habits of foot hygiene must be established. Patients are instructed to wash and dry their feet well each day. The feet are inspected for interdigital cracking, and the condition of the toenails is checked. Nails are trimmed straight

across. Socks are changed daily, and tight socks or large ones that bunch up are avoided. Shoes are replaced often as the child grows. The child should not go barefoot.

Infections. Immunizations against communicable diseases are essential (see Chapter 31).

Emotional upsets. Emotional upsets can be as disturbing to the patient as an infection and may require food adjustments, insulin adjustments, or both. Table 30-5 lists nursing interventions for stress on the child and family related to type I diabetes.

Urine checks. Routine urine checks for sugar are being replaced by the more accurate glucose blood monitoring. However, this procedure does not test for acetone, which the patient may need to determine, particularly during illness and when the blood glucose level is high. Daily urine checks may be advocated for some patients. Saying urine "check" rather than "test" is less confusing to young children.

Glucose-insulin imbalances. The patient is taught to recognize the signs of insulin shock and ketoacidosis (see Table 30-3). Early attention to changes and daily recordkeeping are stressed. Many excellent teaching films and brochures are available. The child should wear a bracelet identifying him or her as a diabetic. Wallet cards are also available. Teachers, athletic coaches, and guidance personnel are informed about the disease and should have the telephone numbers of the patient's parents and health care provider.

Travel. With planning, children can enjoy travel with their families, and older adolescents can travel alone. Before leaving, the child should be seen by the physician for a checkup and prescriptions for supplies. A written statement and a card identifying the child as diabetic should be carried. Time changes may affect meals. Additional supplies of insulin, sugar, and food are kept with the child. These are never checked with luggage, especially on an airplane, because they may be lost. If foreign travel is planned, parents must become familiar with the food in the area so that dietary requirements can be met. Local chapters of the American Diabetes Association or the Juvenile Diabetes Foundation can help vacationing families in an emergency.

Follow-up care. The child must see the physician regularly. The child should also be taught to visit the dentist regularly for cleaning of teeth and gums. Brushing and flossing daily are essential. Eyes should be examined regularly; blurry vision must not be disregarded. There are many brochures, books, and journals that offer excellent suggestions and guidance at an age-appropriate level.

Surgery. The patient with diabetes usually tolerates surgery well. Insulin may be given before, during, or after the operation. If the patient is restricted to nothing

table 30-5 *Nursing Interventions for Predictable Types of Stress on a Child with Type I Diabetes and on the Family*

AGE	ISSUE	NURSING INTERVENTIONS
Infant	Trust versus mistrust Onset and diagnosis particularly difficult during infancy; anxiety can be transmitted to infant	Stress consistency in fulfilling needs. Involve both parents in education. Avoid information overload. Instill hope and confidence. Focus on child rather than disease. Review normal growth and development of infancy. Assist in problem solving (e.g., baby-sitters, difficulty in obtaining specimens, baby food exchange lists).
Toddler	Autonomy versus shame and doubt Is this a temper tantrum or high or low blood sugar?	Prepare child for procedures or separations. Encourage exploration of environment. Stress limit setting as a form of love. Admit it is difficult to distinguish temper tantrums from symptoms. If behavior worsens or is prolonged or if physical symptoms appear, check blood sugar level. Provide 24-hour telephone number for advice nurse.
Preschool	Initiative versus guilt May view injections as punishment May view denial of sweets as lack of love "Picky eater"	Foster sense of competence. Educate parents to provide consistent warmth, reassurance, and love. Discuss feelings about child's life and diabetes. Avoid negative connotation by words, such as, "bad blood test," "cheating." Help parents sort out child's fantasies. Plan favorite party dishes on occasion. Invite a playmate for lunch. Suggest alternative nutritious snacks.
Elementary school	Industry versus inferiority Patients may feel they will be cured by hospitalization Grief over lack of cure Rebellion over treatment regimen Rebellion over food plan Anxiety about disclosure of condition to friends Embarrassed about reactions in school, missed days Unpredictable effects of exercise	Assist child in how to respond to teasing from peers ("Yecch, needles"). Explain "honeymoon" stage of disease. Accept child's disappointment. Gradually assume self-management of insulin and specimen tests; this increases feelings of mastery and control. Provide lists of fast-food exchanges. Provide group-related education with diabetic peers. Promote open dialogue among health personnel and teachers, school nurse, and fellow students. Continually reinforce treatment principles with specific regard to hypoglycemia or hyperglycemia and emergencies.
Puberty	"Bouncing" blood sugar levels may make child feel out of control Anger at the disease: "Why must I be different?"	Explain that growth and sex hormones affect blood sugar levels. Girls, in particular, experience difficulties about the time of menstruation.

table 30-5 *Nursing Interventions for Predictable Types of Stress on a Child with Type I Diabetes and on the Family—cont'd*

AGE	ISSUE	NURSING INTERVENTIONS
	More frequent hospitalizations	Adjustments in insulin and food are common for most diabetics at this stage. Assist patient in acceptable ways of expressing anger; discuss anger with parents, because they are often its target. Provide encouragement and support; be alert to marital stress and sibling deprivation.

table 30-6 *Diet Therapy in Pediatric Metabolic Disorders*

DISORDER	MAJOR SIGNS AND SYMPTOMS	DIETARY REGIMEN
Phenylketonuria (PKU)	Mental retardation	Low phenylalanine diet, Lofenalac formula for infants
Celiac disease	Chronic diarrhea, irritability, distention, failure to thrive	Eliminate gluten; use corn flour and vitamin B supplements
Cystic fibrosis	Thick mucus causes obstruction of pancreatic enzymes and poor absorption of nutrients, flatulence, and foul-smelling stools	Pancreatic enzyme replacement with normal meals
Lactose intolerance	Abdominal distension, cramps, diarrhea, failure to thrive	Lactose-free diet; use Prosobee, soy formulas; avoid milk/milk products
Galactose intolerance	Jaundice, vomiting, convulsions, lethargy, blindness	No galactose or lactose in diet; use milk substitutes
Fructose intolerance	Vomiting, diarrhea, failure to thrive	Fructose-free diet; avoid honey, fruit, sorbitol, and sucrose; offer vitamin C and vegetables
Maple syrup urine disease	Acidosis, convulsions	Low-leucine and low-valine diet
Urea cycle defect	Lethargy	Low-protein diet
Acidemia	Seizures, elevated ammonia levels	May need to restrict meat proteins
Diabetes insipidus	Inability to concentrate urine, diuresis	Unrestricted water intake
Diabetes mellitus	Inability to produce insulin to metabolize sugar, protein, and fat	Controlled sugar intake regulated with insulin administration; high-fiber, balanced diet

by mouth, calories may be supplied by intravenous glucose. Details vary according to the procedure and the patient's treatment for diabetes. Careful review of the patient's history helps in formulating nursing care plans and provides a basis for teaching.

Prospects for the Future

Diabetic research is being conducted on many fronts. Geneticists have determined how diabetes is inherited, and soon they will be able to limit who will inherit the disease. Pancreas transplantation has been performed, and the success rate continues to improve. Beta cell transplantation in animals has resulted in their cure. An artificial pancreas is another possibility; its precursors might be the insulin pumps used today. Noninvasive glucose monitors are already in use. Administration of insulin via nasal spray or inhalation is in pilot research. The laser beam has aided the treatment for complicated eye conditions. Such advances hold promise for resolving or eradicating the dilemma of diabetes. Diet therapy for various types of endocrine disorders is reviewed in Table 30-6.

key points

- The two major systems that control and monitor the functions of the body are the nervous system and the endocrine system.
- The term *inborn error of metabolism* refers to a group of inherited biochemical disorders that affect body metabolism.
- Screening programs for early detection of inborn errors are important because some conditions can cause irreversible neurological damage.
- Diabetes mellitus type I (IDDM) is the most common endocrine disorder of children. The body is unable to use carbohydrates properly because of a deficiency of insulin, an internal secretion of the pancreas.
- The symptoms of diabetes appear more rapidly in children. Three symptoms are polydipsia, polyuria, and polyphagia.
- The mainstays of the management of diabetes are insulin replacement, diet, and exercise.
- Diabetic ketoacidosis is a serious complication that may become life threatening.
- Self-management to maintain glucose control and to prevent complications is a major goal of education of the child with diabetes.
- The glycosylated hemoglobin test (HgbA1c) reflects glucose control over a period of months.
- Excess intake of sugar substitutes such as sorbitol can cause diarrhea.
- A child with diabetes insipidus requires unlimited access to water.
- Growth hormone is administered at bedtime to stimulate the natural time of hormone release.
- A deficiency in the secretion of the thyroid gland is termed hypothyroidism. It may be congenital or acquired and requires lifelong treatment by oral administration of a synthetic thyroid hormone.

ONLINE RESOURCES

Diabetes Public Health Resource:
http://www.cdc.gov/diabetes/index.htm
International Society of Pediatric and Adolescent Diabetes:
http://www.ispad.org/clin-2.html

REVIEW QUESTIONS   *Choose the most appropriate answer.*

1. Which of the following is an important aspect of a teaching plan for the parent of a child with hypopituitarism?
   1. The child should be enrolled in a special education program at school
   2. The routine administration of growth hormone should be carried out at bedtime
   3. All family members should have an endocrine work-up
   4. The routine medication should be administered before the school day starts

2. A child who has diabetes mellitus asks why he cannot take insulin orally instead of by subcutaneous injection. The best response of the nurse would be:
   1. Pills are only for adults
   2. Insulin is destroyed by digestive enzymes
   3. Insulin can cause a stomach ulcer
   4. Insulin interacts with food in the stomach

3. Which of the following may indicate a need for insulin in a diabetic child?
   1. Diaphoresis and tremors
   2. Red lips and fruity odor to the breath
   3. Confusion and lethargy
   4. Headache and pallor

4. The nurse teaches the diabetic child to rotate sites of insulin injection in order to:
   1. Prevent subcutaneous deposit of the drug
   2. Prevent lipoatrophy of subcutaneous fat
   3. Decrease the pain of injection
   4. Increase absorption of insulin

5. Kussmaul respirations are seen in diabetic children with
   1. Neuropathy
   2. Ketoacidosis
   3. Hypoglycemia
   4. Retinopathy

objectives

1. Define each key term listed.
2. Discuss three principles involved in standard precautions used to prevent the transmission of communicable diseases in children.
3. Discuss national and international immunization programs.
4. Describe the nurse's role in the immunization of children.
5. Interpret the detection and prevention of common childhood communicable diseases.
6. Discuss the characteristics of common childhood communicable diseases.
7. Formulate a nursing care plan for a child with acquired immunodeficiency syndrome (AIDS).
8. Demonstrate a teaching plan for preventing sexually transmitted diseases (STDs) in an adolescent.

key terms

acquired immunity (p. 748)
active immunity (p. 748)
body substance (p. 747)
communicable disease (kŏ-MŪ-nĭ-kă-b'l dĭ-ZĒZ, p. 747)
endemic (ĕn-DĔM-ĭk, p. 747)
epidemic (ĕp-ĭ-DĔM-ĭk, p. 747)
erythema (ĕr-ĭ-THĒ-mă, p. 749)
fomite (FŌ-mīt, p. 747)
incubation period (p. 747)
macule (MĂK-ūl, p. 749)
natural immunity (p. 748)
nosocomial infection (nŏ-sō-KŌ-mē-ăl ĭn-FĔK-shŭn, p. 748)
opportunistic infection (ŏp-pŏr-tū-NĬS-tĭk ĭn-FĔK-shŭn, p. 748)
pandemic (păn-DĔM-ĭk, p. 747)
papule (PĂP-ūl, p. 750)
passive immunity (p. 748)
pathogens (PĂTH-ō-jĕn, p. 747)
pathognomonic (păth-ŏg-nŏ-MŎN-ĭk, p. 750)
portal of entry (p. 747)
portal of exit (p. 747)
prodromal period (prŏ-DRŌ-măl, p. 747)
pustule (PŬS-tūl, p. 750)
reservoir for infection (p. 747)
scab (p. 750)
standard precautions (p. 749)
vector (VĔK-tĕr, p. 747)
vesicle (VĔS-ĭ-k'l, p. 750)

COMMUNICABLE DISEASE

There have been only a few brief periods in history when infectious disease did not dominate the attention of health care professionals. Despite immunization, sanitation, antibiotics, and other controls, the world continues to face infectious agents such as human immunodeficiency virus (HIV), hepatitis, tuberculosis, and sexually transmitted diseases (STDs). Despite our knowledge of immunizations, some children still suffer from common communicable diseases (Table 31-1). Antibiotic-resistant organisms are increasing, and immunocompromised patients are threatened by nonpathogenic organisms. Prevention and control are key factors in managing infectious disease.

COMMON CHILDHOOD COMMUNICABLE DISEASES

The incidence of common childhood communicable diseases has dramatically decreased as immunological agents have been developed. Diseases such as smallpox have declined to a point worldwide that routine immunizations are no longer recommended. (A brief review of smallpox is presented in this chapter because the nurse must be able to identify a smallpox lesion and promptly refer for follow-up care to avoid an outbreak of this deadly illness.) Providing all children with the appropriate immunizations is the health care challenge of today. Air travel is commonplace, and rapid transmission of contagious diseases from around the world requires alert assessment by the nurse and all health care workers.

Text continued on p. 748

Table 31-1 *Communicable Diseases of Childhood*

DISEASE	CAUSATIVE ORGANISM	SIGNS AND SYMPTOMS	INCUBATION PERIOD	PREVENTION/TREATMENT	HOW LONG CONTAGIOUS	NURSING INTERVENTIONS
Chickenpox (varicella) (Figure 31-1)	Varicella zoster virus	Prodromal signs include mild fever followed by macules, papules, vesicles, pustules, and scabs. All stages of lesion are present on the body at the same time.	2-3 weeks (13-17 days average)	Vaccine available; acyclovir (Zovirax) or immune globulin (VZIG) is given to immunosuppressed children who are exposed.	6 days after appearance of rash	Trim fingernails to prevent scratching. (Removal of scabs may cause scars.) Calamine lotion may reduce itching. Isolate from others.
Smallpox (variola)	Virus	Child appears toxic. Macules, papules, vesicles, pustules, and scabs appear. Only one stage of the lesion at a time is present on the body.	6-18 days (12 days average)	Routine smallpox vaccination is no longer recommended unless patient is traveling into high-risk country.	Highly contagious; CDC notification required	This is a toxic illness with a high mortality rate. Strict isolation is required, preferably in a negative pressure room and with restricted caregivers.
German measles (rubella) (Figure 31-2)	Rubella virus	Mild fever and cold symptoms precede a rose-colored, maculo-papular rash. Glands at ears and back of neck are enlarged.	2-3 weeks (18 days average)	All infants should receive vaccine, with boosters at preschool age.	Until rash fades (5 days)	Provide symptomatic treatment and comfort measures. Avoid exposing any woman who might be in the early months of pregnancy, because rubella can cause fetal anomalies.

Disease	Cause	Signs and Symptoms	Incubation	Immunity/Prevention	Period of Communicability	Nursing Care
Measles (rubeola) (Figure 31-3)	Virus	Fever, cough, and conjunctivitis is followed by small white (Koplik) spots on inner cheeks (enanthem); maculopapular rash (exanthem) then erupts.	1-2 weeks (10 days average)	All infants should receive vaccine at 15 months and boosters at preschool age. Gamma globulin may be given after exposure. Vitamin A is recommended to reduce morbidity.	From 4 days before to 5 days after rash appears	Provide symptomatic care. Isolate and provide quiet activities. Use measures to reduce eyestrain caused by photophobia. Give detailed oral care.
Fifth disease (erythema infectiosum)	Human parvovirus B19 (HPV)	Child has "slapped cheek" appearance. Generalized rash appears, subsides, and reappears if skin is irritated by sun or heat.	4-14 days	None.	During incubation period	This is a benign condition unless child is immunocompromised. Isolation is not required. Condition may last 1-3 weeks.
Roseola (exanthem subitum) (sixth disease)	Herpesvirus 6 (HSV-6)	Persistent high (39.4° to 40.5° C [103° to 105° F]) fever is present, then drops rapidly as the rash appears. The maculopapular rash is nonpruritic and blanches easily.	2 weeks	None; high fever may precipitate convulsions.	Until rash fades	Rest and quiet should be provided. Teach parents temperature-reducing techniques and prevention of seizures.
Mumps (parotitis)	Paramyxovirus	Fever, headache, glands near ear and toward jawline ache and develop painful swelling. Parotid gland is enlarged. Condition may be bilateral.	14-21 days (18 days average)	Vaccine (MMR) is given after 15 months of age.	Until swelling subsides	Encourage fluids, apply ice compresses to neck for comfort. Isolate.

Continued

table 31-1 *Communicable Diseases of Childhood—cont'd*

DISEASE	CAUSATIVE ORGANISM	SIGNS AND SYMPTOMS	INCUBATION PERIOD	PREVENTION/TREATMENT	HOW LONG CONTAGIOUS	NURSING INTERVENTIONS
Whooping cough (pertussis)	*Bordetella pertussis*	Fever, cold, and cough are present. Spells of coughing are accompanied by a noisy gasp for air that creates a "whoop."	5-21 days (10 days average)	Vaccinate all infants with series (DPT). Exposed unvaccinated child may be given erythromycin. Cool mist tent and antibiotics are used for treatment.	Several weeks	Isolate, bed rest, provide abdominal support during coughing spell. Refeed child if he or she vomits. Observe for airway obstruction.
Polio (infantile paralysis; poliomyelitis)	Enterovirus	Fever, headache, stiff neck and stiff back, paralysis.	1-2 weeks	Start complete series of polio vaccines in infancy. May require respirator care.	1 week for throat secretions; 4 weeks for feces	Isolate, bed rest, observe for respiratory distress. Provide positioning, physiotherapy, and range-of-motion exercises.
Infectious mononucleosis (glandular fever)	Epstein-Barr virus (EBV)	Low-grade fever, malaise, jaundice, enlarged spleen.	2-6 weeks	Limit contact with saliva. Do not share eating utensils.	(Spread by direct contact only)	Provide rest and supportive treatment. Isolation is not required. Provide school tutoring to maintain grade level.
Hepatitis A	Enterovirus 72	Fever, anorexia, headache, abdominal pain, malaise, jaundice, dark urine, and chalklike stools.	15-45 days	Hepatitis A vaccine is recommended for children traveling to endemic areas. Gamma globulin is given if child is exposed.	Virus may be shed for up to 6 months in neonates	Educate family and community concerning the ingestion of contaminated water or shellfish from contaminated water or swimming in contaminated water. Proper handwashing is essential. Standard precautions are essential.

Disease	Causative Agent	Incubation	Signs and Symptoms	Period of Communicability	Treatment	Prevention/Nursing Care
Hepatitis B	HBV virus	30-180 days	Symptoms are the same as type A. Can manifest liver pathology.	May persist in carrier state	Hepatitis B vaccine (HBV) series is given during newborn period or for health care workers or travelers. Interferon or reverse transcriptase inhibitors may be an effective treatment. Liver transplant may be necessary. Immune globulin may be indicated for exposed, susceptible children.	Prevent contact with blood or blood products. Identify high-risk mothers and newborns. Educate concerning need for vaccination.
Lyme disease	*Borrelia burgdorferi*	3-32 days	Skin lesions at site of tick bite. Macule with raised border and clear center. May "burn." Fever, arthralgia. May lead to heart and neurological involvement.	Spread by infected tick	Wear protective clothing in wooded area. Inspect for ticks after play when camping. Light-colored clothing makes tick more noticeable. Remove tick with tweezer. Inspect pets. Treat with amoxicillin or doxycycline.	Educate concerning the prevention of exposure.
Tuberculosis	*Mycobacterium tuberculosis*	2-10 weeks airborne droplet infection	Low-grade fever, malaise, anorexia, weight loss, cough, night sweats. Children are often asymptomatic. Adenopathy, pneumonia, and positive tuberculin skin test.	After treatment when cough subsides	Early detection is through routine PPD skin test. Examine contacts. Exposed children may receive isoniazid (INH) and rifampin, which inhibits growth of the organism.	Isolate newborn from infected mother. Identify contacts. Isolate, using special mask (see Appendix A).

Continued

table 31-1 *Communicable Diseases of Childhood—cont'd*

DISEASE	CAUSATIVE ORGANISM	SIGNS AND SYMPTOMS	INCUBATION PERIOD	PREVENTION/TREATMENT	HOW LONG CONTAGIOUS	NURSING INTERVENTIONS
Diphtheria	*Corynebacterium diphtheriae*	Common cold with purulent nasal discharge. Malaise, sore throat. White or gray membrane forms in throat, causing respiratory distress.	2-5 days	DPT vaccine is given to all infants. Intravenous antibiotics and antitoxin, tracheotomy required. Provide oxygen and suction as needed.	During incubation and clinical illness; may become a carrier	Observe for respiratory, cardiac, and central nervous system involvement. Isolate. Identify contacts for treatment.
Scarlet fever	Group A beta-hemolytic *Streptococcus*	Tachycardia, strawberry tongue, pinpoint rash, circumoral pallor, desquamation.	2-5 days	Penicillin therapy is given for 10 days. Culture/treat streptococcal infections.	During incubation and clinical illness; may become a carrier	Respiratory precautions; bed rest; quiet activity. Teach regarding prevention of streptococcal infections.

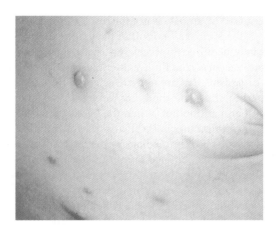

FIGURE **31-1** Chickenpox.

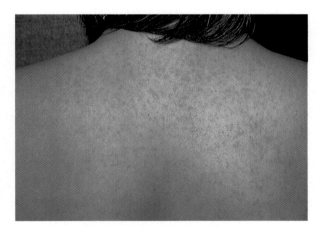

FIGURE **31-2** German measles.

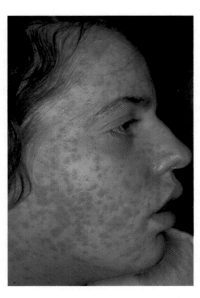

FIGURE **31-3** Measles.

REVIEW OF TERMS

A communicable disease is one that can be transmitted, directly or indirectly, from one person to another. Organisms that cause disease are called pathogens.

The incubation period is the time between the invasion by the pathogen and the onset of clinical symptoms. The prodromal period refers to the initial stage of a disease: the interval between the earliest symptoms and the appearance of a typical rash or fever. Children are often contagious during this time, but because the symptoms are not specific they may attend preschool or another group program and spread the disease. A fomite is any inanimate material that absorbs and transmits infection. A vector is an insect or animal that carries and spreads a disease. A pandemic is a worldwide high incidence of a communicable disease. An epidemic is a *sudden* increase of a communicable disease in a localized area. An endemic is an expected *continuous* incidence of a communicable disease in a localized area.

Body substance refers to moist secretions or parts of the body that can contain microorganisms. Emesis, saliva, sputum, semen, urine, feces, and blood are examples of body substances. Body substance precautions indicate the need to wear disposable protective gloves and/or garments when coming in contact with these body substances. A portal of entry is a route by which the organisms enter the body (e.g., a cut in the skin). A portal of exit is the route by which the organisms exit the body (e.g., feces or urine). A reservoir for infection is a place that supports the growth of organisms (e.g., standing, stagnant water). The *chain of infection* refers to the way in which organisms spread and infect the individual (Figure 31-4). Standard precautions are found in Appendix A. Careful handwashing is basic and essential to contain infection.

HOST RESISTANCE

Many factors contribute to the virulence of an infectious disease. The age, sex, and genetic makeup of the child have a bearing on the degree of resistance. The nutritional status of the person, as well as physical and emotional health, is also important. The efficiency of the blood-forming organs and of the immune systems affects resistance. Important factors in host resistance to disease include the following:

- *Intact skin and mucous membranes:* a break in the skin can be a portal of entry for an organism that can cause illness.
- *Phagocytes* in the blood attack and destroy organisms.

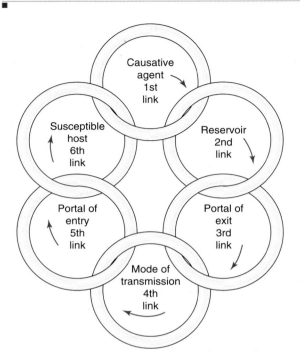

FIGURE **31-4** The chain of infection. The process by which pathogens are transmitted from the environment to a host, invade the host, and cause infection.

- The functioning *immune system* in the body responds to fight infection. Some factors in this immune response include interferon, T-cells, B-cells, and antibodies. Vaccinations assist the body to manufacture antibodies that can help the child to resist infections.

The child who has an underlying condition such as diabetes, cystic fibrosis, burns, or sickle cell disease may be more susceptible to certain organisms. Children with acquired immunodeficiency syndrome (HIV/AIDS) or cancer and children receiving steroid or immunosuppressive drugs often have depressed immune systems. This makes them very susceptible to opportunistic infections (an *opportunistic infection* is caused by organisms *normally* found in the environment that the immune-suppressed individual cannot resist or fight). An infection acquired in a health care facility during hospitalization is termed a nosocomial infection.

TYPES OF IMMUNITY

Immunity is *natural* or *acquired* resistance to infection. In natural immunity, resistance is inborn. Some races apparently have a greater natural immunity to certain diseases than others. Immunity also varies from person to person. If two persons are exposed to the same disease, one may become very ill and the other may have no evidence of the disease.

Acquired immunity is not the result of inherited factors but is acquired as a result of having the disease or is artificially acquired by receiving vaccines or immune serums. Vaccines contain live attenuated (weakened) or dead organisms that are not strong enough to cause the disease but stimulate the body to develop an immune reaction and antibodies. When the person produces his or her own immunity, it is called active immunity.

If a person needs immediate protection from a disease, *antibodies* can be obtained in immune serums; most are from animals, but some are from humans. For example, tetanus serum (used to prevent lockjaw) is procured from the horse, but gamma globulin, which is rich in antibodies, is obtained from human blood. This type of immunity, known as passive immunity, acts immediately but does not last as long as immunity actively produced by the body. Passive immunity *provides* the antibody. It does not stimulate the system to produce its own antibodies.

A *carrier* is a person who is capable of spreading a disease but does not show evidence of it. Typhoid fever is an example of a disease spread by a carrier.

TRANSMISSION OF INFECTION

Infection can be transmitted from one person to another by *direct* or *indirect* means. *Direct transmission* involves contact with the person who is infected (the body fluids of that person, such as nasal discharge or an open lesion). *Indirect transmission* involves contact with objects that have been contaminated by the infected person. These objects are called *fomites*. Doorknobs, used tissues, countertops, and toys are examples of fomites. For example, the respiratory syncytial virus (RSV) lives on dry soap for several hours. Therefore picking up soap used by a person infected with RSV transmits the organism. This is one of the reasons why liquid soap is advocated. The chain of infection transmission is shown in Figure 31-4. Preventing the spread of infection depends on breaking the chain.

Various tests are available to determine whether an individual is susceptible to a particular disease. Examples are the *Schick test* for diphtheria, the *Dick test* for scarlet fever, and the *Mantoux intradermal PPD skin test* for tuberculosis.

MEDICAL ASEPSIS AND STANDARD PRECAUTIONS

The purpose of medical aseptic techniques used with *all* patients is to prevent the spread of infection from one child to another or from the child to the nurse. A person or object is considered *contaminated* if he, she, or it has touched the infected patient or any equipment or fomite that has come in contact with the patient. People or articles that have had no contact with the patient are considered *clean.*

Articles that have come in direct contact with the patient must be disinfected before they can be used by others. When something is disinfected, the microorganisms in or on it are killed by physical or chemical means. The autoclave, which uses steam under pressure, is considered effective in killing most germs when the article is adequately exposed and sterilized for the proper length of time.

All children suspected of having a communicable disease who are admitted to the hospital are placed on isolation (standard) precautions until a definite diagnosis is established. A private room or negative-pressure room (prevents air from flowing out of the room when the door is opened) is assigned. (See Appendix A for specific precautions and practices involved.)

Disposable items are used whenever possible and include diapers, tissues, needles, suction catheters, thermometers, suture sets, dishes, nursing bottles, and utensils. They are double-bagged and disposed of according to hospital procedure.

The nurse must understand the importance of protecting himself or herself and others from the contagious patient. This is accomplished by specific precautions, called standard precautions. The Centers for Disease Control and Prevention (CDC) recommend *standard* precautions for *all* patients; these involve handwashing and the use of disposable gloves. In addition to these precautions, *transmission-based* precautions are designed according to the method of spread of infection, such as large droplet, airborne droplet, or contact with a wound or drainage.

Large droplet infection precautions are used with diseases such as pertussis and influenza. When the patient coughs or sneezes, the droplets can contaminate an area 3 feet around the patient. Beyond 3 feet, a mask and gown are not necessary.

Airborne infection precautions are used for patients with conditions such as tuberculosis, varicella (chickenpox), and rubeola (measles). Small airborne particles caught on floating dust in the room can be inhaled any place in the room. The use of negative-pressure rooms and of masks and gowns when entering the room is recommended.

Contact precautions are used when the condition transmits organisms via skin-to-skin contact or through indirect touch of a contaminated fomite. Gloves and a gown are worn for close contact with patients with RSV, patients with hepatitis A who are incontinent, patients with contagious skin diseases such as impetigo, or patients with wound infections. Some diseases may have more than one mode of spread and therefore require more than one precaution technique.

Because isolation procedures vary from hospital to hospital and from hospital to home, a minimum of specific procedures are presented. Standard precautions are discussed in Appendix A and describe the protocols for the use of gowns, masks, and other protective clothing. Disposable gloves should be worn whenever touching any body substance. You should be wearing gloves if you are touching something that is moist and not yours.

PROTECTIVE ISOLATION

Protective isolation (also called *reverse isolation* or barrier technique) is used for patients who are *not* communicable but have a lowered resistance and are highly susceptible to infection. This simple procedure reduces the incidence of nosocomial (hospital) infections. The patient is placed in a private room with the door closed. It is recommended that all persons wear a gown, a mask, and gloves when attending the child in reverse isolation. Paper disposable gowns are used. Soiled linen is placed in a plastic isolation laundry bag held by a metal stand. Protective isolation units, such as life islands, are also available. Both the child and the family need adequate explanations.

HANDWASHING

The nurse must wash his or her hands between patients and after removing gloves. Antibacterial soaps are used in some units, but overuse can irritate skin and may promote the development of resistant strains of bacteria. Self-contained liquid soap dispensers are preferable to bar soap, which can harbor organisms.

FAMILY EDUCATION

Education of family members must be ongoing. Factors to be emphasized include the necessity for immunization of children, proper storage of food (particularly perishables), use of pasteurized milk, proper cooking of meats, cleanliness in food preparation, and proper handwashing. The nurse must review the ways in which infectious diseases are spread. Children must be taught to avoid using community hand towels. Other modes of transmission, such as crowded living conditions, insects, rodents, and sandboxes, may also be discussed.

RASHES

Many infectious diseases begin with a rash. Rashes tend to be itchy (pruritic) and uncomfortable. Symptomatic care is provided by prescribing acetaminophen (Tylenol) and diphenhydramine (Benadryl) or topical lotions. Rashes can be described as follows:

- Erythema: a diffused reddened area on the skin
- Macule: a circular reddened area on the skin

- **Papule:** a circular reddened area on the skin that is elevated
- **Vesicle:** a circular reddened area on the skin that is elevated and contains fluid
- **Pustule:** a circular reddened area on the skin that is elevated and contains pus
- **Scab:** a dried pustule that is covered with a crust
- **Pathognomonic:** a term used to describe a lesion or symptom that is *characteristic* of a specific illness (e.g., Koplik spots are pathognomonic for measles)

> **NURSING TIP**
> Apply lotions to open lesions sparingly to avoid absorption that could lead to drug toxicity.

WORLDWIDE IMMUNIZATION PROGRAMS

HEALTHY PEOPLE 2010

The United States Public Health Service has made immunizing 95% of all children in the United States against childhood communicable diseases a goal to achieve by the year 2010. Some reasons for the current low vaccination rate include a knowledge deficit in parents, a lack of accessibility to vaccination clinics, the cost of vaccinating children, a fear of adverse reactions, misunderstandings about contraindications, and failure to track or follow-up on immunization records. Federally funded programs to provide the vaccine and to educate are already in place. The effort of the World Health Organization (WHO) and United Nations Children's Fund (UNICEF) have resulted in dramatic declines in vaccine-preventable illnesses worldwide, especially in third world countries. New vaccines are developed and assessed for routine use in endemic areas. The influenza vaccine, the pneumococcal vaccine, varicella vaccine, and RSV immune globulin (RespiGam) are available for children. Vaccines for cholera and yellow fever are available for families traveling to endemic areas. The CDC provides advice concerning vaccinations needed for persons traveling to various parts of the world.

THE NURSE'S ROLE

Worldwide immunization practices have eliminated smallpox as a threat. However, nurses must remain alert to signs and symptoms because bioterrorism may involve a new smallpox threat. Measles is rarely seen in developed countries. Current vaccinations against varicella, hepatitis, influenza (for high-risk children), and pneumonia (for children over 2 years of age) are available, and the challenge is to make them accessible. The

nurse is a vital link in educating parents about the need for immunizations.

The Vaccine

Correct *storage* of vaccines is essential to ensure potency. The nurse should check the label to determine what type of refrigeration is needed. The correct *route of administration* is important to achieve immunization. The oral, subcutaneous, and intramuscular routes are used for various vaccines. Multiple doses of a vaccine at predetermined intervals may be needed to achieve an immunity status. The nurse can educate parents and school personnel about immunization schedules and should assess the immunization status of each child at every clinic visit (Figure 31-5).

> **NURSING TIP**
> The earliest age a vaccine can be administered is the youngest age the infant can respond by developing antibodies to that illness.

Vaccine Storage and Handling

Proper storage and handling of vaccines ensure that potency is maintained. Vaccines should not be stored in

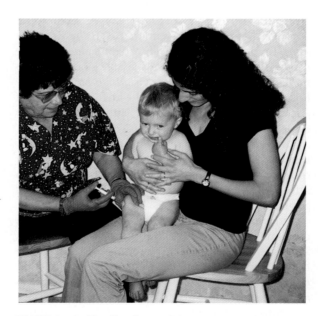

FIGURE **31-5** The "hug" restraining position for administration of vaccinations. Note that the arms are restrained by the mother and that the chld's legs are restrained between the mother's knees. The mother comforts the child during the procedure and may breastfeed after the procedure. The site for intramuscular injections in infants is the thigh, and the nurse wears a protective glove. The use of aerosol sprays or EMLA cream may reduce the pain of multiple injections in infants and children.

the doors of refrigerators or freezers. Most vaccines are stored inside the refrigerator at 1.6° to 7.7° C (35° to 46° F). Varicella vaccine (Varivax) is very fragile. It must be stored in the freezer at $-15°$ C (5° F) or lower and used within 30 minutes of reconstitution. The vaccine cannot be refrozen after it has thawed. Inactivated vaccines can be harmed if frozen and live vaccines are harmed by heat and light. This information is especially important to know when participating in outdoor mass immunization programs.

Emergency Preparedness

Most parts of the United States are threatened at times by sudden and unexpected power outages caused by storms, earthquakes, and other events. To minimize the potential for vaccine loss, preventive steps should be taken in preparation for such an emergency. These steps include keeping several bottles of water and cold packs in the freezer to help maintain the temperature of the vaccines if power is disrupted.

Allergy to Vaccines

Children who have a history of allergy to neomycin should notify the health care provider before receiving the inactivated poliovirus vaccine (IPV), measles-mumps-rubella vaccine (MMR), and varicella vaccine. An allergy to gelatin or eggs should also be reported before receiving MMR or varicella vaccine. Epinephrine should be available in the unit where vaccines are administered.

A serious allergy to baker's yeast should be reported to the health care provider before receiving hepatitis B immunization, and an allergy to aluminum hydroxide may be a contraindication to receiving hepatitis A vaccine. The influenza vaccine should not be given to persons who are allergic to eggs.

Varicella vaccine, if not given on the same day as MMR, must be given *no less* than 28 days later. A tuberculin test should not be given within 6 weeks of receiving an MMR or varicella immunization, because the results will not be accurate.

Mercury toxicity. The American Academy of Pediatrics recommends that Comvax, the only thimerosal-free hepatitis B vaccine, be used for infants born to women who test negative for hepatitis B; this should begin at the 2-month clinic visit. If Comvax is not available, the hepatitis B vaccination should begin at 6 months of age. Recombivax HB can be ordered preservative free for use in infants younger than 2 months of age. Thimerosal is a mercury-containing preservative used in some vaccines, and there is some concern over the rise of mercury toxicity in children.

The U.S. Food and Drug Administration (FDA) is urging the reduction of this substance in vaccines and medical equipment such as thermometers and blood-pressure machines. Research is ongoing. Parents should be counseled about reducing exposures to other sources of mercury (Atkinson et al., 2002). Rotavirus vaccine is no longer recommended because it is associated with the development of intussusception.

The PCV pneumococcal vaccine (Prevnar) does not contain thimerosal and is effective in preventing common childhood pneumonia and otitis media. The hepatitis A vaccine is not licensed to be used before 2 years of age (Behrman, Kliegman, & Jenson, 2000).

Reducing pain at the site of injection, especially when multiple injections are required, should be considered. The use of vapocoolant sprays or EMLA cream is effective. Using the proper technique of injection of vaccines is important. The *Haemophilus influenzae* type b (Hib) vaccine must be given in a separate syringe from other vaccines given at the same clinic visit. The varicella vaccine is given subcutaneously, whereas the diphtheria-pertussis-tetanus (DPT) vaccine causes significant tissue irritation if given subcutaneously, and careful IM technique is essential.

The immunization program in the United States is recommended by the CDC and the American Academy of Pediatrics (AAP). Advances in the field of immunology may change recommendations for existing policies and recommend new policies. (See the websites at the end of this chapter for updates.)

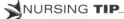

NURSING **TIP**

The pertussis vaccine is not given to children older than 7 years of age.

IMMUNIZATION SCHEDULE FOR CHILDREN

Informed consent concerning the potential risks and documentation of immunization is essential. Parents should have copies of their child's immunization records. The immunization program for children in the United States is described in Figure 31-6.

Contraindications to live virus vaccine administration may include the following:

- Immunocompromised state
- Pregnancy
- Bacteremia or meningitis

Recommended Childhood Immunization Schedule
United States, 2002

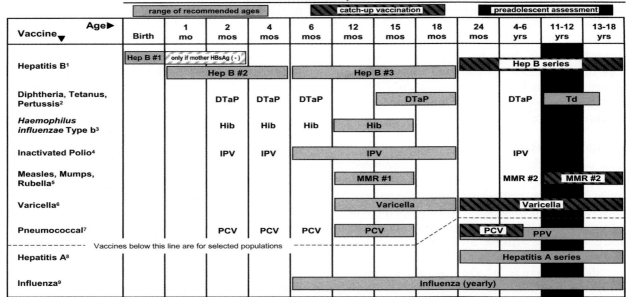

Vaccine	Age ► Birth	1 mo	2 mos	4 mos	6 mos	12 mos	15 mos	18 mos	24 mos	4-6 yrs	11-12 yrs	13-18 yrs
			range of recommended ages			catch-up vaccination				preadolescent assessment		
Hepatitis B¹	Hep B #1 only if mother HBsAg (-)										Hep B series	
		Hep B #2			Hep B #3							
Diphtheria, Tetanus, Pertussis²			DTaP	DTaP	DTaP		DTaP			DTaP	Td	
Haemophilus influenzae Type b³			Hib	Hib	Hib	Hib						
Inactivated Polio⁴			IPV	IPV		IPV				IPV		
Measles, Mumps, Rubella⁵						MMR #1				MMR #2	MMR #2	
Varicella⁶						Varicella					Varicella	
Pneumococcal⁷			PCV	PCV	PCV	PCV				PCV	PPV	
Hepatitis A⁸	Vaccines below this line are for selected populations										Hepatitis A series	
Influenza⁹						Influenza (yearly)						

This schedule indicates the recommended ages for routine administration of currently licensed childhood vaccines, as of December 1, 2001, for children through age 18 years. Any dose not given at the recommended age should be given at any subsequent visit when indicated and feasible. ▨ Indicates age groups that warrant special effort to administer those vaccines not previously given. Additional vaccines may be licensed and recommended during the year. Licensed combination vaccines may be used whenever any components of the combination are indicated and the vaccine's other components are not contraindicated. Providers should consult the manufacturers' package inserts for detailed recommendations.

1. Hepatitis B vaccine (Hep B). All infants should receive the first dose of hepatitis B vaccine soon after birth and before hospital discharge; the first dose may also be given by age 2 months if the infant's mother is HBsAg-negative. Only monovalent hepatitis B vaccine can be used for the birth dose. Monovalent or combination vaccine may be used to complete the series; four doses of vaccine may be administered if combination vaccine is used. The second dose should be given at least 4 weeks after the first dose, except for Hib-containing vaccine which cannot be administered before age 6 weeks. The third dose should be given at least 16 weeks after the first dose and at least 8 weeks after the second dose. The last dose in the vaccination series (third or fourth dose) should not be administered before age 6 months.

Infants born to HBsAg-positive mothers should receive hepatitis B vaccine and 0.5 mL hepatitis B immune globulin (HBIG) within 12 hours of birth at separate sites. The second dose is recommended at age 1-2 months and the vaccination series should be completed (third or fourth dose) at age 6 months.

Infants born to mothers whose HBsAg status is unknown should receive the first dose of the hepatitis B vaccine series within 12 hours of birth. Maternal blood should be drawn at the time of delivery to determine the mother's HBsAg status; if the HBsAg test is positive, the infant should receive HBIG as soon as possible (no later than age 1 week).

2. Diphtheria and tetanus toxoids and acellular pertussis vaccine (DTaP). The fourth dose of DTaP may be administered as early as age 12 months, provided 6 months have elapsed since the third dose and the child is unlikely to return at age 15-18 months. **Tetanus and diphtheria toxoids (Td)** is recommended at age 11-12 years if at least 5 years have elapsed since the last dose of tetanus and diphtheria toxoid-containing vaccine. Subsequent routine Td boosters are recommended every 10 years.

3. *Haemophilus influenzae* type b (Hib) conjugate vaccine. Three Hib conjugate vaccines are licensed for infant use. If PRP-OMP (PedvaxHIB® or ComVax® [Merck]) is administered at ages 2 and 4 months, a dose at age 6 months is not required. DTaP/Hib combination products should not be used for primary immunization in infants at ages 2, 4 or 6 months, but can be used as boosters following any Hib vaccine.

4. Inactivated polio vaccine (IPV). An all-IPV schedule is recommended for routine childhood polio vaccination in the United States. All children should receive four doses of IPV at ages 2 months, 4 months, 6-18 months, and 4-6 years.

5. Measles, mumps, and rubella vaccine (MMR). The second dose of MMR is recommended routinely at age 4-6 years but may be administered during any visit, provided at least 4 weeks have elapsed since the first dose and that both doses are administered beginning at or after age 12 months. Those who have not previously received the second dose should complete the schedule by the 11-12 year old visit.

6. Varicella vaccine. Varicella vaccine is recommended at any visit at or after age 12 months for susceptible children, i.e. those who lack a reliable history of chickenpox. Susceptible persons aged ≥ 13 years should receive two doses, given at least 4 weeks apart.

7. Pneumococcal vaccine. The heptavalent **pneumococcal conjugate vaccine (PCV)** is recommended for all children age 2-23 months. It is also recommended for certain children age 24-59 months. **Pneumococcal polysaccharide vaccine (PPV)** is recommended in addition to PCV for certain high-risk groups. See *MMWR* 2000;49(RR-9);1-35.

8. Hepatitis A vaccine. Hepatitis A vaccine is recommended for use in selected states and regions, and for certain high-risk groups; consult your local public health authority. See *MMWR* 1999;48(RR-12);1-37.

9. Influenza vaccine. Influenza vaccine is recommended annually for children age ≥ 6 months with certain risk factors (including but not limited to asthma, cardiac disease, sickle cell disease, HIV, diabetes; see *MMWR* 2001;50(RR-4);1-44), and can be administered to all others wishing to obtain immunity. Children aged ≤12 years should receive vaccine in a dosage appropriate for their age (0.25 mL if age 6-35 months or 0.5 mL if aged ≥ 3 years). Children aged ≤ 8 years who are receiving influenza vaccine for the first time should receive two doses separated by at least 4 weeks.

For additional information about vaccines, vaccine supply, and contraindications for immunization, please visit the National Immunization Program Website at www.cdc.gov/nip or call the National Immunization Hotline at 800-232-2522 (English) or 800-232-0233 (Spanish).

Approved by the Advisory Committee on Immunization Practices (www.cdc.gov/nip/acip), the American Academy of Pediatrics (www.aap.org), and the American Academy of Family Physicians (www.aafp.org).

OSP 02 64574

FIGURE **31-6** Immunization schedule for infants and children in the United States. Hib is given intramuscularly. MMR and IPV are given subcutaneously. *Var,* Varicella vaccine; *Hep,* hepatitis; *DPT or DtaP,* diphtheria and tetanus toxoids and acellular pertussis vaccine; *HBV,* hepatitis B vaccine; *Hib, Hemophilus influenzae* B vaccine.

- Immunocompromised caregiver in the home
- Corticosteroid therapy (requires individual evaluation)
- History of high fever (40.5° C [105° F]) after previous vaccinations

✳NURSING **TIP**_____
An interrupted vaccination series can usually continue without restarting the entire series.

THE FUTURE OF IMMUNOTHERAPY

Research concerning the development of new vaccines and the refinement of established vaccines continues at an amazing pace. The use of transgenic plants for oral administration of bacterial and viral antigens would enable low-cost, effective distribution. Research in the field of transcutaneous immunization involves the application of an antigen with an adjuvant to the intact skin. Recombinant DNA technology and the use of adjuvants are being developed for rheumatic fever and malaria. Alum is an adjuvant currently used in the vaccine against hepatitis B to increase its effectiveness. RNA and DNA viruses are being developed for use as carriers (vectors) of other antigens. Bacterial DNA are also being developed as carriers of antigens. A "gene gun" that blasts the vaccine through intact skin is also in the development stage. The techniques in research may hold promise for developing effective vaccines against influenza A virus, HIV-1, malaria, and Ebola. A catalogue of genes that code for viruses and potential immunogens is being studied.

The most exciting development in immunology is the use of immunotherapy for noncommunicable diseases. An example would be the mucosal administration of myelin in multiple sclerosis and a type 2 collagen for rheumatic arthritis. The possibility of preventing specific types of cancer has been recognized, and the challenge of developing tumor antigens that lyse tumor cells is also a clear possibility. In Alzheimer's disease the formation of neurotoxic plaques in the brain causes the loss of mental function. Early immunization with amyloid B may prevent or lyse the plaque formation and avoid the devastating problem of this disease.

The use of immunotherapy for autoimmune diseases is promising. The greatest achievement of the twentieth century was the eradication of smallpox and the development of many safe vaccines for children. Perhaps the achievement of the twenty-first century will be the development of immunotherapy for noncommunicable diseases such as Alzheimer's disease and cancer.

BIOTERRORISM AND THE PEDIATRIC PATIENT

A NEW TYPE OF CHILDHOOD TRAUMA
Physiological Effects

Children are generally more vulnerable to biological warfare because their immune systems are not fully developed. They are also closer to the ground so that heavy particles from an aerosol-propelled agent may reach them in higher doses than a taller adult. All new drugs are tested on adults as they are being developed, and it sometimes takes many years to determine safety for the pediatric patient. Therefore, in effect, a new drug that is developed to treat a bioterror chemical agent may be more harmful to the pediatric patient. The large head and body surface area in relation to weight and low fat content in the body makes the child more vulnerable to develop hypothermia, which can be life threatening in the pediatric age-group. Therefore the routine "haz mat" decontamination procedure of stripping and total body washing may not be suitable for the pediatric patient.

Table 31-2 lists common diseases (and their symptoms) that are spread through bioterrorism. Chemical agents that may be used in bioterrorist attacks may include *pulmonary* agents such as chlorine, *cyanide* agents such as sulfur mustard, *nerve* agents such as sarin, or *incapacitating* agents such as BZ, a glycolate anticholinergic compound. The CDC should be contacted concerning the management of victims.

Psychological Effects

Terrorist acts in the form of chemical warfare or physical assaults such as bombings can be brought into the home via television from remote locations in the United States, thus violating a child's personal feeling of safety. Children listen to television and to their trusted adults expressing fears, perhaps lose loved ones or friends, and may play out their own fears in toys, art, or altered behavior.

INITIAL OBSERVATION

Although the "ABCs" of emergency triage for adults apply to children, a pediatric quick examination involves the following:

- *Appearance:* alert, aware of surroundings, interacts
- *Respiratory effort:* tachypnea may indicate shock, whereas retractions may indicate a lung problem
- *Skin color:* circulatory problems causing cyanosis, pallor, mottling, capillary refill time (CFT) more than 2 seconds

The initial examination of a patient after suspected exposure to a biological agent may be delayed between expo-

| table 31-2 | *Common Diseases Spread Through Bioterrorism* |

BIOLOGICAL AGENTS USED AS WEAPONS	SYMPTOMS	INCUBATION PERIOD
Anthrax	Flu-like symptoms that improve, then respiratory and circulatory collapse occurs; chest x-ray shows widened mediastinum caused by thoracic edema; skin lesions involve vesicles with a black eschar center and enlarged adjacent lymph nodes	1 to 45 days
Botulism	Difficulty speaking and swallowing, blurred or double vision; respiratory distress; descending muscular paralysis NOTE: Inhaled form has *no* gastrointestinal symptoms	1 to 5 days
Ebola virus (*Filovirus*)	Abrupt onset of fever, headache, muscle pain, gastrointestinal upset, maculopapular rash on the trunk, petechiae, and progressive bleeding	4 to 10 days
Lassa fever (*Arenavirus*)	Fever, retrosternal pain, tremor of tongue and hands, hearing loss	7 to 16 days
Plague	Fever; mucopurulent sputum, chest pain, hemoptysis, purpura	2 to 3 days
Smallpox	"Chickenpox-like" lesions starting on the face and extremities, with each stage of the lesions progressing from one state to the next *together*	12 days (average)
Tularemia	Fever, pneumonitis, nonproductive cough, periorbital edema	3 to 5 days

sure and the development of symptoms (incubation period). Tentative triage categories for victims of bioterrorist attacks may include *immediate* (requiring prompt intervention), *delayed* (care can wait for a short time), *minimal* (only outpatient care is required), and *expectant* (moribund victims unlikely to survive lifesaving measures (Armstrong, 2002).

A heightened awareness by health care professionals plays a critical role in facilitating early recognition of the release of a biological agent as a weapon. The health care professional must immediately notify the infection control department of the hospital. The CDC in Atlanta must also be notified. They now have a 24-hour hotline number. Both phone numbers should be available to the health care professional.

SEXUALLY TRANSMITTED DISEASES

OVERVIEW

Sexually transmitted disease (STD) is the general name given to infections spread through direct sexual activity. This term replaces the term *venereal disease*. STDs can be transmitted by a pregnant woman to her unborn child and cause serious problems in the fetus such as blindness, birth defects, or death (Table 31-3). The occurrence of an STD in a prepubertal patient should always prompt investigation into the possibility of sexual abuse.

> **NURSING TIP**
> The use of condoms to prevent STDs, although recommended, is not considered 100% effective because condoms are apt to slip or break during intercourse and can be damaged by oil-based lubricants.

NURSING CARE AND RESPONSIBILITIES

Regardless of the medical professional's feelings about the changes in society and sexual permissiveness, the consequences of these changes must be recognized and managed. Nurses who wish to help adolescents with STDs must create an environment in which the adolescent feels safe and at ease. What adolescents need is emotional support, which the nurse can provide through listening and through a nonjudgmental attitude.

table 31-3 *Nursing Care to Prevent and Treat Sexually Transmitted Diseases*

NURSING GOALS

To provide anticipatory guidance concerning sexuality at a level that the child or young person can comprehend throughout developmental cycle

To prevent infection

To identify early symptoms and provide prompt treatment if infection occurs

To prevent sequelae

OBSERVATION	NURSING INTERVENTIONS
Children under 12 years of age	Provide age-appropriate instruction concerning sexuality; also explore expected patterns that might occur before next visit.
Puberty and adolescence	Review structure and function of reproductive systems; review personal hygiene; discuss values and decision making, possible sexual behavior and consequences, and prevention of pregnancy and STDs.
Self-concept: anticipate evidence of fear, embarrassment, anger, and decreased self-esteem upon suspicion of infection	Create nonjudgmental atmosphere; listen, assess level of knowledge, observe nonverbal behavior, establish confidentiality; provide privacy when assisting with pelvic or genital examination; provide appropriate draping of patient; realize anger is often a mask for depression, grief—do not take personally.
Skin and hair	It is not uncommon to see skin rashes, "crabs" (pubic lice), or scabies (mites).
Sexual partners	Determine sexual preference; investigate and direct to treatment; persons with multiple sexual partners, homosexuals, persons with new partners, and those with history of prior STD are at particular risk.
Sexual intercourse	Abstain during treatment; use condom to prevent reinfection.
Medication	Take all of prescribed medication; if taking tetracycline, advise to take 1 hour before or 2 hours after meals (on empty stomach); avoid dairy products, antacids, iron, and sunlight.
Compliance with treatment	Stress importance of follow-up and routine annual Papanicolaou (Pap) smears.
Sequelae	Discuss the possible complications of specific disorders such as birth defects and infertility.

The nurse approaches the patient with sensitivity and recognizes that the adolescent is embarrassed and in need of privacy, especially during examinations. Girls are often afraid and always nervous about a pelvic examination. This is true even when their outward manner may seem otherwise. Careful explanations are needed. The patient is draped appropriately, and the nurse remains during the examination to provide reassurance. The findings are discussed with the patient, and questions are encouraged. Most adolescents need to be drawn out and do not readily ask questions, even when they do not understand.

The requirement to report sexual contacts is an emotionally charged topic that often prevents patients from seeking help. The person who is assured of confidentiality and who has been treated in a dignified manner is more apt to cooperate. Girls who are sexually active must be taught to take responsibility for their own health. Young people must be made aware of the fact that sex with only one partner does not eliminate the risk because this partner may have had contact with others; the partner needs only one sexual experience with one infected person to transmit disease.

The nurse assesses the person's level of knowledge and provides information at an understandable level. Many young people have little knowledge of their body and their developing sexuality. Others have mild to deep-seated emotional problems that must be addressed. They may be using sex to escape from reality, to express hostility or rebellion, or to call attention to themselves. They may be involved in relationships they no longer desire and therefore need help in formulating positive attitudes toward themselves. They also need help understanding their behavior and that of others. In particular, adolescents must learn that they are responsible for their own actions if they choose to be sexually active. Prevention of STDs is discussed in Chapter 11.

> **⭑NURSING TIP**
> Sex education is not limited to the mechanics of intercourse but rather includes the feelings involved in a sexual experience: expectations, fantasies, fulfillments, and disappointments.

HIV/AIDS IN CHILDREN

Pediatric HIV/AIDS is a worldwide public health problem with a devastating outcome. Children usually acquire the AIDS infection in the following ways:

- Contact with an infected mother at birth (approximately 90% of cases in infants)
- Sexual contact with an infected person
- Use of contaminated needles or contact with infected blood

Educating the public about the role of unprotected sex and intravenous drug abuse in increasing the risk of AIDS infection is a public health challenge.

AIDS is caused by a retrovirus known as the human immunodeficiency virus type 1 (HIV-1) that attacks lymphocytes (the white blood cells that protect against disease). It appears to cause an imbalance between the helper T-cells (CD4+) that support the immune system and the suppressor T-cells that shut it down. In a person not infected with HIV, the number of CD4+ cells remains constant over time. In an HIV-infected person, the number of $CD4^+$ cells drops as months and years go by. The CD4+ cell count is a measure of the damage to the immune system caused by HIV and of the body's ability to fight infection. A physician uses the CD4+ cell count to help determine the best medical treatments for the individual.

A series of terms for this disorder have been developed, but the disease is now classified along a continuum by the CDC. The categories include the following:

- *Asymptomatic infection.* This refers to a latent period. Individuals in this category have positive antibody tests, indicating exposure to the virus, but they are not ill.
- *Symptomatic HIV infection.* Many individuals have this earlier and milder condition (compared with AIDS). This was formerly referred to as AIDS-related complex (ARC).
- *AIDS.* This refers to the most advanced involvement, which includes the finding of HIV antibodies in the patient's blood, the presence of complicating opportunistic infections, and other criteria.

Children do not get AIDS from casual relationships at schools and medical facilities or through family living. The virus is infectious but not highly contagious, and the circumstances for acquiring it are specific, as previously indicated. Improved attention to hygiene practices in response to this disease can only be applauded.

Because passive transmission of antibodies from the mother occurs, infants are born with antibodies that crossed the placenta. Some infants' systems become clear of antibodies in about 15 months, whereas other infants eventually experience the infection. Because of the transference of antibodies, the standard enzyme-linked immunosorbent assay (ELISA) and Western blot tests used to diagnose HIV infection in older children and adults are less reliable until the child is at least 15 months of age.

Manifestations. Criteria for the disease in children have been outlined by the CDC. Initial symptoms in infancy are vague and include failure to thrive, lymphadenopathy (enlarged lymph glands), chronic sinusitis, and nonresponse to the treatment of infections. The patient becomes subject to overwhelming infection. Opportunistic infections such as oral thrush, *Pneumocystis carinii* pneumonia, herpes viruses, and cytomegalovirus take advantage of the body's depressed immune system. Kaposi's sarcoma, a rare type of skin cancer, appears to be less common in children than in adults. Serious bacterial infections such as meningitis, impetigo, and urinary tract problems are reported in children. In general, the symptoms of HIV infection develop more rapidly in infants, and this may be attributed to the infant's immature immune system.

Treatment and nursing care. Treatment and nursing care are supportive because there is no cure for HIV/AIDS at this time. Assessment and care of the child with HIV/AIDS are critically important. Education concerning long-term compliance with prescribed medication and supportive care to promote growth and development are essential. Nursing Care Plan 31-1 provides selected nursing diagnoses and interventions for a newborn or infant with HIV/AIDS.

Psychological support for these children is paramount. Sensory stimulation and touching are especially

NURSING CARE PLAN 31-1

The Newborn/Infant with AIDS

PATIENT DATA: A new mother who is HIV-positive is rooming-in with her infant son who has been admitted with an upper respiratory infection.

SELECTED NURSING DIAGNOSIS   *Risk for infection related to HIV attack on T cells and the suppression of antibody function*

Outcomes	Nursing Interventions	Rationales
Patient will be free from infection as evidenced by intact skin, absence of respiratory distress, and normal laboratory findings.	1. Anticipate opportunistic infections because patient's immune system is depressed.	1. Opportunistic infections are those that occur because of the opportunity afforded by poor health of patient. Newborns and preterm infants have immature immune systems and are particularly susceptible; once infected, they have few reserves to fight illness.
	2. Monitor respiratory status closely; watch for restlessness, apprehension.	2. Lungs are a target for infection; patients are subject to pneumonia, particularly *Pneumocystis carinii*.
	3. Examine patient regularly for infection (puncture sites, mouth, rectum, pierced ears).	3. Thrush and herpes simplex are common in children; the perianal region is in danger of secondary infection from feces.
	4. Reposition frequently.	4. Frequent repositioning reduces pooling of secretions in lungs.
	5. Administer antipyretics and antibiotics as prescribed.	5. These will increase patient comfort and may help to ward off infection. Pneumonia requires aggressive efforts to identify pathogen; fever is common.

SELECTED NURSING DIAGNOSIS   *Imbalanced nutrition: less than body requirements related to anorexia, anemia, thrush*

Outcomes	Nursing Interventions	Rationales
Nutrition will be maintained as evidenced by normal healing, muscle tone, and body weight.	1. Offer small portions of high-calorie, bland foods often.	1. Infant has poor appetite and may have mouth sores.
	2. Provide oral formula to infants as prescribed.	2. Infant must have sufficient nutrients to meet growth and development and to maintain body expenditures.
	3. Administer nasogastric tube feedings if ordered.	3. Preterm and weakened infants may require nasogastric feedings.
	4. Provide hyperalimentation therapy if ordered.	4. Nutritional supplements may be necessary as disease progresses; prognosis is poor despite aggressive management.
	5. Provide for mobility to ensure muscle strength.	5. Immobility contributes to wasted muscles; toddlers need to be up and around as condition permits.
	6. Chart intake and output, daily weights.	6. These patients become easily dehydrated. Daily weights will determine nutritional progress.

Continued

NURSING CARE PLAN 31-1—cont'd

SELECTED NURSING DIAGNOSIS *Risk for injury related to changes in central nervous system and from decreased blood components*

Outcomes	Nursing Interventions	Rationales
Parents will become aware of potential sources of injury; parents will recognize signs of bleeding. Child will not show signs of injury as evidenced by absence of petechiae.	1. Provide developmentally safe environment.	1. Children are accident prone; normal cuts and abrasions become easily infected; impetigo can be very dangerous for this child.
	2. Observe skin for petechiae and bruising; explain to parents.	2. Thrombocytopenia is common. Kaposi's sarcoma, a form of skin cancer, is rare in children but may be seen in adolescents; looks like bruise in early stages.
	3. Monitor laboratory reports (e.g., prothrombin times, hematocrit).	3. Cultures of blood, urine, throat, and stool may be ordered; child may be unable to generate a white cell response great enough to be detected in laboratories, and there may also be an abnormal response of cells.

SELECTED NURSING DIAGNOSIS *Risk for impaired skin integrity related to immunosuppression*

Outcomes	Nursing Interventions	Rationales
Skin will remain intact; patient is able to eat without discomfort.	1. Inspect mouth often for lesions (*Candida albicans*).	1. Mouth sores may prevent child from eating.
	2. Observe frequently for diaper rash; apply prescribed ointment; maintain skin intactness by thorough, gentle cleansing.	2. Skin is subject to breakdown and infection.
	3. Apply nystatin suspension if ordered.	3. Nystatin may soothe and promote healing.

SELECTED NURSING DIAGNOSIS *Deficient knowledge of family related to care of the infant after hospitalization*

Outcomes	Nursing Interventions	Rationales
Family will verbalize understanding of the disease process, transmission, and necessary precautions.	1. Clarify misconceptions about the disease.	1. Misconceptions create anxiety; there are many misconceptions about AIDS.
	2. Help to prepare parents for possible need for long-term follow-up care.	2. Prognosis involves remissions and exacerbations; zidovudine (AZT) is showing promise for delaying onset of AIDS if used after positive serological testing; much controversy about testing exists.
	3. Prepare parents adequately for discharge from hospital.	3. Children should remain with their families and, if possible, should be managed out of the hospital with medical and social supports.
	4. Encourage parents to stay abreast of current, unfolding information.	4. Newer developments may change picture of disease; this instills some hope in family.
	5. Provide ongoing support services.	5. Because of the stigma, possible length, and prognosis of this disease, families require much support.

NURSING CARE PLAN 31-1—cont'd

SELECTED NURSING DIAGNOSIS	*Fear (parents and patient) related to loss of normal life or possible death*	

Outcomes	Nursing Interventions	Rationales
Parents will verbalize fears; family will develop coping skills that assist them in managing stress related to life-threatening disease.	1. Encourage family to support one another and keep lines of communication open.	1. Fear is reduced if it can be shared.
	2. Alert parents to self-help groups.	2. AIDS support groups or hospice can be helpful. Discuss the value of life support measures; families may be faced with such difficult decisions.
	3. Acquire accurate knowledge about disease.	3. There is much inaccurate information about how AIDS is acquired and transmitted.
	4. Dispel inordinate fears of the general public.	4. It is important that pediatric nurses be well informed about the disease.

?CRITICAL THINKING QUESTION

A new mother has been diagnosed with AIDS and is rooming-in with her infant in the pediatric unit. The mother states she wants to breastfeed her infant because she feels well enough. Her CD4+ levels are high. She states she wants herself and the infant to adhere to normal routine practices like other healthy newborns. What nursing response is appropriate?

---

important for infants. The effects of isolation can be physically and emotionally devastating to the developing child. Many infants are abandoned, outlive their mothers, or must live in foster care. Unique programs such as Children's AIDS Program (CAP) provide a homelike respite care environment and day care. The goal of the program is to help families living with HIV/AIDS infection to stay together.

The nurse anticipates interventions related to the care of the child with a life-threatening disease. Efforts to support families in crisis are particularly pertinent. Often the extended family must take over. Many families have few financial resources and are exhausted from the child's frequent hospitalizations and physical care. They need to be introduced to such agencies as social service, financial aid, HIV/AIDS and grief support groups, home health, nutritional programs such as Women, Infants, and Children (WIC), and hospice.

Several medications are used to manage HIV/AIDS in children. A fungal infection called *Pneumocystis carinii* may be the first opportunistic infection to affect the pediatric patient. Prophylactic medications are available. The nurse should be alert for central nervous system involvement such as motor deficits or a failure to achieve developmental milestones. RSV, pneumonia, renal failure, and gastrointestinal malfunction often plague the child with HIV/AIDS.

Children with HIV/AIDS should be assessed for the need to update routine immunizations. Tuberculosis testing is done routinely and as needed. Several antiviral drugs are being tested in children. Early diagnosis and treatment can improve the quality and length of life for many children.

key points

- *Standard precautions* are techniques recommended by the CDC to prevent the transmission of communicable diseases.
- *Body substance* refers to moist secretions of the body that can contain microorganisms.
- An *opportunistic infection* is caused by organisms normally found in the environment that the immunosuppressed child cannot fight.
- Immunization programs in the United States provide *active* immunity for children.
- Proper handwashing is the basic essential factor to prevent the transmission of infection.
- Proper storage of vaccines and appropriate routes of administration are essential to ensure the potency of the vaccine.
- Education of parents about the need for immunizations against common childhood communicable diseases is a primary nursing responsibility.

- Koplik spots are white spots on the mucous membrane of the oral cavity that occur before a skin rash and are indicative of measles (rubeola) infection.
- In chickenpox (varicella), all stages of the skin lesions are present on the skin at the same time.
- A child with German measles (rubella) should not be cared for by a woman in the early months of pregnancy because the virus can cause fetal anomalies.
- In children with roseola, a persistently high fever *suddenly* drops as the rash erupts.
- Gamma globulin offers *passive* immunity for exposed children who are immunosuppressed.
- Listening skills and a nonjudgmental attitude is essential when caring for adolescents with sexually transmitted diseases (STDs).
- Children acquire the HIV/AIDS infection by contact with an infected mother at birth, sexual contact with an infected person, or use of contaminated needles during drug use.

- The long-term nursing goals in the care for a child with AIDS are to promote compliance for long-term drug therapy and to provide support to maintain optimum growth and development.

ONLINE RESOURCES

Vaccine Fact Finder: http://www.immunofacts.com

National Immunization Program: http://www.cdc.gov/nip

Child Health Statistics: http://www.childstats.gov

Response to Disasters:
http://www.aap.org/policy/re9813.html

Public Health Emergency Preparedness and Response:
http://www.bt.cdc.gov

Smallpox Vaccine Recommendations:
http://www.cdc.gov/mmwr/preview/mmwrhtml/
rr5010a1.htm

REVIEW QUESTIONS   *Choose the most appropriate answer.*

1. The nurse is caring for a newborn with HIV/AIDS. Which of the following is a priority goal?
   1. Encourage breastfeeding
   2. Prevent infections
   3. Provide initial immunizations
   4. Notify social services

2. An adolescent diagnosed with AIDS asks about the mode of transmission for the illness. An accurate response is that it was most likely:
   1. A casual contact with a friend who is HIV-positive
   2. A latent response to an inherited predisposition
   3. Use of a contaminated toilet seat
   4. Contact with contaminated body substance through sex or intravenous needle use

3. When providing play therapy for a child with a communicable disease who is in an isolation room, a priority principle or rationale for toy selection would include:
   1. The toy should be selected from the hospital playroom
   2. Most children love books
   3. It is best to bring the child's favorite toy from home
   4. The toy should be washable

4. A parent brings a 2-month-old infant to the clinic for the second in the immunization series. The nurse should prepare for administration of which of the following immunizations?
   1. DPT, Hib, polio
   2. DPT, polio, MMR
   3. DPT, polio, varicella
   4. Td, hepatitis, MMR

5. The DPT immunization is administered:
   1. Orally
   2. Subcutaneously
   3. Intramuscularly
   4. Intravenously

32 The Child with an Emotional or Behavioral Condition

objectives

1. Define each key term listed.
2. Discuss the impact of early childhood experience on a person's adult life.
3. List the symptoms of potential suicide in children and adolescents.
4. Discuss immediate and long-range plans for the suicidal patient.
5. Differentiate among the following terms: psychiatrist, psychoanalyst, clinical psychologist, and counselor.
6. List five criteria for referring a child to a mental health counselor or agency.
7. List four behaviors that may indicate substance abuse.
8. Name two programs for members of families of alcoholics.
9. Discuss the problems facing children of alcoholics.
10. List four symptoms of attention deficit-hyperactivity disorder.
11. Describe techniques of helping children with attention deficit-hyperactivity disorder to adjust to the school setting.
12. Compare and contrast the characteristics of bulimia and anorexia nervosa.

key terms

art therapy (p. 762)
behavior modification (p. 762)
bibliotherapy (p. 762)
Diagnostic and Statistical Manual of Mental Disorders IV (DSM-IV) (p. 770)
dysfunctional (p. 772)
family therapy (p. 762)
intervention (p. 762)
milieu therapy (mēl-yoo THĔR-ă-pē, p. 762)
play therapy (p. 762)
psychosomatic (sī-kō-sō-MĂ-tĭk, p. 762)
recreation therapy (p. 762)
sibling rivalry (p. 773)

THE NURSE'S ROLE

The nurse is often the person who has the greatest amount of contact with the family. Assessing child-parent relations is an important and ongoing aspect of care. To work effectively with the disturbed child, nurses first must understand the types of behavior considered within normal range. Nurses are valuable members of the multidisciplinary health care team in that they work closely with hospitalized acutely ill children, long-term chronically ill children, and children in school. Nurses should keep a careful record of behavior and note relationships with members of the family. Such notations are meaningful to the physician and other staff members, who are as concerned with preventing problems from arising as they are with treating them.

Everyday, everywhere, children are trying to cope with stress. Many succeed and grow stronger; some do not. Early childhood intervention programs are helpful in preventing major problems that impact growth and development. Parenting classes teach what to expect at various ages and stages. They also stress the importance of age-appropriate discipline and guidance. Parent groups provide education, socialization, and support. Other agencies provide a variety of services. Some services include the National Alliance for the Mentally Ill (NAMI), Family Service Association of America, Inc., Toughlove, and the Youth Suicide National Center. Nurses must be aware of such resources to guide parents appropriately (see Appendix B).

When parents request guidance, the nurse encourages them to seek help from their family physician or pediatrician or from a community mental health center. In the hospital, a psychiatric clinical nurse specialist (CNS) is an excellent resource. If the child is in school, the services of the school psychologist or guidance counselor may prove valuable. Some religious centers employ counselors who are available free of charge to parishioners. Families who lack adequate financial resources can be directed to the appropriate agencies.

Some agencies not only provide emergency funds but can also set up a budgeting system for those receiving minimum wages. This is particularly helpful when the parents are young adolescents.

No matter how dysfunctional the parent-child relationship, most children consciously and unconsciously identify with parental values. Discrediting the parents threatens the child's security and creates anxiety. The nurse reassures parents and helps them regain or maintain confidence in their parenting role. In addition, because children do not seek treatment on their own, the nurse should assist parents in becoming invested in the treatment modality. Finally, as a professional, the nurse supports organizations concerned with mental health, votes on issues that are pertinent to the welfare of children in the community, and offers services when needed.

✦NURSING **TIP**

Parents provide important assessment data about the child that the young child cannot provide. They are also important in bringing the child to therapy. Discrediting parents threatens the child and is not therapeutic.

TYPES AND SETTINGS OF TREATMENT

The basic staff of the modern child guidance clinic is composed of a psychiatrist, a psychologist, a social worker, a pediatrician, and the nurse. Usually the child guidance clinic provides diagnostic and treatment services. It may be part of a hospital, school, court, or public health or welfare service, or it may be an independent agency.

The *psychiatrist* is a medical doctor who specializes in mental disorders. The *psychoanalyst* is usually a psychiatrist but may be a psychologist; all psychoanalysts have advanced training in psychoanalytic theory and practice. The *clinical psychologist* has an advanced degree in clinical psychology from a recognized university. Many of these specialists work in the school system with children, teachers, and families to prevent or resolve problems. A *counselor* is a professional with a master's degree from an accredited institution. Many counselors specialize in a specific area, such as substance abuse or counseling of children. In most states, counselors must be licensed.

Children who do not respond well to individual outpatient therapy may require the type of care provided in residential treatment centers. Their home situations may be so disruptive that they might benefit from a change of environment. This alternative also provides a cooling-down period for the family. Family therapy is

begun and includes all family members. The length of stay for the child varies from 1 to 3 weeks. Partial hospitalization programs in which the child attends therapy during the day and returns home at night are popular. Intervention may involve individual, family, or group therapy; behavior modification; or milieu therapy. It may also involve a combination of these therapies. Behavior modification focuses on modifying specific behaviors by means of stimulus and response conditioning. Milieu therapy refers to the physical and social environment provided for the child. Art therapy, music therapy, and play therapy are particularly helpful in dealing with younger children who have difficulty expressing themselves. Recreation therapy is also valuable. Bibliotherapy, the reading of stories about children in a situation similar to the child's, is also therapeutic. Creating an *emotionally safe environment* is basic to all forms of therapy.

ORIGINS OF EMOTIONAL AND BEHAVIORAL CONDITIONS

Early childhood experiences are critical to personality formation. Situations that disrupt family patterns can have a lasting impact on the child. Children who come from dysfunctional families may experience any of the following: failure to develop a sense of trust (in their caregivers and environment), excessive fears, misdirected anger manifested as behavior problems, depression, low self-esteem, lack of confidence, and feelings of lack of control over themselves and their environment. These and other manifestations may make children feel negative about themselves and the world. They experience guilt and may blame themselves when confronted with disappointment and failure.

Growing up can be painful even under the best circumstances. It is difficult for the child in the early school years to live up to so many rapidly developing standards. Guilt and anxiety develop. Finger sucking, nail biting, excessive fears, stuttering, and conduct problems are reflections of nervous tension.

The current trend toward prevention by identifying risk factors and advocating early intervention is a major goal of children's mental health services. The term psychosomatic has come to refer to the bodily dysfunctions that seem to have an emotional or a mental basis. Each person has a different potential for coping with life. Truancy, lying, stealing, failure in school, and a crisis such as death or divorce of parents are but a few of the difficulties that may require intervention. Box 32-1 summarizes some of the disorders that can affect behavior and appear during infancy, childhood, and adoles-

Summary of Disorders Usually First Evident in Infancy, Childhood, and Adolescence

Adjustment disorders
Anxiety disorders (separation, obsessive-
    compulsive)
Attention deficit–hyperactivity disorder
Autistic disorder
Bipolar depression
Conduct disorder
Developmental disorders (e.g., language, math)
Eating disorders (anorexia, bulimia, pica)
Encopresis
Enuresis
Major depression
Mental retardation
Oppositional disorder
Schizophrenia
Sleep disorders
Stereotyped movement disorders (tics, Tourette's
    syndrome)
Stuttering
Substance abuse

Data from American Psychiatric Association. (1994). *Diagnostic and statistical manual of disorders (DSM-IV)* (4th ed.). Washington D.C.: Author.

cence. Some behavioral disorders are caused by genetic factors; for example, autism is thought to have autosomal recessive inheritance.

ORGANIC BEHAVIOR DISORDERS

CHILDHOOD AUTISM

Autism is a developmental disorder manifested by motor-sensory, cognitive, and behavioral dysfunctions. It involves impaired social interaction, communication, and interests. It may be caused by a defect in neurogenesis in the early weeks of fetal life. It may also involve an abnormal neurochemical status with some abnormalities in catecholamine pathways and increased serotonin levels. It occurs in three to four of every 10,000 children and is more common in males.

Autism is usually diagnosed by 4 years of age, although symptoms appear earlier. Failure to make eye contact and look at others, poor attention behavior, and poor orientation to one's name are significant signs of dysfunction by 1 year of age. Research has shown that cognitive delays, if present, do not always occur early. Peer-related social behavior normally develops early in the preschool period, with symbolic play normally emerging by 2 years of age. Autistic children do not show interest in other children and have difficulty engaging in pretend play. Solitary play is the preference for the autistic child.

Early identification and intervention may help the autistic child. The nurse who is alert to identify dysfunctions in the social behavior of young children can facilitate early referral, which may result in more meaningful social advances for the autistic child. Treatment of autism involves providing well-structured home and school environments, behavioral modification, and in some cases the use of specific drugs to deal with specific behavior problems.

Drug therapy in autism is not curative. The goal of drug therapy is to reduce behavioral symptoms that interfere with cognitive development and family interactions. Haloperidol calms the child without sedating, but it offers no help with learning abilities. Stimulants such as amphetamines decrease hyperactivity, but they impair cognition and may increase self-injurious behavior. A multidisciplinary approach to care is essential. The nurse's role is to identify abnormal behavior as early as possible, refer for follow-up care, and monitor the side effects of prescribed medications.

During hospitalization, the nurse should provide a highly structured environment with few distractions. A normal homelike routine should be maintained whenever possible, with safety a priority. Communication should be at the child's developmental level, using one request at a time in a slow and friendly manner.

The development of meaningful language by 5 years of age is a favorable prognosis, although most autistic children require long-term care.

OBSESSIVE-COMPULSIVE DISORDERS IN CHILDREN

With obsessive-compulsive disorder (OCD), a recurrent, persistent, repetitive thought invades the conscious mind (*obsession*) or a ritual movement or activity (not related to adapting to the environment) assumes inordinate importance (*compulsion*). The rituals or movements may involve touching an object, saying a certain word, or washing the hands repetitively. OCD in children differs from OCD in adults in that the symptoms are not usually part of an obsessive personality. The behavior may start as early as 4 years of age but may not be noticed as interfering with daily functioning until 10 years of age or older. Children usually are aware of their compulsive behavior and may voluntarily control themselves while in school with peers. Untreated, the problem grows to interfere with total functioning. OCD is related to depression and other psychiatric disorders such as Tourette's syndrome; suicidal behavior is a high risk for adolescents with OCD.

OCD does not involve an impairment of cognitive function or interpersonal relationships. OCD has a genetic origin. Some research studies show involvement of the basal ganglia of the frontal lobe and a problem with neurohormonal system. Children often become withdrawn and isolated from their peers and family. Poor school performance is related to compulsive repetitive behavior rather than a deficit in intelligence. Family conflicts arise to compound the problem. Clomipramine is one medication used to control behavior. Fluoxetine and fluvoxamine alter serotonin and are effective for OCD problems.

Behavior therapy combined with medication provides the best results. The treatment involves "exposure and response prevention." For behavior therapy to be successful, however, the child must be motivated and capable of following directions. Parent and sibling involvement and support are essential. The nurse's role is to assess normal growth and development and understand that ritualistic behavior that is normal at 3 years of age is normally replaced by hobbies of collecting and special interests by 8 years of age. Prolonged ritualistic behavior should be referred for follow-up care. Assessing the response to and side effects of medications used to treat OCD is an important nursing role.

ENVIRONMENTAL OR BIOCHEMICAL BEHAVIOR DISORDERS

DEPRESSION

Depression in a child is not as easy to identify as depression in an adult. Many children have difficulty expressing their feelings and often "act out" their concerns. Depression is an emotion common to childhood. Sadness over grades, moving to a new community, or the loss of a pet may trigger a depressive mood that results in either a dependent-type or disruptive-type behavior. These manifestations are resolved in a short time and are considered perfectly normal.

A major depressive or mood disorder is usually characterized by a prolonged behavioral change from baseline that interferes with schooling, family life, and/or age-specific activities. Symptoms can include loss of appetite, sleep problems, lethargy, social withdrawal, and sudden decrease in grades. In young children, head banging, truancy, lying, and stealing can occur. If left untreated, depressive behavior can lead to substance abuse and/or suicide. Inheritance factors, organic factors, and environmental factors all contribute to major depressive disorders in children. Treatment of depressive disorders is often on an outpatient basis and may include prescribed drugs.

Nursing responsibilities include recognizing the signs of depression and initiating appropriate and prompt referral (Nursing Care Plan 32-1). Educating parents and school personnel concerning the identification of children at risk is an important nursing function in the community and in the hospital setting.

SUICIDE

Suicide is the third leading cause of death in adolescents after accidents and homicide. Completed suicides are more common in boys than in girls, but girls make more attempts. Many adolescent suicides are not intended to end in death but instead are a cry for help that may end tragically. The risk of a successful suicide increases when there is a plan of action, a means to carry out the plan, and an absence of obvious resources to turn to for help. The breakdown of family ties, pressure to succeed, or foiled relationships may trigger a low self-esteem or frustration that results in the turning of feelings of hostility or hopelessness inward.

Suicidal behaviors can be identified as *suicidal ideation,* which involves thoughts about suicide; *suicidal gestures,* which are an attempt at a suicidal action that does not result in injury; and a *suicidal attempt,* which is an action that is seriously intended to cause death (although it may be unsuccessful). Some adolescents may exhibit rage behavior or an emotional outburst that results in an *impulsive act* that can result in accidental death. Some adolescents display a chronic type of high-risk behavior that can lead to serious injury or death. The nurse's role lies in education, prevention, and identification of those children at risk and prompt referral for follow-up care.

Some manifestations of suicidal behavior include a flat affect or "fixed" facial expression; a deterioration in school performance; isolation from friends and family; changes in physical appearance; giving away of cherished possessions; and talk of death. The nurse is a vital link in working with school personnel to develop peer support groups and educate families concerning the available community resources. Mental health associations, hotlines, drop-in centers, safe houses, and free clinics are community resources that can be used.

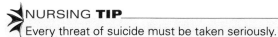

NURSING TIP
Every threat of suicide must be taken seriously.

NURSING TIP
When an adolescent feels hopeless and talks about feeling useless or worthless, do not contradict what he or she is saying. Instead listen, indicate your understanding, and encourage the expression of feelings.

NURSING CARE PLAN 32-1

The Depressed Adolescent

PATIENT DATA: An adolescent is admitted with a diagnosis of depression after a failed suicide attempt.

SELECTED NURSING DIAGNOSIS   *Risk for self-directed violence related to depression and stress*

Outcomes	Nursing Interventions	Rationales
Adolescent will state whether suicide is contemplated. Adolescent does not harm self and states two healthy coping measures. Adolescent will verbalize acceptance of protective measures. Family will verbalize seriousness of suicidal threats.	1. Ask adolescent if suicidal thoughts are present.	1. This information is important to know because it will determine intervention; most depressed adolescents are filled with contradictory feelings; talking honestly about them helps to clarify them.
	2. Inquire about precipitating event: broken romance, poor grades, and so on.	2. Suicidal reactions are associated with feelings of hopelessness often related to the loss of a significant or valued relationship or to a disappointment.
	3. Determine if the adolescent has specific suicidal plan.	3. How person plans to take his or her life is one of most significant criteria of assessing suicidal potential; more specific plans are a more dangerous threat.
	4. Determine if the adolescent has a history of suicidal attempts.	4. The situation is considered more critical if the adolescent has made serious attempts in the past.
	5. Determine if the adolescent has a history of emotional instability.	5. A history of emotional instability is more dangerous.
	6. Determine if the adolescent has the means available to injure himself or herself.	6. If the means to commit suicide are available (i.e., drugs, gun), the threat is imminent and more serious.
	7. Provide supervision as outlined by the physician or institution.	7. Surveillance and support by staff and family are important.
	8. Determine if a "safe contract" has been signed and discussed with the adolescent.	8. This is a written agreement that the adolescent will contact a nurse, counselor, or crisis line or go to an emergency room before harming self.
	9. The family will attend team conferences as appropriate.	9. It is wise to have available as many persons as possible to support one another and share the stress of the situation.
	10. Administer antidepressants if ordered.	10. Antidepressants elevate the mood of the patient; unfortunately, most antidepressants must be taken for 3 to 4 weeks before a therapeutic response is evident; some require monitoring of blood values.
	11. Monitor room for potentially dangerous articles.	11. Belts, glasses, rope, and other materials may be used to self-destruct.

Continued

NURSING CARE PLAN 32-1—cont'd

Outcomes	Nursing Interventions	Rationales
	12. Explain precautions to the adolescent and family members.	12. Explanations will lessen fear and increase compliance.
	13. Reinforce to parents the seriousness of the adolescent's suicidal threat.	13. *All* suicidal threats need to be taken seriously.

SELECTED NURSING DIAGNOSIS *Ineffective coping related to poor self-esteem, isolation, inability to deal with painful feelings*

Outcomes	Nursing Interventions	Rationales
Adolescent will make a positive statement about self. Adolescent will accept positive statements from others. Adolescent will accept the presence of the nurse, peers, or significant others. Adolescent will gradually deal with painful feelings by sharing and expressing them either verbally or nonverbally. Adolescent will speak in future terms.	1. Have the adolescent list two positive things about self and reinforce daily. 2. Instruct the adolescent to draw "how I see myself" and "how others see me."	1. Determines adolescent's strengths so the nurse can build on them. 2. Provides valuable information about the adolescent's self-esteem. Self-destructive behavior reflects underlying depression related to low self-esteem and anger directed inward. Drawing offers a release from feelings, helps to clarify emotions, and is a vehicle for discussion between the patient and the nurse.
	3. Build extra time into visits so that the adolescent does not feel rushed; give your undivided attention.	3. This indicates that you are truly interested; a ringing telephone and personal interruptions devalue the visit.
	4. Instruct the adolescent to draw a box and put things that bring happy feelings in the box; then instruct to draw another box and place things that cause sadness in that box. Encourage the adolescent to verbalize feelings about drawings; respect the adolescent's wish not to talk should this occur.	4. Drawings help adolescents distance themselves from the problem and see it more clearly.
	5. Review methods of coping.	5. Discovering how the adolescent coped in the past when he or she was less distressed is of importance so that these methods can be reinforced.
	6. Suggest healthy methods of coping such as exercise, relaxation tapes, and talking things out with parents or peers.	6. Many adolescents are not aware of healthy coping methods.

?CRITICAL THINKING QUESTION

An adolescent, recently discharged from an inpatient psychiatric facility with a diagnosis of depression, comes to the clinic complaining of headache and stomachache and states that no one will believe she is sick. Her parents believe her medical and psychiatric problems are just a means of getting attention. What interviewing techniques by the nurse would be appropriate?

SUBSTANCE ABUSE

Substance abuse is the illegal use of drugs, alcohol, or tobacco for the purpose of producing an altered state of consciousness. Substances may be ingested, injected, or inhaled to produce the desired effect. Four levels of substance abuse have been established: *experimentation, controlled use, abuse,* and *dependence.* Although there is often a fine line between controlled use and abuse, frequency may be a major signal. This is especially true when accompanied by inappropriateness, such as "getting stoned" at the weekend party versus on the way to school.

There are two types of dependence: *psychological* and *physical.* Psychological dependence includes a craving for and a compulsive need to use a substance. Physical dependence occurs with drugs such as heroin and alcohol. People become "hooked on the drug" and experience physical withdrawal symptoms in addition to psychological dependence. *Tolerance* develops when a user's body becomes accustomed to certain drugs. The person must then increase the dose each time to maintain its effect. Table 32-1 summarizes the characteristics of some of the more commonly abused drugs and the adolescent's reactions to them. Table 32-2 lists street names for some of these drugs.

Alcohol

Experimentation with alcohol has traditionally been accepted as a normal part of growing up. All states have legal drinking age laws that are well defined and implemented. However, studies have shown that eighth-grade children have experimented with beverages containing alcohol. Nurses must educate the public that alcoholism is a disease with established criteria that are both treatable and preventable. The devastating physical consequences of alcohol abuse as well as the increased risk of accidents and injury should be discussed with children as early as elementary school age. School nurses and parent-teacher associations can work together to prevent alcohol abuse and identify alcohol abusers who can be referred for follow-up care. Al-Anon, Alateen, and Alcoholics Anonymous (AA) are programs listed in most local telephone directories in the United States and welcome the young adolescent seeking help with an alcohol problem. Alcoholism is often a family disease. Adults often serve alcohol freely at social events in the home and therefore offer mixed messages about alcohol use to their children.

Cocaine

The easy availability of cocaine and the affordability of "crack" cocaine are the causes of increased experimentation by children. The drug can be "snorted," smoked, or used intravenously. The drug can cause life-threatening systemic responses as well as aggressive, antisocial behavior. Acute overdose can result in death. Treatment usually requires inpatient residential care.

Gateway substances are common household products and alcohol that can be abused to achieve an altered state of consciousness, or "high" (Figure 32-1). A feeling of euphoria can be followed by central nervous system depression, seizures, and cardiac arrest. "Huffing" substances include cleaning fluid, glue, lighter fluid, paints, shoe polish, various aerosols, and gasolines that are inhaled in various ways. They are called gateway substances because their use often leads to the abuse of stronger drugs (such as cocaine) and drug addiction.

> ➤NURSING **TIP**_____
> It has been estimated that more than 2 million people use cocaine on a regular basis. "Crack" is a popular form of cocaine and can be extremely addictive.

Marijuana

Marijuana is a hemp plant (*Cannabis sativa*). Hashish, the portion of the plant that is most potent, is smoked or ingested and rapidly absorbed by the body and metabolized by the liver. Asthmatic children can have serious reactions due to the bronchoconstriction that occurs when smoking this substance. A loss of inhibitions, euphoria, and a loss of coordination and of goal-direction are associated with the use of this substance. Users should be referred for professional counseling.

Opiates

Heroin is the most common opiate abused by adolescents. Because opiate users often drop out of school, statistics concerning use by children in school are lacking. The main consequence of heroin abuse is related to the sharing of unsterile needles, which places the adolescent at risk for human immunodeficiency virus (HIV) infection. Hepatitis and other infections are also common among heroin users. Long-term treatment programs are the therapy of choice for adolescents.

Prevention and Nursing Goals

The prevention of substance abuse begins by helping expectant parents to develop good parenting skills. It is imperative that children learn to feel good about themselves very early in life. They need a safe environment and adults whom they can trust and who serve as good role models. As orderly development proceeds, the growing child learns to interact with others and develops a sense of identity. A positive self-image and feelings of self-worth help adolescents fine-tune their adaptive coping skills. In time they rely on their own problem-solving

table 32-1 | *Characteristics of Abused Drugs and Their Acute Reactions in Adolescents*

CLASS	EXAMPLE	ROUTE	BEHAVIORAL SIGNS	PHYSICAL SIGNS	MEDICAL COMPLICATIONS
Opiates	Heroin, methadone, morphine	Subcutaneous, intranasal, intravenous	Euphoria, lethargy to coma	Constricted pupils, respiratory depression, cyanosis, rales, needle marks	Injection site infection, hepatitis, bacterial endocarditis, amenorrhea, peptic ulcer, pulmonary edema, tetanus
Hypnotics Sedatives	Barbiturates, glutethimide	Oral, intravenous	Slurred speech, ataxia, short attention span, drowsiness, combativeness, violence	Constricted pupils (barbiturates), dilated pupils (glutethimide), needle marks	Injection site infection, hepatitis, endocarditis
	Alcohol	Oral	As above		Gastritis, CNS infection, depression
Stimulants	Amphetamines	Oral, subcutaneous, intravenous	Hyperactivity, insomnia, anorexia, paranoia, personality change, irritability	Hypertension, weight loss, dilated pupils	Injection site infection, hepatitis, endocarditis, psychosis, depression
	Cocaine	Intravenous, intranasal	Restlessness, hyperactivity, occasional depression or paranoia	Hypertension, tachycardia	Nausea, vomiting, inflammation or perforation of nasal septum
Hallucinogens	LSD, THC, PCP, STP (DOM), mescaline, DMT	Oral Inhaled	Euphoria, dysphoria, hallucinations, confusion, paranoia	Dilated pupils, occasional hypertension, hyperthermia, piloerection	Primarily psychiatric with high risk to individuals with unrecognized or previous psychiatric disorder
Hydrocarbons, fluorocarbons	Glue (toluene)	Inhalant	Euphoria, confusion, general intoxication	Nonspecific	Secondary trauma, asphyxiation from plastic bag used to inhale fumes
	Cleaning fluid (trichloroethylene)	Inhalant	Euphoria, confusion, general intoxication, vomiting, abdominal pain	Oliguria, jaundice	Hepatitis, renal injury
	Aerosol sprays, Freon	Inhalant	Euphoria, dysphoria, slurred speech, hallucinations	Nonspecific	Psychiatric
Cannabis	Marijuana, hashish, THC	Smoke, oral	Mild intoxication and simple euphoria to hallucination (dose-related)	Occasional tachycardia, delayed response time, poor coordination	Occasionally psychiatric, with depressive or anxiety reactions

Modified from Behrman, R., & Kliegman, R. (1998). *Nelson essentials of pediatrics* (3rd ed.). Philadelphia: W.B. Saunders.
LSD, Lysergic acid diethylamide; *THC*, tetrahydrocannabinol; *PCP*, phencyclidine piperidine; *STP (DOM)*, 2,5-dimethoxy-4-methylamphetamine; *DMT*, dimethyltryptamine.

table 32-2	**Street Names for Commonly Abused Drugs***
STREET NAME	**DRUG**
A's	Amphetamines
Acid	Lysergic acid diethylamide (LSD)
Angel dust	Dimethyltryptamine (DMT) or phencyclidine piperidine (PCP) sprinkled over parsley or tobacco
Barbs	Barbiturates
Bennies	Benzedrine (amphetamine sulfate)
Black	LSD
Bullets	Secobarbital (Seconal)
Charlie	Cocaine
Coke	Cocaine
Crack	A form of cocaine
Crap	Heroin
Downers	Barbiturates or tranquilizers
Goofballs	Barbiturates
Hash	Hashish
Horse	Heroin
Joint	Marijuana cigarette
Mickey	Combination of alcohol and a hypnotic drug
Pot	Marijuana
PG	Paregoric
Rainbows	Tuinal (secobarbital sodium and amobarbital sodium)
Smack	Heroin
Speed	Methamphetamine
Uppers	Central nervous system stimulants
Yellow jackets	Pentobarbital

*These names often change and vary within subcultures.

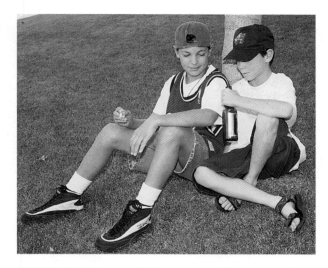

FIGURE **32-1** Beer and cigarettes used by young adolescents are considered "gateway" substances that can lead to other illegal substances.

abilities and ideally do not need chemicals to manage the complexities of life. Nurses in their various settings can contribute to this process. They can also educate their patients about the seriousness of substance abuse.

Although it is generally true that problem drinkers cannot be helped unless they want to be, more *intervention* is now being done. Most adolescents involved in substance abuse do not choose to enter treatment but are coerced by family members or the juvenile justice system. Although the issue is controversial, clinical experience in substance abuse treatment settings has shown that many adolescents become interested in treatment and make behavioral changes after they have been required to enter a treatment program.

Children of Alcoholics

Pathophysiology. Until recently, little attention has been given to children of alcoholics. This trend is changing, and support groups such as Adult Children of Alcoholics are more numerous. This discussion is directed to young children of alcoholics, although unresolved issues are similar in adults. Pediatric nurses are in an excellent position to recognize and intervene in cases in which physical or emotional neglect exists because of parental alcoholism. These problems stem from the parents' preoccupation with the disease. It is not unusual for both parents to be users.

Children of alcoholics are often confused by the unpredictability of family life. They do not understand why their needs are not being met. In some families there is a role reversal, with the child being forced to act maturely and make decisions ordinarily assumed by a parent. Often these children believe they are responsible for the disruptive environment. They are at high risk for emotional or physical abuse, including sexual abuse. Children of alcoholics are also strong candidates for becoming alcoholics as adults. Role models are distorted or lacking. A parent may try to cover up for the drinking partner by lying to employers and relatives but may punish the child for the same behavior. The child may become isolated from peers while trying to avoid embarrassment at home.

Four predominant coping patterns of children of alcoholics are flight, fight, the perfect child, and the super coper or family savior (Figure 32-2). The child who flees may do so literally or emotionally. The goal is to get away; as the child grows older, more and more time is

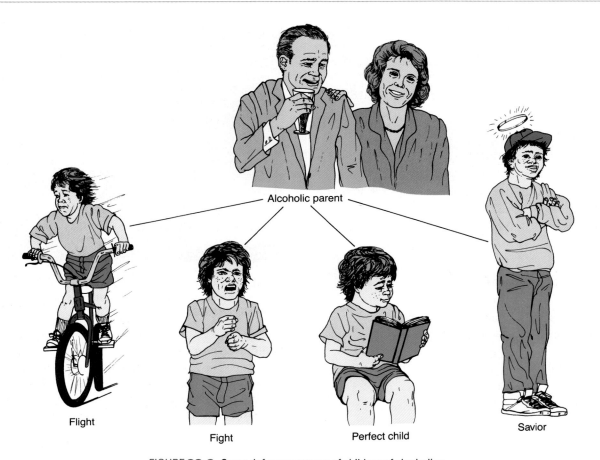

FIGURE **32-2** Some defense patterns of children of alcoholics.

spent away from home. Feelings are buried and left un-expressed. The child fighter is aggressive and displays acting-out behavior. The perfect child tries to gain love by never causing any trouble; he or she is obedient and is generally a good student. The savior or super coper feels overly responsible, often has a job to help out, and tries to do everything perfectly.

Manifestations, nursing care, and treatment. Early recognition of and intervention for children of alco-holics are paramount. The astute nurse with a height-ened awareness of alcoholism can expand admission observations and nursing history. Some clues that may or may not be related to this problem include a refusal to talk about family life, poor school grades or over-achievement, an unusual need to please, fatigue, passive or acting-out behavior, or maturity beyond the child's years. Treatment is multifold. One immediate priority is to teach the child how to get help in an emergency and to put him or her in touch with someone from the ex-tended family, school, or other suitable agency. Cultural diversities must be incorporated into treatment plans.

ATTENTION DEFICIT–HYPERACTIVITY DISORDER

Pathophysiology. The term *attention deficit–hyper-activity disorder (ADHD)* refers to a developmentally in-appropriate degree of gross motor activity, impulsivity, and inattention in the school or home setting that be-gins before age 7 years, lasts more than 6 months, and is not related to the existence of any other central nervous system illness. It is more common in boys than in girls. It occurs more often in some families, which suggests a genetic connection. The Diagnostic and Statistical Manual of Mental Disorders IV (DSM-IV) has defined the condition precisely and has established specific cri-teria for diagnosis.

Learning disability is an educational term; however, learning disabilities often occur in children with ADHD. Although these children may have average or above-average intellectual ability, they experience difficulties in areas such as the following:

- *Receptive language* such as listening and understanding

- *Expressive language* such as an inability to express ideas
- *Information processing* such as differentiating words that look or sound alike
- *Memory* such as remembering personal information or spelling
- *Motor coordination* such as copying forms, printing, writing
- *Orientation* such as confusing left and right
- *Behavior problem* such as difficulty in concentrating, impatient

A quick office tool used to identify children who have learning disabilities has been developed and is called the "Einstein Evaluation of School Related Skills." It tests reading, math, auditory memory, language, visual function, and motor function. It can be given as a screening tool in the clinic to kindergartners through fifth graders. Early intervention can help the child reach his or her full potential.

Dyslexia (reading difficulties) and *dysgraphia* (writing difficulties) may be apparent. These children may transpose letters; for example, they may read "pot" for "top." They may also have difficulty in expressing themselves.

✦ NURSING **TIP**
ADHD is characterized by inattention, hyperactivity, impulsivity, and distractibility.

Manifestations. The symptoms of ADHD as defined by the *DSM-IV* usually occur before 7 years of age and are summarized as follows:

- *Inattention* (at least three of the following). Is easily distracted, needs a calm atmosphere in which to work, fails to complete work, does not appear to listen, has difficulty concentrating unless instruction is one-to-one, needs information repeated
- *Impulsivity* (at least three of the following). Is disruptive with other children, talks out in class, is extremely excitable, cannot wait turn, is overly talkative, requires a lot of supervision
- *Hyperactivity* (at least two of the following). Climbs on furniture, fidgets, is always "on the go," cannot stay seated, does things in a loud and noisy way

The history involves a description of the child's behavior and responses, an observation of parenting style, and an understanding of the existing family stresses. The coping strategies of the child should be observed, and input from schoolteachers is sought. Psychologists may interpret behavior rating scales administered to the child.

| box 32-2 | *Strategies for Managing Children with ADHD in the Classroom* |

> Seat the child in the front of the classroom to minimize distraction.
> Remind the child to focus his or her attention whenever necessary.
> Give clear instructions, and repeat them often.
> Provide breaks between periods of work or study.

Modified from Berkowitz, C. (2000). *Pediatrics, a primary care approach.* Philadelphia: W.B. Saunders.

The management of ADHD is multidisciplinary. Family education to deal with their knowledge deficit about the condition, counseling to help the family and child deal with the problems encountered, and medication to help control some symptoms are the core of therapy. Medications such as methylphenidate (Ritalin) and dextroamphetamine (Dexedrine) may be prescribed but may interfere with alertness and cognitive ability. *Emphasizing the strengths of the child rather than the problems is essential to any plan of care.* Various support groups can aid parents in their coping skills. The school nurse can help teachers develop strategies for managing children with ADHD in the classroom (Box 32-2). Increasing positive interactions, providing tutoring, giving computer assistance, and using behavioral management strategies under the supervision of a professional psychologist are helpful approaches to care. ADHD is a chronic, long-term condition that can persist through adulthood. Some children who are "labeled" in school develop low self-esteem and antisocial behavior.

ANOREXIA NERVOSA

Pathophysiology. Anorexia nervosa (*anorexia,* "want of appetite" and *nervosa,* "nervous") is a form of self-starvation seen mostly in adolescent girls. Only 10% of patients with eating disorders are male. The criteria for this disorder are well outlined in the *DSM-IV.* It is characterized by the following:

- Failure to maintain the minimum normal weight for age and height (less than 85% of expected weight)
- An intense fear of gaining weight
- Excess influence of body weight on self-evaluation
- Amenorrhea

The etiology of anorexia nervosa may be genetic. The adolescents characteristically have average to superior intelligence and are overachievers who expect to be perfect in all areas. For young people with the disorder, their own emerging sexuality is very threatening. They experience anxiety and guilt over an imagined or a real fear of intimacy. They have low self-esteem, are obedient, and are nonassertive and shy.

Families of these young people are often dysfunctional. They may exhibit such abnormal behaviors as overprotectiveness, rigidity, lack of privacy, and inability to resolve conflicts. Affluent families may be at high risk when the concept of being thinner rules and the focus is on diet and exercise.

Manifestations. The primary symptom of anorexia nervosa is severe weight loss. Adolescents who wish to be fashion models or actresses or who participate in sports, dance, or gymnastics activities may be at risk for developing an eating disorder. On physical examination, some of the following conditions may be evident: dry skin, amenorrhea, lanugo hair over the back and extremities, cold intolerance, low blood pressure, abdominal pain, and constipation.

Adolescents with anorexia experience feelings of helplessness, lack of control, low self-esteem, and depression. Socialization with peers diminishes. Mealtime becomes a family battleground. The body image becomes increasingly disturbed (Figure 32-3), and there is a lack of self-identity. The young person remains egocentric and unable to complete normal adolescent tasks.

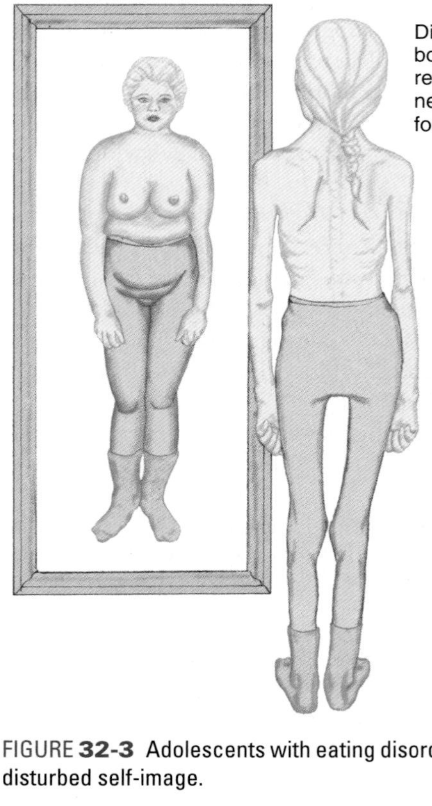

Distorted body image results in extreme need to control food intake.

Amenorrhea
Lanugo
Fatigue
Constipation
Dry, flaky skin
Severe caries
Dull, brittle hair
Muscle wasting

FIGURE **32-3** Adolescents with eating disorders often have a disturbed self-image.

Although eating less, the anorexic individual is preoccupied with food and its preparation. Hunger is denied. The patient complains of bloating and abdominal pain after ingesting small amounts of food.

Treatment and nursing care. The treatment of anorexia nervosa is complex and involves several modalities. Some hospitals have eating disorder units. A brief period of hospitalization may be necessary to correct electrolyte imbalance, establish a minimum restoration of nutrients, and stabilize the patient's weight. It also provides a time-out from a dysfunctional home environment.

Therapies include individual and family psychotherapy, behavioral therapy, and pharmacological therapy. Antidepressant medications may be helpful. The nurse plays an important role in ensuring that the atmosphere is relaxed and nonpunitive. Follow-up after discharge from the unit is essential. Individual and family therapy is continued.

Nurses working with adolescents in any capacity must be alert to the symptoms of this condition; a lack of recognition is one of the biggest obstacles to treatment. In the early stages, dissatisfaction with body image, amenorrhea, and social isolation are suspect. Young people must be educated about the seriousness of the disorder. Educational materials, referral sources, and counseling are available from the National Association of Anorexia Nervosa and Associated Disorders. Encouragement and support from self-help groups are also valuable.

Prognosis. Most patients gain weight in the hospital regardless of the type of therapy. However, this may not predict future success. Complications include gastritis, cardiac arrhythmias, inflammation of the intestine, and kidney problems. Fatalities do occur, particularly in untreated persons. Approximately 50% of patients are cured, approximately 30% improve but continue to have dysfunctional eating problems and a distorted body image (although they function well in school and at work), and approximately 15% remain chronically ill through adulthood.

BULIMIA

Bulimia, or compulsive eating, is recognized by the *DSM-IV* as a separate eating disorder. It has been estimated that as many as 5% of college women and 1% of college men have this condition. It is characterized by recurrent episodes of uncontrolled binge eating followed by self-induced vomiting and the misuse of laxatives and/or diuretics.

Family dysfunctions are usually present in children with bulimia; unlike with anorexia, however, the mother-daughter relationship is usually distant or strained. Depression and alcoholism may be a family problem. The binge-purge cycle is thought to be a coping mechanism for dealing with guilt, depression, and low self-esteem. Impulsive behaviors are characteristic of adolescents with bulimia.

Persistent vomiting can cause erosion of tooth enamel and eventual tooth loss. The use of laxatives and self-induced vomiting can cause electrolyte imbalance. Muscle weakness will result if ipecac is routinely used to induce vomiting. The HEADSSS (*H*ome, *E*mployment or *E*ducation, *A*ctivities, *D*rugs, *S*exual activity, *S*uicidal ideas, *S*afety) format of interviewing adolescents is helpful in obtaining a detailed assessment.

. . .

The nursing role in dealing with adolescents with eating disorders is to educate, prevent, identify, and refer. It is very difficult to identify an adolescent with a weight obsession in a society in which weight and thinness define beauty. This concept is reinforced in movies and magazines. A supportive and respectful but firm manner should be maintained by the nurse. Establishing trust with the adolescent is the first step in education, referral, and treatment. Adolescents with eating disorders must maintain a sense of control in their therapy for success to be achieved. Compromise and contracts must replace authoritative restrictions on diet and activity. A referral to support groups and child and family counseling groups is helpful. A multidisciplinary approach with the nurse, pediatrician, nutritionist, psychiatrist, and social worker helps to achieve a positive outcome.

MINIMIZING THE IMPACT OF BEHAVIOR DISORDERS IN CHILDREN

EFFECT OF THE ILLNESS ON GROWTH AND DEVELOPMENT

Children respond to traumatic events in their life and to stressors within the family, in the school, and within the peer or social group. The duration and intensity of the stressful event and the child's coping skills determine the impact on the growth and development process. Knowledge of normal growth and development throughout childhood combined with good observation and listening skills can enable the nurse to play a major role in minimizing the negative impact of behavior problems on growth and development. Because outpatient services play a significant role in health care today, nurses must be aware of agencies and support groups available to children with behavior disorders and their parents. Prompt, early referral and treatment can improve the prognosis of emotional and behavioral dis-

orders, enabling the children to reach their potential in growth and development.

Children's behavior problems require a total family approach to care. Education of the community (school personnel), family (parents and siblings), and child is an essential nursing responsibility. Patient advocacy with a focus on prevention and long-term management are goals of care. A knowledgeable, caring, understanding, and supportive nature is valuable for any nurse caring for children with behavior disorders.

EFFECT OF THE ILLNESS ON SIBLINGS

Most siblings of children with emotional disorders either suffer emotional scars or develop protective coping mechanisms to deal with their experiences. Siblings of children with long-term illness are at risk for developing poor self-esteem and problems with their own peer relationships. Some siblings, however, are resilient and develop strength and positive coping mechanisms. Sibling rivalry, a competition between siblings for the attention or love of parents, is a normal part of growth and development, but guilt on the part of the other sibling enters the picture when one sibling becomes ill. Sibling rivalry teaches interactive social skills that will be used with friends and at work later in life. A child who is left at home with a baby-sitter while the parents tend to an ill sibling in the hospital may feel abandoned and often is burdened with extra household responsibilities that may add to the stress. Some children may react negatively to the stress of making dinner for the rest of the family, whereas other children react positively and develop positive self-esteem, knowing they are trusted with such a task.

The nurse can provide support for the family system, identify available resources, and collaborate with the health care team to meet total family needs.

key points

- Early childhood experiences are critical to personality formation.
- The child's environment must be safe, and the child must be able to trust caretakers.
- Nurses play an important role in the mental and emotional assessment of children because they often have the most contact with the hospitalized child and family.
- Talk of suicide must always be taken seriously.
- The risk of suicide increases when there is a definite plan of action, the means are available, and the person has few resources for help and support.
- Substance abuse is the number one problem of American adolescents.

- Al-Anon and Alateen are two excellent resources for family members of alcoholics.
- The *Diagnostic and Statistical Manual of Mental Disorders IV (DSM-IV)* lists specific criteria for various mental conditions seen in children and adults.
- Attention deficit-hyperactivity disorder is characterized by a developmentally inappropriate degree of gross motor activity, impulsivity, distractibility, and inattention in school or at home.
- Behavior problems can be caused by the stresses accompanying the transition from childhood to adulthood or genetic or biochemical factors.
- Autistic children do not show interest in other children, do not make eye contact, and do not engage in "pretend" play.
- Obsessive-compulsive disorders in children do not involve impaired cognitive functioning.
- Ritualistic behavior may interfere with daily activities.
- A major depressive disorder is characterized by a prolonged behavioral change from baseline that interferes with school or age-specific activities.
- Substances abused by children and adolescents may be inhaled, injected, or ingested. The practice of sharing unsterile needles may lead to HIV infection.

- Emphasizing the strengths of the child rather than the weaknesses is essential when caring for a child with a behavioral disorder.
- Anorexia nervosa can lead to starvation and death.
- Bulimia is an eating disorder that involves bingeing and purging and can result in deterioration of teeth and electrolyte imbalance.
- Education, prevention, identification, and referral are essential nursing functions in the care of the child with a behavior disorder.

ONLINE RESOURCES

National Center for Learning Disabilities: http://www.ncld.org/

International Dyslexia Association: http://www.interdys.org

Agency for Healthcare Research and Quality: http://ahrq.gov/clinic/index.html

Autism Society of America: http://www.autism-society.org

Chronic Constipation and Encopresis in Children: http://www.med.virginia.edu/cmc/tutorials/constipation/

Medicine Net: http://www.medicinenet.com

REVIEW QUESTIONS   *Choose the most appropriate answer.*

1. The adolescent with anorexia nervosa has a body self-image characteristically expressed by:
   1. Wearing tight clothing to emphasize thinness
   2. Increasing elation as weight is lost
   3. Feeling "fat" even when appearing thin
   4. Efforts to achieve specific figure measurements

2. A priority goal in the approach to a child with anorexia nervosa is to:
   1. Encourage weight gain
   2. Prevent depression
   3. Limit exercise
   4. Correct malnutrition

3. A child with suspected bulimia should be assessed for:
   1. Abnormal weight gain
   2. Abnormal weight loss
   3. Erosion of tooth enamel
   4. Amenorrhea

4. An important approach to the care for a 7-year-old child diagnosed with attention deficit—hyperactivity disorder (ADHD) is to encourage:
   1. A diet high in processed foods
   2. Regular use of sedatives
   3. Strict discipline
   4. A structured, one-on-one environment

5. When assessing an 8-year-old child with obsessive-compulsive disorder (OCD), the nurse would expect to find:
   1. An intelligence deficit
   2. Ritualistic behavior
   3. Antisocial behavior
   4. Combative behavior

CHAPTER 33 Complementary and Alternative Therapies in Maternity and Pediatric Nursing

objectives

1. Define each key term listed.
2. Define complementary and alternative medicine (CAM) therapy.
3. Describe the involvement of the federal government in CAM therapy.
4. Discuss the acceptance of CAM therapy in nursing practice.
5. Discuss the impact on nursing care of patients who use CAM therapy.
6. Identify the role of the nurse in CAM therapy.
7. State three herbal products contraindicated in pregnancy.
8. State three herbal products commonly used in pediatrics.
9. State popular herbs used during menopause.
10. State three herbs that should be discontinued 2 weeks before surgery.
11. State the use of meridians, dermatomes, and reflexology lines in CAM therapy.
12. State five types of CAM therapy in common use.

key terms

alternative therapy (p. 775)
aromatherapy (p. 779)
coin-rubbing (p. 778)
complementary therapy (p. 775)
dermatome (DĔR-mă-tōm, p. 780)
herbal medicine (p. 781)
hyperbaric oxygen therapy (HBOT) (p. 784)
meridian (mĕ-RĬD-ē-ăn, p. 780)
reflexology lines (p. 780)
Rolfing (RŌL-fĭng, p. 778)
shiatsu (shē-ĂT-soo, p. 779)

DEFINITION OF CAM THERAPIES

Complementary therapy refers to nontraditional therapy that is used *with* traditional or conventional therapy. An example would be the treatment of hyperten-sion with medication *plus* relaxation or biofeedback techniques. Alternative therapy refers to unconventional or nontraditional therapy that *replaces* conventional or traditional therapy. An example would be the use of soy products instead of hormone replacement therapy in menopause.

Complementary and alternative medicine (CAM) therapies are also known as *integrative therapies, integrative healing,* and *holistic healing.* Although CAM therapy is used throughout the lifespan, this unit focuses only on the common gynecological, obstetric, and pediatric practices.

THE NURSE'S ROLE IN CAM THERAPY

Many CAM therapies are based on accepted theories such as the gate control theory of pain relief (see p. 160). Nurses have used complementary therapies such as imagery, journaling, therapeutic touch, humor, and support groups and therefore have an integral role in the development and assessment of CAM therapy. Studies have shown that 70% to 90% of people worldwide use some sort of CAM therapy for adults and children, with complementary therapy readily accepted in Europe. Knowledge concerning CAM therapy expands knowledge about health care practices used in many cultures. *Cultural competence* is a sensitivity and respect for practices and philosophies different from one's own; the awareness and understanding of CAM therapy can enhance the cultural competence of nurses.

The focus of health care has changed, moving the patient from the hospital into the home. The hospital setting is somewhat of a controlled environment, but nursing care in the home brings new challenges. As nurses enter this health care environment within the community, they will no longer be surrounded by familiar equipment, practices, and support personnel. Instead they will encounter some *alternative health care* practices involving patients who want increasing control over their health problems, need to be a part of the decision-making process, and want to incorporate cul-

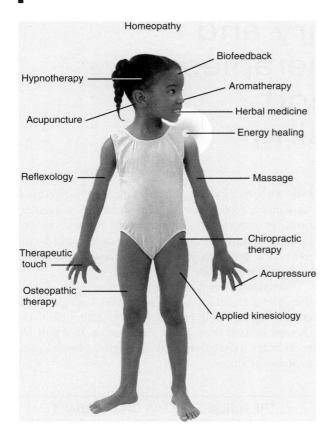

FIGURE **33-1** Alternative health care.

tural beliefs and traditions in their care. In addition to accepting treatment prescribed by a traditional health care provider, the patient may also be consulting other healing authorities such as holistic practitioners, naturopaths, and nutritional consultants (Figure 33-1). Food therapy, vitamin and mineral supplements, herbal therapy, and acupressure are common forms of alternative therapies practiced in many homes. Box 33-1 lists popular folk healers.

The greater acceptance of CAM therapies by the layperson and the inclusion of CAM therapies in medical curricula and practice has resulted in the need for nurses to understand CAM therapy, how it can be used, and how it may interact with or enhance traditional medical or nursing care (Table 33-1). It is important to note that not all alternative therapists are licensed, not all alternative medicines are regulated, and much of the practice is not scientifically (research) based.

In a survey of pharmacists, 73% sold herbal medications but only 45% had continuing education concerning herbal products (Chang, Kennedy, Holdford, & Small, 2000). This may indicate knowledge of the use of herbal medications but a need for increased understanding of possible adverse interactions and side effects.

Box 33-2 lists some cautions concerning the use of CAM therapy. However, some CAM practices have filtered into accepted nursing practice (e.g., massage, imagery, and aromatherapy). CAM therapy is not currently viewed as part of routine health care, which is evidenced by the lack of health insurance coverage for that type of health care. It is likely that nurses today and in the future will encounter CAM therapy as part of the health care delivery system. Therefore it is essential that nurses understand basic underlying philosophies and beliefs concerning CAM interventions. The nurse's role is not to promote the acceptance of CAM therapy but to recognize and respect its use in patients and to use critical thinking skills to determine interactions with traditional therapy. Healing is best achieved with the patient as a partner and consideration given to the cultural and environmental influences that impact the overall health and wellness of the patient and family.

FEDERAL REGULATIONS

There are more than 1800 identified CAM therapies practiced in the United States. The practices are not standardized, and often there is a lack of research-based

table **33-1** | *Herbs That Should Be Discontinued 2 Weeks Before Surgery*

HERB	SIDE EFFECTS	PROBLEMS DURING SURGERY
Echinacea	Unpleasant taste sensation, potential liver toxicity	May potentiate barbiturate toxicity
Garlic	Increased bleeding time, hypotension	Increased risk of intraoperative hemodynamic instability
Ginger	Increased bleeding time	Increased risk of intraoperative hemodynamic instability
Gingko biloba	Platelet dysfunction	Increased intraoperative/postoperative bleeding tendencies; may decrease effectiveness of intravenous barbiturates
St. John's wort	Dry mouth, dizziness, constipation, nausea	Pseudoephedrine, monoamine oxidase inhibitors (MAOIs), selective serotonin reuptake inhibitors (SSRIs) should be avoided
Ginseng	Hypertension, insomnia, headache, vomiting, epistaxis, prolonged bleeding time, hypoglycemia	Increased risk of intraoperative hemodynamic instability
Kava kava	Characteristic scaling of the skin	May potentiate the effect of barbiturates/ benzodiazepine, thereby causing excessive sedation (lethargy)
Feverfew	Mouth ulcers, gastrointestinal irritability, headache	Increased risk of intraoperative hemodynamic instability
Ephedra (Ma huang)	Hypertension, tachycardia, stroke, dysrhythmias	May interact with volatile anesthetic agents (e.g., halothane) to cause fatal cardiac dysrhythmias; profound intraoperative hypotension

The nurse must be alert to the effects of CAM therapy on traditional medical or nursing care.

evidence concerning their mechanism of action, effectiveness, or safety.

In 1938 the Federal Food, Drug and Cosmetic Act required all drugs, including herbs, to be safe before sale. In 1962 the Kefauver-Harris Drug Amendment required proof to the Food and Drug Administration (FDA) of drug effectiveness before placing agents on the market for sale. Herbal manufacturers declared their products to be "dietary supplements" and therefore were not included under this law. In 1976 the Proxmire amendment prevented the FDA from regulating supplement potency. In 1994 the Dietary Supplement Health and Education Act defined the term *dietary supplement* and prohibited claims of medicinal value. There have been requests by many health groups for closer regulation of dosages, warnings, and contraindications for dietary supplements but the FDA has not yet regulated the herbal industry. For this reason, many dietary supplements and herbal remedies vary in their strengths and ingredients.

In 1992 the National Institutes of Health (NIH) created the Office of Alternative Medicine to evaluate the various CAM therapies. It has since been renamed the National Center for Complementary and Alternative Medicine (NCCAM). This Center serves as a public clearinghouse and resource for research concerning CAM therapies. There are 11 university or medical center-affiliated research facilities for alternative medicine in the United States today. The more popular herbs and oils are the first to be researched in centers such as the University of California, Los Angeles (UCLA) and the University of Chicago.

In 1994 the Dietary Supplement Health and Education Act (DSHEA) required regulations in the marketing of dietary supplements that include plant extracts, vitamins, minerals, and herbs that are available to consumers without a prescription. Claims on labels must reveal they are *not* FDA approved.

In 1999 the NIH directed the NCCAM to work together with the Office of Dietary Supplements in research programs concerning the safety and efficacy of alternate medications. A journal, *The Scientific Review of Alternative Medicine,* is an example of publications dedicated to evaluating CAM therapies based on review of medical studies.

OVERVIEW OF COMMON ALTERNATIVE HEALTH CARE PRACTICES

MASSAGE

An underlying premise of alternate healing techniques is that the symptoms are the result of a problem in the body that may not be related to the specific symptom manifested. The body is thought to have a self-healing ability that can be aided by spinal or energy manipulation. Soft-tissue massage is thought to bolster the immune response. Fascia pressure, stretching and manipulation, known as Rolfing, are thought to improve muscle and bone function. "Cao-Gio" or coin-rubbing is a form of skin manipulation thought to help bring the body into healthy alignment (Figure 33-2). Neuromuscular massage helps to relieve muscle tension and trigger points of pain and generally improves circulation. Perineal massage during pregnancy and before delivery may avoid the need for an episiotomy during delivery, thereby reducing perineal trauma. *Effleurage* is a form of massage used during labor (see Figure 7-3).

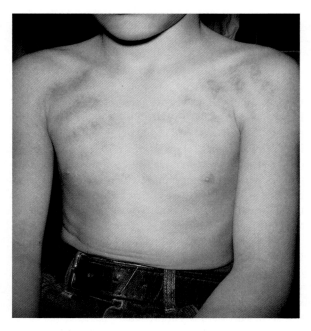

FIGURE **33-2** "Cao-gio" (coin-rubbing) is a form of fascial manipulation believed to bring the body in alignment with gravity. It is a form of CAM therapy that can easily be mistaken for child abuse because of the lingering marks on the skin after treatment.

Massage therapy is often used for children with asthma, arthritis, and eating disorders. Gentle touch massage therapy has had positive effects on premature infants. Massage and manipulative therapy is contraindicated in patients with cancer, osteoporosis, localized infection, and cardiac and circulatory disorders because of the increased blood flow to affected areas. Children with Down's syndrome are particularly prone to cervical spine anomalies and may be injured by manual manipulative therapy. Children who have a history of sexual abuse do not usually respond favorably to touch therapy.

OSTEOPATHY

Osteopaths combine manipulative therapy with traditional (allopathic) medicine. Pressure point therapy is based on the theory that certain areas of the body are connected to specific identified pressure points such as the feet, hands, and ears. It is believed that channels conduct vital energy through the body. The osteopath can guide a woman with previous back problems to select a birthing position that will not aggravate the problem. Many osteopaths currently practice in the mainstream of western medicine.

ENERGY HEALING

Energy healing involves the belief that an electromagnetic flow emerges from the therapist's hands and can funnel energy into the patient. Some believe that repatterning a patient's own energy field can aid in healing. The body, mind, spirit, and emotions are usually involved in this type of therapy.

A wristband that uses transcutaneous electrical nerve stimulation (TENS) can prevent nausea and vomiting during chemotherapy (Figure 33-3). TENS, "shen," "reiki," and the use of magnets are other forms of energy therapy.

REFLEXOLOGY

Reflexology deals with reflex points in the hands and feet that are thought to correspond to every organ or part of the body. The foot or hand represents a map of the entire body linked by energy pathways (Figure 33-4). Massaging these reflex points can relieve specific problems.

ACUPUNCTURE AND ACUPRESSURE

Acupuncture is an ancient oriental practice that works on the principle that the body has complex meridians that are pathways to specific organs or parts of the body. These meridians surface at specific locations called acupuncture points. It is at these points that positive or negative energy can be realigned. "Chi" energy is thought to regulate proper body function, and acupuncture or acupressure is applied to restore a balance of chi energy. In acupuncture, hair-thin needles are applied to specific meridians and may stimulate nerve cells to release endorphins.

Acupressure uses finger pressure and massage on the meridian sites (see Figure 33-4) rather than needles. Acupuncture and acupressure have achieved popularity in the Western world and can be used during pregnancy to control nausea, backache, and pain. Acupressure

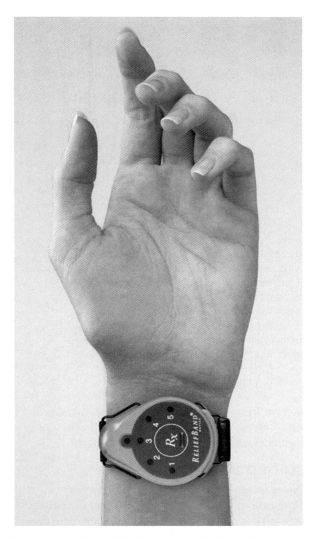

FIGURE **33-3** The ReliefBand is a watchlike device worn on the ventral side of the wrist where the median nerve is closest to the surface of the skin. When activated, the device emits a low-level electrical current across two small electrodes on its underside. A green light verifies function. A red light warns of low battery. The ReliefBand is indicated for the treatment of nausea and vomiting caused by pregnancy, postoperative nausea, chemotherapy, and motion sickness.

wristbands are available for use to prevent nausea and vomiting during travel or pregnancy. These techniques have also been useful for minor postpartum problems such as constipation. Acupoints to avoid during pregnancy include the bottom of the foot, the inner lower leg, the base of the thumb, and most areas over the abdomen because pressure here may result in negative outcomes, such as premature labor. Shiatsu is a finger pressure used with an emphasis on preventing disease rather than treating symptoms. Pressure is applied to achieve a level of sensation between pain and pleasure in the individual.

HOMEOPATHY

Homeopathy accounts for approximately 25% of pediatric visits to alternative health practitioners. Homeopathy uses plants, herbs, and earth minerals that are thought to stimulate the body's immune system to deal with specific health problems. The homeopathic philosophy involves the belief that disease is an energy imbalance and that prescribed remedies assist the body to reestablish correct balance. Homeopathic remedies are taken sublingually and should not be combined with caffeine, alcohol, or traditional Western medications. Some homeopathic medicines are alcohol based, and some contain mercury or arsenic bases that can cause toxicity or allergic responses in children. Only one remedy is administered at a time, and minimum dosage is the principle of most practitioners.

AYURVEDA

Ayurveda is an ancient Hindu healing regimen that deals with the biological rhythms of nature and can include music, herbs, massage, aromatherapy, and a diet tailored to the specific body type.

AROMATHERAPY

Aromatherapy is an ancient practice that involves concentrated fluid or the essence of specific herbs that are combined with steams or baths to inhale or bathe the skin. Essential oils are concentrated and, if undiluted, are usually used in 2- to 5-drop doses. Often a few drops of the herbal oil are added to soaps or regular lotions immediately before use. Concentrated oils are volatile and must be freshly prepared and stored properly. Some essential oils are contraindicated during pregnancy because of the effect on the mother or fetus; these include anise, juniper, thyme, wintergreen, nutmeg, pennyroyal, and mugwort. Aromatherapy under the supervision of a trained aromatherapist with oils such as jasmine, citrus, clary sage, lavender, and peppermint, has been useful during labor and delivery to relieve anxiety, reduce nausea, and improve the general feeling of well-being.

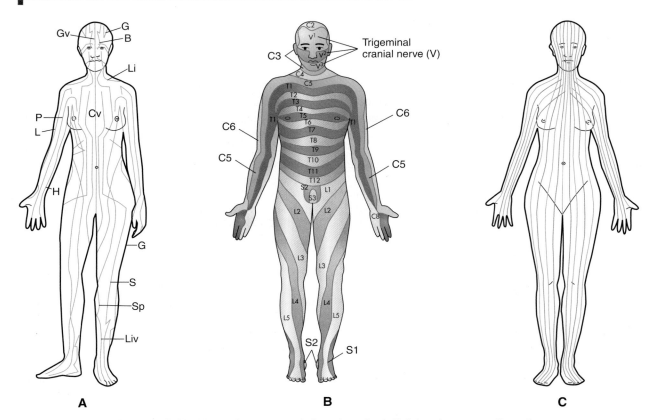

FIGURE **33-4 A,** Meridians. Acupuncture is based on the belief that the correct flow of energy through meridians (invisible tracks running through the body) control the health of all vital organs. Stimulating any of the 14 meridians with heat, electricity, needles, or pressure can affect corresponding parts of the body. **B,** Dermatomes. The areas of the skin innervated by the dorsal roots of the spinal cord are called a dermatome. Obstructing one dermatome line can anesthetize that segment of the skin and adjacent structures (although some dermatome lines from adjacent dorsal roots of the spine can overlap). **C,** Reflexology lines. Reflexology lines divides the body into 10 zones of longitudinal lines. Blockage of the lines is thought to obstruct vital energy pathways. Stimulating the area around the ankle bone can affect the uterus and pelvic organs and relieve pain during labor.

> **NURSING TIP**
> Lavender, chamomile, and sandalwood essential oils are useful in aromatherapy for children with chronic pain.

HYPNOTHERAPY

In *hypnotherapy,* the patient enters a hypnotic state of induced sleep. Under the guidance of the practitioner, specific and potentially long-lasting suggestions are given to the patient. Smoking cessation and pain control has been successfully achieved using this method. Some patients resist the trance state and are not candidates for hypnotherapy.

HYDROTHERAPY

Hydrotherapy is the therapeutic use of water to promote relaxation. It is often used during labor in the form of

showers. In some independent birthing centers, delivery is accomplished underwater under the direction of certified nurse midwives (CNMs). See Chapter 7.

GUIDED IMAGERY

Guided imagery is based on the ancient Greek belief that the mind can influence the body. Asking the patient to focus on a specific image can result in the reduction of stress and increased performance. This technique is most often combined with breathing and relaxation techniques to manage the discomforts of labor. See Chapter 7.

BIOFEEDBACK

Biofeedback is a type of relaxation therapy that enables the patient to recognize tension in the muscles via responses on an electronic machine and visual electromyography responses. The process is also used by traditional health care providers for drug addiction and chronic pain control.

CHIROPRACTIC CARE

Chiropractic care deals with the relationship between the spinal column and nervous system and involves nerve energy thought responsible for restoring and maintaining health. During pregnancy, circulating hormones such as relaxin increase the mobility of joint capsules and pelvic joint structures that affect the musculoskeletal system. Vigorous manipulation should be avoided between the twelfth and sixteenth weeks of pregnancy to avoid stimulating a miscarriage or premature labor.

Most chiropractors also use massage, diet, nutritional, and enzyme therapy for a more comprehensive approach. Chiropractors offer well-child care by preventive manipulation.

HERBAL REMEDIES

The World Health Organization (WHO) reports that herbal remedies are often used worldwide and are the first-line treatment for most children in Third World countries. Herbal medicine has been used for thousands of years in many countries. Herbs are powerful nutritional agents, and most are safe to ingest. Occasionally an allergic-type reaction is encountered, possibly because of differences in processing or storing of the product. Herbal products are sold in stores, but the growth, processing, storage, and prescription are not regulated the way they are for traditional drugs. However, there are general guidelines for their use, including dosages and the recommendation that herbal mixtures are preferred to single-herb products.

Many current medications are related to herbal remedies. Digitalis originates from foxglove, opiates originate from poppy flowers, and quinine originates from the cinchona trees. However, some herbs, such as ephedra, can be fatal to children. Herbal remedies consumed during pregnancy can reach the fetus. Breastfeeding mothers who use herbal remedies can pass the substance to their nursing infants. Home-grown herbs, such as chamomile used for tea, can be contaminated with botulism. Taking time to elicit an accurate history from parents may reveal their practice of using herbal remedies for the family.

Herbal capsules are about four times stronger than herbal teas, and *herbal extracts* are about four to eight times stronger than capsules. Most extracts should not be taken longer than 6 consecutive days. *Herbal tinctures* contain a high amount of alcohol and are not often recommended. *Herbal baths* are relaxing and soothing, and herbal salves, oils, compresses, and poultices use the skin as the body's organ of ingestion. Most practitioners emphasize that herbal dosage is determined by body weight and that megadoses can be harmful.

Herbs and Obstetrics

CAM therapy for obstetrics helps some women feel a sense of control over their well-being. Because many women view CAM therapy and herbal remedies as "natural remedies," they may not be aware of the possible dangers to themselves or their growing fetus. The patient may have been using herbal products before becoming pregnant, and the question of whether or not to continue during pregnancy, labor, and delivery must be discussed with the health care provider. Table 33-2 lists commonly used herbs that are contraindicated during pregnancy.

In general, herbs that promote menstruation are contraindicated in pregnancy (Box 33-3). It should be remembered that tannic acid and bran decrease the absorption of iron from foods, and therefore tea with meals should be avoided during pregnancy when blood volume increases and hemoglobin levels may fall into the anemic zone. The use of herbal products for neonates is contraindicated unless carefully monitored by a licensed herbalist and neonatalogist. The ingestion of high levels of vitamin C by a breastfeeding mother can result in colic in the newborn infant.

Herbs and Pediatrics

The use of CAM therapy has increased for children with various chronic diseases. Chiropractic, biofeedback, homeopathy, and herbal-food supplements are popular treatments for children. Parents sometimes prefer "natural remedies" such as herbs to prescription medicines for their children diagnosed with attention deficit-hyperactivity disorder (ADHD). Herbal treatments focus on improving cognition, producing sedation, or alleviating anxiety. These herbs are obtained without a prescription, and their use is often not supported by scientific studies concerning effectiveness or safety. Some herbs are contained in flavored tea sold in the supermarket. Parents often do not discuss CAM therapy used with their children unless directly asked by the nurse or health care provider. Table 33-3 reviews herbs commonly used for children. The Online Resources section at the end of this chapter can be used to help parents find reliable information.

Herbs and Menopause

Menopause is a stage of *health* within the health-illness continuum in a woman's life. It is not approached as a disease or illness but rather as a unique stage of life and as a normal, healthy process. The physiological alterations

table **33-2** │ *Common Herbs Contraindicated in Pregnancy and Lactation*

HERB	USE	CONTRAINDICATION
Aloe vera	Treats constipation Aids wound healing	Causes engorgement of pelvic vessels that can result in increased bleeding and spontaneous abortion; avoid during pregnancy.
Garlic, ginger, ginkgo	Decreases cholesterol Prevents motion sickness Lessens depression	Avoid in pregnancy; do not use with other antiplatelet medications.
St. John's wort	Lessens depression	Avoid exposure to sun. Increases tone of uterus. Use with caution in pregnancy. Interacts with alcohol, cold and flu medications, chocolate, aged cheese, and beer.
Angelica (Dong quai)	Used for gynecological disorders, menstrual discomfort, and postmenopausal symptoms	Avoid in pregnancy and breastfeeding because of uterine stimulation. Prolongs prothrombin time and causes poor glycemic control in diabetics.
Chamomile	Prevents urinary tract infections, gastrointestinal spasms; used for sedation	Avoid in pregnancy. May cause abortion and teratogenic effects on fetus.
Feverfew	Used for migraine headache and menstrual problems	Avoid use during pregnancy and lactation. Can cause withdrawal symptoms.
Flax (flaxseed)	Used for bowel problems	Contraindicated in pregnancy; potential for toxicity. Must be refrigerated.
Ginseng	Antistress Used to increase stamina	Avoid in pregnancy and breastfeeding. May be toxic. Central nervous system effects increase when used with coffee or tea. Interacts with St. John's wort and monoamine oxidase (MAO) inhibitors.
Kava kava	Reduces anxiety and stress	Avoid in pregnancy and lactation. May cause nutritional deficiencies or blood dyscrasias.
Ma huang (Ephedra)	Used as central nervous system stimulant	Avoid use during pregnancy. Can cause cardiac arrhythmia, urinary retention, and uterine contractions.
Nettle	Used as diuretic	Diuresis can cause electrolyte imbalance.

Data from Hadley, S., & Petry, J. (1999). Medicinal herbs: A primer for primary care. *Hospital Practice 34*(6), 105-106, 109-112, 115-116; O'Neil, C., Avila, J., & Ferroco, C. (1999). Herbal medicines: Getting beyond the hype. *Nursing 1999 28*(4), 58; and Spencer, J., & Jacobs, J. (1999). *Complementary and alternative medicine: An evidence-based approach.* St. Louis: Mosby.

that occur as a woman reaches and enters menopause result in minor discomforts such as hot flashes, night sweats, and insomnia. Traditionally, hormone replacement therapy (HRT) has been the most popular approach to managing menopausal symptoms. Recently, more "natural" paths of management have developed, including the following:

- Exercise, such as weight-bearing or water aerobic exercise programs

box **33-3** │ *Herbs That Promote Menstruation May Cause Miscarriage If Used During Pregnancy*

Cascara	Mugwort
Cohosh	Pennyroyal
Goldenseal	Sage
Juniper	Senna
Marjoram	Wormwood
Motherwort	

table 33-3 | *Herbs Commonly Used in Pediatrics*

HERB	USE	TOXICITY OR CAUTIONS
Blue-green algae (*Cyanobacteria spirulina*)	Stimulates tumor necrosis Antiinflammatory Antiviral Antifungal Used in children with ADHD	There are no clinical studies supporting cognitive improvement in children. Contaminated source of collection can cause toxicity, liver failure, and cholera. Should not be used in children with phenylketonuria. Nutritional value is limited in humans.
Chamomile (Manzanilla)	Used to calm infants with colic	Use with caution if allergic to ragweed.
Ephedra (Ma huang)	Used for asthma, decongestant, central nervous system stimulant	Often used by adolescents as an illegal stimulant. Can cause hypertension, anxiety, and toxic psychosis. Overdose can be deadly.
Echinacea	Immune enhancer	Increases barbiturate toxicity. Do not use with immunosuppressant therapy.
Evening primrose oil (*Oenothera biennis*)	Relieves eczema, asthma, and diabetic retinopathy	Nausea, diarrhea, and headache can occur.
Feverfew (*Tanacetum parthenium*)	Migraine relief	Contraindicated in pregnancy, lactation, and children under 2 years of age. Can cause mouth ulcers; may interact with antithrombotic drugs.
Fish oil	Improves visual processing and coordination Reduces asthma risk	Flatus, bad breath can occur. Do not use with anticoagulants or in bleeding disorders.
Ginkgo biloba	Improves alertness and memory Possibly decreases hypoxia damage to brain	Headache, dizziness can occur. Decreases the effectiveness of barbiturates. Do not use with aspirin or bleeding disorders.
Ginseng (*Eleutherococcus senticosus*)	Stimulant Aids resistance to stress Used in ADHD	Potentiates the effect of caffeine and other stimulants. Not to be taken with steroids or hormones.
Kava kava (*Piper methysticum*)	Reduces anxiety	Scaly skin rash can occur. Enhances barbiturate levels. Can cause oculomotor problems. Do not use with sedatives or anticoagulants. Increases high-density lipoproteins (HDLs).
Kombucha (Kargasok tea)	Used for children with cancer, multiple sclerosis	Can cause metabolic acidosis.
Lemon balm (*Melissa officinalis*)	Sleep disorders	May inhibit thyroid hormones.
Licorice (*Glycyrrhiza glabra*)	Treatment of asthma and stomach problems	Contraindicated in hypertension, kidney, and heart disease.
Melatonin (*N*-acetyl-5-methoxytryptamine)	Antioxidant Sleep cycle disorders	Reduced alertness, headache, irritability, possible suppression of puberty can occur. Use with caution in children with seizures.

Continued

table 33-3	*Herbs Commonly Used in Pediatrics—cont'd*	
HERB	**USE**	**TOXICITY OR CAUTIONS**
Pycnogenol (Oligomeric proanthocyanidin; OPC)	Antioxidant Improves behavior in ADHD	Avoid use in bleeding disorders. Do not use with anticoagulants.
Siete Jarabes	Used as expectorant and laxative Relieves asthma and congestion	Is a combination of sweet almond, castor oil, licorice, honey, and other products. May cause diarrhea or hypertension.
St. John' wort *(Hypericum perforatum)*	Antidepressant	Can cause photosensitivity. Do not use with nasal decongestants, asthma medications, monoamines, or drugs with phenylalanine content. Can cause high blood pressure.
Valerian *(Valeriana officinalis)*	Sleep disorders Antianxiety	Gastrointestinal upset, headache can occur. Do not use with other sedatives.

Data from Chan, E., Gardner, P., & Kempero, K. (2000). Herbs and dietary supplements in ADHD. *Contemp Pediatr,* 17 (9), 116; Lininger, S. et al. (1999). *A-Z guide to drug, vitamin, and herb interactions.* Roseville, CA: Prima Publishing; and *PDR for Herbal Medicines.* (2000). Oradell, NJ: Medical Economics. *ADHD,* Attention deficit–hyperactivity disorder.

- Relaxation techniques, including breathing, biofeedback, and hypnosis
- A low-fat, high-fiber and soy diet
- Herbs (Table 33-4)

HYPERBARIC OXYGEN THERAPY

Hyperbaric oxygen therapy (HBOT) uses an airtight enclosure to provide compressed air or oxygen under increased pressure. HBOT is used to revive children with carbon monoxide poisoning, to aid wound healing, and to treat the diving syndrome known as decompression illness. Many hospitals currently use hyperbaric oxygen therapy as a standard treatment for wound healing and other specific problems. HBOT is also used as CAM therapy in private centers. HBOT is contraindicated during pregnancy, because the increased oxygen saturation can cause the ductus arteriosus to close, resulting in fetal death. Research concerning the use and effects of HBOT is ongoing.

SAUNA/HEAT THERAPY

Overheating the body has long been used to speed up metabolism and inhibit the replication of viruses and bacteria. The sweating that results from the sauna is thought to help eliminate body waste. Patients should monitor their pulse during treatment. Some medical conditions can inhibit the ability to perspire, and heat can adversely affect the cardiac status of some patients. Therefore medical guidance should be sought before using this type of therapy. Sauna/heat therapy is contraindicated during pregnancy.

table 33-4	*Popular Herbs Used in Menopause*
HERB	**USES/CONTRAINDICATIONS**
Black cohosh *(Cimicifuga racemosa)*	Diminishes hot flashes by reducing luteinizing hormone; reduces joint pain, hot flashes, and other menopausal discomforts
Sage *(Salvia officinalis)*	Contains phytosterols and bioflavonoids; effective for night sweats and hot flashes and has been used to dry lactating breasts
Dong quai *(Angelica sinensis)*	Contains phytoestrogens; contraindicated with midcycle spotting and fibroids
Chasteberry (Vitex Agnus-Castus)	Reduces hot flashes and dizziness caused by high levels of follicle-stimulating hormone (FSH); balances hormonal fluctuations when combined with other herbs
Motherwort *(Leonurus cardiaca)*	Relieves hot flashes and moodiness; reduces anxiety and insomnia

Data from Learn, C. D., & Higgins, P. G. (1999). Harmonizing herbs: Managing menopause with help from Mother Earth. *AWHONN Lifelines* 3(5): 39-43; and Lindsay, S. (1999). Menopause naturally: Exploring alternatives to traditional hormone replacement therapy. *AWHONN Lifelines* 3(5): 32-38.

key points

- To promote positive outcomes, nurses must be well informed about the use and validity of complementary and alternative medicine (CAM) practices and understand the potential interactions with prescribed medications and treatments.
- Complementary therapies are treatments used in *conjunction* with traditional medicine.
- Alternative therapies are treatments that *replace* traditional medical therapy.
- The National Center for Complementary and Alternative Medicine, part of the National Institutes of Health, was created to conduct and review research concerning the efficacy and dangers of CAM therapy.
- Many herbal preparations do not have research-based data to determine safe dosage and use.
- Some CAM therapies, such as guided imagery, massage, and therapeutic touch, have been used successfully by nurses for many years.
- It is likely that nurses today and in the future will encounter some form of CAM therapy as part of the health care delivery system.
- Transcutaneous electrical nerve stimulation (TENS) is a form of energy therapy used to prevent nausea in labor, after surgery, and during chemotherapy.
- Nurses must use critical thinking skills to determine the interactions between CAM therapy and traditional prescribed treatments.
- Coin-rubbing is a type of CAM therapy that can be mistaken for child abuse because of lingering skin marks after treatment.
- Meridians are invisible (imaginary) lines running through the body that are thought to control the health of vital organs. Stimulation of any of the 150 pressure points on the 14 meridian sites is the basis of acupressure/acupuncture.
- Dermatomes are areas of the skin that are innervated by the dorsal roots of the spinal cord and affect specific segments of the skin and adjacent structures. These areas are manipulated by chiropractors.
- Reflexology lines divide the body into 10 zones of longitudinal lines. Blockage is thought to obstruct energy pathways and is the basic concept of reflexology.
- As part of routine history data collection, nurses should ask all patients if they use a form of CAM therapy; this information should be recorded on the chart.

ONLINE RESOURCES

Five-Year Plan: National Center for Complementary and Alternative Medicine: http://www.nccam.nih.gov/health

Attention Deficit-Hyperactivity Disorder: http://www.adhd.org

Herbs and Supplements: http://www.mcp.edu/herbal/default.htm

National Center for Complementary and Alternative Medicine: http://www.nccam.nih.gov

Nursing Center: http://www.nursingcenter.com

CRITICAL THINKING QUESTIONS

Explain the way in which complementary and alternative therapies can be used during labor.

Identify complementary and alternative techniques taught to women during most prenatal classes.

1. The nurse should communicate to parents that herbal medicines sold over-the-counter:
   1. Are harmless to children
   2. Are effective substitutes for traditional medication
   3. Can interact with prescribed medications and produce adverse effects
   4. Should never be given to children

2. Which of the following instructions would a nurse give a patient who is using an herbal product?
   1. Encourage the patient to use high doses of single herb to maximize effectiveness
   2. Depend on the label for claims of benefits of use
   3. Buy the least expensive brand of the product
   4. Inform the health care provider of all herbal products used

3. A patient in the prenatal clinic asks the nurse about the use of alternative or complementary therapies during her pregnancy. The most appropriate response of the nurse would be:
   1. Discussing CAM therapy is not within the scope of practice of the LVN/LPN
   2. All CAM therapies should be stopped during pregnancy, labor, and delivery
   3. Many complementary therapy techniques are taught in prenatal classes; some forms of alternative therapies may be contraindicated during pregnancy, labor, and delivery
   4. Only those herbs approved by the FDA should be used during pregnancy, labor, or delivery

4. The branch of the federal government that conducts research concerning the safety and efficacy of specific CAM therapies is:
   1. Department of Health and Human Services
   2. National Center for Complementary and Alternative Medicine (NCCAM)
   3. Food and Drug Administration (FDA)
   4. Drug Enforcement Agency (DEA)

5. The role of the nurse in CAM therapy is to:
   1. Encourage the use of CAM therapy in maternity/pediatric patients
   2. Discourage the use of CAM therapy in maternity/pediatric patients
   3. Discuss the impact or interaction of the CAM therapy with prescribed therapy
   4. Provide a resource of certified CAM therapists for maternity/pediatric patients

A Standard Precautions and Body Substance Isolation Precautions

All health care providers must apply Standard Precautions to all patients regardless of diagnosis, disease, or infection status. The health care provider should perform appropriate barrier precautions to prevent exposure to skin or mucous membranes, especially when contact with blood, body fluids, secretions, and excretions is anticipated:

- Wash hands thoroughly before and immediately after performing a task/procedure.
- Clean gloves should be worn whenever touching blood, body fluids, secretions, and excretions. They should also be worn when handling items or surfaces soiled with blood or body fluids and when performing venipuncture/vascular access. Gloves must be changed and hands washed after contact with each and every patient.
- Personal protective equipment (PPE) such as face masks, protective eyewear (goggles)/face shields, and fluid-repelling gowns should be worn for procedures that are likely to generate droplets of blood or exposure to body fluids, secretions, and/or excretions. If mouth-to-mouth resuscitation is needed, always use a resuscitation mask or bag to avoid direct contact with the patient's mucous membranes.
- All health care providers should take precautions to prevent injuries that can be caused from inappropriate handling of needles, scalpels, and other sharp instruments. After sharp items are used, they must be placed in **PUNCTURE-RESISTANT** containers nearby.

Transmission-based precautions (TBPs) are for patients with a suspected and/or diagnosed infection by an organism with a high risk of transmission. In such cases, both standard precautions and transmission-based precautions must be used. There are three types of transmission-based precautions:

1. *Airborne precautions* (5 microns or smaller in size) must be used whenever working with a patient who has tuberculosis (TB), chickenpox (varicella), or measles (rubeola). These infecting organisms can be inhaled by the health care provider or others in the room. Therefore face masks must be worn, and special ventilation and air-handling protocols must be used to prevent transmission of the organism. Patients are placed in a private room, and specific air-circulation requirements and/or filtration of air particles must be followed. All health care providers coming in contact with the TB-positive patient **MUST** be fitted for and wear a Hepa-Filter or N-95 face mask.

2. *Droplet precautions* (5 microns or larger) are used when the infection is spread through talking, coughing, or sneezing. *Haemophilus influenzae* type B, pertussis (whooping cough), scarlet fever, pneumonia, and rubella fall into this category. Transmission of these large droplets require contact within 3 feet, because the large size does not stay suspended in the air for an extended time. Droplet precautions require a separate room but do not require special ventilation or air handling. When working within 3 feet of a patient with a droplet infection, using standard precautions and wearing a disposable face mask are recommended.

3. *Contact precautions* are used to reduce the spread of infectious organisms by direct or indirect contact. Contact precautions are to be used when skin-to-skin contact may occur, such as turning or bathing a patient. When possible, these patients are placed in a private room or in a room with someone who has the same infection. On entering the room, the health care providers should wear clean gloves. While performing care on this patient, gloves should be changed after having any contact with blood, body fluids, secretions, or excretions that may have a high concentration of the infecting organism. Health care providers must be sure to remove their gloves **BEFORE** leaving the patient's room and to wash their hands thoroughly and dry them. They must be careful not to touch anything in the patient's room as they leave. If the potential for clothing to be exposed to contaminates is high, a cover gown is worn and is put on **BEFORE** enter-

ing the patient's room. Once care has been completed, gloves are removed **BEFORE** removing the cover gown.

All patients on TBP should be transported from the room only for essential purposes. Patients with airborne precautions should wear a mask during transport.

The Centers for Disease Control and Prevention (CDC) in Atlanta, Georgia, provides guidelines for infection control, and the Occupational Health and Safety Commission (OSHA) establishes legal requirements for infection control. Employers are mandated to provide equipment and employee protection measures.

Internet Website for Maternal-Child Health Organizations and Foundations

The following website has several hyperlinks to a large number of supplemental maternal, child, and family health websites. These websites include various organizations, foundations, and health education programs available on the state and federal level. This website is very easy to navigate and is in an easy-to-read format. Using the website address provided here, point and click on the division or service you are interested in and follow the directions provided. This website is provided by the Health Resources and Services Administration Maternal and Child Health Bureau and is updated regularly.

http://www.mchb.hrsa.gov

C NANDA-Approved Nursing Diagnoses 2001-2002

Activity intolerance
Activity intolerance, risk for
Adjustment, impaired
Airway clearance, ineffective
Anxiety
Anxiety, death
Aspiration, risk for
Body image, disturbed
Body temperature, imbalanced, risk for
Bowel incontinence
Breastfeeding, effective
Breastfeeding, ineffective
Breastfeeding, interrupted
Breathing pattern, ineffective
Cardiac output, decreased
Caregiver role strain
Caregiver role strain, risk for
Comfort, impaired
Communication, impaired verbal
Conflict, decisional
Confusion, acute
Confusion, chronic
Constipation
Constipation, perceived
Constipation, risk for
Coping, defensive
Coping, ineffective community
Coping, family, compromised
Coping, family, disabled
Coping, ineffective
Coping, readiness for enhanced community
Coping, readiness for enhanced family
Denial, ineffective
Dentition, impaired
Development, delayed risk for
Diarrhea
Disuse syndrome, risk for

Diversional activity, deficient
Dysreflexia, autonomic
Dysreflexia, autonomic, risk for
Energy field, disturbed
Environmental interpretation syndrome, impaired
Failure to thrive, adult
Falls, risk for
Family processes, dysfunctional: alcoholism
Family processes, interrupted
Fatigue
Fear
Fluid volume, deficient
Fluid volume, deficient, risk for
Fluid volume excess
Fluid volume imbalance, risk for
Gas exchange, impaired
Grieving
Grieving, anticipatory
Grieving, dysfunctional
Growth, disproportionate, risk for
Growth and development, delayed
Health maintenance, ineffective
Health-seeking behaviors
Home maintenance, impaired
Hopelessness
Hyperthermia
Hypothermia
Incontinence, urinary, functional
Incontinence, urinary, reflex
Incontinence, urinary, stress
Incontinence, urinary, total
Incontinence, urinary, urge
Incontinence, urinary urge, risk for
Infant behavior, disorganized
Infant behavior, disorganized, risk for
Infant behavior, organized, readiness for enhanced

Infant feeding pattern, ineffective
Infection, risk for
Injury, perioperative positioning, risk for
Injury, risk for
Intracranial adaptive capacity, decreased
Knowledge, deficient
Latex allergy response
Latex allergy response, risk for
Loneliness, risk for
Memory, impaired
Mobility, impaired bed
Mobility, impaired physical
Mobility, impaired wheelchair
Nausea
Noncompliance
Nutrition, imbalanced: less than body requirements
Nutrition, imbalanced: more than body requirements
Nutrition, imbalanced: risk for more than body requirements
Oral mucous membrane, impaired
Pain, acute
Pain, chronic
Parent/infant/child attachment, impaired, risk for
Parental role conflict
Parenting, impaired
Parenting, impaired, risk for
Peripheral neurovascular dysfunction, risk for
Personal identity, disturbed
Poisoning, risk for
Post-trauma syndrome
Post-trauma syndrome, risk for
Powerlessness
Powerlessness, risk for
Protection, ineffective

Rape-trauma syndrome

Rape-trauma syndrome: compound reaction

Rape-trauma syndrome: silent reaction

Relocation stress syndrome

Relocation stress syndrome, risk for

Role performance, ineffective

Self-care deficit, bathing/hygiene

Self-care deficit, dressing/grooming

Self-care deficit, feeding

Self-care deficit, toileting

Self-esteem, chronic low

Self-esteem, situational low

Self-esteem, situational low, risk for

Self-mutilation

Self-mutilation, risk for

Sensory perception, disturbed

Sexual dysfunction

Sexuality patterns, ineffective

Skin integrity, impaired

Skin integrity, impaired, risk for

Sleep deprivation

Sleep pattern, disturbed

Social interaction, impaired

Social isolation

Sorrow, chronic

Spiritual distress

Spiritual distress, risk for

Spiritual well-being, readiness for enhanced

Suffocation, risk for

Suicide, risk for

Surgical recovery, delayed

Swallowing, impaired

Therapeutic regimen management, effective

Therapeutic regimen management, community, ineffective

Therapeutic regimen management, family, ineffective

Therapeutic regimen management, ineffective

Thermoregulation, ineffective

Thought processes, disturbed

Tissue integrity, impaired

Tissue perfusion, ineffective

Transfer ability, impaired

Trauma, risk for

Unilateral neglect

Urinary elimination, impaired

Urinary retention

Ventilation, impaired spontaneous

Ventilatory weaning response, dysfunctional

Violence, risk for: other-directed

Violence, risk for: self-directed

Walking, impaired

Wandering

North American Nursing Diagnosis Association: *Nursing diagnoses: definitions and classification 2001-2002,* Philadelphia, 2001, NANDA.

	OUNCES															
POUNDS	**0**	**1**	**2**	**3**	**4**	**5**	**6**	**7**	**8**	**9**	**10**	**11**	**12**	**13**	**14**	**15**
0	—	28	57	85	113	142	170	198	227	255	283	312	336	369	397	425
1	454	482	510	539	567	595	624	652	680	709	737	765	794	822	850	879
2	907	936	964	992	1021	1049	1077	1106	1134	1162	1191	1219	1247	1276	1304	1332
3	1361	1389	1417	1446	1474	1503	1531	1559	1588	1616	1644	1673	1701	1729	1758	1786
4	1814	1843	1871	1899	1928	1956	1984	2013	2041	2070	2098	2126	2155	2183	2211	2240
5	2268	2296	2325	2353	2381	2410	2438	2466	2495	2523	2551	2580	2608	2637	2665	2693
6	2722	2750	2778	2807	2835	2863	2892	2920	2948	2977	3005	3033	3062	3090	3118	3147
7	3175	3203	3232	3260	3289	3317	3345	3374	3402	3430	3459	3487	3515	3544	3572	3600
8	3629	3657	3685	3714	3742	3770	3799	3827	3856	3884	3912	3941	3969	3997	4026	4054
9	4082	4111	4139	4167	4196	4224	4252	4281	4309	4337	4366	4394	4423	4451	4479	4508
10	4536	4564	4593	4621	4649	4678	4706	4734	4763	4791	4819	4848	4876	4904	4933	4961
11	4990	5018	5046	5075	5103	5131	5160	5188	5216	5245	5273	5301	5330	5358	5386	5415
12	5443	5471	5500	5528	5557	5585	5613	5642	5670	5698	5727	5755	5783	5812	5840	5868
13	5897	5925	5953	5982	6010	6038	6067	6095	6123	6152	6180	6209	6237	6265	6294	6322
14	6350	6379	6407	6435	6464	6492	6520	6549	6577	6605	6634	6662	6690	6719	6747	6776
15	6804	6832	6860	6889	6917	6945	6973	7002	7030	7059	7087	7115	7144	7172	7201	7228
	0	**1**	**2**	**3**	**4**	**5**	**6**	**7**	**8**	**9**	**10**	**11**	**12**	**13**	**14**	**15**
	OUNCES															

To convert the weight known in grams to pounds and ounces, for example, of a baby weighing 3717 gm, glance down columns to find the figure closest to 3717, which is 3714. Refer to the number to the far left or right of the column for pounds and the number at the top or bottom for ounces to get 8 pounds, 3 ounces.

Conversion formulas:

___ Pounds $\times$ 453.6 = grams

___ Ounces $\times$ 28.35 = grams

___ Grams $\div$ 453.6 = pounds

___ Grams $\div$ 28.35 = ounces

Temperature Equivalents

Celsius	Fahrenheit
34.0	93.2
34.2	93.6
34.4	93.9
34.6	94.3
34.8	94.6
35.0	95.0
35.2	95.4
35.4	95.7
35.6	96.1
35.8	96.4
36.0	96.8
36.2	97.1
36.4	97.5
36.6	97.8
36.8	98.2
37.0	98.6
37.2	98.9
37.4	99.3
37.6	99.6
37.8	100.0
38.0	100.4
38.2	100.7
38.4	101.1
38.6	101.4
38.8	101.8
39.0	102.2
39.2	102.5
39.4	102.9
39.6	103.2
39.8	103.6
40.0	104.0
40.2	104.3
40.4	104.7
40.6	105.1
40.8	105.4
41.0	105.8
41.2	106.1
41.4	106.5
41.6	106.8
41.8	107.2
42.0	107.6
42.2	108.0
42.4	108.3
42.6	108.7
42.8	109.0
43.0	109.4

Conversion formulas:
___ Fahrenheit to Celsius: $(°F - 32) \times (5/9) = °C$
___ Celsius to Fahrenheit: $(°C) \times (9/5) + 32 = °F$

Common Spanish Phrases for Maternity and Pediatric Nurses

Is there someone with you who speaks English?

¿Hay alguien con usted que hable inglés?
*Ah-ee **ahl**-gee-ehn kohn oos-**tehd** keh **ah**-bleh een-**glehs?***

I am the nurse.

Soy la enfermera.
*Soy lah ehn-fehr-**meh**-rah.*

Sit down, please.

Siéntese, por favor.
*See-**ehn**-teh-seh, pohr fah-**bohr.***

Lie down.

Asuéstese.
*Ah-**kwehs**-teh-seh.*

Turn on your right (left) side.

Voltéese del lado derecho (izquierdo).
*Bohl-**teh**-eh-seh dehl **lah**-doh deh-**reh**-choh (ees-kee-**her**-doh).*

Lie on your back.

Acuéstese boca arriba.
*Ah-kwehs-**teh-seh boh**-kah ah-**ree**-bah.*

Lie on your stomach.

Acuéstese boca abajo.
*Ah-**kwehs**-teh-seh **boh**-kah ah-**bah**-hoh.*

You need to take medicine/medication.

Usted necesita tomar medicina.
*Oos-**tehd** neh-seh-**see**-tah toh-**mahr** meh-dee-**see**-nah.*

Show me with one finger where you have the pain.

Enséñeme con un solo dedo dónde tiene el dolor.
*Ehn-**seh**-nyeh-meh kohn oon **soh**-loh **deh**-doh **dohn**-deh tee-**eh**-neh ehl doh-**lohr.***

Do you have nausea?

¿Tiene náusea?
*Tee-eh-neh **nah**-oo-seh-ah?*

Do you have vomiting?

¿Tiene vómito?
*Tee-**eh**-neh **boh**-mee-toh?*

When was the last time that you ate?

¿Cuándo fue la últim a vez que comió?
*Kwahn-do fweh lah **ool**-tee-mah behs **keh** koh-mee-**oh?***

Do you have diarrhea?

¿Tiene diarrea?
*Tee-**eh**-neh dee-ah-**reh**-ah?*

Are you constipated?

¿Está estreñido/-a?
*Ehs-**tah** ehs-treh-**nyee**-doh/-dah?*

Are you passing gas?

¿Está pasando gas?
*Ehs-**tah** pah-**sahn**-doh gahs?*

Does it burn when you urinate?

¿Le arde cuando orina?
*Leh **ahr**-deh **kwahn**-doh oh-**ree**-nah?*

Bend your knees.

Doble las rodillas.
***Doh**-bleh lahs roh-**dee**-yahs.*

Do you have pain here?

¿Tiene dolor aquí?
*Tee-**eh**-neh doh-**lohr** ak-**kee?***

Breathe deeply.

Respire profundo.
*Rehs-**pee**-reh proh-**foon**-doh.*

Drink clear liquids.

Tome líquidos claros.
*Toh-meh **lee**-kwee-dohs **klah**-rohs.*

Can you give us a stool sample?

¿Puede darnos una muestra de excremento?
*Pweh-deh **dahr**-nohs **oo**-nah **mwehs**-trah deh eks-kreh-**mehn**-toh?*

When was the last time you had a bowel movement?

¿Cuándo fue la última vez que obró (que usó el baño)?
*Kwahn-doh fweh lah **ool**-tee-mah behs keh oh-**broh** (keh oo-**soh** ehl **bah**-nyoh)?*

Drink eight glasses of water a day.

Tome ocho vasos de agua al día.
*Toh-meh **oh**-choh **bah**-sohs deh **ah**-gwah ahl **dee**-ah.*

Do you have sexual relations with men (women, prostitutes)?

¿Tiene usted relaciones sexuales con hombres (mujeres, prostitutas)?
*Tee-**eh**-neh oos-**tehd** rel-lah-see-**oh**-nehs sek-soo-**ah**-lehs kohn **ohm**-brehs (moo-**heh**-rehs, prohs-tee-**too**-tahs)?*

Are you allergic to any medicine or food?

¿Es alérgica a alguna medicina o alimento?
*Ehs ah-**lehr**-hee-kah ah al-**goo**-nah meh-dee-**see**-nah oh ah-lee-**mehn**-toh?*

Do you take medicine?

¿Toma usted medicina?
*Toh-mah oos-**tehd** meh-dee-**see**-nah?*

Do you have the medicine with you?

¿Trae la medicina con usted?
*Trah-eh lah meh-dee-**see**-na kohn oos-**tehd**?*

Take your medication.

Tome su medicina.
*Toh-meh soo meh-dee-**see**-nah.*

I am going to give you pain medicine.

Le voy a dar medicina para el dolor.
*Leh boy ah dahr med-dee-**see**-nah **pah**-rah ehl doh-**lohr**.*

Do you have shortness of breath?

¿Tiene falta del aire?
*Tee-**ehn**-eh **fahl**-tah deh **ay**-reh?*

We need a urine sample.

Necesitamos una muestra de orina.
*Neh-seh-see-**tah**-mohs oo-nah **mwehs**-trah deh oh-**ree**-nah.*

You need a catheter in your bladder.

Usted necesita una sonda en la vejiga.
*Oos-**tehd** neh-seh-**see**-tah oo-nah **sohn**-dah ehn lah beh-**hee**-gah.*

Have you lost weight?

¿Ha perdido peso?
*Ah pehr-**dee**-doh **peh**-soh?*

How long have you had the discharge?

¿Cuánto tiempo tiene con el deshecho/flujo?
*Kwahn-toh tee-**ehm**-poh tee-**eh**-neh kohn ehl dehs-**eh**-choh/**floo**-hoh?*

What do you use to prevent pregnancy?

¿Qué clase de anticonceptivo usa para prevenir el embarazo?
*Keh **klah**-seh deh ahn-tee-kohn-sept-**tee**-boh **oo**-sah **pah**-rah preh-beh-**neer** ehl ehm-bah-**rah**-soh?*

When was your last period?

¿Cuándo fue su última regla/menstruación?
*Kwahn-do fweh soo **ool**-tee-mah **reh**-glah/mehns-troo-ah-see-**ohn**?*

Are your periods regular?

¿Sus reglas/menstruaciones son regulares?
*Soos **rehs**-glahs/mehns-troo-ah-see-**oh**-nehs sohn reh-goo-**lah**-rehs?*

Are you pregnant?

¿Esta embarazada?
*Ehs-**tah** ehm-bah-rah-**sah**-dah?*

How many times have you been pregnant?

¿Cuántas veces ha esado embarazada?
*Kwahn-tahs **beh**-sehs ah ehs-**tah**-doh ehm-bah-rah-**sah**-dah?*

How many children do you have?

¿Cuántos hijos tiene?
*Kwahn-tohs **ee**-hohs tee-**eh**-neh?*

Have you received prenatal care?

¿Ha recibido cuidado prenatal?
*Ah reh-see-**bee**-doh kwih-**dah**-doh preh-nah-**tahl**?*

When was the last time you visited your doctor?

¿Cuándo fue la última vez que visitó a su médico?
*Kwahn-doh fweh lah **ool**-tee-mah behs keh bee-see-**toh** ah soo **meh**-dee-koh?*

How long have you had vaginal bleeding?

¿Por cuánto tiempo ha tenido sangrado vaginal?
*Pohr **kwahn**-toh te-**ehm**-poh ah teh-**nee**-doh sahn-**grah**-doh bah-hee-**nahl**?*

How many sanitary pads did you use today?

¿Cuántas toallas femininas usó hoy?
*Kwhan-tahs toh-**ah**-yahs feh-meh-**nee**-nahs oo-**soh** oh-ee?*

Are you having contractions?

¿Tiene contracciones?
*Tee-**eh**-neh kohn-trahk-see-**ohn**-ehs?*

How many minutes do the contractions last?

¿Cuántos minutos le duran las contracciones?
Kwahn-tohs mee-noo-tohs leh doo-rahn lahs kohn-trakh-see-ohn-ehs?

Did your bag of water break?

¿Se le rompió la fuente del agua?
Seh leh rohm-pee-oh lah fwehn-teh dehl ah-gwah?

When did your bag of water break?

¿Cuándo se le reventó la fuente del agua?
Kwahn-doh seh leh reh-behn-toh lah fwehn-teh dehl ah-gwah?

(Don't) push.

(No) Empuje.
(Noh) Ehm-poo-heh.

I am going to listen to the baby's heartbeat.

Voy a escuchar los latidos del corazón del bebé.
Boh-ee ah ehs-koo-chahr lohs lah-tee-dohs dehl koh-rah-sohn dehl beh-beh.

Do you want me to call a friend or relative for you?

¿Quiere que yo le llame a una amistad o pariente?
Kee-eh-reh keh yoh leh yah-meh ah oo-nah ah-mees-tahd oh pah-ree-ehn-teh?

I need to comb your hair.

Necesito peinarle el pelo.
Neh-seh-see-toh peh-ee-nahr-leh ehl peh-loh.

Do you know if you have diabetes?

¿Usted sabe si tiene diabetes?
Oos-tehd sah-beh see tee-eh-neh dee-ah-beh-tehs?

Do you take insulin (diabetic pills)?

¿Toma insulina (píldoras para la diabetes)?
Toh-mah een-soo-lee-nah (peel-doh-rahs pah-rah lah dee-ah-beh-tehs)?

What type of insulin do you take? Regular? NPH? Humulin 70/30?

¿Qué tipo de insulina toma? ¿Regular? ¿NPH? ¿Humulina 70/30?
Keh tee-poh deh een-soo-lee-nah toh-mah? Reh-goo-lahr? Eh-neh Peh Ah-cheh? Oo-moo-lee-nah seh-tehn-tah treh-een-tah?

How many units of insulin do you take in the morning (evening)?

¿Cuántas unidades de insulina toma en la mañana (tarde)?
Kwahn-tahs oo-nee-dah-dehs deh een-soo-lee-nah toh-mah ehn lah mah-nyah-nah (tahr-deh)?

Do you check your blood sugar level at home?

¿Usted revisa en casa el nivel de azúcar de la sangre?
Oos-tehd reh-bee-sah ehn kah-sah ehl nee-behl deh ah-soo-kahr deh lah sahn-greh?

What was the blood sugar when you checked it?

¿Cuánto fue el azúcar cuándo lo revisó?
Kwahn-toh fweh ehl ah-soo-kahr kwan-doh loh reh-bee-soh?

When was the last time you took your medicine?

¿Cuándo fue la última vez que tomó su medicina?
Kwahn-doh fweh lah ool-tee-mah behs keh toh-moh soo meh-dee-see-nah?

(X) hours (days, weeks) ago.

(X) hora (días, semanas).
(X) oh-rahs (dee-ahs, seh-mah-nahs).

Have you eaten breakfast?

¿Ha desayunado?
Ah dehs-ah-yoo-nah-doh?

Have you eaten lunch?

¿Ha almorzado (merendado, tomado el lonche)?
Ah ahl-mohr-sah-doh (meh-rehn-dah-doh, toh-mah-doh ehl lohn-cheh)?

Have you eaten dinner/supper?

¿He cenado (tomado la comida)?
Ah seh-nah-doh (toh-mah-doh lah koh-mee-dah)?

When did the accident occur?

¿Cuándo ocurrió el accidente?
Kwahn-doh oh-koo-ree-oh ehl ak-see-dehn-teh?

Did you lose consciousness?

¿Perdió el conocimiento?
Pehr-dee-oh ehl koh-noh-see-mee-ehn-toh?

When was the last time you received a tetanus vaccine?

¿Cuándo fue la última vez que recibió una vacuna del tétano?
Kwahn-doh fweh lah ool-tee-mah behs keh reh-see-bee-oh oo-nah bah-koo-nah dehl teh-tah-noh?

Does the baby sleep more than usual?

¿El/La bebé duerme más de lo normal?
Ehl/Lah beh-beh dwehr-meh mahs deh loh nohr-mahl?

Does the baby cry more than usual?

¿El/La bebé llora más de lo normal?
Ehl/Lah be-beh yoh-rah mahs deh loh nohr-mahl?

Do you have difficulty waking up the child?

¿Tiene dificultad para despertar al niño (a la niña)?
*Tee-**eh**-neh dee-fee-kool-**tahd** **pah**-rah dehs-pehr-**tahr** ahl nee-nyoh (ah lah **nee**-nyah)?*

When was the last time you gave him/her medicine for the fever?

¿Cuándo fue la última vez que le dio medicina para la fiebre?
*Kwahn-doh fweh lah **ool**-tee-mah behs keh leh dee-**oh** meh-dee-**see**-nah **pah**-rah lah fee-**eh**-breh?*

Be sure he/she drinks plenty of fluids.

Asegure que tome muchos líquidos.
*Ah-seh-**goo**-reh keh **toh**-meh moo-chohs lee-kee-dohs.*

Give him/her Tylenol every four hours.

Dele Tylenol cada cuatro horas.
*Deh-leh **tay**-leh-nohl **kah**-dah koo-**ah**-troh **oh**-rahs.*

Is he/she acting normally?

¿Está actuando normalmente?
*Ehs-**tah** ahk-too-**ahn**-doh nohr-mahl-**mehn**-teh?*

When he/she vomits, does the emesis shoot out in projectile form?

Cuándo vomita, ¿sale disparado el vómito en forma proyectil?
*Kwahn-doh boh-**mee**-tah, **sah**-leh dees-pah-**rah**-doh ehl **boh**-mee-toh en **fohr**-mah proh-yek-**teel?***

When was the last time he/she vomited?

¿Cuándo fue la última vez que vomitó?
*Kwahn-doh fweh lah **ool**-tee-mak behs keh-boh-mee-**toh?***

Has the baby lost weight?

¿Ha perdido peso el/la bebé?
*Ah pehr-**dee**-doh **peh**-soh ehl/lah   beh-**beh**?*

Have you recently traveled outside the country?

¿Recientemente ha viajado fuera del país?
*Reh-see-ehn-teh-**mehn**-teh ah bee-ah-**hah**-doh **fweh**-rah dehl pah-**ees**?*

Have you changed his/her formula?

¿Le ha cambiado la fórmula?
*Leh ah kahm-bee-**ah**-doh lah **fohr**-moo-lah?*

What brand of formula does he/she take?

¿Qué marca de fórmula toma?
*Keh **mahr**-kah deh **fohr**-moo-lah **toh**-mah?*

Do you give him/her cow's milk?

¿Le da leche de vaca?
*Leh dah **leh**-chech deh **bah**-kah?*

Does the baby vomit only when you give him/her milk?

¿El/La bebé vomita solamente cuándo le da leche?
*Ehl/Lah beh-**beh** boh-**mee**-tah soh-lah-**mehn**-teh **kwahn**-doh leh dah **leh**-cheh?*

Is there another person in the house with the same symptoms?

¿Hay otra persona en casa con los mismos síntomas?
*Ah-ee **oh**-trah pehr-**soh**-nah ehn **kah**-sah kohn lohs **mees**-mohs **seen**-toh-mahs?*

Does he/she have a history of asthma?

¿Tiene una historia de asma?
*Tee-**eh**-neh oo-nah ees-**toh**-ree-ah deh **ahs**-mah?*

We need to do an x-ray of his/her chest.

Necesitamos hacerle una radiografia del pecho.
*Neh-seh-see-**tah**-mohs ah-**sehr**-leh oo-nah rah-dee-oh-grah-**fee**-ah dehl **peh**-choh.*

When did the convulsion occur?

¿Cuándo le ocurrió la convulsión?
*Kwahn-doh leh oh-koo-ree-**oh** lah kohn-bool-see-**ohn**?*

How long did the convulsion last?

¿Cuánto tiempo duró la convulsión?
*Kwahn-toh tee-**ehm**-poh doo-**roh** lah kohn-bool-see-**ohn**?*

Did the child lose consciousness?

¿Perdió el ninó/la niná el conocimiento?
*Pehr-dee-**oh** ehl **nee**-nyoh/lah **nee**-nyah ehl koh-noh-see-mee-**ehn**-toh?*

When did the rash appear?

¿Cuándo empezó la erupción?
*Kwahn-doh ehm-peh-**soh** lah eh-roop-see-**ohn**?*

Do you have a new dog or cat at home?

¿Tienen un nuevo perro o gato en casa?
*Tee-**eh**-nehn oon **nweh**-boh **peh**-roh oh **gah**-toh ehn **kah**-sah?*

Have you used a new soap, shampoo, detergent, or lotion?

¿Ha usado un nuevo jabón, champú, detergente, o loción?
*Ah oo-**sah**-doh oon **nweh**-boh hah-**bohn**, chahm-**poo**, deh-tehr-**hehn**-teh, oh loh-see-**ohn**?*

Are your child's shots up to date?

¿Está al corriente con sus vacunas su hijo/-a?
*Ehs-**tah** ahl koh-ree-**ehn**-teh kohn soos bah-**koo**-nahs soo **ee**-hoh/-hah?*

How long has he/she had trouble walking?

¿Cuánto tiempo lleva con dificultad al caminar?
*Kwahn-toh tee-**ehm**-poh yeh-bah kohn dee-fee-kool-**tad** ahl kah-mee-**nahr**?*

Is he/she teething?

¿Le están saliendo los dientes?
*Leh ehs-**tahn** sah-lee-**ehn**-doh lohs dee-**ehn**-tehs?*

Did he/she fall?

¿Se cayó?
*Seh kah-**yoh**?*

Does he/she have problems swallowing?

¿Tiene problemas al tragar?
*Tee-**eh**-neh proh-**bleh**-mahs ahl trah-**gahr**?*

Modified from Nasr, I., Cordero, M. (1996). *Medical spanish: An instant translator.* Philadelphia: W. B. Saunders.

G Commonly Used Abbreviations in Maternity and Pediatric Nursing

AC	abdominal circumference		EFW	estimated fetal weight
AGA	appropriate for gestational age		EGA	estimated gestational age
AROM	artificial rupture of membranes		ENT	ear, nose, and throat
AB	abortion		FAS	fetal alcohol syndrome
AD	right ear		FB	foreign body
AGE	acute gastroenteritis		FHR	fetal heart rate
AS	auricle sinister (left ear)		FHS	fetal heart sound
AU	both ears		FHT	fetal heart tone
B.S.	breath sounds		FSH	follicle-stimulating hormone
bid	two times a day		FTT	failure to thrive
BCP	birth control pill		FUO	fever of unknown origin
BM	bowel movement		Fx	fracture
BOM	bilateral otitis media		GER	gastroesophageal reflux
BOW	bag of waters		g	gram
Bpd	biparietal diameter		G	gravida (number of pregnancies)
BPD	bronchopulmonary dysplasia (infants)		GDM	gestational diabetes mellitus
bpm	beats per minute		GI	gastrointestinal
BRP	bathroom privileges		GIFT	gamete intrafallopian transfer
BS	bowel sounds		GnRH	gonadotrophin-releasing hormone
BSA	body surface area		GTPAL	gravida, term, premature, abortion, living children
BSE	breast self-examination		gtt	drops
BTB	breakthrough bleeding		GTT	glucose tolerance test
BW	birth weight		H&H	hemoglobin and hematocrit
C/S	cesarean section		H&P	history and physical
CAN	child abuse and neglect		HBO	hyperbaric oxygen
cp	cerebral palsy		HC	head circumference
CNS	central nervous system		hCG	human chorionic gonadotrophin
CNS	clinical nurse specialist		HELLP	hemolysis, elevated liver enzymes, low platelet count
CPD	cephalo-pelvic disproportion		HIB	hemophilus influenza B conjugate vaccine
CRL	crown rump length		HPL	human placental lactogen
CST	contraction stress test		HR	heart rate
CX	cervix		HRT	hormone replacement therapy
D&C	dilation & curettage		I/O	intake and output
DFA	diet for age		I&D	incision and drainage
DOB	date of birth		IM	intramuscular
EBL	estimated blood loss		IUD	intrauterine device
EDC	estimated date of confinement		IUGR	intrauterine growth retardation
EDD	estimated date of delivery		IVF	in vitro fertilization
EFM	external fetal monitor			

KUB	kidneys, ureters, bladder	PR	per rectum
KVO	keep vein open	PROM	premature rupture of membranes
L&D	labor and delivery	PT	prothrombin time
LBW	low birth weight	PTT	partial thromboplastin time
LDR	labor-delivery room	R.A.D.	reactive airway disease
LGA	large for gestational age	RDA	recommended daily allowance
LH	leutinizing hormone	RDI	recommended daily intake
lmp	last menstrual period	RDS	respiratory distress syndrome
LMP	left mentoposterior	REM	rapid eye movement
LNMP	last normal menstrual period	R/O	rule out
LOM	left otitis media	ROM	rupture of membranes
MAS	meconium aspiration syndrome	ROM	range of motion
MDI	metered dose inhaler	S̄	without
med neb	nebulized medication	S/S	signs and symptoms
ml	milliliter	SAT	saturation
mm	millimeter	SC	subcutaneous (also SQ)
N/V/D/C	nausea, vomiting, diarrhea, constipation	SGA	small for gestational age
NCP	nursing care plan	SIDS	sudden infant death syndrome
NKDA	no known drug allergies	SL	sublingual (under the tongue)
NPO	nothing by mouth	SOAP	subjective/objective/assessment and planning
NST	non-stress test	SOB	shortness of breath
NSVD	normal spontaneous vaginal delivery	SPROM	spontaneous premature rupture of membranes
NTT	nasotracheal tube	STAT	at once
NV	neurovascular	STD	sexually transmitted disease
OB	obstetric	TKO	to keep open
OC	oral contraceptive	TO	telephone order
O.D.	ocular dexter (right eye)	TPN	total parenteral nutrition
OE	otitis externa	TRA	to run at
ORIF	open reduction internal fixation	tsp	teaspoon
OTC	over-the-counter (nonprescription drug)	TSS	toxic shock syndrome
O.U.	each eye	UC	uterine contractions
O.S.	left eye	ung.	ointment
os	by mouth	VBAC	vaginal birth after cesarean
PAR	postanesthesia recovery	VDRL	Venereal Disease Research Laboratories
Para	birth of a viable infant	VLBW	very low birth weight
p.c.	post cibum (after meals)	VO	verbal order
PDA	patent ductus arteriosus	W-D	well developed
PEG	percutaneous endoscopic gastrostomy	WIC	women, infants, children
PERRLA	pupils equal, round, reactive to light, and accommodation	wn	well nourished
PICC	peripherally inserted central venous catheter	WNL	within normal limits
PID	pelvic inflammatory disease	y/o	year old
PIH	pregnancy induced hypertension	YOB	year of birth
PKU	phenylketonuria	ZIFT	zygote intrafallopian transfer
PMDD	premenstrual dysphoric disorder	↑	increase
PMS	premenstrual syndrome	↓	decrease
PO	per os (by mouth)	+	positive, plus
P.P.	post prandial (after meals)	<	less than
PP	postpartum	>	greater than
PPD	tuberculin test	~	approximate
		Δ	change

Complete Bibliography and Reader References

Chapter 1 The Past, Present, and Future

Ackley, B., & Ladwig, G. (1999). *Nursing diagnosis handbook: A guide to planning care* (5th ed.). St. Louis: Mosby.

Alfaro-LeFevre, R. (1999). *Critical thinking in nursing: A practical approach* (2nd ed.). Philadelphia: W.B. Saunders.

Behrman, R., Kliegman, R., & Jenson, H. (2000). *Nelson textbook of pediatrics* (16th ed.). Philadelphia: W.B. Saunders.

Berkowitz, C. (2000). *Pediatrics: A primary care approach* (2nd ed.). Philadelphia: W.B. Saunders.

Betz, C. (2002). The Surgeon General's report on health care needs of individuals with mental retardation. *J Pediatr Nurs, 17*(2), 79-81.

Callister, L. (2001). Culturally competent care of women and newborns: Knowledge, attitudes and skills. *J Obstet Gynecol Neonatal Nurs, 30*(2), 209-215.

Committee on Children with Disabilities. (1995). Guidelines for home care of infants, children and adolescents with chronic disease. *Pediatrics, 96*(1 pt 1), 161-164.

Cookfair, J. (1996). *Nursing care in the community* (2nd ed.) St. Louis: Mosby.

Gravely, S. (2001). When your patient speaks Spanish and you don't. *RN, 64*(5), 65-67.

Hamric, A., Sprouse, J., & Hansen, C. (2001). Advanced practice nursing: An integrative approach (2nd ed.). Philadelphia: W.B. Saunders.

Jeng, L., & Robin, N. (2002). Progress in understanding genetics of impaired hearing. *Contemp Pediatr, 19*(6), 79.

Johnson, M., Bulechek, G., Dochterman, J.M., Maas, M., & Moorhead, S. (2001). *Nursing diagnosis outcomes and interventions: NANDA, NOC & NIC linkages.* St. Louis: Mosby.

Johnson, M., Maas, M., & Moorhead, S. (2000). *Nursing outcomes classification (NOC)* (2nd ed.). St. Louis: Mosby.

Kornfeld, J. (1997). Managed care from my perspective. *Hosp Pract, 32*(6), 45-52.

Lloyd-Puryear, M., & Fursman, I. (2002). Newborn screening and genetic testing. *J Obstet Gynecol Neonatal Nurs, 31*(2), 200-207.

McCloskey, J., & Bulechek, G. (2001). *Nursing interventions classification (NIC)* (3rd ed.). St. Louis: Mosby.

National Association for Home Care. (1995). *Basic statistics about home care.* Washington, DC: Author.

North American Nursing Diagnosis Assocation. (2001). *Nursing diagnoses: Definitions and classification 2001-2002.* Philadelphia: Author.

Pachter, L. (1997). Practicing culturally sensitive pediatrics. *Contemp Pediatr, 14*(9), 139.

Schuman, A. (1997). Home sweet home: The best place for pediatric care. *Contemp Pediatr, 14*(3), 79-104.

Tinkle, M., & Cheek, D. (2002). Human genomics: Challenges and opportunities. *J Obstet Gynecol Neonatal Nurs, 31*(2), 178-187.

U.S. Department of Health and Human Services. (2000). *Healthy People 2010: National Health Promotion and Disease Prevention Objectives.* DHHS Pub. No. (PHS) 91-50213. Washington, DC: Government Printing Office.

Ulrich, S., & Canale, S. (2001). *Nursing care planning guides.* (5th ed.) Philadelphia: W.B. Saunders.

U.S. National Commission on the International Year of the Child: Report to the President G.P.O. March 1980 (classic reference).

Wilkinson, J. (1996). *Nursing process: A critical thinking approach.* Reading, MA: Addison-Wesley.

Williams, J. (2000). Impact of genome research on children and families. *J Pediatr Nurs, 15*(4), 207-211.

Chapter 2 Human Reproductive Anatomy and Physiology

Burroughs, A., & Leifer, G. (2001). *Maternity nursing* (8th ed.). Philadelphia: W.B. Saunders.

Creasy, R., & Resnick, R. (1999). *Maternal-fetal medicine* (4th ed.). Philadelphia: W.B. Saunders.

Guyton, A., & Hall, J. (2000). *Textbook of medical physiology* (10th ed.). Philadelphia: W.B. Saunders.

Hacker, N., & Moore, J. (1998). *Essentials of obstetrics and gynecology* (3rd ed.). Philadelphia: W.B. Saunders.

Herlihy, B., & Maebius, N. (2000). *The human body in health and illness.* Philadelphia: W.B. Saunders.

Ladewig, P., London, M., Moberly, S., & Olds, S. (2002). *Maternal-newborn nursing* (5th ed.). Upper Saddle River, NJ: Prentice Hall Health.

Moore, K., & Persaud, T. (1998). *Before we are born: Essentials of embryology and birth defects* (5th ed.). Philadelphia: W.B. Saunders.

Thibodeau, G., & Patton, K. (1999). *Anatomy and physiology* (4th ed.). St. Louis: Mosby.

Thibodeau, G., & Patton, K. (2000). *Structure and function of the body* (11th ed.). St. Louis: Mosby.

Wilson, K., & Waugh, A. (1998). *Ross and Wilson anatomy and physiology in health and illness* (8th ed.). London: Churchill Livingstone.

Wylie, L. (2000). *Essential anatomy and physiology in maternity care.* London: Churchill Livingstone.

Chapter 3 Prenatal Development

Barker, D. (1998). *Mothers, babies and health in later life* (2nd ed.). London: Churchill Livingstone.

Brooks, S., Mitchell, A., & Steffenson, N. (2000). Mothers, infants, and DHA. *MCN, 25*(2), 71-75.

Brundage, S. (2002). Preconception health care. *Am Fam Physician, 65*(12), 2507-2514.

Burroughs, A., & Leifer, G. (2001). *Maternity nursing* (8th ed.). Philadelphia: W.B. Saunders.

Creasy, R., & Resnick, R. (1999). *Maternal-fetal medicine* (4th ed). Philadelphia: W.B. Saunders.

Desposito, F., et al. (2000). American Academy of Pediatrics Committee on Genetics: Folic acid for the prevention of neural tube defects. *Pediatrics, 101*(3), 335.

Faro, S. (2002). Why we shouldn't screen pregnant patients for bacterial vaginosis. *Contemp Obstet Gynecol, 47*(5), 136.

Guyton, A., & Hall, J. (2000). *Textbook of medical physiology* (10th ed.). Philadelphia: W.B. Saunders.

Herlihy, B., & Maebus, N. (2000). The human body in health and illness. Philadelphia: W.B. Saunders.

Ladewig, P., London, M., Moberly, S., & Olds, S. (2002). *Maternal-newborn nursing* (5th ed.). Upper Saddle River, NJ: Prentice Hall Health.

Lapp, T. (2000). ACOG addresses psychosocial screening in pregnant women. *Am Fam Pract, 62*(12), 2701.

Lea, D. (2002). Ahead to the past: How genetics is changing your practice. *Nursing 2002, 32*(6), 48.

Lockwood, C., D'Alton, M., Platt, L., & Bahado-Singh, R. (2001). New developments in ultrasound. *Contemp Obstet Gynecol, 46*(5), 12.

Moore, K., & Persaud, T. (1998). *The developing human: Clinically oriented embryology* (6th ed.). Philadelphia: W.B. Saunders.

Moore, K., & Persaud, T. (1998). *Before we are born: Essentials of embryology and birth defects* (5th ed.). Philadelphia: W.B. Saunders.

Stables, D. (1999). Physiology in childbearing with anatomy and related biosciences. London: Balliere-Tindall.

Thibodeau, G., & Patton, K. (1999). *Anatomy and physiology* (4th ed.). St. Louis: Mosby.

Thibodeau, G., & Patton, K. (2000). *Structure and function of the body* (11th ed.). St. Louis: Mosby.

U.S. Department of Health and Human Services. (2000). *Healthy People 2010: National Health Promotion and Disease Prevention Objectives.* DHHS Pub. No. (PHS) 91-50213. Washington, DC: Government Printing Office.

Walsh, D., & Adzick, S. (2000). Fetal surgical intervention. *Am J Perinatol, 17*(6), 277-283.

Wilcox, A., Weinberg, C., & Baird, D. (1995). Timing of sexual intercourse in relation to ovulation. *N Engl J Med, 333*(23), 1517-1521.

Wilson, K., & Waugh, A. (1998). *Ross and Wilson anatomy and physiology* (8th ed.). London: Churchill Livingstone.

Wylie, L. (2000). *Essential anatomy and physiology in maternity care.* London: Churchill Livingstone.

Chapter 4 Prenatal Care and Adaptations to Pregnancy

American Academy of Pediatrics & American College of Obstetricians and Gynecologists. (1997). Maternal and newborn nutrition. In *Guidelines for perinatal care* (4th ed.). Elk Grove Village, IL: American Academy of Pediatrics.

American College of Obstetricians and Gynecologists. (1994). Exercise during pregnancy and the postpartum period. *ACOG Technical Bulletin 189,* Washington, DC: Author.

Association of Women's Health, Obstetric, and Neonatal Nurses. Mattson, S., & Smith, J. (Eds.) (2000). *Core curriculum for maternal-newborn nursing* (2nd ed.). Philadelphia: W.B. Saunders.

Beckman, C., & Dysart, D. (2000). The challenge of multicultural care. *J Contemp Obstet Gynecol, 45*(2), 12.

Bond, L. (2000). Physiology in pregnancy. In S. Matteson & J. Smith (Eds.), *Core curriculum for maternal and newborn nursing* (2nd ed.). Washington, DC: Association of Women's Health, Obstetric, and Neonatal Nurses.

Briggs, G. (2001, Dec 15). Drugs, pregnancy, and lactation. *Fam Pract News,* p. 16.

Brooks, S., Mitchell, A., & Steffanson, N. (2000). Mothers, infants, and DHA. *MCN, 25*(2), 71-75.

Clapp, J. (2001). Recommending exercise during pregnancy. *J Contemp Obstet Gynecol, 46*(1), 30.

Clapp, J., Stepanchak, W., Tomaselli, J., Kortan, M., & Faneslow, S. (2000). Portal vein blood flow: Effects of pregnancy, gravity, and exercise. *Am J Obstet Gynecol, 183*(1), 167-172.

Creasy, R., & Resnick, R. (1999). *Maternal-fetal medicine* (4th ed.). Philadelphia: W.B. Saunders.

Hacker, N., & Moore, J. (1998). *Essentials of obstetrics and gynecology* (3rd ed.). Philadelphia: W.B. Saunders.

Kent, T., Gregor, J., Deardorff, L., & Katz, V. (1999). Edema of pregnancy: A comparison of water aerobics and static immersion. *Am J Ostet Gynecol, 94*(5 pt 1), 726-729.

Ladewig, P., London, M., Moberly, S., & Olds, S. (2002). *Maternal-newborn nursing* (5th ed.). Upper Saddle River, NJ: Prentice Hall Health.

Lapp, T. (2000). ACOG addresses psychosocial screening in pregnant women. *Am Fam Physician, 62*(12), 701-702.

Littleton, L., & Engelbretson, J. (2002). *Maternal, neonatal, and women's health nursing.* New York: Delmar.

Lowdermilk, D., Perry S., & Bobak, I. (2000). *Maternity and women's healthcare* (7th ed.). St. Louis: Mosby.

Mahan, L.K., & Escott-Stump, S. (2000). *Krause's food, nutrition and diet therapy* (10th ed.). Philadelphia: W.B. Saunders.

Matteson, P. (2001). *Women's health during the childbearing years.* St. Louis: Mosby.

Mattson, S. (2000). Providing culturally competent care. *Lifelines, 4*(5), 37-39.

McKinney, E., Ashwill, J., Murray, S., James, S., Gorrie, T., & Droske, S. (2000). *Maternal-child nursing.* Philadelphia: W.B. Saunders.

Menihan, C. (1996). Intrapartum fetal monitoring. In K.R. Simpson & P.A. Creehan (Eds.), *AWHONN's perinatal nursing* (pp. 187-225). Washington, DC: Association of Women's Health, Obstetric, and Neonatal Nurses.

Mindell, J., & Jacobson, B. (2000). Sleep disturbances during pregnancy. *J Obstet Gynecol Neonatal Nurs, 29*(6), 590-597.

Moore, K., & Persaud, T. (1998). *Before we are born: Essentials of embryology and birth defects* (5th ed.). Philadelphia: W.B. Saunders.

Morbidity and Mortality Weekly Report. (2001). Knowledge and use of folic acid among women of reproductive age. *MMWR, 50*(10), 185-89.

Murray, S., McKinney, E., & Gorrie, T. (2002). *Foundations of maternal-newborn nursing* (3rd ed.). Philadelphia: W.B. Saunders.

Ottani, P. (2002). Embracing global similarities: A framework for cross-cultural obstetrical care. *J Obstet Gynecol Neonatal Nurs, 31*(1), 33-38.

Quilligan, E., & Zuspan, F. (2000). *Current therapies in obstetrics and gynecology* (5th ed.). Philadelphia: W.B. Saunders.

Raychaudhuri, K., & Maresh, M. (2000). Glycemic control throughout pregnancy and fetal growth in insulin dependent diabetes. *Am J Obstet Gynecol, 95*:190-194.

Rubin, R. (1984). *Maternal identity and the maternal experience.* New York: Springer (classic reference).

Russell, R. (2001). *Dietary reference intakes.* USDA Human Nutrition Research Center on Aging, Tufts University, Boston Conference on Jan 9, 2001. Washington, DC: National Academy of Science.

Stables, D. (1999). *Physiology in childbearing with anatomy and related biosciences.* London: Balliere-Tindall.

Swinth, J., Nelson, L., Hadeed, A., & Anderson, G. (2000). Shared kangaroo care for triplets. *MCN, 25*(4), 214-216.

Teschendorf, M., & Evans, C. (2000). Hydrotherapy during labor. *MCN, 25*(4), 798.

Wylie, L. (2000). *Essentials of anatomy and physiology in maternity care.* London: Churchill Livingstone.

Chapter 5 Nursing Care of Women with Complications During Pregnancy

Bebbie, K., & Qureshi, K. (2002). Emergency and disaster preparedness: Core competencies for nurses. *Am J Nurs, 2*(1), 46.

Benirschke, K. (2001). Fetal consequences of amniotic fluid meconium. *Contemp Obstet Gynecol, 48*(6), 76.

Blake, D., & Woods, E. (2001). The future is here: Non-invasive diagnosis of STD in teens. *Contemp Obstet Gynecol, 46*(3), 103.

Briggs, G. (2001, Dec. 15). Drugs, pregnancy, and lactation. *Fam Pract News,* p. 16.

Buchanan, T., & Coustan, D. (1999). Diabetes mellitus. In G.N. Burrow & T.P. Duffy (Eds.), *Medical complications in pregnancy* (5th ed.). Philadelphia: W.B. Saunders.

Chames, M., & Sibai, B. (2001). When chronic hypertension complicates pregnancy. *Contemp Obstet Gynecol, 46*(4), 70.

Collins, T., Saltzman, R., & Jordan, M. (1999). Viral infections. In G.N. Burrow & T.P. Duffy (Eds.), *Medical complications during pregnancy* (5th ed.). Philadelphia: W.B. Saunders.

Control and prevention of rubella: Evaluation and management of suspected outbreaks, rubella in pregnant women and surveillance for congenital rubella syndrome. (2001). *MMWR, 50*(RR-12), 1-23.

Coustan, D. (2001). Oral hypoglycemic agents and OB/GYN. *Contemp Obstet Gynecol, 46*(4), 44.

Creasy, R., & Resnik, R. (1999). *Maternal-fetal medicine* (4th ed.). Philadelphia: W.B. Saunders.

Donahue, D. (2002). Diagnosis and treatment of herpes simplex infection during pregnancy. *J Obstet Gynecol Neonatal Nurs, 31*(1), 99-106.

Ferris, T. (1999). Hypertension and preeclampsia. In G.N. Burrow & T.P. Duffy (Eds.), *Medical complications in pregnancy* (5th ed.). Philadelphia: W.B. Saunders.

Garite, T., & Porreco, R. (2001). Evaluating fetal hypoxia with pulse oximetry. *Contemp Obstet Gynecol, 46*(7), 12.

Garner, E., Lipson, E., Bernstein, M., et al. (2001). Hydatidiform mole: What happens during next pregnancy. *Contemp Obstet Gynecol, 46*(7), 96.

Grose, C. (2000). Viral infections in the fetus and newborn. In R. Behrman, R. Kliegman, & H. Jenson (Eds.), *Nelson textbook of pediatrics* (16th ed.). Philadelphia: W.B. Saunders.

Hacker, N., & Moore, J. (1998). *Essentials of obstetrics and gynecology.* Philadelphia: W.B. Saunders.

Hager, W. (2001). Preventing group B streptococcal infections with targeted therapy. *Contemp Obstet Gynecol, 46*(3), 92.

Haggerty, L., Kelly, U., Hawkins, J., et al. (2001). Pregnant women's perceptions of abuse. *J Obstet Gynecol Neonatal Nursing, 30*(3), 283.

Holzemer, W. (2002). HIV and AIDS: The symptom experience: What cell counts and viral loads won't tell you. *Am J Nurs, 102*(4), 48-52.

Howard-Rubin, R. (2001). Disarm bioterrorism with knowledge and vigilance. *Spectrum, 2*(2), 26W.

Jenkins, T. (2001). Timing cerclage removal when the patient has PROM. *Contemp Obstet Gynecol, 46*(1), 53.

Kenner, C. (1998). Neonatal acquired immunodeficiency syndrome: Human immunodeficiency virus. In C. Kenner, J. Lott, & A. Flandermeyer (Eds.), *Comprehensive neonatal nursing: A physiologic perspective* (2nd ed., pp. 815-837). Philadelphia: W.B. Saunders.

Kurdas, C. (2001). New guidelines for detecting and managing hypertension in pregnancy. *Contemp Obstet Gynecol, 26*(2), 15.

Ladewig, P., London, M., Moberly, S., & Olds, S. (2002). *Maternalnewborn nursing* (5th ed.). Upper Saddle River, NJ: Prentice Hall Health.

Laros, R. (1999). Maternal hematological disorders. In R. Creasy & R. Resnik (Eds.), *Maternal-fetal medicine* (4th ed.). Philadelphia: W.B. Saunders.

Lee, R. (1999). Sexually transmitted infections. In G. Burrow & T. Duffy (Eds.), *Medical complications during pregnancy* (5th ed.). Philadelphia: W.B. Saunders.

Lewis, L. (2000). Which medications are safe in pregnancy. *Patient Care, 34*(24), 19.

Lockwood, C., D'Alton, M., Platt, L., & Bahado-Singh, R. (2001). New developments in ultrasound. *Contemp Obstet Gynecol, 46*(5), 12.

Lowdermilk, D., Perry, S., & Bobak, I. (2000). *Maternity and women's healthcare.* St. Louis: Mosby.

Mahan, L., & Escott-Stump, S. (2000). *Krause's food, nutrition and diet therapy.* Philadelphia: W.B. Saunders.

Matteson, P. (2001). *Women's health during the childbearing years.* St. Louis: Mosby.

Mattson, S., & Smith, J. (2000). *Core curriculum for maternal-newborn nursing* (2nd ed.). Washington, DC: Association of Women's Health, Obstetric, and Neonatal Nurses.

McAnulty, J., Metcalfe, J., & Ueland, K. (1999). Cardiovascular disease. In G. Burrow & T. Duffy (Eds.), *Medical complications during pregnancy* (5th ed.). Philadelphia: W.B. Saunders.

McCarter-Spaulding, D. (2002). Parvovirus B 19 in pregnancy. *J Obstet Gynecol Neonatal Nurs, 31*(1), 107-112.

Moore, T. (1999). Diabetes in pregnancy. In R. Creasy & R. Resnik (Eds.), *Maternal-fetal medicine* (4th ed.). Philadelphia: W.B. Saunders.

Neal, J. (2001). $Rh_o(D)$ isoimmunizations and current management modalities. *J Obstet Gynecol Neonatal Nurs, 30*(6), 589.

Persell, D., Arangie, P., Young, C., Stokes, E., Payne, W., Skorga, P., & Gilbert-Palmer, D. (2002). Preparing for bioterrorism. *Nursing 2002, 32*(2), 36-43.

Pymar, H., & Creinin, M. (2001). Offering mifepristone as an abortion option. *Contemp Obstet Gynecol, 26*(2), 113.

Raychaudhuri, K., & Maresh, M. (2000). Glycemic control throughout pregnancy and fetal growth in insulin dependent diabetes. *J Obstet Gynecol, 95*(2), 190-194.

Repke, T., & Sibai, B. (2001). Should mild preeclampsia be treated with magnesium sulfate. *Contemp Obstet Gynecol, 26*(3), 25.

Tiller, C. (2002). Chlamydia during pregnancy: Implications and impact on perinatal and neonatal outcome. *J Obstet Gynecol Neonatal Nurs, 31*(1), 93-98.

Weiss, J., & Malone, F. (2001). Caring for obese obstetrical patients. *Contemp Obstet Gynecol, 46*(6), 12.

Yost, N. (2001). Diagnosing and managing sickle cell disease in pregnancy. *Contemp Obstet Gynecol, 46*(3), 45.

Chapter 6 Nursing Care During Labor and Birth

American Academy of Pediatrics (AAP) and American College of Obstetricians and Gynecologists (ACOG). (1997). *Guidelines for perinatal care* (4th ed.). Elk Grove Village, IL; Washington, DC: Author.

Calhoun, S. (2000). Focus on fluids: Examining maternal hydration and amniotic fluid volume. *Lifelines, 3*(6), 20.

Callister, L. (1995). Cultural meanings of childbirth. *J Obstet Gynecol Neonatal Nurs 24*(4), 327-331.

Callister, L. (2001). Culturally competent care of women and newborns: Knowledge, attitude and skills. *J Obstet Gynecol Neonatal Nurs, 30*(2), 209-215.

Chamberlain, G., & Simpkins, P. (2000). *A practice of obstetrics and gynecology.* London: Churchill Livingstone.

Clayworth, S. (2000). The nurse's role during oxytocin administration. *MCN, 25*(2), 80-84.

Creasey, R., & Resnick, R. (1999). *Maternal-fetal medicine.* (4th ed.). Philadelphia: W.B. Saunders.

DeVoe, L., & McDaniel, T. (2002). Visual vs. computerized analysis of fetal heart rate changes. *Contemp Obstet Gynecol, 47*(5), 64.

Eason, E., & Feldman, P. (2000). Much ado about a little cut: Is an episiotomy worthwhile. *Obstet Gynecol, 95*(4), 616-618.

Gabbe, S., Niebyl, J., & Simpson, J. (2001). *Obstetrics: Normal and problem pregnancies* (4th ed.). London: Churchill Livingstone.

Green, C. (2000). *Critical thinking in nursing: Case studies across the curriculum.* Upper Saddle River, NJ: Prentice Hall Health.

Greenslate, K., & Creehan, P. (2000). Is there a role for the LPN in the care of women during labor and birth? *MCN, 25*(4), 176-177.

Greer, J., Cameron, I., Kitchner, H., & Prentice, A. (2000). *Mosby's color atlas and textbook of obstetrics.* St. Louis: Mosby

Ladewig, P., London, M., Moberly, S., & Olds, S. (2002). *Maternalnewborn nursing.* (5th ed.). Upper Saddle River, NJ: Prentice Hall Health.

Lipson, J., & Steiger, N. (1996). *Self care nursing in a multicultural context.* Thousand Oaks, CA: Sage Publishers.

Lipson, J., Dibble, S., & Minarik, P. (1998). *Culture and nursing care.* San Francisco: UCSF Nursing Press.

Lowdermilk, D., Perry, S., & Bobak, I. (2000). *Maternity and women's healthcare* (7th ed). St. Louis: Mosby.

Mattson, S. (2000). Striving for cultural competence. *AWHONN Lifelines, 4*(3), 48-52.

Mattson, S., & Smith, J. (Eds.) (2000). *Core curriculum for maternalnewborn nursing* (2nd ed.). Washington, DC: Association of Women's Health, Obstetric, and Neonatal Nurses.

Mayberry, L., Wood, S., Strange, L., Lee, L., Heisler, D., & NeilsonSmith, K. (2000). Managing second stage of labor. *AWHONN Lifelines, 3*(6), 28-34.

Minato, J. (2001). Is it time to push? *AWHONN Lifelines, 4*(6), 20-23.

Morey, S. (2000). ACOG develops guidelines for induction of labor. *Am Fam Physician, 62*(2), 445.

Murasaki, S. (1996). *Diary of Lady Murasaki.* New York: Penguin Press.

Ottani, P. (2002). Embracing global similarities: A framework for cross-cultural obstetrical care. *J Obstet Gynecol Neonatal Nurs, 31*(1), 33-38.

Putta, L., & Spencer, J. (2000). Assisted vaginal delivery using the vacuum extractor. *Am Fam Physician, 62*(6), 1316-1320.

Quilligan, E., & Zuspan, F. (2000). *Current therapy in obstetrics and gynecology* (5th ed.). Philadelphia: W.B. Saunders.

Shilling, T. (2000). Cultural perspectives on childbearing. In F. Nichols & S. Humenick (Eds.), *Childbirth education: practice, research, and theory* (2nd ed.). Philadelphia: W.B. Saunders.

Simpson, K., & Knox, E. (2001). Fundal pressure during the second stage of labor. *MCN, 26*(2), 64-70.

Simpson, K., & Porter, M. (2001). Fetal oxygen saturation monitoring. *AWHONN Lifelines, 5*(2), 26-33.

Teschendorf, M. (2000). Hydrotherapy during labor. *MCN, 25*(4), 198-203.

Thureen, P., Deacon, J., O'Neill, P., & Hernendez, J. (1999). *Assessment and care of the well newborn.* Philadelphia: W.B. Saunders.

VandeVusse, L. (1999). The essential forces of labor revisited. *MCN, 24*(4), 176-184.

Willis, W. (1999). Culturally competent nursing care during the perinatal period. *J Perinat Neonat Nurs, 13*(3), 45-59.

Wong, D., Perry, S., & Hockenberry, M. (2002). *Maternal-child nursing care* (2nd ed.). St. Louis: Mosby.

Chapter 7 Nursing Management of Pain During Labor and Birth

American Academy of Pediatrics and American College of Obstetricians and Gynecologists. (1997). *Guidelines for perinatal care* (4th ed.). Elk Grove Village, IL: Author.

American College of Obstetricians and Gynecologists (1996). ACOG Technical Bulletin Number 225: Obstetric analgesia and anesthesia. *Int J Gynecol Obstet, 54*(3), 281-292.

Callister, L. (2001). Culturally competent care for women and newborns: Knowledge, attitudes, and skills. *J Obstet Gynecol Neonatal Nurs, 30*(2), 209-215.

Creasy, R., & Resnick, R. (1999). *Maternal-fetal medicine* (4th ed.). W.B. Saunders.

Kee, R. (2001). A pre-emptive strike against postoperative pain. *Contemp Obstet Gynecol, 46*(4), 65-75.

Kingsley, C. (2001). Epidural analgesia: Your role. *RN, 64*(3), 53-57.

Ladewig, P., London, M., Moberly, S., & Olds, S. (2002). *Maternal-newborn nursing* (5th ed.). Upper Saddle River, NJ: Prentice Hall Health.

Lowdermilk, D., Perry, S., & Bobak, I. (2000). *Maternity and women's health care* (7th ed.). St. Louis: Mosby.

Managing epidurals: Exploring the nurse's role and AWHONN's newest position statement. (2001). *AWHONN Lifelines, 5*(4), 27-29.

Mattson, S. (2000). Providing culturally competent care. *AWHONN Lifelines, 4*(5), 37-39.

McKinney, E., Ashwill, J., Murray, S., James, S., Garrie, S., & Droske, S. (2000). *Maternal-child nursing.* Philadelphia: W.B. Saunders.

Smiley, R. (2002). Epidural anesthesia: Update 2002. *Contemp Obstet Gynecol, 47*(6), 32.

Quilligan, E., & Zuspan, F. (2000). *Current therapy in obstetrics and gynecology* (5th ed.). Philadelphia: W.B. Saunders.

Chapter 8 Nursing Care of Women with Complications During Labor and Birth

American Academy of Pediatrics and American College of Obstetricians and Gynecologists. (1997). *Guidelines for perinatal care* (4th ed.). Elk Grove Village, IL: Author.

American College of Obstetricians and Gynecologists. (1995a). *Technical Bulletin No. 196: Operative vaginal delivery.* Washington, DC: Author.

American College of Obstetricians and Gynecologists. (1995b). *Technical Bulletin No. 218: Dystocia and the augmentation of labor.* Washington, DC: Author.

Andrews, W., Copper, R., Hauth, J., Goldenberg, R., Neely, C., & Dubard, M. (2000). Second trimester cervix ultrasound. *Obstet Gynecol, 95*(2), 222-226.

Bell, J., Campbell, D., Graham, W., Penney, G., Ryan, M., & Hall, M. (2001). Do obstetric complications explain high cesarean section rates among women over 30? *BMJ, 322*(7291), 894-895.

Briggs, G. (2001, Dec. 15). Drug, pregnancy, and lactation. *Fam Pract News,* p. 16.

Burroughs, A., & Leifer, G. (2001). *Maternity nursing* (8th ed.). Philadelphia: W.B. Saunders.

Creasy, R., & Resnick, R. (1999). *Maternal-fetal medicine* (4th ed.). Philadelphia: W.B. Saunders.

Cunningham, F., MacDonald, P., Gant, N., Leveno, K., Gilstrap, L., Hankins, G., et al. (1997). *Williams' obstetrics* (20th ed.). Norwalk, CT: Appleton & Lange.

Fischer, J., & Newton, W. (2001). Should we use Foley catheter for preinduction cervical ripening. *J Fam Pract, 50*(8), 655.

Hacker, N., & Moore, J. (1998). *Essentials of obstetrics and gynecology* (3rd ed.). Philadelphia: W.B. Saunders.

Hannah, M., Hannah, W., Hewson, S., Hodnett, E., Saigal, S., & Willan, A. (2000). Planned cesarean section vs planned vaginal birth for breech presentation at term. *Lancet. 356*(9239), 1375-1383.

Ladewig, P., London, M., Moberly, S., & Olds, S. (2002). *Maternal-newborn nursing* (5th ed.). Upper Saddle River, NJ: Prentice Hall Health.

Lowdermilk, D., Ferry, S., & Bobak, J. (2000). *Maternity and women's health care* (7th ed.). St. Louis: Mosby.

Mead, P., Dinsmoor, M., & Gibbs, R. (2000). Bacterial vaginosis in pregnancy. *Cont Obstet Gynecol, 45*(12), 37.

Murray, S., McKinney, E., & Gorrie, T. (2002). *Foundations of maternal-newborn nursing* (3rd ed.). Philadelphia: W.B. Saunders.

National Center for Health Statistics. (1996). *Healthy people 2000 review: 1995-1996.* Hyattsville, MD: Author.

National Center for Health Statistics. (2001); http://www.cdc.gov/nchs.

Ramos, L., & Kaunitz, A. (2001). Reassessing the value of maintenance tocolyses in preterm labor. *Contemp Obstet Gynecol, 46*(7), 45.

Sanz, L. (2001). Managing episiotomies and their complications. *Contemp Obstet Gynecol, 46*(5), 51.

Schwartz, M., & O'Grady, J. (2002). The obstetric vacuum extractor: Recent innovations and best practices. *Contemp Obstet Gynecol, 47*(5), 114.

Shipp, T., Zelop, C., Repke, J., Cohen, A., Caughey, A., & Lieberman, E. (2000). Labor after previous cesarean. *Obstet Gynecol, 95*(6 pt 1), 913-916.

Stables, D. (1999). *Physiology in childbearing with anatomy and related biosciences.* London: Builliere-Tindall.

Zamorski, M., & Biggs, W. (2001). Management of suspected fetal macrosomia. *Am Fam Physician, 63*(2), 302-306.

Zuspan, F., & Quilligan, E. (2000). *Current therapy in obstetrics and gynecology* (5th ed.). Philadelphia: W.B. Saunders.

Chapter 9 The Family After Birth

American Academy of Pediatrics and American College of Obstetricians and Gynecologists. (1997). *Guidelines for perinatal care* (4th ed.). Elk Grove Village, IL; Washington, DC: Author.

Barringer, S., & Williams, A. (2000). Perinatal HIV transmission. *Adv Nurse Pract,* 69.

Biancuzzo, M. (1999). *Breastfeeding the newborn: Clinical strategies for nurses.* St. Louis: Mosby.

Britt, R., & Pasero, C. (1999). Using analgesics during breastfeeding. *Am J Nurs, 99*(9), 20.

Cahill, J., & Wagner, C. (2002). Challenges in breastfeeding. *Contemp Pediatr, 19*(5), 94.

Clark, S. et al. (2000). Coumadin derivatives and breastfeeding. *Obstet Gynecol, 95*:938-940.

Control and prevention of rubella: Evaluation and management of suspected outbreaks, rubella in pregnant women and surveillance for congenital rubella syndrome. (2001). *MMWR, 50*(RR-12), 1-23.

Dennis, C., (2002). Breastfeeding initiation and duration: A 1990-2000 literature review. *J Obstet Gynecol Neonatal Nurs, 31*(1), 12-32.

Georgieff, M. (2001). Taking a rational approach to the choice of formula. *Cont Ped, 18*(8), 112.

Hill, P. (2000). Update on breastfeeding. *MCN, 25*(5), 248-251.

Krist, A. (2001). Obstetric care in patients with HIV disease. *Am Fam Physician, 63*(1), 107-116, 121-122.

Lowdermilk, D., Perry, S., & Bobak, I. (2000). *Maternity and women's healthcare.* St. Louis: Mosby.

Lund, C., Osborne, J., Kuller, J., Lane, A., Lott J., & Raines, D. (2001). Neonatal skin care: Clinical outcomes of AWHONN/NANN evidence based clinical practice guideline. *J Obstet Gynecol Neonatal Nurs, 30*(1), 41-51.

Moreland, J., & Coombs, J. (2000). Promoting and supporting breastfeeding. *Am Fam Physician, 61*(7), 2093-2100, 2103-2104.

Mortality and Morbidity Weekly Report. (2001). *50* (RR-12), 1-24.

Mortality and Morbidity Weekly Report. (2002). *51* (RR-2), 1-35.

Murray, S., McKinney, E., & Gorrie, T. (2002). *Foundations of maternal-newborn nursing* (3rd ed.). Philadelphia: W.B. Saunders.

Nikoden, V., Danziger, D., Gebka, N., Gulmezoglu, A., & Hofmeyr, G. (1993). Do cabbage leaves prevent breast engorgement: A randomized control study. *Birth, 20*(2), 61-64.

Ringdahl, E. (2002). Promoting postpartum exercise. *Sportsmedicine, 30*(2), 31.

Riordan, J., & Gil-Hopple, K. (2001). Breastfeeding care in multicultural populations. *J Obstet Gynecol Neonatal Nurs, 30*(2), 216-223.

Schanlen, R. (Ed.). Breastfeeding (2001). *Pediatr Clin North Am 48* (1 & 2), 1-261.

Stables, D. (1999). *Physiology in childbearing with related anatomy and biosciences.* London: Balliere-Tindall.

Thureen, P., Deacon, J., O'Neill, P., & Hernandez, J. (1999). *Assessment and care of the well newborn.* Philadelphia: W.B. Saunders.

Tiedje, L., Schiffman, R., Omar, M., Wright, J., Buzzitta, C., McCann, A., et al. (2002). An ecological approach to breastfeeding. *MCN, 27*(3), 154-161.

Walling, A. (2000). Which oral anticoagulants are safe during breastfeeding. *Am Fam Physician, 62*(12), 2669.

Wilkinson, M., & Murtip. (1996). Effects of storage, time, temperature, and composition of containers on biological components of human milk. *J Hum Lact, 12,* 31-35.

Wilson, A., Forsyth, J., Greene, S., Irvine, L., Hau C., & Howie, P. (1998). Relationship of infant diet to childhood health. *BMJ, 316* (7124), 21-25.

Chapter 10   Nursing Care of Women with Complications Following Birth

Cunningham, F., MacDonald, P., Gant, N., Leveno, K., Gilstrap, L., Hankins, G., et al. (1997). *Williams obstetrics* (20th ed.). Norwalk, CT: Appleton & Lange.

Geissler, I., & Braucht, N. (1999). The health needs of homeless women. In L. Wallis (Ed.), *Textbook of women's health.* Philadelphia: J.B. Lippincott.

Hacker, N., & Moore, J. (1998). *Essentials of obstetrics and gynecology* (3rd ed.). Philadelphia: W.B. Saunders.

Ladewig, P., London, M., Moberly, S., & Olds, S. (2002). *Maternal-newborn nursing* (5th ed.). Upper Saddle River, NJ: Prentice Hall Health.

Lund, C., Osborne, J., Kuller, J., Lane, A., Lott J., & Raines, D. (2001). Neonatal skin care: Clinical outcomes of AWHONN/NANN evidence based clinical practice guideline. *J Obstet Gynecol Neonatal Nurs, 30*(1), 41-51.

Matteson, P. (2001). *Women's health during the childbearing years.* St. Louis: Mosby.

McKinney, E., Ashwill, J., Murray, S., James, S., Gorrie, T., & Droske, S. (2000). *Maternal-child nursing.* Philadelphia: W.B. Saunders.

Mendenhall, A., & Eichenfield, L. (2000). Caring for newborn's skin. *Contemp Pediatr, 17*(8), 98.

Murray, S., McKinney, E., & Gorrie, T. (2002). *Foundations of maternal-newborn nursing* (3rd ed.). Philadelphia: W.B. Saunders.

Rice, M., Records, K., & Williams, M. (2001). Postpartum depression. *Nurse Pract, 5*(4), 1-4.

Singla, A., Berkowitz, R., Saphier, C. (2002). Obstetric hemorrhage in Jehovah's Witness. *Contemp Obstet Gynecol, 47*(4), 32.

Stables, D. (1999). *Physiology in childbearing with anatomy and related sciences.* London: Bailliere-Tindall.

Wong, D., Perry, S., & Hockenberry, M. (2002). *Maternal-child nursing care* (2nd ed.). St. Louis: Mosby.

Chapter 11   The Nurse's Role in Women's Health Care

Alexander, N. (2002). New methods of delivering hormonal contraception. *Contemp Obstet Gynecol, 47,* 44-48.

American Cancer Society. (1999). *Cancer facts and figures 1999.* New York: Author.

American College of Obstetricians and Gynecologists. (1996). *Guidelines for women's health care.* Washington, DC: Author.

American College of Obstetricians and Gynecologists. (1999a) *ACOG Technical Bulletin, 226*(7), 886-893.

American College of Obstetricians and Gynecologists. (1999b). *Primary and preventive care: Periodic assessments: ACOG Committee Opinion.* Washington, DC: Author.

Andrist, L. (2001). Vaginal health and infections. *J Obstet Gynecol Neonatal Nurs, 30*(3), 306-315.

Archer, D., & Utian, W. (2001). Decisions in prescribing HRT. *Contemp Obstet Gynecol, 46*(8), 86.

Bachmann, G., & Nevadunsky, N. (2000). Diagnosis and treatment of atrophic vaginitis. *Am Fam Physician, 61*(10), 3090-3096.

Barnard, N., Scialli, A., Hurlock, D., & Bertron, P. (2000). Diet and sex hormone binding globulin, dysmenorrhea, and PMS. *Obstet Gynecol, 95*(2), 245-250.

Baxter, P. (2001). Midlife changes in sexual response. *Adv Nurs Pract, 9*(3), 67.

Benjamin, S., Gallagher, R., & Helms, J. (2001). Complimentary approaches to chronic pain. *Patient Care, 35*(4), 21.

Blake, D., & Woods E. (2001). The future is here: Non-invasive diagnosis of STDs in teens. *Contemp Obstet Gynecol, 46*(3), 103-121.

Boehm, D. (2001). Women and HIV/AIDS. *J Obstet Gynecol Neonatal Nurs, 30*(3), 342-350.

Boston's Women's Health Book Collective. (1998). *The new our bodies ourselves.* New York: Simon & Schuster.

Budd, B. (2000). Genital herpes in adolescents. *Adv Nurs Pract, 8*(3), 30-34.

Burk, R. (1999). HPV. *Hosp Pract, 34*(12), 103-111.

Cates, W. (2001). Treating STDs to help control HIV infection. *Contemp Obstet Gynecol, 46*(19), 107.

Centers for Disease Control; http://www.cdc.gov.

Choe, J. (2000). Urinary control devices for stress incontinence in women. *Adv Nurs Pract,* p. 65.

Connelly, E. (1999). Are one size fits all prescriptions becoming a thing of the past. *Am J Nurs, 99*(8), 46.

Culligan, P., & Heit, M. (2000). Urinary incontinence in women. *Am Fam Physician, 62*(11), 2433-2452.

Cutson, T., & Meuleman, E. (2000). Managing menopause. *Am Fam Physician, 61*(5), 1391-1406.

Davidson, M. (2001). Managing uterine fibroids: New approach to medication. *Clin Rev, 11*(6), 79.

Dinsmore, M. (2000). Managing HIV infected patient. *Contemp Obstet Gynecol, 45*(12), 52.

Egan, M., & Lipsky, M. (2000). Diagnosis of vaginitis. *Am Fam Physician, 62*(5), 1095-1104.

Foureroy, J. (2001). Overactive bladder. *Adv Nurs Pract, 9*(3), 59.

George, S. (2002). The menopause experience: A woman's perspective. *J Obstet Gynecol Neonatal Nurs, 31*(1), 77-85.

Goldman, M., & Hatch, M. (2000). *Women and health.* San Francisco: Academic Press.

Grimes, D., Hinson, V., & Sandheimer. (2001). New approaches to emergency contraception. *Contemp Obstet Gynecol, 46*(6), 59.

Hill, D., Weiss, N., Beresford, S., Voigt, L., Daling, J., Stanford, J., et al. (2000). Continuous and combined HRT and risk of endometrial cancer. *Am J Obstet Gynecol, 183*(6), 1456-1461.

Isaacson, K. (2001). Endometrial ablation: Is one technique best? *Contemp Obstet Gynecol, 46*(7), 11.

Jones, C. (2001). Premenstrual dysphoric disorder. *Adv Nurs Pract, 9*(3), 87.

Katz, A. (2002). Sexuality after hysterectomy. *J Obstet Gynecol Neonatal Nurs, 31*(3), 256-262.

Kaunitz, A. (2001). Choosing to menstruate or not. *Patient Care, 35*(4), 72.

Keye, W., Chang, R., Rebar, R., & Soules, M. (1995). *Infertility: Evaluation and treatment.* Philadelphia: W.B. Saunders.

Klingman, L. (1999). Assessing the female reproductive system. *Am J Nurs, 99*(8), 37-43.

Lapp, T. (2000). ACOG issues: Recommendations for management of endometriosis. *Am Fam Physician, 62*(6), 1431-1434.

LeBlanc, E., Janowsky, J., Chan, B., & Nelson, H. (2001). Hormone replacement therapy and cognition. *JAMA, 285*(11), 1489-1499.

Lindsay, S. (2000). Menopause naturally: Exploring alternatives to traditional hormone replacement therapy. *AWHONN Lifelines, 3*(5), 32-38.

Lowdermilk, D., Perry, S., & Bobak, I. (2000). *Maternity and women's healthcare* (7th ed.). Mosby.

Mastroianni, L., Ravnikar, V., & Wooten, W. (2001) Assessing and maintaining bone health in the postmenopausal woman. *Contemp Obstet Gynecol, 46*(10), 44.

Matteson, P. (2001). *Women's health during the childbearing years.* St. Louis: Mosby.

Mead, P., Dinsmoor, M., & Gibbs, R. (2000). Bacterial vaginosis in pregnancy. *Contemp Obstet Gynecol, 45*(12), 37.

Merchant, J., Oh, K., & Klerman, L. (1999). Douching: A problem for adolescent girls and young women. *Arch Pediatr Adolesc Med, 153*(8), 834-837.

Miller, K., & Graves, C. (2000). Update on prevention and treatment of STDs. *Am Fam Physician, 61*(2), 379-386.

Morris, B., Young, C., & Kearney, K. (2000). Emergency contraception. *Am J Nurs, 100*(9), 46-48.

Morrow, M. (2000). The evaluation of common breast problems. *Am Fam Physician, 61*(8), 2371-2385.

Murray, S., McKinney, E., & Gorrie, T. (2002). *Foundations of maternal-newborn nursing* (3rd ed.). Philadelphia: W.B. Saunders.

Peters, S. (2000). Condom sense: Reducing condom mistakes. *Adv Nurs Pract, 8*(4), 47-49.

Pirog, E. (2001). Is cervical cancer caused by HPV infection? *Contemp Obstet Gynecol, 46*(7), 69.

Priestley, C., Jones, B., Dhar, J., & Goodwin, L. (1997). What is normal vaginal flora? *Genitourin Med, 13,* 23-28.

Rawlins, S. (2001). Nonviral sexually transmitted infections. *J Obstet Gynecol Neonatal Nurs, 30*(3), 324-331.

Richart, R., Cox, T., Davey, D., & Wright, T. (2001). Bethesda 2001: How the new pap terminology will impact clinical practice. *Contemp Obstet Gynecol, 46*(10), 14.

Richart, R., Cox, T., Twiggs, L., et al. (2002). A sea of change in diagnosis and management of HPV and cervical disorders. *Contemp Obstet Gynecol, 47*(6), 67

Ringdahl, E. (2000). Treatment of recurrent vulvovaginal candidiasis. *Am Fam Physician, 61*(11), 3306-3317.

Saunders, C. (2000). Monitoring HPV infection. *Patient Care,* 142.

Schrager, S. (2002). Abnormal uterine bleeding associated with hormonal contraception. *Am Fam Physician, 65*(10), 2073-2080.

Schwartz, M., Klein, A., & McLucas, B. (2001). Using uterine artery embolization to treat fibroids. *Contemp Obstet Gynecol, 46*(8).

Scott, L., & Hasik, K. (2001). The similarities and differences of endometritis and pelvic inflammatory disease. *J Obstet Gynecol Neonatal Nurs, 30*(3), 332-341.

Shepherd, J., & Muto, M. (2000). Testing for genetic susceptibility to ovarian and breast cancer. *Patient Care 34*(11), 131-153.

Smith, S. (2000). Uterine fibroid embolization. *Am Fam Physician, 61*(12), 3601-3612.

Speroff, L. (2001). Postmenopausal estrogen therapy and ovarian cancer. *Contemp Obstet Gynecol, 46*(5), 77.

Speroff, L., & Mazzaferrie. (2001). HRT. *Hosp Pract, 36*(5), 37-45.

Stamm, C., & McGregor, J. (2001). Diagnosis and treatment of STDs in young women. *Contemp Pediatr, 18*(2), 53.

Stone, M., Westley, E., & Cullens, V. (2002). Emergency contraception. *Contemp Obstet Gynecol, 47*(3), 106.

Stumpf, P. (2001). Screening patients for osteoporosis. *Contemp Obstet Gynecol, 46,* 31.

Swenson, D. (2001). Pap smear testing during pregnancy. *Adv Nurs Pract, 9*(8), 53.

Thomas, D. (2001). Sexually transmitted viral infections: Epidemiology and treatment. *J Obstet Gynecol Neonatal Nurs, 30*(3), 316-323.

Tumolo, J. (2000). Update on contraception. *Adv Nurse Pract, 8*(8), 74-80.

Viera, A., & Larkins-Pettigrew, M. (2000). Practical use of the pessary. *Am Fam Physician, 61*(9), 2719-2729.

Vlastos, A., Richards-Kartum, R., Zuluaga, A., & Fallen, M. (2002). New approaches to cervical cancer screening. *Contemp Obstet Gynecol, 47*(5), 87.

Walsh, C., & Irwin, K. (2002). Combatting the silent chlamydia epidemic. *Contemp Obstet Gynecol, 47*(4), 90.

Weis, B. (2001). HIV in adolescents. *Adv Nurs Pract, 9*(3), 44.

Yen, S., Jaffe, R., & Barbieri, R. (1999). *Reproductive endocrinology: Physiology pathophysiology, and clinical management* (4th ed.). W.B. Saunders.

Zawacki, K., & Phillips, M. (2002). Cancer, genetics, and women's health. *J Obstet Gynecol Neonatal Nurs, 31*(2), 208-216.

Zinger, M., & Thomas, M. (2001). Using the levonorgestrel IUS. *Contemp Obstet Gynecol, 46*(5), 35.

Chapter 12 The Term Newborn

Behrman, R., Kliegman, R., & Jenson, H. (2000). *Nelson textbook of pediatrics* (16th ed.). Philadelphia: W.B. Saunders.

Beyea, S. (1996). *Critical pathways for collaborative nursing care.* Reading, MA: Addison-Wesley.

Brazelton, T.B. (1973). *The neonatal behavioral assessment scale.* Philadelphia: J.B. Lippincott (classic reference).

Cookfair, J. (1996). *Nursing care in the community* (2nd ed.). St. Louis: Mosby.

Kaufman, M., Clark, J., & Castro, C. (2001). Neonatal circumcision: Benefits, risks, family teaching. *MCN, 26*(4), 197-201.

Ladewig, P., London, M., Moberly, S., & Olds, S. (2002). *Maternal-newborn nursing* (5th ed.). Upper Saddle River, NJ: Prentice Hall Health.

Masters-Harte, L., & Abdel-Rahman, S. (2001). Sucrose analgesia for minor procedures in newborn infants. *Ann Pharmacother, 35*(7-8), 947-952.

McCartney, P. (2000). Bulb syringes in newborn care. *MCN, 25*(4), 217.

Mendenhall, A., & Eichenfield, L. (2000). Back to basics: Caring for newborn skin. *Contemp Pediatr, 17*(8), 98.

Moon, R., Patel, K., & Schaefer, S. (2000). Sudden infant death syndrome in child care settings. *Pediatrics, 106,* 295-300.

Murray, S., McKinney, E., & Gorrie, T. (2002). *Foundations of maternal-newborn nursing* (3rd ed.). Philadelphia: W.B. Saunders.

National Center for Health Statistics; http://www.cdc.gov/nchs.

Thureen, P., Deacon, J., O'Neill, P., & Hernandez, J. (1999). *Assessment and care of the well newborn.* Philadelphia: W.B. Saunders.

United States Preventative Service Task Force. (2001). Newborn hearing screening: Recommendations and rationales. *Am Fam Physician, 64*(12), 1995.

U.S. Department of Health and Human Services. (1992). Acute pain management in infants, children, and adolescents: Operative and medical procedures. (AHCPR 92-0020). Washington, DC: U.S. Government Printing Office.

U.S. Department of Health and Human Services. (2000). *Healthy People 2010: National Health Promotion and Disease Prevention Objectives.* DHHS Pub. No. (PHS) 91-50213. Washington, DC: Government Printing Office.

Wong, D., Wilson, D., & Hockenberry-Eaton, M. (2001). *Wong's Essentials of pediatric nursing* (6th ed.). St. Louis: Mosby.

Chapter 13 Preterm and Postterm Newborns

American Academy of Pediatrics Committee on Injury and Poison Prevention and Committee on Newborn. (1996). Safe transportation of premature and LBW infants. *Pediatrics, 97*(5), 758-760.

Barkin, R., & Rosen, P. (1999). *Emergency pediatrics: A guide to ambulatory care* (5th ed.). St. Louis: Mosby.

Behrman, R., Kliegman, R., & Jenson, H. (2000). *Nelson textbook of pediatrics* (16th ed.). Philadelphia: W.B. Saunders.

Blackburn, S., & Loper, D. (1992). *Maternal, fetal, and neonatal physiology.* Philadelphia: W.B. Saunders.

Cerrato, P. (2001). An authoritative voice on antenatal corticosteroids. *Contemp Obstet Gynecol, 46*(3), 125-131.

Creasy, R., & Resnik, R. (1999). *Maternal-fetal medicine* (4th ed.). Philadelphia: W.B. Saunders.

Demasio, K., & Bahado-Singh, R. (2002). Fetal growth restriction: An evidence-based approach. *Contemp Obstet Gynecol, 47*(6), 53.

Engler, A., Ludington-Hoe, S., Cusson, R., Adams, R., Bahnsen, M., Brumaugh, E., et al. (2002). Kangaroo care: National survey of practice, knowledge, barriers, and perceptions. *MCN, 27*(3), 146-153.

Franck, L., Quinn, D., & Zahr, L. (2000). Effect of less frequent bathing on preterm infants skin flora and pathogenic colonization. *J Obstet Gynecol Neonatal Nurs, 29*(6), 584-589.

Gartner, L., & Dixit, R. (2000). The jaundiced newborn: Minimizing the risks. *Patient Care, 34*(6), 89.

Guyton, A., & Hall, J. (2000). Textbook of medical physiology (10th ed.). Philadelphia: W.B. Saunders.

Lund, C., Kuller, D., Lane, A., Lott, J., Raines, D., & Thomas, K. (2001). Neonatal skin care. *J Obstet Gynecol Neonatal Nurs, 30*(1), 41-51.

McCoy, S. (2001). Neonatal sepsis. *Adv Nurs Pract, 9*(6), 89.

Medoff-Cooper, B., McGrath, J., & Bilker, W. (2000). Nutritive sucking and neurobehavioral development in preterm infants from 34 weeks PCA to term. *MCN, 25*(2), 64-70.

Mendenhall, A., & Eichenfield, L. (2000). Caring for newborn's skin. *Contemp Pediatr, 17*(8), 98.

Murray, S., McKinney, E., & Gorrie, T. (2002). *Foundations of maternal-newborn nursing* (3rd ed.). Philadelphia: W.B. Saunders.

Swinth, J., & Nelson, L., Hadeed, A., & Anderson, G. (2000). Shared kangaroo care for triplets. *MCN, 25*(4), 214-216.

Thureen, P., Deacon, J., O'Neill, P., & Hernandez, J. (1999). *Assessment and care of the well newborn.* Philadelphia: W.B. Saunders.

Wong, D., Wilson, D., & Hockenberry-Eaton, M. (2001). *Wong's Essentials of pediatric nursing* (6th ed.). St. Louis: Mosby.

Chapter 14 The Newborn with a Congenital Malformation

Behrman, R., Kliegman, R., & Jenson, H. (2000). *Nelson textbook of pediatrics* (16th ed.). Philadelphia: W.B. Saunders.

Bender, P. (2000). Genetics of cleft lip and palate. *J Pediatr Nurs, 15*(4), 242-249.

Burke, S., Kaufmann, E., Harrison, M., & Wiskin, N. (1999). Assessment of stressors in families with a child who has a chronic condition. *MCN, 24*(2), 98-106.

Dixit, R., & Gartner, L. (2000). The jaundiced newborn. *Patient Care, 34*(2), 45.

Fanaroff, A., & Martin, R. (2001). *Neonatal-perinatal medicine: Diseases of the fetus and infant* (7th ed.). St. Louis: Mosby.

Jackson, P., & Vessey, J. (2000). *Primary care of the child with a chronic condition* (3rd ed.). St. Louis: Mosby.

Johns Hopkins Hospital. (2000). *Harriet Lane handbook* (15th ed.). St. Louis: Mosby.

Krist, A., & Crawford-Faucher, A. (2002). Management of newborns exposed to maternal HIV infection. *Am Fam Physician, 65*(10), 2049-2056.

Ladewig, P., London, M., Moberly, S., & Olds, S. (2002). *Maternal-newborn nursing* (5th ed.). Upper Saddle River, NJ: Prentice Hall Health.

Levine, M., Carey, W., & Crocker, A. (1999). *Developmental-behavioral pediatrics* (3rd ed.). Philadelphia: W.B. Saunders.

Lewis, J. (2001). Understanding genetics in nursing. *Lifelines, 5*(2), 50-56.

March of Dimes Perinatal Data Center. (1997). Statbook: Statistics for monitoring maternal and infant health. Washington, DC: Author.

Metheny, N., & Titler, M. (2001). Assessing placement of feeding tubes. *Am J Nurs, 101*(5), 36-45.

Meyer, K. (1999). Using kangaroo care in a clinical setting with full term infants having feeding problems. *MCN, 24*(4), 190-192.

Newberger, D. (2000). Down's syndrome: Prenatal risk assessment and diagnosis. *Am Fam Physician, 62*(4), 825-838.

Porter, M., & Dennis, B. (2002). Hyperbilirubinemia in the term newborn. *Am Fam Physician, 65*(4), 599-606.

Seidel, H., Rosenstein, B., & Pathak, A. (2001). *Primary care of the newborn* (3rd ed.). St. Louis: Mosby.

Serwint, J., & Rutherford, K. (2000). Sharing bad news with parents. *Contemp Pediatr, 17*(3), 45.

Walsh, D., & Adzick, N. (2000). Fetal intervention: Where we are and where are we going. *Contemp Pediatr, 17*(6), 3.

Wong, D., Wilson, D., & Hockenberry-Eaton, M. (2001). *Wong's Essentials of pediatric nursing* (6th ed.). St. Louis: Mosby.

Chapter 15 An Overview of Growth, Development, and Nutrition

Barker, D. (1998). Mothers, babies, and health in later life. London: Churchill-Livingstone.

Bartholomey, S. (1994). Infant rice cereal: A simple ORT solution. *Pediatr Basic.* Fremont, MI: Gerber Products.

Beall, S. (2000). Addressing the health needs of children in foster care. *Adv Nurs Pract*, 61.

Behrman, R., Kliegman, R., & Jenson, H. (2000). *Nelson textbook of pediatrics* (16th ed.). Philadelphia: W.B. Saunders.

Booth, S., Sallis, J., Rittenbaugh, C., Hill, J., Birch, L., Frank, L., et al. (2001). Environmental and societal factors affect food choice and physical activity: Rationale, influences, and leverage points. *Nutr Rev, 59*(3), 21-40.

Cookfair, J. (1996). *Nursing care in the community* (2nd ed.). St. Louis: Mosby.

Ferrara, L. (2000). Drug therapy for children with ADHD. *Clin Lett Nurse Pract 4*(3), 9.

Griffen, A. (2000). Pediatric oral health. *Pediatr Clin North Am, 47*(5), 975-1188.

Levine, M., Carey, W., & Crocker, A. (1999). *Developmental-behavioral pediatrics* (3rd ed.). Philadelphia: W.B. Saunders.

Macknin, M., Piedmonte, M., Jacobs, J., & Skibinski, C. (2000). Symptoms associated with infant teething: A prospective study. *Pediatrics, 105*(4 pt 1), 747-752.

Mahan, L., & Escott-Stump, S. (2000). *Krause's food, nutrition and diet therapy* (10th ed.). Philadelphia: W.B. Saunders.

Nichols, M., & Livingston, D. (2002). Preventing pediatric obesity: Assessment and management in the primary care setting. *J Am Acad Nurs Pract, 14*(2), 55-62.

Roberts, S., & Dallal, G. (2001). The new childhood growth charts. *Nutrition Rev, 59*(2), 31-36.

Sanchez, O., & Childers, N. (2000). Anticipatory guidance in infant oral health: Rationale and recommendations. *Am Fam Physician, 61*(1), 115-124.

Seibold, E. (2000). A practical guide for developmental screening. *Clinical Lett Nurse Pract, 4*(3), 7.

Smilkstein, G., Ashworth, C., & Montano, D. (1984). The validity and reliability of the family APGAR as a test of family function. *J Fam Pract 15,* 303 (classic reference).

Wetter, A., Goldberg, J., King, A., Sigman-Grant, M., Baer, R., Crayton, E., et al. (2001). How and why do individuals make food and activity choices? *Nutr Rev, 59*(3), 11-21.

Wong, D., Wilson, D., & Hockenberry-Eaton, M. (2001). *Wong's Essentials of pediatric nursing* (6th ed.). St. Louis: Mosby.

Chapter 16 The Infant

American Academy of Pediatrics. (2000). AAP report on thimerosol in childhood vaccines. *Am Fam Physician, 61*(5), 1558.

Behrman, R., Kliegman, R., & Jenson, H. (2000). *Nelson textbook of pediatrics* (16th ed.). Philadelphia: W.B. Saunders.

Brooks, S., Mitchell, A., & Steffenson, N. (2000). Mothers, infants, and DHA: Implications for nursing practice. *MCN, 25*(2), 71-75.

Fleisher, D. (1998). Coping with colic. *Contemp Pediatr, 15*(6), 144.

Fournier, R., & Garpiel, S. (2002). Should parents be advised against bed-sharing with their infants. *MCN, 27*(1), 8-9.

Fowles, E. (1999). The Brazelton Neonatal Behavior Scale and maternal identity. *MCN, 24*(6), 287-293.

Levine, M., Carey, W., & Crocker, A. (1999). *Developmental-behavioral pediatrics* (3rd ed.). Philadelphia: W.B. Saunders.

Lund, C., Kuller, J., Lane, A., Lott, J., Raines, D., & Thomas, K. (2001). Neonatal skin care. *J Obstet Gynecol Neonatal Nurs, 30*(1), 41-51.

Mahan, L., & Escott-Stump, S. (2000). *Krause's food, nutrition, and diet therapy* (10th ed.). Philadelphia: W.B. Saunders.

Moon, R. (2001). Are you talking to your parents about SIDS? *Contemp Pediatr, 18*(3), 122-129.

Olsen, R., Barbaresi, W., & Olsen, G. (1998). Development in the first year of life. *Contemp Pediatr, 15*(7), 81.

Peckenpaugh, N., & Poleman, C. (1999). *Nutrition essentials and diet therapy* (8th ed.). Philadelphia: W.B. Saunders.

Schanler, R. (2001). Breastfeeding 2001: The management of breastfeeding. *Pediatr Clin North Am, 48*(2), 1-261.

Sigman-Grant, M., Bush, G., & Anentheswaran, R. (1992). Microwave heating of infant formula: A dilemma resolved. *Pediatrics, 90*(3), 414.

Wong, D., Wilson, D., & Hockenberry-Eaton, M. (2001). *Wong's Essentials of pediatric nursing* (6th ed.). St. Louis: Mosby.

Woods, A., & Benner, J. (2000). Visiting the CDC on the web. *Nursing 2000, 30*(6), 32.

Zimmerman, R. (2001). The 2001 recommended childhood immunization schedule. *Am Fam Physician, 63*(1), 151-154.

Chapter 17 The Toddler

Behrman, R., Kliegman, R., & Jenson, H. (2000). *Nelson textbook of pediatrics* (16th ed.). Philadelphia: W.B. Saunders.

Biagioli, F. (2002). Proper use of child safety seats. *Am Fam Physician, 65*(10), 2085-2090.

Eden, A. (1999). Helping toddlers eat right. *Contemp Pediatr, 16*(3), 197-201.

Flax, J., & Rapin, I. (1998). Evaluating children with delayed speech and language *Contemp Pediatr, 15*(10), 184.

Huffman, G. (2000). Swimming programs for infants and toddlers. *Pediatrics, 105,* 868-870.

Levine, M., Carey, W., & Crocker, A. (1999). *Developmental-behavioral pediatrics* (3rd ed.). Philadelphia: W.B. Saunders.

Mahan, L., & Escott-Stump, S. (2000). *Krause's food, nutrition and diet therapy* (10th ed.). Philadelphia: W.B. Saunders.

Monsen, R. (2001). Children and pets. *J Pediatr Nurs, 16*(3), 197-198.

Montgomery, T. (1994). When not talking is the chief complaint. *Contemp Pediatr, 11*(9), 49.

Schuman, A. (2001). Pediatric urban legends: Debunking common myths. *Contemp Pediatr, 18*(3), 115-120.

Wong, D., Wilson, D., & Hockenberry-Eaton, M. (2001). *Wong's Essentials of pediatric nursing* (6th ed.). St. Louis: Mosby.

Chapter 18 The Preschool Child

Anderson, J., & Bluestone, N. (2000). Breathholding spells. *Contemp Pediatr, 17*(1), 61.

Behrman, R., Kliegman, R., & Jenson, H. (2000). *Nelson textbook of pediatrics* (16th ed.). Philadelphia: W.B. Saunders.

Blockman, J. (1998). Children who refuse food. *Contemp Pediatr, 15*(10), 198.

Brazelton, T. (1993). *Touchpoints: Your child's emotional and behavioral development.* Reading, MA: Addison-Wesley.

Byrd, R. (1998). School readiness: More than a summer's work. *Contemp Pediatr, 15*(5), 39.

Fierro-Cobas, V., & Chan, E. (2001). Language development in bilingual children. *Contemp Pediatr, 18*(7), 79.

Flax, J., & Kapin, I. (1998). Evaluation of children with delayed speech and language. *Contemp Pediatr, 15*(10), 184.

Gaffney, K., Barndt-Inaglio, B., & Kollar, S. (2002). Early clinical assessment for harsh child discipline strategies. *MCN, 27*(1), 34-40.

Ivey, J. (2001). Children's responses to contact with elders. *MCN, 26*(1), 23-27.

Kelly, D., & Bullock, L. (2000). Grandfather-grandchild bonding. *MCN, 25*(4), 211-213.

Levine, M., Carey, W., & Crocker, A. (1999). *Developmental-behavioral pediatrics* (3rd ed.). Philadelphia: W.B. Saunders.

Montgomery, T. (1994). When children do not talk. *Contemp Pediatr, 11*(9), 49.

Scales, J., Fleisher, A., Sinal, S., & Krowchuk, D. (1999). Skin lesions that mimic abuse. *Contemp Pediatr, 16*(1), 136.

Thiedke, C. (2001). Sleeping disorders in children. *Am Fam Physician, 63*(2), 277-284.

Wong, D., Wilson, D., & Hockenberry-Eaton, M. (2001). *Wong's Essentials of pediatric nursing* (6th ed.). St. Louis: Mosby.

Chapter 19 The School-Age Child

Beck, A., & Meyers, N. (1996). Health enhancement and companion animal ownership. *Am Rev Public Health, 17,* 247-257.

Behrman, R., Kliegman, R., & Jenson, H. (2000). *Nelson textbook of pediatrics* (16th ed.). Philadelphia: W.B. Saunders.

Berlinger, J. (2001). Domestic violence. *Nursing 2000, 31*(8), 58.

Betz, C. (2000). Childhood obesity. *J Pediatr Nurs, 15*(3), 135-136.

Betz, C. (2000). The continuing challenge of empowering children and families. *J Pediatr Nurs, 15*(2), 269-271.

Bush, R., Fodal, R., & Van Metre, T. (1995). Taming your patient's animal allergies. *Patient Care, 29*(7), 71.

Byrd, R. (1998). School readiness: More than a summer's work. *Contemp Pediatr, 15*(5), 39.

Connelly, K. (1997). Advising families about pets. *Contemp Pediatr, 14*(2), 71.

Finan, S. (1997). Promoting healthy sexuality: Guidelines for the school-age child and adolescent. *Nurse Pract, 22*(11), 54-64.

Gershman, K., Socks, J., & Wright, J. (1994). Which dogs bite? A case-controlled study of risk factors. *Pediatrics, 93*(6 pt 1), 913-917.

Gidding, S. (2001). Controlling cholesterol in children. *Contemp Pediatr, 18*(3).

Gottesman, R., & Kelly, M. (2001). You can make a difference with these kids. *RN, 64*(6), 45-49.

Hart, B., & Hart, L. (1995). Selecting pet dogs on the basis of cluster analysis of breed behavior profiles and gender. *J Am Vet Med Assoc, 180*(11), 1181-1185.

Hesman, R., & Kelly, M. (2000). Helping children with disabilities to a brighter adulthood. *Contemp Pediatr, 17*(11), 42.

Jorgensen-Huston, C. (2001). Dogbites. *Nursing 2001, 31*(7), 88.

Le, T., & Dire, D. (2002). Managing human and animal bites. *Clinical Adv Nurs Pract, 5*(4), 27.

Kahn, J., & Emans, S. (1999). Gynecological exam of prepubertal girls. *Contemp Pediatr, 16*(3), 148.

Mahan, L., & Escott-Stump, S. (2000). *Krause's food, nutrition and diet therapy* (10th ed.). Philadelphia: W.B. Saunders.

Mulryan, K., Cathers, P., & Fagin, A. (2000). Combatting abuse: Protecting the child. *Nurs 2000, 30*(7), 39-43.

National Association of State Public Health Veterinarians, Inc. (2000). Compendium of animal rabies control. *MMWR, 46*(RR-4), 1.

Plaut, M., Zimmerman, E., & Goldstein, R. (1996). Health hazards to humans associated with domestic pets. *Am Rev Public Health, 17,* 221-245.

Quinlan, D. (2000). Dogbites in children. *Nursing Spectrum, 20*(3), 28-32.

Seigel, J. (1995). Pet ownership and the importance of pets among adolescents. *Anthrozoos, 8*(4), 217.

Shor, E. (1998). Guiding the family of a school aged child. *Contemp Pediatr, 15*(3), 75.

Simon, J., & Kaw, P. (2001). Commonly missed diagnosis in childhood eye exams. *Am Fam Physician, 64*(4), 623-638.

Steele, R. (1997). Sizing up risks of pet transmitted diseases. *Contemp Pediatr, 14*(9), 43-68.

Twomey, J., Bevis, M., & McGibbon, E. (2001). Association between adult and child bicycle helmet use. *MCN, 26*(5), 272-277.

U.S. Department of Health and Human Services. (2000). *Healthy People 2010: National Health Promotion and Disease Prevention Objectives.* DHHS Pub. No. (PHS) 91-50213. Washington, DC: Government Printing Office.

Wallerstedt, C., & Fletcher, B. (2000). Teaching with toys. *AWHONN Lifelines, 4*(14), 45-46.

Wong, D., Wilson, D., & Hockenberry-Eaton, M. (2001). *Wong's Essentials of pediatric nursing* (6th ed.). St. Louis: Mosby.

Chapter 20 The Adolescent

Alderman, E. (2000). Breast problems in the adolescent. *Patient Care, 34*(6), 56-80.

American Academy of Child and Adolescent Psychiatry. (1998). Practice parameters in assessment and treatment of adolescents with depressive disorders. *J Am Acad Child Adolesc Psychiatry, 37*(10 supp), 63S-83S.

Barnard, N., Eckel, R., & Garza, C. (2001). Cautioning patients about extreme diets. *Patient Care, 35*(15), 28.

Behrman, R., Kliegman, R., & Jenson, H. (2000). *Nelson textbook of pediatrics* (16th ed.). Philadelphia: W.B. Saunders.

Deering, C., & Cody, D. (2002). Communicating with children and adolescents. *Am J Nurs, 102*(3), 34-41.

Griffin, C. (1999). Reframing menarche education: A developmental perspective. *Adv Nurs Pract, 7*(11), 53-57.

Hobart, J., & Smucker, D. (2000). The female athlete triad. *Am Fam Physician, 61*(11), 3357-3364.

Kolasa, K., Poehlman, G., & Peery, A. (2000). Is a vegetarian diet healthy for kids? *Patient Care, 34*(5), 111-128.

Levine, M., Carey, W., & Crocker, A. (1999). *Developmental behavioral pediatrics* (3rd ed.). Philadelphia: W.B. Saunders.

Lyznick, J., Nielsen, N., & Schneider, J. (2000). Cardiovascular screening of young athletes. *Am Fam Physician, 62*(4), 765-774.

Mahan, L., & Escott-Stump, S. (2000). *Krause's food, nutrition and diet therapy* (10th ed.). Philadelphia: W.B. Saunders.

Mansbach, J., & Gordon, C. (2001). Demystifying delayed puberty. *Contemp Pediatr, 18*(4), 43-62.

Maron, B., Thompson, P., Puffer, J., McGrew, C., Strong, W., Douglas, P., et al. (1998). Cardiovascular preparticipation screening for competition athletes: A statement from the health profession from the AHA. *Circulation, 97*(22), 2294.

Preboth, M. (2000). AAP statement on suicide in adolescents. *Am Fam Physician, 62*(12), 2704.

Schwartz, R. (1997). Are you ready to deal with the pot smoking patient. *Contemp Pediatr, 11*(4), 85.

Schwartz, R., Milteer, R., & LeBeau, M. (2000). Drug facilitated sexual assault (date rape). *Am Fam Physician, 93*(6), 558-561.

Shelow, S., Baron, M., Beard, L., et al. (1995). Sexuality, contraception and the media. *Pediatrics, 95,* 298-300.

Stevens-Simon, C. (1997). Reproductive health care for your adolescent female patients. *Contemp Pediatr, 14*(2), 35.

Swartz, M. (1994). Promoting helmet use in recreational sports. *J Pediatr Health Care, 8*(3), 138-139.

U.S. Department of Health and Human Services. (2000). *Healthy People 2010: National Health Promotion and Disease Prevention Objectives.* DHHS Pub. No. (PHS) 91-50213. Washington, DC: Government Printing Office.

White, C. (2001). Adolescent creatinene supplementation. *RN, 64* (1), 55.

Wong, D., Wilson, D., & Hockenberry-Eaton, M. (2001). *Wong's Essentials of pediatric nursing* (6th ed.). St. Louis: Mosby.

Woods, E., & Blake, D. (2001). Noninvasive diagnosis of STDs in teens. *Contemp Pediatr, 18*(2), 71.

Chapter 21 The Child's Experience of Hospitalization

Beckman, C., & Dysart, D. (2000). The challenge of multicultural medical care. *Contemp Obstet Gynecol, 45*(12), 50.

Behrman, R., Kliegman, R., & Jenson, H. (2000). *Nelson texbook of pediatrics* (16th ed.). Philadelphia: W.B. Saunders.

Benjamen, S., Gallagher, R., & Helms, J. (2001). CAM Approaches to chronic pain. *Patient Care, 35*(4), 37.

Betz, C. (2000). The challenge of empowering children and families. *J Pediatr Nurs, 15*(2), 269-271.

Beyea, S. (1996). *Critical pathways for collaborative nursing care.* Philadelphia: W.B. Saunders.

Hallstrom, I., Runesson, I., & Elander, G. (2002). Observed parental needs during their child's hospitalization. *J Pediatr Nurs, 17*(2), 140-148.

Ignatavicius, D., & Hausman, K. (1995). *Clinical pathways for collaborative practice.* Philadelphia: W.B. Saunders.

Jackson, P., & Vessey, J. (2000). Primary care of a child with a chronic condition (3rd ed.). St. Louis: Mosby.

Klenner, S. (2000). Mapping out a clinical pathway. *RN, 63*(6), 33-36.

Kost, M. (1999). Conscious sedation. *Nursing 99, 29*(4), 34-39.

Lynn, A., Ulman, G., & Spreker, M. (1999). Pain control in young infants. *Contemp Pediatr, 16*(11), 39.

Maikler, V. (1998). Pharmacologic pain management in children: A review of intervention research. *J Pediatr Nurs, 1*(1), 3-14.

Mattson, S. (2000). Providing culturally competent care. *AWHONN Lifelines, 4*(5), 37-39.

McCaffery, M., & Pasero, C. (1999). *Pain: A clinical manual* (2nd ed.). St. Louis: Mosby.

McCarthy, A., Cool, V., & Hanrahan, K. (1998). Cognitive behavioral interventions in children during painful procedures: Research challenges and program development. *J Pediatr Nurs, 13*(1), 55-63.

Reif, P., & Niziolek, M. (2001). Troubleshooting tips for PCA. *RN, 64*(4), 33-37.

Varlas, K. (2001). Guided imagery. *Adv Nurs Pract, 9*(3), 51.

Wong, D., Wilson, D., & Hockenberry-Eaton, M. (2001). *Wong's Essentials of pediatric nursing* (6th ed.). St. Louis: Mosby.

Chapter 22 Health Care Adaptations for the Child and Family

Behrman, R., Kliegman, R., & Jenson, H. (2000). *Nelson textbook of pediatrics* (16th ed.). Philadelphia: W.B. Saunders.

Blackwell, J. (2002). Fever of undetermined origin: Outpatient evaluation and management in patients 2 months to 36 months. *J Am Acad Nurse Pract, 14*(2), 51.

Carrol, P. (1998). Closing in on safer suctioning. *RN, 61*(5), 22-26.

Carroll, V. (2000). Abduction: Lowering the Risk. *AWHONN Lifelines, 3*(6), 25-27.

Crenshaw, J., & Winslow, E. (2002). Perioperative fasting. *Am J Nurs, 102*(5), 36.

Kirkpatrick, J., Alexander, J., & Cain, R. (1997). Recovering urine from diapers: Are test results accurate? *MCN, 22*(1), 96-102.

Kraus, D., Stohlmeyer, A., Hannon, P., & Freels, S. (2001). Effectiveness and infant acceptance of the medibottle vs. the oral syringe. *J. Human Pharm Drug Ther, 21*(4), 416-423.

Laskowski, L., & Salati, D. (2001). Responding to pediatric trauma. *Nursing 2001, 31*(9), 36.

Leder, R., Knight, J., & Emans, J. (2001). Sexual abuse: When to suspect: How to assess. *Contemp Pediatr, 18*(5), 59-74.

Maikler, V. (1998). Pharmacologic pain management in children. *J Pediatr Nurs, 13*(1), 3-14.

Metheny, N., Wehrle, M., & Wiersemal, C. (1998). Testing feeding tube placement: Auscultation vs. pH method. *Am J Nurs, 98*(5), 37-42.

Pride, H. (2000). When a rash is more than a rash: Skin signs of systemic disease. *Contemp Pediatr, 17*(11), 104-124.

Prober, C. (2000). No golden rules for managing fever in infants. *Patient Care, 34*(1), 69-91.

Rideout, M., & First, L. (2001). Fever measurement and management. *Contemp Pediatr, 18*(5), 58.

Saunders, C. (2001). Mercury manometers are still the gold standard. *Hypertension, 37,* 185-186.

Schuman, A. (2001). New guidelines for pediatric life support. *Contemp Pediatr, 18*(9), 39-53.

Wedekind, C., & Fidler, B. (2001). Compatability of commonly used IV solutions in pediatrics. *Critical Care Nurse, 21*(4), 45-51.

Wong, D., Wilson, D., & Hockenberry-Eaton, M. (2001). *Wong's Essentials of pediatric nursing* (6th ed.). St. Louis: Mosby.

Chapter 23 The Child with a Sensory or Neurological Condition

Agency of Health Care Planning and Research (1994). *Federal guidelines for treatment of OME in young children.* Pub. No. 94-0620, 94-0623, and 94-0624. Silver Springs, MD: Author.

Bacal, D., & Hertle, R. (1998). Don't be lazy about looking for amblyopia. *Contemp Pediatr, 15*(6), 99.

Behrman, R., Kliegman, R., & Jenson, R. (2000). *Nelson textbook of pediatrics* (16th ed.). Philadelphia: W.B. Saunders.

Benbodis, S., & Tatum, W. (2001). Advances in the treatment of epilepsy. *Am Fam Physician, 64*(1), 91-98.

Betz, C. (2002). The Surgeon General's report on health care needs of individuals with mental retardation. *J Pediatr Nurs, 17*(2), 79-81.

Bolte, R. (2000). Drowning: A preventable cause of death. *Patient Care, 34*(7), 129.

Brillhart, B. (2000). Prevention and assessment of head injuries in infants and small children. *Clin Lett Nurse Pract, 4*(9), 3.

Duchowney, M. (2000). Seizure recurrence in childhood epilepsy. *Ann Neurol, 48*(2), 137-139.

Gill, J., & Gieron-Korthals, M. (2002). What pediatricians and parents need to know about febrile convulsions. *Contemp Pediatr, 19*(5), 139.

Gottesman, R., & Kelly, M. (2000). Helping children with learning disabilities. *Contemp Pediatr, 17*(1), 91.

Jackson, P., & Vessey, J. (2000). *Primary care of the child with a chronic condition* (3rd ed.). St. Louis: Mosby

Kestle, E. (2000). Clinical research in hydrocephalus. *Hydocephal Assoc Newsletter,* Fall 2000.

Leifer, G. (2001). Hyperbaric oxygen therapy: What every nurse should know. *Am J Nurs 101*(8), 36.

Leppik, I., & Baringer, J. (2000). Selecting treatment in patients with epilepsy. *Hospital Pract, 35*(5), 35-47.

Lewis, D. (2002). Headaches in children and adolescents. *Am Fam Physician, 65*(4), 625-632.

Mahan, L., & Escott-Stump, S. (2000). *Krause's food, nutrition and diet therapy* (10th ed.). Philadelphia: W.B. Saunders.

McAbee, G., & Wark, J. (2000). A practical approach to uncomplicated seizures in children. *Am Fam Physician, 62*(5), 1109-1116.

Newell, P., & Churchill, E. (2000). Chronic otitis media in children: Helping families cope. *Adv Nurs Pract, 8*(1), 55-56.

Pagel, J. (2000). Nightmares and disorders of daydreaming. *Am Fam Physician, 61*(7), 2037-2044.

Painter, M., Scher, M., Stein, M., Armatti, S., Wang, Z., Gardiner, J., Paneth, N., Minngh, B., & Alvin, J. (1999). Phenobarbital compared to phenytoin for treatment of neonatal seizures. *N Engl J Med, 341*(7), 485-489.

Pellock, J. (2000). Newer medications in pediatric epilepsy. *Am Fam Physician, 61*(9), 2817.

Pichichero, M. (2000). Acute otitis media. *Am Fam Physician, 61*(8), 2410-2416.

Preboth, M. (1999). AAFP and AAP issue a practice parameter on management of closed head injuries in children. *Am Fam Physician, 60*(9), 2698-2705.

Reece, R., & Sege, R. (2000). Childhood head injuries accidental or inflicted. *Arch Pediatr Adolesc Med, 154*(1), 11-15.

Thiedke, C. (2001). Sleep disorders in children. *Am Fam Physician, 63*(2), 277-284.

Wong, D., Wilson, D., & Hockenberry-Eaton, M. (2001). *Wong's Essentials of pediatric nursing* (6th ed.). St. Louis: Mosby.

Chapter 24 The Child with a Musculoskeletal Condition

Allen-Greiner, K. (2002). Adolescent idiopathic scoliosis. *Am Fam Physician, 65*(9), 1817.

Behrman, R., Kliegman, R., & Jenson, R. (2000). *Nelson textbook of pediatrics* (16th ed.). Philadelphia: W.B. Saunders.

Chaney, S. (2000). Child abuse: Clinical findings and management. *J Am Acad Nurs Pract, 12*(11), 467-471.

Chiocca, E. (1998). Action stat: Shaken baby syndrome. *Nursing 98, 28*(5), 33.

Chiocca, E. (1998). Child abuse and neglect: A status report. *J Pediatr Nurs, 13*(2), 128-130.

Chiocca, E. (1998). The nurse's role in the prevention of child abuse and neglect. *J Pediatr Nurs, 13*(3), 194-195.

Consumer Product Safety Commission. (2001). School-related injuries and deaths in children. *Clin Rev, 11*(6), 116.

Davis, R. (2000). International scene: Cultural health care or child abuse: The practice of Cao Gio. *J Am Acad Nurse Pract, 12*(3), 89-95.

Godley, D. (2002). A practical guide to a child who limps. *Contemp Pediatr, 19*(2), 56.

Jackson, P., & Vessey, J. (2000). *Primary care of the child with a chronic condition* (3rd ed.). St. Louis: Mosby.

Kocher, M., Zurakowski, D., & Kesser, J. (1999). Differentiating between septic arthritis and transient synovitis of the hip in children. *J Bone Joint Surg 81*(12), 1622-1670.

Mulryan, K., Cathers, P., & Fagin, A. (2000). Protecting the child. *Nursing 2000, 30*(7), 39-43.

Pressel, D. (2000). Evaluation of physical abuse in children. *Am Fam Physician, 61*(10), 3057-3064.

Schneider, D., Hofman, M., & Peterson, J. (2002). Diagnosis and treatment of Paget's disease of the bone. *Am Fam Physician, 65*(10), 2069-2072.

Song, E., & Anderson, J. (2001). How violent video games may violate children's health. *Contemp Pediatr, 18*(5), 102-119.

Veenema, T. (2001). Children's exposure to community violence. *J Nurs Scholarsh, 33*(2), 167-173.

Wolfe, M., Uhl, T., & McCluskey, L. (2001). Management of ankle sprains. *Am Fam Physician, 63*(1), 93-104.

Wong, D., Wilson, D., & Hockenberry-Eaton, M. (2001). *Wong's Essentials of pediatric nursing* (6th ed.). St. Louis: Mosby.

Wyshak, G. (2000). Teenage girls, carbonated beverage consumption and bone fractures. *Arch Pediatr Adolesc Med, 154*(6), 610-613.

Chapter 25 The Child with a Respiratory or Cardiovascular Disorder

American Academy of Pediatrics, Peter, G., (Ed.). (2000). *Red Book: Report of the Committee on Infectious Diseases.* Elk Grove Village, IL: Author.

Ball, T., Castro-Rodriguez, J., Griffith, K., Holberg, C., Martinez, F., & Wright, A. (2000). Siblings, day care attendance and the risk of asthma and wheezing during childhood. *N Engl J Med, 343*(8), 538-543.

Behrman, R., Kliegman, R., & Jenson, H. (2000). *Nelson textbook of pediatrics* (16th ed.). Philadelphia: W.B. Saunders.

Bjornson, C., & Johnson, D. (2001). The characteristic cough: When to treat croup and what to use. *Contemp Pediatr, 18*(10), 74.

Griffen, S. (2000). Nebulized steroid is effective treatment for croup in children. *Am Fam Physician, 61*(6), 1808.

Guergen, B. (2000). Inhaled corticosteroids in the treatment of asthma. *Adv Nurs Pract, 8*(10), 51.

Hayden, M. (2000). Leukotreine modifiers: Expanded role may be on the horizon. *Adv Nurs Pract, 8*(10), 42-46.

Kemper, K. (2002). Otitis media: When parents don't want antibiotics or tubes. *Contemp Pediatr, 19*(4), 47.

Koppa, D. (2000). Infants with chronic nasal congestion. *Clin Rev, 10*(3), 107.

Markowitz, G. (2000). Don't be sidelined: Managing exercise induced asthma in children. *Adv Nurs Pract, 8*(4), 77-80.

Miller, C., & Holden, P. (1998). Pediatric liquid ventilation. *RN, 61*(4), 51-54.

Opperwall, B. (2000). Allergies and asthma. *Adv Nurs Pract, 8*(9), 34-38.

Perkin, R., & Young, T. (2000). Obstructive sleep apnea in children. *Adv Nurs Pract, 8*(10), 57-59.

Plaut, T. (1999). The peak flow diary for adults, teens, and children over 5. Amherst, MA: Pediapress.

Pope, B. (2002). A patient education guide for asthma. *Nursing 2002, 32*(5), 44.

Putman, H. (2002). Food allergies: Keeping kids safe. *RN, 65*(6), 26-30.

Rinnard, B., Gossman G., Robbins, R., & Rennard, S. (2000). Chicken soup inhibits neutrophil chemotaxis in vitro. *Chest, 118*(4), 1150-1157.

Smith, P. (2001). Primary care for children with congenital heart disease. *J Pediatr Nurs, 16*(5), 308-319.

Stemplel, D., Pederson, S., et al. (2002). Asthma. *Contemp Pediatr, 19*(2), 62.

Timmons, K. (2000). School and community management of pediatric asthma. *Adv Nurs Pract, 8*(1), 53-54, 74.

Togger, D., & Brenner, P. (2001). Metered dose inhalers. *Am J Nurs, 101*(10), 26-32.

Uzark, K. (2001). Therapeutic cardiac catheterization for congenital heart disease: A new era in pediatric care. *J Pediatr Nurs, 16*(5), 300-307.

Wong, D., Wilson, D., & Hockenberry-Eaton, M. (2001). *Wong's Essentials of pediatric nursing* (6th ed.). St. Louis: Mosby.

Chapter 26 The Child with a Condition of the Blood, Blood-Forming Organs, or Lymphatic System

Abshire, T. (2001). Approaching anemia in children. *Contemp Pediatr, 18*(9), 104.

American Academy of Pediatrics. (2000). Policy statement on childhood bereavement. *Am Fam Physician, 62*(1), 1439.

American Pain Society (1999). *Guidelines for the management of acute and chronic pain in sickle cell disease.* Glenview, IL: Author.

Balling, K., & McCubben, M. (2001). Hospitalized children with chronic illness: Parental caregiving needs and valuing parental expertise. *J Pediatr Nurs, 16*(2), 110-119.

Behrman, R, Kliegman, R., & Jenson, H. (2000). *Nelson textbook of pediatrics* (16th ed.). Philadelphia: W.B. Saunders.

Behrman, R., & Kliegman, R. (1998). *Essentials of pediatrics* (3rd ed.). Philadelphia: W.B. Saunders.

Cordoni, A. (2000). Von Willebrand's disease: Diagnosis and treatment. *Am J Nurs Pract, 4*(3), 9.

Davis, P., Kraus, R., & Willett, W. (2001). The impact of diet on chronic disease. *Patient Care, 35*(15), 51.

Eremita, D. (2001). Dolasteron for chemotherapy nausea. *RN, 64*(3), 38-40.

Glaser, V. (2000). Bone marrow transplant for cancer: Exploring the options. *Patient Care, 34*(5), 75-92.

Goldsmith, C. (2000). Sickle cell anemia. *Nurseweek, 13*(21), 26.

Jackson, P., & Vessey, J. (2000). *Primary care of the child with a chronic condition* (3rd ed.). St. Louis: Mosby.

Johnson, M., & Robin, N. (2000). Pediatrics and the human genome project. *Contemp Pediatr, 17*(5), 100.

Kelly, K. (2000). Acute lymphocytic leukemia in children. *Adv Nurs Pract, 8*(4), 57-58, 61-64, 94.

Kubler-Ross, E. (1969). *On death and dying.* New York: Macmillan (classic reference).

Kubler-Ross, E. (1975). *Death: The final stage of growth.* Englewood Cliffs, NJ: Prentice-Hall (classic reference).

Kubler-Ross, E. (1982). *On child and death.* New York: Macmillan (classic reference).

Leifer, R. (1997). *The happiness project: Transforming the three poisons that cause suffering we inflict on ourselves and others.* Ithaca, NY: Snow Lion Publishers.

Leung, A., & Chan, K. (2001). Evaluating children with purpura. *Am Fam Physician, 4*(3), 419-428.

Lewis, C., Brecker, M., Reaman, G., & Sahler, O. (2002). How can you help meet the needs of dying children. *Contemp Pediatr, 19*(4), 147.

Mahan, C., & Escott-Stump, S. (2000). *Krause's food, nutrition and diet therapy* (10th ed.). Philadelphia: W.B. Saunders.

Miller, S., Sleeper, L., Pegelow, C., Enos, L., Wang, W., Weiner, S., Wethers, D., Smith, J., & Kinney, T. (2000). Prediction of adverse outcomes in children with sickle cell disease. *N Engl J Med, 342*(2), 83-89.

Morgan, E., & Murphy, S. (2000). Care of children who are dying of cancer. *N Engl J Med, 342,* 347-348.

Periyakoil, V., & Hallenbeck, J. (2002). Managing preparatory grief and depression at the end of life. *Am Fam Physician, 65*(5), 883-890.

Rivlin, D. (2001). Books for children when a child's friend dies. *Contemp Pediatr, 18*(10), 134.

Smith-Stoner, M., & Frost, A. (1998). Coping with grief and loss. *Nursing 98, 28*(2), 48-50.

Vanderkieft, G. (2001). Breaking bad news. *Am Fam Physician, 64*(12), 1975-1978.

Wethers, D. (2000). Sickle cell disease in childhood. *Am Fam Physician, 62*(6), 1309-1314.

Wolfe, J., Grier, H., Klar, N., Levin, S., Ellenbogen, J., Sallem-Schatz, S., Emanuel, E., & Weeks, J. (2000). Symptoms and suffering at the end of life for children with cancer. *New Engl J Med, 342*(5), 326-333.

Wong, D., Wilson, D., & Hockenberry-Eaton, M. (2001). *Wong's Essentials of pediatric nursing* (6th ed.). St. Louis: Mosby.

Young, G., Toretsky, J., Campbell, A., & Eskanazi, A. (2000). Recognition of common childhood malignancies. *Am Fam Physician, 61*(7), 2144-2154.

Chapter 27 The Child with a Gastrointestinal Condition

Barkin, R., & Rosen, P. (1999). *Emergency pediatrics: A guide to ambulatory care* (5th ed.). St. Louis: Mosby.

Behrman, R., Kliegman, R., & Jenson, H. (2000). *Nelson textbook of pediatrics* (16th ed.). Philadelphia: W.B. Saunders.

Bradley, R. (2001). Gastroesophageal reflux in children. *Adv Nurs Pract, 9*(8), 40-45.

Castell, D. (1999). A practical approach to heartburn. *Hosp Pract, 34*(12), 89-98.

Jackson, P., & Vessey, J. (2000). *Primary care of the child with a chronic condition* (3rd ed.). St. Louis: Mosby.

Jung, A. (2001). Gasto-esophageal reflux in infants and children. *Am Fam Physician, 64*(11), 1853-1860.

Kimura, K., & Loening-Bauckle, V. (2000). Bilious vomiting in newborns: Rapid diagnosis of intestinal obstruction. *Am Fam Physician, 61*(9), 2791-2798.

Mahan, L., & Escott-Stump, S. (2000). *Krause's food, nutrition and diet therapy* (10th ed.). Philadelphia: W.B. Saunders.

Mays, D. (1995). Turn ABGs into child's play. *RN, 58*(1), 36-39.

Osterhoudt, K. (2000). The toxic toddler: Drugs that can kill in small doses. *Contemp Pediatr, 17*(3), 73.

Pena, B., Mondi, K., Graus, S., et al. (1999). Ultrasound and limited CT in diagnosis and management of appendicitis in children. *JAMA 282,* 1041-1046.

Sadovski, R. (2000). Management of ingested coins in children. *Am Fam Physician, 61*(5), 1513.

Salas, S., Angel, C., Salas, N., Murillo, C., & Swischuk, M. (2000). Sigmoid volvulus in children and adolescents. *J Am Coll Surgeon, 190*(6), 717-723.

Simpson, W., Jr., & Schuman, S. (2002). Recognizing and management of acute pesticide poisoning. *Am Fam Physician, 65*(8), 1599-1604.

Sullivan, L. (2001). Abdominal pain in children. *Adv Nursing Pract, 9*(3), 54.

Van Boxel, A., & Puhl, P. (2001). Pediatric emergency: Assessing gut pain. *RN, 64*(4), 38-42.

Wong, D., Wilson, D., & Hockenberry-Eaton, M. (2001). *Wong's Essentials of pediatric nursing* (6th ed.). St. Louis: Mosby.

Wong, D., Perry, S., & Hockenberry, M. (2002). *Maternal-child nursing care* (2nd ed.). St. Louis: Mosby.

Chapter 28   The Child with a Genitourinary Condition

Behrman, R., Kliegman, R., & Jenson, H. (2000). *Nelson textbook of pediatrics* (16th ed.). Philadelphia: W.B. Saunders.

Bukowski, T., & Zeman, P. (2001). Hypospadias: Of concern but correctable. *Contemp Pediatr 18*(2), 89.

Docimo, S., Silver, R., & Cromie, W. (2000). The undescended testicle: Diagnosis and management. *Am Fam Physician 62*(9), 2037-2044, 2047-2048.

Fisher, M. (1999). Pyelonephritis at home: Why not? *Pediatrics, 104*(1 pt 1), 109-111.

Haberman, A., et al. (1999). Oral versus intravenous therapy for urinary tract infection in young febrile children. *Pediatrics 104,* 79-86.

Hogg, R., et al. (2000). Recognizing and treating nephrotic syndrome. *Contemp Pediatr, 17*(11), 84.

Jackson, P., & Vessey, J. (2000). *Primary care of the child with a chronic condition* (3rd ed.). St. Louis: Mosby.

Mahan, L., & Escott-Stump, S. (2000). *Krause's food, nutrition and diet therapy* (10th ed.). Philadelphia: W.B. Saunders.

Roberts, L. (2000). The American Academy of Pediatrics parameters on urinary tract infections in febrile infants and young children. *Am Fam Physician, 62*(8), 1815-1822.

Sadovsky, R. (2000). Urinary tract infection in children. *Am Fam Physician, 61*(6), 1816.

Sadvosky, R. (2000). Usefulness of clean-catch urine collection in infants. *Am Fam Physician, 61*(8), 2475.

Wong, D., Wilson, D., & Hockenberry-Eaton, M. (2001). *Wong's Essentials of pediatric nursing* (6th ed.). St. Louis: Mosby.

Wong, D., Perry, S., & Hockenberry, M. (2002). *Maternal-child nursing care* (2nd ed.). St. Louis: Mosby.

Chapter 29   The Child with a Skin Condition

Adams, A. (2000). Surgical site infections: Another look at banishing bugs. *Nursing 2000, 30*(6), 50-51.

Behrman, R., Kliegman, R., & Jenson, H. (2000). *Nelson textbook of pediatrics* (16th ed.). Philadelphia: W.B. Saunders.

Brilliant, L. (2000). Perianal streptococcal dermatitis. *Am Fam Physician, 61*(2), 391-397.

Chamlin, S. (2002). Shedding light on moles, melanoma, and the sun. *Contemp Pediatr, 19*(6), 102.

Darmstadt, G. (2000). Skin abscesses in children. *Patient Care 34*(8), 37.

Hilton, G. (2002). Emergency: Thermal burns. *Am J Nurs, 101*(11), 32-34.

Jackson, P., & Vessey, J. (2000). *Primary care of the child with a chronic condition* (3rd ed.). St. Louis: Mosby.

Johnson, B., & Nunley, J. (2000). Use of systemic agents in treating acne vulgaris. *Am Fam Physician, 62*(8), 1823-1830, 1835-1836.

Kaplan, D. (2001). Cutaneous conundrums: Dermatological disguises. *Consultant, 41*(5 supp), 663.

Kjaer, S., Svare, E., Worm, A., Walboomers, J., Meijer, C., & van den Brule, A. (2000). Human papillomavirus infection in Danish female sex workers: Decreasing prevalence with age despite continuously high sexual activity. *Sex Trans Dis, 27*(8), 438-445.

Krafchik, B. (2000). Atopic dermatitis and food allergy: A dermatologists view. *Contemp Pediatr,* April supp, p. 8-11.

Levy, M. (2000). Pediatric dermatology. *Pediatr Clin North Am, 47*(4), 921-935.

Mancini, A. (2000). Acne vulgaris: A treatment update. *Contemp Pediatr, 17*(12), 122-133.

Mazurek, C., & Lee, N. (2000). How to manage head lice. *West J Med 172*(5), 342-345.

Milner, M., Mottar, R., & Smith, C. (2002). The burn wheel. *Am J Nurs, 101*(11), 35-37.

Morgan, L., & Luczon-Peterman, P. (2001). Uncovering the facts: Parental behaviors and knowledge regarding sun protection. *J Med Acad Nurse Pract 16*(6), 285-289.

Parhizgar, B. (2001). Skin signs of systemic disease. *Clin Advis, 11*(8), 33.

Patel, C., Kinsey, G., Koperski-Moen, K., & Bungilm, L. (2000). Vacuum-assisted wound closure. *Am J Nurs, 100*(12), 45-48.

Pongrocic, J. (2000). Is it food allergy? *Contemp Pediatr, 17*(12), 101-117.

Prebath, M. (2000). HIV testing for children in foster care. *Am Fam Physician 62*(11), 2541.

Pride, H. (2000). Skin signs of systemic disease. *Contemp Pediatr, 17*(11), 104.

Rodgers, G. (2000). Reducing the toll of childhood burns. *Contemp Pediatr, 17*(4), 152.

Rudnick, C., & Hoekzema, G. (2002). Neonatal herpes simplex virus infections. *Am Fam Physician, 65*(6), 1138-1142.

Russell, J. (2000). Topical therapy for acne. *Am Fam Physician 61*(2), 357-366.

Shaikh, V., & Nucci, A. (2000). Artificial fingernails: Too hot to handle. *Contemp Pediatr, 17*(11), 99.

Smith, L. (2000). Atopic dermatitis and food allergy: An allergist's view. *Contemp Pediatr,* April (suppl.), pp. 1-8.

Stephens, M. (2000). Controlling head lice. *Patient Care, 34*(10), 37-48.

U.S. Department of Health and Human Services. (1999). Guidelines for isolation precautions in hospitals: Hospital infection control practices advisory committee. *Am J Infect Control, 24*(1), 32-45.

Walling, A. (2000). Resistant perianal diaper rash. *Am Fam Physician 61*(1), 225.

Weinstein, A., & Berman, B. (2002). Topical treatment of common superficial tinea infections. *Am Fam Physician, 65*(10), 2095-2102.

Weston, W., & Morelli, J. (2000). Steroid rosacea in prepubertal children. *Arch Pediatr Adolesc Med, 154*(1), 62-64.

Wiebelhaus, P., & Hansen, S. (2001). Another choice for burn victims. *RN, 64*(9), 34.

Wong, D., Wilson, D., & Hockenberry-Eaton, M. (2001). *Wong's Essentials of pediatric nursing* (6th ed.). St. Louis: Mosby.

Wong, D., Perry, S., & Hockenberry, M. (2002). *Maternal-child nursing care* (2nd ed.). St. Louis: Mosby.

Chapter 30 The Child with a Metabolic Condition

American Diabetes Association. (2000). Type II diabetes in children and adolescents. *Pediatrics, 105,* 671-680.

Behrman, R., Kliegman, R., & Jenson, H. (2000). *Nelson textbook of pediatrics* (16th ed.). Philadelphia: W.B. Saunders.

Calwell, J. (2001). Insulin therapy. *RN, 64*(9), 38.

Clarke, K. (2002). New insulin therapy: No needles needed. *Nursing 2002, 32*(5), 49-51.

Colberg, S., & Walsh, J. (2002). Pumping insulin during exercise. *Sportsmedicine, 30*(4), 33.

Flood, L. & Constance, A. (2002). Diabetes and exercise safety. *Am J Nurs, 102*(6), 67.

Hafeez, W., & Vuguin, P. (2000). Managing diabetic ketoacidosis: A delicate balance. *Contemp Pediatr, 17*(6), 72.

Jackson, P., & Vessey, J. (2000). *Primary care of the child with a chronic condition* (3rd ed.). St. Louis:Mosby.

Kirchner, J. (2000). Use of growth hormone therapy in children. *Am Fam Physician, 61*(5), 1510.

Luna, B., & Feinglos, M. (2001). Oral agents in the management of type 2 diabetes mellitus. *Am Fam Physician, 63*(9), 1747-1756.

Mahan, L., & Escott-Stump, S. (2000). *Krause's food, nutrition and diet therapy* (10th ed.). Philadelphia: W.B. Saunders.

Passanza, C. (2001). Blood glucose monitor options. *RN, 64*(6), 36-43.

Preboth, M. (2000). Diabetes in the school and day care setting. *Am Fam Physician, 62*(5), 1189.

Robertson, C. (2001). Diabetes update: The untold story of disease prevention. *RN, 64*(3), 60-64.

Sadovsky, R. (2000). Growth hormone in children and adolescents of short stature. *Am Fam Physician, 61*(9), 2871.

Saunders, S. (2000). Troglitazone (Rezulin) withdrawn from market. *Patient Care, 34*(10), 12.

Schultz, J. (2000). Type 2 diabetes. *Nurseweek, 13*(20), 22.

Singleton, J., & Vacarro-Olko, J. (2000). Promoting care-of-self in type II diabetes mellitus: The HbA_1c. *Clin Lett Nurse Pract, 4*(6), 4-6.

Watts, S. (2001). New standards for diabetic screening and care. *Adv Nurse Pract, 9*(3), 65.

Wong, D., Wilson, D., & Hockenberry-Eaton, M. (2001). *Wong's Essentials of pediatric nursing* (6th ed.). St. Louis: Mosby.

Wong, D., Perry, S., & Hockenberry, M. (2002). *Maternal-child nursing care* (2nd ed.). St. Louis: Mosby.

Chapter 31 The Child with a Communicable Disease

Ada, G. (2001). Vaccines and vaccinations. *N Engl J Med, 345*(14), 1042-1053.

Armstrong, J. (2002). Chemical warfare. *RN, 65*(4), 32-39.

Arnon, S., Schechter, R., Inglesby, T., Henderson, D., Bartlett, J., Ascher, M., et al. (2001). Botulinum toxin as a biological weapon. *JAMA, 285*(8), 1059-1070.

Ascherio, A., Zhang, S., Hernan, M., Olek, M., Coplan, P., Brodovicz, K., & Walker, A. (2001). Hepatitis B vaccine and the risk of multiple sclerosis. *N Engl J Med, 344*(5), 327-332.

Atkinson, W., Pickerling, L., Schwartz, B., Weniger, B., Iskander, J., & Watson, J. (2002). General recommendations on immunization: Recommendations of the Advisory Committee on Immunization Practices and the American Academy of Family Physicians. *MMWR, 51*(RR-2), 1-35.

Avalos-Block, S. (2001). The hard truth about PPD skin test. *Nursing 2001, 31*(6), 56-57.

Barlow, W., Davis, R., Glasser, J., Rhodes, P., Thompson, R., Mullooly, J., et al. (2001). Risk of seizures after receipt of whole cell pertussis or measles, mumps, and rubella vaccine. *N Engl J Med, 345*(9), 656-661.

Barone, S., Pontrelli, L., & Krilov, L. (2000). The differentiation of classic Kawasaki disease, atypical Kawasaki disease, and acute adenoviral infection. *Arch Pediatr Adolesc Med, 154*(5), 453-456.

Behrman, R., Kliegman, R., & Jenson, H. (2000). *Nelson textbook of pediatrics* (16th ed.). Philadelphia: W.B. Saunders.

Cardor, K., & Weston, W. (2002). Atypical viral exanthems. *Contemp Pediatr, 19*(2), 111.

CDC Update. (2001). Investigation of anthrax associated with intentional exposure and interim public health guidelines. *50*(41), 889-893.

Chasens, E., & Umlauf, M. (2000). Post-polio syndrome. *Am J Nurs, 110*(12), 60-67.

Coffman, S., Peck, J., & Rasmussen, C. (2001). Developing a synagis clinic for respiratory syncytial virus prophylaxis. *MCN, 26*(5), 246-251.

Davidhizar, R., & Shearer, R. (2002). Helping children cope with public disasters: Support given immediately after a traumatic event can counteract or even negate long-term adverse effects. *Am J Nurs, 102*(3), 26-33.

Dennis, D., Inglesby, T., Henderson, D., Bartlett, J., Ascher, M., Eizen, E., et al. (2001). Tularemia as a biological weapon: Medical and public health management. *JAMA, 285*(21), 2763-2773.

Department of Health Services, State of California. (2001, June 16). Vaccine storage and rolling blackouts. *Health Bulletin #1.*

Evers, D. (2001). Teaching mothers about childhood immunizations. *MCN, 26*(5), 253-256.

Fleisher, T., & Ballow, M. (2000). Primary immune deficiencies. *Pediatr Clin North Am, 47*(6), 1197-1403.

Gellin, B., & Schaffner, A. (2001). The risks of vaccination. *N Engl J Med, 334*(5), 372-373.

Henderson, D., et al (1999). Smallpox as a biological weapon. *JAMA, 281,* 2127-2137.

Inglesby, T., et al. (2000). Plague as a biological weapon. *JAMA, 283,* 2281-2290.

Jackson, P., & Vessey, J. (2000). *Primary care of the child with a chronic condition* (3rd ed.). St. Louis: Mosby.

Kilpatrick, J. (2002). Nuclear attacks: A ready response. *RN, 65*(5), 46-51.

Kirchner, J. (2000). Prognosis of children with vertically acquired HCV. *Am Fam Physician, 16*(11), 3394.

Leiberman, J. (2001). Varicella vaccine: What we have learned. *Contemp Pediatr, 18*(1), 50-60.

Lindow, K., & Warren, C. (2001). Understanding rosacea. *Am J Nurs, 101*(10), 44-51.

Mayoral, C., Marino, R., Rosenfeld, W., Greensher, J. (2000). Alternating antipyretics: Is this an alternative? *Pediatrics, 105*(5), 1009-1012.

Minichiello, V. (2002). New vaccine technology: What do you need to know? *J Am Acad Nurse Pract, 14*(2), 73-81.

Montalto N., Gum, K., & Ashley, K. (2000). Updated treatment for influenza A & B. *Am Fam Physician, 62*(11), 2467-2476.

Reilly, J., & Deason, D. (2002). Emergency: Smallpox. *Am J Nurs, 102*(2), 51-55.

Schuman, A. (2001). Preparing children and families to travel overseas. *Contemp Pediatr, 18*(6), 45-59.

Smith, C., & Taylor, D. (2000). Quieting the 100 day cough: A primer on pertussis. *Adv Nurse Pract, 8*(10), 60-62.

Wade, C. (2000). Keeping lyme disease at bay. *Am J Nurs, 100*(7), 26-31.

Waggoner-Fountain, L., & Donowitz, L. (2000). Infection control in the office: Keeping germs at bay. *Contemp Pediatr, 17*(9), 43.

Wong, D., Wilson, D., & Hockenberry-Eaton, M. (2001). *Wong's Essentials of pediatric nursing* (6th ed.). St. Louis: Mosby.

Wong, D., Perry, S., & Hockenberry, M. (2002). *Maternal-child nursing care* (2nd ed.). St. Louis: Mosby.

Chapter 32 The Child with an Emotional or Behavioral Condition

American Academy of Pediatrics, Committee on Quality Improvement. (2000). Clinical practice guidelines: Diagnosis and evaluation of the child with attention deficit/hyperactivity disorder. *Pediatrics, 105*(5),1158-1170.

American Psychiatric Association. (1994). *Diagnostic and statistical manual of mental disorders* (4th ed.). Washington, DC: Author.

Antal-Otong, D. (2001). Overcoming major depression. *Adv Nurse Pract, 9*(3), 71.

Baren, M. (2002). ADHD in adolescents. *Contemp Pediatr, 19*(4), 124.

Behrman, R., Kliegman, R., & Jenson, H. (2000). *Nelson textbook of pediatrics* (16th ed.). Philadelphia: W.B. Saunders.

Courchesne, E. (1997). Brainstem, cerebellar and limbic neuro-anatomical abnormalities in autism. *Curr Opin Neurobiol, 7*(2), 269-278.

Ferrara, L. (2000). Drug therapy for children with ADHD. *Clin Lett Nurse Pract, 4*(3), 9.

Fleitas, J. (2000). When Jack fell down, Jill came tumbling after: Siblings in the web of illness and disability. *MCN, 25*(5), 267-273.

Gordon, A. (2001). Eating disorders: Anorexia nervosa. *Hosp Pract, 36*(2), 36.

Gottesman, R., & Kelly, M. (2000). Helping children with learning disorders. *Contemp Pediatr, 17*(11), 42.

Gottesman, R., & Kelly, M. (2001). You can make a difference with these kids. *RN, 64*(6), 45.

Griswold, K., & Pessar, L. (2000). Management of bipolar disorder. *Am Fam Physician, 62*(6), 1343-1353, 1357-1358.

Huffman, G. (2000). A comparison of treatments in children with ADHD. *Am Fam Physician, 61*(3), 2839.

Jackson, P., & Vessey, J. (2000). *Primary care of the child with a chronic condition* (3rd ed.). St. Louis: Mosby.

Kaplan, E. (2000). Pediatric autoimmune neuropsychiatric disorder association with streptococcus (PANDAS). *Contemp Pediatr, 17*(8), 81.

Leifer, R. (1997). *The happiness project: Transforming the three poisons that cause suffering we inflict on ourselves and others.* Ithaca, NY: Snow Lion Publishers.

LoBuono, C. (2000). Dealing with the alcohol controversy. *Patient Care,* March 15, pp. 211-225.

Longo, L., Parran, T., Johnson, B., & Kinsey, W. (2000). Addiction: Identification and management of the drug-seeking patient. *Am Fam Physician, 61*(8), 2401-2408.

Lynch, A., Glod, C., & Fitzgerald, F. (2001). Psychopharmacologic treatment of adolescent depression. *Arch Psychiatr Nurs, 15*(1), 41-47.

O'Connell, T., Kaye, L., & Plosay, J. (2000). Gamma-hydroxybutyrate (GHB): A newer drug of abuse. *Am Fam Physician, 62*(11), 2478-2483.

Paulk, D. (2001). Munchausen syndrome by proxy. *Clin Rev, 11*(18), 50.

Pinkowish, W. (2000). What keeps depressed patients from committing suicide? *Patient Care, 34*(8), 17.

Seidenfeld, M., & Rickert, V. (2001). Impact of anorexia bulimia and obesity of gynecological health of adolescents. *Am Fam Physician, 64*(3), 445-450.

Son, S., & Kirchner, J. (2000). Depression in children and adolescents. *Am Fam Physician, 62*(10), 2297-2308, 2311-2312.

Teall, A., & Graham, C. (2001). Youth access to tobacco in two communities. *J Nurs Schol, 33*(2), 175-178.

Thiedke, C. (2001). Sleep disorders in children. *Am Fam Physician, 63*(2), 277-284.

Tumolo, J. (2000). Breathing deep and dying. *Adv Nurse Pract, 81*(12), 51.

Walling, A. (2000). A new screening tool for patients with eating disorders. *Am Fam Physician, 61*(7), 2183.

Walling, A. (2000). Antinausea drug promising in treatment of bulimia nervosa. *Am Fam Physician, 62*(5), 1156.

Wong, D., Wilson, D., & Hockenberry-Eaton, M. (2001). *Wong's Essentials of pediatric nursing* (6th ed.). St. Louis: Mosby.

Wong, D., Perry, S., & Hockenberry, M. (2002). *Maternal-child nursing care* (2nd ed.). St. Louis: Mosby.

Zitelli, B., & Davis, H. (1997). *Atlas of pediatric physical diagnosis* (3rd ed.). St. Louis: Mosby.

Chapter 33 Complementary and Alternative Therapies in Maternity and Pediatric Nursing

Anderson, C., Lis-Balchin, M., & Kirk-Smith, M. (2000). Evaluation of massage with essential oils on childhood ectopic eczema. *Phytother Res, 14*(6), 452-456.

Bakerink, J., Gaspe, S., Jr., Dimand, R., & Eldridge, M. (1996). Multiple organ failure after ingestion of pennyroyal oil from herbal tea in two infants. *Pediatrics, 98*(5), 944-947.

Bello, C., & West, D. (2001). Using herbal therapy wisely. *Nurse Pract, 5*(1), 1.

Buckle, J. (1999). Use of aromatherapy as a complimentary treatment for chronic pain. *Altern Ther Health Med, 5*(5), 142-151.

Cady, R. (2002). Are there legal issues for nurses when patients use CAM therapy? *MCN, 27*(3), 119.

Caspi, O., Bell, I., Rychener, D., Gaudet, T., & Weil, A. (2000). The Tower of Babel: Communication and medicine: An essay on medical education and complementary-alternative medicine. *Arch Intern Med, 160*(21), 3193-3195.

Chan, E., Gardiner, P., & Kemper, K. (2000). Herbs and dietary supplements in ADHD. *Contemp Pediatr, 17*(9), 116.

Chang, Z., Kennedy, D., Holdford, D., & Small, R. (2000). Pharmacists knowledge and attitudes toward herbal medicines. *Ann Pharmacother, 34*(6), 710-715.

Colbath, J., & Prawlucki, P. (Ed.). (2001). Holistic nursing care. *Nurs Clin North Am, 36*(1), 1-168.

Cornell, S. (Ed.). (2000, Nov). Alternative medicine. *Adv Nurse Pract,* p. 27.

Fontaine, K. (2000). *Healing practice of alternative therapy for nurses.* Upper Saddle River, NJ: Prentice Hall Health.

Gaster, B., & Holroyd, J. (2000). St. John's wort for depression: A systematic review. *Arch Int Med, 160,* p. 152-155.

Gephart, H., & Green, M. (2001). ADHD resources for parents. *Contemp Pediatr, 17*(9), 133.

Hadley, S., & Petry, J. (1999). Medicinal herbs: A primer for primary care. *Hosp Pract, 34*(6), 105-116.

Hatcher, T. (2001). The proverbial herb. *Am J Nurs, 101*(2), 36-43.

Hornstra, G. (2000). Essential fatty acids in mothers and their neonates. *Am J Clin Nutr, 71*(5), 1262S-1269S.

Huber, N. (2000). Ginko biloba: A CNS enhancer. *Adv Nurs Pract, 8*(11), 26.

Kaler, M., & Ravella, P. (2002). Staying on the ethical high ground with CAM. *Nurse Pract, 27*(7), 38-42.

Kass-Annese, B. (2000). Alternative therapies for menopause. *Clin Obstet Gynecol, 43*(1), 162-183.

Kemper, K. (1996). Seven herbs every pediatrician should know. *Contemp Pediatr, 13*(12), 79.

Kemper, K. (1996). *The holistic pediatrician comprehensive guide to safe and effective therapies for the 25 most common childhood ailments.* New York: Harper Perennial.

Kuhn, M. (1999). Complimentary treatment for health care providers. New York: J.B. Lippincott.

Labrecque, M., Eason, E., Marcoux, S., Lemieux, F., Pinault, J., Feldman, P., & Laperriere, L. (1999). Randomized controlled trial of prevention of perineal trauma by perineal massage during pregnancy, *Am J Obstet Gynecol, 180*(3 pt 1), 593-600.

Learn, C., & Higgins, P. (1999). Harmonizing herbs. *AWHONN Lifelines, 3*(5), 39-43.

Leifer, G. (2001). Hyperbaric oxygen therapy: What every nurse should know. *Am J Nurs 101*(8), 36.

Lindsay, S. (1999). Menopause naturally: Exploring alternatives to traditional hormone replacement therapy. *AWHONN Lifelines, 3*(5), 32-38.

Martin, A., Schauble, P., Rai, S., & Curry, R., Jr. (2001). The effects of hypnosis on the labor process and birth outcome of pregnant adolescents. *J Fam Pract, 50*(5), 441-443.

Moore, S. (1997). *Understanding pain and its relief in labor.* London: Churchill Livingstone.

Nardino, R. (2001). Spirulina (blue green algae) as antiviral, antineoplastic and anti-inflammatory agent. *Alt Med Alert, 4*(6), 67.

National Center for Complimentary and Alternative Medicine. (2000). The 5-year NCCAM Strategic Plan 2001-2005; available from NCCAM.nih.gov/niccam/strategic.

Nurses handbook of alternative and complimentary therapies. (1998). Springhouse, PA: Springhouse.

Olson, G. (2001). When your pregnant patient uses alternative medicine. *Contemp Obstet Gynecol, 46*(9), 45.

O'Neil, C., Avila, J., & Ferroro, C. (1999). Herbal medicines: Getting beyond the hype. *Nursing 99, 28*(4), 58.

Pennachio, D. (Ed.). (2000). Drug herb interactions: How vigilant should you be? *Patient Care, 34*(19), 41-69.

Petry, J., & Hadley, S. (2001). Medicinal herbs: Answers and advice. *Hosp Pract, 36*(7), 57.

Physician's desk reference for herbal medicines. (2002). Montvale, NJ: Medical Economics.

Reed, F., Pettigrew, A., & King, M. (2000). Alternate and complimentary therapies in nursing curricula. *J Nurs Educ, 39*(3), 133-139.

Schulz, V., Hansel, R., Varro, E., & Telger, T. (1998). *Rational phytotherapy: A physician's guide to herbal medicine.* New York: Springer-Verlag.

Snyder, M., & Lindquist, R. (1998). *Complimentary and alternative therapies in nursing* (3rd ed.). NY: Springer.

Spencer, J., & Jacobs, J. (1999). *Complimentary and alternative medicine: An evidence-based approach.* St. Louis: Mosby.

Spigelblatt, L. (1997). Alternative medicine: A pediatric conundrum. *Contemp Pediatr, 14*(8), 57.

Springer, M., & Linquist, R. (2001). Issues in complimentary therapies, *OJIN, 6*(2), 27.

Sutherland, J. (2000). Getting to the point: Meridian therapy is making its way to nursing practice. *Am J Nurs, 100*(9), 40-45.

Tiran, D., & Mack, S. (2000). *Complimentary therapies for pregnancy and childbirth* (2nd ed.). London: Bailliere-Tindall.

Waddell, D., Hummel, E., & Sumners, A. (2001). Three herbs you should get to know. *Am J Nurs, 101*(4), 48-53.

Chapter 1

Figure 1-1, From Harrison, M.R., Globus, M.S., & Filly, R.A. (Eds.). (1991). *The unborn patient: Prenatal diagnosis and treatment* (2nd ed.). Philadelphia: W.B. Saunders. 1-2, From Thibodeau, G.A., & Patton, K.T. (1999). *Anatomy & physiology* (4th ed.). St. Louis: Mosby.

Chapter 2

Figure 2-1, 2-2, 2-3, 2-4, From Herlihy, B., & Maebius, N.K. (2000). *The human body in health and illness.* Philadelphia: W.B. Saunders. 2-5, From Gorrie, T.M., McKinney, E.S., & Murray, S.S. (1998). *Foundations of maternal-newborn nursing* (2nd ed.). Philadelphia: W.B. Saunders. 2-6, Modified from *Stedman's illustrated medical dictionary* (25th ed.). (1990). Baltimore: Williams & Wilkins. 2-7, 2-8, From Thibodeau, G.A., & Patton, K.T. (1999). *Anatomy & physiology* (4th ed.). St. Louis: Mosby.

Chapter 3

Figure 3-1, 3-2, 3-5, From Moore, K.L., & Persaud, T.V.N. (1998). *The developing human: Clinically oriented embryology* (6th ed.). Philadelphia: W.B. Saunders. 3-3, From Herlihy, B., & Maebius, N.K. (2000). *The human body in health and illness.* Philadelphia: W.B. Saunders. 3-4, From Thibodeau, G.A., & Patton, K.T. (2000). *Structure & function of the body* (11th ed.). St. Louis: Mosby. 3-6, From McKinney, E.S., Ashwill, J.W., Murray, S.S., James, S.R., Gorrie, T.M., & Droske, S.C. (2000). *Maternal-child nursing.* Philadelphia: W.B. Saunders. 3-7, From Thibodeau, G.A., & Patton, K.T. (1999). *Anatomy & physiology* (4th ed.). St. Louis: Mosby. Table 3-1: Unn. figs. 3-1, 3-2, 3-3, 3-4, From Moore, K.L., & Persaud, T.V.N. (1998). *The developing human: Clinically oriented embryology* (6th ed.). Philadelphia: W.B. Saunders. Unn. figs. 3-5, 3-6, 3-7, 3-8, From Moore, K.L, Persaud, T.V.N., & Shiota, K. (1994). *Color atlas of clinical embryology.* Philadelphia: W.B. Saunders.

Chapter 4

Figure 4-1, From Swartz, M.H. (2002). *Textbook of physical diagnosis: History and examination* (4th ed.). Philadelphia: W.B. Saunders. 4-3, *A,* From Gorrie, T.M., McKinney, E.S., & Murray, S.S. (1998). *Foundations of maternal-newborn nursing* (2nd ed.). Philadelphia: W.B. Saunders. 4-4, Provided courtesy of MedaSonics, Inc. 4-5, From Matteson, P.S. (2001). *Women's health during the childbearing years: A community-based approach.* St. Louis: Mosby. 4-6, From Moore, K.L., & Persaud, T.V.N. (1998). *The developing human: Clinically oriented embryology* (6th ed.). Philadelphia: W.B. Saunders. 4-7, Courtesy of U.S. Department of Agriculture.

Chapter 5

Figure 5-1, 5-3, From Moore, K.L., & Persaud, T.V.N. (1998). *The developing human: Clinically oriented embryology* (6th ed.). Philadelphia: W.B. Saunders. 5-5, From Thibodeau, G.A., & Patton, K.T. (1999). *Anatomy & physiology* (4th ed.). St. Louis: Mosby. 5-6, From Thibodeau, G.A., & Patton, K.T. (2000). *Structure and function of the body* (11th ed.). St. Louis: Mosby. 5-7, From Zitelli, B.J., & Davis, H.W. (Eds.). (1997). *Atlas of pediatric physical diagnosis* (3rd ed.). St. Louis: Mosby. 5-8, From Clark, D.A. (2000). *Atlas of neonatology: A companion to Avery's diseases of the newborn* (7th ed.). Philadelphia: W.B. Saunders.

Chapter 6

Figure 6-1, *B,* Courtesy Hill-Rom Company, Inc., Batesville, IN. 6-2, 6-5, 6-7, 6-8, 6-10, 6-11, 6-20, From Matteson, P.S. (2001). *Women's health during the childbearing years: A community-based approach.* St. Louis: Mosby. 6-9, From Moore, K.L., & Persaud, T.V.N. (1998). *Before we are born: Essentials of embryology and birth defects* (5th ed.). Philadelphia: W.B. Saunders. 6-12, 6-16, 6-17, 6-24, Courtesy of Loma Linda University Medical Center, Loma Linda, CA. 6-13, 6-14, 6-15, Courtesy of Corometrics Medical Systems, Inc., Wallingford, CT. Redrawn with permission. 6-22, *A-M,* Courtesy of Michael S. Clement, MD, Mesa, AZ. In Lowdermilk, D.L., Perry, S.E., & Bobak, I.M. (2000). *Maternity and women's health care* (7th ed.). St. Louis: Mosby.

Chapter 7

Figure 7-1, 7-4, Courtesy of Loma Linda University Medical Center, Loma Linda, CA. 7-6, 7-7, From Matteson, P.S. (2001). *Women's health during the childbearing years: A community-based approach.* St. Louis: Mosby.

Chapter 8

Figure 8-1, From Matteson, P.S. (2001). *Women's health during the childbearing years: A community-based approach.* St. Louis: Mosby. 8-3, 8-6, 8-8, From Lowdermilk, D.L., Perry, S.E., & Bobak, I.M. (1999). *Maternity nursing* (5th ed.) St. Louis: Mosby. 8-9, From Gorrie, T.M., McKinney, E.S., & Murray, S.S. (1998). *Foundations of maternal-newborn nursing* (2nd ed.). Philadelphia: W.B. Saunders.

Chapter 9

Figure 9-3, From Gorrie, T.M., McKinney, E.S., & Murray, S.S. (1998). *Foundations of maternal-newborn nursing* (2nd ed.). Philadelphia: W.B. Saunders. 9-7, *A,* Courtesy of Prosec Protection Systems, Lakewood, NJ. 9-10, From Herlihy, B., & Maebius, N.K. (2000). *The human body in health and illness.* Philadelphia: W.B. Saunders. 9-11, From Wong, D.L., Perry, S.E., & Hockenberry-Eaton, M.J. (2002). *Maternal-child nursing care* (2nd ed.). St. Louis: Mosby. 9-14, Permission to use and/or reproduce this copyrighted material has been granted by the owner, Hollister Incorporated.

Chapter 10

Figure 10-1, From McKinney, E.S., Ashwill, J.W., Murray, S.S., James, S.R., Gorrie, T.M., & Droske, S.C. (2000). *Maternal-child nursing.* Philadelphia: W.B. Saunders. 10-2, From Swartz, M.H. (1998). *Textbook of physical diagnosis: History and examination* (3rd ed.). Philadelphia: W.B. Saunders.

Chapter 11

Figure 11-3, From Grimes, D.E., & Grimes, R.M. (1994). *AIDS and HIV infection.* St. Louis: Mosby. 11-6, From Herlihy, B., & Maebius, N.K. (2000). *The human body in health and illness.* Philadelphia: W.B. Saunders. Box 11-1: Unn. figs. 11-1, 11-2, 11-3, From Lowdermilk, D.L., Perry, S.E., & Bobak, I.M. (2000). *Maternity and women's health care* (7th ed.). St. Louis: Mosby. Table 11-1: Unn. figs. 11-4, From Grimes, D.E., & Grimes, R.M. (1994). *AIDS and HIV infection.* St. Louis: Mosby. Unn. figs. 11-5, 11-6, From Jarvis, C. (2000). *Physical examination and health assessment* (3rd ed.) Philadelphia: W.B. Saunders. Unn. fig. 11-7, From Callen, J.P., Greer, K.E., Paller, A.S., & Swinyer, L.J. (2000). *Color atlas of dermatology* (2nd ed.). Philadelphia: W.B. Saunders.

Chapter 12

Figure 12-3, *A*, 12-5, *A*, From Gorrie, T.M., McKinney, E.S., & Murray, S.S. (1998). *Foundations of maternal-newborn nursing* (2nd ed.). Philadelphia: W.B. Saunders. 12-3, *B*, From Zitelli, B.J., & Davis, H.W. (1997). *Atlas of pediatric physical diagnosis* (3rd ed.). St. Louis: Mosby. 12-5, *B*, 12-6, From Thureen, P.J., Deacon, J., O'Neill, P., & Hernandez, J.A. (1999). *Assessment and care of the well newborn.* Philadelphia: W.B. Saunders. 12-5, *C,D,* From McKinney, E.S., Ashwill, J.W., Murray, S.S., James, S.R., Gorrie, T.M., & Droske, S.C. (2000). *Maternal-child nursing.* Philadelphia: W.B. Saunders. 12-12, From Wong, D.L., Hockenberry-Eaton, M., Wilson, D., Winkelstein, M., Ahmann, E., & DiVito-Thomas, P.A. (1999). *Whaley & Wong's nursing care of infants and children* (6th ed.). St. Louis: Mosby. 12-14, Redrawn from *Clinical Education Aid #3.* Courtesy of Ross Labs, 1978. Table 12-2: Unn. figs. 12-1, 12-2, 12-3, 12-6, From Eichenfield, L.F., Frieden, I.J., & Esterly, N.B. (2001). *Textbook of neonatal dermatology.* Philadelphia, W.B. Saunders. Unn. figs. 12-4, 12-7, From Zitelli, B.L., & Davis, H.W. (1997). *Atlas of pediatric physical diagnosis* (3rd ed.). St. Louis: Mosby. 12-5, From Thureen, P.J., Deacon, J., O'Neill, P., & Hernandez, J.A. (1999). *Assessment and care of the well newborn.* Philadelphia: W.B. Saunders. Unn. fig. 12-8, Courtesy Jane Deacon, MS, RN, NNP, The Children's Hospital, Denver, CO. In Gorrie, T.M., McKinney, E.S., & Murray, S.S. (1998). *Foundations of maternal-newborn nursing* (2nd ed.). Philadelphia: W.B. Saunders. Unn. fig. 12-9, From Swartz, M.H. (1998). *Textbook of physical diagnosis: History and examination* (3rd ed.) Philadelphia: W.B. Saunders.

Chapter 13

Figure 13-1, 13-3, *B,C,* From Zitelli, B.L., & Davis, H.W. (1997). *Atlas of pediatric physical diagnosis* (3rd ed.). St. Louis: Mosby. 13-2, From Ballard, J.L., Khoury, J., Wedig, K., et al. (1991). New Ballard score expanded to include extremely premature infants. *J Pediatr, 119,* 417-423. St. Louis: Mosby. 13-3, *D,* From Gorrie, T.M., McKinney, E.S., & Murray, S.S. (1998). *Foundations of maternal-newborn nursing* (2nd ed.). Philadelphia: W.B. Saunders. 13-6, Reprinted by permission of Nellcor Puritan Bennett Inc., Pleasanton, CA.

Chapter 14

Figure 14-1, 14-13, From Herlihy, B., & Maebius, N.K. (2000). *The human body in health and illness.* Philadelphia, W.B. Saunders. 14-2, Courtesy of Dr. Albert Biglan, Children's Hospital of Pittsburgh. In Zitelli, B.L., & Davis, H.W. (1997). *Atlas of pediatric physical diagnosis* (3rd ed.). St. Louis: Mosby. 14-5, 14-7, Courtesy of Dr. A.E. Chudlely, Section of Genetics and Metabolism, Department of Pediatrics and Child Health, Children's Hospital and University of Manitoba, Winnipeg, Manitoba, Canada. From Moore, K.L., & Persaud, T.V.N. (1998). *The developing human: Clinically oriented embryology* (6th ed.). Philadelphia: W.B. Saunders. 14-8, From Bowden, V.R., Dickey, S.B., & Greenberg, S.C. (1998). *Children and their families: The continuum of care.* Philadelphia, W.B. Saunders. 14-9, From Ross Laboratories. (1986). *Clinical education Aid No. 15.* Columbus, OH: Author. Reproduced with permission of Ross Laboratories. 14-10, Wheaton Pavlik Harness. Courtesy of Wheaton Brace Company. 14-12, From Zitelli, B.L., & Davis, H.W. (1997). *Atlas of pediatric physical diagnosis* (3rd ed.). St. Louis: Mosby. 14-15, © 2002 Medela, Inc. Used with permission of Medela, Inc., McHenry, IL. 14-16, Courtesy of Ohmeda Medical, Laurel, MD.

Chapter 15

Figure 15-2, *A,* From Seidel, H.M., Benedict, G. W., Ball, J. W., & Dains, J.E. (1999). *Mosby's guide to physical examination* (4th ed.). St. Louis: Mosby. 15-2, *B,* Redrawn from *Human growth and growth disorders: An update,* South San Francisco, 1989, Genentech. In Wong, D.L., Hockenberry-Eaton, M., Wilson, D., Winkelstein, M.L.,

Ahmann, E., & DiVito-Thomas, P.A. (1999). *Whaley & Wong's nursing care of infants and children* (6th ed.). St. Louis: Mosby. 15-3, From McKinney, E.S., Ashwill, J.W., Murray, S.S., James, S.R., Gorrie, T.M., & Droske, S.C. (2000). *Maternal-child nursing.* Philadelphia: W.B. Saunders. 15-4, Developed by the National Center for Health Statistics in collaboration with the National Center for Chronic Disease Prevention and Health Promotion (2000). 15-6, *A,* Courtesy of the Health Connection, 55 W Oak Ridge Drive, Hagerstown, MD 21740. Reprinted with permission. 15-6, *B,* Courtesy of U.S. Department of Agriculture Center for Nutrition Policy and Promotion. 15-11, From Swartz, M.H. (1998). *Textbook of physical diagnosis: History and examination* (3rd ed.). Philadelphia: W.B. Saunders.

Chapter 16

Figure 16-5, Modified from Mahan, L.K., & Escott-Stump, S. (1996). *Krause's food, nutrition and diet therapy* (9th ed.). Philadelphia: W.B. Saunders.

Chapter 17

Figure 17-5, *A,* Bravo Forward-Facing Car Seat. Courtesy of Graco Children's Products, Inc., Macedonia, OH. 17-7, From Harkreader, H. (2000). *Fundamentals of nursing: Caring and clinical judgement.* Philadelphia: W.B. Saunders.

Chapter 20

Figure 20-3, Art overlay courtesy of Observatory Group, Cincinnati, OH. 20-4, Redrawn from photographs of J.M. Tanner, M.D., Institute of Child Health, Department of Growth and Development, University of London, England.

Chapter 21

Figure 21-2*(3),* From Bowden, V.R., Dickey, S.B., & Greenberg, C.S. (1998). *Children and their families: The continuum of care.* Philadelphia: W.B. Saunders. 21-3, Courtesy of AstraZeneca Pharmaceuticals LP, Wilmington, DE. 21-6, Courtesy of Providence General Medical Center, Everett, WA. Created by Randall De Jong. 21-7, Courtesy of Children's Medical Center, Dallas, TX.

Chapter 22

Figure 22-1, Courtesy of Prosec Protection Systems Inc., Lakewood, NJ. 22-3, Courtesy of Hard Manufacturing Company, Buffalo, NY. 22-5*A,* 22-11, 22-13, 22-23, 22-24, 22-27, From Wong, D.L., Hockenberry-Eaton, M., Wilson, D., Winkelstein, M.L., Ahmann, E., & DiVito-Thomas, P.A. (1999). *Whaley & Wong's nursing care of infants and children* (6th ed.). St. Louis: Mosby. 22-5, *B,* From Zitelli, B.J., & Davis, H.W. (Eds.) (1997). *Atlas of pediatric physical diagnosis* (3rd ed.). St. Louis: Mosby. 22-6, From McKinney, E.S., Ashwill, J.W., Murray, S.S., James, S.R., Gorrie, T.M., & Droske, S.C. (2000). *Maternal-child nursing.* Philadelphia: W.B. Saunders. 22-7, Courtesy of Medical Indicators, Carlsbad, CA. 22-8, Braun ThermoScan® Pro 3000. Courtesy of Welch Allyn, Inc. 22-9, Permission to reproduce this copyrighted material has been granted by the owner, Hollister, Inc., Libertyville, IL. 22-10, From Wong, D.L., Wilson, D., & Hockenberry-Eaton, M. (2001). *Wong's essentials of pediatric nursing* (6th ed.). St. Louis: Mosby. 22-12, Nomogram modified from data of E. Boyd by C. D. West. From Behrman, R., & Kliegman, R. (1998). *Nelson's essentials of pediatrics* (3rd ed.). Philadelphia: W.B. Saunders. 22-14, Courtesy of The Medicine Bottle Co., Inc. 22-16, Courtesy of Becton, Dickinson & Co., Franklin Lakes, NJ. 22-20, Courtesy of the Medi-Kids Company, PO Box 5398 Hemet CA, (888)463-3543, www.medi-kid. com. 22-25, From Ashwill, J.W., & Droske, S.C. (1997). *Nursing care of children: Principles and practice.* Philadelphia: W.B. Saunders. 22-26, From Guidelines for cardiopulmonary resuscitation and emergency cardiac care. (1992). *JAMA, 268,* 2172-2302.

Copyright 1992, American Medical Association. Box 22-1: Unn. fig. 22-1, From Leifer, G. (1982). *Principles and techniques in pediatric nursing* (4th ed.). Philadelphia: W.B. Saunders.

Chapter 23

Figure 23-1, Art overlay courtesy of Observatory Group, Cincinnati, OH. 23-2, 23-11, From Zitelli, B.J., & Davis, H.W. (Eds.). (1997). *Atlas of pediatric physical diagnosis* (3rd ed.). St. Louis: Mosby. 23-3*A*, From Wong, D.L., Hockenberry-Eaton, M., Wilson, D., Winkelstein, M.L., Ahmann, E., DiVito-Thomas, P.A. (1999). *Whaley & Wong's nursing care of infants and children* (6th ed.). St. Louis: Mosby. 23-3, *B*, From Seidel, H.M., Benedict, G.W., Ball, J.W., Dains, J.E. (1999). *Mosby's guide to physical examination* (4th ed.). St. Louis: Mosby. 23-4, From Behrman, R.E., & Kliegman, R.M. (1992). *Nelson textbook of pediatrics* (14th ed.). Philadelphia, W.B. Saunders. 23-5, 23-6*A*, From Thibodeau, G.A., & Patton, K.T. (1999). *Anatomy & physiology* (4th ed.). St. Louis: Mosby. 23-6, *B*, From Thibodeau, G.A., & Patton, K.T. (2000). *Structure and function of the body* (11th ed.). St. Louis: Mosby. 23-8, From Behrman, R., Kliegman, R., & Jenson, H.B. (2000). *Nelson textbook of pediatric* (16th ed.). Philadelphia: W.B. Saunders. 23-10, From Callen, J.P., Greer, K.E., Paller, A.S., & Swinyer, L.J. (2000). *Color atlas of dermatology* (2nd ed.). Philadelphia: W.B. Saunders. 23-12, 23-13, From Wong, D.L., Wilson, D., & Hockenberry-Eaton, M. (2001). *Wong's essentials of pediatric nursing* (6th ed.). St. Louis: Mosby.

Chapter 24

Figure 24-1, Art overlay courtesy of Observatory Group, Cincinnati, OH. 24-2, Redrawn from deWit, S.C. (1992). *Keane's essentials of medical-surgical nursing* (3rd ed.). Philadelphia: W.B. Saunders. 24-4, 24-6, 24-7, From Bowden, V.R., Dickey, S.B., & Greenberg, S.C. (1998). *Children and their families: The continuum of care.* Philadelphia: W.B. Saunders. 24-9, From Leifer, G. (1982). *Principles and techniques in pediatric nursing.* Philadelphia: W.B. Saunders. 24-10, Courtesy of Bert Oppenheim. 24-11, From Thibodeau, G.A., & Patton, K.T. (1999). *Anatomy and physiology* (4th ed.). St. Louis: Mosby.

Chapter 25

Figure 25-1, 25-12, Art overlay courtesy of Observatory Group, Cincinnati, OH. 25-3, 25-11, From Ashwill, J.W., & Droske, S.C. (1997). *Nursing care of children: Principles and practice.* Philadelphia: W.B. Saunders. 25-6, From Bowden, V.R., Dickey, S.B., & Greenberg, S.C. (1998). *Children and their families: The continuum of care.* Philadelphia: W.B. Saunders. 25-7, Courtesy of Keller Medical Specialties. 25-8, © 1996 Pedipress, Inc. All rights reserved. Thomas F. Plaut, M.D. Pedipress, Inc., 125 Red Gate Lane, Amherst, MA 01002 (800) 611-6081, www.pedipress.com. 25-10, From Swartz, M.H. (1998). *Textbook of physical diagnosis: History and examination* (3rd ed.) Philadelphia: W.B. Saunders. 25-15, Redrawn from Pillitteri, A. (1992). *Maternal and child health nursing: Care of the childbearing and childrearing family.* Philadelphia: J.B. Lippincott. 25-17, From Zitelli, B.J., & Davis, H.W. (Eds.). (1997). *Atlas of pediatric physical diagnosis* (3rd ed.). St. Louis: Mosby.

Chapter 26

Figure 26-1, Art overlay courtesy of Observatory Group, Cincinnati, OH. 26-2, From Thibodeau, G.A., & Patton, K.T. (1999). *Anatomy and physiology* (4th ed.). St. Louis: Mosby. 26-3, 26-5, From Zitelli, B.J., & Davis, H.W. (Eds.) (1997). *Atlas of pediatric physical diagnosis* (3rd ed.). St. Louis: Mosby. 26-6, From Bluefarb, S.M. (1984): *Dermatology.* Kalamazoo, MI, Upjohn.

Chapter 27

Figure 27-1, Art overlay courtesy of Observatory Group, Cincinnati, OH. 27-2, From Betz, C., Hunsburger, M., & Wright, S. (1994).

Family-centered nursing care of children (2nd ed.). Philadelphia: W.B. Saunders. 27-3, 27-9, From Zitelli, B.J., & Davis, H.W. (Eds.) (1997). *Atlas of pediatric physical diagnosis* (3rd ed.). St. Louis: Mosby. 27-5, From Bowden, V.R., Dickey, S.B., & Greenberg, S.C. (1998). *Children and their families: The continuum of care.* Philadelphia: W.B. Saunders.

Chapter 28

Figure 28-1, 28-3, Art overlay courtesy of Observatory Group, Cincinnati, OH. 28-2, From Thibodeau, G.A., & Patton, K.T. (1999). *Anatomy and physiology* (4th ed.). St. Louis: Mosby. 28-6, From Ashwill, J.W., & Droske, S.C. (1997). *Nursing care of children: Principles and practice.* Philadelphia: W.B. Saunders. 28-8, From Zitelli, B.J., & Davis, H.W. (Eds.). (1997). *Atlas of pediatric physical diagnosis* (3rd ed.). St. Louis: Mosby.

Chapter 29

Figure 29-1, Art overlay courtesy of Observatory Group, Cincinnati, OH. 29-2, 29-5, 29-18, From Zitelli, B.J., Davis, H.W. (Eds.) (1997). *Atlas of pediatric physical diagnosis* (3rd ed.). St. Louis: Mosby. 29-3, From Swartz, M.H. (1998). *Textbook of physical diagnosis: history and examination* (3rd ed.). Philadelphia: W.B. Saunders. 29-4, From Weston, W.L., Lane, A.T., & Morelli, J.G. (1996). *Color textbook of pediatric dermatology* (2nd ed.). St. Louis: Mosby. 29-6, 29-7, 29-9, 29-10, 29-11, 29-12, 29-13, From Hurwitz, S. (1993). *Clinical pediatric dermatology: A textbook of skin disorders of childhood and adolescence* (2nd ed.). Philadelphia: W.B. Saunders. 29-8, From Bowden, V.R., Dickey, S.B., & Greenberg, S.C. (1998). *Children and their families: The continuum of care.* Philadelphia: W.B. Saunders. 29-14, Courtesy Dr. Michael Sherlock. In Zitelli, B.J., & Davis, H.W. (Eds.). (1997). *Atlas of pediatric physical diagnosis* (3rd ed.). St. Louis: Mosby. 29-15, From Wong, D.L., Perry, S.E., & Hockenberry-Eaton, M.J. (2002). *Maternal child nursing care* (2nd ed.). St. Louis: Mosby. 29-16, From Ignatavicius, D.D., Workman, M.L. (2002). *Medical-surgical nursing: Critical thinking for collaborative care* (4th ed.). Philadelphia: W.B. Saunders.

Chapter 30

Figure 30-1, Art overlay courtesy of Observatory Group, Cincinnati, OH. 30-2, Courtesy of Dr. T.P. Foley, Jr., Pittsburgh. In Zitelli, B.J., & Davis, H.W. (Eds.). (1997). *Atlas of pediatric physical diagnosis* (3rd ed.). St. Louis: Mosby. 30-3, Modified from Waechter, E.H., & Blake, F.G. (1976). *Nursing care of children* (9th ed.). Philadelphia: J.B. Lippincott. 30-4, AtLast® Blood Glucose System. Courtesy of Amira Medical, Scotts Valley, CA. 30-5, Courtesy of Disetronic Medical Systems, Inc., Minneapolis, MN. 30-6, From Betz, C., Hunsberger, M., & Wright, S. (1994). *Family-centered nursing care of children* (2nd ed.). Philadelphia: W.B. Saunders. 30-7, From McKinney, E.S., Ashwill, J.W., Murray, S.S., James, S.R., Gorrie, T.M., & Droske, S.C. (2000). *Maternal-child nursing.* Philadelphia: W.B. Saunders. 30-8, From Bowden, V.R., Dickey, S.B., & Greenberg, S.C. (1998). *Children and their families: The continuum of care.* Philadelphia: W.B. Saunders. 30-9, From Price, M.J. (1983). Insulin and oral hypoglycemic agents. *Nurs Clin North Am, 18,* 687-706.

Chapter 31

Figure 31-1, From Feigin, R.D., & Cherry, J.D. (1987). *Textbook of pediatric infectious diseases* (2nd ed.). Philadelphia: W.B. Saunders. 31-2, 31-3, From Hurwitz, S. (1993). *Clinical pediatric dermatology: A textbook of skin disorders of childhood and adolescence* (2nd ed.). Philadelphia: W.B. Saunders. 31-4, From Leahy, J., & Kizilay, P. (1998). *Foundations of nursing practice: A nursing process approach.* Philadelphia: W.B. Saunders.

Chapter 32

Figure 32-1, From Bowden, V.R., Dickey, S.B., & Greenberg, S.C. (1998). *Children and their families: The continuum of care.* Philadelphia: W.B. Saunders. 32-3, From McKinney, E.S., Ashwill, J.W., Murray, S.S., James, S.R., Gorrie, T.M., & Droske, S.C. (2000). *Maternal-child nursing.* Philadelphia: W.B. Saunders.

Chapter 33

Figure 33-1, Art overlay courtesy of Observatory Group, Cincinnati, OH. 33-2, From Shah, B.R., & Laude, T.A. (2000). *Atlas of pediatric clinical diagnosis.* Philadelphia: W.B. Saunders. 33-3, Courtesy of Woodside Biomedical, Inc., Carlsbad, CA. 33-4, *A,C,* From Moore, S. (Ed.). (1997). *Understanding pain and its relief in labour.* Churchill Livingstone. 33-4, *B,* From Thibodeau, G.A., & Patton, K.T. (2000). *Structure and function of the body* (11th ed.). St. Louis: Mosby.

A

abdominal delivery A cesarean birth.

abduction A movement away from the midline of the body.

abortion The end of a pregnancy before the fetus is viable, whether spontaneous or elective.

abruptio placentae A premature separation of a normally implanted placenta.

abstinence Voluntarily refraining from participation in sexual intercourse.

abuse To attack or cause injury—physical, sexual, emotional, or spiritual. This term includes nonaccidental injury and neglect.

acceleration Heart rate increases over the baseline rate of at least 15 beats/min for at least 15 seconds.

acidosis A condition in which there is either a marked increase in the level of acids in the blood or body tissues or a marked decrease in the alkaline reserve (bicarbonate). The pH in the blood is low.

acini cells Cells that secrete a substance that helps with digestion in the alimentary tract and with breathing in the respiratory tract.

acme The peak, or period of greatest strength, of a uterine contraction.

acrocyanosis A peripheral blueness of the hands and feet due to reduced peripheral circulation (normal in newborns).

adduction A movement toward the midline of the body.

adolescence A period of human development beginning with puberty and ending with young adulthood.

advocacy Speaking or acting in support of a person's rights and needs.

afterbirth The placenta and membranes delivered during the third stage of labor.

afterpains Painful contractions of the uterus that occur for several days after delivery; they occur most often in multiparas and are more painful during breastfeeding.

AIDS Acquired immunodeficiency syndrome; caused by HIV, characterized by depressed immune system, and involves a deficiency in the CD4+ and T-lymphocytes.

airway management A positioning of the head and neck to ensure patency of the airway; may include interventions to ensure adequate oxygenation.

albuminuria The presence of a type of protein in the urine.

allergy An abnormal immune response to a substance that causes an inflammatory response resulting in hypersensitivity.

alternative treatment Methods to maintain health in the treatment of disease that differ from the traditionally accepted westernized practice of medicine.

alveoli The area in the lungs where the exchange of carbon dioxide and oxygen occurs.

amenorrhea The absence or suppression of menstruation; normal before puberty, during pregnancy and lactation, and after menopause.

amniocentesis Transabdominal puncture of the amniotic sac (fetal membranes) to obtain a sample of amniotic fluid for study.

amnioinfusion The infusion of warmed saline into the uterus to relieve cord compression or to wash meconium out of the cavity to prevent aspiration at birth.

amnion The inner of the two fetal membranes; thin and transparent; holds the fetus suspended in amniotic fluid.

amnionitis An inflammation or infection of the membrane closest to the developing fetus.

amniotic fluid A transparent, almost colorless fluid contained in the fetal membranes/amnion; it protects the fetus from injury, maintains an even temperature, and allows fetal movement.

amniotic sac The sac formed by the amnion and chorion that contains fluid and the fetus; it is commonly known as the "bag of waters."

amniotomy A surgical procedure in which the amniotic sac is ruptured to facilitate delivery of the fetus.

analgesic A drug that relieves pain but does not produce unconsciousness.

androgen A substance that stimulates masculinization, such as the male hormones testosterone and androsterone.

android pelvis A female pelvis that resembles a masculine size and shape.

anemia A decrease in the amount of hemoglobin or red blood cells circulating within the body.

anesthesia A partial or complete loss of sensation, especially of pain, with or without the loss of consciousness.

angioma A tumor, usually benign, that is made up chiefly of blood and lymph vessels.

animism A period of cognitive development in which the child attributes life to inanimate objects.

anomaly Not normal in form, structure, or position; a congenital anomaly is an abnormality present at birth.

anorexia nervosa A syndrome most often seen in adolescent girls and characterized by an extreme form of self-starvation. Although its onset may be acute, the underlying emotional problem develops over a relatively long time.

anoxia A complete absence of oxygen in the blood.

antenatal Before birth.

antepartum Before the onset of labor.

anterior Pertaining to the front or top of the body.

anterior fontanel A diamond-shaped area between the two frontal and two parietal bones of the newborn's head; also called the *soft spot*.

anthropoid pelvis A female pelvis with a transverse diameter that is equal to or smaller than the anteroposterior diameter.

antibody A specific protein substance that is formed in the body in response to antigens and restricts or destroys antigens.

antigen A substance that precipitates an immune response, resulting in the formation of antibodies. Antigen-antibody reactions form the basis for immunity.

anuria The lack of urine formation by the kidneys.

Apgar score An evaluation tool with a maximum score of 10; used to assess a newborn at 1 minute and 5 minutes after delivery. Five factors (scored 0, 1, or 2) are heart rate, color, muscle tone, reflex irritability, and respiratory effort.

apnea A cessation of respirations.

areola The pigmented circle of tissue around the nipple of the breast.

AROM An artificial rupture of (amniotic) membranes with a sterile instrument, such as an Amnihook or Allis clamp.

aromatherapy The absorption of essential oils or their aromas by the lungs or skin for systemic effects.

artificial insemination The mechanical injection of viable semen into the vagina for the purpose of impregnation.

ascariasis Roundworm infestation.

asphyxia An inadequate amount of oxygen or an increased amount of carbon dioxide in the blood and tissues of the body.

asynchrony The lack of concurrence in time. A growing child may look gangling because of asynchrony of growth (i.e., different body parts mature at different rates).

ataractics A tranquilizing agent.

atelectasis An incomplete expansion of the lungs or a collapse of the alveoli after expansion.

atony A lack of muscle tone or strength.

attachment A strong psychological bond of affection between an infant and a significant other.

attitude In obstetrics, the position of the fetus in the uterus (normally one of flexion of the head and extremities).

augmentation of labor The enhancement of labor after it has begun.

autoimmunity A condition in which the body produces antibodies against its own tissues.

autolysis The breakdown or endogenous destruction of cells due to enzymes in the body.

autonomy Functioning independently; self-control.

autosomal inheritance Characteristics transmitted on a chromosome other than a sex chromosome.

autosome A chromosome within the body that does not determine sexuality.

B

bacteriuria The presence of bacteria in the urine.

bag of waters The membrane containing the amniotic fluid and the fetus.

ballottement In obstetrics, the fetus floats away when palpated and then returns to touch the examiner's fingers.

barrier technique A method of medical asepsis using various types of isolation precautions or standard precautions as recommended by the Centers for Disease Control and Prevention. In contraception, a method in which sperm are prevented from entering the cervix.

Bartholin's glands Two small mucous glands situated on each side of the vaginal orifice that secrete small amounts of mucus during coitus (intercourse).

basal body temperature chart A written graphic chart of daily body temperatures, usually taken on awakening. The temperature usually drops at the beginning of ovulation.

bilirubin An orange or yellowish pigment in bile; a breakdown product of hemoglobin carried by the blood to the liver, where it is chemically changed and excreted in bile or is conjugated and excreted in the stools.

Billing's method A method used to check cervical mucus for elasticity, stickiness, wetness, and lubrication.

biofeedback A method of training designed to help an individual control his or her autonomic (involuntary) nervous system.

biophysical profile (BPP) A system of estimating the status of a fetus by evaluating heart rate, respiratory movement, muscle movement and tone, and amniotic fluid volume. Low scores require prompt delivery.

Bishop's score A scoring system that uses cervical dilation, effacement, fetal station, cervical consistency, and position to determine if labor can be safely induced.

blastocyst A stage in embryonic development that follows the morula. Implantation in the uterus generally occurs at this stage.

blastula A phase of the fertilized ovum in which all its cells are arranged into a hollow ball or cavity.

bleb An irregularly shaped elevation of the epidermis; a blister or bulla.

bloody show A mixture of blood and mucus from the cervix that often precedes labor.

bonding Attachment; the process whereby a unique relationship is established between two people; used in conjunction with parent-newborn attachment.

bone marrow transplant A transplantation of bone marrow from one person to another; currently used to treat aplastic anemia and leukemia.

booster injection The administration of a substance to renew or increase the effectiveness of a prior immunization injection (e.g., a tetanus booster).

bradycardia A heart rate slower than the expected rate for age. In a newborn, a heart rate lower than 110 beats/min; in a child, a heart rate less than 70 beats/min; in an adult, a heart rate less than 60 beats/min.

Braxton-Hicks contractions Intermittent contractions of the uterus; they occur more frequently toward the end of pregnancy and are sometimes mistaken for true labor contractions.

breech presentation A birth in which the buttocks or feet (or both) present instead of the head; occurs in approximately 3% of all deliveries.

Broviac catheter A central venous line used in small children who require total parenteral or continuous intravenous infusion.

brown fat Also called *brown adipose tissue;* forms in the fetus around the kidneys, adrenals, and neck; between the scapulae; and behind the sternum. Its dark brown hue is a result of its density, enriched blood supply, and abundant nerve supply. Its main purpose is heat production in the neonate.

Bryant traction A type of skin traction apparatus commonly used for toddlers with a fractured femur. Vertical suspension is used.

C

café-au-lait spots Light brown patch spots on the skin that may be characteristic of neurofibromatosis (a condition of tumors of various sizes on the peripheral nerves).

calendar method A natural method of birth control that uses the calendar to determine which phase of the menstrual cycle the woman is in.

caput The head; the occiput of the fetal head, which appears at the vaginal introitus before delivery of the head.

caput succedaneum A swelling or edema occurring in the newborn scalp that crosses the suture lines. Usually simply called *caput.* It is self-limiting and requires no treatment.

cardiac decompensation Heart failure.

cardinal movement *See* Mechanisms of labor.

carpal tunnel syndrome Occurs when pressure is placed on the median nerve as it goes through the carpal tunnel into the hand. When compressed, it can cause pain and numbness of the affected extremity.

It can occur in pregnancy and/or with repetitive motion (typing, frequent twisting of the wrist).

cephalic presentation A birth in which the fetal head presents against the cervix.

cephalocaudal The orderly development of muscular control, which proceeds from head to foot.

cephalohematoma A subperiosteal swelling containing blood; found on the head of a newborn. The swelling does not cross suture lines and therefore often appears unilateral. Usually disappears within a few weeks to 2 months without treatment.

cephalopelvic disproportion (CPD) A condition in which the fetus cannot pass through the maternal pelvis. Also called *fetopelvic disproportion.*

cerclage Closing the cervix with a suture to prevent early dilation and spontaneous abortion.

certified nurse-midwife (CNM) A registered nurse who has completed special training approved by the American College of Nurse-Midwives and passed a certification test. The CNM provides care to women who have a normal, uncomplicated pregnancy and delivery.

cerumen Ear wax.

cervical cap A contraceptive device that fits over the cervix.

cervical os The small opening of the cervix that dilates during the first stage of labor.

cervix The lower part of the uterus.

cesarean birth Delivery of the fetus by means of an incision into the abdominal wall and the uterus; abdominal delivery.

Chadwick's sign A violet-blue color of vaginal mucous membrane caused by increased vascularity; it is visible about the fourth week of pregnancy.

chignon A newborn scalp edema created by a vacuum extractor.

chloasma gravidarum A yellow-brown pigmentation over the bridge of the nose and cheeks during pregnancy and in some women who are taking oral contraceptives; also known as the *mask of pregnancy.*

chordee A congenital anomaly in which a fibrous strand of tissue extends from the scrotum to the penis, preventing urination with the penis in the normal elevated position; commonly associated with hypospadias.

chorion The fetal membrane closest to the interior uterine wall; it gives rise to the placenta and continues as the outer membrane surrounding the amnion.

chorionic villi Threadlike projections on the chorionic surface of the placenta; they help to form the placenta and secrete human chorionic gonadotropin.

chromosome A structure composed of tightly packed DNA; it is found in the nuclei of plant and animal cells and is responsible for the transmission of hereditary characteristics.

circumcision The surgical removal of the foreskin of the penis.

cleansing breath A slow, deep breath that is taken at the beginning and end of each contraction of labor.

clitoris The female organ that is homologous to the male penis; a small oval body of erectile tissue situated at the anterior junction of the vulva.

coitus Sexual intercourse.

coitus interruptus Removal of the erect penis from the vagina before ejaculation.

colostrum A secretion from the breast before the onset of true lactation; it has a high protein content, provides some immune properties, and cleanses the newborn's intestinal tract of mucus and meconium.

colposcopy A special type of scope used to examine the vagina and cervix for unusual changes or neoplasms.

comedo A skin lesion caused by a plug of keratin, sebum, and bacteria; there are two types: blackheads and whiteheads.

complementary therapies A nontraditional treatment method or methods used to maintain health or treat disease; used in conjunction with traditional medical therapy or treatment.

conception The union of the male sperm and female ovum; fertilization.

conceptus The products of conception.

condom A sheath or covering that is usually made from rubber or latex and is placed over an erect penis to prevent the ejaculate from entering the vagina. The female condom is inserted into the vagina before penetration and is fitted over the cervix with an inner ring to help hold it in place.

congenital Present at birth.

congenital malformation An anomaly present at birth.

contraception The prevention of conception or impregnation.

contraction A tightening and shortening of uterine muscles during labor, causing effacement and dilation of the cervix; contributes to downward and outward movement of fetus.

contraction stress test (CST) Manual manipulation of the nipple of the breast to stimulate the production of oxytocin and test the fetal response to uterine contractions; used for high-risk pregnancies. *See also* Oxytocin challenge test (OCT).

convection The loss of heat from a warm surface to air currents that are much cooler.

Coomb's test A blood test to determine if Rh+ antibodies are present in the blood of the mother or neonate.

coping Dealing effectively with stress and problems.

corpus luteum A small endocrine structure that develops inside a ruptured ovarian follicle and secretes both estrogen and progesterone.

couvade A syndrome in which the father experiences the symptoms of the pregnant partner.

craniosynostosis A premature closure of the cranial sutures that produces a head deformity and damage to the brain and eyes; craniostenosis.

crowning The appearance of the presenting fetal part (head) at the vaginal orifice during labor.

culdocentesis A fluid aspiration from the cul-de-sac of the posterior vagina, either for diagnostic or therapeutic reasons.

culture The symbols, ideas, values, traditions, and practices shared by a group of people; can also mean the growth of organisms in a special medium.

cyanosis A condition in which the skin takes on a blue, gray, or slate cast/color due to a lack of oxygen in the blood.

cystic hygroma A lymphangioma most commonly seen in the neck and axillae.

D

DDST Denver Developmental Screening Test. Assesses the developmental status of a child during the first 6 years of life in five areas: personal, social, fine motor adaptive, language, and gross motor activities.

deceleration A periodic decrease in baseline fetal heart rate; can be early, late, or variable.

decidua basalis The part of the decidua that unites with the chorion to form the placenta. It is shed in lochial discharge after delivery.

deciduous teeth Baby teeth.

decrement A decrease or stage of decline, as of a contraction.

delivery The expulsion of infant (with the placenta and membranes) from the woman at birth.

Denis Browne splint Two separate footplates attached to a crossbar and fitted to a child's shoes; sometimes used to correct clubfeet.

developmental task A skill that occurs at a particular time or age range and, when accomplished, provides the basis for future tasks.

diagonal conjugate The distance between the sacral promontory and the lowest border of the symphysis pubis; the pelvic diameter.

diaphoresis Profuse sweating.

diaphragm A contraceptive device that is used with a spermicide to prevent sperm from entering the uterus.

dilation of the cervix An expansion of the cervical os that allows for passage of the fetus.

diploid Containing a set of maternal and a set of paternal chromosomes. In humans, the diploid number of chromosomes is 46.

disproportion A term used to define whether the pelvis of the mother is too small or the fetal head is too large for safe delivery.

dizygotic twins Fetuses that develop from two fertilized ova; fraternal twins.

duration In obstetrics, the elapsed time from the beginning of a contraction until the end of the same contraction.

dyscrasia A synonym for "disease."

dysfunctional Inadequate, abnormal.

dysmenorrhea Menstruation that is painful.

dyspareunia Painful sexual intercourse.

dystocia Difficult labor due to mechanical factors produced by the fetus or the maternal pelvis or due to inadequate uterine or other muscular activity.

E

early decelerations A fetal heart rate decrease during a contraction as a result of head compression.

eclampsia Pregnancy-induced hypertension complicated by one or more seizures.

ectoderm The outer layer of cells in the developing embryo that give rise to the skin, nails, and hair.

ectopic pregnancy Implantation of a fertilized ovum outside uterine cavity; the most common ectopic site is the fallopian tube.

effacement A thinning and shortening of the cervix that occurs late in pregnancy and during labor.

effleurage Using the tips of the fingers to lightly stroke the abdomen in a patterned movement; a distraction method used to help cope with the pain of active labor.

egocentrism A type of thinking in which a child has difficulty seeing anyone else's point of view; this self-centering is normal in young children.

ejaculation The expulsion of semen and sperm from the penis.

embryo The early stage of development. In humans, the period from about 3 to 8 weeks' gestation.

empowerment Providing tools and knowledge to the family to enable informed participation in decision making about health care.

encephalitis An inflammation of the brain.

encopresis The passage of stools in a child's underwear or in other inappropriate places after 4 years of age. Some children display concurrent behavioral problems.

endoderm The inner layer of cells in a developing embryo that give rise to internal organs such as the intestines.

endometriosis A medical condition in which endometrial tissue is found in the body other than the uterus.

endometritis An inflammation or infection of the uterine lining, usually from bacterial invasion.

endometrium The mucous membrane that lines the inner surface of the uterus.

endorphins A natural body substance secreted by the pituitary gland that is similar in action to morphine. Levels of endorphins increase during pregnancy and peak during the labor process.

en face A position in which the parent and infant have eye-to-eye contact at no more than a 9- to 10-inch distance.

engagement The entrance of the fetal presenting part into the pelvis (e.g., the leading edge of the fetal head is at the level of the maternal ischial spines in a vertex presentation).

engorgement A vascular congestion or distention. In obstetrics, the swelling of breast tissue brought about by an increase in blood and lymph supply to the breast, preceding true lactation.

enuresis The abnormal inability to control urine; may be due to organic, allergic, or psychological problems.

epididymis A structure on the posterior border of the testis, where coiled storage ducts provide for maturation and transport of the spermatozoa.

epidural block A regional anesthetic block achieved by injecting a local anesthetic agent in the space overlying the dura of the spinal cord.

episiotomy An incision of the perineum to facilitate delivery and to avoid laceration of the perineum.

epispadias A congenital anomaly in which the urethral meatus is located on the dorsal surface of the penis.

Epstein's pearls An accumulation of yellow-white epithelial cells on the hard palate of a newborn. They usually disappear within a few weeks of delivery.

estrogen A substance produced by the ovaries; during puberty it increases its production and helps to produce the secondary sex characteristics.

ethic A system of moral principles or standards that guides behavior.

ethnic Groups of people within a culture classified according to religious, racial, national, or physical characteristics.

external os The lower cervical opening.

F

facies Pertaining to the appearance or expression of the face; certain congenital syndromes typically present with a specific facial appearance.

fallopian tubes The tubes that extend from the uterus to the ovaries. They serve as a passageway for ova from the ovary to the uterus and for spermatozoa from the uterus toward the ovary; oviducts; uterine tubes.

false labor Contractions of the uterus (regular or irregular) that may be strong enough to be interpreted as true labor but do not dilate the cervix.

family Apgar A screening test that reveals how a member of the family perceives its function.

fern test a.k.a., *ferning.* A palm-leaf pattern seen on a glass slide that contains dried cervical mucus. Can be used to determine what phase of the menstrual cycle the woman is in. *See* Billing's method.

fertilization The union of an ovum and a sperm.

fetal alcohol syndrome A syndrome that causes prenatal and postnatal growth retardation, mental retardation, and facial abnormalities, including a flat, thin upper lip border and down-slanting eyes.

fetal attitude A position of the fetus in the uterus, normally one of flexion, with the head flexed forward and the arms and legs flexed.

fetal blood sampling A sample of blood taken from the fetus while in the uterine cavity.

fetal heart rate (FHR) The number of times the fetal heart beats per minute; the normal range is 110 to 160 beats/min at term.

fetal heart tones (FHTs) The fetal heartbeat as heard through the mother's abdominal wall.

fetal lie Describes how the spine of the fetus is oriented in relation to the mother's spine.

fetal position Refers to how a reference point on the fetal presenting part is oriented within the mother's pelvis.

fetoscope A stethoscope specially adapted to facilitate listening to the fetal heart.

fetus A term used for the developing structure from the eighth week after fertilization until birth.

fibrinogen A component found in the blood that aids in blood clotting.

fibrocystic breast A benign disorder of the breast in which cysts arise from glandular tissues.

first stage of labor The stage that begins with the first contractions of true labor and is completed when the cervix is fully dilated to 10 cm.

flexion In obstetrics, a situation that occurs when resistance to the descent of the infant down the birth canal causes its head to flex or bend, with the chin approaching the chest, thus reducing the diameter of the presenting part.

fontanels Openings at the point of union of skull bones, often referred to as *soft spots.*

footling A breech presentation in which one foot or both feet present.

foramen ovale The opening between the left and right atria in the fetal heart.

forceps Obstetric instruments occasionally used to aid in birth by assisting fetal rotation and/or descent.

foreskin The fold of loose skin covering the end of the penis; prepuce.

fourth trimester The first 12 weeks following birth when family adaptation occurs.

frequency In labor, the period of time from the beginning of one contraction to the beginning of the next.

Friedman graph A method of describing and recording the progress of labor.

fulminating Occurring rapidly; usually said of a disease.

fundus The upper portion of the uterus between the fallopian tubes.

G

gamete A mature germ cell; an ovum or sperm.

gate control theory The stimulation of larger sensory nerves to obstruct the path of pain stimuli from reaching the central nervous system; a method used to cope with pain.

gavage Feeding the patient by means of a stomach tube or a tube passed through the nose, pharynx, and esophagus into the stomach.

gene The smallest unit of inheritance; genes are located on the chromosomes.

genetic code A component in the DNA structure that determines the amino acid sequence within each DNA strand.

genetics The study of heredity.

genotype The genetic makeup of a living being.

geographic tongue Unusual patterns of papilla formation and denuded areas on the tongue.

gestation The period of intrauterine development from conception through birth; pregnancy.

gestational age The actual time, from conception to birth, that the fetus remains in the uterus.

gestational diabetes mellitus An endocrine disorder that occurs only when the woman is pregnant.

gestational trophoblastic disease Hydatidiform mole; occurs when the chorionic villi abnormally increase and develop small sacs that resemble small grapes. Chromosomal abnormalities are found in many cases.

glucometer A meter used to measure blood glucose.

glucosuria Glucose in the urine (glycosuria).

gonad A sex gland; ovaries in the female and testes in the male.

Goodell's sign A softening of cervix that occurs during the second month of pregnancy.

graafian follicle The ovarian cyst containing the ripe ovum; it secretes estrogens.

grasp reflex When lightly stimulating the palm of a neonate, the hand grasps the stimulus; used in determining the maturity of the newborn infant.

gravid Pregnant.

gravida The number of times a woman has been pregnant; a pregnant woman.

guided imagery An alternative therapy that uses pleasant mental images of events, feelings, or sensations; used as a distraction method of coping with the pain of labor.

gynecologist A health care provider who specializes in the care and treatment of female reproductive issues including, but not limited to, menstruation, pregnancy, menopause, and various forms of cancer.

H

habilitation A term used to describe a treatment on a patient who is handicapped from birth and therefore is *learning,* not relearning, a task.

habituation In an infant, the ability to become accustomed to certain noises, voices, etc., within the environment.

heart failure A decrease in cardiac output necessary to meet the metabolic needs of the body.

heel stick (heel puncture) A method of obtaining neonate blood from the heel for testing.

Hegar's sign A softening of the lower uterine segment found upon palpation in the second or third month of pregnancy.

hemangioma A benign tumor of the skin that consists of blood vessels.

herbal medicine An alternative and/or complementary method for treating various ailments using herbs and plants.

holism An approach to caring for a person that recognizes and adapts to his or her physical, intellectual, emotional, and spiritual nature; a way of relating to the patient as a whole or biopsychosocial individual rather than just a person with an ailment.

Homan's sign On dorsiflexion of the foot, the patient experiences pain in the calf of the leg; used as an indication of thrombophlebitis.

hormone A substance produced in an organ or gland and conveyed by blood to another part of the body to exert an effect.

hot flash A facial flushing related to vasomotor response to hormonal changes in the perimenopausal woman.

human chorionic gonadotropin (hCG) The hormone produced by chorionic villi and found in the urine of pregnant women.

human immunodeficiency virus (HIV) The organism that causes AIDS.

hydramnios Polyhydramnios; an excess of amniotic fluid, leading to overdistention of the uterus. Often seen in diabetic pregnant women even if there is no coexisting fetal anomaly.

hydrops fetalis A condition of the fetus in which there is cardiac decompensation, hepatosplenomegaly, and respiratory distress or failure. Usually due to erythroblastosis fetalis, infection, or multisystem organ failure of the fetus in utero.

hymen A membranous fold that normally partially covers the entrance to the vagina in a female who has not had vaginal penetration.

hyperbilirubinemia An excessive amount of bilirubin in the blood; more commonly seen in hemolytic disorders of the newborn, infection, and extreme cold stress.

hypercapnia An increased amount of carbon dioxide in the blood.

hyperemesis gravidarum Excessive vomiting during pregnancy, leading to dehydration and starvation.

hyperglycemia An excess amount of glucose in the blood. Seen most often in diabetic patients.

hypernatremia Excess sodium in the blood.

hypokalemia A potassium deficit in the blood.

hypospadias A developmental anomaly in which the urethra opens on the lower surface of the penis.

hypotension Low blood pressure. Can cause dizziness to actual syncopal episodes.

hypoxia Inadequate oxygenation of the tissues.

hysterectomy The surgical removal of the uterus only.

I

icterus neonatorum Jaundice in the newborn.

immune response The body's response to a substance it deems as foreign.

immunoglobulin A protein within the body that can act as an antibody.

implantation The embedding of a fertilized ovum in the uterine mucosa 6 or 7 days after fertilization.

impotence The inability to achieve and/or maintain an erection in the male.

impregnate To make pregnant or to fertilize.

inborn error of metabolism A deficiency of specific enzymes that are needed for normal metabolism and growth. Develops in utero; may be inherited.

incarcerated Confined, constricted.

incest Sexual activities among family members. Often seen in father-daughter relationships, less often in mother-son or sibling relationships.

incompetent cervix A mechanical defect in the cervix, making it unable to remain closed throughout pregnancy and resulting in spontaneous abortion.

increment An increase or addition; to build up, as of a contraction.

induction Artificial initiation of labor.

infant mortality rate The number of deaths that occur in the first 12 months of life per 1000 live births.

infertility The inability to produce offspring.

inlet of the pelvis The upper opening into the pelvic cavity.

innominate bone The hipbone, ilium, ischium, and pubis.

integrative therapy Combines complementary and alternative therapy with traditional medicine to facilitate healing. A biopsychosocial approach to care.

internal os The opening found between the cervix and uterus.

intrapartum The time of onset of true labor, followed by the delivery of the neonate and finally the placenta.

in vitro fertilization Test tube fertilization in which the ripe ovum is collected and fertilized in vitro (in glass) by sperm. The embryo is then transferred to a woman's uterus.

involution Rolling or turning inward; reduction in the size of the uterus following delivery.

K

kangaroo care The use of skin-to-skin contact between the neonate/infant and the caregiver; used to promote bonding between the parent and infant.

karyotype The chromosomal makeup of a body cell, arranged from largest to smallest. The normal number of chromosomes in humans is 46.

Kegel exercise The tightening and relaxing of the pubococcygeal muscles. Helps to strengthen the pelvic floor muscles.

kernicterus A grave form of jaundice of the newborn, accompanied by brain damage.

kilogram A unit of measure. One kilogram (kg) is equal to 2.2 pounds, or 1000 mg.

L

labia In obstetrics, the external folds of skin on either side of the vulva.

labia majora The larger outer folds of skin on either side of the vulva.

labia minora The smaller inner folds of skin on either side of the vulva.

labor The process by which the fetus is expelled from the uterus; childbirth; confinement; parturition.

laceration In obstetrics, a tear in the perineum, vagina, or cervix.

lactase The enzyme that breaks down lactose.

lactation The process of producing and supplying breast milk.

lactiferous ducts Tiny tubes within the breast that conduct milk from the acini cells to the nipple.

lactose intolerant The inability to adequately digest milk products.

laminaria A type of kelp or seaweed that can be used to help dilate the cervical canal to aid in delivery of the products of conception (neonate).

lanugo Fine, downy hair seen on all parts of the fetus, except the palms of the hands and soles of the feet, by the end of 20 weeks' gestation.

late deceleration The slowing of the fetal heart during a uterine contraction that continues after the contraction ends.

Leopold's maneuver A method of abdominal palpation used to determine fetal position or placement within the uterus.

let-down reflex A pattern of stimulation, hormone release, and muscle contraction that forces milk into the lactiferous ducts, making it available to the infant; milk ejection reflex.

letting go A phase in the development of the parental role.

libido The sexual drive, be it unconscious or conscious.

lie The position of the fetus described by the relationship of the long axis of the fetus to the long axis of the mother.

lightening The moving of the fetus and uterus downward into the pelvic cavity.

linea nigra A line of darker pigmentation extending from the pubis to the umbilicus noted in some women during the later months of pregnancy.

lochia The maternal discharge of blood, mucus, and tissue from the uterus; may last for several weeks after birth.

lochia alba White vaginal discharge that follows lochia serosa and lasts from about the tenth to the twenty-first day after delivery.

lochia rubra Red, blood-tinged vaginal discharge that occurs following delivery and lasts 2 to 4 days.

lochia serosa Pink, serous, and blood-tinged vaginal discharge that follows lochia rubra and lasts until the seventh to tenth day after delivery.

L/S ratio The ratio of the phospholipids lecithin and sphingomyelin produced by the fetal lungs; useful in assessing fetal lung maturity.

lunar month A 28-day cycle corresponding to the phases of the moon. A normal pregnancy lasts 10 lunar months.

luteinizing hormone (LH) The anterior pituitary hormone responsible for stimulating ovulation and developing the corpus luteum.

M

macrocephaly An abnormally large skull. Can be found in infants with hydrocephalus.

macrosomia An abnormally large infant, or a neonatal birth weight above the 90th percentile.

mammary glands Compound glandular elements of the breast that in the female secrete milk to nourish the infant.

mastectomy Surgical removal of a breast.

maternal mortality rate A number reflecting the amount of maternal deaths, which occur within 42 days after termination of a pregnancy or delivery of a live fetus within 1 year.

McDonald's sign A probable sign of pregnancy in which the examiner can easily flex the body of the uterus against the cervix.

mechanisms (cardinal movements) of labor The positional changes of the fetus as it moves through the birth canal during labor and delivery.

meconium The first stool of the newborn; a mixture of amniotic fluid and secretions of the intestinal glands.

meconium aspiration syndrome The aspiration of meconium in utero. The presence of meconium in the trachea or its appearance on a chest x-ray film helps to establish this diagnosis.

meconium ileus A deficiency of pancreatic enzymes in the intestinal tract in which the meconium of the fetus becomes excessively sticky and adheres to the intestinal wall, causing obstruction. Occasionally seen in babies born with cystic fibrosis.

meconium-stained fluid Amniotic fluid that contains meconium.

megacolon Hirschsprung's disease; a congenital absence of ganglionic cells in a segment of the large bowel that results in massive dilation of the bowel.

meiosis Cell division to halve the number of chromosomes in the ova and sperm to 23.

menarche The beginning of menstrual and reproductive function in girls.

meningomyelocele A sacklike cyst containing the meninges, spinal cord, and fluid that has herniated through the spinal column, usually via some form of anatomical defect of the bony spinal canal.

menopause The permanent cessation of menses.

menstrual cycle The cyclic buildup of uterine lining, ovulation, and sloughing of the lining occurring approximately every 28 days in nonpregnant females.

menstruation (menses) The shedding of uterine lining at the end of the menstrual cycle, resulting in a bloody discharge from the vagina.

meridian An imaginary line that encircles the body. Used in some forms of alternative or complementary therapies (see Chapter 33).

mesoderm The intermediate layer of germ cells in the embryo that gives rise to connective tissue, bone marrow, muscles, blood, lymphoid tissue, and epithelial tissue.

metered dose inhaler (MDI) A device that delivers measured puffs of medication for inhalation.

microcephaly A congenital anomaly in which the head of the newborn is abnormally small.

milia Very small, white, keratin-filled cysts or papules normally found on an infant's face. They generally disappear if left alone.

miliaria Prickly heat; inflammation of the skin caused by sweating.

miscarriage Lay term for spontaneous abortion.

mitosis Cell division in all body cells other than the gametes (ova and sperm).

molding The shaping of the fetal head to facilitate movement through the birth canal during labor.

mongolian spot A benign, blue-hued pigmentation usually found around the lower back or buttock. Seen most often in dark-skinned infants.

monozygotic twins Two fetuses that develop from a single divided fertilized ovum; identical twins.

mons veneris The fleshy tissue over the female symphysis pubis from which hair develops at puberty.

Montgomery's glands (tubercles) Small nodules located around the nipples that enlarge during pregnancy and lactation. They produce moisturizing secretion.

morbidity Pertains to illness, disease.

morning sickness Nausea and vomiting occurring during the first trimester of pregnancy; may occur at any time during the day.

Moro reflex When a newborn is jarred, the legs draw up and the arms fold across the chest.

mortality Pertains to death.

morula A solid mass of cells that developed from the fertilized ovum.

mucous plug A collection of thick mucus that blocks the cervical canal during pregnancy.

multifetal pregnancy A pregnancy in which the woman is carrying two or more fetuses; also called *multiple gestation*. Can be twins, triplets, etc.

multigravida A woman who has previously been pregnant.

multipara A woman who has had more than one pregnancy in which the fetus(es) was viable (20 weeks' gestation).

murmur A sound heard when listening to the heart; caused by blood leaking through openings that have not closed as they should before birth.

mutation A change in genetic material.

N

Nägele's rule A method of determining the estimated date of delivery (EDD); after obtaining the first day of the last menstrual period, subtract 3 months and add 7 days.

narcotic agonist A drug that is used to reverse narcotic effects.

neonate An infant between the age of birth and 28 days of life.

nesting The provision of an enclosed space, bounded by a small blanket roll encircling the preterm infant. It helps to provide a calm, supportive environment for the infant.

neutral thermal environment An environment that is neither too hot nor too cold, thus the body does not need overwork itself to deliver oxygen or increase its metabolic rate to maintain a normal body temperature.

nevus (pl, *nevi*) A congenital discoloration of an area of the skin, such as a strawberry mark or mole.

nitrazine paper A specially treated type of paper that turns a specific color in the presence of amniotic fluid.

nonnutritive sucking Any sucking activity that is not related to the intake of nutrients.

nonshivering thermogenesis The oxidation of brown fat in the neonate to produce heat to keep warm.

NST Nonstress test; an assessment method by which the reaction (or response) of the fetal heart rate to fetal movement is evaluated.

nuchal Pertaining to the neck.

nuchal cord A term to describe a situation in which the umbilical cord is wrapped around the fetus's neck.

nuclear family A family group that consists of one or more adults and one or more children.

nulligravida A female who has never been pregnant.

nullipara A female who has not delivered a live fetus.

O

obstetrics The branch of medicine concerned with the care of women during pregnancy, childbirth, and the postpartum period.

occiput The posterior part of the skull.

oligohydramnios A decreased amount of amniotic fluid.

oliguria A decrease in urine secretion by the kidney.

omphalocele A herniation of abdominal contents at the umbilicus.

ophthalmia neonatorum Acute conjunctivitis of the newborn, often caused by *Gonococci* or *Chlamydia*.

opportunistic infection An infection caused by bacteria normally found in the environment that become pathogenic to the body due to a defective immune system; usually seen in immunosuppressed individuals whose CD4+ count has dropped to a critical level, such as patients with cancer or AIDS.

oral contraceptive A medication, usually a combined progesterone and estrogen pill, used to prevent pregnancy.

orgasm Occurs at the peak or climax of sexual and emotional excitement. In the male, ejaculation generally occurs during orgasm.

orthopnea A condition in which the patient must sit up to breathe.

orthostatic hypotension A decrease in either systolic or diastolic blood pressure when moving from a supine or sitting position to a fully upright position.

Ortolani's maneuver An examination maneuver on a newborn to determine the presence or absence of congenital hip malformation.

osteoporosis A decrease in the overall mass of bones due to an increase in the trabeculae of the bone. Can be caused by age, sedentary lifestyle, smoking, diet, and many other factors.

ovarian cycle The changes that the ovarian follicles undergo throughout the menstrual cycle. Days 1 to 14 are the follicular phase, and days 15 to 28 are the luteal phase.

ovulation The normal process of discharging a mature ovum from an ovary approximately 14 days before the onset of menses.

ovum The female reproductive cell; egg.

oxytocics Drugs that intensify uterine contractions to hasten birth or control postpartum hemorrhage.

oxytocin challenge test (OCT) A method of assessing the fetal response to labor by administering an oxytocic drug to stimulate a few labor contractions. Used in high-risk pregnancies. *See* Contraction stress test (CST).

P

paced breathing A breathing technique used during labor to help the woman relax and to increase her pain tolerance.

para A woman who has borne offspring who reached the age of viability (20 to 24 weeks' gestation).

paraphimosis Impaired circulation of the uncircumcised penis due to improper retraction of the foreskin.

parenteral A medication route other than the gastrointestinal tract. Can be intravenous, intramuscular, etc.

parity The condition of having borne offspring who attained the age of viability. The number of pregnancies ending after the age of viability.

parturient Pertaining to the act of childbirth. A woman giving birth.

parturition The process of giving birth.

passive acquired immunity Antibodies to a communicable disease are given to the patient.

pelvic rocking (tilt) An exercise to help strengthen abdominal muscles and reduce the strain on the lower back.

pelvis The lower portion of the trunk of the body, bounded by the hipbones, coccyx, and sacrum.

penis The male organ of copulation, reproduction, and urination.

perinatal mortality rate The number of fetal and neonatal deaths in a given time period per 1000 live births.

perineum The area of tissue between the anus and the scrotum in males or between the anus and the vagina in females.

Pfannenstiel incision A low, transverse incision into the abdomen that is nearly invisible when healed; often used for cesarean section (surgical) deliveries.

phenotype The entire physical, biochemical, and physiologic makeup of an individual as determined both genetically and environmentally.

phimosis A tightening of the prepuce of the uncircumcised penis.

phocomelia The absence or incomplete formation and development of the arms, forearms, thighs, and legs. The hands and feet are present but may be abnormally developed.

phototherapy The treatment of disease by exposure to light; often used to treat hyperbilirubinemia in the newborn.

pica The eating of substances not ordinarily considered edible or to have nutritive value.

pincer grasp The use of the index finger and thumb to grasp an object.

PKU (phenylketonuria) A genetic disorder caused by the faulty metabolism of phenylalanine, an amino acid essential to life and found in all protein foods. If left untreated, mental retardation can occur.

placenta A specialized disk-shaped organ that connects the fetus to the uterine wall for gas, nutrient, and waste exchanges; also called *afterbirth*.

placenta previa The abnormal placental implantation in the lower uterine segment.

placental souffle Soft-blowing sounds produced by blood coursing through the dilated arteries of the uterus; has the same rate as the maternal pulse.

polydactyly A developmental anomaly characterized by the presence of extra fingers or toes.

polyhydramnios An excessive amount of amniotic fluid within the placenta.

postpartum After childbirth.

postpartum hemorrhage A blood loss greater than 500 ml after vaginal birth or 1000 ml after cesarean birth.

precipitate birth A birth that occurs without a trained attendant present.

precipitate labor A rapid progression of labor that lasts fewer than 3 hours.

pregnancy The condition of having a developing embryo or fetus in the body after fertilization of the female egg by the male sperm.

prehension The use of the hands to pick up small objects; grasping.

prenatal Before birth.

presentation The fetal body part that enters the maternal pelvis first.

presenting part The fetal part that first enters the maternal pelvis.

presumptive signs of pregnancy Symptoms that suggest pregnancy but do not confirm it, such as cessation of menses, quickening, Chadwick's sign, and morning sickness.

preterm infant Premature infant; an infant born before 37 weeks' gestation.

primigravida A woman who is pregnant for the first time.

primipara A woman who has given birth to her first child (past the point of viability), whether or not that child is living or was alive at birth.

prodrome The initial symptoms indicating an approaching disease.

progesterone A hormone produced by the adrenal cortex, the corpus luteum, and the placenta. Its function is to stimulate the development of the mammary glands and growth of the endometrium and to maintain a pregnancy.

projectile vomiting Vomiting that occurs with force (vomitus landing 2 to 4 feet away).

prolactin A hormone produced by the anterior pituitary gland that stimulates lactation or milk production.

prolapsed cord An umbilical cord that becomes trapped between the fetal presenting part and the maternal pelvis.

prostaglandin (PG) In obstetrics, PGE_2 gel is used on the cervix to help induce labor. PG is mistakenly referred to as a hormone but is actually an autacoid because it acts only on the tissue in which it was formed.

proteinuria The presence of protein in the urine.

pseudocyesis A condition in which the woman has symptoms of pregnancy but in which hormonal pregnancy test results are negative; false pregnancy.

psychoprophylaxis Psychophysical training aimed at preparing the expectant parents to cope with the processes of labor and to avoid concentration on the discomforts associated with childbirth.

puberty The period of time during which the secondary sexual characteristics develop and the ability to procreate is attained.

pudendal block The injection of an anesthetizing agent at the pudendal nerve to produce numbness of the external genitals and the lower one third of the vagina.

puerperal morbidity Postpartum fever; a temperature of 38° C (100.4° F) or higher after the first 24 hours and continuing for at least 2 days during the first 10 days after delivery.

puerperium The period of time after delivery until involution of the uterus is complete, usually 6 weeks.

pulmonary vascular resistance (PVR) In the fetus, PVR is the resistance to the flow of blood in the fetal lung tissue.

pulse oximeter Equipment that determines the level of blood oxygen saturation by means of a sensor placed on the skin.

Q

quickening The first fetal movements felt by the pregnant woman, usually between 16 and 18 weeks' gestation.

R

radiation Heat loss from the body to a cooler object within the environment. The object does not necessarily need to be touching the body. Can also refer to a mode of therapy used for cancer.

rapport Harmonious relation.

reflexology An integrative therapy that uses varying degrees of pressure, usually to the hands or feet, to promote relaxation.

reflux A backward flow of fluid (e.g., vesico-ureteral reflux [urine is forced from the bladder into the ureters], gastric reflux [stomach contents flow into the esophagus]). It may or may not enter the oral cavity.

regression Behavior that is more appropriate to an earlier stage of development. Often occurs in children as a response to stress.

relaxin A water-soluble protein secreted by the corpus luteum that causes relaxation of the symphysis pubis and facilitates cervical dilation during birth.

retractions Abnormal "sucking in" of the chest wall during inspiration. Can be substernal or intercostal; indicates respiratory distress.

retrolental fibroplasia Blindness usually found in the preterm infant that is associated with oxygen concentrations and in which the blood vessels of the retina become damaged.

Rh factor An antigen present on the surface of blood cells that make the blood cell incompatible with blood cells that do not have the antigen.

rhabdomyosarcoma An extremely malignant neoplasm originating in skeletal muscle.

RhoGAM An immune globulin given to the mother (not the infant) after the delivery of an Rh+ infant to an Rh− mother.

rhythm method A natural form of birth control that requires the woman to chart her menstrual cycles for several months on a calendar. This method is based on the woman ovulating about 14 days *before* the next menstrual cycle begins. Enables proper utility of contraception during fertile period or abstinence.

rickets A disease of the bones caused by a lack of calcium or vitamin D.

ritualism A need to maintain strict structure and routine.

rooting reflex An infant's tendency to turn the head and open the lips to suck when one side of the mouth or cheek is touched or stroked.

S

sacrum Five fused vertebrae that form a triangle of bone just beneath the lumbar vertebrae and between the hipbones.

salpingitis Inflammation or infection of a fallopian tube.

scoliosis Lateral curvature of the spine.

second stage of labor The stage lasting from complete dilation of the cervix to expulsion of the fetus.

semen Thick, whitish fluid ejaculated by the male during orgasm; contains the spermatozoa and their nutrients.

separation anxiety Distress that occurs when strangers separate the infant from the parents.

sex chromosomes The X and Y chromosomes that are responsible for sex determination; women have two X chromosomes; men have one X and one Y chromosome.

sexually transmitted disease (STD) Refers to diseases ordinarily transmitted by direct sexual contact with an infected individual.

shunt A bypass.

Skene's ducts (paraurethral ducts) The ducts located on either side of the urethra; provide lubrication of the urethra.

smegma A cheeselike substance secreted by the sebaceous glands near the clitoris in the female and under the prepuce of an uncircumcised male.

Snellen alphabet chart A device used to measure near and far vision; a variation of the Snellen E chart.

spermatogenesis The process by which mature spermatozoa are formed and during which the number of chromosomes is reduced by half.

spermatozoa Mature sperm cells produced by the testes.

spina bifida A congenital embryonic neural tube defect in which there is an imperfect closure of the spinal vertebrae. There are two types: occulta (hidden) or cystic (sac or cyst).

spinnbarkeit Elasticity seen in cervical mucus at the time of ovulation.

spontaneous abortion The loss of the products of conceptions before 20-weeks' gestation; miscarriage.

standard precautions Infection control guidelines established by the Centers for Disease Control and Prevention to prevent the spread of infection (see Appendix A).

station The relationship of the presenting fetal part to an imaginary line drawn between the pelvic ischial spines.

sterility The inability of the male to impregnate a female. The inability of a female to conceive. Can also refer to the absence of live organisms on an object.

stillbirth The delivery of a dead fetus.

strabismus (cross-eye or squint) A condition in which the child is not able to direct both eyes toward an object at the same time due to lack of muscle coordination.

striae gravidarum Stretch marks; shiny reddish lines that appear on the abdomen, breasts, thighs, and buttocks of pregnant women as a result of stretching the skin.

stridor A shrill sound heard during respiration caused by air passing through a narrowed portion of the respiratory tract.

subinvolution A slower-than-expected return of the uterus to its nonpregnant condition. Infection or retained placenta are the usual causes.

supine hypotension syndrome The lowering of blood pressure when in a supine position. Occurs due to pressure or weight of the pregnant uterus on the inferior vena cava.

surfactant A surface-active mixture of lipoproteins secreted in the alveoli and air passages that reduces the surface tension of pulmonary fluids and contributes to the elasticity of pulmonary tissue.

surrogate mother A fertile woman who is impregnated for the purpose of producing a child for another (infertile) couple.

sutures Separation between fetal skull bones that permit molding during the birth process.

syndactyly The webbing together of two or more fingers/toes. Most often this is an inherited anomaly.

T

taking hold The second phase of maternal adaptation in which the mother assumes control of herself and the infant.

taking in The initial maternal adaptation following birth in which passive acceptance of care occurs.

talipes equinovarus Clubfoot.

teratogen A nongenetic factor that can produce malformations of the fetus.

term infant A live-born infant of 38 to 42 weeks' gestation.

testes The male gonads, in which sperm and testosterone are produced.

testosterone The male hormone; responsible for the development of secondary male characteristics.

therapeutic play Guided play that results in physical or psychological well-being.

third stage of labor The time from delivery of the fetus to the time when the placenta has been completely expelled.

thrombophlebitis Inflammation or the formation of a blood clot in or along a vein.

thrombus A blood clot that moves within the circulation.

tissue perfusion Nutrition and oxygenation of tissue resulting from adequate blood flow.

tocodynamometer External device that can be used to identify the pressure of uterine contractions during labor.

tocolytic A drug that inhibits uterine contractions.

tocotransducer An electronic monitoring device used to measure uterine contractions.

TORCH Acronym used to describe a group of infections that represent potentially severe fetal problems if infection occurs during pregnancy. *TO,* Toxoplasmosis; *R,* rubella; *C,* cytomegalovirus; and *H,* herpesvirus.

toxic shock syndrome (TSS) An infection usually caused by *Staphylococcus aureus* and found most often in women of reproductive age who use tampons.

transition The period of labor in which the cervix is approximately 8 cm dilated, the contractions are very strong, and the laboring woman feels the urge to push.

transplacental Through the placenta (i.e., the exchange of nutrients, waste products, drugs, and hormones).

triage A process used to determine the urgency of illness to prioritize care.

trimester One third of the gestational time for pregnancy.

trophoblast Comprises the nutrient relationship with the endometrium of the uterus.

true labor Changes in the cervix are the key distinctions between true and false labor. The contractions gradually develop a regular pattern, becoming more frequent and stronger and causing effacement and dilation of the cervix.

turgor Normal elasticity of the skin.

tympanometry The measurement of mobility of the tympanic membrane of the ear and the estimation of middle-ear pressure.

U

ultrasound High-frequency sound waves that may be directed (through the use of a transducer) into the maternal abdomen. The ultrasonic sound waves reflected by the underlying structures of varying densities allow maternal and fetal tissues, bones, and fluids to be identified.

umbilical cord The structure connecting the placenta to the umbilicus of the fetus through which nutrients from the woman are exchanged for wastes from the fetus.

umbilicus The navel or "belly button" on the abdomen that formed the attachment of the umbilical cord during fetal life.

uterine dysfunction A pattern of labor that interferes with the normal progression of labor and delivery.

uterus A hollow muscular organ in which the fertilized ovum is implanted and the developing fetus is nourished until birth.

V

vacuum extractor A device to assist the birth of fetal head using suction.

vagina The musculomembranous tube or passageway located between the external female genitals and the uterus.

Valsalva's maneuver Holding one's breath or bearing down as though passing stool, thereby increasing intra-abdominal and intra-thoracic pressure.

variability Describes the fluctuations, or constant changes, in the baseline heart rate. Has a fine, sawtooth appearance on the recording strip of a heart monitor.

varicella Chickenpox.

varicose veins Permanently distended veins.

variola Smallpox.

vas deferens A duct that aids in the transport of sperm and semen into the male urethra.

vasectomy A form of male sterilization in which the vas deferens are cut and ligated.

vector A carrier that transmits an infective agent from one host to another.

ventriculography An x-ray examination of the ventricles of the brain following the injection of air into the ventricles.

vernix caseosa A protective, cheeselike, whitish substance made up of sebum and desquamated epithelial cells that is present on fetal skin and the skin of newborn.

version A turning of the position of the fetus in the uterus before birth. Can be spontaneously or manually induced.

vertex The top or crown of the head.

viable Capable of living.

volvulus A twisting of the loops of the small intestine, causing obstruction.

vulva The external structure of the female genitals, lying between the mons veneris and anus.

W

Wharton's jelly Yellow-white gelatinous material that surrounds and protects the vessels of the umbilical cord.

wheal A large, slightly raised, red or blistered area of skin; may itch.

WIC Woman-infant-children; a subsidized supplemental food program for mothers and children.

womb A lay term referring to the gravid uterus.

X

X chromosome The female sex chromosome.

Y

Y chromosome The male sex chromosome.

Z

zygote A fertilized ovum.

Index

A

Abbreviations, 799-800
Abdomen
  compression during pregnancy, 57f
  enlargement as probable sign of pregnancy, 53
Abdominal pain
  in abruptio placentae, 93
  in ectopic pregnancy, 89
  in encephalitis, 548
Abdominal pregnancy, 89f
Abdominal striae, 52f, 53-54
Abdominal tightening exercise, 210-211
Abducens nerve, 544f, 545t, 561b
Abnormal labor, 188-196
Abnormal uterine bleeding, 254
ABO incompatibility, 339b
Abortion, 50, 84-86, 85f, 86t, 87t
Abruptio placentae, 91f, 93
  in amniotomy, 177
  placenta previa versus, 92t
Abscess in acute otitis media, 536
Absence seizure, 549-552, 550-551t
Absorption of nutrients, 371f
Abstinence method of contraception, 261
Abstract reasoning, 456, 463
Abuse
  child, 585-588, 587b, 588f
  during pregnancy, 116
Acceleration, fetal heart rate pattern and, 139
Accessory glands of male, 23
Accident prevention
  preschooler and, 432-433, 433f
  toddler and, 416, 417-418t, 419f, 420f
Accidental drowning, 563
Accidental needle stick, 516, 516f
Accolate. See Zafirlukast.
Accutane. See Isotretinoin.
Acetaminophen
  for child, 479
  for fever in nasopharyngitis, 594
  overdose of, 678-679
Acetylsalicylic acid poisoning, 679-680
ACHES acronym, 263
Acid poisoning, 679t
Acidemia, 739t
Acidosis, 673
Acme of contraction, 124, 126f
Acne vulgaris, 705f, 705-706
Acoustic nerve, 544f, 545t, 561b
Acquired immunity, 748
Acquired immunodeficiency syndrome, 257, 260t
  adolescent and, 466
  breastfeeding and, 225
  education for school-age child, 441
  pediatric, 756-759
  in pregnancy, 110

Acquired immunodeficiency syndrome—cont'd
  prenatal screening for, 49t
  risk factors for, 110b
Acrocyanosis, 152, 289, 292, 294t
Activated charcoal, 677
Activated partial thromboplastin time, 107
Active immunity, 748
Active phase of labor, 145t
Activity restriction
  in pregnancy-induced hypertension, 96
  in preterm labor, 198
Acupressure, 778-779
Acupuncture, 778-779
Acute bronchiolitis, 596-597
Acute bronchitis, 596
Acute coryza, 591
Acute croup, 595-596, 596f
Acute cystitis, 690
Acute glomerulonephritis, 693t, 693-694
Acute laryngotracheobronchitis, 594
Acute otitis media, 535-537
Acute pharyngitis, 594
Acute spasmodic laryngitis, 594
Addison's disease, 726t
Adenoiditis, 599-600
ADHD. See Attention-deficit hyperactivity disorder.
Adipose tissue, 701
Adjunctive drugs in labor pain management, 167
Adjustment phase, fathers during pregnancy and, 72
Admission
  to hospital or birth center, 133-136
  during labor, 134b, 134-135
  to pediatric unit, 483-484, 494-496, 495-497f, 498b
  to postpartum or nursery unit, 217-221, 218t, 219f, 221f
Adolescence, 455
Adolescent, 455-474
  administration of medications, 509b
  after birth care of, 203
  anorexia nervosa in, 771-772, 772f
  behavior conditions in, 763t
  bulimia in, 772-773
  career plans of, 464-465, 465f
  childbirth preparation class for, 158
  chronic illness in, 646t
  cognitive development of, 463
  daydreams and, 465
  depression in, 472, 764, 765-766
  developmental theories of adolescence and, 364t
  diabetes mellitus in, 738-739t
  general characteristics of, 455-456, 456b, 457f
  heart-healthy guidelines for, 628b
  hospitalization of, 490-491
  intravenous therapy for, 522-523t
  nursing approach to, 472, 472f
  nutrition for, 376, 376t, 468-470
  oxygen therapy for, 526b
  parenting of, 467-468, 468f, 469t
  peer relationships of, 463-464, 464f
  personal care and, 470
  physical development of, 456-460, 458t, 459f, 460b, 461f, 467f

Page numbers followed by *f* indicate figures; *b* indicates boxes, and *t* indicates tables.

Adolescent—cont'd
psychological adaptations to pregnancy, 72-73
psychosocial development of, 460-463, 462f
response to death, 651t
responsibility and, 465
safety issues of, 470-471, 471f
sexual behavior of, 465-467, 467t
substance abuse and, 471-472, 767, 768t, 769t
suicide and, 764
weight gain during pregnancy, 60
Adoption, 274
Adrenal disorders, 726t
Adult *versus* child growth and development, 349-351f, 349-352
Advanced practice nurse, 12, 12b
Advanced reproductive techniques, 273t, 273-274
Advocate, 7
Aerosol spray, 710t
abuse of, 768t
AFP. *See* Alpha-fetoprotein.
African-American family
cultural influences on, 358-359t
food patterns of, 368t
labor and delivery and, 121t
Afterpains, 205
AFV. *See* Amniotic fluid volume.
Aganglionic megacolon, 661-662, 662f
Age
fertility and, 271
older couple pregnancy and, 73
pregnant adolescent and, 73
recommended dietary allowances and, 372t
Age of viability, 37, 50
Agency for Healthcare Research and Quality, 774
Ages and Stages Questionnaire, 397
Aggression, toddler and, 413t
Aid to Families with Dependent Children, 377t
AIDS. *See* Acquired immunodeficiency syndrome.
Air ring for perineal pain, 208
Airborne infection precautions, 749
Airway
asthma and, 602, 602f, 603f
burn and, 717
epiglottitis and, 596
nasopharyngitis and, 592-593
obstruction of, 528, 529f
Albumin, 505
Albuminuria. *See* Proteinuria.
Alcohol
adolescent and, 767, 768t
children of alcoholics and, 769-770, 770f
use during lactation, 65
use during pregnancy, 114t
Aldomet. *See* Methyldopa.
Algo hearing screening test, 286
Alkaline poisoning, 679t
Alkalosis, vomiting and, 664, 673t
Allergen, 707
Allergic conjunctivitis, 541
Allergic rhinitis, 591, 600-602, 602f
Allergic salute, 602f
Allergy
pet ownership and, 451-452
spina bifida and, 327
to vaccine, 751
Alliance for Children and Families, 453
Aloe vera, 782t
Alopecia, 711
chemotherapy-associated, 643

Alpha-adrenergic blockers for pregnancy-induced hypertension, 94
Alpha-fetoprotein testing, 82t
Altered level of consciousness, 564-565
Alternative family, 355t
Alternative therapy, 775-786
acupuncture and acupressure as, 778-779
aromatherapy as, 779
ayurveda as, 779
biofeedback as, 780-781
chiropractic care as, 781
definition of, 775
energy healing as, 778, 779f
federal regulations and, 776-778
guided imagery as, 780
herbal remedies as, 781-784, 782b, 782-784t
homeopathy as, 779
hydrotherapy as, 780
hyperbaric oxygen therapy as, 784
hypnotherapy as, 780
massage as, 778, 778f
nurse's role in, 775-776, 776b, 776f, 777t
osteopathy as, 778
reflexology as, 778, 780f
sauna as, 784
Alveolus
breast, 28, 29f
lung, 598
Ambivalence
of father in pregnancy, 72
in first trimester, 70
Amblyopia, 540
Ambulation
pharmacological labor pain management and, 174
postpartum, 210
after cesarean birth, 213
for prevention of thrombosis, 244
Amenorrhea, 51, 254
Americaine. *See* Benzocaine.
American Cancer Society, 253b
American Indian, labor and delivery for, 121t
American Nurses Association standards of care, 10
Amethopterin, 115t
Aminoglycosides
interactions with food, 512t
magnesium sulfate and, 96, 197
Amniocentesis, 81f, 83t
before cesarean birth, 184
in prenatal laboratory test, 49t
in Rh and ABO incompatibility, 100
Amnioinfusion, 140, 176
Amnion, 36
Amniotic fluid
assessment of, 141
fetal maturity and, 177
version and, 180
Amniotic fluid embolism, 201
Amniotic fluid volume, 82t
Amniotic membrane, 134
Amniotic sac, 36
Amniotomy, 141, 176-177
for hypotonic labor, 188
in labor induction, 178
Amphetamines, 768t
Ampicillin, 112
Ampulla of fallopian tube, 26
Amylase, 370
Anabolic steroids, 469-470
Analgesic potentiators, 165t

Analgesics
    after cesarean birth, 213
    for afterpains, 206
    for episiotomy-associated pain, 182
    during labor and birth, 164, 167
    for mastitis, 247
Anaphylactic shock, 237
Anasarca, 338, 672
Anastomosis in intussusception, 663
Androgens, 23, 456
Androgynous, term, 440
Android pelvis, 27, 27f
Anemia, 107-108, 108b, 633-639
    in abruptio placentae, 92t, 93
    after postpartum hemorrhage, 238
    in erythroblastosis fetalis, 338, 340
    heart disease and, 106
    in hemophilia, 640
    iron-deficiency, 633-634, 635
    in previa placenta, 92, 92t
    in sickle cell disease, 634-638, 636f, 637f, 638t
    in thalassemia, 638-639, 639f
Anencephaly, 82t
Anesthesia for childbirth, 164, 166t
Angelica, 782t
Angiocardiography, 618t
Angiotensin-converting enzyme inhibitors, 115t
Animal bite, 418t
Animism, 423
Ankle sprain, 584t
Announcement phase, fathers during pregnancy and, 72
Anorexia
    in acute pharyngitis, 594
    in diabetes mellitus, 728
    in nasopharyngitis, 594
Anorexia nervosa, 771-772, 772f
Antacids, 512t
Antepartum, term, 47
Anterior chamber, 539f
Anterior fontanel, 127, 127f, 285
Anterior pituitary disorders, 726t
Anteroposterior diameter, 27, 28f, 28t
Anthrax, 754t
Anthropoid pelvis, 27, 27f
Antibiotics
    for acute pharyngitis, 594
    for mastitis, 247
    for osteomyelitis, 577
    during pregnancy, 113, 114t
    for premature rupture of membranes, 196
    tocolytic therapy and, 197
Antibody, 748
Antibody screen, 49t
Anticipatory guidance for school-age child, 442, 443b
Anticoagulants
    during pregnancy, 114t
    for venous thrombosis, 243
Anticonvulsants, 115t, 552t
Antidiuretic hormone, 725
Antiembolic stockings, 244
Antiemetics, 84
Antigen, 338b
Antihemophilic globulin, 640
Antihistamines, 601
Antihypertensives
    interactions with food, 512t
    for pregnancy-induced hypertension, 96-97

Antiinflammatory drugs
    for asthma, 604-605
    for child, 479
    for rheumatic fever, 626
Antipyretics
    for acute otitis media, 536
    for encephalitis, 548
Antiviral medications, 597-598
Anus
    female, 24f
    imperforate, 658
    male, 22f
Anxiety
    human immunodeficiency virus and, 110
    in hypertonic labor, 188
    in leukemia, 644
    pregnant adolescent and, 72
    psyche of labor and, 130
Aortocaval compression, 55
Aortography, 618t
Apgar score, 152, 153t, 288, 288f
Apical pulse of newborn, 290, 290f
Aplastic crisis, 638t
Apnea in preterm newborn, 309-310
Appendicitis, 675-676
Appetite, 378
Approximation of perineum, 207
Apricot pit poisoning, 678t
aPTT. See Activated partial thromboplastin time.
AquaMEPHYTON, 153
Arab family, labor and delivery for, 121t
AROM. See Artificial rupture of membranes.
Aromatherapy, 779
Arousal awareness, 560b
Art therapy, 435, 762
Arterial blood gases, 673t
Arthropod bites, 679t
Arthroscopy, 569
Articulation disorder, 427t
Artificial insemination, 273
Artificial rupture of membranes, 176
Artificial sweeteners, 733
Artificialism, 423
Ascariasis, 677
Aschoff's bodies, 625
Ascites, 690
ASD. See Atrial septal defect.
Asepsis, 748-749
Asian family, cultural influences on, 359-360t
Aspartame, 371, 733
Aspiration
    general anesthesia and, 170
    pregnancy and, 165
Aspiration pneumonitis, 170
Aspirin
    for Kawasaki disease, 629
    poisoning with, 679-680
    postpartum use of, 205
    for rheumatic fever, 626
Assay
    cervical fibronectin, 49t
    enzyme-linked immunosorbent, 756
    pregnancy test and, 54
Assessment of hospitalized child, 496-505
    basic data collection in, 496-497
    blood pressure in, 499-500, 500f, 501t, 502t
    body temperature in, 501-503, 503f, 503t
    head circumference in, 505

Assessment of hospitalized child—cont'd
  height in, 505
  history survey in, 497
  pulse and respirations in, 499, 499*t*
  weight in, 503-505
Associative play, 427
Asthma, 602-606
  dental health in, 382*t*
  medications for, 603-605, 604*t*
  metered-dose inhaler for, 604, 606, 606*b*, 607*f*
  pathophysiology of, 602, 602*f*, 603*f*
Asthma diary, 607*f*
Asymmetry, 583
Asymptomatic bacteriuria, 112
Asynchrony, 456
Ataractics, 165*t*
Ataxia, 562*b*
Ataxic cerebral palsy, 555*t*
Atelectasis, 609
Athetoid cerebral palsy, 555*t*
Athetosis, 554-555
Athlete's foot, 711-712
Atonic seizure, 551*t*
Atony, uterine, 240-241, 241*t*, 242*f*
Atopic dermatitis, 706-710, 707*f*, 710*t*
Atresia, esophageal, 657-658
Atrial septal defect, 618-619, 619*f*
Atrophy in cystic fibrosis, 609
Attachment
  bonding and, 223*f*, 223-224
  postpartum care and, 205*b*
Attention-deficit hyperactivity disorder, 770-771, 771*b*
Attitude, fetal, 128
Auditory association area of brain, 543*f*
Auditory brainstem response, 286
Auditory nerve, 544*f*, 545*t*, 561*b*
Auditory stimulation, toys and, 403*t*
Augmentation of labor, 177-180, 178*t*, 188
Aura, 549
Aurantoin, 581
Auscultation
  of fetal heart rate, 136
  of pediatric blood pressure, 499-500, 500*f*, 501*t*, 502*t*
Autism, 411*b*, 763
Autism Society of America, 774
Autograft, 719
Automobile accident during pregnancy, 115
Automobile safety, toddler and, 417*t*
Autonomy, toddler and, 411
Autosome, 33
Autosyringe, 644-645
Avulsed tooth, 381, 440
Axillary temperature, 502-503
  neonatal, 220
Ayurveda, 779
Azalea poisoning, 678*t*

B

Babinski reflex, 284*t*
Baby blues, 214, 214*b*
Baby teeth, 378-379, 379*f*
Bacitracin, 720*b*
Back labor, 160
Back pain
  in abnormal labor, 192
  during pregnancy, 58, 68
Bacteremia, 545-546, 546*b*

Bacteria in urine, 686*t*
Bacterial infection
  in acute otitis media, 535
  in acute pharyngitis, 594
  in conjunctivitis, 541, 541*f*
  cutaneous, 710
  in epiglottitis, 596
  in meningitis, 546-547, 547*f*
  in osteomyelitis, 577
  in pneumonia, 598
  during pregnancy, 111
  in rheumatic fever, 625
  in toxic shock syndrome, 256
Bacterial vaginosis, 258*t*
Bacteriuria, 688
Balance, pregnancy and, 58
Ballard scoring system, 306, 307*f*, 567
Ballet, injury risks in, 585*t*
Ballottement, 53
Baptism, 215
Barbiturates
  abuse of, 768*t*
  drug interactions with, 512*t*
Barium swallow, 618*t*
Barlow's test, 331
Barotrauma, 538
Barrier methods of contraception, 264-265, 266*b*, 267*f*
Barrier technique, 749
Bartholin gland, 24, 25*f*, 31
Barton tongs, 571
Basal body temperature, 267*f*, 267-268
Basal thermometer, 267
Baseline rate, fetal heart rate pattern and, 137
Basketball, injury risks in, 585*t*
Basophil, 633*f*
Bath oils, 710*t*
Bathing of newborn, 218, 295
Battered child syndrome, 585
Battering during pregnancy, 115-116
Becker muscular dystrophy, 579
Bed rest
  for pregnancy-induced hypertension, 96, 97
  in rheumatic fever, 626
Bed-wetting, 412*t*, 431-432
Bedtime habits of preschooler, 427
Beer, 769*f*
Behavior
  of adolescent, 458*t*
  from age 1 to 5 years, 347*b*
  dehydration and, 670*t*, 672*t*
  during mealtime, 400*t*
  toddler and, 412-413*t*
Behavior modification, 762
Behavior therapy in obsessive-compulsive disorder, 764
Behavioral disorders, 761-774
  anorexia nervosa in, 771-772, 772*f*
  attention-deficit hyperactivity disorder in, 770-771, 771*b*
  autism in, 763
  bulimia in, 772-773
  depression in, 764, 765-766
  impact on growth and development, 773
  nurse's role in care of, 761-762
  obsessive-compulsive disorder in, 763-764
  origins of, 762-763, 763*b*
  substance abuse and, 767-770, 768*t*, 769*t*
  suicide and, 764
  types and settings of treatment, 762

Benign crouplike conditions, 595
Benign fibroids, 195
Benign paroxysmal vertigo, 554
Benzathine penicillin, 626
Benzocaine
    for perineal pain, 208
    toxicity of, 678t
Best friend interaction, 463
Beta-blockers
    for pregnancy-induced hypertension, 94
    in tocolytic therapy, 197
Beta-thalassemia, 108, 638
Betamethasone, 198
Bi-ischial diameter, 28, 28t
Bibliotherapy, 762
Bicarbonate, 673t
Bikini skin incision in cesarean birth, 184
Biliblanket Plus High Output Phototherapy System, 344f
Bilirubin
    neonatal jaundice and, 312
    of newborn, 288
Billings method, 268, 268f
Biofeedback, 780-781
Biological dressings, 719
Biophysical profile, 83t, 180
Biopsy, renal, 686
Bioterrorism, 112-114, 113b, 753-754, 754t
Biotin, 372t
Biparietal diameter, 127, 127f
Bipolar disorder, 249
Birth, 119-155
    admission to hospital or birth center, 133-136
        assessments in, 134b, 134-135
        false labor and, 135-136, 136t
        procedures in, 135
    complications following, 237-250
        hemorrhage and, 237-243, 241t, 242f
        homeless mother and, 249
        mood disorders and, 248-249
        puerperal infection and, 244-247, 245t
        shock and, 237
        subinvolution of uterus and, 247-248
        thromboembolic disorders and, 243t, 243-244
    components of labor and, 124-130
        passage in, 126-127
        passenger in, 127f, 127-129, 128b, 128f, 129f, 130f
        powers in, 124-125, 125f, 126f
        psyche in, 130-131
    cultural influences on, 119-120, 121-123t
    diabetes mellitus and, 105
    dysfunctional, 188
    emergency, 134b
    heart disease and, 106, 107
    high-risk pregnancy and, 117
    induction of
        for premature rupture of membranes, 196
        for prolonged pregnancy, 198
    mechanisms of, 131-133, 132-133f
    nurse role in, 145-146t
    nursing care before birth, 136-143
        coping and, 142-143, 143f, 144f
        fetal monitoring and, 136-141, 137b, 138-140f, 140b
        maternal monitoring and, 141f, 141-142, 142b
    nursing care during, 144-148, 147-150f
    nursing care immediately after birth, 148-154
        infant and, 151f, 151-154, 152f, 153t, 154f
        mother and, 148-151

Birth—cont'd
    pain in, 158-161
    pregnancy-induced hypertension and, 94, 96
    prenatal classes in, 156-158, 157b, 158f, 159b
    settings for, 120, 120f
    sickle cell disease and, 108
    signs of, 131
    stages and phases of, 144, 145-146t
    vaginal birth after cesarean birth and, 144
Birth control, 261-269
    barrier methods of, 264-265, 266b, 267f
    basal body temperature in, 267f, 267-268
    calendar method of, 268
    cervical mucous method of, 268, 268f
    emergency contraception and, 269
    hormonal contraceptives in, 261-264, 262f, 263f
    intrauterine device in, 264
    natural methods of, 267
    spermicides for, 266-267
    sterilization in, 268f, 268-269
Birth defects, 320-345
    assessment of, 219-220
    cleft lip in, 327f, 327-328
    cleft palate in, 328-329
    clubfoot in, 329-330, 330f
    developmental hip dysplasia in, 330-334, 331f, 332f, 334b
    diabetic mother and, 344
    Down syndrome in, 336f, 336-338, 337t
    emotional support for grieving parents, 215
    erythroblastosis fetalis in, 338-339b, 338-343, 339-340f, 343-344f, 344b
    galactosemia in, 335-336
    hydrocephalus in, 321-324, 322f, 323f
    intracranial hemorrhage in, 343-344
    maple syrup urine disease in, 335
    myelodysplasia and spina bifida in, 324-327, 325-327f
    phenylketonuria in, 334-335
Birth injury, 219-220
Birth rate, 9t, 10b
Birthing center, 5
Birthing room, 120
Bisacodyl, 210
Bishop's score, 177, 178t
Black cohosh, 275, 784t
Black mountain laurel poisoning, 678t
Blackhead, 705
Bladder
    after birth, 150
    descent of fundus and, 205
    distended, 688
    exstrophy of, 688
    female, 24f
    male, 22, 22f
    postpartum care and, 205b
    postpartum infection of, 210
    soft tissue obstruction during labor and, 195
    urinary tract infection and, 112
    uterine atony and, 241, 242f
Bladder training, 413-414, 414f
Blalock-Taussig surgical procedure, 621
Blastocyst, 34, 36f
Blastomere, 34
Bleeding
    abnormal uterine, 254
    in abruptio placentae, 92t, 93
    fetal size and, 192
    intracranial, 343-344

Bleeding—cont'd
  in leukemia patient, 644
  lochia and, 206
  other than bloody show, 133
  in placenta previa, 92*t*
  postpartum, 210, 237-243
    anemia in, 238
    early, 238-242, 241*t*, 242*f*
    hypovolemic shock in, 238
    late, 242-243
    observation of, 149-150
  pregnancy-induced hypertension and, 96
  in previa placenta, 92
  tendency in preterm newborn, 311
  from umbilical cord, 221
  vaginal birth after cesarean and, 144
Bleeding disorders, 639-641
  of early pregnancy, 84-91
  of late pregnancy, 91-93, 92*t*
Blended family, 355*t*, 356
Bleomycin, 512*t*
Blood
  formed elements of, 633*f*
  incompatibility between pregnant woman and fetus, 99-100, 100*f*
  normal values during infancy and childhood, 633*t*
  normal values in nonpregnant and pregnant women, 56*t*
  postpartum changes in values, 209
Blood clotting
  in abruptio placentae, 92*t*
  in placenta previa, 92*t*
  preeclampsia and, 95
Blood disorders, 320, 321*b*, 631-646
  hemophilia in, 639-641
  Hodgkin's disease in, 645*t*, 645-646
  immune thrombocytopenic purpura in, 641
  iron-deficiency anemia in, 633-634, 635
  leukemia in, 641-645, 642*f*, 643*f*, 644*b*
  platelet disorders in, 641
  sickle cell disease in, 634-638, 636*f*, 637*f*, 638*t*
  thalassemia in, 638-639, 639*f*
Blood dyscrasias, 631
Blood flow
  for late deceleration, 140
  in postpartum hemorrhage, 238
  in pregnancy-induced hypertension, 96
Blood glucose
  in diabetes mellitus, 102, 728
  exercise and, 105
  in neonatal hypoglycemia, 221
  prenatal screening of, 49*t*, 50
  self-monitoring of, 730, 732*f*
Blood patch, 170, 170*f*
Blood pressure
  in admission assessment, 134
  after birth, 150
  dehydration and, 670*t*
  of hospitalized child, 499-500, 500*f*, 501*t*, 502*t*
  of infant, 386*f*
  labor pain management and, 173
  of newborn, 220
  postpartum hemorrhage and, 238
  in pregnancy, 55
  in pregnancy-induced hypertension, 94, 95, 96
  of preschooler, 422-423
  of toddler, 408
Blood specimen, 506, 507*f*

Blood tests
  in cesarean birth, 184
  in dehydration, 670*t*
  in diabetes mellitus, 728-729, 729*f*
  in musculoskeletal disorders, 569
  prenatal, 49*t*
Blood transfusion
  for ectopic pregnancy, 89
  in leukemia, 644-645
  reaction to, 644
  in thalassemia, 639
Blood typing
  in cesarean birth, 184
  prenatal, 49*t*
Blood urea nitrogen, 686*t*
Blood volume, postpartum changes in, 209
Bloody show, 131
Blue-green algae, 783*t*
Blunt trauma during pregnancy, 115
Body image
  of adolescent, 458*t*, 463
  anorexia nervosa and, 772, 772*f*
  pregnant adolescent and, 64
Body lice, 712*f*, 712-713
Body proportions
  adult *versus* child, 350, 351*f*
  of toddler, 405-408, 408*f*
Body substance, 747
Body substance isolation precautions, 787-788
Body surface area, 510, 714*f*
Body temperature
  in admission assessment, 134
  after birth, 150
  amniotomy and, 177
  dehydration and, 670*t*
  exercise during pregnancy and, 65-67
  fever and
    in acute otitis media, 536
    in acute pharyngitis, 594
    chills and, 209
    in hospitalized child, 501-503, 503*f*, 503*t*
    in Kawasaki disease, 628
    in meningitis, 546
    in nasopharyngitis, 594
    nursing care plan for, 504
    in pneumonia, 598
    postpartum, 244
    in rheumatic fever, 625
    in sepsis, 545
  hypothermia and, 151, 218, 617
  of infant, 386*f*
  of mother before birth, 141
  neonatal, 220, 289-290, 290*f*
  premature rupture of membranes and, 196
  of preterm newborn, 310, 313*f*, 313-314, 316*f*
Boggy uterus, 240-241, 242*f*
Bonding and attachment
  maternal-infant, 153
  newborn care and, 222-224, 223*f*
Bone
  adult *versus* child growth of, 352
  fracture of, 570-574, 571-574*f*, 578*f*
  osteomyelitis and, 574-579
Bone marrow aspiration, 632, 642, 643*f*
Bone marrow transplantation, 644
Bone scan, 569

Bony pelvis
   abnormal labor and, 194-195
   in passage of labor, 126-127
Boron, 64t
Bottle feeding, 233f, 233-234, 398-399, 399t
Bottle-mouth caries, 380, 381f
Botulinum toxin, 555
Botulism, 754t
Bowel
   function in newborn, 218-219
   postpartum care and, 205b
Bowel training, 413-414, 414f
Bowlegged, 568-569
BPD. See Bronchopulmonary dysplasia.
BPP. See Biophysical profile.
Bra for adolescent girl, 459-460
Braces in cerebral palsy, 555
Brachial artery, pediatric blood pressure and, 500f
Bradley method of childbirth preparation, 161
Bradycardia
   in apneic episode, 310
   exercise during pregnancy and, 67
   in hospitalized child, 497
Brain
   functional areas of, 543f
   of newborn, 283
   role in ventilation, 591
   of toddler, 408
   tumor of, 548f, 548-549
Brainstem auditory evoked response, 537
BRAT diet, 666
Braxton Hicks contraction, 53, 131
Brazelton Neonatal Behavioral Assessment Scale, 287, 397, 538
Breakthrough bleeding, 254
Breast, 28, 29t
   assessment in newborn, 220
   changes as presumptive sign of pregnancy, 51-52
   development of, 459f, 461b
   postpartum care and, 205b
   postpartum changes in, 208-209
   reproductive changes in pregnancy and, 55
   self-examination of, 252, 253b
Breast milk, 371, 398t
   oral contraceptive-associated decrease in, 262
   phases of production of, 226
   for preterm newborn, 314
   storing and freezing of, 231-232
Breast milk jaundice, 312, 312f
Breast pump, 231, 231f
Breastfeeding, 224-232, 398-399, 399t
   afterpains and, 205
   assisting mother in, 226-229, 227t, 228b, 228f, 229f
   for contraception, 269
   contraceptives and, 208
   diabetes mellitus in pregnancy and, 106
   in galactosemia, 336
   herpes virus lesion and, 109
   human immunodeficiency virus and, 110
   of hypoglycemic newborn, 221
   lochia and, 206
   mastitis and, 246-247, 247f
   maternal-infant bonding and, 153
   in phenylketonuria, 335
   physiology of lactation and, 225-226, 226f
   postpartum analgesia and, 213-214
   postpartum immunization for rubella and, 211

Breastfeeding—cont'd
   prenatal class in, 157b
   preventing problems with, 229b, 229-230, 230f
   special situations in, 230-231, 231f
   substance abuse and, 115
   weaning from, 402
Breath-holding spell, 554
Breath sounds after cesarean birth, 213
Breathing exercises
   in cystic fibrosis, 614
   in labor pain management, 163-164
Breech birth, 194f
Breech presentation, 128, 128b, 192
Brethine. See Terbutaline.
Bribe, 430
Bright's disease, 693
Broad ligament, 25, 25f
Broca's area, 543f
Bronchiolitis, 596-597
Bronchitis, 596
Bronchodilators, 603-604, 604t
Bronchopulmonary dysplasia, 309, 615
Broviac catheter, 517-518
Brow presentation of fetus, 128
Bruising
   in child abuse, 587
   of perineum, 207
   in platelet disorders, 641
Bryant traction, 569, 570, 572f
Buck extension, 569, 570
Bulb suctioning of mucus, 288, 288f
Bulbourethral gland, 22f, 23
Bulging fontanel, 497
Bulimia, 382t, 772-773
Burn, 713-720
   classification of, 713-715, 714f
   electrical, 715, 716f
   emergency care in, 716-717
   nursing care in, 719-720, 720b
   pathophysiology of, 713
   preschooler and, 433
   toddler and, 417t
   wound care in, 717-719, 718f
Burner, 584t
Burping of newborn, 229, 230f, 233
Butorphanol, 165t
Buttercup poisoning, 678t

C

Caffeine
   athlete and, 469
   postpartum intake of, 232
   use during pregnancy and lactation, 63
Calcium
   during lactation, 65
   for menopausal symptoms, 275
   postpartum intake of, 232
   during pregnancy and lactation, 61
   recommended dietary allowance of, 372t
Calcium channel blockers
   for pregnancy-induced hypertension, 94
   in tocolytic therapy, 197
Calcium disodium edetate, 681
Calcium gluconate
   for hypocalcemia in preterm newborn, 311
   for pregnancy-induced hypertension, 96

Calcium lactate, 311
Calculating pediatric drug doses, 510, 512*f*
Calculating safe drug dose, 510-511, 512*b*
Calender method of contraception, 268
Caloric intake
    during pregnancy, 60
    of toddler, 414
Camellia seed poisoning, 678*t*
Camphor toxicity, 678*t*
Cancer
    dental health in, 382*t*
    Hodgkin's disease and, 645*t*, 645-646
    leukemia and, 641-645, 642*f*, 643*f*, 644*b*
    nursing care plan for chemotherapy, 647-649
Candidiasis
    cutaneous, 704*f*
    oral, 676
    sexually transmitted, 258*t*
    vaginal, 55
Canine, 379*f*
Cao-gio, 778, 778*f*
Capillary refill, 574*f*
Captopril, 115*t*
Caput succedaneum, 192, 284, 285*f*
Car safety
    for infant, 402-403, 403*t*
    for toddler, 416, 419*f*
Car seat
    for infant, 235, 235*f*, 402
    for toddler, 419*f*
Carbamazepine, 115*t*, 552*t*
Carbohydrates for athlete, 469
Carbon dioxide narcosis, 591
Carbon monoxide, 679*t*
Cardiac catheterization, 618*t*
Cardiac output
    adult *versus* child, 351
    exercise during pregnancy and, 67
    postpartum changes in, 209
Cardiac surgery, 622
Cardinal ligaments, 25
Cardinal movements, 131, 132*f*
Cardiogenic shock, 237
Cardiorespiratory function of newborn, 152
Cardiovascular disorders, 616-629
    congenital heart disease in, 616-622, 618*t*
        atrial septal defect in, 618-619
        coarctation of aorta in, 620
        hypoplastic left heart syndrome in, 622
        patent ductus arteriosus in, 620
        tetralogy of Fallot in, 620-621, 621*f*
        ventricular septal defect in, 619-620
    congestive heart failure in, 622-624, 623*f*
    hyperlipidemia and, 627, 627*t*, 628*b*
    hypertension and, 627
    Kawasaki disease in, 628*f*, 628-629
    rheumatic fever in, 624-627, 625*f*, 626*b*
Cardiovascular system
    adult *versus* child, 351, 617*f*
    changes in pregnancy, 55-56, 56*f*, 56*t*
    postpartum changes in, 209
Carditis, 625
Care map, 6
Care plan, 13-15, 15*b*
Career plans of adolescent, 464-465, 465*f*
Caries, 380
Carrier, 748

Case study, 13-15, 15*b*
Cast
    for clubfoot, 329-330
    for developmental dysplasia of hip, 331-334, 332*f*
    renal, 686*t*
Cat allergy, 451-452
Catheterization
    abnormal labor and, 195
    in amnioinfusion, 176
    in electronic fetal monitoring, 137
    postpartum, 206
    in uterine inversion, 201
Cat's eye reflex, 542
CD4+ cell count, 756
Celiac disease, 659*f*, 659-660, 739*t*
Cell differentiation, 34-36, 37*b*
Cell division, 33-34, 35*f*
Celsius temperature, 793
Center of gravity in pregnancy, 58
Centering, 423
Central abruptio placentae, 92*t*
Central nervous system
    adult *versus* child, 351
    congenital malformations of, 321-327
        hydrocephalus in, 321-324, 322*f*, 323*f*
        myelodysplasia and spina bifida in, 324-327, 325*f*, 326*f*, 327*f*
    neonatal, 283, 283*f*, 284*f*, 284*t*
    pain modification and, 160
    preeclampsia and, 95
Central sulcus, 543*f*
Central venous access device, 517-518
Cephalic brow presentation, 129*f*
Cephalic face presentation, 129*f*
Cephalic presentation, 128, 131*b*
Cephalic vertex presentation, 129*f*
Cephalocaudal development, 349, 349*f*
Cephalohematoma, 284, 285*f*
Cephalopelvic disproportion
    cesarean birth and, 183
    in trauma during pregnancy, 116
Cerclage, 84
Cerebral edema, 563
Cerebral palsy, 554
Cerebrospinal fluid, hydrocephalus and, 321, 322*f*
Certified nurse-midwife, 7
Cervical cap, 256, 264-265
Cervical culture, 49*t*
Cervical dilation, 124, 125*f*, 126*f*, 195
Cervical effacement, 124, 125*f*, 197
Cervical fibronectin assay, 49*t*
Cervical mucous method, 268, 268*f*
Cervical ripening, 178
Cervical traction, 573*f*
Cervix, 24*f*, 25*f*, 26
    contractions and, 124
    induction of labor and, 177
    infertility and, 271
    laceration during labor and birth, 242
    menstruation and, 461*f*
    in placenta previa, 91
    postpartum changes in, 207
    reproductive changes in pregnancy and, 55
Cesarean birth, 183-188, 185*t*, 186-187*f*
    for abruptio placentae, 93
    breech presentation and, 128
    forceps or vacuum extraction birth *versus*, 182
    herpes virus lesion and, 109

Cesarean birth—cont'd
  multifetal pregnancy and, 194
  nursing care plan for, 212
  postpartum changes after, 211-214
  for premature rupture of membranes, 196
  preparatory classes in, 156
  for previa placenta, 93
  for prolapsed umbilical cord, 199
  vaginal birth after, 144
Chadwick's sign, 53
Chafing, 704, 704*f*
Chain of infection, 748*f*
Chalasia, 665
Chamomile, 782*t*, 783*t*
Charting issues, 17-18
Chasteberry, 784*t*
Cheiloplasty, 327
Chelating agents, 681
Chemical burn, 713
Chemicals, infertility and, 271-272
Chemoprophylaxis for rheumatic fever, 626
Chemoreceptor, 591
Chemotherapy
  dental health during, 381, 382*t*
  for Hodgkin's disease, 645
  in leukemia, 643
  nursing care plan for, 647-649
Chest circumference
  of newborn, 221
  of toddler, 408
Chest-clapping therapy, 609
Chest pain in pneumonia, 598
Chest radiography, 618*t*
CHF. *See* Congestive heart failure.
Chiari malformation, 321
Chickenpox, 742*t*, 747*f*
Chignon, 183
Chilblain, 720
Child
  adult growth and development *versus,* 349-351*f,* 349-352
  assessment of length, 350*f*
  chronically ill, 646*t,* 646-650
  dying, 650-654, 651*t,* 654*b*
  hospitalized. *See* Hospitalized child.
  immunization schedule for, 751, 752*f*
  normal blood values of, 633*t*
  recommended dietary allowances for, 372*t*
  respiratory distress in, 595, 595*f*
  response to death, 651, 651*t*
Child abuse, 585-588, 587*b,* 588*f*
Child Abuse Prevention and Treatment Act, 4
Child care, toddler and, 415-416, 416*f*
Child Care Food Program, 377*t*
Childbirth, 119-155
  admission to hospital or birth center, 133-136
    assessments in, 134*b,* 134-135
    false labor and, 135-136, 136*t*
    procedures in, 135
  complications following, 237-250
    hemorrhage and, 237-243, 241*t,* 242*f*
    homeless mother and, 249
    mood disorders and, 248-249
    puerperal infection and, 244-247, 245*t*
    shock and, 237
    subinvolution of uterus and, 247-248
    thromboembolic disorders and, 243*t,* 243-244

Childbirth—cont'd
  components of labor and, 124-130
    passage in, 126-127
    passenger in, 127*f,* 127-129, 128*b,* 128*f,* 129*f,* 130*f*
    powers in, 124-125, 125*f,* 126*f*
    psyche in, 130-131
  cultural influences on, 119-120, 121-123*t*
  diabetes mellitus and, 105
  dysfunctional, 188
  heart disease and, 106
  induction of
    for premature rupture of membranes, 196
    for prolonged pregnancy, 198
  mechanisms of, 131-133, 132-133*f*
  nurse role in, 145-146*t*
  nursing care before birth, 136-143
    coping and, 142-143, 143*f,* 144*f*
    fetal monitoring and, 136-141, 137*b,* 138-140*f,* 140*b*
    maternal monitoring and, 141*f,* 141-142, 142*b*
  nursing care during, 144-148, 147-150*f*
  nursing care immediately after birth, 148-154
    infant and, 151*f,* 151-154, 152*f,* 153*t,* 154*f*
    mother and, 148-151
  pain in, 158-161
  prenatal classes in, 156-158, 157*b,* 158*f,* 159*b*
  settings for, 120, 120*f*
  sickle cell disease and, 108
  signs of, 131
  stages and phases of, 144, 145-146*t*
  vaginal birth after cesarean birth and, 144
Childproofing of home, 420, 420*f*
Children's Bureau, 3-4
Children's Charter of 1930, 5
Children's Food Pyramid, 369*f*
Children's Health Topics, 436
Children's hospital unit, 476
Chills immediately after birth, 209
Chinese American family
  culture influences on, 359-360*t*
  food patterns of, 368*t*
  labor and delivery for, 121*t*
Chiropractic care, 781
Chlamydia trachomatis, 257, 258*t*
  newborn and, 153, 154*f*
  in pneumonia, 598
Chloasma, 52
Chlorothiazide, 624
Choking, toddler and, 417-418*t*
Cholesteatoma, 536
Cholesterol, 373, 373*b*
  diabetes mellitus and, 733
  hyperlipidemia and, 627, 627*t*
Choline, 372*t*
Chordee, 688
Chorea, 625
Chorioamnionitis, 196, 197
Chorion, 34-36
Chorionic villous sampling, 83*t*
Choroid, 539*f*
Christmas disease, 640
Chromosomal abnormalities, 320, 321*b*
  alpha-fetoprotein testing and, 82*t*
  Down syndrome in, 336-338, 337*t*
Chronic diarrhea, 666
Chronic hypertension in pregnancy, 94*t,* 96*b*
Chronically ill child, 646*t,* 646-650
Cilia, fallopian tube, 26

Cineangiocardiography, 618*t*
Circulation
    fetal, 42-43, 44*f*
    neonatal, 288
Circumcision, 291-292, 292*f*
Classic incision for cesarean birth, 184, 185*f*
Classic phenylketonuria, 334
Clavicle fracture, 192
Clean-catch specimen, 505
Cleaning fluid abuse, 768*t*
Cleansing breath, 163
Cleavage, 34
Cleft lip, 327*f*, 327-328
Cleft palate, 328-329
Climacteric, 26, 29, 275
Clinical Linguistic and Auditory Milestone Scale, 397
Clinical nurse specialist, 12
Clinical pathway, 6
    for hospitalized child, 484-486, 486*f*
    for pyloric stenosis, 660
    for term newborn, 298-301
Clinical psychologist, 762
Clique, 463
Clitoris, 24, 24*f*, 31
Clonazepam, 552*t*
Clonic movement, 549
Cloning, 274
Clothing
    for newborn, 302-303, 303*f*
    for preschooler, 432
    for toddler, 412
Clubbing of fingers, 609, 621
Clubfoot, 329-330, 330*f*
CNS. *See* Clinical nurse specialist or Central nervous system.
Coagulation
    amniotic fluid embolism and, 201
    in cesarean birth, 184
    lochia and, 206
    postpartum changes in, 209
Coarctation of aorta, 619*f*, 620
Cocaine, 767, 768*t*, 769*f*
    infertility and, 272
    use during pregnancy, 114*t*
Coccyx, 27
Cochlear implant, 537-538
Cognition, 363
Cognitive development, 363, 365*t*
    of adolescent, 458*t*, 463
    of preschooler, 423, 424-425*t*
    of toddler, 406-407*t*, 408-409
Cognitive impairment, 557*b*, 557-559, 558*b*, 559*t*
Cohabitation family, 355*t*
Coin-rubbing, 778, 778*f*
Colace. *See* Docusate sodium.
Cold sore, 706, 706*f*
Cold stress, 289*t*
    in newborn, 151
    in preterm newborn, 310
Cold therapy
    in episiotomy care, 181, 208
    for soft tissue injury, 570
Colic, 389*t*, 395, 395*f*, 396
Colitis, 664
Collagen diseases, 624
Colon
    gastroenteritis and, 664, 664*b*
    Hirschsprung's disease and, 661-662, 662*f*
Colon conduit, 689*t*

Colonoscopy, 657
Color
    in Apgar scoring, 153*t*
    in neurovascular assessment, 574
Colostrum, 55
Coma
    in encephalitis, 548
    in meningitis, 546
Comedo, 705
Comminuted fracture, 571*f*
Common cold, 591
Communicable disease, 741-746*t*, 741-760
    bioterrorism and, 753-754, 754*t*
    host resistance and, 747-748
    human immunodeficiency virus in, 756-759
    immunization programs for, 750*f*, 750-753, 752*f*
    immunotherapy in, 753
    medical asepsis and standard precautions in, 748-749
    rashes in, 749-750
    sexually transmitted disease in, 754-756, 755*t*
    terminology in, 747
Communicating hydrocephalus, 321
Communication
    intercultural, 482-483
    between parent and child, 442
    parenthood and, 216
Communication disorder, toddler and, 410*t*
Community, family as part of, 356, 357-362*t*
Community-based care of infant, 388, 395
Community-based nursing, 18
Community Mental Health Center, 4
Compartment syndrome, 573, 574
Competitive play, 382*t*
Complementary therapy, 775-786
    acupuncture and acupressure as, 778-779
    aromatherapy as, 779
    ayurveda as, 779
    biofeedback as, 780-781
    chiropractic care as, 781
    definition of, 775
    energy healing as, 778, 779*f*
    federal regulations and, 776-778
    guided imagery as, 780
    herbal remedies as, 781-784, 782*b*, 782-784*t*
    homeopathy as, 779
    hydrotherapy as, 780
    hyperbaric oxygen therapy as, 784
    hypnotherapy as, 780
    massage as, 778, 778*f*
    for menopausal symptoms, 275
    nurse's role in, 775-776, 776*b*, 776*f*, 777*t*
    osteopathy as, 778
    reflexology as, 778, 780*f*
    sauna as, 784
Complete abortion, 86*t*
Complete blood count
    in cesarean birth, 184
    in musculoskeletal disorders, 569
    in prenatal laboratory test, 49*t*
Complete breech presentation, 128, 129*f*
Complete prolapsed umbilical cord, 198, 199*f*
Complete uterine rupture, 199
Complex partial seizure, 551*t*
Complications during labor and birth, 176-202
    abnormal labor and, 188-196
        duration in, 195-196
        fetus in, 192-194, 194*f*
        pelvis and soft tissues in, 194-195

Complications during labor and birth—cont'd
  abnormal labor and—cont'd
    powers of labor in, 188-192, 190*b*
    psyche in, 195
  emergencies and, 198-201
    amniotic fluid embolism in, 201
    prolapsed umbilical cord in, 198-199, 199*f*, 200*f*
    uterine inversion in, 200-201
    uterine rupture in, 199-200
  obstetric procedures and, 176-188
    amnioinfusion in, 176
    amniotomy in, 176-177
    cesarean birth in, 183-188, 185*t*, 186-187*f*
    episiotomy and lacerations in, 180-182, 181*f*
    forceps and vacuum extraction births in, 182*f*, 182-183
    induction or augmentation of labor in, 177-180, 178*t*
    version in, 180
  premature rupture of membranes and, 196
  preterm labor and, 196-198, 197*b*
    signs of impending labor in, 196-197
    stopping, 197-198
    tocolytic therapy in, 197
  prolonged pregnancy and, 198
Complications following birth, 237-250
  hemorrhage in, 237-243, 241*t*, 242*f*
  homeless mother and, 249
  mood disorders in, 248-249
  puerperal infection in, 244-247, 245*t*
  shock in, 237
  subinvolution of uterus in, 247-248
  thromboembolic disorders in, 243*t*, 243-244
Compound fracture, 570, 571*f*
Compression, aortocaval, 55
Compulsion, 763
Compulsive eating, 772-773
Computed tomography
  in appendicitis, 675
  in musculoskeletal disorders, 569
Concentrated liquid infant formula, 233
Concrete operations, 438-439
Concrete phase of thinking, 463
Concussion, 559, 584*t*
Conditioned responses of newborn, 287
Condom
  female, 265, 267*f*
  male, 265, 266*b*
  to prevent sexually transmitted disease, 754
Conductive heat loss, 218, 218*t*
Condylomata acuminata, 260*t*
Confidentiality, child hospitalization and, 491
Conformity, adolescent and, 456, 466-467
Congenital deafness, 537
Congenital disorders, 320-345
  celiac disease in, 659*f*, 659-660
  cleft lip in, 327*f*, 327-328
  cleft palate in, 328-329
  clubfoot in, 329-330, 330*f*
  developmental hip dysplasia in, 330-334, 331*f*, 332*f*, 334*b*
  diabetic mother and, 344
  Down syndrome in, 336*f*, 336-338, 337*t*
  erythroblastosis fetalis in, 338-339*b*, 338-343, 339-340*f*, 343-344*f*, 344*b*
  esophageal atresia in, 657-658
  galactosemia in, 335-336
  hernia in, 663*f*, 663-664
  Hirschsprung's disease in, 661-662, 662*f*
  hydrocephalus in, 321-324, 322*f*, 323*f*
  imperforate anus in, 658

Congenital disorders—cont'd
  intracranial hemorrhage in, 343-344
  intussusception in, 662-663, 663*f*
  maple syrup urine disease in, 335
  Meckel's diverticulum in, 663
  myelodysplasia and spina bifida in, 324-327, 325-327*f*
  phenylketonuria in, 334-335
  pyloric stenosis in, 658-659, 659*f*, 660
Congenital heart disease, 616-622, 618*t*
  atrial septal defect in, 618-619
  coarctation of aorta in, 620
  hypoplastic left heart syndrome in, 622
  patent ductus arteriosus in, 620
  tetralogy of Fallot in, 620-621, 621*f*
  ventricular septal defect in, 619-620
Congenital laryngeal stridor, 595
Congestive heart failure
  pediatric, 622-624, 623*f*
  during pregnancy, 106, 106*b*
Conjoined twins, 44
Conjunctiva, 539*f*
Conjunctivitis, 541, 541*f*
  in acute pharyngitis, 594
  in Kawasaki disease, 628
Conscious sedation, pediatric, 480
Consent before hospitalization, 494
Consistency, parenting and, 430
Constipation, 666
  high-fiber foods for, 370*t*
  neonatal, 297
  postpartum, 210, 234
  during pregnancy, 56, 68-69
Consumer education in toddler injury prevention, 416, 419*f*
Consumerism, 7
Contact precautions, 749
Continuous electronic monitoring in labor induction, 179
Contraception, 261-269
  barrier methods of, 264-265, 266*b*, 267*f*
  basal body temperature method of, 267*f*, 267-268
  breastfeeding and, 208
  calendar method of, 268
  cervical mucous method of, 268, 268*f*
  emergency, 269
  hormonal contraceptives in, 261-264, 262*f*, 263*f*
  intrauterine device in, 264
  natural methods of, 267
  postpartum use of, 208, 234
  spermicides for, 266-267
  sterilization in, 268*f*, 268-269
Contraceptive diaphragm, 256, 265
Contraction, 124-125, 126*f*, 133
  amniotomy and, 177
  assessment by palpation, 142*b*
  Braxton Hicks, 131
  fetal heart rate pattern and, 137
  labor induction and, 180
  in maternal monitoring before birth, 141
  in precipitate birth, 195
  in trauma during pregnancy, 116
  version and, 180
Contraction stress test, 83*t*
Contracture in cerebral palsy, 555
Contusion, 569
Convective heat loss, 218, 218*t*
Convulsion
  in encephalitis, 548
  in pregnancy-induced hypertension, 96

Cooley's anemia, 108, 639, 639*f*
Cooley's Anemia Foundation, 655
Coombs' test, 100, 338*b*
Cooperative play, 382*t*, 420
Coping
    during labor and birth, 142-143, 143*f*, 144*f*
    with pregnancy-induced hypertension, 97
Copper, 64*t*
Copper intrauterine device, 264
Cor pulmonale, 609
Cord care, 221, 221*f*
Core body temperature, 503
Cornea, 539*f*
Coronal suture, 127*f*
Corporal punishment, 411
Corpus, uterine, 26
Corpus luteum, 55
Corticosteroids for asthma, 604-605
Corticotropin-releasing hormone, 196
Coryza, 591
Cost containment, 5, 10-12
Cotyledon, 41
Cough
    in acute bronchitis, 596
    in acute pharyngitis, 594
    after cesarean birth, 213
    in asthma, 603
    in croup, 594
    in epiglottitis, 596
    in pneumonia, 598
    in sinusitis, 594
Cough syncope, 554
Coumadin. *See* Warfarin.
Counseling
    in Down syndrome, 338
    in human immunodeficiency virus, 110
Counselor, 762
Cowper's glands, 22*f*, 23
Cow's milk-based formula, 232-233
CPD. *See* Cephalopelvic disproportion.
Crabs, 712
Cradle cap, 704, 704*f*
Cradle hold
    for breastfeeding, 227
    in transporting hospitalized child, 497*f*
Cranberry juice, 112
Cranial nerves, 544*f*, 545*t*, 560*b*
Cream, 710*t*
Creatinine, 686*t*
Creative play, 382*t*
Crepitus, 192
CRH. *See* Corticotropin-releasing hormone.
Crib, 302
    radiant heat, 314
    safety issues, 496, 496*f*
Crib death, 615-616
Critical pathway, 6
Critical periods, 352
Critical thinking, 15-16, 16*b*
Cromolyn sodium, 604
Cross-cultural considerations, 7
Cross-eye, 540-541
Croup syndromes, 594-597, 595*f*, 596*f*
Croupette, 595
Crowning, 144, 149*f*
Crust, 702*b*
Crutchfield tongs, 571

Crying
    of hospitalized child, 482, 489
    of newborn, 224
Cryptorchidism, 291, 694-697
CST. *See* Contraction stress test.
Cuban family
    cultural influences on, 357*t*
    labor and delivery for, 121*t*
Culdocentesis, 89
Cultural competence, 775
Cultural considerations, 7
    in abnormal labor, 195
    in adolescence, 462, 463*f*
    in assessing child for abuse, 588, 588*f*
    effects of cultural practices on preschooler, 423, 423*f*
    in family care after birth, 203-204
    in family influences, 357-362*t*
    in father role, 72
    in group B streptococcus infection, 111
    in impending preterm labor, 197
    in infertility, 270
    influences on birth practices, 119-120, 121-123*t*
    in menopause, 276
    in nutrition, 367, 368*t*
    in pain management, 280
    in pain modification, 161
    in pediatric hospitalization, 480-483
    in postpartum care, 204, 204*f*, 205*b*
    in premature rupture of membranes, 196
Curettage, 243
Curling's ulcer, 717
Currant jelly stools, 662
Cushingoid appearance, 344
Cushing's disease, 726*t*
Cutis marmorata, 294*t*
Cyanide, 679*t*, 753
Cyanosis
    in bronchopulmonary dysplasia, 615
    in congestive heart failure, 623
    in cystic fibrosis, 609
    in tetralogy of Fallot, 620
Cyclic hormone therapy, 275
Cyst, ovarian, 280
Cystic fibrosis, 608*f*, 608-615
    diet therapy in, 739*t*
    lung involvement in, 608-609, 609*f*
    nursing care plan for, 610-611
    pancreatic involvement in, 609
    postural drainage in, 609, 612-613*f*, 614
Cystitis, 112, 688, 690
Cystocele, 278-279
Cystometrogram, 686
Cystoscopy, 686
Cytomegalovirus, 109

D

Daily nursing care of newborn, 224
Dancing reflex, 283, 284*t*
Dander allergy, 451-452
Dandy-Walker syndrome, 321
Data collection, 496-497
Dating, 465-466
Dawn phenomenon, 737
Day care, 415-416, 416*f*
Daydreams, 465
Daytime wetting, 431
D&C. *See* Dilation and curettage.

Deafness, 537-538

Death

child response to, 650, 651, 651*t*

physical changes before, 654

preschooler concept of, 428

stages of dying and, 654, 654*b*

Debridement of wound, 717-718

Decerebrate posturing, 560, 560*f*

Decidua, 34, 55, 204

Deciduous teeth, 378-379, 379*f*

Decorticate posturing, 560, 560*f*

Decrement of contraction, 124, 126*f*

Deep partial-thickness burn, 715*t*

Deep vein thrombosis, 243*t*, 243-244

Deferoxamine mesylate, 639

Dehiscence of uterus, 199

Dehydration, 670-672, 671*t*, 672*t*

in diarrhea, 666

fluid and electrolyte imbalance and, 669, 669*f*, 670*t*

in hyperemesis gravidarum, 81

in postpartum fever, 244

in pyloric stenosis, 659

in sickle cell disease, 108

vomiting and, 664

Delirium

in encephalitis, 548

in meningitis, 546

Deltoid muscle as injection site, 515, 515*f*

Demerol. *See* Meperidine.

Denial

in child reaction to hospitalization, 477

pregnant adolescent and, 72

Dental caries, 380

adolescent and, 470

bottle feeding and, 234

cleft palate and, 329

Dental hygiene, 380*b*, 380-381, 381*f*, 382*t*, 470

Denver Home Screening Questionnaire, 397

Denver II, 352, 397

Depakene. *See* Valproic acid.

Depo-Provera, 263-264

Depression

in adolescent, 472, 764, 765-766

postpartum, 214, 248

as reaction to infertility, 270

Depth perception, 539

Dermabrasion, 706

Dermatitis

atopic, 706-710, 707*f*, 710*t*

diaper, 704-705, 705*f*

seborrheic, 704, 704*f*

Dermatome, 780*f*

Dermis, 700

Dermoplast. *See* Benzocaine.

DES. *See* Diethylstilbestrol.

Descent, 132*f*

labor and, 131

of uterine fundus after birth, 205

Descriptive word pain scale, 478*f*

Desferal. *See* Deferoxamine mesylate.

Desmopressin

for diabetes insipidus, 726

for enuresis, 432

for hemophilia, 640

Desquamation, 294*t*, 295

Detachment, child reaction to hospitalization, 477

Development, 349, 349*b*. *See also* Growth and development.

Developmental disabilities, 650

Developmental hip dysplasia, 330-334, 331*f*, 332*f*, 334*b*

Developmental milestones

Down syndrome and, 337*t*

in first year, 389-394*t*

Developmental screening, 352

Dexedrine. *See* Dextroamphetamine.

Dextroamphetamine, 771

Diabetes insipidus, 725-727, 739*t*

Diabetes mellitus

maternal, 100-106, 102*f*, 105*t*

effects in pregnancy, 101*b*

pathophysiology of, 101

tocolytic therapy and, 197

pediatric, 727-740

blood glucose self-monitoring in, 730, 732*f*

diabetic ketoacidosis and, 729, 729*t*

diagnostic blood tests in, 728-729, 729*f*

etiology and classification of, 727

future prospects in, 739-740

insulin management of, 733*f*, 733-737, 734*f*, 735*t*, 736*f*

nursing care plan for, 731-732

nutritional management of, 732-733, 739*t*

stress and, 737, 738-739*t*

type I, 727*t*, 728

Diabetic diet, 371

Diabetic ketoacidosis, 729, 729*t*

Diagnosis-related groupings, 10

Diagnostic and Statistical Manual of Mental Disorders, 770

Diagnostic testing

for congenital heart defects, 618*t*

in diabetes mellitus, 728-729, 729*f*

fetal, 82-84*t*

in musculoskeletal disorders, 569

Diagonal conjugate, 27, 28*t*

Dialysis, 680

Diaper dermatitis, 704-705, 705*f*

Diapers, 302

Diaphoresis, postpartum, 209

Diaphragm, 591, 592*f*

contraceptive, 256, 265

Diaphragmatic hernia, 591

Diarrhea, 665-666

in acute otitis media, 536

nursing care plan for, 667-668

Diastasis recti, 210

DIC. *See* Disseminated intravascular coagulation.

Dick-Read method of childbirth preparation, 161

Dick test, 748

Diet

cultural influence on postpartum, 204

in cystic fibrosis, 614

for diabetes mellitus, 102

for diarrhea, 666

fertility and, 271

in galactosemia, 336

infant and, 389-394*t*

ketogenic, 553

in nephrotic syndrome, 690

in pediatric diabetes mellitus, 732-733

in pediatric metabolic disorders, 739*t*

in phenylketonuria, 225

postpartum self-care teaching and, 234

for pregnancy-induced hypertension, 95-96

role in dysmenorrhea, 255

substance abuse and, 114

Dietary supplement, 373, 777

Diethylstilbestrol, 115*t*
Differential relaxation, 159*b*
Digestion, neonatal, 297
Digitoxin, 624
Digoxin, 624
Dilantin. *See* Phenytoin.
Dilation, 55
    cervical, 124
Dilation and curettage
    for hydatidiform mole, 91
    for pregnancy termination, 85, 87*t*
Dilation and effacement, 145*t*
Dilutional anemia, 56
Dimensional analysis, 511, 511*b*
Diphenoxylate, 678*t*
Diphenylhydantoin. *See* Dilantin.
Diphtheria, 746*t*
Diphtheria-pertussis-tetanus vaccine, 751, 752*f*
Diploid, 33
Diplopia, 541
Direct Coombs' test, 340
Direct transmission of infection, 748
Directional patterns of growth, 349, 349*f*
Discharge
    from perineum, 207
    vaginal
        impending labor and, 131
        during pregnancy, 68
Discharge planning
    after birth, 234-235
    in child hospitalization, 491-492
    for newborn, 302
    pediatric tracheostomy and, 525
Discipline
    preschooler and, 429-430
    toddler and, 410-411, 412*t*
Diseases transmitted by pets to humans, 452*t*
Dislocation of hip, 330-331
Disposable diapers, 302
Disseminated intravascular coagulation
    in abruptio placentae, 93
    in trauma during pregnancy, 116
Distraction as pain relief measure, 159*b*, 162-163
Diuresis, postpartum, 209
Diuretics
    for congestive heart failure, 624
    pregnancy and, 64
Diuril. *See* Chlorothiazide.
Diurnal wetting, 431
Diversion as pain relief measure, 159*b*, 162-163
Diverticulum, Meckel's, 663
Diving accident, 470-471
Divorce, 356
Dizygotic twins, 44, 45*f*
DKA. *See* Diabetic ketoacidosis.
Docosahexaenoic acid-omega 3 fatty acids, 58
Documentation
    in abortion, 85
    issues in, 17-18
    of pharmacological labor pain management, 174
Docusate calcium, 210
Docusate sodium, 210
Dog allergy, 452
Dong quai, 782*t*, 784*t*
Donor area in graft, 719
Donor oocyte, 273*t*
Dopamine, 116

Doppler transducer
    in electronic fetal monitoring, 137
    in fetal heart rate assessment, 54, 137*b*
Doppler ultrasound blood flow assessment, 82*t*
Dorsal pedal artery, pediatric blood pressure and, 500*f*
Dorsogluteal muscle as injection site, 515
Douching
    for contraception, 269
    risk for pelvic inflammatory disease, 261
Down syndrome, 336*f*, 336-338, 337*t*
Drainage after cesarean birth, 213
Dressing after cesarean birth, 213
Dressing of newborn, 302-303, 303*f*
DRGs. *See* Diagnosis-related groupings.
Drop attack, 551*t*
Drowning, 418*t*, 563
Drug abuse, 767-770, 768*t*, 769*t*
    adolescent and, 471-472
    during pregnancy, 113*f*, 113-115, 114-115*t*
Drug dependence, 767
Drug-drug interactions, 378, 511, 512*t*
Drug-environment interactions, 378, 511, 511*t*
Drug-food interactions, 378, 512*t*, 513
Drug-induced disorders, infertility and, 271-272
Drug tolerance, 767
Drugs. *See* Medications.
Dual career family, 355*t*
Duchenne's muscular dystrophy, 579
Ductus arteriosus, 43, 44*f*, 197
Ductus venosus, 43, 44*f*
Dulcolax. *See* Bisacodyl.
Duncan delivery of placenta, 147, 148*t*
Dural puncture, 168
Duration
    of abnormal labor, 195-196
    of contraction, 124, 126*f*
Dust, asthma and, 605
Dwyer instrument, 582
Dying child, 650-654, 651*t*, 654*b*
Dysfunctional, term, 772
Dysfunctional family, 762
Dysfunctional labor, 188
Dysgraphia, 771
Dyslexia, 540, 771
Dysmenorrhea, 254-255
Dyspareunia, 24, 255
Dysphagia, 594
Dyspnea
    in congestive heart failure, 623
    in cystic fibrosis, 609
    in pregnancy, 55, 69
Dystocia, 188
Dysuria, 686
DZ. *See* Dizygotic.

E

E chart, 539, 540*f*
Ear, 533-538, 534*f*, 535*f*
    acute otitis media and, 535-537
    barotrauma and, 538
    cleft palate and, 329
    hearing impairment and, 537-538
    of newborn, 220, 286, 286*f*
    otitis externa and, 535
    positioning child for examination of, 498*f*
Eardrops, 514, 514*b*
Early deceleration, fetal heart rate pattern and, 139

Early Language Milestone Scale, 397
Early postpartum hemorrhage, 238-242, 241*t*, 242*f*
Eating disorders, 771-773, 772*f*
Ebola virus, 754*t*
Ecchymosis, 702*b*
in child abuse, 587
of perineum, 207
in platelet disorders, 641
Echinacea, 777*t*, 783*t*
Echo/Doppler scan, 82*t*
Echocardiography, 618*t*
Echolalia, 424*t*
Eclampsia, 94, 94*t*, 95
Ectoderm, 36, 37*b*, 683
Ectopic pregnancy, 86-90, 89*f*, 90*b*
Eczema, 706-710, 707*f*, 710*t*
EDD. *See* Estimated date of delivery.
Edema
cerebral, 563
in congestive heart failure, 623, 624
of lower extremities, 69-70
of mucous membrane, 55
in nephrotic syndrome, 690
in overhydration, 672
of perineum, 207
postpartum, 209
in pregnancy, 57
in pregnancy-induced hypertension, 95
pulmonary, 198
Education
in childbearing, 156-158, 157*f*
in coping with labor, 142-143
in diabetes mellitus in pregnancy, 105-106
in heart disease, 107
in hyperemesis gravidarum, 84
in nonpharmacological labor pain management, 164
in pediatric diabetes mellitus, 730
in postpartum self-care, 234-235
in substance abuse during pregnancy, 113-114
in urinary tract infection, 112
Education for All Handicapped Children Act, 4, 397
Effacement, 55, 124
Effleurage, 159*b*, 162, 162*f*, 778
Egocentric thinking, 420
Egocentrism, 423
Ejaculation, 31, 271
Ejaculatory duct, 22*f*, 23
Elderberry poisoning, 678*t*
Elective abortion, 86*t*
Electric shock injury
during pregnancy, 117
toddler and, 418*t*
Electrical burn, 713, 715, 716*f*
Electrocardiography, 618*t*
Electrolyte imbalance, 666
Electrolytes
for amniotic fluid embolism, 201
in impending preterm labor, 197
vomiting and, 664
Electronic fetal monitoring, 116, 136-137, 138*f*
Electronic measurement of pediatric blood pressure, 500
Electronic Medical Library, 532
Elemental iron, 107
Emancipated minor, 491
Emancipation, 460
Embolism, pulmonary, 243, 243*t*, 244
Embolization of uterine fibroid, 280

Embryo, 25, 37, 38-40*t*
Embryonic disc, 36
Emergency care
in burn, 716-717
during labor and birth, 134*b*, 198-201
Emergency contraception, 269
Emergency delivery kit, 134
Emergency preparedness, 113, 751
Emission, 29
EMLA. *See* Eutectic mixture of local anesthetics.
Emotional abuse, 585
Emotional care
in abortion, 85-86
of burn victim, 720, 721*f*
in cesarean birth, 185
in cystic fibrosis, 614-615
in diabetes mellitus in pregnancy, 106
of family after birth, 214-216
during hypotonic labor, 188
in pediatric diabetes mellitus, 737, 738*t*
postpartum, 205*b*
Emotional development
of infant, 386
of preschooler, 424-425*t*
of school-age child, 444-446*f*, 444-447, 448-450*t*
Emotional disorders, 761-774
anorexia nervosa in, 771-772, 772*f*
attention-deficit hyperactivity disorder in, 770-771, 771*b*
autism in, 763
bulimia in, 772-773
depression in, 764, 765-766
impact on growth and development, 773
nurse's role in care of, 761-762
obsessive-compulsive disorder in, 763-764
origins of, 762-763, 763*b*
substance abuse and, 767-770, 768*t*, 769*t*
suicide and, 764
types and settings of treatment, 762
Emotional neglect, 585
Emotionally safe environment, 762
Empowerment, 2
Enalapril, 115*t*
Encephalitis, 547-548
Encephalomyelitis, 547
Encephalopathy, 542
Encopresis, 666, 684
Endemic, term, 747
Endocrine dysfunction, 723-740
diabetes insipidus and, 725-727
diabetes mellitus and, 727-740
blood glucose self-monitoring in, 730, 732*f*
diabetic ketoacidosis and, 729, 729*t*
diagnostic blood tests in, 728-729, 729*f*
etiology and classification of, 727
future prospects in, 739-740
insulin management of, 733*f*, 733-737, 734*f*, 735*t*, 736*f*
nursing care plan for, 731-732
nutritional management of, 732-733, 739*t*
stress and, 737, 738-739*t*
type I, 727*t*, 728
hypothyroidism and, 725, 725*f*
Tay-Sachs disease and, 724-725
Endocrine tests in fertility screening, 272
Endoderm, 36, 37*b*, 683
Endometrial cycle, 30*f*
Endometriosis, 255
Endometritis, 244, 245*t*

Endometrium, 25f, 26, 34, 36f, 204
  menstruation and, 461f
Endorphins, 160
Endoscopy, gastrointestinal, 656-657
Endovaginal ultrasound, 49t
Enema
  as admission procedure, 135
  pediatric, 519
Energy healing, 778, 779f
Energy level
  before labor, 131
  older couple pregnancy and, 73
Energy requirements, 372t
Engagement, 131, 132f
Engorgement, 208, 229, 230, 232
Engrossment, 214
Enterobiasis, 676-677
Enterocolitis, 661, 664
Enucleation, 542
Enuresis, 431-432, 686
Environment
  growth and development and, 355
  labor pain management and, 164
Environmental hazard during pregnancy, 112-117
Enzyme-linked immunosorbent assay, 756
Eosinophil, 633f, 633t
Ephedra, 777t, 782t, 783t
Ephedrine, 604t
Epicanthal folds, 539
Epidemic, 747
Epidermis, 700
Epididymis, 22f, 23
Epidural anesthesia, 169f
  after cesarean birth, 213
  in labor pain management, 166t, 167, 168-169
  maternal pushing and, 125
  subarachnoid block versus, 168
Epidural blood patch, 170, 170f
Epidural space, regional analgesics and anesthetics and, 167
Epifoam. See Pramoxine.
Epiglottitis, 596
Epilepsy, 549-554, 550-551t, 552t, 553f
Epimetrium, 25f
Epinephrine, 604t
Epiphyseal closure, 460
Epiphyseal fusion, 352
Epiphysis, 570
Episiotomy, 135, 180-182, 181f
  fetal size and, 192
  perineum and, 207-208
Episodic dyscontrol syndrome, 554
Epispadias, 687f, 687-688
Epstein's pearls, 292, 294t
Erection, 29
  adolescent and, 459
  male infertility and, 271
Erikson's stages of child development, 363-365, 364t, 365-366t
  adolescent and, 456b
  school-age child and, 439b
Erythema, 749
Erythema infectiosum, 743t
Erythema marginatum, 625
Erythema toxicum, 294t
Erythroblastosis fetalis, 100, 100f, 338-339b, 338-343, 339-340f, 343-344f, 344b
Erythrocyte, 632, 633f
Erythrocyte sedimentation rate, 569

Erythromycin
  drug interactions with, 512t
  for ophthalmia neonatorum and Chlamydia trachomatis infection, 153, 154f
Erythropoietin, 631
Eschar, 717
Escharotomy, 717
Esophageal atresia, 657-658
Essential hypertension, 627
Estimated date of delivery, 48, 51, 51b
Estimation of gestational age, 82t
Estrogen, 42
  hormone replacement therapy and, 274-275
  menopause and, 276
  puberty and, 456
Ethambutol, 111
Ethanol poisoning, 679t
Ethical issues in assisted reproduction, 274
Ethinyl estradiol, 269
Ethosuximide, 552t
Etretinate, 115t
Eustachian tube, 534, 535f
Eutectic mixture of local anesthetics, 479f, 480, 515
Evaporation, 218, 218t
Evening primrose oil, 783t
Evil eye, 482
Evoked otoacoustic emissions, 537
Ewing's sarcoma, 580
Exanthem, 702-703
Exanthem subitum, 743t
Exchange transfusion in erythroblastosis fetalis, 340
Excretory function, 685f
Exercise
  childbirth preparation class and, 158
  diabetes mellitus and, 102-105, 737
  fertility and, 271
  infant and, 389-394t
  lochia and, 206
  perimenopausal symptoms and, 278
  postpartum, 210-211
  during pregnancy, 56, 65-68, 66-67f, 157b
Exhaustion, maternal pushing and, 125
Expressive language, 409t, 426t
Expressive language delay, 427t
Expulsion, 132f, 133, 146t, 149f
Exstrophy of bladder, 688
Extended family, 355, 355t
Extension, 132f, 133
Extensor posturing, 560, 560f
External ear, 535f
External fetal monitor, 137b
External genitalia
  female, 23-24, 24f
  male, 22, 22f
External os, 26
External rotation, 132f, 133, 149f
External version, 180, 192
Extrauterine life, 282-283
Extremities, postpartum care and, 205b
Extrusion reflex, 398
Extubation, 525
Eye, 538-542, 539f
  amblyopia and, 540
  conjunctivitis and, 541, 541f
  dehydration and, 670t
  dyslexia and, 540
  hyphema and, 541-542

Eye—cont'd
    neonatal, 153
    neurological assessment and, 562*b*
    preeclampsia and, 95
    retinoblastoma and, 542
    strabismus and, 540-541
    visual acuity tests and, 539, 540*f*
Eye contact, 482
Eye patch
    in amblyopia, 540
    in strabismus, 541
Eye prosthesis, 542
Eyedrops, 514, 514*b*
Eyelid, 539*f*
Eyestrain, 541

F

Face presentation of fetus, 128
FACES pain scale, 478*f*
Facial nerve, 544*f*, 545*t*, 561*b*
Factor VIII deficiency, 639-641
Fahrenheit temperature, 793
Failure to thrive, 621, 673-674
Fair Labor Standards Act of 1938, 3
Fallopian tube, 24*f*, 25*f*, 26
    infertility and, 271
    menstruation and, 461*f*
Falls
    infant and, 402
    during pregnancy, 115
    toddler and, 417*t*
False labor, 135-136, 136*t*
False pelvis, 27, 126
Family, 203-236
    adolescent and, 458*t*
    attachment, 223
    bonding, 223
    care for specific groups and cultures of, 203-204
    of child with cleft lip and palate, 329
    child's hospitalization and, 483
    cultural influences on postpartum care and, 204, 204*f*
    discharge planning and, 234-235
        newborn care in, 235, 235*f*
        postpartum self-care teaching in, 234-235
    of Down syndrome child, 337
    emotional care of, 214*b*, 214*f*, 214-216, 215*t*
    family care plan and, 216-217
    growth and development and, 355*f*, 355-356, 357-362*t*
    high-risk pregnancy and, 117
    infection control and, 749
    newborn care and, 217-224
        admission to postpartum or nursery unit in, 217-221, 218*t*, 219*f*, 221*f*
        bonding and attachment in, 222-224, 223*f*
        daily care in, 224
        security and, 222
    of preterm newborn, 317, 317*f*
Family APGAR, 356
Family care plan, 18, 216-217
Family-centered care, 2
Family day care center, 432
Family planning, 261-269
    barrier methods in, 264-265, 266*b*, 267*f*
    basal body temperature in, 267*f*, 267-268
    calendar method in, 268
    cervical mucous method in, 268, 268*f*
    emergency contraception and, 269
    hormonal contraceptives in, 261-264, 262*f*, 263*f*

Family planning—cont'd
    intrauterine device in, 264
    natural methods in, 267
    spermicides in, 266-267
    sterilization in, 268*f*, 268-269
Family therapy, 762
Family violence, 584, 584*b*
Fantasy play, 382*t*
FAS. *See* Fetal alcohol syndrome.
Fascia pressure, 778
Fasting blood glucose, 728
Fat intake of infant, 401
Father
    bonding and attachment and, 223
    developmental stages of fatherhood, 72*b*
    emotional care after birth, 214, 214*f*
    psychological adaptations to pregnancy, 72, 72*b*, 72*f*
Fatigue
    ineffective maternal pushing and, 192
    pain modification and, 160
    parenthood and, 216
    in pregnancy, 52, 68
Fear
    pediatric hospitalization and, 480, 481-482
    toddler and, 411
Febrile seizure, 549
Federal regulations in complementary therapies, 776-778
Feeding
    behavior of infant during, 400*t*, 401*f*
    breastfeeding and, 224-232, 398-399, 399*t*
        afterpains and, 205
        assisting mother in, 226-229, 227*t*, 228*b*, 228*f*, 229*f*
        for contraception, 269
        contraceptives and, 208
        diabetes mellitus in pregnancy and, 106
        in galactosemia, 336
        herpes virus lesion and, 109
        human immunodeficiency virus and, 110
        of hypoglycemic newborn, 221
        mastitis and, 246-247, 247*f*
        maternal-infant bonding and, 153
        in phenylketonuria, 335
        physiology of lactation and, 225-226, 226*f*
        postpartum analgesia and, 213-214
        postpartum immunization for rubella and, 211
        prenatal class in, 157*b*
        preventing problems with, 229*b*, 229-230, 230*f*
        special situations in, 230-231, 231*f*
        substance abuse and, 115
        weaning from, 402
    cerebral palsy and, 556, 556*b*, 556*f*
    cleft lip and, 328
    difficulties in congestive heart failure, 623
    formula, 232-234, 233*f*
    of fussy infant, 230
    of healthy child, 374*f*, 374-376, 377*t*
    of ill child, 376-378, 378*f*
    Piaget's theory of development in relation to, 365*t*
Female
    adolescent growth and development, 459*f*, 459-460, 460*b*
    pediatric blood pressure readings, 502*t*
    physiology of sex act, 31
    puberty and, 22
    recommended dietary allowances for, 372*t*
    reproductive system of, 23-28
        breasts and, 28, 29*f*, 459*f*
        external genitalia and, 23*f*, 23-24
        internal genitalia and, 24*f*, 24-26, 25*f*

Female—cont'd
  reproductive system of—cont'd
    menstruation and, 28-29, 30*f*
    of newborn, 292
    pelvis and, 26-28, 27*f*, 28*f*, 28*t*
  sterilization of, 268*f*, 269
Female condom, 265, 267*f*
Femoral fracture, 570, 578*f*
Femoral head, Legg-Calvé-Perthes disease and, 579
Fentanyl
  anesthesia and, 168
  for child, 480
  intrapartum, 165*t*
Fern test, 141
Fertility, 271-272
Fertility awareness method of contraception, 267
Fertility rate, 10*b*
Fertilization, 33-34, 36*f*
Fertilization age, 50
Fetal alcohol syndrome, 113*f*
Fetal attitude, 128
Fetal circulation, 42-43, 44*f*
Fetal circulatory shunt, 43
Fetal compromise
  in abruptio placentae, 92*t*
  oxytocin labor induction and, 179
  in placenta previa, 92*t*
Fetal heart rate
  in abruptio placentae, 93
  in admission assessment, 134
  amniotomy and, 177
  assessment and documentation of, 137*b*
  before birth, 136
  in cesarean birth, 184
  in labor induction, 180
  prenatal visit and, 50
  in placenta previa, 93
  recurrent pregnancy loss and, 84
  in second trimester, 71
Fetal lie, 127
Fetal monitoring
  before birth, 136-141, 137*b*, 138*f*, 139*f*, 140*b*, 140*f*
  indomethacin and, 197
  labor pain management and, 173
Fetal mortality, 10*b*
Fetal movement
  decreased, 133
  as positive sign of pregnancy, 54
  in second trimester, 71
Fetal oxygenation
  biophysical profile and, 83*t*
  in precipitate birth, 195-196
Fetal position, 128-130, 130*f*, 131*b*, 160, 192
Fetal presentation, 128, 129*f*, 131*b*, 160, 192
Fetal surgery, 10*f*
Fetoscope, 54, 137*b*, 138*f*
Fetus, 21, 37
  abnormal labor and, 192-194, 194*f*
  abruptio placentae and, 92*t*
  acidosis in, 166
  admission assessment and, 134
  assessment of, 80-81, 81*f*, 82-84*t*
  development of, 38-40*t*
  diabetic mother and, 105
  diagnostic testing of, 82-84*t*
  head of, 127
  induction of labor and, 177
  lung maturation of, 84*t*, 197

Fetus—cont'd
  maternal substance abuse and, 114
  percutaneous umbilical blood sampling and, 83*t*
  placenta previa and, 92*t*
  pregnancy-induced hypertension and, 96
  premature rupture of membranes and, 196
  prolonged labor and, 195
  prolonged pregnancy and, 198
  skull of, 127*f*
Fever
  in acute otitis media, 536
  in acute pharyngitis, 594
  chills and, 209
  in hospitalized child, 501-503, 503*f*, 503*t*
  in Kawasaki disease, 628
  in meningitis, 546
  in nasopharyngitis, 594
  nursing care plan for, 504
  in pneumonia, 598
  postpartum, 244
  in rheumatic fever, 625
  in sepsis, 545
Fever blister, 706, 706*f*
Feverfew, 777*t*, 782*t*, 783*t*
FHR. *See* Fetal heart rate.
Fiber, 367
  postpartum intake of, 210
Fibrinogen
  for amniotic fluid embolism, 201
  in nonpregnant and pregnant women, 56*t*
  in trauma during pregnancy, 116
Fibroid, uterine, 279-280
Fibronectin test, 196
Fibular fracture, 578*f*
Fifth disease, 743*t*
Fight-or-flight reaction, 195
Fimbriae, 25*f*, 26
Fine motor skills of toddler, 406-407*t*
Fingerprints, infant identification and, 152
Firm contraction, 124
First-degree burn, 715*t*
First-stage breathing, 163-164
Fish oil, 783*t*
Fistula, tracheoesophageal, 657-658
Five-year-old preschooler, 428-429
Flat nipple, 230
Flaxseed, 782*t*
Flexion, 131-133, 132*f*
Flexor posturing, 560, 560*f*
Fluid and electrolyte balance, 666-670, 669*f*, 670*t*, 671*b*
  in overhydration, 672, 673*t*
  pediatric, 666-669, 668*f*
  urinary changes in pregnancy and, 57
  vomiting and, 664
Fluids
  for burn victim, 717, 719-720
  for dehydration, 671-672
  for hyperemesis gravidarum, 84
  for hypotonic labor, 188
  infant intake of, 400
  for nasopharyngitis, 594
  postpartum intake of, 210, 232
  during pregnancy and lactation, 63
  for urinary tract infection, 112
Fluoride
  ingestion of, 382*t*
  recommended dietary allowance of, 372*t*
Fluorocarbons, 768*t*

Foam stability index, 84t
Focal point, 159b, 162
Folate, 372t
Foley catheter, 184
Folic acid, 61, 107, 108b, 324
Folic acid antagonists, 115t
Folic acid deficiency anemia, 107
Folk healer, 776b
Follicle-stimulating hormone
    menstruation and, 28-29
    testosterone production and, 23
Follicular ovarian cyst, 280
Follow-up appointment, 234
Fomite, 747, 748
Fontanel, 284-286
    dehydration and, 670t, 672t
    fetal, 127
    of hospitalized child, 497
    neurological assessment and, 562b
Food
    allergy in spina bifida, 327
    buying, storing, and serving of baby food, 402, 402b
    for infant, 399-400, 401f
    newborn responses to, 284t
    recommendations in pregnancy, 108b
Food, Drug, and Cosmetic Act, 777
Food additives, 371
Food-drug interactions, 378, 512t, 513
Food guide pyramid, 58f
Food labels, 664b
Food stamps, 377t
Foot
    assessment in newborn, 220
    care in diabetes mellitus, 737
Football, injury risks in, 585t
Football hold
    for breastfeeding, 227, 228f
    in transporting hospitalized infant, 496, 497f
Footling breech presentation, 128, 129f
Footprints, infant identification and, 152
Foramen ovale, 43, 44f
Forceps birth, 182f, 182-183
Forceps marks, 295t
Foregut, 656
Foreign body, gastrointestinal, 681
Foremilk, 226
Foreskin, 22, 22f, 291
Formal operations, 463
Formula feeding, 232-234
Foster parent family, 355t
Four-year-old preschooler, 428
Fourchette, 23, 24f
Fowler's sling, 665f
Foxglove poisoning, 678t
Fracture, 570-574, 571-574f, 578f
    clavicle, 192
    skull, 560
Frank breech presentation, 128, 129f
Fraternal twins, 44, 45f
Freestanding birth center, 120
Frejka splint, 332
Freon abuse, 768t
Frequency
    of contraction, 124, 126f
    urinary, 686
Freud's theory of development, 364t
    adolescent and, 456b
    school-age child and, 439b

Friedman curve, 195
Frontal bone of fetal skull, 127f
Frontal suture, 127f
Frostbite, 720-721
Fructosamine, 729
Fructose intolerance, 739t
FTT. See Failure to thrive.
Full breech presentation, 128, 129f
Full inclusion, 11
Full-thickness burn, 715t
Functional murmur, 288
Functional scoliosis, 582
Fundal height
    during gestation, 53f
    prenatal visit and, 50
Fundal massage, 201
Fundus, 205f
    after cesarean birth, 187
    assessing and massaging of, 207b, 207f
    descent after birth, 205
    lochia and, 206
    postpartum care and, 205b
    uterine, 25f, 26
Fungal infection, 676, 711-712, 712f
Funic souffle, 54
Furosemide, 624
Fussy infant, 230

G

Gabapentin, 552t
Gait, 568-569
Galactagogues, 226
Galactose intolerance, 739t
Galactosemia, 335-336
Gamete intrafallopian transfer, 273, 273t
Gametogenesis, 33-34, 34, 35f
Gardnerella vaginalis, 258t
Garlic, 777t, 782t
Gastric influences on pediatric drug absorption, 508
Gastrocolic reflex, 297
Gastroenteritis, 664, 664b, 667-668
Gastroesophageal reflux, 665, 665f
Gastrointestinal disorders, 656-682
    appendicitis in, 675-676
    celiac disease in, 659f, 659-660
    constipation in, 666
    dehydration in, 670-672, 671t, 672t
    diarrhea in, 665-668
    esophageal atresia in, 657-658
    failure to thrive in, 673-674
    fluid and electrolyte imbalance in, 666-670, 669f, 670t, 671b
    foreign bodies in, 681
    gastroenteritis in, 664, 664b
    gastroesophageal reflux in, 665, 665f
    hernias in, 663f, 663-664
    Hirschsprung's disease in, 661-662, 662f
    imperforate anus in, 658
    intussusception in, 662-663, 663f
    kwashiorkor in, 674-675
    Meckel's diverticulum in, 663
    overhydration in, 672, 673t
    pinworms in, 676-677
    poisoning in, 677-681
        drugs in, 677-680, 678t, 679b
        general concepts in, 677, 677t
        lead, 680-681
        poisonous plants in, 677, 678t
    pyloric stenosis in, 658-659, 659f, 660

Gastrointestinal disorders—cont'd
  rickets in, 675
  roundworms in, 677
  scurvy in, 675
  thrush in, 676
  vomiting in, 664-665
Gastrointestinal system
  changes in pregnancy, 56-57, 57f
  cleft lip and, 327f, 327-328
  cystic fibrosis and, 609
  excretory function of, 685f
  neonatal, 295-297, 296f
  postpartum changes in, 210
  preeclampsia and, 95
Gastroschisis, 82t
Gastrostomy, 519, 524b, 524f
Gate control theory of pain, 160
Gateway substances, 767, 769f
Gavage feeding, 519
  in burn victim, 720
  in preterm newborn, 314
Gay, 467
Gel, 710t
Gender
  determination of, 684
  growth and development and, 355
Gender identity, 440
Gender role, 456
Gene therapy, 11f
General anesthesia for childbirth, 164, 166t, 170
General thinking, 15-16
Generalized seizure, 549-552, 550-551t
Genetic anemia, 108
Genetic counseling in phenylketonuria, 335
Genitalia
  neonatal, 220, 291-292
  Tanner's stages of sexual maturity and, 461b
  trauma during labor, 242
Genitourinary system, 683-699
  acute glomerulonephritis and, 693t, 693-694
  assessment of, 686, 686t
  cryptorchidism and, 694-697
  development of, 683-684, 684f
  exstrophy of bladder and, 688
  hydrocele and, 694, 697f
  hypospadias and epispadias and, 687f, 687-688
  impact of surgery on, 698
  neonatal, 291-292, 292f
  nephrotic syndrome and, 690-693
  obstructive uropathy and, 688, 689t
  phimosis and, 686-687, 687f
  urinary tract infection and, 688-690, 689f
  Wilms' tumor and, 694
Gentamycin, 512t
Genu valgum, 568-569
Genu varum, 568-569
Germ layers, 34, 36, 37b
German measles, 742t, 747f
Gestational age, 50, 306
  assessment of, 219-220
  new Ballard scale and, 307f
  premature rupture of membranes and, 196
Gestational diabetes, 100, 101
  nutrition in pregnancy and, 65
  prenatal class in, 157b
Gestational surrogate, 273t
Gestational trophoblastic disease, 82t, 90, 90f

Ginger, 777t, 782t
Gingivitis, 381
Ginkgo biloba, 777t, 782t, 783t
Ginseng, 777t, 782t
Glandular fever, 744t
Glans penis, 22, 22f, 291
Glasgow Coma Scale, 562, 563t
Global language delay, 427t
Glomerulus, 690
Glossopharyngeal nerve, 544f, 545t, 561b
Glucagon, 736
Glucocorticoids, 197
Glucometer, 730, 732f
Glucose
  effect of pregnancy on, 56-57, 101
  in impending preterm labor, 197
  urinary, 686t
Glucose-insulin imbalance, 737
Glucose tolerance test, 728, 729f
Glucosuria, 728
Glue sniffing, 768t
Gluten enteropathy, 659
Glutethimide, 768t
Glyburide, 102
Glycemic index, 733
Glycosuria, 728
  diabetes mellitus and, 101
  in pregnancy, 57
Glycosylated hemoglobin, 102, 728
Goals of adolescent, 458t
Goldenrod poisoning, 678t
Gomco clamp, 291
Gonadotropin cycle, 30f
Gonorrhea, 257, 259t
Goodell's sign, 53
Government influences in maternity and pediatric care, 3
Gower's maneuver, 579
Grand mal seizure, 549-552, 550-551t
Grandparent
  emotional care after birth for, 215, 215t
  prenatal class for, 157b
  psychological adaptations to pregnancy, 74
Granular leukocyte, 633f
Grasp reflex, 283, 283f, 284t, 386
Gravida, 50
Greenstick fracture, 570, 571f
Grieving parent
  emotional care after birth, 215-216
  sudden infant death syndrome and, 616
Groshong catheter, 517-518
Gross motor skills of toddler, 406-407t
Group B streptococcus infection
  in acute pharyngitis, 594
  in pregnancy, 111
  in rheumatic fever, 625
Group therapy, pediatric, 476
Growth, term, 349, 349b
Growth and development, 346-365
  of adolescent, 456-460, 458t, 459f, 460b, 461f, 467f
  child versus adult, 349-351f, 349-352
  developmental screening and, 352
  directional patterns of, 349, 349f
  factors influencing, 352-356, 355t, 357-362t
  growth standards in, 352, 353f
  impact of illness on, 773
  impact on nursing care, 346-348, 348b
  of infant, 387-388, 389-394t

Growth and development—cont'd
  of mealtime behavior, 400*t*
  of parent, 363-365, 365-366*t*
  personality development and, 356, 363, 363*f*, 364*t*, 365*t*
  play and, 382*t*, 382-383
  of school-age child, 444*f*, 444-447, 445*f*, 446*f*
  terminology in, 349, 349*b*
Growth chart, 352, 353-354*f*
Growth spurt, 346, 456
Guarding, 675
Guided imagery, 780
Gums, phenytoin-induced hyperplasia of, 553*f*
Guthrie blood test, 334-335
Gymnastics, injury risks in, 585*t*
Gynecoid pelvis, 27, 27*f*, 194
Gynecologic infections, 255-261
  normal vagina and, 256, 256*b*
  toxic shock syndrome in, 256
Gynecological age, 64

H

Habilitation after spina bifida surgery, 325-326
Habituation in effleurage, 159*b*, 162
Haemophilus influenzae
  in acute otitis media, 535
  in acute pharyngitis, 594
  in epiglottitis, 596
  in osteomyelitis, 577
  in pneumonia, 598
Haemophilus influenzae type b vaccine, 751, 752*f*
Hair
  examination of, 701
  head lice and, 712*f*, 712-713
  neonatal, 219
Haitian family, 358*t*
Hallucinogens, 768*t*
Halo traction, 582, 583*f*
Handicapped child, play and, 434-435
Handwashing, 302, 749
Haploid, 33
Hard palate, cleft, 328-329
Harelip, 327*f*, 327-328
Harlequin color change, 295*t*
Harrington rod, 582
Hashish, 767, 768*t*
Hay fever, 600-602, 602*f*
HBOT. *See* Hyperbaric oxygen therapy.
hCG. *See* Human chorionic gonadotropin.
hCS. *See* Human chorionic somatomammotropin.
Head
  hydrocephalus and, 321-324, 322*f*, 323*f*
  neonatal, 283-286, 285*f*
Head circumference, 351
  of hospitalized child, 505
  of newborn, 221, 283, 285*f*
  of toddler, 408
Head injury, 559-563, 560*f*, 561-562*b*, 563*t*
Head lag, 283, 283*f*, 284*t*
Head lice, 712*f*, 712-713
Head lift exercise, 211
Headache
  in acute otitis media, 536
  dural puncture and, 168
  in encephalitis, 547
  in meningitis, 546
Health, nutrition and, 370-371
Health care delivery systems, 10-12, 12*b*

Health care reform, 16-17
Health examination for school-age child, 447-451, 448-450*t*
Health maintenance of infant, 395*f*, 395-397
Health maintenance organization, 11, 12*b*
Health promotion, 11
Healthy People 2010, 17, 17*b*
  goals for women's health, 251
  immunizations and, 750
  prenatal development and, 43
Hearing, neonatal, 286, 286*f*
Hearing aid, 538
Hearing impairment, 536, 537-538
Heart, adult *versus* child, 351
Heart disease, 106*b*, 106-107
  congenital, 616-622, 618*t*
    atrial septal defect in, 618-619
    coarctation of aorta in, 620
    hypoplastic left heart syndrome in, 622
    patent ductus arteriosus in, 620
    tetralogy of Fallot in, 620-621, 621*f*
    ventricular septal defect in, 619-620
  congestive heart failure in, 622-624, 623*f*
Heart murmur
  in newborn, 288
  in patent ductus arteriosus, 620
Heart rate
  adult *versus* child, 351
  in Apgar scoring, 153*t*
  neonatal, 220
  in postpartum hemorrhage, 238
Heartburn, 69
Heat loss, neonatal, 218*t*
Heat production, fluid and electrolyte imbalance and, 666
Heat therapy, 784
  in episiotomy care, 182
  for postpartum perineum care, 208
Heel-to-ear maneuver, 308*f*
Hegar's sign, 53
Height, 352
  child *versus* adult, 349, 350*f*
  of hospitalized child, 505
  of preschooler, 422
  of school-age child, 439
  of toddler, 408
Heimlich maneuver, 528, 529*f*
HELLP syndrome, 94*t*, 95
Hemangioma, 703, 703*f*
Hemarthrosis, 640
Hematocrit
  neonatal, 288
  in nonpregnant and pregnant women, 56*t*
  normal values of, 633*t*
  postpartum changes in, 209
  prenatal, 49*t*
Hematoma
  fetal presentation and position and, 192
  in hemophilia, 640
  in platelet disorders, 641
  postpartum, 242
Hematopoiesis, 631
Hematuria, 640
Hemodynamics, 617
Hemoglobin
  anemia and, 633
  neonatal, 288
  in nonpregnant and pregnant women, 56*t*
  prenatal, 49*t*
  thalassemia and, 638

Hemoglobin electrophoresis, 49*t*

Hemoglobin S, 634

Hemolytic disease of newborn, 338-339*b*, 338-343, 339-340*f*, 343-344*f*, 344*b*

Hemophilia, 382*t*, 639-641

Hemorrhage
  in abruptio placentae, 92*t*, 93
  fetal size and, 192
  intracranial, 343-344
  lochia and, 206
  in placenta previa, 92*t*
  postpartum, 210, 237-243
    anemia in, 238
    early, 238-242, 241*t*, 242*f*
    hypovolemic shock in, 238
    late, 242-243
    observation of, 149-150
  pregnancy-induced hypertension and, 96
  in placenta previa, 92
  vaginal birth after cesarean and, 144

Hemorrhoids
  postpartum, 207
  during pregnancy, 56, 69

Hemosiderosis
  in sickle cell disease, 637
  in thalassemia major, 639

Heparin
  for heart disease, 107
  for venous thrombosis, 243

Heparin lock, 517

Hepatitis A, 225, 744*t*

Hepatitis A vaccine, 752*f*

Hepatitis B, 257, 745*t*
  high risk for, 110*b*
  in pregnancy, 109
  prenatal screening for, 49*t*

Hepatitis B vaccine, 751, 752*f*

Hepatitis C, 225

Herbal medicine, 781-784, 782*b*, 782-784*t*

Hereditary traits, 353

Hernia
  diaphragmatic, 591
  umbilical, 663*f*, 663-664

Herniorrhaphy, 664

Heroin, 114*t*, 767, 768*t*

Herpes simplex virus
  breastfeeding and, 225
  in cutaneous infection, 706, 706*f*
  in genital infection, 257, 259*t*
  in pregnancy, 109

Heterograft, 719

Hexosaminidase deficiency, 724-725

Hiccups (Hiccoughs)
  infant and, 389*t*
  neonatal, 297

Hickman catheter, 517-518

High-fiber foods, 367, 370*t*

High-risk newborn
  postterm, 306, 317-318
  preterm, 305-317
    causes of prematurity, 306
    close observation of, 314, 316*t*
    family reaction to, 317, 317*f*
    hypoglycemia and hypocalcemia in, 310-311
    immature kidneys in, 312
    inadequate respiratory function in, 306-310, 309*f*
    increased tendency to bleed in, 311

High-risk newborn—cont'd
  preterm—cont'd
    jaundice in, 312*t*, 312-313
    necrotizing enterocolitis in, 312
    nursing care plan for, 315
    physical characteristics of, 306
    poor control of body temperature in, 310, 313*f*, 313-314, 316*f*
    poor nutrition in, 312, 314
    positioning and skin care of, 314, 316*f*
    prognosis for, 314-317
    retinopathy of prematurity in, 311*f*, 311-312
    sepsis in, 310
  transporting of, 318

High-risk pregnancy, 80

Hindgut, 656

Hindmilk, 226

Hindu family, 122*t*

Hindu healing regimen, 779

Hip, developmental dysplasia of, 330-334, 331*f*, 332*f*, 334*b*

Hirschsprung's disease, 661-662, 662*f*

Hispanic American family
  cultural influences on, 357*t*
  food patterns of, 368*t*
  labor and delivery and, 123*t*

History survey of hospitalized child, 497

History taking
  infant, 397
  in pharmacological labor pain management, 170-173
  prenatal, 48

HIV. *See* Human immunodeficiency virus infection.

Hives, 702

HMO. *See* Health maintenance organization.

Hmong family
  cultural influences on, 360*t*
  labor and delivery for, 122*t*

Hoarseness, 594

Hockey, injury risks in, 585*t*

Hodgkin's disease, 645*t*, 645-646

Holistic healing, 775

Homans' sign, 209

Home care, 476
  after pediatric hospitalization, 492
  of chronically ill child, 650
  in cleft lip and palate, 329
  in juvenile rheumatoid arthritis, 581
  of newborn, 302-303, 303*f*

Home phototherapy, 340-343

Home preparation of infant foods, 402*b*

Home setting for childbirth, 120-124

Homeless family, 356

Homeless mother, 249

Homeopathy, 779

Homeostasis, 670

Homosexuality, 355*t*, 467, 467*t*

Hordeolum, 703*f*

Hormonal contraceptives, 261-262

Hormonal injection, 263-264

Hormone implants, 263, 263*f*

Hormone replacement therapy, 274-275

Hormones, 723
  exercise during pregnancy and, 67
  infertility and, 271
  in lactation, 225-226

Hospice, 476

Hospital
  safety measures in, 495*f*, 495-496, 496*f*
  setting for childbirth, 120

Hospital-acquired infection, 749
Hospitalized child, 475-532
  admission to pediatric unit, 494-496, 495-497f, 498b
  adolescent, 490-491
  airway obstruction management in, 528, 529f
  appetite of, 378
  assessment of, 496-505
    basic data collection in, 496-497
    blood pressure in, 499-500, 500f, 501t, 502t
    body temperature in, 501-503, 503f, 503t
    head circumference in, 505
    height in, 505
    history survey in, 497
    pulse and respirations in, 499, 499t
    weight in, 503-505
  blood specimens and, 506, 507f
  clinical pathways for, 484-486, 486f
  confidentiality and legal issues, 491
  cultural needs of family and, 480-483
  development of nursing care plan, 484, 485f, 486f
  discharge planning and, 491-492
  drug physiology and, 479f, 479-480
  enema for, 519
  fear and, 480, 481-482
  feeding of, 376-378, 378f
  gastrostomy in, 519, 524b, 524f
  home care and, 492
  infant, 486-487, 487f
  lumbar puncture and, 506-507, 507f
  medication administration to, 508-519, 509b
    avoiding drug interactions in, 511t, 511-513, 512t
    calculating pediatric drug doses in, 510, 512f
    calculating safe drug dose in, 510-511, 512b
    intravenous medications in, 516-518, 517f, 518f
    nosedrops, eardrops, and eyedrops in, 414b, 514
    oral medications in, 513f, 513-514
    parenteral fluids and, 518, 520-523t
    rectal medications in, 514
    subcutaneous and intramuscular injections in, 514-516, 515f, 516f
    total parenteral nutrition and, 518-519, 524f
  nurse role in admission, 483-484
  outpatient clinic and, 475-476
  oxygen therapy for, 525-527, 526b, 527f, 528f
  pain and, 478f, 478-479
  parent reaction to, 482
  physiologic responses to medications, 507-508
  preoperative and postoperative care of, 528-531, 529f, 530t, 531t
  preparation for surgery, 529f, 530t
  preschooler, 435-436, 489
  regression and, 480
  school-age child, 489-490
  separation anxiety and, 477-478
  stool specimens and, 505-506
  toddler, 487-489, 488b
  tracheostomy care in, 519-525, 525f
  urine specimens and, 505, 506f, 506t
Host resistance, 747-748
Hot Fast low-angle shot imaging, 276
HPV. See Human papilloma virus.
HRT. See Hormone replacement therapy.
Human chorionic gonadotropin, 42
  in hydatidiform mole, 91
  pregnancy tests and, 54
  recurrent pregnancy loss and, 84
Human chorionic somatomammotropin, 42

Human immunodeficiency virus infection, 257, 260t
  adolescent and, 466
  breastfeeding and, 225
  education for school-age child, 441
  pediatric, 756-759
  in pregnancy, 110
  prenatal screening for, 49t
  risk factors for, 110b
Human insulin, 733
Human leukocyte antigen B-27, 569
Human papilloma virus, 257, 260t
Human placental lactogen, 42
Humeral fracture, 578f
Humidity, asthma and, 605
Humulin, 735t
Hunger
  after labor and delivery, 210
  behavior in infant, 400t
  neonatal, 229b
Hyaline membrane disease, 308-309, 309f
Hydatidiform mole, 82t, 90f, 90-91
Hydralazine, 96
Hydramnios, 177
Hydrocarbons, 768t
Hydrocele, 694, 697f
Hydrocephalus, 321-324, 322f, 323f
Hydrocortisone, 208
Hydronephrosis, 688
Hydrops fetalis, 338
Hydrotherapy, 159b, 780
Hydroxyzine, 165t, 167
Hygiene
  adolescent and, 470
  in cystic fibrosis, 614
  postpartum self-care teaching and, 234
Hymen, 24
Hyperactivity, 771
Hyperalimentation, 518, 520-523t
Hyperbaric oxygen therapy, 784
Hyperbilirubinemia, 312, 340
Hyperemesis gravidarum, 81-84
Hyperglycemia, 729t
  in diabetes mellitus, 728
  hypoglycemia versus, 105t
  pregnancy and, 101
  Somogyi phenomenon and, 736-737
Hyperhemolytic crisis, 638t
Hyperinsulinism, 344
Hyperkalemia, 693
Hyperlipidemia, 627, 627t, 628b
Hyperopia, 540
Hyperparathyroidism, 726t
Hyperpigmentation, 210
Hyperpituitarism, 726t
Hypertension, 93-99, 94b, 94t, 95t, 96b, 627
Hypertonic dehydration, 670t, 671
Hypertonic labor dysfunction, 188, 190b
Hypertonic uterine infusion, 87t
Hyperventilation, 163, 164b
Hypervolemia, 55
Hyphema, 541-542
Hypnotherapy, 780
Hypnotics abuse, 768t
Hypoalbuminemia, 690
Hypocalcemia, 310-311
Hypoglossal nerve, 544f, 545t, 561b

Hypoglycemia, 729t
  gestational diabetes and, 65
  hyperglycemia *versus,* 105t
  in infant of diabetic mother, 344
  neonatal hypothermia and, 151, 218
  newborn care and, 221-222
  pregnancy and, 101
  in preterm newborn, 310-311
  Somogyi phenomenon and, 737
Hypoglycemic drugs, 102
Hypoparathyroidism, 726t
Hypopituitarism, 726t
Hypoplastic left heart syndrome, 622
Hypospadias, 271, 291, 687f, 687-688
Hypostatic pneumonia, 598
Hypotension
  in amniotic fluid embolism, 201
  epidural block and, 169
  exercise during pregnancy and, 67
  in hospitalized child, 497
  pregnancy and, 165
  in sepsis, 545
  subarachnoid block and, 170
Hypothermia, 617
  neonatal, 151, 218
Hypothyroidism, 725, 725f
Hypotonia, 725
Hypotonic dehydration, 670t, 671
Hypotonic labor dysfunction, 188-190
  hypertonic *versus,* 190b
  macrosomia and, 192
Hypotonicity in Down syndrome, 337
Hypovolemia, 95
Hypovolemic shock, 237
  abortion and, 85
  in abruptio placentae, 93
  in dehydration, 671-672
  in ectopic pregnancy, 89
  in postpartum hemorrhage, 238
  in placenta previa, 92
  signs and symptoms of, 90b
  uterine rupture and, 200
Hypoxia
  in erythroblastosis fetalis, 338
  exercise during pregnancy and, 67, 105
  neonatal, 151
  pregnancy and, 165
  pregnancy-induced hypertension and, 95
  in previa placenta, 92
Hysterectomy
  for abnormal uterine bleeding, 254
  hormone replacement therapy after, 275
  for uterine fibroids, 280
  for uterine inversion, 201
  for uterine rupture, 200
Hysterosalpingography, 272
Hysteroscopic myomectomy, 280
Hysteroscopy, 272

I

Ibuprofen
  for child, 479
  for fever in nasopharyngitis, 594
Icterus, 312
Icterus neonatorum, 295
Identical twins, 44, 45f

Identification
  bracelet for hospitalized child, 494-495, 495f
  of embryo or fetus, 54
  of newborn, 219, 219f, 222
Identity *versus* role confusion, 460
Idiopathic epilepsy, 549
Idiopathic scoliosis, 582
Idiopathic thrombocytopenia purpura, 641
Ileal conduit, 689t
Iletin 1 insulin, 735t
Ileus, 717
Ilium, 26
Illness
  nutrition and, 371-374, 373b, 376-378, 378f
  prevention in infant, 397-402, 399b, 399t, 400t, 401f, 402b
Imagery in labor pain management, 159b, 162-163
Imaginary playmate, 434
Imaging
  in appendicitis, 675
  in congenital heart defects, 618t
  in musculoskeletal disorders, 569
  three-dimensional, 82t
Immobility in abnormal labor, 195
Immune system, postpartum changes in, 211
Immune thrombocytopenic purpura, 641
Immunity, 351, 748
Immunization, 750f, 750-753, 752f
  for hepatitis B in newborn, 109-110
  for infant, 389-394t, 398
  newborn discharge care and, 234
  during pregnancy, 113
  for preschooler, 435
  rubella in pregnancy and, 109
  for viral infection, 109
Immunocompromised child, pet ownership and, 451
Immunoglobulin A, 297
Immunoglobulin G, 297
Immunoglobulin M, 297
Immunotherapy, 753
Impending birth, 134
Impending labor, 196-197
Imperforate anus, 658
Impetigo, 710-711, 711f
Implantation of zygote, 34
Implanted port, 518
Impulsive act, 764
Impulsivity, 771
In-toeing, 568
In vitro fertilization, 273, 273t
Inattention, 771
Inborn errors of metabolism, 320, 334-336, 724-725
Incarcerated hernia, 663
Incision in cesarean birth, 184
Incisor, 379f
Incompetent cervix, 84
Incomplete abortion, 85f, 86t
Incomplete uterine rupture, 199
Incontinence, 279
  spina bifida and, 326, 327f
Increased intracranial pressure
  after hydrocephalus surgery, 324
  in head injury, 560
  in intracranial hemorrhage, 344
  pediatric, 548f
  in Reye's syndrome, 542
Increment of contraction, 124, 126f
Incubation period, 747

Incubator, 313, 313f
Indirect Coombs' test, 339
Indirect transmission of infection, 748
Individuals with Disabilities Education Act, 553
Indomethacin, 197
Induced abortion, 86t
Induction of labor, 177-180, 178t
Ineffective maternal pushing, 190-192
Inevitable abortion, 85f, 86t
Infant, 385-404
    administration of medications, 509b
    behavior conditions in, 763t
    car safety for, 402-403, 403t
    chronic illness in, 646t
    community-based care of, 388, 395
    dental hygiene for, 380b
    developmental milestones of, 389-394t
    developmental theories of infancy, 364t
    diabetes mellitus in, 738t
    of diabetic mother, 344
    emotional development of, 386
    fall prevention in, 402
    Glasgow Coma Scale for, 563t
    health maintenance of, 395f, 395-397
    heart-healthy guidelines for, 628b
    hospitalization of, 486-487, 487f
    identification of, 152-153
    illness prevention in, 397-402, 399b, 399t, 400t, 401f, 402b
    immediately after birth, 151f, 151-154, 152f, 153t, 154f
    intravenous therapy for, 520-521t
    length of, 350f
    motor development of, 386, 387-388f
    need for constant care and guidance, 386-387
    normal blood values of, 633t
    nutrition for, 374, 374f, 375t
    oral stage of, 386f, 396
    oxygen therapy for, 526b
    recommended dietary allowances for, 372t
    respiratory distress in, 595, 595f
    response to death, 651t
    toy safety for, 403, 403t
Infant formula, 232-233, 398-399, 399t
Infant mortality rate, 8t, 10b, 282
Infantile eczema, 706-710, 707f, 710t
Infantile paralysis, 744t
Infantile spasm, 552
Infarct, 634
Infection, 108-112, 110b
    abruptio placentae and, 92t, 93
    after cesarean birth, 213
    after hydrocephalus surgery, 323-324
    in amniotomy, 177
    in appendicitis, 675-676
    beta-thalassemia minor and, 108
    cesarean birth and, 184
    chain of, 748f
    in diabetic patient, 737
    episiotomy and, 181
    fungal, 676
    in leukemia patient, 644
    nephrotic syndrome and, 692-693
    premature rupture of membranes and, 196
    in preterm newborn, 310
    prevention in newborn, 297-302
    in previa placenta, 92
    prolonged labor and, 195

Infection—cont'd
    puerperal, 244-247, 245t
    transmission of, 748
    worm, 676-677
Infectious diarrhea, 666
Infectious disease, 741-746t, 741-760
    bioterrorism and, 753-754, 754t
    breastfeeding and, 225
    host resistance and, 747-748
    human immunodeficiency virus in, 756-759
    immunization programs for, 750f, 750-753, 752f
    immunotherapy in, 753
    medical asepsis and standard precautions in, 748-749
    rashes in, 749-750
    sexually transmitted disease in, 754-756, 755t
    terminology in, 747
Infectious mononucleosis, 744t
Infertility, 269-274
    evaluation of, 272
    factors influencing fertility and, 271-272
    female factors in, 271
    male factors in, 270-271
    social and psychological implications of, 270
    therapies for, 272-274, 273t
Influenza vaccine, 751, 752f
Informed consent before hospitalization, 494
Infundibulum, fallopian tube, 25f, 26
Infusion port, 518
Infusion pump, 645
Inguinal hernia, 663, 694
Injury prevention
    preschooler and, 432-433, 433f
    toddler and, 416, 417-418t, 419f, 420f
Inner ear, 535f
Innervation of female reproductive system, 26
Insect sting, 679t
Insulin shock, 735-737
Insulin therapy, 102, 733f, 733-737, 734f, 735t, 736f
Insulin, types of
    Iletin 1, 735t
    Lente, 735t
Intake and output
    after cesarean birth, 213
    after hydrocephalus surgery, 324
    in amniotic fluid embolism, 201
    in congestive heart failure, 624
    hyperemesis gravidarum and, 84
    in labor induction, 180
    in maternal monitoring before birth, 142
    in meningitis, 547
    in nephrotic syndrome, 690-691
    preterm labor and, 198
    preterm newborn and, 312
    in respiratory syncytial virus, 597
Intal. See Cromolyn sodium.
Integration of skills, 352
Integrative healing, 775
Integrative therapies, 775
Integumentary system, 700. See also Skin.
    changes in pregnancy, 57-58
    excretory function of, 685f
    neonatal, 292f, 292-295, 294-295t
    postpartum changes in, 210
Intellectual competency of school-age child, 448-450t
Intensity of contraction, 124, 126f
Intercostal muscles, 591
Intermediate-acting insulin, 735t

Intermittent auscultation of fetal heart rate, 136
Internal genitalia
    female, 24f, 24-26, 25f
    male, 22-23
Internal os, 26
Internal rotation, 132f, 133
Internal version, 180
International Dyslexia Association, 774
International Year of Child, 4, 6b
Internet websites, 789
Intertrigo, 704, 704f
Interval of contraction, 125, 126f
Intervention, 762, 769
Intestinal influences on pediatric drug absorption, 508
Intimacy, 455, 462, 462f
Intra-cytoplasmic sperm injection, 273t, 274
Intracranial hemorrhage, 196, 343-344
Intracranial pressure
    after hydrocephalus surgery, 324
    head injury and, 560
    intracranial hemorrhage and, 344
    in Reye's syndrome, 542
Intramuscular injection, pediatric, 514-516, 515f, 516f
Intrapartum analgesics, 165t
Intrathecal narcotics, 167
Intrauterine device, 89, 264
Intrauterine growth restriction, 95
Intravenous immunoglobulin, 598
Intravenous infusion
    as admission procedure, 135
    care during, 518, 520-523t
Intravenous medications, pediatric, 516-518, 517f, 518f
Intuitive thought stage, 423
Intussusception, 662-663, 663f
Inverted nipple, 230
Involution, 204, 247
Iodine
    preset upper limit for daily adult intake of, 64t
    recommended dietary allowances of, 372t
Ipecac syrup, 677
Iris, 539f
Irish-American family, cultural influences on, 361t
Iron
    preset upper limit for daily adult intake of, 64t
    recommended dietary allowances of, 372t
    supplements of
        for anemia after postpartum hemorrhage, 238
        interactions with food, 512t
        for iron-deficiency anemia, 106, 107
        during pregnancy and lactation, 61, 65, 108b
Iron-deficiency anemia, 107, 633-635
Irritable infant, 395
Ischemia
    exercise during pregnancy and, 105
    in neurovascular assessment, 573
Ischial spine, station and, 131
Ischium, 26, 27
Isocarboxazid, 512t
Isograft, 719
Isoimmunization, 99, 338, 338b
Isolation precautions, 787-788
Isoniazid
    drug interactions with, 512t
    for tuberculosis, 111
Isotonic dehydration, 670t, 671
Isotretinoin, 115t, 706
Isthmus of fallopian tube, 26

Italian American family
    cultural influences on, 361-362t
    food patterns of, 368t
Itching, 657
    in atopic dermatitis, 707
    body cast and, 334
    in miliaria, 703
    in pregnancy, 57
ITP. See Immune thrombocytopenic purpura.
IUD. See Intrauterine device.

J

Jacksonian seizure, 550t
Jamaican family, 123t
Japanese American family
    cultural influences on, 360t
    food patterns of, 368t
    labor and delivery for, 122-123t
Jaundice
    in erythroblastosis fetalis, 340
    newborn discharge care and, 234
    in preterm newborn, 312t, 312-313
Jealousy, preschooler and, 430f, 430-431
Jewish American family, 368t
Jimsonweed poisoning, 678t
Jitteriness, epidural block and, 168
Jock itch, 712
Jock strap, 459
Joint instability, 58
Jones criteria, 626, 626b
Juvenile hypothyroidism, 725, 725f
Juvenile rheumatoid arthritis, 382t, 580-581

K

Kanamycin, 114t
Kangaroo care, 314, 316f
Kardex, 485f
Kargasok tea, 783t
Kava kava, 777t, 782t, 783t
Kawasaki disease, 628f, 628-629
Kegel exercises, 211, 279
Kernicterus, 312, 340
Ketoacidosis
    in diabetes mellitus, 101, 102
    in maple syrup urine disease, 335
Ketogenic diet, 553
Ketone, 686t
Ketonemia, 727
Ketonuria, 102
Ketorolac, 479
Kick count, 82t
Kidney, 683
    adult versus child, 351
    neonatal, 291
    postpartum changes in, 210
    postpartum infection of, 210
    of preterm newborn, 312
    urinary tract infection and, 112
    Wilms' tumor and, 694
Kidney, ureter, and bladder x-ray study, 675
Kirschner wire, 571
Knee-chest position, 199, 200f
Knee injury, 584t
Knock-kneed, 568-569
Kohlberg's theory of moral development, 363, 364t
Kombucha, 783t
Korean family, 123t

Kubler-Ross stages of dying, 654
Kwashiorkor, 674-675
Kyphosis, 582*f*

L

Labetalol
    breastfeeding and, 99
    for pregnancy-induced hypertension, 94, 96
Labia majora, 23, 24*f*
Labia minora, 23, 24*f*
Labor and birth, 119-155
    admission to hospital or birth center, 133-136
        assessments in, 134*b*, 134-135
        false labor and, 135-136, 136*t*
        procedures in, 135
    complications following, 237-250
        hemorrhage in, 237-243, 241*t*, 242*f*
        homeless mother and, 249
        mood disorders and, 248-249
        puerperal infection in, 244-247, 245*t*
        shock in, 237
        subinvolution of uterus in, 247-248
        thromboembolic disorders in, 243*t*, 243-244
    components of, 124-130
        passage in, 126-127
        passenger in, 127*f*, 127-129, 128*b*, 128*f*, 129*f*, 130*f*
        powers in, 124-125, 125*f*, 126*f*
        psyche in, 130-131
    cultural influences on, 119-120, 121-123*t*
    diabetes mellitus and, 105
    dysfunctional, 188
    heart disease and, 106
    induction of
        for premature rupture of membranes, 196
        for prolonged pregnancy, 198
    mechanisms of, 131-133, 132-133*f*
    nurse role in, 145-146*t*
    nursing care before birth, 136-143
        coping and, 142-143, 143*f*, 144*f*
        fetal monitoring and, 136-141, 137*b*, 138-140*f*, 140*b*
        maternal monitoring and, 141*f*, 141-142, 142*b*
    nursing care during, 144-148, 147-150*f*
    nursing care immediately after birth, 148-154
        infant and, 151*f*, 151-154, 152*f*, 153*t*, 154*f*
        mother and, 148-151
    pain in, 158-161
    prenatal classes in, 156-158, 157*b*, 158*f*, 159*b*
    settings for, 120, 120*f*
    sickle cell disease and, 108
    signs of, 131
    stages and phases of, 144, 145-146*t*
    vaginal birth after cesarean birth and, 144
Labor-delivery-recovery-postpartum room, 120
Labor-delivery-recovery room, 4-5, 120, 120*f*
Laboratory testing
    as admission procedure, 135
    in musculoskeletal disorders, 569
    for pregnancy-induced hypertension, 95*t*
    prenatal, 49*t*
Laceration in labor and birth, 180-182, 181*f*, 242
Lactated Ringer's solution in amnioinfusion, 176
Lactation, 55
    oral contraceptive-associated decrease in, 262
    physiology of, 225-226, 226*f*
Lactation reflex arc, 226*f*
Lactiferous duct, 29*f*
Lactiferous sinus, 29*f*

Lactose intolerance, 65, 739*t*
Lacuna, 41, 41*f*
Lamaze method of childbirth preparation, 161
Lambdoid suture, 127*f*
Lamictal. *See* Lamotrigine.
Laminaria for cervical ripening, 178
Lamotrigine, 552*t*
Language
    preschooler and, 423*f*, 423-424, 424*t*, 426*t*, 427*t*
    toddler and, 406-407*t*, 409*f*, 409-410, 410*t*, 411*b*
Language disorder, 427*t*
Language loss, 427*t*
Lanoxin. *See* Digoxin.
Lantana poisoning, 678*t*
Lanugo, 292, 306, 701
Laotian American family
    food patterns of, 368*t*
    labor and delivery and, 122*t*
Laparoscopic surgery
    in ectopic pregnancy, 89
    in female sterilization, 269
    in fertility testing, 272
    for uterine fibroids, 280
Large droplet infection precautions, 749
Large-for-gestational-age, 306
Laryngeal spasm, 595
Laryngitis, 594, 595
Laryngomalacia, 595
Laryngotracheobronchitis, 594, 595-596, 596*f*
Larynx, 592*f*
Laser ablation for abnormal uterine bleeding, 254
Lasix. *See* Furosemide.
Lassa fever, 754*t*
Last normal menstrual period, 48
Latch-on, 228
Latchkey children, 443-444, 444*b*
Late deceleration, fetal heart rate pattern and, 140, 140*f*
Late postpartum hemorrhage, 242-243
Latent phase of labor, 145*t*
Lateral canthus, 539*f*
Latex allergy, 327
Laurel poisoning, 678*t*
Laxatives, postpartum use of, 210
Lazy eye, 540
LDR. *See* Labor-delivery-recovery room.
LDRP. *See* Labor-delivery-recovery-postpartum room.
Lead poisoning, 679*t*, 680-681
Learning disability, 770
Lecithin, 591
Lecithin/sphingomyelin ratio, 84*t*, 591
Left-to-right shunt, 617
Leg cramps, 69
Leg exercises after cesarean birth, 213
Leg pain, 192
Legal issues
    in assisted reproduction, 274
    in child hospitalization, 491
Legg-Calvé-Perthes disease, 579
Leiomyoma, 279-280
Lemon balm, 783*t*
Length, 352
    assessment in infant and child, 350*f*
    of newborn, 221, 290, 291*f*
Lens, 539*f*
Lente insulin, 735*t*
Leopold's maneuvers, 50
Lesbian, 467

Letdown reflex, 225, 226f
Lethargic infant, 395-397
Lethargy
　postictal, 549
　in sepsis, 545
Leukemia, 641-645, 642f, 643f, 644b
Leukocyte, 632, 633f, 633t
Leukocytosis, 640
Leukokoria, 542
Level of consciousness, 545b, 554
　altered, 564-565
　head injury and, 562
　neurological assessment and, 560b
Level of maturation, 306
Levonorgestrel, 263, 263f, 269
Levothyroxine, 725
Leydig cell, 23
Libido, menopause and, 276
Lice, 712f, 712-713
Licorice, 783t
Lie, fetal, 127, 128f
Life-support infant-transport incubator, 313
Lightening, 55
Limit setting
　preschooler and, 429-430
　toddler and, 411
Lip, cleft, 327f, 327-328
Lip reading, 538
Lipase, 370
Lipoatrophy, 734
Lipohypertrophy, 734
Lipoid pneumonia, 598
Lithium, 115t
Liver
　preeclampsia and, 95
　Reye's syndrome and, 542
　thalassemia major and, 639
LNMP. See Last normal menstrual period.
Lobule of breast, 28
Local anesthetics
　for child, 480
　for childbirth, 166t, 167
Lochia
　estimating volume of, 206f
　postpartum care and, 205b
　postpartum changes in mother, 205-207, 211
　uterine atony and, 240
Lochia alba, 206
Lochia rubra, 205, 240
Lochia serosa, 206
Long-acting insulin, 735t
Long-term memory, 426t
Longitudinal fracture, 571f
Longitudinal lie, 127, 128f
Lordosis, 582f
Lordotic curve, 58
Lotion, 710t
Low back pain, 93
Low blood sugar, prolonged pregnancy and, 198
Low-flow oxygen, 527, 528f
Low transverse incision in cesarean birth, 184, 185f
Low vertical incision in cesarean birth, 184, 185f
Lumbar lordosis, 408
Lumbar puncture, pediatric, 506-507, 507f
Luminal. See Phenobarbital.
Lung, neonatal, 287-288
Lung sounds after cesarean birth, 213

Lutein cyst, 280
Luteinizing hormone
　in control of testosterone, 458-459
　menstruation and, 28-29
　testosterone production and, 23
Lyme disease, 745t
Lymphadenopathy, 632
Lymphatic system, 631-632
Lymphocyte, 633f, 633t
Lysergic acid diethylamide, 768t

M

Ma huang, 777t, 782t, 783t
Macrosomia, 102f, 192, 344
　gestational diabetes mellitus and, 101
　hypotonic labor dysfunction and, 192
　prolonged pregnancy and, 198
Macula, 539f
Macule, 702b, 749
Mafenide acetate, 720b
Magnesium, 372t
Magnesium sulfate, 116-117
　for pregnancy-induced hypertension, 96
　in tocolytic therapy, 197
Magnetic resonance imaging, 82t
　for congenital heart defects, 618t
　in musculoskeletal disorders, 569
Mainstream, term, 12
Major burn, 717
Major depression, 249
Malabsorption in celiac disease, 662f
Male
　adolescent growth and development, 458-459, 459f, 460b
　newborn genitalia of, 291
　pediatric blood pressure readings, 501t
　physiology of sex act, 29-31
　puberty and, 21-22
　recommended dietary allowances for, 372t
　reproductive system of, 22t, 22-23
　sterilization of, 268f, 268-269
Male condom, 265, 266b
Male factor infertility, 270-271
Mammography, 252
Managed care, 12b
Manganese, 64t
Manipulative therapy, 778
Mantoux skin test, 748
Maple syrup urine disease, 335, 739t
Marasmus, 674f
Marginal abruptio placentae, 92t
Marginal placenta previa, 91, 92t
Marigold poisoning, 678t
Marijuana, 114t, 767, 768t
Maslow's hierarchy of basic needs, 363, 363f
Massage, 159b, 778, 778f
Mastitis, 232, 245t
Masturbation, 426-427
Maternal and Child Health, 377t, 789
Maternal condition
　in admission assessment, 134
　pain modification and, 160
Maternal diabetes mellitus, 344
Maternal-fetal circulation, 41f
Maternal-infant bonding, 153
Maternal monitoring before birth, 141f, 141-142, 142b
Maternal mortality rate, 10b
Maternal nutrition, breastfeeding and, 232

Maternal pushing, 125
    ineffective, 190-192
    patterned paced breathing and, 164
Maternity nursing, 1-19
    abbreviations used in, 799-800
    advanced practice nurses and, 12, 12*b*
    child care and, 7-10, 8*t*, 9*t*, 10*b*, 10*f*, 11*f*
    community-based nursing and, 18
    critical thinking in, 15-16, 16*b*
    documentation and, 17-18
    health care delivery systems and, 10-12, 12*b*
    health care reform and, 16-17
    Healthy People 2010 and, 17, 17*b*
    historical background of, 2-4, 5*b*, 6*b*
    nursing care plans in, 13-15, 15*b*
    nursing process in, 12-13, 13*t*
    present issues in, 4-7
Maturation, 349, 349*b*
Maturity-onset diabetes of youth, 727
McBurney's point, 675
McDonald's sign, 53
MDI. *See* Metered-dose inhaler.
Measles, 743*t*, 747*f*
Measles-mumps-rubella vaccine, 751, 752*f*
Measurement of newborn, 220-221
Mebendazole, 677
Mechanical ventilation, 201
Mechanisms of labor, 132*f*
Meckel's diverticulum, 663
Meconium, 295, 296*f*
    amniotomy and, 177
    newborn passage of, 153, 219
    prolonged pregnancy and, 198
Meconium ileus, 609
Medial canthus, 539*f*
Median episiotomy, 181
Medibottle, 513, 513*f*
Medical asepsis, 748-749
Medical diagnosis, 13*t*
Medications
    for asthma, 603-605, 604*t*
    hospitalized child and, 508-519, 509*b*
        avoiding drug interactions in, 511*t*, 511-513, 512*t*
        calculating pediatric drug doses in, 510, 512*f*
        calculating safe drug dose in, 510-511, 512*b*
        intravenous medications in, 516-518, 517*f*, 518*f*
        nosedrops, eardrops, and eyedrops in, 414*b*, 514
        oral medications in, 513*f*, 513-514
        parenteral fluids and, 518, 520-523*t*
        rectal medications in, 518, 520-523*t*
        subcutaneous and intramuscular injections in, 514-516, 515*f*, 516*f*
        total parenteral nutrition and, 518-519, 524*f*
    for infertility, 272
    during lactation, 65
    for leukemia, 643-644, 644*b*
    newborn and, 153
    overdose of, 677-680, 678*t*, 679*b*
    pediatric physiology and, 479*f*, 479-480, 507-508
    phototoxicity of, 511, 512*t*
    poisoning and, 679*t*
    for pregnancy-induced hypertension, 97
Medicine dropper, 514
Medicine Net, 774
Mediolateral episiotomy, 181, 181*f*
Medroxyprogesterone, 263-264
Megacolon, 661-662, 662*f*

Megaloblastic anemia, 107
Meiosis, 33-34
Melatonin, 783*t*
Membranes rupture, 184
    artificial, 176
    premature, 196
    spontaneous, 177
Memory of toddler, 409
Menarche, 22, 29, 459
Meninges, 167
Meningitis, 546-547, 547*f*
Meningocele, 324
Meningococcal meningitis, 546
Meningomyelocele, 324, 325*f*
Menopause, 26, 29, 275-278
    herbal medicine and, 781-784, 784*t*
Menstrual cycle, 30*f*
Menstrual disorders, 254-255
Menstruation, 28-29, 30*f*, 461*f*
    herbs and, 782*b*
    pain during, 254-255
    postpartum changes in, 208
    puberty and, 459
Mental development of school-age child, 444-446*f*, 444-447, 448-450*t*
Mental disorders, 761-774
    anorexia nervosa in, 771-772, 772*f*
    attention-deficit hyperactivity disorder in, 770-771, 771*b*
    autism in, 763
    bulimia in, 772-773
    depression in, 764, 765-766
    impact on growth and development, 773
    nurse's role in care of, 761-762
    obsessive-compulsive disorder in, 763-764
    origins of, 762-763, 763*b*
    substance abuse and, 767-770, 768*t*, 769*t*
    suicide and, 764
    types and settings of treatment, 762
Mental retardation, 557*b*, 557-559, 558*b*, 559*t*
    play and, 434-435
Meperidine, 165*t*
Mercury toxicity, 751
Meridians, 779, 780*f*
Mescaline, 768*t*
Mesoderm, 36, 37*b*, 683
Metabolic acidosis, 166
Metabolic disorders, 334-336, 723-740
    diabetes insipidus in, 725-727
    diabetes mellitus in, 727-740
        blood glucose self-monitoring in, 730, 732*f*
        diabetic ketoacidosis and, 729, 729*t*
        diagnostic blood tests in, 728-729, 729*f*
        etiology and classification of, 727
        future prospects in, 739-740
        insulin management of, 733*f*, 733-737, 734*f*, 735*t*, 736*f*
        nursing care plan for, 731-732
        nutritional management of, 732-733, 739*t*
        stress and, 737, 738-739*t*
        type I, 727*t*, 728
    hypothyroidism in, 725, 725*f*
    Tay-Sachs disease in, 724-725
Metabolic rate
    adult *versus* child, 350
    fluid and electrolyte imbalance and, 666
Metered-dose inhaler, 604, 606, 606*b*, 607*f*
Methadone, 768*t*
Methergine. *See* Methylergonovine.
Methicillin-resistant *Staphylococcus aureus*, 710

Methotrexate
  for ectopic pregnancy, 89
  during pregnancy, 115*t*
  for pregnancy termination, 87*t*
Methyl salicylate, 678*t*, 679-680
Methyldopa
  breastfeeding and, 99
  for pregnancy-induced hypertension, 94
Methylergonovine
  for subinvolution of uterus, 247
  for uterine atony, 241
  for uterine contraction, 206
Methylphenidate, 771
Mexican American family
  cultural influences on, 357*t*
  food patterns of, 368*t*
  labor and delivery and, 123*t*
Microwave heating of infant formula, 233, 399*b*
Micturition, 686
Middle ear, 535*f*
Midgut, 656
Midline episiotomy, 181, 181*f*
Midwife, 6-7
Mifepristone
  for emergency contraception, 269
  for pregnancy termination, 87*t*
Migratory polyarthritis, 625
Mild contraction, 124
Milestones, 385
Milk. *See* Breast milk, Cow's milk, Formula.
Milia, 292, 295*t*
Miliaria, 703, 704*f*
Milieu therapy, 762
Military presentation of fetus, 128
Milligrams per kilogram, 510-511, 511*b*
Milwaukee brace, 582, 582*t*
Minilaparotomy, 269
Minimal change nephrotic syndrome, 690
Missed abortion, 86*t*
Missing Children's Act, 4
Mist tent, 527
Mitosis, 33
Mitral stenosis, 625
Mittelschmerz, 254
Mixed cerebral palsy, 555*t*
Modeling, 430
Moderate contraction, 124
Modified Jones criteria, 626, 626*b*
Modified paced breathing, 163, 163*f*
Molar, 379*f*
Molar pregnancy, 90
Molding of newborn head, 127, 283-284, 285*f*
Molybdenum, 64*t*
Mongolian spot, 292-295, 295*t*
Monoamine oxidase inhibitors, 512*t*
Monocyte, 633*f*, 633*t*
Monozygotic twins, 44, 45*f*
Mons pubis, 23, 24*f*
Montgomery tubercle, 28
Mood
  postpartum, 214
  in third trimester, 71
Mood disorders, 248-249
MOPP regimen, 645
Morbidity, 282
Morbidity rate, 2
Moro reflex, 283, 284*f*, 284*t*

Morphine abuse, 768*t*
Mortality rate, 2
Morula, 34, 36*f*
Mosaicism, 337
Motherwort, 784*t*
Motility disorders, 664-672
  constipation in, 666
  dehydration in, 670-672, 671*t*, 672*t*
  diarrhea in, 665-668
  fluid and electrolyte imbalance in, 666-670, 669*f*, 670*t*, 671*b*
  gastroenteritis in, 664, 664*b*
  gastroesophageal reflux in, 665, 665*f*
  overhydration in, 672, 673*t*
  vomiting in, 664-665
Motor control, 426*t*
Motor development of infant, 386, 387-388*f*
Motor response
  in head injury, 562-563
  neurological assessment and, 560*b*
Motor speech area of brain, 543*f*
Mouth lesions in leukemia, 642, 642*f*
Movement
  in head injury assessment, 562-563
  neonatal, 290
  in neurovascular assessment, 574
MRI. *See* Magnetic resonance imaging.
MRSA. *See* Methicillin-resistant *Staphylococcus aureus.*
Mucocutaneous lymph node syndrome, 628*f*, 628-629
Mucous membranes, dehydration and, 670*t*, 672*t*
Mucous plug, 55
Mucus suctioning in newborn, 288, 288*f*
Multidisciplinary action plan, 6
Multigravida, 50
Multipara, 50
Multiple birth, 43-45, 45*f*, 193-194
  after birth care in, 203-204
  breastfeeding and, 230-231, 231*f*
  weight gain and, 60
Mummy restraint, 496, 497*b*, 497*f*
Mumps, 743*t*
Murmur
  in newborn, 288
  in patent ductus arteriosus, 620
Muscle cramps, 584*t*
Muscle tone
  in Apgar scoring, 153*t*
  observation of, 569
Musculoskeletal disorders, 567-589
  child abuse and, 585-588, 587*b*, 588*f*
  clubfoot in, 329-330, 330*f*
  Duchenne's muscular dystrophy in, 579
  Ewing's sarcoma in, 580
  family violence and, 584, 584*b*
  fractures in, 570-574, 571-574*f*, 578*f*
  gait observation in, 568-569
  juvenile rheumatoid arthritis in, 580-581
  Legg-Calvé-Perthes disease in, 579
  muscle tone observation in, 569
  osteomyelitis in, 574-579
  osteosarcoma in, 579-580
  scoliosis in, 582*f*, 582-583, 583*f*
  sports injuries in, 583-584, 584*t*, 585*t*
  torticollis in, 581
  trauma in, 569-570
Musculoskeletal system
  assessment of, 567-570, 568*f*
  neonatal, 290
  postpartum changes in, 210-211

Music as nonpharmacological pain relief measure, 159b, 163
Muslim family, 122t
Myelodysplasia, 324-327, 325-327f
Myelogram, 579
Myoclonic spasm, 552
Myofibroma, 279-280
Myolysis, 280
Myoma, 279-280
Myomectomy, 280
Myometrium, 25f, 26
Myringotomy, 536
Mysoline. *See* Primidone.
MZ. *See* Monozygotic.

N

Nagele's rule, 51, 51b
Nalbuphine, 165t
Naloxone
    for child, 480
    intrapartum analgesics and, 165t
    in labor pain management, 167
    for narcotic-induced respiratory depression, 152
    for opioid reversal after cesarean birth, 213
NANDA. *See* North American Nursing Diagnosis Association.
Narcan. *See* Naloxone.
Narcissism, 71
Narcissistic, term, 490
Narcotics, 167
    in cesarean birth recovery, 188
    intrapartum, 165t
Nasal congestion
    in allergic rhinitis, 601
    during pregnancy, 69
Nasal discharge
    in acute bronchiolitis, 597
    in nasopharyngitis, 582
Nasogastric tube, 513
Nasopharyngitis, 591-594
National Association for Retarded Citizens, 558
National Center for Complementary and Alternative Medicine, 777,
    785
National Center for Learning Disabilities, 774
National Cholesterol Evaluation Program, 373b
National Hydrocephalus Foundation, 565
National School Lunch Program, 377t
Nationality, growth and development and, 353-354
Native American family
    cultural influences on, 362t
    food patterns of, 368t
Natural family planning, 267
Natural immunity, 748
Nausea
    in hyperemesis gravidarum, 81
    in pregnancy, 51, 68
Near-drowning, 563
Nebulizer, 606
Necrosis, 721
Necrotizing enterocolitis, 312
Nedocromil, 604
Needle stick, 516, 516f
Negative variance, 6
Negativism, toddler and, 405
Neisseria gonorrhoeae, 259t
    in ophthalmia neonatorum, 153
Neonatal Behavioral Assessment Scale, 287
Neonatal intensive care unit, 305
Neonatal mortality, 10b, 282

Neonate, 282. *See also* Newborn.
Nephron, 683, 693
Nephrostomy, 689t
Nephrotic syndrome, 690-693
Nerve agents, 753
Nerve damage
    in fracture, 578f
    precipitate birth and, 196
Nerve supply to female reproductive system, 26
Nervous system
    adult *versus* child, 351
    congenital malformations of, 321-327
        hydrocephalus in, 321-324, 322f, 323f
        myelodysplasia and spina bifida in, 324-327, 325f, 326f, 327f
    neonatal, 283, 283f, 284f, 284t
Nesting, 314, 316f
Nettle, 782t
Neural tube defect, 61
Neurodevelopmental therapy, 397
Neurologic conditions, 533-566
    brain tumor and, 548f, 548-549
    cerebral palsy and, 554-557, 555b, 555f, 556b, 556f, 557b
    ear and, 533-538, 534f, 535f
        acute otitis media and, 535-537
        barotrauma and, 538
        hearing impairment and, 537-538
        otitis externa and, 535
    encephalitis and, 547-548
    eye and, 538-542, 539f
        amblyopia and, 540
        conjunctivitis and, 541, 541f
        dyslexia and, 540
        hyphema and, 541-542
        retinoblastoma and, 542
        strabismus and, 540-541
        visual acuity tests and, 539, 540f
    head injuries and, 559-563, 560f, 561-562b, 563t
    meningitis and, 546-547, 547f
    mental retardation and, 557b, 557-559, 558b, 559t
    near-drowning and, 563
    Reye's syndrome and, 542-545, 546b
    seizure disorders and, 549b, 549-554
        epilepsy in, 549-554, 550-551t, 552t, 553f
        febrile seizures in, 549
    sepsis and, 545-546, 546b
Neurological check, 542, 561-562b
Neurological examination, 569
Neuromuscular dissociation, 159b
Neuromuscular scoliosis, 582
Neurovascular assessment, 573-574
Neurovascular checks, 573
Neutral thermal environment, 151-152, 313
Neutropenia, 690
Neutrophil, 633f, 633t
Nevus, 295t, 703, 703f
Nevus flammeus, 295t
New Ballard scoring system, 306, 307f
Newborn, 282-304
    adjustment to extrauterine life, 282-283
    discharge planning for, 302
    general anesthesia effects on, 170
    home care of, 302-303, 303f
    homeless, 249
    incontinence in, 327f
    infection prevention and, 297-302
    nursery unit care of
        admission care in, 217-221, 218t, 219f, 221f
        bonding and attachment and, 222-224, 223f

Newborn—cont'd
  nursery unit care of—cont'd
    daily care in, 224
    hypoglycemia and, 221-222
    initial care of skin and, 222
    screening tests in, 222
    security and, 222
  oxygen therapy for, 526b
  physical assessment of, 283-297
    Apgar score in, 288, 288f
    circulatory system in, 288
    conditioned responses and, 287
    gastrointestinal system in, 295-297, 296f
    genitourinary system in, 291-292, 292f
    head in, 283-286, 285f
    hearing in, 286, 286f
    integumentary system in, 292f, 292-293, 294-295t
    length and weight in, 290, 291f
    musculoskeletal system in, 290
    Neonatal Behavioral Assessment Scale in, 287
    nervous system and reflexes in, 283, 283f, 284f, 284t
    pain and, 287, 287f
    providing warmth and, 289, 289f
    respiratory system in, 287-288
    sleep and, 286-287
    temperature, pulse, and respirations in, 289-290, 290f
    visual stimuli and sensory overload in, 286
  postterm, 317-318
  preterm, 305-317
    causes of prematurity, 306
    close observation of, 314, 316t
    family reaction to, 317, 317f
    hypoglycemia and hypocalcemia in, 310-311
    immature kidneys in, 312
    inadequate respiratory function in, 306-310, 309f
    increased tendency to bleed in, 311
    jaundice in, 312t, 312-313
    necrotizing enterocolitis in, 312
    physical characteristics of, 306
    poor control of body temperature in, 310, 313f, 313-314, 316f
    poor nutrition in, 312, 314
    positioning and skin care of, 314, 316f
    prognosis for, 314-317
    retinopathy of prematurity in, 311f, 311-312
    sepsis in, 310
    transporting of, 318
  weight conversions for, 792
Niacin, 372t
NIC. See Nursing Interventions Classification.
Nicaraguan family, 121t
Nickel, 64t
Nifedipine
  for pregnancy-induced hypertension, 94
  in tocolytic therapy, 197
Night terrors, 554
Night wandering, 428
Nightshade poisoning, 678t
Nighttime wetting, 431
Nipple
  flat or inverted, 230
  trauma to, 230
Nipple confusion, 230
Nipple stimulation
  contraction and, 159b
  hypotonic labor and, 190
  of labor, 179
  of nonnursing mother, 209

Nitrazine test, 141, 196
NOC. See Nursing Outcome Criteria.
Nociceptor, 287
Nocturia, 686
Nocturnal emission, 22, 459
Nocturnal enuresis, 431
Nomogram, 510, 510f
Noncommunicating hydrocephalus, 321
Nondisjunction of chromosome, 337
Nonintentional abortion, 86t
Nonnutritive sucking, 378, 378f, 431
Nonorganic failure to thrive, 673
Nonparalytic strabismus, 540
Nonpharmacological pain management, 159b, 161-164
Nonsteroidal antiinflammatory drugs, 479
Nonstress test, 83t, 180
Norms, 385
Norplant contraception system, 263, 263f
North American Nursing Diagnosis Association (NANDA), 15, 790-791
Nosedrops, 514, 514b
Nosocomial infection, 749
Nothing by mouth status, 378
Novolin, 735t
NPH insulin, 735t
NST. See Nonstress test.
Nubain. See Nalbuphine.
Nuchal cord, 140
Nuchal rigidity
  in encephalitis, 548
  in head injury, 563
  in meningitis, 546
Nuclear family, 355t
Nulligravida, 50
Nullipara, 50
Nurse role
  in behavioral conditions, 761-762
  in complementary and alternative therapies, 775-776, 776b, 776f, 777t
  in family coping with dying child, 654b
  in immunizations, 750
  in labor process, 145-146t
  in pain management during labor and birth, 164, 170-174
  in pediatric admission, 483-484
Nursery school, 432
Nursery unit care of newborn, 217-224
  admission care in, 217-221, 218t, 219f, 221f
  bonding and attachment and, 222-224, 223f
  daily care in, 224
  hypoglycemia and, 221-222
  initial care of skin and, 222
  screening tests in, 222
  security and, 222
Nursing activity, 13b
Nursing care plan, 13-15, 15b
  for adolescent depression, 765-766
  for altered level of consciousness, 564-565
  for cancer chemotherapy, 647-649
  for cesarean birth, 212
  for child undergoing renal surgery, 695-697
  for clinical pathway. See Clinical pathway.
  for colic, 396
  for cystic fibrosis, 610-611
  for dying child, 652-653
  for eczema, 708-709
  family care plan, 217
  for gastroenteritis, 667-668

Nursing care plan—cont'd
    for hospitalized child, 481-482, 484, 485f, 486f
    for iron deficiency anemia, 635
    for pediatric diabetes mellitus, 731-732
    for pediatric fever, 504
    for pediatric human immunodeficiency virus, 757-759
    for perimenopausal symptoms, 277-278
    in phototherapy, 341-342
    for pictorial pathway. See Pictorial pathway.
    for postpartum hemorrhage, 239-240
    for postpartum infection, 246
    for preterm newborn, 315
    for spica cast, 333
    for stress caused by cultural diversity, 14-15
    in traction, 575-577
    for urinary tract infection, 691-692
Nursing caries, 380, 381f
Nursing diagnosis, 13b, 13t, 790-791
Nursing intervention, 13b
Nursing Interventions Classification, 15
Nursing Outcome Criteria, 15
Nursing process, 12-13, 13t
    application to growth and development, 348b
    critical thinking and, 16, 16b
    in sex education, 441t, 467t
NutraSweet, 733
Nutrients
    digestion of, 371f
    prolonged pregnancy and, 198
Nutrition, 367-381
    for adolescent, 376, 376t, 468-470
    for burn victim, 720
    cleft palate and, 329
    cultural patterns in, 367, 368t
    in diabetes mellitus, 732-733, 739t
    family and, 367, 369-371f, 372t
    food-drug interactions and, 378
    health and, 370-371
    illness and, 371-374, 373b, 376-378, 378f
    for impending preterm labor, 196-197
    for infant, 374, 374f, 375t, 398-402, 399b, 399t, 400t, 401f, 402b
    nutritional care plan and, 370
    Piaget's theory of development in relation to, 365t
    postpartum infection and, 245
    for pregnancy and lactation, 58f, 58-65, 62t, 63b, 63t
    prenatal visit and, 50
    for preschooler, 375t, 376
    for preterm newborn, 312, 314
    for school-age child, 375t, 376, 448-450t
    teeth and, 378-380, 379f, 380b, 381f, 382t
    for toddler, 374, 375t, 414-415, 415t
Nutritional anemia, 107
Nutritional care plan, 370
Nutritional deficiencies, 672-675
    failure to thrive in, 673-674
    kwashiorkor in, 674f, 674-675
    rickets in, 675
    scurvy in, 675
Nystagmus, 548

O

Object permanence, 403, 409
Oblique diameter, 27, 28f, 28t
Oblique fracture, 571f
Oblique lie, 127
Observation of preterm newborn, 314, 316t
Obsession, 763

Obsessive-compulsive disorder, 763-764
Obstetric conjugate, 27, 28t
Obstetric procedures
    for complications during labor and birth, 176-188
        amnioinfusion in, 176
        amniotomy in, 176-177
        cesarean birth in, 183-188, 185t, 186-187f
        episiotomy and lacerations in, 180-182, 181f
        forceps and vacuum extraction births in, 182f, 182-183
        induction or augmentation of labor in, 177-180, 178t
        version in, 180
    herbal medicine and, 781, 782b, 782t
Obstetrician, 1
Obstetrics, 1
Obstruction, soft tissue, 195
Obstructive emphysema, 609
Obstructive uropathy, 688, 689t
Occipital bone, 127f
Occipito-frontal diameter, 127f
Occiput, 127f
Occiput fetal position, 129
Occiput posterior position, 192
Occult prolapse of cord, 198, 199f
OCD. See Obsessive-compulsive disorder.
Oculomotor nerve, 544f, 545t, 561b
O.D., 514
Odor
    of lochia, 206
    of vomitus, 677t
Oil of wintergreen, 679-680
Ointment, 710t
    pediatric absorption of, 508
Oleander poisoning, 678t
Olfactory nerve, 544f, 545t, 561b
Oligohydramnios
    amnioinfusion for, 176
    amniotic fluid volume and, 82t
    premature rupture of membranes and, 196
Oligomeric proanthocyanidin, 784t
Oliguria, 686
Oncologist, 641
Oocyte, 26
Oogenesis, 33
Open glottis pushing, 164
Ophthalmia neonatorum, 153, 154f, 541
Ophthalmic medications, 514
Opioid analgesics
    abuse of, 767, 768t
    for child, 479-480
    for labor pain management, 167
Opisthotonos position, 546, 547f, 562b
Opportunistic infections, 748
Optic disc, 539f
Optic nerve, 539f, 544f, 545t
Oral candidiasis, 676
Oral care, 380b, 380-381, 381f, 382t
    cleft palate and, 329
Oral contraceptives, 262f, 262-263
Oral hydration solutions
    for dehydration, 669-670
    for gastroenteritis, 664, 664b
Oral lesions in leukemia, 642, 642f
Oral medications, 513f, 513-514
Oral rehydration solution, 374, 666
Oral stage of infancy, 386f, 396
Oral temperature, 502
Orchiopexy, 697

Ordinal position in family, 354-355
Organic behavior disorders, 763-764
Organic failure to thrive, 673
Organic murmur, 288
Orgasm, 31
Orthodontic appliance, 381, 470
Orthodox Jewish family, 122*t*
Orthopedic surgery in cerebral palsy, 555-556
Orthopnea, 595
Orthostatic hypotension
    postpartum, 209
    in pregnancy, 55
Ortolani's sign, 331
O.S., 514
Ossification, 352
Osteochondrosis, 579
Osteomyelitis, 574-579
Osteopathy, 778
Osteoporosis
    menopause and, 276
    therapy for, 275
Osteosarcoma, 579-580
Otitis externa, 535
Otitis media, 535-537
Otoscope, 534-535
O.U., 514
Outpatient clinic, 475-476
Ovarian cycle, 30*f*
Ovarian cyst, 280
Ovary, 24*f*, 25*f*, 26
    changes in pregnancy, 55
    infertility and, 271
    menstruation and, 461*f*
Over-the-counter drugs poisonous to toddler, 678*t*
Over-the-counter skin products, 710
Overfeeding, 374
Overhydration, 672, 673*t*
Overnutrition, 371
Oviduct, 26
Ovulation, 26, 29, 30*f*, 36*f*
    infertility and, 271
    postpartum changes in, 208
Ovum, 26
Oxygen
    prolonged pregnancy and, 198
    respiratory changes in pregnancy and, 55
    saturation, 527
Oxygen therapy
    in acute croup, 595-596
    for late deceleration, 140
    pediatric, 525-527, 526*b*, 527*f*, 528*f*
    in pneumonia, 599
    in pregnancy-induced hypertension seizure, 97
    for placenta previa, 93
    for prolapsed umbilical cord, 199
    for respiratory distress syndrome, 309
Oxytocin, 225
    abortion and, 85
    for labor induction, 178, 179
    late deceleration and, 141
    for pregnancy-induced hypertension, 96
    for prolonged pregnancy, 198
    for uterine atony, 241
    for uterine contraction, 206
    for uterine inversion, 201
    uterine rupture and, 200

P

PACE interview, 471-472
Pacifier, 230, 386, 386*f*
Packed red blood cells, 201
Pain
    in abnormal labor, 195
    in abruptio placentae, 92*t*, 93
    in acute otitis media, 536
    in appendicitis, 675
    in ectopic pregnancy, 89
    in encephalitis, 548
    in hospitalized child, 478*f*, 478-479
    during injection, 515-516
    in intussusception, 662
    during labor and birth, 160
    during menstrual cycle, 254-255
    neurological assessment and, 560*b*, 573
    in newborn, 287, 287*f*
    physical factors in, 160
    in placenta previa, 92*t*
    in pneumonia, 598
    postpartum care and, 205*b*
    in postpartum hematoma, 242
    in sickle cell disease, 637
    at vaccination site, 751
Pain assessment tool, 478*f*
Pain management
    in acute otitis media, 536
    after cesarean birth, 213-214
    cultural aspects of, 280
    during labor and birth, 156-175
        childbirth pain *versus* other pain, 158
        education for childbearing and, 156-158, 157*b*, 157*f*, 158*f*, 159*b*
        factors in, 158-161
        nonpharmacological, 161-164, 162*f*, 163*f*, 164*b*
        pharmacological, 164-174, 165-166*t*, 168-170*f*
    pediatric, 479*f*, 479-480
Pain Resource Center, 492
Pain threshold, 158
Pain tolerance, 158-160
Pakistani family, 122*t*
Palate, cleft, 328-329
Pallor, 574
Palm, 58
Palmar grasp reflex, 283, 283*f*, 284*t*
Palpated prolapsed umbilical cord, 198
Palpation for pediatric blood pressure, 500
Palpebral fissure, 539*f*
Palpitations, 55
PALS. *See* Pediatric Advanced Life Support.
Pancreas, cystic fibrosis and, 609
Pancrease, 614
Pancrelipase, 614
Pandemic, 747
Panic, precipitate birth and, 196
Pantothenic acid, 372*t*
Papanicolaou test, 49*t*, 252-253, 684
Papilledema, 548
Papule, 702*b*, 750
Para, 50
Parachute reflex, 386
Paradione. *See* Paramethadione.
ParaGard, 264
Parallel play, 382*t*, 415, 416*f*, 420, 427
Paralytic ileus, 717
Paralytic strabismus, 540-541

Paramethadione, 115*t*
Paraphimosis, 686-687, 687*f*
Parathyroid disorders, 726*t*
Paraurethral duct, 24
Parent
    of adolescent, 467-468, 468*f*, 469*t*
    consistency and, 430
    growth and development of, 363-365, 365-366*t*
    reaction to child hospitalization, 482
Parenteral fluids
    for fluid and electrolyte imbalance, 670
    for hospitalized child, 518, 520-523*t*
Parenteral medications, pediatric, 514-519
    absorption of, 508
    nosedrops, eardrops, and eyedrops, 514, 514*b*
    rectal, 514
    subcutaneous and intramuscular injections, 514-516, 515*f*, 516*f*
Parenthood, 216
Parents Without Partners, 453, 473
Parietal bone, 127*f*
Parotitis, 743*t*
Paroxysmal epilepsy, 549
Paroxysmal hypercyanotic episode, 621, 621*f*
Partial abruptio placentae, 92*t*
Partial placenta previa, 91, 92*t*
Partial pressure of carbon dioxide, 673*t*
Partial seizure, 550*t*, 552
Partial-thickness burn, 715*t*
Partial thromboplastin time
    in heart disease, 107
    in hemophilia, 640
Passage of labor, 126-127
Passenger of labor, 127-129, 127-130*f*, 128*b*
Passive immunity, 748
Patent ductus arteriosus, 619*f*, 620
Pathogen, 747
Pathognomonic, term, 750
Pathologic fraction, 571*f*
Pathological jaundice, 312, 312*f*, 340
Patient, 13*b*
Patient-controlled analgesia, 188, 213
Patterned paced breathing, 163*f*, 164
Pavlik harness, 331, 331*f*
PCA. *See* Patient-controlled analgesia.
Peach pit poisoning, 678*t*
Peak flowmeter, 605, 605*f*
Peak of contraction, 124, 126*f*
Pearson attachments, 571
Pediatric Advanced Life Support, 624
Pediatric nurse, 7
Pediatric nurse practitioner, 12
Pediatric nursing, 7-10, 8*t*, 9*t*, 10*b*, 10-11*f*
    abbreviations used in, 799-800
    herbal medicine and, 781, 783-784*t*
    impact of growth and development on, 346-348, 348*b*
Pediatric research center, 475
Pediatric unit, 476
Pediatrics, 2
Pediculosis, 712*f*, 712-713
Peer relationships, 458*t*, 463-464, 464*f*
Pelvic examination, 48, 252-254
Pelvic floor dysfunction, 278-279
Pelvic inflammatory disease, 261
Pelvic inlet, 27, 28*f*
Pelvic outlet, 27-28
Pelvic tilt exercise, 211

Pelvis
    abnormal labor and, 194-195
    female, 26-28, 27*f*, 28*f*, 28*t*
    menstruation and, 461*f*
    pain modification and, 160
Penetrating trauma during pregnancy, 115
Penicillin
    for acute pharyngitis, 594
    for group B streptococcus infection, 111
    interactions with food, 512*t*
    for rheumatic fever, 626
Penis, 22, 22*f*
    hypospadias and epispadias, 687*f*, 687-688
    neonatal, 291
    phimosis and, 686-687, 687*f*
Perception, infant and, 387-388*f*
Percutaneous umbilical blood sampling, 83*t*, 100
Perimenopausal symptoms, 275-278
Perimetrium, 25*f*, 26
Perinatal damage, 320, 321*b*
Perinatal mortality, 10*b*, 282
Perinatology, 282
Perineal care, 207*b*, 208, 234
Perineal massage, 181
Perineal scrub preparation, 147*f*
Perineum, 24, 24*f*
    laceration during labor and birth, 242
    postpartum care of, 205*b*, 208
    postpartum changes in, 207-208
Periodic changes in fetal heart rate pattern, 139
Peripheral venous device, 517
Peripherally inserted central venous catheter, 517
Peritoneal dialysis, 680
Periurethral laceration, 242
Permanent contraception, 268*f*, 268-269
Permanent teeth, 379
Personal space, 482
Personality development, 356
Pertussis, 744*t*
Pessary, 279
Pet ownership, 451-452, 452*b*, 452*t*
Petechiae, 632
    in immune thrombocytopenic purpura, 641
    in leukemia, 642
Petit mal seizure, 549-552, 550-551*t*
Petroleum distillates, 679*t*
Pfannenstiel skin incision in cesarean birth, 184
PG. *See* Phosphatidylglycerol.
pH, 673*t*
    urine, 686*t*
    vaginal, 25, 256
Phantom limb pain, 580
Pharyngitis, 594
Pharynx, 592*f*
Phencyclidine hydrochloride, 768*t*
Phenelzine, 512*t*
Phenergan. *See* Promethazine.
Phenobarbital, 552*t*
Phenylketonuria, 222, 334-335, 739*t*
Phenylpropanolamine, 678*t*
Phenytoin, 552*t*
    drug interactions with, 512*t*
    effects on gums, 553*f*
    during pregnancy, 115*t*
Phimosis, 686-687, 687*f*
Phlebitis, intravenous medications and, 516

Phonological processing, 426*t*

Phosphatidylglycerol, 84*t*

Phosphatidylinositol, 84*t*

Phosphorus, 372*t*

Photograph, infant identification and, 152-153

Phototherapy in erythroblastosis fetalis, 340*f*, 340-343, 343*f*, 344*f*

Phototoxicity of drugs, 511, 512*t*

Physical abuse, 585

Physical activity, heart disease and, 106

Physical dependence, 767

Physical development
    of adolescent, 456-460, 458*t*, 459*f*, 460*b*, 461*f*, 467*f*
    of infant, 389-394*t*
    of preschooler, 422-423
    of school-age child, 439-440, 444-446*f*, 444-447, 448-450*t*
    of toddler, 405-408, 408*f*

Physical examination
    in admission assessment, 135
    of infant, 398
    neonatal, 283-297
        Apgar score in, 288, 288*f*
        circulatory system in, 288
        conditioned responses and, 287
        gastrointestinal system in, 295-297, 296*f*
        genitourinary system in, 291-292, 292*f*
        head in, 283-286, 285*f*
        hearing in, 286, 286*f*
        integumentary system in, 292*f*, 292-293, 294-295*t*
        length and weight in, 290, 291*f*
        musculoskeletal system in, 290
        Neonatal Behavioral Assessment Scale in, 287
        nervous system and reflexes in, 283, 283*f*, 284*f*, 284*t*
        pain and, 287, 287*f*
        providing warmth and, 289, 289*f*
        respiratory system in, 287-288
        sleep and, 286-287
        temperature, pulse, and respirations in, 289-290, 290*f*
        visual stimuli and sensory overload in, 286
    prenatal, 48

Physical neglect, 585

Physical survey of hospitalized child, 497-505, 506*f*
    blood pressure in, 499-500, 500*f*, 501*t*, 502*t*
    body temperature in, 501-503, 503*f*, 503*t*
    head circumference in, 505
    height in, 505
    pulse and respirations in, 499, 499*t*
    weight in, 503-505

Physician's Desk Reference, 509

Physiologic jaundice, 285

Physiological and psychological changes in pregnancy, 74-78*t*

Physiological anemia, 351

Physiological jaundice, 312, 312*f*, 340

Physiology of lactation, 225-226, 226*f*

PI. *See* Phosphatidylinositol.

Piaget's theory of development
    adolescent and, 456*b*
    school-age child and, 439*b*

Pica, 65, 680, 681

Pictorial pathway, 486, 486*f*

PID. *See* Pelvic inflammatory disease.

Pigmentation changes, 52

Pincer grasp, 386

Pinkeye, 541, 541*f*

Pinworms, 676-677

Pitocin
    abortion and, 85
    for labor induction, 178, 179

Pitocin—cont'd
    late deceleration and, 141
    for uterine contraction, 206

Pituitary gland
    disorders of, 726*t*
    menstruation and, 461*f*

PKU. *See* Phenylketonuria.

Placenta, 34, 40-42, 42*f*
    cesarean birth and, 184, 187*f*
    expulsion in labor, 146*t*
    retained fragments of, 242-243

Placenta previa, 91*f*, 91-93, 92*t*

Placental hormones, 41-42

Placental transfer, 41

Plague, 754*t*

Plants, poisonous, 677, 678*t*

Plasma cholesterol, 627*t*

Plastibell clamp, 291

Plastic strip thermometer, 502

Platelet, 632, 633*f*
    disorders of, 641
    transfusion in amniotic fluid embolism, 201

Platelet count
    in heart disease, 107
    in immune thrombocytopenic purpura, 641

Platypelloid pelvis, 27, 27*f*

Play, 382*t*, 382-383
    preschooler and, 425, 433*f*, 433-435
    school-age child and, 443, 443*f*, 448-450*t*
    toddler and, 419-420, 420*f*

Play therapy, 433, 435, 762

Plumbism, 680-681

PMDD. *See* Premenstrual dysphoric disorder.

PMS. *See* Premenstrual syndrome.

Pneumococcal vaccine, 751, 752*f*

Pneumocystis carinii pneumonia, 598, 756, 759

Pneumonia, 598-599
    following hydrocephalus surgery, 322-323
    Pneumocystis carinii, 598, 756, 759

Pneumonitis, aspiration, 170

PNP. *See* Pediatric nurse practitioner.

POC. *See* Products of conception.

Poinsettia poisoning, 678*t*

Poison control center, 677

Poisoning, 677-681
    drugs in, 677-680, 678*t*, 679*b*
    general concepts in, 677, 677*t*
    lead, 680-681
    poisonous plants in, 677, 678*t*
    preschooler and, 433
    toddler and, 418*t*

Poisonous plants, 677, 678*t*

Poker chip pain assessment tool, 478*f*

Polio, 744*t*

Polio vaccine, 752*f*

Poliomyelitis, 744*t*

Polyarthritis, 625

Polycystic kidney, 688

Polycythemia, 621

Polydipsia
    in diabetes insipidus, 726
    in diabetes mellitus, 101, 728

Polygamous family, 355*t*

Polyhydramnios
    amniotic fluid volume and, 82*t*
    tracheoesophageal fistula and, 658

Polyphagia, 101, 728

Polyuria, 686
    in diabetes insipidus, 726
    in diabetes mellitus, 101, 728
Popliteal artery, pediatric blood pressure and, 500f
Porcine xenograft, 719
Port-wine stain, 295t, 703, 703f
Portal of entry, 747
Portal of exit, 747
Position
    fetal, 128-130
    for variable deceleration, 140
Positioning
    for breastfeeding, 227-228, 228f
    of child
        after hydrocephalus surgery, 324
        for blood specimen, 506, 507f
        for ear examination, 498f
        for lumbar puncture, 507f
        in mist tent, 527f
        in nephrotic syndrome, 690
        preterm newborn, 314, 316f
        in spina bifida, 326
    for fetal presentation and position, 192
    for hypotonic labor, 188-190
    for ineffective maternal pushing, 192
    as nonpharmacological pain relief measure, 159b, 162, 173
    for preterm labor, 198
    for prolapsed umbilical cord, 199, 200f
    Fowler's sling, 665f
Positive signs of pregnancy, 54, 54f
Postage stamp graft, 719
Postcentral gyrus, 543f
Posterior fontanel, 127, 127f, 285
Posterior pituitary disorders, 726t
Posterior tibial artery, pediatric blood pressure and, 500f
Posthealing care of burn, 719-720, 720b
Postictal lethargy, 549
Postmaturity, 317-318
Postoperative nursing care
    in cheiloplasty, 328
    in cleft palate repair, 329
    in hydrocephalus, 323-324
    pediatric, 528-531, 529f, 530t, 531t
    in spina bifida, 326-327
Postpartum blues, 214, 214b
Postpartum depression, 214, 248
Postpartum hemorrhage, 237-243
    anemia in, 238
    early, 238-242, 241t, 242f
    hypovolemic shock in, 238
    late, 242-243
Postpartum period
    care during
        cultural influences on, 204, 204f
        in pregnancy-induced hypertension, 97-99
        changes in mother, 204-214, 205b
        complications during, 237-250
            abruptio placentae and, 92t
            hemorrhage in, 237-243, 241t, 242f
            homeless mother and, 249
            mood disorders in, 248-249
            placenta previa and, 92t
            puerperal infection in, 244-247, 245t
            shock in, 237
            subinvolution of uterus in, 247-248
            thromboembolic disorders in, 243t, 243-244

Postpartum period—cont'd
    heart disease and, 106
    self-care in, 234-235
Postpartum psychosis, 248-249
Postterm newborn, 306, 317-318
Postural drainage, 609, 612-613f, 614
Posture
    pregnancy and, 58
    of toddler, 412-413
Posturing, 560, 560f, 560-561b
Potty-chair, 413-414, 414f
Powdered infant formula, 233
Powers of labor, 124-125, 125-126f, 188-192, 190b
PPO. See Preferred provider organization.
PPROM. See Preterm premature rupture of membranes.
Pramoxine, 208
Preadolescence, 446f, 446-447
Precentral gyrus, 543f
Precipitate birth, 195-196
Preconception care, 48
Preconceptual stage, 423
Preeclampsia, 93-94, 94t, 95
Preferred provider organization, 11, 12b
Prefrontal area of brain, 543f
Pregnancy
    adolescent, 64
    diagnosis of, 51-54, 52b
    high-risk, 80
    multifetal, 43-45, 45f
    prolonged, 198
    termination of, 87t
Pregnancy-induced hypertension, 94t
    laboratory tests for, 95t
    risk factors for, 94b
Pregnancy loss, 87t
Pregnancy-related complications, 80-118, 81b
    anemia and, 107-108, 108b
    assessment of fetal health and, 80-81, 81f, 82-84t
    bleeding disorder of early pregnancy and, 84-91
        abortion as, 84-86, 85f, 86t, 87t
        ectopic pregnancy as, 86-90, 89f, 90b
        hydatidiform mole as, 90f, 90-91
    bleeding disorders of late pregnancy and, 91-93, 92t
    blood incompatibility between pregnant woman and fetus and, 99-100, 100f
    diabetes mellitus and, 100-106, 101b, 102f, 105t
    environmental hazards and, 112-117
        bioterrorism and, 112-114, 113b
        substance abuse and, 113f, 113-115, 114-115t
        trauma and, 115-117
    family and, 117
    heart disease and, 106b, 106-107
    hyperemesis gravidarum and, 81-84
    hypertension and, 93-99, 94b, 94t, 95t, 96b
    infections and, 108-112, 110b
Pregnancy test, 54
    in ectopic pregnancy, 89
Prehension, 386, 387-388f
Premature newborn. See Preterm newborn.
Premature rupture of membranes, 196
Premenstrual dysphoric disorder, 255
Premenstrual syndrome, 255
Premolar, 379f
Premotor area of brain, 543f
Prenatal care, 47-79
    cardiovascular system and, 55-56, 56f, 56t
    common discomforts in pregnancy and, 68-70

Prenatal care—cont'd
  definition of terms in, 50-51, 51*b*
  determining estimated date of delivery, 51, 51*b*
  diagnosis of pregnancy and, 51-54, 52*b*
    positive signs for, 54, 54*f*
    presumptive signs for, 51-53, 52*f*
    probable signs for, 53*f*, 53-54
  exercise during pregnancy and, 65-68, 66-67*f*
  gastrointestinal system and, 56-57, 57*f*
  integumentary and skeletal systems and, 57-58
  nursing interventions in, 74-78*t*
  nutrition during lactation and, 65
  nutritional requirements and, 60-63, 62*t*, 63*b*, 63*t*
  physiological changes in pregnancy and, 74-78*t*
  pregnancy-induced hypertension and, 97
  prenatal education and, 74, 157*b*
  prenatal visits and, 48-50, 49*t*
  psychological adaptations to pregnancy and, 70-74, 71*f*, 72*b*, 72*f*
  recommended dietary allowances and intakes and, 63-64, 64*t*
  reproductive system and, 54-55
  respiratory system and, 55
  special nutritional considerations and, 64-65
  urinary system and, 57
  weight gain and, 60, 61*t*
Prenatal development, 33-46
  cell differentiation in, 34-36, 37*b*
  cell division and gametogenesis in, 33-34, 35*f*
  fetal circulation and, 42-43, 44*f*
  Healthy People 2010 and, 43
  implantation of zygote and, 34
  milestones in, 37-40, 38-40*f*
  multifetal pregnancy and, 43-45, 45*f*
  placenta and, 40-42, 42*f*
  sex determination and, 34, 37*f*
  tubal transport of zygote and, 34, 41*f*
  umbilical cord and, 42
Preoperational period, 365*t*
Preoperational phase, 423
Preoperative nursing care, 528-531, 529*f*, 530*t*, 531*t*
  in hydrocephalus, 322-323
Preschool program, 432
Preschooler, 422-437
  accident prevention for, 432-433, 433*f*
  administration of medications, 509*b*
  bedtime habits of, 427
  behavior patterns of, 347*b*
  chronic illness in, 646*t*
  clothing for, 432
  cognitive development of, 423, 424-425*t*
  dental hygiene for, 380*b*
  developmental theories and, 364*t*
  diabetes mellitus in, 738*t*
  discipline and limit setting for, 429-430
  effects of cultural practices on, 423, 423*f*
  enuresis and, 431-432
  five-year-old, 428-429
  four-year-old, 428
  heart-healthy guidelines for, 628*b*
  hospitalization of, 435-436, 489
  intravenous therapy for, 520-521*t*
  jealousy and, 430*f*, 430-431
  language development of, 423*f*, 423-424, 426*t*, 427*t*
  nursery school and, 432
  nutrition for, 375*t*, 376
  oxygen therapy for, 526*b*
  physical development of, 422-423

Preschooler—cont'd
  play and, 425, 433*f*, 433-435
  response to death, 651*t*
  sexual curiosity and, 425-427
  spiritual development of, 425
  three-year-old, 427-428
  thumb sucking and, 431
Presentation, fetal, 128
Pressure point therapy, 778
Presumptive signs of pregnancy, 51-53, 52*f*
Preterm labor, 196-198, 197*b*
  abortion and, 84
  exercise during pregnancy and, 67
Preterm newborn, 305-317
  breastfeeding of, 231
  causes of prematurity, 306
  close observation of, 314, 316*t*
  family reaction to, 317, 317*f*
  hypoglycemia and hypocalcemia in, 310-311
  immature kidneys in, 312
  inadequate respiratory function in, 306-310, 309*f*
  increased tendency to bleed in, 311
  jaundice in, 312*t*, 312-313
  necrotizing enterocolitis in, 312
  nursing care plan for, 315
  physical characteristics of, 306
  poor control of body temperature in, 310, 313*f*, 313-314, 316*f*
  poor nutrition in, 312, 314
  positioning and skin care of, 314, 316*f*
  prognosis for, 314-317
  retinopathy of prematurity in, 311*f*, 311-312
  sepsis in, 310
  transporting of, 318
Preterm premature rupture of membranes, 196
Prevention of substance abuse, 767-769
Preventive health care, 251-254, 253*b*
  for infant, 300*b*, 397-402, 399*t*, 400*t*, 401*f*, 402*b*
  in pediatric trauma, 570
Previability, term, 306
Prickly heat, 703, 704*f*
Primary hypertension, 627
Primidone, 552*t*
Primigravida, 50
Primipara, 50
Probable signs of pregnancy, 53*f*, 53-54
Procardia. *See* Nifedipine.
Processus vaginalis, 694
Prodromal labor, 135
Prodromal period, 747
Products of conception, 87*t*
Progesterone, 42
Progesterone-releasing intrauterine device, 264
Progestin, 275
Program for Children with Special Health Needs, 377*t*
Progress of labor, 141
Progressive relaxation, 159*b*
Projectile vomiting, 658-659, 659*f*, 660
Prolactin, 225
Prolapse
  umbilical cord, 177, 198-199, 199*f*, 200*f*
  uterine, 279
  vaginal wall, 278-279
Prolonged labor, 195
Prolonged pregnancy, 198
Prolonged QT syndrome, 554
Promethazine, 165*t*

Propranolol, 197
Proprioception, 426t
Prostaglandin synthesis inhibitors, 197
Prostaglandins
    amniotomy and, 177
    for cervical ripening, 178
    for pregnancy termination, 87t
    for prolonged pregnancy, 198
    role in dysmenorrhea, 254-255
Prostate gland, 22f, 23
Prosthesis, eye, 542
Protective isolation, 749
Protein
    kwashiorkor and, 674-675
    during lactation, 61, 65
    during pregnancy, 61
    recommended dietary allowances of, 372t
    urinary, 686t
Protein hydrolysate, 233
Proteinuria, 690
    in preeclampsia, 94t
    in pregnancy, 57
    in pregnancy-induced hypertension, 95, 96
Proximodistal development, 349, 349f
Pruritus, 657
    in atopic dermatitis, 707
    body cast and, 334
    in miliaria, 703
    in pregnancy, 57
Pseudoanemia, 56
Pseudohypertrophic muscular dystrophy, 579
Pseudomenstruation, 292
Psyche of labor, 130-131
    abnormal labor and, 195
Psychiatrist, 762
Psychoanalyst, 762
Psychologic considerations
    in adaptation to pregnancy, 70-74, 71f, 72b, 72f
    in bioterrorism, 753
    in cleft lip and palate, 329
    in infertility, 270
    in menopause, 276
Psychological dependence, 767
Psychomotor seizure, 551t
Psychoprophylactic method of childbirth preparation, 161
Psychosis, postpartum, 248-249
Psychosocial development of adolescent, 460-463, 462f
Psychosomatic, term, 762
PTT. *See* Partial thromboplastin time.
Ptyalism, 56
Puberty, 21-22, 456
    diabetes mellitus and, 738-739t
    female and, 459f, 459-460, 460b
Pubic hair, 459f, 460b
Pubic lice, 712
Pubis, 26
Public Health Department, 4
Pudendal block, 166t, 167-168, 168f
Pudendal nerve, 168, 168f
Puerperal infection, 244-247, 245t
Puerperium, 1, 203
Puerto Rican American family
    cultural influences on, 357t
    food patterns of, 368t
    labor and delivery for, 123t
Pulmonary edema, 198

Pulmonary embolism, 243, 243t, 244
Pulse
    in admission assessment, 134
    after birth, 150
    in congestive heart failure, 623, 624
    dehydration and, 670t
    of hospitalized child, 499, 499t
    of infant, 386f
    in neurovascular assessment, 573
    of newborn, 289-290, 290f
    postpartum, 209
Pulse oximetry
    in amniotic fluid embolism, 201
    pharmacological labor pain management and, 174
    in retinopathy of prematurity, 311, 311f
Pulse pressure, 500, 620
Pupil, 539f
    head injury and, 560f
Pure Food and Drug Act, 4
Purified protein derivative skin test, 748
Purpura, 632, 642
Pursed-lip breathing
    in asthma, 606
    in cystic fibrosis, 614
Pustule, 702b, 750
Pycnogenol, 784t
Pyelonephritis, 112, 688
Pyloric stenosis, 658-659, 659f, 660
Pyloromyotomy, 659
Pyridoxine, 111
Pyrosis, 56

Q

Quality of life, 12
Quickening, 52-53

R

Race, growth and development and, 353-354
Radial artery, pediatric blood pressure and, 500f
Radial fracture, 578f
Radiant heat crib, 314
Radiation burn, 713
Radiation exposure during pregnancy, 115t
Radiation heat loss, 218, 218t
Radiation treatment in brain tumor, 548
Radiography in musculoskeletal disorders, 569
Radioimmunoassay, 54
Radionuclide angiocardiography, 618t
Rage attack, 554
Range of motion exercise during pregnancy, 67
Rapid-acting insulin, 735t
Rapid antigen detection, 113
Rapid eye movement sleep, 287
Rapid plasma reagin, 49t
Rash, 702-703, 749-750
    chickenpox, 742t, 747f
    diaper, 303
    in Kawasaki disease, 628, 628f
    measles, 743t, 747f
    rubella, 742t, 747f
RDS. *See* Respiratory distress syndrome.
Reactive airway disease, 598
Ready-to-feed formula, 233
Real-time ultrasonography, 49t
Rebound hyperglycemia, 736-737
Rebound tenderness, 675

Receptive language, 409*t*, 426*t*

Recommended dietary allowances, 62*t*, 372*t*
  for pregnancy and lactation, 63-64, 64*t*

Recovery from labor, 146*t*

Recovery room assessments, 185

Recreation therapy, 762

Rectal medication, 514

Rectal sphincter, episiotomy and, 181

Rectal temperature, neonatal, 220

Rectocele, 279

Rectum, female, 24*f*

Recurrent abortion, 86*t*

Recurrent pregnancy loss, 84

Red blood cell, 631, 633*f*
  in nonpregnant and pregnant women, 56*t*
  normal values of, 633*t*
  yolk sac and, 36

Reed-Sternberg cell, 645

REEDA, 208

Reflective listening, 469*t*

Reflex irritability, 153*t*

Reflexes of newborn, 283, 283*f*, 284*f*, 284*t*

Reflexology, 778, 780*f*

Reflexology lines, 780*f*

Reflux, gastroesophageal, 665, 665*f*

Refresher class in childbirth preparation, 156

Regional analgesics and anesthetics, 164, 167-170, 168-170*f*

Regression, pediatric hospitalization and, 480

Regular insulin, 735*t*

Regurgitation, general anesthesia and, 170

Relaxation, 780-781
  for ineffective maternal pushing, 192
  in nonpharmacological labor pain management, 159*b*, 161-162

Relief Band, 779*f*

Renal biopsy, 686

Renal function
  adult *versus* child, 351
  neonatal, 218-219

Renal surgery, 695-697, 698

Reporting of child abuse, 586

Reproduction, 21-32
  cystic fibrosis and, 609
  female reproductive system and, 23-28
    breasts and, 28, 29*f*
    changes during pregnancy, 54-55
    cystic fibrosis and, 609
    development of, 684, 686*f*
    external genitalia and, 23*f*, 23-24
    internal genitalia and, 24*f*, 24-26, 25*f*
    menstruation and, 28-29, 30*f*
    pelvis and, 26-28, 27*f*, 28*f*, 28*t*
    postpartum changes in, 204-209, 205*f*, 206*f*, 207*b*, 207*f*
  female sex act and, 31
  male reproductive system and, 22*t*, 22-23
  male sex act and, 29-31
  puberty and, 21-22

Reservoir for infection, 747

Respiration, 591, 592*f*
  in admission assessment, 134
  adult *versus* child, 350
  after birth, 150
  Apgar scoring and, 153*t*
  in congestive heart failure, 623
  dehydration and, 670*t*
  of hospitalized child, 499, 499*t*
  of infant, 386*f*
  of newborn, 289-290, 290*f*

Respiration—cont'd
  of preschooler, 422
  in respiratory distress syndrome, 309
  of toddler, 408

Respiratory care
  after cesarean birth, 213
  pediatric tracheostomy and, 519-525, 525*f*

Respiratory depression, general anesthesia and, 170

Respiratory disorders, 591-616
  acute pharyngitis in, 594
  allergic rhinitis in, 600-602, 602*f*
  asthma in, 602-606
    medications for, 603-605, 604*t*
    metered-dose inhaler for, 604, 606, 606*b*, 607*f*
    pathophysiology of, 602, 602*f*, 603*f*
  bronchopulmonary dysplasia in, 615
  croup syndromes in, 594-597, 595*f*, 596*f*
  cystic fibrosis in, 608*f*, 608-615
    lung involvement in, 608-609, 609*f*
    nursing care plan for, 610-611
    pancreatic involvement in, 609
    postural drainage in, 609, 612-613*f*, 614
  nasopharyngitis in, 591-594
  pneumonia in, 598-599
  respiratory syncytial virus in, 597-598
  sudden infant death syndrome and, 615-616
  tonsillitis and adenoiditis in, 599-600

Respiratory distress
  in acute bronchiolitis, 597
  in amniotic fluid embolism, 201
  in asthma, 605
  in bronchopulmonary dysplasia, 615
  in croup, 595, 595*f*
  neonatal hypothermia and, 218
  in newborn, 152
  in respiratory syncytial virus, 597

Respiratory distress syndrome, 308-309, 309*f*

Respiratory rate
  neonatal, 220
  in pneumonia, 598
  of toddler, 408

Respiratory syncytial virus, 597-598

Respiratory system
  adult *versus* child, 593*b*
  changes in pregnancy, 55
  development of, 591
  excretory function of, 685*f*
  neonatal, 287-288
  preeclampsia and, 95
  of preterm infant, 306-310, 309*f*

Respiratory tract infection
  acute otitis media and, 536
  congestive heart failure and, 623

Respite care, 492, 650

Responsibility, adolescent and, 465

Rest
  in nasopharyngitis, 582
  in rheumatic fever, 626

Restraints, pediatric, 498*b*

Resuscitation of newborn, 152

Retina, 539*f*

Retinoblastoma, 542

Retinopathy of prematurity, 311*f*, 311-312

Retrograde ejaculation, 271

Retrolental fibroplasia, 311

Reverse isolation, 749

Reward, preschooler and, 429-430

Reye's syndrome, 542-545, 546b
Rh and ABO incompatibility, 99-100, 100f
Rh factor, 49t
Rheumatic carditis, 625
Rheumatic fever, 624-627, 625f, 626b
Rhinitis
    in acute pharyngitis, 594
    allergic, 600-602, 602f
Rhinovirus, 591
Rho immune globulin, 338, 338b, 339
    abortion and, 85
    postpartum dose of, 211
    for Rh and ABO incompatibility, 100
Rhythm method of contraception, 268
Rib, 591, 592f
Ribavirin, 597-598
Riboflavin, 372t
RICE therapy, 570
Rickets, 675
Rifampin, 111
Rights of child, 6
Ringworm, 711
Ritalin. See Methylphenidate.
Rite of passage, 21
Ritodrine, 197
Ritualism, 405
Rivotril. See Clonazepam.
Role disruption, high-risk pregnancy and, 117
ROM. See Range of motion.
Rooming-in, 483, 487-488
Roommate selection in adolescent hospitalization, 491
Rooting reflex, 283, 284t
Roseola, 743t
Round ligament, 25
Roundworms, 677
RPR. See Rapid plasma reagin.
RU486, 269
Rubella, 742t, 747f
    postpartum immunization for, 211
    in pregnancy, 109
    titer in prenatal laboratory test, 49t
Rubeola, 743t, 747f
Rubin's psychological changes of puerperium, 214b
Rugae, 25, 25f, 207
Running, injury risks in, 585t
Rupture
    of membranes, 133
        artificial, 176
        in cesarean birth, 184
        false labor and, 136
        before labor, 131
        premature, 196
        spontaneous, 177
    uterine
        during labor and birth, 199-200
        oxytocin labor induction and, 179
Russell traction, 569, 570-571, 572f

S

Sacral pressure as pain relief measure, 159b, 162
Sacrum, 27
    fetal position and, 129
Safety
    adolescent and, 470-471, 471f
    hospitalized child and, 495f, 495-496, 496f
    of infant, 389-394t
    in pediatric oxygen therapy, 525-527

Safety—cont'd
    in pharmacological labor pain management, 173
    preschooler and, 435
    school-age child and, 442, 444b, 448-450t
    toddler and, 418t
    toys and, 403, 403t, 434
Safety Syringe Products, 492
Sage, 784t
Sagittal diameter, 28, 28t
Sagittal suture, 127f
St. John's wort, 777t, 782t, 784t
Salicylate poisoning, 679-680
Saline lock, 517
Salivation
    dehydration and, 670t
    neonatal, 297
Sarcoptes scabiei, 713
Sarin, 753
Satellite clinic, 475
Satiety, infant and, 399
Sauna, 784
Scab, 750
Scabies, 713
Scald burn, 721
Scalded skin syndrome, 710
Scalp vein distention, 562b
Scar tissue, abnormal labor and, 195
Scarf sign, 290, 308f
Scarlet fever, 746t
Schick test, 748
School-age child, 438-454
    administration of medications, 509b
    cholesterol and, 373b
    chronic illness in, 646t
    dental hygiene for, 380b
    developmental theories and, 364t
    diabetes mellitus in, 738t
    gender identity and, 440
    general characteristic of, 438-439, 439b, 439f
    growth and development of, 444f, 444-447, 445f, 446f
    health examination for, 447-451, 448-450t
    heart-healthy guidelines for, 628b
    hospitalization of, 489-490
    intravenous therapy for, 522-523t
    latchkey, 443-444, 444b
    nutrition for, 375t, 376
    oxygen therapy for, 526b
    pet ownership and, 451-452, 452b, 452t
    physical growth of, 439-440
    play and, 443, 443f
    response to death, 651t
    school-related tasks of, 441-442, 442t, 443b
    sex education for, 440-441, 441t
School Breakfast Program, 377t
School-related tasks, 441-442, 442t, 443b
Schultze delivery of placenta, 147, 148t
Sclera, 539f
Scoliosis, 582f, 582-583, 583f
Scope of practice, 13b, 16
Screening
    developmental, 352
    for Down syndrome, 337
    for hepatitis B, 109
    of newborn, 222
Scrotum, 22, 22f, 459
    hydrocele and, 694, 697f
Scurvy, 675

Seborrheic dermatitis, 704, 704f
Sebum, 705
Second-degree burn, 715t
Second-stage breathing, 164
Security in newborn care, 222
Sedatives
    abuse of, 768t
    for encephalitis, 548
    for hypertonic labor, 188
Seizure
    in acute otitis media, 536
    in eclampsia, 94t
    in epilepsy, 549-554, 550-551t, 552t, 553f
    febrile, 549
    pregnancy-induced hypertension and, 97
Selective attention, 426t
Selenium
    preset upper limit for daily adult intake of, 64t
    recommended dietary allowances of, 372t
Self-concept of adolescent, 458t, 462
Self-consoling behaviors, 411
Self-examination
    of breast, 252, 253b
    vulvar, 252
Self-help skills, Down syndrome and, 337t
Semen, 23, 272
Semilente insulin, 735t
Seminal fluid, 271
Seminal vesicle, 22f, 23
Sensation in neurovascular assessment, 573
Sense of identity, 460-462
Sense of intimacy, 462, 462f
Sensitization to Rh antibody, 338, 338b
Sensorimotor development of toddler, 408-409
Sensorimotor period, 365t
Sensorimotor stimulation, toys and, 403t
Sensory conditions
    ear and, 533-538, 534f, 535f
        acute otitis media and, 535-537
        barotrauma and, 538
        hearing impairment and, 537-538
        otitis externa and, 535
    eye and, 538-542, 539f
        amblyopia and, 540
        conjunctivitis and, 541, 541f
        dyslexia and, 540
        hyphema and, 541-542
        retinoblastoma and, 542
        strabismus and, 540-541
        visual acuity tests and, 539, 540f
Sensory overload, newborn and, 286
Separation anxiety, 385
    hospitalization and, 477-478
    preschooler and, 435-436
    toddler and, 409, 413t
Sepsis, 545-546, 546b
    premature rupture of membranes and, 196
    in preterm newborn, 310
Septic abortion, 86t
Septic shock, 237
Septicemia, 710
Sequencing, 426t
Serum alpha-fetoprotein, 49t
Setting sun sign, 321, 323f
Sex determination, 34, 37f
Sex education
    for adolescent, 466
    for school-age child, 440-441, 441t

Sex hormones, 30f, 458
Sex Information and Education Council of United States, 440
Sexual abuse, 585
Sexual behavior of adolescent, 460, 463f, 465-467, 467t
Sexual curiosity, preschooler and, 425-427
Sexual development of adolescent, 458t, 460f, 461b
Sexual intercourse
    after birth, 207
    postpartum self-care teaching and, 234
    in second trimester, 71
    urinary tract infection and, 112
Sexual latency, 438
Sexual maturity ratings, 459f, 468
Sexuality Information and Education Council of U.S., 436
Sexually transmitted disease, 257-261, 258-260t, 754-756, 755t
    adolescent and, 466
    during pregnancy, 111
Shaken baby syndrome, 560
Shave prep, 135
Sheppard-Towner Act of 1921, 3
Shiatsu, 779
Shin splints, 584t
Shock
    in abruptio placentae, 93
    in dehydration, 671-672
    in hemophilia, 640
    in hospitalized child, 497
    postpartum, 237
    pregnancy and, 165
    in trauma during pregnancy, 116
    uterine inversion and, 201
Shoes for toddler, 412
Shoulder dystocia, 192
Shoulder pain in ectopic pregnancy, 89
Shoulder presentation, 127, 129f
Shunt, 617
    fetal circulatory, 43
    ventriculoperitoneal, 322, 323f
Shyness, toddler and, 413t
SIADH, 726t
Sibling
    child hospitalization and, 483
    death of, 651t
    emotional care of, 214-215
    prenatal class for, 157b
Sibling rivalry, 413t, 773
Sickle cell disease, 108, 634-638, 636f, 637f, 638t
Sickle cell trait, 634, 636
Sickledex, 636
Side-lying position
    for breastfeeding, 227
    for prolapsed umbilical cord, 199
SIDS. See Sudden infant death syndrome.
SIECUS. See Sex Information and Education Council of United States.
Siete Jarabes, 784t
Sight and Hearing Association, 565
Sigmoidoscopy, 657
Sign language, 538
Significant hypertension, 627
Signs of impending preterm labor, 196-197
Silver nitrate, 720b
Silver sulfadiazine cream, 720b
Simian crease, 336f, 337
Simple fracture, 570, 571f
Simple partial seizure, 550t
Single father, 73
Single mother, 73, 203

Single parent family, 355*t*
Sinusitis, 594
Sitting, perineal pain and, 208
Sitz bath
    in episiotomy care, 182
    for perineal pain, 208
Sixth disease, 743*t*
Skeletal system changes in pregnancy, 57-58
Skeletal traction, 571, 573*f*
Skene's duct, 24
Skiing, injury risks in, 585*t*
Skin, 700-722
    assessment in newborn, 219
    burns and, 713-720
        classification of, 713-715, 714*f*
        electrical, 715, 716*f*
        emergency care in, 716-717
        nursing care in, 719-720, 720*b*
        pathophysiology of, 713
        wound care in, 717-719, 718*f*
    cystic fibrosis and, 609
    dehydration and, 670*t*, 672*t*
    development and function of, 700-701, 701*f*
    disorders of, 701-713
        acne vulgaris in, 705*f*, 705-706
        diaper dermatitis in, 704-705, 705*f*
        fungal infections in, 711-712, 712*f*
        herpes simplex virus in, 706, 706*f*
        impetigo in, 710-711, 711*f*
        infantile eczema in, 706-710, 707*f*, 710*t*
        intertrigo in, 704, 704*f*
        miliaria in, 703, 704*f*
        pediculosis in, 712*f*, 712-713
        port-wine nevus in, 703, 703*f*
        scabies in, 713
        seborrheic dermatitis in, 704, 704*f*
        staphylococcal infection in, 710
        strawberry nevus in, 703, 703*f*
        terms in, 702*b*
    excretory function of, 685*f*
    frostbite and, 720-721
    of newborn, 292*f*, 292-293, 294-295*t*
    of postterm newborn, 318
    of preterm newborn, 306, 308*f*, 314, 316*f*
    prolonged pregnancy and, 198
    rheumatic fever and, 625
    stimulation in nonpharmacological labor pain management, 162
    of toddler, 408
Skin care
    in cerebral palsy, 555
    in diabetes mellitus, 737
    in nasopharyngitis, 594
    in newborn, 222
    in spina bifida, 326-327
Skin graft, 718-719
Skin rash, 702-703
    diaper, 303
    in Kawasaki disease, 628, 628*f*
Skin sensor thermometer, 503*f*
Skin turgor. *See* Turgor.
Skull fracture, 560
Sleep
    adult *versus* child patterns of, 351-352
    infant and, 389-394*t*, 397
    newborn and, 286-287
    toddler and, 412*t*
Slow-paced breathing, 163, 163*f*
Smallpox, 742*t*, 754*t*

Smegma, 24, 291
Smiling, 482
Smoke detector, 416
Smoking
    fertility and, 271
    during pregnancy, 114*t*
Snake bite, 679*t*
Snellen chart, 539, 540*f*
Social behavior
    of infant, 389-394*t*
    of toddler, 406-407*t*
Social considerations
    in infertility, 270
    in parenthood, 216
Social development of school-age child, 444-446*f*, 444-447, 448-450*t*
Social norms, 464
Sodium intake during pregnancy, 64
Sodium nitroprusside, 97
Soft tissue
    abnormal labor and, 194-195
    injuries of, 570
    in passage of labor, 127
Sole crease, 220
Solid foods for infant, 399-400, 401*f*
Somatic sensory association area of brain, 543*f*
Somogyi phenomenon, 736-737
Sore throat, 594
Sound, newborn responses to, 284*t*
Soy formula, 233
Soy products, 275
Spanish phrases, 794-798
Spasm
    infantile, 552
    laryngeal, 595
Spasmodic croup, 595
Spasmodic laryngitis, 594, 595
Spastic cerebral palsy, 555*t*
Spasticity
    in cerebral palsy, 554
    neurological assessment and, 562*b*
Special Milk Program, 377*t*
Special Olympics, 558
Specific gravity, 686*t*
Speech
    cleft palate and, 329
    development in toddler, 409*t*, 409-410, 410*t*, 411*b*
Sperm, 31, 270-271
Spermatogenesis, 22, 33
Spermicide, 266-267
SPF. *See* Sun protective factor.
Sphingomyelin, 591
Spica cast for developmental dysplasia of hip, 331-334, 332*f*
Spider bite, 679*t*
Spider nevus, 57
Spina bifida, 82*t*, 324-327, 325-327*f*
Spinal accessory nerve, 544*f*, 545*t*, 561*b*
Spinal anesthesia
    in cesarean birth, 184, 186*f*
    for childbirth, 166*t*, 169*f*, 169-170
Spinal tap, 506-507, 507*f*
Spine, scoliosis and, 582*f*, 582-583, 583*f*
Spinnbarkeit, 256, 268, 268*f*
Spiral fracture, 570, 571*f*
Spirituality
    adolescent and, 462, 463*f*
    preschooler and, 425
Spleen, 632

Splenectomy
  in Hodgkin's disease, 645-646
  in sickle cell disease, 638
Splenic sequestration, 638*t*
Split Russell traction, 571
Spongiosis, 707
Spontaneous abortion, 86*t*
Spontaneous rupture of membranes, 177
Sports
  injuries in, 471, 583-584, 584*t*, 585*t*
  nutrition and, 469-470
Sports bra, 460
Sprain, 569, 584*t*
Sprue, 659
Squint, 540-541
SROM. *See* Spontaneous rupture of membranes.
Stadol. *See* Butorphanol.
Stage of industry, 438
Standard precautions, 748-749, 787-788
Standards of care, 13*b*
Staphylococcal infection
  cutaneous, 710
  in osteomyelitis, 577
  in toxic shock syndrome, 256
Startle reflex, 537
Station, 131, 133*f*
Statistics, 7, 8*t*, 9*t*, 10*b*
Status asthmaticus, 606
Status epilepticus, 553-554
STD. *See* Sexually transmitted disease.
Steinmann pin, 571
Stenosis, pyloric, 658-659, 659*f*, 660
Sterilization, 268*f*, 268-269
Sternal retractions in pneumonia, 598
Steroids
  for asthma, 604-605
  for premature rupture of membranes, 196
  for speeding fetal lung maturation, 197
Stillborn infant, 215-216
Stimulants abuse, 768*t*
Stinger, 584*t*
Stomach
  influences on pediatric drug absorption, 508
  of preterm newborn, 312
Stool, neonatal, 295-297, 296*f*
Stool softener, 210
Stool specimen, 505-506
Stork bite, 292, 295*t*
Strabismus, 540-541
Strain, 570, 584*t*
Strangulated hernia, 663-664
Strawberry nevus, 703, 703*f*
Strawberry tongue, 628
Street names for abused drugs, 769*t*
Strep throat, 594
Streptococcal infection
  in acute otitis media, 535
  in acute pharyngitis, 594
  during pregnancy, 111
  in rheumatic fever, 625
Streptomycin, 114*t*
Stress
  in abnormal labor, 195
  heart disease and, 107
  hyperemesis gravidarum and, 84
  infertility and, 270
  labor and, 166

Stress—cont'd
  in pediatric diabetes mellitus, 737, 738*t*
  pediatric hospitalization and, 477
  reduction for impending preterm labor, 196-197
Stress incontinence, 279
Stress ulcer, 717
Stretch marks, 210
Stretching, episiotomy and, 181
Striae
  abdominal, 52*f*, 53-54
  postpartum fading of, 210
Stridor
  in croup, 594
  in laryngomalacia, 595
Stroke volume in congestive heart failure, 623
Structural scoliosis, 582
Student athlete, 471
Stye, 702*b*, 703*f*
Subacute bacterial endocarditis, 626
Subarachnoid block, 166*t*, 167, 168, 169-170
Subarachnoid space, 167
Subcutaneous gland, 701
Subcutaneous injection
  of insulin, 734*f*
  pediatric, 514-516, 515*f*, 516*f*
Subdural space, 167
Subinvolution of uterus, 247-248
Sublimaze. *See* Fentanyl.
Submentobregmatic diameter of fetal skull, 127*f*
Suboccipitobregmatic diameter of fetal skull, 127*f*
Substance abuse, 767-770, 768*t*, 769*t*
  adolescent and, 471-472
  during pregnancy, 113*f*, 113-115, 114-115*t*
Sucking
  nonnutritive, 378, 378*f*
  oral stage of infancy and, 386, 386*f*
Suckling, 225, 228
Suctioning
  of mucus, 288, 288*f*
  of tracheostomy tube, 523-524
Sudden infant death syndrome, 615-616
Suffocation, toddler and, 417-418*t*
Suicidal attempt, 764
Suicidal gestures, 764
Suicidal ideation, 764
Suicide, 764
Sulfasalazine, 581
Sulfur mustard, 753
Sullivan's theory of development, 364*t*
Summer Food Service Programs, 377*t*
Sun protective factor, 470
Sunbathing, 470
Sunken fontanel, 497
Superficial burn, 715*t*
Superficial vein thrombosis, 243, 243*t*
Supine hypotension syndrome, 55, 56*f*, 93
Supine vena caval syndrome, 67
Supplemental feeding of newborn, 230
Supplements for anemia during pregnancy, 108
Support
  in abnormal labor, 195
  of partner in labor, 143
  single mother pregnancy and, 73
Suppository, pediatric, 514
Supraoccipital diameter of fetal skull, 127*f*
Suprapubic tube placement, 689*t*
Surfactant, 39, 308, 591, 592*f*

Surfak. *See* Docusate calcium.
Surgery
    for cleft lip, 327
    for cleft palate, 328
    for clubfoot, 330
    in diabetic child, 737-739
    discontinuation of herbal remedies before, 777*t*
    for ectopic pregnancy, 90
    genitourinary, 698
    for hydrocephalus, 322
    for infertility, 272
    for otitis media, 536
    preparation of child for, 529*f*, 530*t*
    in sickle cell disease, 638
    for spina bifida, 324-325
    in tetralogy of Fallot, 621
Surrogate parenting, 273, 273*t*
Suspensory ligaments of Cooper, 29*f*
Suture of fetal head, 127
Swaddling, 497*f*
Sweat gland, cystic fibrosis and, 609
Sweat test, 609
Sweet pea poisoning, 678*t*
Sweets, 380
Swimmer's ear, 535
Swimming safety, 470-471
Sydenham's chorea, 625
Symbolic functioning, 423
Symbolic group play, 382*t*
Symphysis pubis, 27
    fetal size and, 192
Syndrome of inappropriate antidiuretic hormone (SIADH), 726*t*
Syphilis, 257, 259*t*
Systematic inflammatory response syndrome, 545
Systems theorist, 363

T

Tachycardia
    in congestive heart failure, 623, 624
    in postpartum hemorrhage, 238
    preterm labor and, 198
    in respiratory syncytial virus, 597
    in sepsis, 545
Tachypnea
    in congestive heart failure, 623
    in respiratory distress syndrome, 309
    in respiratory syncytial virus, 597
    in sepsis, 545
Talipes equinovarus, 329
Tampon, toxic shock syndrome and, 256
Tanner mesh graft, 719
Tanner's stages of sexual maturity, 460*b*
Target organ, 723
Tay-Sachs disease, 724-725
Tearing, dehydration and, 670*t*, 672*t*
Technology advances, 10, 10*f*, 11*f*
Teeth, 378-380, 379*f*, 380*b*, 381*f*, 382*t*
Tegretol. *See* Carbamazepine.
Telangiectatic nevus, 292
Telecommunication devices for deaf, 538
Temper tantrum, 411, 412*t*
Temperature
    in admission assessment, 134
    after birth, 150
    amniotomy and, 177
    dehydration and, 670*t*
    exercise during pregnancy and, 65-67

Temperature—cont'd
    fever and
        in acute otitis media, 536
        in acute pharyngitis, 594
        chills and, 209
        in hospitalized child, 501-503, 503*f*, 503*t*
        in Kawasaki disease, 628
        in meningitis, 546
        in nasopharyngitis, 594
        nursing care plan for, 504
        in pneumonia, 598
        postpartum, 244
        in rheumatic fever, 625
        in sepsis, 545
    hypothermia and, 151, 218, 617
    of infant, 386*f*
    of mother before birth, 141
    neonatal, 220, 289-290, 290*f*
    premature rupture of membranes and, 196
    of preterm newborn, 310, 313*f*, 313-314, 316*f*
Temperature cycle, 30*f*
Temperature equivalents, 793
Temporal lobe seizure, 551*t*
Temporary contraception, 261-268
    barrier methods of, 264-265, 266*b*, 267*f*
    basal body temperature method of, 267*f*, 267-268
    calendar method of, 268
    cervical mucous method of, 268, 268*f*
    hormonal contraceptives in, 261-264, 262*f*, 263*f*
    intrauterine device in, 264
    natural methods of, 267
    spermicides for, 266-267
TENS. *See* Transcutaneous electrical nerve stimulation.
Teratogen, 33, 112
Terbutaline
    for hypertonic labor, 188
    in tocolytic therapy, 197
Testicular torsion, 697
Testis, 22*f*, 23, 459
    cryptorchidism and, 694-697
Testosterone, 458
    male puberty and, 21-22
    testicular production of, 23
Tet spell, 621, 621*f*
Tetracycline
    interactions with food, 512*t*
    during pregnancy, 114*t*
Tetrahydrozoline hydrochloride, 678*t*
Tetralogy of Fallot, 619*f*, 620-621, 621*f*
Thalassemia, 108, 638-639, 639*f*
Theophylline
    drug interactions with, 604*t*
    interactions with food, 512*t*
Therapeutic abortion, 86*t*
Therapeutic insemination, 273, 273*t*
Therapeutic play, 435
Thermal burn, 713, 717
Thermal stimulation for pain management, 159*b*, 162
Thermometer, 502
Thermoregulation
    in newborn, 151-152, 218, 218*t*, 289-290, 290*f*
    in preterm newborn, 310, 313*f*, 313-314, 316*f*
Thiamine, 372*t*
Third-degree burn, 715*t*
Thirst, dehydration and, 670*t*, 672*t*
Thomas splint, 571
Thoracotomy, 616-617

Threatened abortion, 85f, 86t
Three-dimensional imaging, 82t
Three-year-old preschooler, 427-428
Thrombocyte, 632, 633f
Thrombocytopenia, 644
Thrombophlebitis
   after cesarean birth, 213
   in pregnancy, 56
   trauma-related, 116
Thrombosis, 634
   deep vein, 243t, 243-244
   postpartum, 209
   in pregnancy, 106
Thrush, 676
Thumb sucking, 431
Thyroid hormones
   hypothyroidism and, 725, 725f
   for speeding fetal lung maturation, 198
Thyroid-releasing hormone, 198
Tibial fracture, 578f
Tilade. See Nedocromil.
Time-out period, 411, 429
Tinea capitis, 711
Tinea corporis, 711, 712f
Tinea cruris, 712
Tinea pedis, 711-712
Tinnitus, 168
Tissue turgor in newborn, 292f, 292
Title V of Social Security Act, 3
Title XIX of Medicaid, 3
Titmus machine, 539
Tobacco use
   fertility and, 271
   during pregnancy, 114t
Tocolytic therapy, 197
   for hypertonic labor, 188
   labor induction and, 178
   during pregnancy, 116
   for prolapsed umbilical cord, 199
   for version, 180
Toddler, 405-421
   administration of medications, 509b
   behavior patterns of, 347b
   chronic illness in, 646t
   daily care of, 411-413
   day care for, 415-416, 416f
   dental hygiene for, 380b
   developmental theories and, 364t
   diabetes mellitus in, 738t
   general characteristics of, 405-410, 406-407t
     physical development and, 405-408, 408f
     sensorimotor and cognitive development and, 408-409
     speech development and, 409t, 409-410, 410t, 411b
   guidance and discipline for, 410-411, 412t
   heart-healthy guidelines for, 628b
   hospitalization of, 487-489, 488b
   injury prevention and, 416, 417-418t, 419f, 420f
   intravenous therapy for, 520-521t
   nutrition for, 374, 375t, 414-415, 415t
   over-the-counter drugs poisonous to, 678t
   oxygen therapy for, 526b
   toys and play and, 419-420, 420f
Toilet independence, 412t, 413-414, 414f
Toluene, 768t
Tonic-clonic seizure, 95, 550t
Tonic movement, 549
Tonic neck reflex, 283, 284f, 284t

Tonsillectomy, 599
Tonsillitis, 599-600
Tooth, avulsed, 440
Toothbrushing, 381
Topamax. See Topiramate.
Topical anesthetics, 480
Topical medications, 508, 710t
Topiramate, 552t
TORCH infection, 108
Torsion, testicular, 697
Torticollis, 581
Total abruptio placentae, 92t
Total body surface area, 713, 714f
Total parenteral nutrition
   for hyperemesis gravidarum, 84
   pediatric, 518-519, 524f
   for preterm newborn, 314
Total placenta previa, 91, 92t
Touch
   in bonding and attachment, 223
   cultural considerations in, 482
   as pain relief measure, 159b
Toxemia, 94
Toxic shock syndrome, 256
Toxicity of supplements and food fortification, 63
Toxoplasmosis, 110-111
Toys, 419-420, 420f
TPALM system, 51b
TPN. See Total parenteral nutrition.
Trachea, 592f
Tracheal stoma, 525
Tracheoesophageal fistula, 657-658
Tracheostomy care, 519-525, 525f
Tracheotomy, 596
Traction, 570-574, 571-574f, 578f
   Buck extension, 569, 570
   halo, 582, 583f
   Russell, 569, 570-571, 572f
Transcutaneous electrical nerve stimulation, 778
TransCyte, 719
Transfusion
   for ectopic pregnancy, 89
   in leukemia, 644-645
   in thalassemia, 639
Transfusion reaction, 644
Transient gestational hypertension, 94t
Transillumination, 321
Transition phase of labor, 145t
Transitional object, 487
Transitional stools, 295, 296f
Translator, 204
Translocation of chromosome, 337
Transmission-based precautions, 749
Transmission of infection, 748
Transplantation, bone marrow, 644
Transport
   of high-risk newborn, 318
   of hospitalized child, 496, 497f, 498b
Transvaginal ultrasound
   in ectopic pregnancy, 89
   impending labor and, 196
Transverse diameter, 27-28, 28f, 28t
Transverse fracture, 571f
Transverse gyrus, 543f
Transverse lie, 127, 128f
Transverse skin incision in cesarean birth, 184
Tranylcypromine, 512t

Trauma
  head, 559-563, 560f, 561-562b, 563t
  musculoskeletal, 569-570
  nipple, 230
  during pregnancy, 115-117
  to teeth, 381
Tremor, neonatal, 290
Trendelenburg position, 199, 200f
Treponema pallidum, 259t
tRH. See Thyroid-releasing hormone.
Trichloroethylene, 768t
Trichomoniasis, 258t
Tridione. See Trimethadione.
Trigeminal nerve, 544f, 545t, 561b
Triglyceride levels, 627t
Trimester, 51
Trimethadione, 115t
Trisomy 21, 337
Trochlear nerve, 544f, 545t, 561b
Trophoblast, 34
True labor, 136t
True pelvis, 27, 126-127
TSS. See Toxic shock syndrome.
Tubal embryo transfer, 273, 273t
Tubal ligation, 268f, 269
Tubal pregnancy, 86, 89f
Tubal transport of zygote, 34, 41f
Tuberculin skin test, 49t
Tuberculosis, 745t
  breastfeeding and, 225
  in pregnancy, 111
Tularemia, 754t
Tulip poisoning, 678t
Tumor
  brain, 548f, 548-549
  Ewing's sarcoma, 580
  osteosarcoma, 579-580
  retinoblastoma, 542
Turgor
  dehydration and, 670t, 672t
  in newborn, 292f, 292
Turning child in body cast, 334b
24-hour urine specimen, 505, 506t
Twins
  after birth care of, 203-204
  breastfeeding and, 230-231, 231f
Tympanic membrane, 533-534, 535f
Tympanic thermometer, 502, 503f
Tympanometry, 537
Type I diabetes mellitus, 100, 727t, 728
Type II diabetes mellitus, 100, 727t

U

Ulcer
  Curling's, 717
  in leukemia, 642, 642f
Ulnar fracture, 578f
Ultralente insulin, 735t
Ultrasound, 82t
  in fertility testing, 272
  for fetal maturity, 177
  in impending preterm labor, 197
  in measurement of pediatric blood pressure, 500
  in musculoskeletal disorders, 569
  in pregnancy diagnosis, 54
  prenatal, 49t
  during version, 180

Umbilical clamp, 219, 219f
Umbilical cord, 42
  care of, 221, 221f
  cutting of, 152f
  prolapse of, 198-199, 199f, 200f
Umbilical hernia, 663
Underfeeding, 374
Undernutrition, prenatal development and, 43
Undescended testes, 291, 694-697
Unilateral Moro reflex, 192
United Nations Declaration of Rights of Child, 6
United States Consumer Product Safety Commission, 419
Upper respiratory tract infection, 535
Upright position in transporting hospitalized child, 497f
Urea cycle defect, 739t
Ureter, 683
Ureteritis, 688
Ureterostomy, 689t
Urethra
  female, 683
  male, 22, 22f
Urethral meatus
  female, 24, 24f
  male, 22, 22f
Urethritis, 688
Urge incontinence, 279
Urgency, 686
Uric acid, 686t
Urinalysis, 686
  in impending preterm labor, 197
  prenatal, 49t, 50
Urinary bladder, 683
  after birth, 150
  descent of fundus and, 205
  distended, 688
  distention in uterine atony, 241, 242f
  exstrophy of, 688
  female, 24f
  male, 22, 22f
  postpartum care and, 205b
  postpartum changes in, 210
  postpartum infection of, 210
  soft tissue obstruction during labor and, 195
  urinary tract infection and, 112
Urinary catheter after cesarean birth, 213
Urinary diversion, 688, 689t
Urinary frequency, 52, 57
Urinary incontinence, 279
Urinary retention, 169, 170
Urinary system, 683-699
  acute glomerulonephritis and, 693t, 693-694
  assessment of, 686, 686t
  changes in pregnancy, 57
  cryptorchidism and, 694-697
  development of, 683-684, 684f
  excretory function of, 685f
  exstrophy of bladder and, 688
  hydrocele and, 694, 697f
  hypospadias and epispadias and, 687f, 687-688
  impact of surgery on, 698
  neonatal, 153, 218-219, 291
  nephrotic syndrome and, 690-693
  obstructive uropathy and, 688, 689t
  phimosis and, 686-687, 687f
  postpartum changes in, 210
  preeclampsia and, 95

Urinary system—cont'd
  urinary tract infection and, 688-690, 689f
  Wilms' tumor and, 694
Urinary tract infection
  after cesarean birth, 213
  nursing care plan for, 691-692
  pediatric, 688-690, 689f
  postpartum, 210, 245t
  in pregnancy, 57, 111-112
Urine
  average daily excretion of, 671t
  dehydration and, 670t
  pediatric volumes of, 506t
Urine casts, 686t
Urine checks, 737
Urine glucose, 686t
Urine ketones, 102
Urine output
  in burn victim, 717
  edema and, 95
  postpartum, 210
  in respiratory syncytial virus, 597
  in trauma during pregnancy, 116
Urine pH, 686t
Urine protein, 686t
Urine red blood cells, 686t
Urine specific gravity, 686t
Urine specimen, 505, 506f, 506t
Urine stasis in pregnancy, 57
Urine white blood cells, 686t
Uroflow, 686
Urologic monitoring in spina bifida, 326
Uterine atony, 192, 240-241, 241t, 242f
Uterine contraction, 124-125, 126f, 133
  amniotomy and, 177
  assessment by palpation, 142b
  Braxton Hicks, 131
  fetal heart rate pattern and, 137
  labor induction and, 180
  in maternal monitoring before birth, 141
  in precipitate birth, 195
  in trauma during pregnancy, 116
  version and, 180
Uterine fibroid, 279-280
Uterine hyperstimulation, cervical ripening and, 178
Uterine incision in cesarean birth, 184
Uterine souffle, 54
Uterine tube, 26, 271
Uteroplacental insufficiency, 140
Uterosacral ligaments, 25
Uterus, 25f, 25-26
  abnormal uterine bleeding and, 254
  abruptio placentae and, 92t, 93
  after birth, 149
  infertility and, 271
  inversion during labor and birth, 200-201
  menstruation and, 461f
  overdistention in hypotonic labor, 188
  placenta previa and, 92t
  postpartum changes in, 204-205, 211
  premature rupture of membranes and, 196
  probable signs of pregnancy and, 53
  prolapse of, 279
  reproductive changes in pregnancy, 54
  rupture of
    during labor and birth, 199-200
    oxytocin labor induction and, 179

Uterus—cont'd
  subinvolution of, 247-248
  trauma during pregnancy and, 116

V

Vaccination, 750f, 750-753, 752f
  for hepatitis B in newborn, 109-110
  for infant, 389-394t, 398
  newborn discharge care and, 234
  during pregnancy, 113
  for preschooler, 435
  rubella in pregnancy and, 109
  for viral infection, 109
Vacuum aspiration
  for hydatidiform mole, 91
  for pregnancy termination, 87t
Vacuum curettage, 87t
Vacuum extraction, 182f, 182-184
Vacuum extractor, 182
Vagina, 24f, 24-25, 25f
  female sex act and, 31
  laceration during labor and birth, 242
  menstruation and, 461f
  normal, 256, 256b
  postpartum changes in, 207
  reproductive changes in pregnancy and, 55
Vaginal birth after cesarean, 144
  childbirth preparation and, 156-158, 157b
  uterine rupture and, 200
Vaginal bleeding
  after birth, 149-150
  in ectopic pregnancy, 89
  in placenta previa, 91
  in uterine inversion, 201
Vaginal discharge
  impending labor and, 131
  in pregnancy, 68
Vaginal examination
  in admission assessment, 135
  amniotomy and, 177
  false labor and, 135
  in progress of labor, 141
Vaginal hematoma, 168
Vaginal infection, 255-261
  normal vagina and, 256, 256b
  toxic shock syndrome in, 256
Vaginal introitus, 24
Vaginal ring, 264
Vaginal vestibule, 24, 24f
Vaginal wall prolapse, 278-279
Vagus nerve, 544f, 545t, 561b
Valerian, 784t
Valgus, term, 568
Valproic acid, 115t, 552t
Vanadium, 64t
Variability, fetal heart rate pattern and, 137-139
Variable deceleration, fetal heart rate pattern and, 139f, 139-140
Variance, 6
Varicella, 742t, 747f
Varicella vaccine, 751, 752f
Varicella zoster, 225
Varicocele, 271
Varicose vein, 56, 69
Variola, 742t
Varus, term, 568
Vas deferens, 22f, 23
Vasectomy, 268, 268f

Vasoocclusive crisis, 638*t*
Vasopressin, 725
Vasospasm, 94
Vastus lateralis muscle as injection site, 515, 515*f*
VBAC. *See* Vaginal birth after cesarean.
Vector, 747
Vegetarian diet, 367, 468-469
Vegetarian Food Pyramid, 370*f*
Vehicle accident, 470
Vena caval syndrome. *See* Supine hypertension.
Venereal disease, 754
Venereal Disease Research Laboratory, 49*t*
Venous access device, 517-518
Venous thrombosis, 106, 243*t*, 243-244
Ventilation, 591, 593*t*
Ventricular septal defect, 619*f*, 619-620
Ventriculoperitoneal shunt, 322, 323*f*
Ventrogluteal muscle as injection site, 515, 515*f*
Vernix caseosa, 292, 700-701
    assessment in newborn, 219
    of preterm newborn, 306
Version, 180
Vertex presentation, 128
Vertical incision in cesarean birth, 184, 186*f*
Vesicle, 702*b*, 750
Vesicostomy, 689*t*
Vesicoureteral reflux, 688, 689, 689*f*
Vibroacoustic stimulation test, 83*t*
Vietnamese American family
    cultural influences on, 359*t*
    food patterns of, 368*t*
    labor and delivery for, 123*t*
Villus, chorionic, 36
Violence, family, 584, 584*b*
Violet poisoning, 678*t*
Viral infection
    cytomegalovirus, 109
    herpes simplex virus
        breastfeeding and, 225
        in cutaneous infection, 706, 706*f*
        in genital infection, 257, 259*t*
        during pregnancy, 109
    human immunodeficiency virus, 257, 260*t*
        adolescent and, 466
        breastfeeding and, 225
        education for school-age child, 441
        pediatric, 756-759
        in pregnancy, 110
        prenatal screening for, 49*t*
        risk factors for, 110*b*
    in pregnancy, 108-110
    varicella zoster, 225
Virazole. *See* Ribavirin.
Vision
    reflexes of, 284*t*
    of toddler, 408-409
Vistaril. *See* Hydroxyzine.
Visual acuity test, 539, 540*f*
Visual analog pain scale, 478*f*
Visual analysis, 426*t*
Visual association area of brain, 543*f*
Visual cortex, 543*f*
Visual disturbance, epidural block and, 168
Visual stimulation
    newborn assessment and, 286
    toys and, 403*t*

Vital signs
    in abortion, 85
    in abruptio placentae, 93
    in cesarean birth, 184
    in head injury, 562
    of infant, 386*f*
    in labor induction, 179
    in maternal monitoring before birth, 141
    in meningitis, 547
    neonatal, 220
    pharmacological labor pain management and, 174
    postpartum, 205*b*, 209
    prenatal visit and, 48-50
    in preterm labor, 198
    in placenta previa, 93
    of school-age child, 440
    tocolytic therapy and, 197
    in trauma during pregnancy, 116
    in uterine inversion, 201
Vitamin A
    preset upper limit for daily adult intake of, 64*t*
    recommended dietary allowances of, 372*t*
Vitamin A derivatives, 115*t*
Vitamin B6, 372*t*
Vitamin B12, 372*t*
Vitamin C
    for anemia during pregnancy, 108
    interactions with air, 512*t*
    interactions with food, 512*t*
    for iron-deficiency anemia, 107
    for newborn, 297
    in pregnancy, 108*b*
    recommended dietary allowances of, 372*t*
    scurvy and, 675
Vitamin D
    for menopausal symptoms, 275
    for newborn, 297
    recommended dietary allowance of, 372*t*
    rickets and, 675
Vitamin E
    for menopausal symptoms, 275
    recommended dietary allowances of, 372*t*
Vitamin K
    to control bleeding in salicylate poisoning, 680
    newborn and, 153
    recommended dietary allowances of, 372*t*
Vitamins for newborn, 297
Voiding cystourethrography, 686
Volkmann's ischemia, 572
Volleyball, injury risks in, 585*t*
Volume expanders for amniotic fluid embolism, 201
Vomiting, 664-665
    in acute otitis media, 536
    in bulimia, 773
    in encephalitis, 548
    in hyperemesis gravidarum, 81
    in intussusception, 662
    in meningitis, 546
    nursing care plan for, 667-668
    odor of vomitus in poisoning, 677*t*
    in pregnancy, 51, 68, 165
    projectile, 658-659, 659*f*, 660
VSD. *See* Ventricular septal defect.
Vulva, 23-24, 24*f*
    precipitate birth and, 196
    self-examination of, 252
Vulvovaginal gland, 24

W

Walking
  for contraction stimulation, 179
  hypotonic labor and, 190
Warfarin
  use during pregnancy, 114*t*
  for venous thrombosis, 243
Water, 63
Water hemlock poisoning, 678*t*
Water intoxication, 57, 179
Weaning from breastfeeding, 232, 402
Weight
  change in second trimester, 71
  child *versus* adult, 349-350
  fertility and, 271
  of hospitalized child, 503-505
  neonatal, 220-221, 290, 291*f*
  nephrotic syndrome and, 692
  pregnancy-induced hypertension and, 96
  prenatal visit and, 50
  of preschooler, 422
  of school-age child, 439
  of toddler, 408
Weight conversions, 792
Weight gain
  in congestive heart failure, 623
  distribution in pregnancy, 61*t*
  edema and, 95
  heart disease and, 106
  nutrition for pregnancy and lactation and, 60, 61*t*
  substance abuse and, 114
Weight loss
  dehydration and, 670*t*, 672*t*
  impending labor and, 131
  postpartum, 234
Wernicke's area, 543*f*
Western blot test, 756
Wet dream, 22
Wharton's jelly, 42
Wheal, 702*b*
Wheezing
  in asthma, 603
  in bronchopulmonary dysplasia, 615
  in cystic fibrosis, 609
  in respiratory syncytial virus, 597
White blood cell, 632
  disorders of, 641-646
    Hodgkin's disease in, 645*t*, 645-646
    leukemia in, 641-645, 642*f*, 643*f*, 644*b*
  in nonpregnant and pregnant women, 56*t*
  postpartum changes in, 209
White blood cell count
  in leukemia, 642
  neonatal, 288
  in puerperal infection, 244
White House conferences, 4, 5*b*
Whitehead, 705
Whooping cough, 744*t*
WIC. *See* Women, Infants and Children.
Wilms' tumor, 694
Wisdom tooth, 379*f*
Witch hazel, 208
Withdrawal method of contraception, 269
Women, Infants, and Children, 377*t*
Women's health care, 251-281
  abnormal uterine bleeding and, 254
  amenorrhea and, 254

Women's health care—cont'd
  breast care in, 252, 253*b*
  cultural aspects of pain control and, 280
  endometriosis and, 255
  family planning and, 261-269
    barrier methods in, 264-265, 266*b*, 267*f*
    basal body temperature in, 267*f*, 267-268
    calendar method in, 268
    cervical mucous method in, 268, 268*f*
    emergency contraception and, 269
    hormonal contraceptives in, 261-264, 262*f*, 263*f*
    intrauterine device in, 264
    natural methods in, 267
    spermicides in, 266-267
    sterilization in, 268*f*, 268-269
  goals of *Healthy People 2010* and, 251
  hormone replacement therapy and, 274-275
  infertility and, 269-274
    evaluation of, 272
    factors influencing fertility and, 271-272
    female factors in, 271
    male factors in, 270-271
    social and psychological implications of, 270
    therapies for, 272-274, 273*t*
  menopause and, 275-278
  menstrual cycle pain and, 254-255
  normal vagina and, 256, 256*b*
  ovarian cyst and, 280
  pelvic examination in, 252-254
  pelvic floor dysfunction and, 279
  pelvic inflammatory disease and, 261
  premenstrual dysphoric disorder and, 255
  sexually transmitted diseases and, 257-261, 258-260*t*
  toxic shock syndrome and, 256
  urinary incontinence and, 279
  uterine fibroids and, 279-280
  uterine prolapse and, 279
  vaginal wall prolapse and, 278-279
  vulvar self-examination in, 252
Wood's light, 711
Worms, 676-677
Wound care in burn, 717-719, 718*f*
Wound infection, postpartum, 245*t*
Wrestling, injury risks in, 585*t*
Wristband identification of infant, 152
Wry neck, 581

X

Xenograft, 719

Y

Y chromosome, 684
Yam root, 275
Yeast infection, 258*t*
Yolk sac, 36
Yutopar. *See* Ritodrine.

Z

Zafirlukast, 605
Zarontin. *See* Ethosuximide.
Zileuton, 605
Zinc
  preset upper limit for daily adult intake of, 64*t*
  recommended dietary allowances of, 372*t*
Zyflo. *See* Zileuton.
Zygote, 26, 34, 36*f*, 37
Zygote intrafallopian transfer (ZIFT), 273, 273*t*

Skills, Techniques, and Clinical Tips

Steps in Preparing a Care Plan, 15

Process of Critical Thinking, 16

TPALM System to Describe Parity, 51

Nägele's Rule to Determine the Estimated Date of Delivery (EDD), 51

Isolation Precautions Required for Common Bioterrorist Agents, 113

Assisting with an Emergency Birth, 134

When to Auscultate and Document the Fetal Heart Rate, 137

Procedure for Determining Fetal Heart Rate, 137

Placement of Fetoscope or Sensors for Fetal Heart Rate Monitoring, 138

Reading the Fetal Heart Monitor, 139-140

Procedure for Determining Contractions by Palpation, 142

Perineal Scrub Preparation, 147

Thermoregulation in Newborn Care, 151

Cardiorespiratory Support in Newborn Care, 152

Applying Ointment to the Eyes of the Newborn, 154

Foot Massage, 158

Effleurage, 162

Applying Sacral Pressure to the Woman in Labor, 162

Hands-and-Knees Position, 194

Positioning of the Mother When the Umbilical Cord Has Prolapsed, 200

Postpartum Nursing Assessments, 205

Estimating the Volume of Lochia, 206

Procedure for Observing and Massaging the Uterine Fundus and for Giving Perineal Care, 207

Weighing and Measuring the Newborn, 220-221, 291

Teaching the New Mother How to Breastfeed, 227

Football Hold for Breastfeeding, 228

Removing the Infant from the Breast, 229

Burping the Infant, 230

Bottle Feeding the Newborn, 233

Teaching Breast Self-Examination, 253

Teaching Use of the Male Condom, 266

Measuring Head Circumference, 285

Bulb Suctioning, 288

Assessing the Apical Pulse, 290

Testing Skin Turgor, 292

Dressing the Newborn, 303

The Incubator, 313

Infant Nesting, 316

Technique for Turning the Child in a Body Cast, 334

Phototherapy Bilibed, 343

The Nursing Process Applied to Growth and Development, 348

Assessing the Length and Height of Infants and Children, 350

The Colic Carry, 395

Heating Refrigerated Formula in a Microwave Oven, 399

Directions for Home Preparation of Infant Foods, 402

Approximate Serving Sizes per Meal for Children, 415

Using the Nursing Process in Sex Education of the School-Age Child, 441

Guidance for Latchkey Families, 444

Teaching Ten Ways to Protect Immunocompromised Children from Pet-Transmitted Disease, 452

Using the Nursing Process in Sex Education for the Adolescent, 467

Four Pain Assessment Tools for Children, 478

Applying EMLA Cream, 480

Teaching Crib Safety, 496

Carrying the Infant: Cradle, Football, Upright, 497

Positioning the Child for an Ear Examination, 498

The Mummy Restraint, 498

Assessing Pulse and Respirations, 499

Sites for Measuring Blood Pressure in Children, 500

Measuring Oral Temperature, 502

Measuring Axillary Temperature, 502

Measuring Body Temperature: Skin Sensor and Tympanic, 503

Measuring the Weight of a Child, 503

Measuring the Height of a Child, 505

Measuring the Head Circumference of a Child, 505

Obtaining a Urine Specimen, 505

Obtaining a Stool Specimen, 505

Positioning the Infant for a Femoral Venipuncture, 507

Positioning the Child for a Lumbar Puncture, 507

Age-Appropriate Techniques for Giving Medication to Children, 509

Using the Nomogram for Estimating Body Surface Area, 510

Formula for Dimensional Analysis, 511

Administering Oral Medications, 513

Administering Nosedrops, 514

Administering Eardrops, 514

Administering Eyedrops, 514

Administering Rectal Medications, 514

Appropriate Sites for Intramuscular Injections in Children, 515

Suctioning, 523

Procedure for Gastrostomy Tube Feeding, 524

Blow-by Oxygen Therapy, 528

General Modifications/Precautions in Pediatric Feeding Techniques for Children with Cerebral Palsy, 556

Feeding the Disabled Child, 556

The Response of the Pupil of the Eye to a Flashlight Beam, 560

Neurological Monitoring of Infants and Children, 561-562

Principles of Managing Soft Tissue Injury, 570

Checklist for Traction Apparatus, 571

Checklist for the Patient in Traction, 572

Nursing Interventions/Patient Teaching for Abused and Neglected Children and Adolescents, 587

Teaching the Use of a Metered Dose Inhaler, 606

Tet Position for Infants with Tetralogy of Fallot, 621

Teaching Heart-Healthy Guidelines for Children, 628

Fowler's Sling, 665

Subcutaneous Injection of Insulin, 734

Sites for Injection of Insulin, 734

Mixing Insulin, 736

The Hug Restraining Position for Administering Vaccinations, 750

Strategies for Managing Children with ADHD in the Classroom, 771